NEUROVASCULAR MEDICINE

Neurovascular Medicine

Pursuing Cellular Longevity for Healthy Aging

Kenneth Maiese, MD

*Division of Cellular and Molecular
 Cerebral Ischemia
Departments of Neurology and Anatomy &
 Cell Biology
Barbara Ann Karmanos Cancer Institute
Center for Molecular Medicine and Genetics
Institute of Environmental Health Sciences
Wayne State University School of Medicine
Detroit, MI*

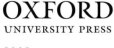

OXFORD
UNIVERSITY PRESS

2009

OXFORD
UNIVERSITY PRESS

Oxford University Press, Inc., publishes works that further
Oxford University's objective of excellence
in research, scholarship, and education.

Oxford New York
Auckland Cape Town Dar es Salaam Hong Kong Karachi
Kuala Lumpur Madrid Melbourne Mexico City Nairobi
New Delhi Shanghai Taipei Toronto

With offices in
Argentina Austria Brazil Chile Czech Republic France Greece
Guatemala Hungary Italy Japan Poland Portugal Singapore
South Korea Switzerland Thailand Turkey Ukraine Vietnam

Copyright © 2009 by Oxford University Press, Inc.

Published by Oxford University Press, Inc.
198 Madison Avenue, New York, New York 10016

www.oup.com

Library of Congress Cataloging-in-Publication Data

Neurovascular medicine: pursuing cellular longevity for
healthy aging / [edited by] Kenneth Maiese.
p. ; cm.
Includes bibliographical references and index.
ISBN 978-0-19-532669-7
1. Pathology, Cellular.   2. Pathology, Molecular.   3. Nervous system—Degeneration.
4. Inflammation—Mediators. I. Maiese, Kenneth, 1958- [DNLM: 1. Nervous System Physiology.
2. Aging—physiology.   3. Cell Physiology.   4. Neurodegenerative
Diseases—prevention & control.   5. Neurons—physiology. WL 102 N5122 2008]
RB113.N48 2008
616.07—dc22   2008006253

9 8 7 6 5 4 3 2 1
Printed in China
on acid-free paper

Preface

It is estimated that more than 500 million individuals suffer from nervous and vascular system disorders in the world. These disorders can comprise both acute and chronic degenerative diseases that involve hypertension, cardiac insufficiency, stroke, traumatic brain injury, presenile dementia, Alzheimer's disease, and Parkinson's disease. In regards to metabolic disorders such as diabetes mellitus, diabetes itself is present in more than 165 million individuals worldwide, and by the year 2030, it is predicted that more than 360 million individuals will be affected by diabetes mellitus. Of potentially greater concern is the incidence of undiagnosed diabetes that consists of impaired glucose tolerance and fluctuations in serum glucose levels that can increase the risk for acute and long-term complications in the vascular and cardiac systems.

Considering the significant risks that can be presented to the nervous and vascular systems, it is surprising to learn that organs such as the brain are highly susceptible to loss of cellular function and have only limited capacity to avert cellular injury. A variety of observations support this premise. For example, the brain possesses the highest oxygen metabolic rate of any organ in the body, consuming 20% of the total amount of oxygen in the body and enhancing the possibility for the aberrant generation of free radicals. In addition, the brain is composed of significant amounts of unsaturated fats that can readily serve as a source of oxygen free radicals to result in oxidative stress. Although a number of mechanisms can account for the loss of neuronal and vascular cells, the generation of cellular oxidative stress represents a significant component for the onset of pathological complications. Initial work in this field by early pioneers observed that increased metabolic rates could be detrimental to animals in an elevated oxygen environment. More current studies outline potential aging mechanisms and accumulated toxic effects for an organism that are tied to oxidative stress. The effects of oxidative stress are linked to the generation of oxygen free radical species in excessive or uncontrolled amounts during the reduction of oxygen. These oxygen free radicals are usually produced at low levels during normal physiological conditions and are scavenged by a number of endogenous antioxidant systems such as superoxide dismutase; glutathione peroxidase; and small molecule substances such as vitamins C, E, D_3, and B_3.

Yet, the brain and vascular system may suffer from an inadequate defense system against oxidative stress despite the increased risk factors for the generation of elevated levels of free radicals in the brain. Catalase activity in the brain, an endogenous antioxidant, has been reported to exist at levels markedly below those in the other organs of the body, sometimes approaching catalase levels as low as 10% in other organs such as the liver. Free radical species that are not scavenged can ultimately lead to cellular injury and programmed cell death, also known as apoptosis. Interestingly, it has recently been shown that genes involved in the apoptotic process are replicated early during processes that involve cell replication and transcription, suggesting a much broader role for these genes than originally anticipated. Apoptotically induced oxidative stress can contribute to a variety of disease states, such as diabetes, cardiac insufficiency, Alzheimer's disease, trauma, and stroke and lead to the impairment or death of neuronal and vascular endothelial cells.

It is clear that disorders of the nervous and vascular systems continue to burden the planet's population not only with increasing morbidity and mortality but also with a significant financial drain through increasing medical care costs coupled to a progressive loss in economic productivity. With the varied nature of diseases that can develop and the multiple cellular pathways that must function together to lead to a specific disease pathology, one may predict that the complexity that occurs inside a cell will also define the varied relationships that can result among different cells that involve neuronal, vascular, and glial cells. For example, activated inflammatory microglia may assist during the recovery phase in the brain following an injury, such as with the removal of injured cells and debri following cerebral hemorrhage. Yet, under different conditions, these cellular scavengers of the brain may also be the principal source for escalating tissue inflammation and promoting apoptotic cell injury in otherwise functional and intact neighboring cells of the brain.

Given the vulnerability of the nervous and vascular systems during development, acute injury, and aging, identifying the cellular pathways that determine cellular function, injury, and longevity may significantly assist in the development of therapeutic strategies to either prevent or at least reduce disability from crippling degenerative disorders. With this objective, *Neurovascular Medicine: Pursuing Cellular Longevity for Healthy Aging* is intended to offer unique insights into the cellular and molecular pathways that can govern neuronal, vascular, and inflammatory cell function and provide a platform for investigative perspectives that employ novel "bench to bedside" strategies from internationally recognized scientific leaders. In light of the significant and multifaceted role neuronal, vascular, and inflammatory cells may play during a variety of disorders of the nervous and vascular systems, novel studies that elucidate the role of these cells may greatly further not only our understanding of disease mechanisms but also our development of targeted treatments for a wide spectrum of diseases. The authors of this book strive to lay the course for the continued progression of innovative investigations, especially those that examine previously unexplored pathways of cell biology with new avenues of study for the maintenance of healthy aging and extended cellular longevity.

Kenneth Maiese
Editor

Contents

Contributors

Henrik Ahlenius, MSc
Laboratory of Neural Stem Cell Biology
Section of Restorative Neurology
Lund Strategic Research Center for Stem
  Cell Biology and Cell Therapy
Lund, Sweden

Maria Antonietta Ajmone-Cat, MSc
Department of Cell Biology
  and Neuroscience
Division of Experimental Neurology
Istituto Superiore di Sanità
Rome, Italy

Tak Yee Aw, PhD
Department of Molecular &
  Cellular Physiology
Louisiana State University
  Health Science Center
Shreveport, LA

Julien S. Baker, PhD, FRSM
Health and Exercise Science Research Unit
Faculty of Health Sport and Science
University of Glamorgan, Pontypridd
Wales, UK

Chandrakumar Balaratnasingam, MD
Centre for Ophthalmology and Visual
  Science and the ARC Centre of Excellence
  in Vision Science
The University of Western Australia
Nedlands, Perth, Australia

Adrian Balseanu, MD
University of Medicine and Pharmacy
Craiova, Romania

Noureddine Brakch, PhD
Service d'Angiologie
Hopital Nestlé
CHUV
Lausanne, Switzerland

Emanuele Cacci, PhD
Department of Cell and Developmental Biology
"La Sapienza" University
Rome, Italy

Massimiliano Castellazzi, BS
Laboratorio di Neurochimica
Sezione di Clinica Neurologica
Dipartimento di Discipline Medico Chirurgiche
  della Comunicazione e del Comportamento
Università degli Studi di Ferrara
Ferrara, Italy

Kokona Chatzantoni, PhD
Division of Hematology
Department of Internal Medicine
Medical School
University of Patras
Patras, Greece

Zhao Zhong Chong, MD, PhD
Division of Cellular and Molecular
  Cerebral Ischemia
Wayne State University School of Medicine
Detroit, MI

Magdalena L. Circu, PhD
Department of Molecular and
  Cellular Physiology
Louisiana State University Health
  Science Center
Shreveport, LA

Adriana Simon Coitinho, PhD
Centro Universitário Metodista IPA
Porto Alegre, RS, Brazil

Stephen J. Cringle, PhD
Centre for Ophthalmology and
  Visual Science and the ARC Centre
  of Excellence in Vision Science
The University of Western Australia
Nedlands, Perth, Australia

Bruce Davies, PhD, FACSM, FRSM
Health and Exercise Science Research Unit
Faculty of Health Sport and Science
University of Glamorgan, Pontypridd
Wales, UK

Mario Di Napoli, MD
Neurological Section, SMDN
Center for Cardiovascular Medicine and
  Cerebrovascular Disease Prevention
Sulmona (AQ), Italy

Peter Evans, MBChB, MD, FRCP
Royal Gwent Hospital
Newport, Gwent, UK

Enrico Fainardi MD, PhD
Unità Operativa di Neuroradiologia
Dipartimento di Neuroscienze
Azienda Ospedaliera Universitaria
Arcispedale S. Anna
Ferrara, Italy

Gabriella Gárdián, MD, PhD
Department of Neurology
University of Szeged
Szeged, Hungary

Michael R. Graham, MBChB, PhD, JCPTGP, FRSM
Health and Exercise Science
  Research Unit
Faculty of Health Sport and Science
University of Glamorgan, Pontypridd
Wales, UK

Steven J. Greco, PhD
Department of Medicine-Hematology/Oncology
UMDNJ-New Jersey Medical School
Newark, NJ

Wenyi Guo, MD, PhD
China-Australia Link Laboratory
EENT Hospital, Fudan University
China

Glaucia N. M. Hajj, PhD
Ludwig Institute For Cancer Research,
  São Paulo Branch
Cellular and Molecular
  Biology Laboratory
São Paulo, SP, Brazil

Christian Humpel, PhD
Laboratory of Psychiatry &
  Exp. Alzheimer's Research
Department of Psychiatry
Innsbruck, Austria

Raouf A. Khalil, MD, PhD
Harvard Medical School
Brigham and Women's Hospital
Division of Vascular Surgery
Boston, MA

Eugene A. Kiyatkin, MD, PhD
Behavioral Neuroscience Branch
National Institute on Drug Abuse - Intramural
  Research Program
National Institutes of Health, DHHS
Baltimore, MD

Zaal Kokaia, PhD
Laboratory of Neural Stem Cell Biology
Section of Restorative Neurology
Lund Strategic Research Center for Stem Cell
  Biology and Cell Therapy
Lund, Sweden

J. Will Langston, PhD
Department of Molecular and Cellular Physiology
Louisiana State University Health
  Science Center
Shreveport, LA

Fuad Lechin, MD, PhD
Departments of Neurophysiology, Neurochemistry,
  Neuropharmacology and Neuroimmunology
Instituto de Medicina Experimental
Faculty of Medicine
Universidad Central de Venezuela
Caracas, Venezuela

Faqi Li, MD, PhD
Division of Cellular and Molecular
  Cerebral Ischemia
Wayne State University School of Medicine
Detroit, MI

Kenneth Maiese, MD
Division of Cellular and Molecular
  Cerebral Ischemia
Departments of Neurology and Anatomy &
  Cell Biology
Barbara Ann Karmanos Cancer Institute
Center for Molecular Medicine
  and Genetics
Institute of Environmental Health Sciences
Wayne State University School of Medicine
Detroit, MI

Takanori Matsui, PhD
Division of Cardiovascular Medicine
Department of Medicine, Kurume University
  School of Medicine
Kurume, Japan

Luisa Minghetti, PhD
Department of Cell Biology and Neuroscience
Division of Experimental Neurology
Istituto Superiore di Sanità
Rome, Italy

Lisamarie Moore, MS
Department of Medicine- Hematology/Oncology
UMDNJ-New Jersey Medical School
Newark, NJ

William H. Morgan, MD, PhD, FRANZCO
Centre for Ophthalmology and Visual Science
The University of Western Australia
Nedlands, Perth, Australia

Ryuichi Morishita, MD, PhD
Division of Clinical Gene Therapy
Osaka University Graduate School of Medicine
Suita, Japan

Athanasia Mouzaki, PhD
Division of Hematology
Department of Internal Medicine
Medical School
University of Patras
Patras, Greece

Hironori Nakagami, MD, PhD
Division of Clinical Gene Therapy &
Division of Gene Therapy Science
Osaka University Graduate School of Medicine
Suita, Japan

Noritaka Nakamichi, PhD
Laboratory of Molecular Pharmacology
Division of Pharmaceutical Sciences
Kanazawa University Graduate School
of Natural Science and Technology
Kanazawa, Japan

Kazuo Nakamura, MD, PhD
Division of Cardiovascular Medicine
Department of Medicine, Kurume University
School of Medicine
Kurume, Japan

Mariana Kiomy Osako, MS
Division of Clinical Gene Therapy &
Department of Geriatric Medicine
Osaka University Graduate School of Medicine
Suita, Japan

Aurel Popa-Wagner, PhD
Department of Neurology
University of Greifswald
Greifswald, Germany

Xiaoying Qiao, MD, PhD
Brigham and Women's Hospital
Division of Vascular Surgery
Boston, MA

Pranela Rameshwar, PhD
Department of Medicine-
Hematology/Oncology
UMDNJ-New Jersey Medical School
Newark, NJ

Mohamed Rholam, PhD
Laboratoire de Biologie et Biochimie
Cellulaire du Vieillissement
Université Paris7 - Denis
Diderot
Paris, France

Katalin Sas, MD
Department of Neurology
University of Szeged
Szeged, Hungary

Imtiaz M. Shah, MD
Mansionhouse Unit
Victoria Infirmary
Glasgow, Scotland, UK

K. S. Sidhu, PhD
Stem Cell Laboratory
School of Psychiatry
The University of New South Wales
NSW, Australia

Er-Ning Su, MD, PhD
Centre for Ophthalmology and
Visual Science and the ARC Centre
of Excellence in Vision Science
The University of Western Australia
Nedlands, Perth, Australia

Xinghuai Sun, MD, PhD
China-Australia Link Laboratory
EENT Hospital, Fudan University
China

Philippe Taupin, PhD
National Neuroscience Institute
National University of Singapore
Nanyang Technological University
Singapore, Singapore

József Toldi, PhD, DSc
Department of Physiology
Anatomy and Neuroscience
University of Szeged
Szeged, Hungary

Katarzyna A. Trzaska, PhD
Department of Medicine-
  Hematology/Oncology
UMDNJ-New Jersey Medical School
Newark, NJ

Bertha van der Dijs, MD
Departments of Neurophysiology,
  Neurochemistry, Neuropharmacology
  and Neuroimmunology
Instituto de Medicina Experimental
Faculty of Medicine
Universidad Central de Venezuela
Caracas, Venezuela

László Vécsei, MD, PhD, DSc
Department of Neurology
Neurology Research Group of the Hungarian
  Academy of Sciences
University of Szeged
Szeged, Hungary

Sho-ichi Yamagishi MD, PhD,
Division of Cardiovascular Medicine
Department of Pathophysiology
  and Therapeutics of Diabetic
  Vascular Complications
Kurume University School of Medicine
Kurume, Japan

Yukio Yoneda, PhD
Laboratory of Molecular Pharmacology
Division of Pharmaceutical Sciences

Kanazawa University Graduate School
  of National Science and Technology
Kanazawa, Japan

Dao-Yi Yu, MD, PhD
Centre for Ophthalmology and Visual Science and
  the ARC Centre of Excellence in Vision Science
The University of Western Australia
Nedlands, Perth, Australia

Paula K. Yu, PhD
Centre for Ophthalmology and Visual Science and
  the ARC Centre of Excellence in Vision Science
The University of Western Australia
Nedlands, Perth, Australia

Xiao-Bo Yu, MD
China-Australia Link Laboratory
EENT Hospital, Fudan University
China

Leon Zagrean MD, PhD
Department of Physiology and Neuroscience
"Carol Davila" University of Medicine and Pharmacy
Bucharest, Romania

Min Zhuo, PhD
Department of Physiology
Faculty of Medicine
University of Toronto Centre for the Study of Pain
University of Toronto
Medical Science Building
Toronto, Ontario, Canada

PART I

Unraveling Pathways of Clinical Function and Disability

Chapter *1*

ROLE OF PRION PROTEIN DURING NORMAL PHYSIOLOGY AND DISEASE

Adriana Simon Coitinho and Glaucia N. M. Hajj

ABSTRACT

Prions are infectious particles composed only of proteins. Their importance resides in the concept that information transmission between two organisms can be devoid of nucleic acid. Prions are also well known as the etiological agents of several neurodegenerative diseases of animals and man called *transmissible spongiform encephalopathies* (TSEs).

Literature on prion-associated diseases, transmission mechanisms, and the related normal isoform of the protein has grown impressively in the last few years (the entry prion in the Web-based search mechanism PubMed gave 8578 hits in July 2007), making it very difficult to cover all aspects of prion in depth in this chapter. We will therefore focus on the history, symptoms, mechanisms of transmission and diagnosis of prion diseases, and currently proposed therapies. There will also be a short discussion on the physiological roles of the normal isoform of the prion.

Keywords: cellular prion protein, prion protein, physiological function, prion diseases, transmissible spongiform encephalopathies, neurodegeneration.

HISTORY

Studies on prions and related diseases date from the beginning of the 20th century, but several questions remain unresolved. Table 1.1 lists the most important scientific reports that have contributed to the current prion hypothesis. The first disease studied was scrapie, a naturally occurring neurodegenerative disease of sheep that can be transmitted experimentally from one sheep to another (Cuille, Chelle 1939) and even to mice (Chandler 1961). In experimental models of scrapie, researchers attempted to isolate the pathological agent from brain extracts of affected animals. In 1980, Stanley Prusiner and coworkers succeeded in isolating a brain fraction enriched with the pathological agent (Prusiner, Groth, Cochran et al. 1980). This material had amyloid characteristics that were seen as small fibrilar aggregates, known as scrapie associated fibrils (SAF) or "prion rods," in electron micrographs (Merz, Somerville, Wisniewski et al. 1981; Prusiner, McKinley, Bowman et al. 1983). The same aggregates were purified from the brain extracts of Creutzfeldt–Jakob disease (CJD) and kuru patients (Merz, Rohwer,

Table 1.1 Historical Overview of Prion Research

Year	Discovery
1898	First scientific description of scrapie (Besnoit, Morel 1898)
1920	First scientific description of CJD (Creutzfeldt 1920, Jakob, 1921)
1939	Experimental transmission of scrapie (Cuille, Chelle 1939)
1957	First scientific description of kuru (Gajdusek, Zigas 1957)
1959	Similarities between kuru and scrapie are observed (Hadlow 1959)
1961	Several strains of the etiological agent of scrapie (Pattison, Millson 1961)
1961	Scrapie experimentally transmitted to mice (Chandler 1961)
1963	Experimental transmission of kuru to chimps (Gajdusek et al. 1966)
1966	Scrapie agent is resistant to UV irradiation (Alper et al. 1966; Alper et al. 1967)
1967	Protein only hypothesis (Griffith, 1967)
1968	CJD transmission to chimps (Gibbs, Jr. et al. 1968)
1980	Scrapie extract is protein rich and proteolysis resistant (Prusiner et al. 1980)
1982	Prion concept (Prusiner 1982)
1985	PrP^C gene discovered Chesebro et al. 1985; Oesch et al. 1985)
1986	PrP^C and PrP^{Sc} come from the same gene (Basler et al. 1986)
1987	First scientific description of BSE (Wells et al. 1987)
1989	PrP^C mutations cause GSS Hsiao et al. 1989)
1992	PrP^C knockout mice (Bueler et al. 1992)
1993	PrP^C knockout mice are resistant to scrapie (Bueler et al. 1993)
1993	Structural differences between PrP^C and PrP^{Sc} (Pan et al. 1993)
1994	PrP^C to PrP^{res} conversion in a noncellular system (Kocisko et al. 1994)
1996	First scientific description of vCJD (Will et al. 1996)
1996	PrP^{Sc} from BSE has a unique glycosylation pattern (Collinge et al. 1996)
1996	PrP^C protein structure described (Riek et al. 1996)
1997	vCJD is caused by BSE infection (Bruce et al. 1997; Hill et al. 1997a)
2000	Experimental BSE transmission through blood (Houston et al. 2000)
2003	PrP^C depletion in neurons reverses TSEs symptoms (Mallucci et al. 2003)
2004	Recombinant PrP^C converted to PrP^{Sc} in vitro (Legname et al. 2004)

Adapted from Aguzzi, Polymenidou 2004.

BSE, Bovine spongiform encephalopathy; CJD, Creutzfedt–Jakob disease; GSS, Gerstmann–Sträussler–Scheinker syndrome; TSE, transmissible spongiform encephalopathy; UV, ultraviolet; vCJD, variant of Creutzfedt–Jakob disease.

Kascsak et al. 1984). The material was partially resistant to proteolysis, generating a protein fragment with a molecular weight of 27 to 30 kDa (Bolton, McKinley, Prusiner 1982; McKinley, Bolton, Prusiner 1983). However, the infectivity of the material was sensitive to treatments that destroyed nucleic acids (DNA and RNA) (Alper, Cramp, Haig et al. 1967). These findings led Prusiner to propose the hypothesis of an infection mediated only by proteins, the "protein only hypothesis," which stated that the etiological agent of scrapie was a "proteinaceous infectious particle" or prion (Prusiner 1982). Although this hypothesis had been suggested a decade earlier by other researchers (Griffith 1967; Gibbons, Hunter 1967), it was credited only after the infectious agent of scrapie was purified by the Prusiner laboratory.

The purified infectious agent was used to produce antibodies that recognized the infectious protein in brain extracts of infected animals. Curiously, the antibody could also identify a protein in brain extracts from uninfected animals, indicating that a homologue of the infectious agent was present in normal brain tissue (Oesch, Westaway, Walchli et al. 1985). The normal protein was sequenced and the encoding gene (*Prnp*) was discovered. The infectious protein was subsequently named scrapie prion protein, or PrP^{Sc}, and the normal form was called *cellular prion protein*, or PrP^C (Basler, Oesch, Scott et al. 1986).

Researchers later found that both proteins had the same amino acid sequence (Turk, Teplow, Hood et al. 1988) but had different three dimensional structures; while PrP^C had a large α-helical content, PrP^{Sc} was predominantly composed of β-sheets (Pan, Baldwin, Nguyen et al. 1993). The difference in structure explains why PrP^C is a soluble molecule susceptible to proteolysis and PrP^{Sc} is insoluble and resistant to proteolysis (Meyer, McKinley, Bowman et al. 1986). The structural properties of PrP^{Sc} favor the formation of insoluble aggregates and amyloid plaques, leading to the hypothesis that PrP^{Sc} might dimerize with PrP^{C}, altering the structure of the normal protein and leading to progressive plaque deposition. In this model, PrP^{Sc} molecules would be exponentially generated from PrP^{C}, a process that would slowly and progressively lead to neuronal death (Prusiner 1989).

Support for the infectious protein theory was found in animals in which the PrP^{C} gene had been removed. These animals that did not express PrP^{C} (PrP^{C} knockouts) also did not exhibit PrP^{Sc} deposition or present neurodegenerative symptoms when inoculated with scrapie (Bueler, Aguzzi, Sailer et al. 1993). Additional experiments were performed in mice that did not express PrP^{C} in neurons (conditional knockouts). When inoculated with the scrapie agent, these mice produced amyloid plaques and PrP^{Sc} deposits but did not display neurological symptoms or neurodegeneration (Mallucci, Dickinson, Linehan et al. 2003). The final line of evidence supporting the prion hypothesis came from the in vitro conversion of PrP^{C} expressed in bacteria (recombinant PrP^{C}) into a form resistant to proteolysis (PrP^{res}) (Kocisko, Come, Priola et al. 1994). More important was the ability to convert PrP^{C} in vitro into an infectious isoform able to produce disease (Legname, Baskakov, Nguyen et al. 2004; Castilla, Saa, Hetz et al. 2005a).

Prion disease can vary substantially in a single host species in terms of incubation period, lesion distribution, and amyloid plaque formation, leading us to the concept of prion strains. Interestingly, prion molecules isolated from distinct types of disease are also structurally distinct (Aucouturier, Kascsak, Frangione et al. 1999). The original strain, when transmitted to the host, will reproduce the original characteristics of the inoculum, so that one animal can reproduce several strains and present the symptoms of each disease (Telling, Parchi, DeArmond et al. 1996).

PRION DISEASES

The discovery of prion diseases was a very intriguing event because the pathogenic agent causes a group of lethal neurodegenerative diseases mediated by a new transmission mechanism (Prusiner 1998). These diseases affect several animal species, including humans (Table 1.2), and are called *spongiform encephalopathies* because of the sponge-like aspect of brain degeneration (Glatzel, Aguzzi 2001; Fornai, Ferrucci, Gesi et al. 2006).

The oldest prion disease known is scrapie, which occurs naturally in goat and sheep. Although the disease was recognized more than 300 years ago, the first scientific description dates from 1898 (Besnoit, Morel 1898). The affected animals present behavioral disturbances, excitability, ataxia, and paralysis, leading to death shortly after the appearance of symptoms (Narang 1987). Scrapie is incurable and fatal in all cases, as are all prion diseases. The nervous system presents histological modifications, with large vacuole formation, intense gliosis, and neuronal loss. Amyloid deposits can also be observed. Scrapie was the first prion disease that was proved to be infectious (Cuille, Chelle 1939), although transmissibility to humans has never been demonstrated. The presence of PrP^{Sc} can be observed in preclinical stages in the nervous system and in lymphoid tissues (Taraboulos, Jendroska, Serban et al. 1992).

In 1986, a neurological disease with clinical signs of rapid progression in behavioral impairment, ataxia, and disestesy was found in cattle in the United Kingdom (Wells, Scott, Johnson et al. 1987). Autopsies found histological alterations in the brains that resembled those found in scrapie (Narang 1996). Therefore, the disease was named *bovine spongiform encephalopathy* (BSE), popularly known as "mad cow disease." The number of cases increased every year, until an epidemic surfaced in Great Britain in the 1980s, with nearly 400,000 animals affected (Wells, Wilesmith 1995).

Table 1.2 Transmissible Spongiform Encephalopathies

Prion Disease	*Host*	*References*
Scrapie	Sheep and Goat	Besnoit, Morel 1898
Transmissible mink encephalopathy (TME)	Mink	Hartsough, Burger 1965
Chronic wasting disease (CWD)	Deer and Elk	Williams, Young 1980
Feline spongiform encephalopathy (FSE)	Cats	Wyatt et al. 1991
Bovine spongiform encephalopathy (BSE)	Cattle	Wells et al. 1987
Kuru	Humans	Gajdusek, Zigas 1957
Creutzfedt–Jakob disease (CJD)	Humans	Jakob 1921; Creutzfeldt 1920
new variant of CJD (nvCJD)	Humans	Will et al. 1996
Gerstmann–Sträussler–Scheinker (GSS) syndrome	Humans	Gerstmann 1928
Fatal familial insomnia (FFI)	Humans	Medori et al. 1992

In the search for the origin of this new disease, researchers found that the cattle had received a dietary protein supplement from meat and bone meal (MBM) from the offal of sheep, cows, and pigs. In the 1970s, an alteration in the MBM manufacturing process and the use of scrapie-contaminated sheep carcasses led to the introduction of prions into cattle diets (Wilesmith, Ryan, Atkinson 1991). The greatest concern was the long asymptomatic phase of this disease. The average incubation time of 5 years is associated with the risk of contaminated cattle being used for human consumption for a prolonged duration before the appearance of any clinical signs.

Other animal species can also be affected by transmissible spongiform encephalopathies (TSEs). Domestic cats and large captive felines have been found with transmissible feline encephalopathy that was probably acquired from prion-contaminated food (Wyatt, Pearson, Smerdon et al. 1991). Wild deer and elk suffer from chronic wasting disease (CWD), a TSE of unknown origin that is endemic to some wild and captive populations of the United States. The disease was first recognized in the 1960s and was initially thought to be a nutritional deficiency related to stress or intoxication. It was recognized as a spongiform encephalopathy (Williams, Young 1980) in 1977 and has since been experimentally transmitted to a variety of animal species.

Minks are also susceptible to a form of TSE called *transmissible mink encephalopathy* (TME) (Sigurdson, Miller 2003). TME, a rare sporadic disease of ranched mink, hypothetically arose from the feeding of scrapie- or BSE-contaminated products (Hartsough, Burger 1965). Affected minks present behavioral alterations, weight loss, and progressive debilitation until death (Marsh, Hadlow 1992).

In humans, the first infectious neurodegenerative disease connected to prions was kuru, a disease observed in the 1950s among the natives of Papua New Guinea. Kuru is considered a cerebellar syndrome, and the symptoms include progressive ataxia, trembling, and loss of movement control, but no dementia. Histopathological alterations are typical of TSEs and include vacuolization, astrogliosis, and amyloid plaque deposition (Gajdusek, Zigas 1957). The similarity of the neuropathological findings between kuru and scrapie (Hadlow 1959) led to the proposal that kuru might also be transmissible, and experimental transmission was accomplished in 1966 (Gajdusek, Gibbs, Alpers 1966). Epidemiological evidence pointed to an association between cannibalism and the emergence of disease. At the time, it was common practice for members of the Fore tribe to eat the brains of dead relatives (Gajdusek, Zigas 1957). It is believed that the disease spread through the ingestion of brain tissue from a sporadic or hereditary case of prion disease.

The extinction of cannibalistic funeral practices in the 1960s has drastically reduced the incidence of kuru (Gajdusek 1977).

The most common human TSE is certainly CJD, with an incidence of one to two cases per million per year. It was first described by Creutzfeldt in 1920 and Jakob in 1921 (Masters, Gajdusek, Gibbs 1981). Symptoms include cognitive deficit, cerebellar signs, sleep disturbance, and behavioral abnormalities with the possibility of peripheral neuropathies, leading to rapid and progressive dementia and death within 12 months. As the disease progresses, pyramidal and extrapyramidal symptoms, ataxia, and visual disturbances are seen, and the patient may develop myoclonus. Histological data (Fig. 1.1) include tissue "sponging," astrocyte proliferation associated with neuronal loss, and amyloid plaques of PrP^{Sc}. The incidence peak is around 55 to 65 years of age (Glatzel, Stoeck, Seeger et al. 2005).

CJD can be of hereditary, iatrogenic, or sporadic origin. The sporadic form of CJD represents 85% of all CJD cases and is believed to develop because of spontaneous alterations in PrP^{C}. It cannot be related to any genetic alteration, environmental risk, or exposure to the infectious agent (Will 2003). There is great variation in the symptoms between individual cases, but the disease typically evolves rapidly in multiple cerebral areas.

Successful experimental transmission of CJD soon followed the recognition of kuru as infectious, leading to a new scientific interest in prion diseases

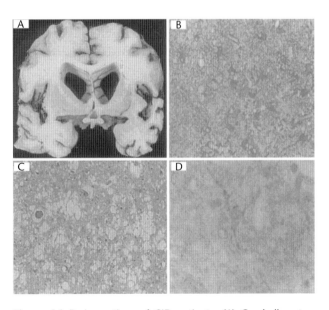

Figure 1.1 Brain sections of CJD patients. (A) Cerebellar atrophy, enlargement of ventricular system, and cortex atrophy. (B) Reactive astrocytic gliosis. (C) Sponge-like lesions, gliosis, and neuronal death. (D) Immunohistochemistry: intraneuronal and extraneuronal immunopositive reactions for PrP^{Sc}.

(Gibbs, Jr., Gajdusek, Asher et al. 1968). The fact that CJD could be experimentally transmitted raised the hypothesis that it could be transmitted from one person to another during medical procedures. In fact, the iatrogenic form of CJD can be caused by PrP^{Sc} exposure during surgical procedures such as human dura mater implantation and corneal grafts (Lang, Heckmann, Neundorfer 1998; Croes, Jansen, Lemstra et al. 2001) with prion-infected tissues, or treatment with human growth hormone (hGH) purified from contaminated pituitaries (Collinge, Palmer, Dryden 1991). hGH injections and dura mater implants have resulted in 267 cases of iatrogenic CJD over the last 20 years (Flechsig, Hegyi, Enari et al. 2001). The incubation time depends on the inoculation site of PrP^{Sc}. Intracerebral exposure is associated with short incubation periods (16 to 28 months), whereas peripheral exposure results in long incubation periods (5 to 30 years). Evidence indicates that the form of exposure has an influence on clinical presentation of the disease. Ataxia is common in cases of infection acquired through the dura mater or hGH. In cases where PrP^{Sc} is directly inoculated into the central nervous system (CNS), dementia is the first symptom (Glatzel, Stoeck, Seeger et al. 2005). Recently, CJD transmission has also been demonstrated through blood or its derivatives (Llewelyn, Hewitt, Knight et al. 2004; Peden, Head, Ritchie et al. 2004).

A relatively novel presentation is the new variant of CJD (nvCJD), which was first described in 1996. Recent studies indicate that nvCJD emerged through BSE transmission to humans, as the molecular characteristics of nvCJD (electrophoretic migration pattern) are very different from classic CJD but are strikingly similar to those of BSE experimentally transmitted to mice and monkeys (Collinge, Sidle, Meads et al. 1996). Oral transmission of BSE had already been documented (Prusiner, Cochran, Alpers 1985; Bons, Mestre-Frances, Belli et al. 1999; Herzog, Sales, Etchegaray et al. 2004) and symptoms were identical to those of nvCJD (Asante, Linehan, Desbruslais et al. 2002). From 1996 to 2001, the incidence of nvCJD in the United Kingdom rose gradually, bringing the fear of a large epidemic. However, incidence has been stable since 2001, and only a small number of countries—the United Kingdom, France, and Ireland—have reported new nvCJD cases (Cousens, Zeidler, Esmonde et al. 1997). The fact that nvCJD has distinct clinical and pathological features makes defining diagnosis criteria easier. Compared to sporadic CJD, the mean duration of nvCJD is 14 months, and patients are younger (mean 29 years of age) and show psychiatric symptoms. Histologically, nvCJD patients show abundant amyloid plaque deposition surrounded by vacuoles ("florid plaques"), and spongiform degeneration is less evident (Ironside, Bell 1997).

Genetic forms of the human prion diseases give rise to three distinct phenotypes: the CJD familial form, Gerstmann–Sträussler–Scheinker syndrome (GSS), and fatal familial insomnia (FFI). All of these diseases are related to one of the 55 recognized pathogenic mutations in the PrP^C gene (*Prnp*) (Table 1.3). The features of familial CJD vary with the underlying mutation, but in general symptoms are the same as those of sporadic CJD, with the exception that onset is at an earlier age and the duration of the illness is prolonged. The first authentic familial case of CJD was reported in 1924 (Kirschbaum 1924). GSS is characterized by progressive cerebellar ataxia that appears in the fifth or sixth decade of life, accompanied by cognitive decline. As opposed to other genetic diseases, GSS consists of specific neuropathological features of multicentric PrP^{Sc} plaques spread over brain tissue (McKintosh, Tabrizi, Collinge 2003). The experimental transmission of familial CJD and GSS (Masters, Gajdusek, Gibbs 1981) was the first known instance in medical science of diseases that are both infectious and heritable.

FFI appears in average at age 48 and causes disturbances in circadian rhythm, motor function, and the endocrine system. A mutation at residue 178 Asp→Asn (D178N) of PrP is responsible for this disease. Interestingly, the same mutation can lead to CJD, depending on a polymorphism at amino acid 129. CJD results when the D178N mutation is accompanied by two valines (Val/Val homozygote) or a valine and a methionine (Val/Met heterozygote) in position 129. When the D178N mutation is accompanied a homozygous Met/Met genotype at amino acid 129, the patient will present with FFI (Medori, Tritschler, LeBlanc et al. 1992). The large amount of data generated in the last 20 years has clearly established the participation of PrP^{Sc} and PrP^C in prion diseases. Nevertheless, the physiological functions of PrP^C are still the subject of intense debate.

CELLULAR PRION PROTEIN

Prion research has evolved immensely in the last 10 years, and today the normal isoform of the infectious prion protein occupies a large part of this research. The next section describes PrP^C and the multiple cellular functions proposed for this protein, demonstrating how its loss of function could be prejudicial to cells.

PrP^C is a constitutively expressed glycoprotein found on the outer plasma membrane of many tissues. The protein is expressed at high levels in the CNS and in low levels in muscle, immune cells, and so on (Table 1.4) (Glatzel, Aguzzi 2001). It is anchored to the cell membrane by a glycosylphosphatidylinositol

Table 1.3 PrP^C Gene Mutations Associated to Prion Diseases

Codon	Mutation	Associated Diseases	References
51–90	Insertion of 48–216 bp	CJD/GSS	Goldfarb et al. 1993
102	Pro/Leu	GSS	Doh-ura et al. 1989
105	Pro/Leu	GSS	Yamada et al. 1993
117	Ala/Val	GSS	Doh-ura et al. 1989
131	Gly/Val	GSS	Panegyres et al. 2001
145	Tyr/STOP	GSS	Ghetti et al. 1996
171	Asn/Ser	Schizophrenia	Samaia et al. 1997
178	Asp/Asn	FFI/CJD	Medori et al. 1992
180	Val/Ile	CJD	Kitamoto et al. 1993
183	Thr/Ala	CJD	Nitrini et al. 1997
187	His/Arg	GSS	Cervenakova et al. 1999
188	Thr/Lys	Dementia	Finckh et al. 2000
196	Glu/Lys	CJD	Peoc'h et al. 2000
198	Phe/Ser	GSS	Hsiao et al. 1992
200	Glu/Lys	CJD	Inoue et al. 1994
202	Asp/Asn	GSS	Piccardo et al. 1998
208	Arg/His	CJD	Mastrianni et al. 1996
210	Val/Ile	CJD	Pocchiari et al. 1993
211	Glu/Gln	CJD	Peoc'h et al. 2000
212	Gln/Pro	GSS	Piccardo et al. 1998
217	Gln/Arg	GSS	Hsiao et al. 1992
232	Met/Arg	CJD	Kitamoto et al. 1993

CJD, Creutzfedt–Jakob disease; FFI, fatal familial insomnia; GSS, Gerstmann–Sträussler–Scheinker syndrome.

Table 1.4 PrP^C Tissue Expression

PrP^C Expression	References
Neurons	Harris et al. 1993; Sales et al. 2002; Ford et al. 2002a
Immune cells	Durig et al. 2000; Kubosaki et al. 2003
Lung	Fournier et al. 1998; Ford et al. 2002b
Muscles	Kovacs et al. 2004
Blood and bone marrow	Mabbott, Turner 2005; Ford et al. 2002b
Stomach	Fournier et al. 1998; Ford et al. 2002b
Kidney	Fournier et al. 1998; Ford et al. 2002b
Spleen	Fournier et al. 1998; Ford et al. 2002b

(GPI) anchor (Prusiner 1998). The physiological role of this protein is not completely understood, but owing to its conservation among species, it is believed to have a key role in many physiological processes (Martins, Mercadante, Cabral et al. 2001; Martins, Brentani 2002).

PrP^C has been implicated in several phenomena such as proliferation, neural differentiation, neuritogenesis, and synaptogenesis. For example, PrP^C expression is positively correlated to proliferative areas in the subventricular zone of the dentate gyrus in the brain (Steele, Emsley, Ozdinler et al. 2006).

On the other hand, PrP^C expression also correlates with neural differentiation (Steele, Emsley, Ozdinler et al. 2006), and its abundance in synaptic boutons suggests a role in axon guidance and synaptogenesis (Sales, Hassig, Rodolfo et al. 2002). The addition of PrP^C to cultured neurons stimulates neuritogenesis and synaptogenesis (Chen, Mange, Dong et al. 2003; Santuccione, Sytnyk, Leshchyns'ka et al. 2005), both markers of neuronal differentiation (Table 1.5).

The PrP^C gene (*Prnp*) contains three exons in the mouse and rat and two exons in the hamster and humans, with the third and second exons, respectively, encoding the entire protein of approximately 250 amino acids (Fig. 1.2). Two signal peptides are present in the molecule, one at the N-terminus, which is cleaved during the biosynthesis of PrP^C in the rough endoplasmic reticulum, and a second at the C-terminus that contains an attachment site for a GPI anchor (Prusiner 1998). The *Prnp* promoter has been identified, and the region that controls the majority of transcription was found upstream of the transcription initiation site. While PrP^C is often referred to as a housekeeping gene and the protein is expressed under most cellular conditions, the chromatin condensation state is also known to alter *Prnp* promoter activity (Cabral, Lee, Martins 2002). In addition, nerve growth factor (NGF), copper, and heat shock all increase PrP^C expression (Shyu, Harn, Saeki et al. 2002; Zawlik, Witusik, Hulas-Bigoszewska et al. 2006; Varela-Nallar, Toledo, Larrondo et al. 2006).

The internalization of PrP^C from the plasma membrane into endocytic organelles has been demonstrated in cell culture (Prado, Alves-Silva, Magalhaes et al. 2004). The majority is recycled back to the plasmalemma without degradation. In neurons, the endocytosis takes place through caveolae- and clathrine-mediated pathways. PrP^C can also be internalized in response to copper and accumulates in the perinuclear region, particularly in the Golgi network (Lee, Magalhaes, Zanata et al. 2001; Brown, Harris 2003).

PrP^C Interaction with Copper Ions and Oxidative Stress

Many reports indicate that PrP^C interacts with copper ions (Cu^{2+}), but the physiological role of this interaction is still a matter of controversy (Brown, Qin,

Herms et al. 1997a). Copper is an essential element that, as an enzymatic cofactor, plays important roles in the biochemical pathways of all aerobic organisms. Cu^{2+} can catalyze the formation of dangerous reactive oxygen species such as the hydroxyl radical, which makes it extremely toxic when present in excess. Some reports show that PrP^C can bind Cu^{2+} through an octapeptide in the N-terminus of the molecule (Fig. 1.3), which is extremely conserved among mammals (Miura, Hori-i Takeuchi 1996; Brown, Qin, Herms et al. 1997a). This binding is consistent with a transport function, in which PrP^C might bind extracellular copper and release it in acidic vesicles inside the cell (Pauly, Harris 1998; Whittal, Ball, Cohen et al. 2000; Miura, Sasaki, Toyama et al. 2005). This action could have a direct impact on the regulation of the presynaptic concentration of Cu^{2+}, in the conformational stability of PrP^C and in the cellular response to oxidative stress. Nevertheless, direct evidence that PrP^C does in fact transport Cu^{2+} is still lacking.

Perhaps the most accepted physiological function of PrP^C is a protective role against oxidative stress (Brown, Qin, Herms et al. 1997a; Herms, Tings, Gall et al. 1999; Klamt, Dal Pizzol, Conte da Frota et al. 2001; Rachidi, Vilette, Guiraud et al. 2003). The capacity of PrP^C to bind Cu^{2+} could alter the activity of the major antioxidant enzyme, Cu/Zn superoxide dismutase (SOD), and, as a consequence, modulate cellular protection against oxidative stress (Brown, Besinger 1998). Neuron cultures from PrP^C knockout mice (*Prnp$^{-/-}$*) have displayed 50% lower SOD-1 activity than that found in wild-type mice, and cell cultures in which PrP^C was overexpressed showed an increase of 20% in SOD activity (Brown, Schulz-Schaeffer, Schmidt et al. 1997b; Klamt, Dal Pizzol, Conte da Frota et al. 2001). The low SOD activity in PrP^C knockout mice could be due to a copper deficiency. Remarkably, it has been suggested that the loss of antioxidant defenses plays a major role in scrapie-infected cells (Milhavet, McMahon, Rachidi et al. 2000) and

Table 1.5 PrP^C Functions

PrP^C Functions	References
Cellular protection from oxidative stress	Brown 2005; Brown et al., 2002
Adhesion and neuritogenesis	Graner et al. 2000a; Graner et al. 2000b; Chen et al. 2003; Lopes et al. 2005; Santuccione et al. 2005
Neuroprotection	Chiarini et al. 2002; Zanata et al. 2002; Lopes et al. 2005
Memory consolidation	Coitinho et al. 2003; Criado et al. 2005; Coitinho et al. 2006; Coitinho et al. 2007
Immune response	Aguzzi et al. 2003
Anti-apoptotic events	Bounhar et al. 2001; Roucou, LeBlanc 2005; Li, Harris 2005
Pro-apoptotic events	Paitel et al. 2003b; Solforosi et al. 2004

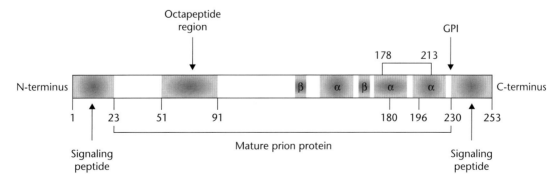

Figure 1.2 Schematic of the prion protein precursor. A signaling peptide present in the N-terminus region is cleaved during synthesis, and another at the C-terminus is the site of glycosylphosphatidylinositol linkage. Glycosylation can occur on residues 180 and 196. A disulfide bridge (178–213) links two of the alpha-helices in this region. α, alpha-helical domain; β, beta-sheet domain.

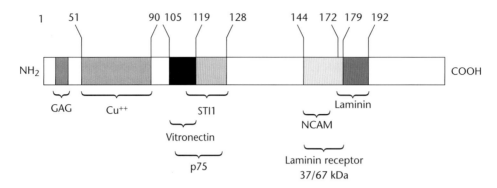

Figure 1.3 Localization of ligand-binding domains in PrP^C. The binding sites for glycosaminoglycans (GAG; 23–35), Cu^{++} ions (51–90), Vitronectin (105–119), neurotrophin p75 receptor (p75; 106–126), stress-inducible protein 1 (STI1; 113–128), laminin (173–192), neural cell adhesion molecule (NCAM; 144–154), and laminin receptor 37/67 kDa (144–179) are indicated. Adapted from Hajj, Lopes, Mercadante et al. 2007.

prion diseases (Guentchev, Voigtlander, Haberler et al. 2000; Wong, Brown, Pan et al. 2001). Other studies have failed to find decreased SOD activity in PrP^C knockout mice (Waggoner, Drisaldi, Bartnikas et al. 2000), and studies in crosses between mice that over-express PrP^C and strains in which SOD is upregulated or downregulated, argue against a protective role for PrP^C against oxidative stress (Hutter, Heppner, Aguzzi 2003).

In some studies, the cellular prion protein itself has exhibited SOD-like activity (Brown, Wong, Hafiz et al. 1999; Brown 2005). Conversion of this protein to the protease-resistant isoform would be accompanied by a loss of antioxidant activity, suggesting a mechanism for neurodegeneration in prion diseases. Nevertheless, this is also controversial, since some studies were not able to detect PrP^C SOD activity (Jones, Batchelor, Bhelt et al. 2005). Therefore, although the binding of copper to PrP^C appears to impart cellular resistance to oxidative stress, the mechanisms associated with this function are still controversial.

PrP^C and the Extracellular Matrix

PrP^C binds two extracellular matrix proteins, laminin and vitronectin, in addition to its interaction with glycosaminoglycans (Fig. 1.3). Laminin is an extracellular heterotrimeric 800 kDa glycoprotein involved in cell proliferation, differentiation, migration, and death (Beck Hunter, Engel 1990). PrP^C is a saturable and high-affinity, specific receptor for laminin. This interaction may be important in a variety of tissues where PrP^C and distinct laminin isoforms are found. The PrP^C–laminin interaction is characterized by cell adhesion and neurite formation and extension (Graner, Mercadante, Zanata et al. 2000a; Graner, Mercadante, Zanata et al. 2000b). PrP^C also interacts with a 37 kDa/67 kDa laminin receptor that may

participate in PrP^C internalization in the plasma membrane (Gauczynski, Peyrin, Haik et al. 2001). The binding of vitronectin leads to axonal growth of dorsal root ganglia neurons. In PrP^C knockout mice, axon growth is compensated by increased activation of other vitronectin receptors, the integrins (Hajj, Lopes, Mercadante et al. 2007). While PrP^C interacts with glycosaminoglycans, the implications of these interactions have not yet been established (Warner, Hundt, Weiss et al. 2002; Pan, Wong, Liu et al. 2002).

STI1, NCAM, and p75NTR Binding

PrP^C is able to form other important interactions with stress-inducible protein (STI1), neural cellular adhesion molecule (NCAM), and p75 neurotrophic receptor to produce more established biological functions (Fig. 1.3). STI1 is a heat shock protein, first described in a macromolecular complex with the Hsp70 and Hsp90 chaperone protein family. STI1 binds PrP^C with high affinity and specificity (Zanata, Lopes, Mercadante et al. 2002). The PrP^C–STI1 interaction shows a neuroprotective response, rescuing neurons from apoptosis through the cAMP-dependent protein kinase (cAMP/PKA) signaling pathway in both retinal and hippocampal neurons (Chiarini, Freitas, Zanata et al. 2002; Lopes, Hajj, Muras et al. 2005). Furthermore, STI1 induces neuritogenesis in hippocampal cells in an extracellular signal–regulated kinase (ERK1/2)-mediated pathway (Chiarini, Freitas, Zanata et al. 2002; Lopes, Hajj, Muras et al. 2005). The PrP^C interaction site with STI1 differs from the laminin-binding site (Coitinho, Freitas, Lopes et al. 2006), indicating that PrP^C could be a component of a macromolecular complex, formed between the cell surface and extracellular proteins, that is composed of at least laminin, STI1, and PrP^C. The interaction between PrP^C and

NCAM recruits the latter to lipid raft compartments in the plasma membrane and induces Fyn phosphorylation. The association between PrP^C and NCAM ultimately leads to neuritogenesis (Santuccione, Sytnyk, Leshchyns'ka et al. 2005). Conversely, the interaction between PrP^C and p75 neurotrophin receptor appears to promote cell death. The neurotoxicity induced by a PrP^C peptide (amino acids 106–126) is a mechanism dependent on its interaction with p75 (la-Bianca, Rossi, Armato et al. 2001).

Role of PrP^C in Memory

PrP^C knockout mice initially presented no apparent phenotypic aberrations (Bueler, Fischer, Lang et al. 1992). However, upon closer examination, these animals suffered from increased sensitivity to pharmacologically induced epilepsy (Walz, Castro, Velasco et al. 2002), increased locomotor activity (Roesler, Walz, Quevedo et al. 1999), and alterations in the glutamatergic system (Coitinho, Dietrich, Hoffmann et al. 2002) and circadian rhythm (Tobler, Gaus, Deboer et al. 1996). Also, PrP^C knockout animals show normal hippocampal memory at 3 months of age but display a deficit at 9 months of age (Coitinho, Roesler, Martins et al. 2003). It was also shown that PrP^C knockout animals are impaired in hippocampus-dependent spatial learning, while nonspatial learning remained intact. These deficits were rescued by the introduction of PrP^C into neurons (Criado, Sanchez-Alavez, Conti et al. 2005).

The PrP^C–laminin interaction is necessary for long-term memory via PKA and MAPK signaling, which are classic pathways for memory consolidation (Coitinho, Freitas, Lopes et al. 2006). Long-term memory, as opposed to short-term memory, depends on continuous protein synthesis and changes in the molecular components of the neuronal synapse (Izquierdo, Medina, Vianna et al. 1999). Moreover, the PrP^C interaction with STI1 demonstrated a pivotal role in memory formation (short-term memory) and consolidation (long-term memory) (Coitinho, Lopes, Hajj et al. 2007).

In humans, mutations in the PrP^C gene have also been involved in the alteration of cognitive processes. For example, a rare polymorphism at codon 171 is linked to psychiatric alterations in humans (Samaia, Mari, Vallada et al. 1997). Furthermore, cognitive performance is impaired in elderly persons (Berr, Richard, Dufouil et al. 1998; Kachiwala, Harris, Wright et al. 2005) and Down syndrome patients (Del Bo, Comi, Giorda et al. 2003) when valine is codified at codon 129. Young individuals with at least one methionine allele in this position were reported to have better long-term memory than control subjects with two valine alleles (Papassotiropoulos, Wollmer, Aguzzi et al. 2005).

PrP^C in the Immune System

Although the nervous system is the main focus of research in prion biology, PrP^C expression is widespread and developmentally regulated in other cell types. In the immune system, PrP^C is expressed in hematopoietic progenitors and mitotic lymphocytes (Ford, Burton, Morris et al. 2002b).

In T lymphocytes, PrP^C expression varies depending on cell activation. T lymphocytes from PrP^C knockout mice show abnormal proliferation and altered cytokine levels after activation, suggesting a role for PrP^C in T-cell mitogenesis-mediated proliferation, activation, and antigenic response (Bainbridge, Walker 2005). Moreover, PrP^C overexpression generates an antioxidant context that leads to differential T-cell development (Jouvin-Marche, Attuil-Audenis, Aude-Garcia et al. 2006). PrP^C knockout mice injected with inflammation-stimulating compounds experience a reduction in leukocyte infiltration and fewer polymorphonuclear cells when compared to wild-type controls (de Almeida, Chiarini, da Silva et al. 2005).

Despite the involvement of specific immune cell types in the accumulation of PrP^{Sc}, little is known about PrP^C in these cells and the possible consequences for immune responses. Mounting evidence indicates that PrP^C may be important for the development and maintenance of the immune system and immunological responses, suggesting a possible loss of immune function in prion diseases.

PrP^C in Cell Death

The role of PrP^C in cell death is controversial because of conflicting results from a number of studies, which can vary depending on the cellular context under observation (Westaway, DeArmond, Cayetano-Canlas et al. 1994; Paitel, Sunyach, Alves et al. 2003b; Solforosi, Criado, McGavern et al. 2004). PrP^C has been implicated in protection against Bax-mediated cell death. Bax is a cytoplasmic pro-apoptotic protein that, in response to apoptotic signals, activates cell death cascades. Bcl-2, a protein that interacts with Bax and inhibits its apoptotic effects, has similarity to the N-terminal region of PrP^C, suggesting a major role for PrP^C in protection against cell death (Li, Harris 2005). In fact, PrP^C suppression of Bax-mediated cell death in neuron cultures depends on the PrP^C N-terminal region domain (Bounhar, Zhang, Goodyer et al. 2001). Familial mutations (D178N and T183A) in this region, which are associated with prion diseases, suppress the anti-Bax function of PrP^C (Roucou, LeBlanc 2005).

On the other hand, some studies have identified PrP^C as a pro-apoptotic protein. Degeneration of skeletal muscle, peripheral nerves, and the CNS is found in mice that overexpress wild-type PrP^C (Westaway, DeArmond, Cayetano-Canlas et al. 1994). PrP^C transfection also enhances cell susceptibility to apoptotic stimuli such as staurosporine, in a p53-dependent pathway (Paitel, Fahraeus, Checler 2003a). Furthermore, the cross-linking of two PrP^C molecules by antibodies in vivo induces cell death in the hippocampus and cerebellum, suggesting that PrP^C functions in the control of neuronal survival. The promotion of neuronal death through PrP^C cross-linking provides a model that explains PrP^{Sc} neurotoxicity (Solforosi, Criado, McGavern et al. 2004).

PrP^C Signaling

Activation of signal transduction pathways is essential to all cell phenomena. PrP^C activation of signal transduction pathways has been demonstrated through the engagement of PrP^C with ligands or antibodies, as well as exposure of cells to recombinant PrP^C (Table 1.6).

Neuroprotection associated with the engagement of STI1 with PrP^C mediates activation of the cAMP/PKA pathway (Chiarini, Freitas, Zanata et al. 2002; Lopes, Hajj, Muras et al. 2005). The basal activity levels of both intracellular cAMP and PKA are higher in PrP^C knockout neurons than in the wild type, which likely represents a compensatory response to the lack of PrP^C (Chiarini, Freitas, Zanata et al. 2002). The PKA pathway has also been implicated in the neurite outgrowth and neuronal survival of cerebellar granule cells that are induced by recombinant PrP^C (Chen, Mange, Dong et al. 2003).

PrP^C interaction with STI1 (Chiarini, Freitas, Zanata et al. 2002; Lopes, Hajj, Muras et al. 2005), antibody-induced clustering of PrP^C (Schneider, Mutel, Pietri et al. 2003; Monnet, Gavard, Mege et al. 2004), or cell treatment with recombinant PrP^C (Chen, Mange, Dong et al. 2003) also leads

to Erk activation, which is associated with neuron differentiation. Basal Erk activation was also higher in PrP^C knockout neurons than in wild-type cells (Brown, Nicholas, Canevari 2002; Lopes, Hajj, Muras et al. 2005). Thus, engagement of PrP^C at the cell surface and exposure to extracellular PrP^C induces Erk activation, and expression of PrP^C affects the basal level of Erk activity.

Another important cell signaling pathway, Fyn, is also triggered by antibody cross-linking of PrP^C (Mouillet-Richard, Ermonval, Chebassier et al. 2000). The same signaling pathway appears to be essential for the axon outgrowth induced by recombinant PrP^C (Kanaani, Prusiner, Diacovo et al. 2005). Furthermore, functional studies have provided strong evidence that PrP^C is able to recruit and stabilize N-CAMs into lipid rafts and activate Fyn (Santuccione, Sytnyk, Leshchyns'ka et al. 2005).

The phosphatidylinositol 3-kinase (PI3-K) signal cascade is a pathway associated with PrP^C neuronal treatment. Activation of PI3-K mediates axon outgrowth (Kanaani, Prusiner, Diacovo et al. 2005) and neuronal survival (Chen, Mange, Dong et al. 2003). This pathway is inhibited in PrP^C knockout mice (Weise, Sandau, Schwarting et al. 2006).

PrP^C is also associated with calcium-mediated cellular events, and calcium channels may be transmembrane partners of PrP^C-mediated signaling (Herms, Tings, Dunker et al. 2001; Korte, Vassallo, Kramer et al. 2003; Fuhrmann, Bittner, Mitteregger et al. 2006). However, no evidence of direct physical interaction of PrP^C with calcium channels at the plasma membrane is available to date.

It is important to note that PrP^C has several functions in cells that depend on its ability to initiate certain signal transduction pathways. More studies of the compensatory mechanisms that stem from PrP^C removal in knockout animals are needed. Almost all signal transduction pathways studied to date are upregulated or inhibited in PrP^C knockout mice, indicating the importance of this protein in the regulation of signaling pathway activation. Studies of pathway regulation alert to the dangers of prion therapeutics based on the removal of PrP^C, since they may affect neurons in unexpected ways.

Table 1.6 Cellular Pathways Induced by PrP^C

Cellular Pathway	References
cAMP/PKA	Chiarini et al. 2002; Lopes et al. 2005
ERK	Chiarini et al. 2002; Lopes et al. 2005
PI3-K	Chen et al. 2003; Vassallo et al. 2005
Fyn	Mouillet-Richard et al. 2000; Santuccione et al. 2005

NEUROINVASION AND PATHOGENICITY

A very important point that is still under discussion is how the prions get to the brain after ingestion. It is believed that the lymphoreticular system is a reservoir for prion replication, playing a major role in PrP^{Sc} replication. After peripheral PrP^{Sc} inoculation, animals lacking B lymphocytes do not develop prion disease, an indication of the importance of this cell type in the transport of PrP^{Sc} to the CNS. Furthermore, it is possible to find the infectious agent in the spleen of infected patients, and PrP^{Sc} transport from the spleen to the CNS appears to depend on the peripheral nerves (Aguzzi, Miele 2004; Glatzel, Giger, Braun et al. 2004; Caramelli, Ru, Acutis et al. 2006). On the other hand, there is evidence that PrP^{Sc} might directly cross the blood–brain barrier (Banks, Niehoff, Adessi et al. 2004).

Neurodegeneration plays a central role in pathogenesis, but the mechanism is still controversial (Fig. 1.4). Two mechanistic hypotheses have been postulated for the action of prion diseases. In the gain-of-function hypothesis, neuronal death is due to PrP^{Sc} toxicity and amyloid formation. The drawback to this hypothesis is that amyloid plaque deposition does not correlate to neuron death in some forms of prion disease (Chretien, Dorandeu, Adle-Biassette et al. 1999). Furthermore, when a transgenic mouse model in which PrP^{C} was ablated only in the neurons was infected with scrapie, there was extensive deposition of amyloid plaques but no neurodegeneration (Mallucci, Dickinson, Linehan et al. 2003). In light of these findings, a loss-of-function mechanism was proposed in which an important cellular function of PrP^{C} would be lost upon its conversion to PrP^{Sc}. Critics of this theory point out that PrP^{C} knockout animals present no apparent phenotype (Bueler, Fischer, Lang et al. 1992), which apparently negates the premise that PrP^{C} is an essential protein for prion disease. Alternatively, a combination of both factors could contribute to the disease.

DIAGNOSIS AND THERAPEUTIC APPROACHES

Initial diagnosis is based on clinical symptoms that include multifocal neurological dysfunction, involuntary myoclonic movements, and rapid progression. In nvCJD, the age of onset is also a very important diagnostic factor. Although routine hematological and biochemical indices are usually normal in prion disease patients, some other examinations may prove helpful. Electroencephalography (EEG) shows triphasic generalized periodic complexes in two-thirds of patients (Will, Matthews 1984), although these patterns are also found in other conditions, such as toxic states (Will 1991). It has been noted that a protein called 14–3-3 is present in the cerebrospinal fluid of 90% of cases (Hsich, Beckett, Collinge et al. 1996), but it can also be present in high concentrations in other diseases such as encephalitis and brain stroke. Neuroimaging techniques, especially magnetic resonance imaging (MRI), may also be useful in prion disease detection. In classical CJD, there is an increase in signal in the caudate and putamen regions of the brain (Finkenstaedt, Szudra, Zerr et al. 1996), whereas in nvCJD there is a signal increase in the pulvinar region of the posterior thalamus (Collie, Sellar, Zeidler et al. 2001).

Detection of PrP^{Sc} by brain biopsy is the most accurate method, although a negative result does not exclude a sampling error. Furthermore, the procedure has an inherent risk of hemorrhage and abscess formation. Tonsil biopsy may also be of diagnostic

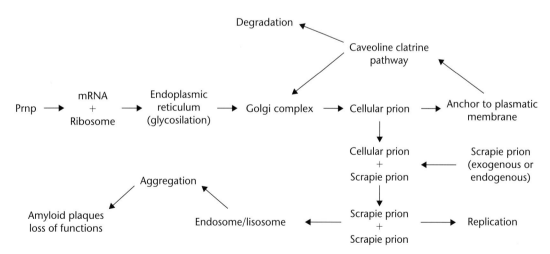

Figure 1.4 Schematic of cellular pathways involved in prion biology and diseases. The cellular prion protein (PrP^{C}) is synthesized, folded, and glycosylated in the endoplasmic reticulum, where a glycosylphosphatidylinositol anchor is added before further modifications in the Golgi complex. The mature protein is transported to the plasma membrane, after which it cycles between the membrane, vesicles, and the Golgi complex. Introduction of the scrapie prion (PrP^{Sc}) into a normal cell leads to the conversion of PrP^{C} into the PrP^{Sc} conformation. The accumulation of insoluble PrP^{Sc} and the loss of function of PrP^{C} are probably involved in disease development.

value in nvCJD cases, although it too presents risks for the patients (Hill, Zeidler, Ironside et al, 1997b).

The diagnostic option for familial diseases is the sequencing of *Prnp* in DNA extracted from peripheral blood and identification of one of the described mutations. Sequencing can also detect a codon 129 polymorphism (valine or methionine), where methionine homozygosity is a risk factor for sporadic CJD and nvCJD. The biochemical analysis of brain samples, through proteinase K digestion followed by Western blotting, allows the classification of the prion strain within the infected tissue (Glatzel, Stoeck, Seeger et al. 2005).

Additionally, new methods have been developed for PrP^{Sc} detection, such as conformation-dependent immunoassay, dissociation-enhanced lanthanide fluorescent immunoassay, capillary gel electrophoresis, fluorescence correlation spectroscopy, and flow microbead immunoassay. All of these methods are awaiting further clinical validation but promise easier and more reliable diagnostic methods for prion diseases (Sakudo, Nakamura, Ikuta et al. 2007).

Recent diagnostic tools include protein misfolding cyclic amplification (PMCA), which is able to detect small concentrations of PrP^{Sc} in blood and can be potentially automated and optimized for highly efficient PrP^{Sc} amplification. In hamsters, PMCA showed 89% sensitivity and 100% specificity, raising the hope for an effective and noninvasive blood diagnostic for PrP^{Sc} (Castilla, Nakamura, Ikuta et al. 2005b; Supattapone, Geoghegan, Rees 2006). However, the most conclusive diagnosis remains the postmortem histopathological analysis, where defined lesions can be observed and immunohistochemistry can detect PrP^{Sc} deposits using specific antibodies (Glatzel, Aguzzi 2001; Glatzel, Stoeck, Seeger et al. 2005). Today, a combination of detection methods has been suggested for differential prion diagnosis: 14–3-3 and other brain-derived proteins in cerebrospinal fluid such as total tau; EEG; and cerebral MRI, including diffusion-weighted images (Heinemann, Krasnianski, Meissner et al. 2007).

Despite many attempts, there is still no effective treatment for prion diseases. However, the knowledge of these diseases has increased tremendously, and disease models provide tools for the development of new therapeutic approaches. Several methods are now used to search for therapeutic compounds, including empirical analysis with screens based on the current knowledge of prion biology. Research-based trials search for compounds that block PrP^{Sc} formation in several ways: by blocking its interaction with PrP^{C}; changing its conformation and allowing its degradation; or reducing the availability of PrP^{C}, thus reducing the amount of substrate available for conversion.

Pharmacological treatments with a variety of compounds, including polysulfated anions, dextrans, Congo Red, oligonucleotides, and cyclic tetrapyrroles, have been proposed. These compounds increase the survival of mice infected with scrapie when administered at the time of infection, but not if administered a month or more after inoculation. Other compounds also clear up infection in cells, but have proved ineffective in mice and humans (Glatzel, Aguzzi 2001; Prusiner, May, Cohen 2004). Derivatives of acridine and the phenothiazine psychotropics have been proposed as possible therapies because of their activity in cellular models; however, neither class was able to affect the protease resistance of preexisting PrP fibrils. More encouragingly, in animal models of prion disease, tetracyclines were found to reduce prion infectivity by direct inactivation of PrP^{Sc} (Caramelli, Ru, Acutis et al. 2006).

The utilization of immunotherapy-based treatment has not achieved successful results in vivo. Antibodies, when injected directly into the brain, give rise to cross-reactions with PrP^{C}, causing neurotoxicity (Heppner, Aguzzi 2004). In contrast, passive immunization studies with PrP^{C}-specific antibodies have indicated that immunotherapeutic strategies directed against PrP^{C} can prevent prion disease (Buchholz, Bach, Nikles et al. 2006).

There is a concern, however, that current methods that might be used to destroy amyloid plaques would do more harm than good. In a recent work, small oligomers of PrP^{Sc} were much more toxic than the plaques themselves. If so, plaque formation would be a natural route of clearance, and the reversal of this process would be even more harmful (Silveira, Raymond, Hughson et al. 2005). The inactivation of PrP^{C} as a therapeutic method also raises concerns. As discussed in the last section, PrP^{C} may have fundamental roles in the nervous system, and its inactivation could prejudice normal function of the nervous system. These reservations show that any therapeutic measure should be studied carefully before validation for human use.

An alternative to disease treatment is the development of a postexposure prophylaxis, where the aim is to avoid PrP^{Sc} transportation from peripheral regions to the CNS. Palliative attempts are also envisioned, and the large cell loss from progressive disease could be regenerated through stem cell implants (Prusiner, May, Cohen 2004; Glatzel, Stoeck, Seeger et al. 2005). Nevertheless, with the advances in the comprehension of physiological functions and pathogenicity mechanisms of prion protein, it is likely that more effective treatments will be developed in the near future (Glatzel, Stoeck, Seeger et al. 2005).

FUTURE PERSPECTIVES

Since the mad cow disease crisis in the 1980s, much has been learned about the mechanisms of prion diseases. As a result, BSE has been practically eradicated. Now the focus has shifted to the biology of the cellular prion protein, the identification of new means of transmission, and the development of efficient diagnostic tools and therapies.

Although prion diseases affect the nervous system, the immune system is also involved in pathogenesis, especially after peripheral inoculations. Animal experiments show that the infection is detectable in lymphoid tissues and suggest the possibility of transmission through blood, tissues, or contaminated surgical materials. Two recent cases confirmed the risk of transmission through blood transfusion (Peden, Head, Ritchie et al. 2004; Mabbott, Turner 2005) and laryngoscopic slides used in tracheal intubations. These instruments are potential vectors, since PrP^{Sc} is highly resistant to inactivation through common methods and has an affinity for metallic materials (Hirsch, Beckett, Collinge et al. 2005). The spread of spongiform encephalopathies through blood and contaminated surgical materials is a public health matter and an economic concern. Further progress will require rapid and efficient diagnostic methods and new strategies of treatment and prevention (Glatzel, Aguzzi 2001; Mabbott, Turner 2005).

The knowledge based on prion proteins has developed rapidly over the last few years; however, efforts are still needed to attain a better understanding of the mechanisms involved in these diseases. Comprehension of the physiological role of PrP^{C} and the pathological process of spongiform encephalopathies could also improve our understanding of other, more common amyloid neurodegenerative diseases, such as Alzheimer's disease.

REFERENCES

Aguzzi A, Heppner FL, Heikenwalder M et al. 2003. Immune system and peripheral nerves in propagation of prions to CNS. *Br Med Bull.* 66:141–159.

Aguzzi A, Miele G. 2004. Recent advances in prion biology. *Curr Opin Neurol.* 17:337–342.

Aguzzi A, Polymenidou M. 2004. Mammalian prion biology: one century of evolving concepts. *Cell.* 116:313–327.

Alper T, Haig DA, Clarke MC. 1966. The exceptionally small size of the scrapie agent. *Biochem Biophys Res Commun.* 22:278–284.

Alper T, Cramp WA, Haig DA, Clarke MC. 1967. Does the agent of scrapie replicate without nucleic acid? *Nature.* 214:764–766.

Asante EA, Linehan JM, Desbruslais M et al. 2002. BSE prions propagate as either variant CJD-like or sporadic CJD-like prion strains in transgenic mice expressing human prion protein. *EMBO J.* 21:6358–6366.

Aucouturier P, Kascsak RJ, Frangione B, Wisniewski T. 1999. Biochemical and conformational variability of human prion strains in sporadic Creutzfeldt–Jakob disease. *Neurosci Lett.* 274:33–36.

Bainbridge J, Walker KB. 2005. The normal cellular form of prion protein modulates T cell responses. *Immunol Lett.* 96:147–150.

Banks WA, Niehoff ML, Adessi C, Soto C. 2004. Passage of murine scrapie prion protein across the mouse vascular blood-brain barrier. *Biochem Biophys Res Commun.* 318:125–130.

Basler K, Oesch B, Scott M et al. 1986. Scrapie and cellular PrP isoforms are encoded by the same chromosomal gene. *Cell.* 46:417–428.

Beck K, Hunter I, Engel J. 1990. Structure and function of laminin: anatomy of a multidomain glycoprotein. *FASEB J.* 4:148–160.

Berr C, Richard F, Dufouil C, Amant C, Alperovitch A, Amouyel P. 1998. Polymorphism of the prion protein is associated with cognitive impairment in the elderly: the EVA study. *Neurology.* 51:734–737.

Besnoit C, Morel C. 1898. Note sur les lesions nervoses de la tremblante du mouton. *Revue Veter Toulouse.* 23:397–400.

Bolton DC, McKinley MP, Prusiner SB. 1982. Identification of a protein that purifies with the scrapie prion. *Science.* 218:1309–1311.

Bons N, Mestre-Frances N, Belli P, Cathala F, Gajdusek DC, Brown P. 1999. Natural and experimental oral infection of nonhuman primates by bovine spongiform encephalopathy agents. *Proc Natl Acad Sci. U.S.A.* 96:4046–4051.

Bounhar Y, Zhang Y, Goodyer CG, LeBlanc A. 2001. Prion protein protects human neurons against Bax-mediated apoptosis. *J Biol Chem.* 276:39145–39149.

Brown DR. 2005. Neurodegeneration and oxidative stress: prion disease results from loss of antioxidant defence. *Folia Neuropathol.* 43:229–243.

Brown DR, Qin K, Herms JW et al. 1997a. The cellular prion protein binds copper in vivo. *Nature.* 390:684–687.

Brown DR, Schulz-Schaeffer WJ, Schmidt B, Kretzschmar HA. 1997b. Prion protein-deficient cells show altered response to oxidative stress due to decreased SOD-1 activity. *Exp Neurol.* 146:104–112.

Brown DR, Besinger A. 1998. Prion protein expression and superoxide dismutase activity. *Biochem J.* 334 Pt 2:423–429.

Brown DR, Wong BS, Hafiz F, Clive C, Haswell SJ, Jones IM. 1999. Normal prion protein has an activity like that of superoxide dismutase. *Biochem J.* 344 Pt 1:1–5.

Brown DR, Nicholas RS, Canevari L. 2002. Lack of prion protein expression results in a neuronal phenotype sensitive to stress. *J Neurosci Res.* 67:211–224.

Brown LR, Harris DA. 2003. Copper and zinc cause delivery of the prion protein from the plasma membrane to a subset of early endosomes and the Golgi. *J Neurochem.* 87:353–363.

Bruce ME, Will RG, Ironside JW et al. 1997. Transmissions to mice indicate that 'new variant' CJD is caused by the BSE agent. *Nature.* 389:498–501.

Buchholz CJ, Bach P, Nikles D, Kalinke U. 2006. Prion protein-specific antibodies for therapeutic intervention of transmissible spongiform encephalopathies. *Expert Opin Biol Ther.* 6:293–300.

Bueler H, Fischer M, Lang Y et al. 1992. Normal development and behaviour of mice lacking the neuronal cell-surface PrP protein. *Nature*. 356:577–582.

Bueler H, Aguzzi A, Sailer A et al. 1993. Mice devoid of PrP are resistant to scrapie. *Cell*. 73:1339–1347.

Cabral AL, Lee KS, Martins VR. 2002. Regulation of the cellular prion protein gene expression depends on chromatin conformation. *J Biol Chem*. 277:5675–5682.

Caramelli M, Ru G, Acutis P, Forloni G. 2006. Prion diseases: current understanding of epidemiology and pathogenesis, and therapeutic advances. *CNS Drugs*. 20:15–28.

Castilla J, Saa P, Hetz C, Soto C. 2005a. In vitro generation of infectious scrapie prions. *Cell*. 121:195–206.

Castilla J, Saa P, Soto C. 2005b. Detection of prions in blood. *Nat Med*. 11:982–985.

Cervenakova L, Buetefisch C, Lee HS et al. 1999. Novel PRNP sequence variant associated with familial encephalopathy. *Am J Med Genet*. 88:653–656.

Chandler RL. 1961. Encephalopathy in mice produced by inoculation with scrapie brain material. *Lancet*. 1:1378–1379.

Chen S, Mange A, Dong L, Lehmann S, Schachner M. 2003. Prion protein as trans-interacting partner for neurons is involved in neurite outgrowth and neuronal survival. *Mol Cell Neurosci*. 22:227–233.

Chesebro B, Race R, Wehrly K et al. 1985. Identification of scrapie prion protein-specific mRNA in scrapie-infected and uninfected brain. *Nature*. 315:331–333.

Chiarini LB, Freitas AR, Zanata SM, Brentani RR, Martins VR, Linden R. 2002. Cellular prion protein transduces neuroprotective signals. *EMBO J*. 21:3317–3326.

Chretien F, Dorandeu A, Adle-Biassette H et al. 1999. A process of programmed cell death as a mechanisms of neuronal death in prion diseases. *Clin Exp Pathol*. 47:181–191.

Coitinho AS, Dietrich MO, Hoffmann A et al. 2002. Decreased hyperlocomotion induced by MK-801, but not amphetamine and caffeine in mice lacking cellular prion protein (PrP(C)). *Brain Res Mol Brain Res*. 107:190–194.

Coitinho AS, Roesler R, Martins VR, Brentani RR, Izquierdo I. 2003. Cellular prion protein ablation impairs behavior as a function of age. *Neuroreport*. 14:1375–1379.

Coitinho AS, Freitas AR, Lopes MH et al. 2006. The interaction between prion protein and laminin modulates memory consolidation. *Eur J Neurosci*. 24:3255–3264.

Coitinho AS, Lopes MH, Haj GN et al. 2007. Short-term memory formation and long-term memory consolidation are enhanced by cellular prion association to stress-inducible protein 1. *Neurobiol Dis*. 26:282–290.

Collie DA, Sellar RJ, Zeidler M, Colchester AC, Knight R, Will RG. 2001. MRI of Creutzfeldt–Jakob disease: imaging features and recommended MRI protocol. *Clin Radiol*. 56:726–739.

Collinge J, Palmer MS, Dryden AJ. 1991. Genetic predisposition to iatrogenic Creutzfeldt–Jakob disease. *Lancet*. 337:1441–1442.

Collinge J, Sidle KC, Meads J, Ironside J, Hill AF. 1996. Molecular analysis of prion strain variation and the aetiology of 'new variant' CJD. *Nature*. 383:685–690.

Cousens SN, Zeidler M, Esmonde TF et al. 1997. Sporadic Creutzfeldt–Jakob disease in the United Kingdom: analysis of epidemiological surveillance data for 1970–96. *Br Med J*. 315:389–395.

Creutzfeldt H. 1920. Über eine eigenartige herdförmige Erkrankung des Zentralnervensystems. *Z ges Neurol Psychiatr*. 57:1–19.

Criado JR, Sanchez-Alavez M, Conti B et al. 2005. Mice devoid of prion protein have cognitive deficits that are rescued by reconstitution of PrP in neurons. *Neurobiol Dis*. 19:255–265.

Croes EA, Jansen GH, Lemstra AW, Frijns CJ, van Gool WA, van Duijn CM. 2001. The first two patients with dura mater associated Creutzfeldt–Jakob disease in the Netherlands. *J Neurol*. 248:877–880.

Cuille J, Chelle PL. 1939. Experimental transmission of trembling to the goat. *Comptes Rendus des Seances de l'Academie des Sciences*. 208:1058–1160.

de Almeida CJ, Chiarini LB, da Silva JP, PM ES, Martins MA, Linden R. 2005. The cellular prion protein modulates phagocytosis and inflammatory response. *J Leukoc Biol*. 77:238–246.

Del Bo R, Comi GP, Giorda R et al. 2003. The 129 codon polymorphism of the prion protein gene influences earlier cognitive performance in Down syndrome subjects. *J Neurol*. 250:688–692.

Doh-ura K, Tateishi J, Sasaki H, Kitamoto T, Sakaki Y. 1989. Pro—leu change at position 102 of prion protein is the most common but not the sole mutation related to Gerstmann–Straussler syndrome. *Biochem Biophys Res Commun*. 163:974–979.

Durig J, Giese A, Schulz-Schaeffer W, Rosenthal C et al. 2000. Differential constitutive and activation-dependent expression of prion protein in human peripheral blood leucocytes. *Br J Haematol*. 108:488–495.

Finckh U, Muller-Thomsen T, Mann U et al. 2000. High prevalence of pathogenic mutations in patients with early-onset dementia detected by sequence analyses of four different genes. *Am J Hum Genet*. 66:110–117.

Finkenstaedt M, Szudra A, Zerr I et al. 1996. MR imaging of Creutzfeldt–Jakob disease. *Radiology*. 199:793–798.

Flechsig E, Hegyi I, Enari M, Schwarz P, Collinge J, Weissmann C. 2001. Transmission of scrapie by steel-surface-bound prions. *Mol Med*. 7:679–684.

Ford MJ, Burton LJ, Li H et al. 2002a. A marked disparity between the expression of prion protein and its message by neurones of the CNS. *Neuroscience*. 111:533–551.

Ford MJ, Burton LJ, Morris RJ, Hall SM. 2002b. Selective expression of prion protein in peripheral tissues of the adult mouse. *Neuroscience*. 113:177–192.

Fornai F, Ferrucci M, Gesi M et al. 2006. A hypothesis on prion disorders: are infectious, inherited, and sporadic causes so distinct? *Brain Res Bull*. 69:95–100.

Fournier JG, Escaig-Haye F, Billetted V et al. 1998. Distribution and submicroscopic immunogold localization of cellular prion protein (PrPc) in extracerebral tissues. *Cell Tissue Res*. 292:77–84.

Fuhrmann M, Bittner T, Mitteregger G et al. 2006. Loss of the cellular prion protein affects the Ca(2+) homeostasis in hippocampal CA1 neurons. *J Neurochem*. 98:1876–1885.

Gajdusek DC. 1977. Unconventional viruses and the origin and disappearance of kuru. *Science*. 197:943–960.

Gajdusek DC, Zigas V. 1957. Degenerative disease of the central nervous system in New Guinea; the endemic occurrence of kuru in the native population. *N Engl J Med*. 257:974–978.

Gajdusek DC, Gibbs CJ, Alpers M. 1966. Experimental transmission of a Kuru-like syndrome to chimpanzees. *Nature*. 209:794–796.

Gauczynski S, Peyrin JM, Haik S et al. 2001. The 37-kDa/67-kDa laminin receptor acts as the cell-surface receptor for the cellular prion protein. *EMBO J*. 20:5863–5875.

Gerstmann J. 1928. Uber ein noch nicht beschriebenes Reflexphanomen bei einer Ekrankung des zerebellaren Systems. *Wien Med Wochenschr*. 78:906–908.

Ghetti B, Piccardo P, Spillantini MG et al. 1996. Vascular variant of prion protein cerebral amyloidosis with tau-positive neurofibrillary tangles: the phenotype of the stop codon 145 mutation in PRNP. *Proc Natl Acad Sci U.S.A.* 93:744–748.

Gibbons RA, Hunter GD. 1967. Nature of the scrapie agent. *Nature*. 215:1041–1043.

Gibbs CJ Jr., Gajdusek DC, Asher DM et al. 1968. Creutzfeldt–Jakob disease (spongiform encephalopathy): transmission to the chimpanzee. *Science*. 161:388–389.

Glatzel M, Aguzzi A. 2001. The shifting biology of prions. *Brain Res Brain Res Rev*. 36:241–248.

Glatzel M, Giger O, Braun N, Aguzzi A. 2004. The peripheral nervous system and the pathogenesis of prion diseases. *Curr Mol Med*. 4:355–359.

Glatzel M, Stoeck K, Seeger H, Luhrs T, Aguzzi A. 2005. Human prion diseases: molecular and clinical aspects. *Arch Neurol*. 62:545–552.

Goldfarb LG, Brown P, Little BW et al. 1993. A new (two-repeat) octapeptide coding insert mutation in Creutzfeldt–Jakob disease. *Neurology*. 43:2392–2394.

Graner E, Mercadante AF, Zanata SM et al. 2000a. Cellular prion protein binds laminin and mediates neuritogenesis. *Brain Res Mol Brain Res*. 76:85–92.

Graner E, Mercadante AF, Zanata SM, Martins VR, Jay DG, Brentani RR. 2000b. Laminin-induced PC-12 cell differentiation is inhibited following laser inactivation of cellular prion protein. *FEBS Lett*. 482:257–260.

Griffith JS. 1967. Self-replication and scrapie. *Nature*. 215:1043–1044.

Guentchev M, Voigtlander T, Haberler C, Groschup MH, Budka H. 2000. Evidence for oxidative stress in experimental prion disease. *Neurobiol Dis*. 7:270–273.

Hadlow WJ. 1959. Scrapie and kuru. *Lancet*. 2:289–290.

Hajj GN, Lopes MH, Mercadante AF et al. 2007. Cellular prion protein interaction with vitronectin supports axonal growth and is compensated by integrins. *J Cell Sci*. 120:1915–1926.

Harris DA, Lele P, Snider WD. 1993. Localization of the mRNA for a chicken prion protein by in situ hybridization. *Proc Natl Acad Sci U.S.A.* 90:4309–4313.

Hartsough GR, Burger D. 1965. Encephalopathy of mink. I. Epizootiologic and clinical observations. *J Infect Dis*. 115:387–392.

Heinemann U, Krasnianski A, Meissner B, Gloeckner SF, Kretzschmar HA, Zerr I. 2007. Molecular subtype-specific clinical diagnosis of prion diseases. *Vet Microbiol*. 123:328–335.

Heppner FL, Aguzzi A. 2004. Recent developments in prion immunotherapy. *Curr Opin Immunol*. 16:594–598.

Herm J, Tings T, Gall S et al. 1999. Evidence of presynaptic location and function of the prion protein. *J Neurosci*. 19:8866–8875.

Herms JW, Tings T, Dunker S, Kretzschmar HA. 2001. Prion protein affects Ca2+-activated K+ currents in cerebellar purkinje cells. *Neurobiol Dis*. 8:324–330.

Herzog C, Sales N, Etchegaray N et al. 2004. Tissue distribution of bovine spongiform encephalopathy agent in primates after intravenous or oral infection. *Lancet*. 363:422–428.

Hill AF, Desbruslais M, Joiner S et al. 1997a. The same prion strain causes vCJD and BSE. *Nature*. 389:448–50,526.

Hill AF, Zeidler M, Ironside J, Collinge J. 1997b. Diagnosis of new variant Creutzfeldt–Jakob disease by tonsil biopsy. *Lancet*. 349:99–100.

Hirsch N, Beckett A, Collinge J, Scaravilli F, Tabrizi S, Berry S. 2005. Lymphocyte contamination of laryngoscope blades--a possible vector for transmission of variant Creutzfeldt–Jakob disease. *Anaesthesia*. 60:664–667.

Houston F, Foster JD, Chong A, Hunter N, Bostock CJ. 2000. Transmission of BSE by blood transfusion in sheep. *Lancet*. 356:999–1000.

Hsiao K, Baker HF, Crow TJ et al. 1989. Linkage of a prion protein missense variant to Gerstmann–Straussler syndrome. *Nature*. 338:342–345.

Hsiao K, Dlouhy SR, Farlow MR et al. 1992. Mutant prion proteins in Gerstmann–Straussler–Scheinker disease with neurofibrillary tangles. *Nat Genet*. 1:68–71.

Hsich G, Kenney K, Gibbs CJ, Lee KH, Harrington MG. 1996. The 14-3-3 brain protein in cerebrospinal fluid as a marker for transmissible spongiform encephalopathies. *N Engl J Med*. 335:924–930.

Hutter G, Heppner FL, Aguzzi A. 2003. No superoxide dismutase activity of cellular prion protein in vivo. *Biol Chem*. 384:1279–1285.

Inoue I, Kitamoto T, Doh-ura K, Shii H, Goto I, Tateishi J. 1994. Japanese family with Creutzfeldt–Jakob disease with codon 200 point mutation of the prion protein gene. *Neurology*. 44:299–301.

Ironside JW, Bell JE. 1997. Florid plaques and new variant Creutzfeldt–Jakob disease. *Lancet*. 350:1475.

Izquierdo I, Medina JH, Vianna MR, Izquierdo LA, Barros DM. 1999. Separate mechanisms for short- and long-term memory. *Behav Brain Res*. 103:1–11.

Jakob A. 1921. Über einenartige Erkrankungen des Zentralnervensystems mit bemerkenswertem anatomischem Befunde (Spastische Pseudosklerose-Encephalomyelopathie mit disseminierten Degenerationsherden). *Z ges Neurol Psychiatr*. 64:147–228.

Jones S, Batchelor M, Bhelt D, Clarke AR, Collinge J, Jackson GS. 2005. Recombinant prion protein does not possess SOD-1 activity. *Biochem J*. 392:309–312.

Jouvin-Marche E, Attuil-Audenis V, Aude-Garcia C et al. 2006. Overexpression of cellular prion protein induces an antioxidant environment altering T cell development in the thymus. *J Immunol*. 176:3490–3497.

Kachiwala SJ, Harris SE, Wright AF et al. 2005. Genetic influences on oxidative stress and their association with normal cognitive ageing. *Neurosci Lett*. 386:116–120.

Kanaani J, Prusiner SB, Diacovo J, Baekkeskov S, Legname G. 2005. Recombinant prion protein induces rapid polarization and development of synapses in embryonic rat hippocampal neurons in vitro. *J Neurochem*. 95:1373–1386.

Kirschbaum WR. 1924. Zwei eigenartige Ekrankung des Zentralnervensystems nach Art der spatischen Pseudosklerose (Jakob). *Z Neurol Psychiatr*. 92:175–220.

Kitamoto T, Ohta M, Doh-ura K, Hitoshi S, Terao Y, Tateishi J. 1993. Novel missense variants of prion protein in Creutzfeldt–Jakob disease or Gerstmann–Straussler syndrome. *Biochem Biophys Res Commun*. 191:709–714.

Klamt F, Dal Pizzol F, Conte da Frota ML JR et al. 2001. Imbalance of antioxidant defense in mice lacking cellular prion protein. *Free Radic Biol Med*. 30:1137–1144.

Kocisko DA, Come JH, Priola SA et al. 1994. Cell-free formation of protease-resistant prion protein. *Nature*. 370:471–474.

Korte S, Vassallo N, Kramer ML, Kretzschmar HA, Herms J. 2003. Modulation of L-type voltage-gated calcium channels by recombinant prion protein. *J Neurochem*. 87:1037–1042.

Kovacs GG, Lindeck-Pozza E, Chimelli, L et al. 2004. Creutzfeldt–Jakob disease and inclusion body myositis: abundant disease-associated prion protein in muscle. *Ann Neurol*. 55:121–125.

Kubosaki A, Nishimura-Nasu Y, Nishimura T et al. 2003. Expression of normal cellular prion protein (PrP(c)) on T lymphocytes and the effect of copper ion: Analysis by wild-type and prion protein gene-deficient mice. *Biochem Biophys Res Commun*. 307:810–813.

la-Bianca V, Rossi F, Armato U et al. 2001. Neurotrophin p75 receptor is involved in neuronal damage by prion peptide-(106–126). *J Biol Chem*. 276:38929–38933.

Lang CJ, Heckmann JG, Neundorfer B. 1998. Creutzfeldt–Jakob disease via dural and corneal transplants. *J Neurol Sci*. 160:128–139.

Lee KS, Magalhaes AC, Zanata SM et al. 2001. Internalization of mammalian fluorescent cellular prion protein and N-terminal deletion mutants in living cells. *J Neurochem*. 79:79–87.

Legname G, Baskakov IV, Nguyen HO et al. 2004. Synthetic mammalian prions. *Science*. 305:673–676.

Li A, Harris DA. 2005. Mammalian prion protein suppresses Bax-induced cell death in yeast. *J Biol Chem*. 280:17430–17434.

Llewelyn CA, Hewitt PE, Knight RS et al. 2004. Possible transmission of variant Creutzfeldt–Jakob disease by blood transfusion. *Lancet*. 363:417–421.

Lopes MH, Hajj GN, Muras AG et al. 2005. Interaction of cellular prion and stress-inducible protein 1 promotes neuritogenesis and neuroprotection by distinct signaling pathways. *J Neurosci*. 25:11330–11339.

Mabbott N, Turner M. 2005. Prions and the blood and immune systems. *Haematologica*. 90:542–548.

Mallucci G, Dickinson A, Linehan J, Klohn PC, Brandner S, Collinge J. 2003. Depleting neuronal PrP in prion infection prevents disease and reverses spongiosis. *Science*. 302:871–874.

Marsh RF, Hadlow WJ. 1992. Transmissible mink encephalopathy. *Rev Sci Tech*. 11:539–550.

Martins VR, Mercadante AF, Cabral AL, Freitas AR, Castro RM. 2001. Insights into the physiological function of cellular prion protein. *Braz J Med Biol Res*. 34:585–595.

Martins VR, Brentani RR. 2002. The biology of the cellular prion protein. *Neurochem Int*. 41:353–355.

Masters CL, Gajdusek DC, Gibbs CJ Jr. 1981. The familial occurrence of Creutzfeldt–Jakob disease and Alzheimer's disease. *Brain*. 104:535–558.

Mastrianni JA, Iannicola C, Myers RM, DeArmond S, Prusiner SB. 1996. Mutation of the prion protein gene at codon 208 in familial Creutzfeldt–Jakob disease. *Neurology*. 47:1305–1312.

McKinley MP, Bolton DC, Prusiner SB. 1983. A protease-resistant protein is a structural component of the scrapie prion. *Cell*. 35:57–62.

McKintosh E, Tabrizi SJ, Collinge J. 2003. Prion diseases. *J Neurovirol*. 9:183–193.

Medori R, Tritschler HJ, LeBlanc A et al. 1992. Fatal familial insomnia, a prion disease with a mutation at codon 178 of the prion protein gene. *N Engl J Med*. 326:444–449.

Merz PA, Somerville RA, Wisniewski HM, Iqbal K. 1981. Abnormal fibrils from scrapie-infected brain. *Acta Neuropathol (Berl)*. 54:63–74.

Merz PA, Rohwer RG, Kascsak R et al. 1984. Infection-specific particle from the unconventional slow virus diseases. *Science*. 225:437–440.

Meyer RK, McKinley MP, Bowman KA, Braunfeld MB, Barry RA, Prusiner SB. 1986. Separation and properties of cellular and scrapie prion proteins. *Proc Natl Acad Sci U.S.A*. 83:2310–2314.

Milhavet O, McMahon HE, Rachidi W et al. 2000. Prion infection impairs the cellular response to oxidative stress. *Proc Natl Acad Sci U.S.A*. 97:13937–13942.

Miura T, Hori-i A, Takeuchi H. 1996. Metal-dependent alpha-helix formation promoted by the glycine-rich octapeptide region of prion protein. *FEBS Lett*. 396:248–252.

Miura T, Sasaki S, Toyama A, Takeuchi H. 2005. Copper reduction by the octapeptide repeat region of prion protein: pH dependence and implications in cellular copper uptake. *Biochemistry*. 44:8712–8720.

Monnet C, Gavard J, Mege RM, Sobel A. 2004. Clustering of cellular prion protein induces ERK1/2 and stathmin phosphorylation in GT1–7 neuronal cells. *FEBS Lett*. 576:114–118.

Mouillet-Richard S, Ermonval M, Chebassier C et al. 2000. Signal transduction through prion protein. *Science*. 289:1925–1928.

Narang H. 1996. Origin and implications of bovine spongiform encephalopathy. *Proc Soc Exp Biol Med*. 211:306–322.

Narang HK. 1987. Scrapie, an unconventional virus: the current views. *Proc Soc Exp Biol Med*. 184:375–388.

Nitrini R, Rosemberg S, Passos-Bueno MR et al. 1997. Familial spongiform encephalopathy associated with a novel prion protein gene mutation. *Ann Neurol*. 42:138–146.

Oesch B, Westaway D, Walchli M et al. 1985. A cellular gene encodes scrapie PrP 27–30 protein. *Cell*. 40:735–746.

Paitel E, Fahraeus R, Checler F. 2003a. Cellular prion protein sensitizes neurons to apoptotic stimuli through Mdm2-regulated and p53-dependent caspase 3-like activation. *J Biol Chem.* 278:10061–10066.

Paitel E, Sunyach C, Alves DC, Bourdon JC, Vincent B, Checler F. 2004. Primary cultured neurons devoid of cellular prion display lower responsiveness to staurosporine through the control of p53 at both transcriptional and post-transcriptional levels. *J Biol Chem.* 279: 612–618 .

Pan KM, Baldwin M, Nguyen J et al. 1993. Conversion of alpha-helices into beta-sheets features in the formation of the scrapie prion proteins. *Proc Natl Acad Sci U.S.A.* 90:10962–10966.

Pan T, Wong BS, Liu T, Li R, Petersen RB, Sy MS. 2002. Cell-surface prion protein interacts with glycosaminoglycans. *Biochem J.* 368:81–90.

Panegyres PK, Toufexis K, Kakulas BA et al. 2001. A new PRNP mutation (G131V) associated with Gerstmann–Straussler–Scheinker disease. *Arch Neurol.* 58:1899–1902.

Papassotiropoulos A, Wollmer MA, Aguzzi A, Hock C, Nitsch RM, de Quervain DJ. 2005. The prion gene is associated with human long-term memory. *Hum Mol Genet.* 14:2241–2246.

Pattison IH, Millson G. 1961. Scrapie produced experimentally in goats with special reference to the clinical syndrome. *J Comp Pathol.* 71:101–109.

Pauly PC, Harris DA. 1998. Copper stimulates endocytosis of the prion protein. *J Biol Chem.* 273:33107–33110.

Peden AH, Head MW, Ritchie DL, Bell JE, Ironside JW. 2004. Preclinical vCJD after blood transfusion in a PRNP codon 129 heterozygous patient. *Lancet.* 364:527–529.

Peoc'h K, Manivet P, Beaudry P et al. 2000. Identification of three novel mutations (E196K, V203I, E211Q) in the prion protein gene (PRNP) in inherited prion diseases with Creutzfeldt–Jakob disease phenotype. *Hum Mutat.* 15:482.

Piccardo P, Dlouhy SR, Lievens PM et al. 1998. Phenotypic variability of Gerstmann–Straussler–Scheinker disease is associated with prion protein heterogeneity. *J Neuropathol Exp Neurol.* 57:979–988.

Pocchiari M, Salvatore M, Cutruzzola F et al. 1993. A new point mutation of the prion protein gene in Creutzfeldt–Jakob disease. *Ann Neurol.* 34:802–807.

Prado MA, Alves-Silva J, Magalhaes AC et al. 2004. PrPc on the road: trafficking of the cellular prion protein. *J Neurochem.* 88:769–781.

Prusiner SB. 1982. Novel proteinaceous infectious particles cause scrapie. *Science.* 216:136–144.

Prusiner SB. 1989. Scrapie prions. *Annu Rev Microbiol.* 43:345–374.

Prusiner SB. 1998. Prions. *Proc Natl Acad Sci U.S.A.* 95:13363–13383.

Prusiner SB, Groth DF, Cochran SP, Masiarz FR, McKinley MP, Martinez HM. 1980. Molecular properties, partial purification, and assay by incubation period measurements of the hamster scrapie agent. *Biochemistry.* 19:4883–4891.

Prusiner SB, McKinley MP, Bowman KA, Bolton DC, Bendheim PE, Groth DF. 1983. Scrapie prions aggregate to form amyloid-like birefringent rods. *Cell.* 35:349–358.

Prusiner SB, Cochran SP, Alpers MP. 1985. Transmission of scrapie in hamsters. *J Infect Dis.* 152:971–978.

Prusiner SB, May B, Cohen F. 2004. Therapeutic approaches to prion diseases. In Prusiner SB, ed. *Prion biology and diseases.* New York, NY: Cold Spring Harbor Laboratory Press, 961–1015.

Rachidi W, Vilette D, Guiraud P et al. 2003. Expression of prion protein increases cellular copper binding and antioxidant enzyme activities but not copper delivery. *J Biol Chem.* 278:9064–9072.

Riek R, Hornemann S, Wider G, Billeter M, Glockshuber R, Wuthrich K. 1996. NMR structure of the mouse prion protein domain PrP(121–321). *Nature.* 382:180–182.

Roesler R, Walz R, Quevedo J et al. 1999. Normal inhibitory avoidance learning and anxiety, but increased locomotor activity in mice devoid of PrP(C). *Brain Res Mol Brain Res.* 71:349–353.

Roucou X, LeBlanc AC. 2005. Cellular prion protein neuroprotective function: implications in prion diseases. *J Mol Med.* 83:3–11.

Sakudo A, Nakamura I, Ikuta K, Onodera T. 2007. Recent developments in prion disease research: diagnostic tools and in vitro cell culture models. *J Vet Med Sci.* 69:329–337.

Sales N, Hassig R, Rodolfo K et al. 2002. Developmental expression of the cellular prion protein in elongating axons. *Eur J Neurosci.* 15:163–1177.

Samaia HB, Mari JJ, Vallada HP, Moura RP, Simpson AJ, Brentani RR. 1997. A prion-linked psychiatric disorder. *Nature.* 390:241.

Santuccione A, Sytnyk V, Leshchyns'ka I, Schachner M. 2005. Prion protein recruits its neuronal receptor NCAM to lipid rafts to activate p59fyn and to enhance neurite outgrowth. *J Cell Biol.* 169:341–354.

Schneider B, Mutel V, Pietri M, Ermonval M, Mouillet-Richard S, Kellermann O. 2003. NADPH oxidase and extracellular regulated kinases 1/2 are targets of prion protein signaling in neuronal and nonneuronal cells. *Proc Natl Acad Sci U.S.A.* 100:13326–13331.

Shyu WC, Harn HJ, Saeki K et al. 2002. Molecular modulation of expression of prion protein by heat shock. *Mol Neurobiol.* 26:1–12.

Sigurdson CJ, Miller MW. 2003. Other animal prion diseases. *Br Med Bull.* 66:199–212.

Silveira JR, Raymond GJ, Hughson AG et al. 2005. The most infectious prion protein particles. *Nature.* 437:257–261.

Solforosi L, Criado JR, McGavern DB et al. 2004. Cross-linking cellular prion protein triggers neuronal apoptosis in vivo. *Science.* 303:1514–1516.

Steele AD, Emsley JG, Ozdinler PH, Lindquist S, Macklis JD. 2006. Prion protein (PrPc) positively regulates neural precursor proliferation during developmental and adult mammalian neurogenesis. *Proc Natl Acad Sci U.S.A.* 103:3416–3421.

Supattapone S, Geoghegan JC, Rees JR. 2006. On the horizon: a blood test for prions. *Trends Microbiol.* 14:149–151.

Taraboulos A, Jendroska K, Serban D, Yang SL, DeArmond SJ, Prusiner SB. 1992. Regional mapping of prion proteins in brain. *Proc Natl Acad Sci. U.S.A.* 89:7620–7624.

Telling GC, Parchi P, DeArmond SJ et al. 1996. Evidence for the conformation of the pathologic isoform of the prion protein enciphering and propagating prion diversity. *Science.* 274:2079–2082.

Tobler I, Gaus SE, Deboer T et al. 1996. Altered circadian activity rhythms and sleep in mice devoid of prion protein. *Nature.* 380:639–642.

Turk E, Teplow DB, Hood LE, Prusiner SB. 1988. Purification and properties of the cellular and scrapie hamster prion proteins. *Eur J Biochem.* 176:21–30.

Varela-Nallar L, Toledo EM, Larrondo LF, Cabral AL, Martins VR, Inestrosa NC. 2006. Induction of cellular prion protein gene expression by copper in neurons. *Am J Physiol Cell Physiol.* 290:C271–C281.

Vassallo N, Herms J, Behrens C et al. 2005. Activation of phosphatidylinositol 3-kinase by cellular prion protein and its role in cell survival. *Biochem Biophys Res Commun.* 332:75–82.

Waggoner DJ, Drisaldi B, Bartnikas TB et al. 2000. Brain copper content and cuproenzyme activity do not vary with prion protein expression level. *J Biol Chem.* 275:7455–7458.

Walz R, Castro RM, Velasco TR et al. 2002. Cellular prion protein: implications in seizures and epilepsy. *Cell Mol Neurobiol.* 22:249–257.

Warner RG, Hundt C, Weiss S, Turnbull JE. 2002. Identification of the heparan sulfate binding sites in the cellular prion protein. *J Biol Chem.* 277:18421–18430.

Weise J, Sandau R, Schwarting S et al. 2006. Deletion of cellular prion protein results in reduced Akt activation, enhanced postischemic caspase-3 activation, and exacerbation of ischemic brain injury. *Stroke.* 37:1296–1300.

Wells GA, Scott AC, Johnson CT et al. 1987. A novel progressive spongiform encephalopathy in cattle. *Vet Rec.* 121:419–420.

Wells GA, Wilesmith JW. 1995. The neuropathology and epidemiology of bovine spongiform encephalopathy. *Brain Pathol.* 5:91–103.

Westaway D, DeArmond SJ, Cayetano-Canlas J et al. 1994. Degeneration of skeletal muscle, peripheral nerves, and the central nervous system in transgenic mice overexpressing wild-type prion proteins. *Cell.* 76:117–129.

Whittal RM, Ball HL, Cohen FE, Burlingame AL, Prusiner SB, Baldwin MA. 2000. Copper binding to octarepeat peptides of the prion protein monitored by mass spectrometry. *Protein Sci.* 9:332–343.

Wilesmith JW, Ryan JB, Atkinson MJ. 1991. Bovine spongiform encephalopathy: epidemiological studies on the origin. *Vet Rec.* 128:199–203.

Will RG. 1991. Epidemiological surveillance of Creutzfeldt–Jakob disease in the United Kingdom. *Eur J Epidemiol.* 7:460–465.

Will RG. 2003. Acquired prion disease: iatrogenic CJD, variant CJD, kuru. *Br Med Bull.* 66:255–265.

Will RG, Matthews WB. 1984. A retrospective study of Creutzfeldt–Jakob disease in England and Wales 1970–79. I: clinical features. *J Neurol Neurosurg Psychiat.* 47:134–140.

Will RG, Ironside JW, Zeidler M et al. 1996. A new variant of Creutzfeldt–Jakob disease in the UK. *Lancet.* 347:921–925.

Williams ES, Young S. 1980. Chronic wasting disease of captive mule deer: a spongiform encephalopathy. *J Wildl Dis.* 16:89–98.

Wong BS, Brown DR, Pan T et al. 2001. Oxidative impairment in scrapie-infected mice is associated with brain metals perturbations and altered antioxidant activities. *J Neurochem.* 79:689–698.

Wyatt JM, Pearson GR, Smerdon TN, Gruffydd-Jones TJ, Wells GA, Wilesmith JW. 1991. Naturally occurring scrapie-like spongiform encephalopathy in five domestic cats. *Vet Rec.* 129, 233–236.

Yamada M, Itoh Y, Fujigasaki H et al. 1993. A missense mutation at codon 105 with codon 129 polymorphism of the prion protein gene in a new variant of Gerstmann–Straussler–Scheinker disease. *Neurology.* 43:2723–2724.

Zanata SM, Lopes MH, Mercadante AF et al. 2002. Stress-inducible protein 1 is a cell surface ligand for cellular prion that triggers neuroprotection. *EMBO J.* 21:3307–3316.

Zawlik I, Witusik M, Hulas-Bigoszewska K et al. 2006. Regulation of PrPC expression: nerve growth factor (NGF) activates the prion gene promoter through the MEK1 pathway in PC12 cells. *Neurosci Lett.* 400:58–62.

Chapter **2**

ROLE OF PROTEIN KINASE C AND RELATED PATHWAYS IN VASCULAR SMOOTH MUSCLE CONTRACTION AND HYPERTENSION

Xiaoying Qiao and Raouf A. Khalil

ABSTRACT

Intracellular signaling activities in vascular smooth muscle (VSM) are central in the control of blood vessel diameter and the regulation of peripheral vascular resistance and blood pressure (BP). Several studies have examined the molecular mechanisms underlying VSM contraction under physiological conditions and the pathological alterations that occur in vascular diseases such as hypertension. Vasoconstrictor stimuli activate specific cell surface receptors and cause an increase in intracellular free Ca^{2+} concentration ($[Ca^{2+}]_i$), which forms a complex with calmodulin, activates myosin light chain (MLC) kinase and leads to MLC phosphorylation, actin–myosin interaction and VSM contraction. In unison, activation of protein kinase C (PKC) increases the myofilament force sensitivity to $[Ca^{2+}]_i$ and MLC phosphorylation, and maintains VSM contraction. PKC comprises a family of Ca^{2+}-dependent and Ca^{2+}-independent isoforms, which have different distributions in vascular tissues and cells, and undergo translocation from the cytosol to the periphery or the center of the cell depending on the type of stimulus. PKC translocation to the VSM cell surface triggers a cascade of events leading to activation of mitogen-activated protein kinase (MAPK) and MAPK kinase (MEK), a pathway that ultimately induces the phosphorylation of the actin-binding protein caldesmon, and enhances actin–myosin interaction and VSM contraction. PKC translocation to central locations in the vicinity of the nucleus induces transactivation of various proteins and promotes VSM cell growth and proliferation. Several forms of experimental and human hypertension are associated with increased expression/activity of PKC and other related pathways such as inflammatory cytokines, reactive oxygen species, and matrix metalloproteinases (MMPs) in VSM as well as the endothelium and extracellular matrix. Identifying the subcellular location of PKC may be useful in the diagnosis and prognosis of VSM hyperactivity states associated with hypertension. Targeting of vascular PKC using isoform-specific PKC inhibitors may work in concert with cytokine antagonists, antioxidants, and MMPs inhibitors, and thereby provide new approaches in the treatment of VSM hyperactivity states and certain forms of hypertension that do not respond to Ca²⁺-channel blockers.

Keywords: vascular biology, calcium, vasoconstriction, blood pressure.

Vascular smooth muscle (VSM) constitutes a significant component of the blood vessel wall. The ability of VSM to contract and relax plays an important role in the regulation of the blood vessel diameter and the blood flow to various tissues and organs. It is widely accepted that Ca²⁺ is a major determinant of VSM contraction. Activation of VSM by various physiological and pharmacological stimuli triggers an increase in intracellular free Ca²⁺ concentration ([Ca²⁺]ᵢ) due to initial Ca²⁺ release from the intracellular stores in the

sarcoplasmic reticulum and sustained Ca²⁺ influx from the extracellular space through excitable Ca²⁺ channels. Four Ca²⁺ ions bind to the regulatory protein calmodulin (CAM) and form a Ca²⁺–CAM complex. Ca²⁺–CAM then activates myosin light chain (MLC) kinase, which in turn promotes the phosphorylation of the 20-kDa MLC, stimulates the cross-bridge cycling of the actin and myosin contractile myofilaments, and leads to VSM contraction (Fig. 2.1). The reverse process occurs during VSM relaxation. Removal of the activating stimulus is associated with a decrease in [Ca²⁺]ᵢ due to Ca²⁺ extrusion via the plasmalemmal Ca²⁺ pump and the Na⁺–Ca²⁺ exchanger, as well as Ca²⁺ reuptake by the sarcoplasmic reticulum. The decrease in [Ca²⁺]ᵢ also favors the dissociation of the Ca²⁺–CAM complex, and the remaining phosphorylated MLC is dephosphorylated by MLC phosphatase, leading to detachment of the actin and

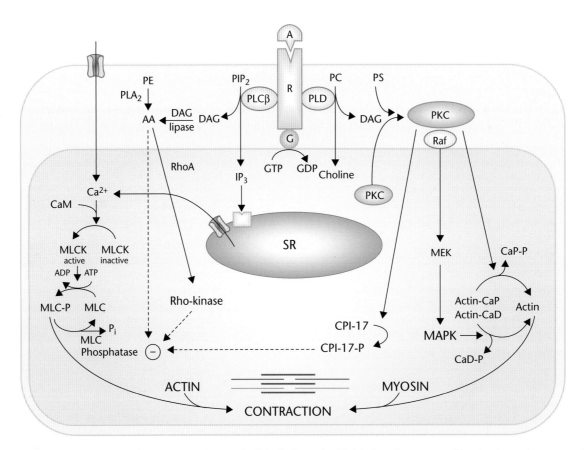

Figure 2.1 Cellular mechanisms of VSM contraction. A physiological agonist (A) binds to its receptor (R), stimulates plasma membrane PLC-β, and increases production of IP₃ and DAG. IP3 stimulates Ca²⁺ release from the sarcoplasmic reticulum (SR). At the same time, the agonist stimulates Ca²⁺ influx through Ca²⁺ channels. Ca²⁺ binds calmodulin (CAM), activates MLC kinase (MLCK), causes MLC phosphorylation, and initiates VSM contraction. DAG activates PKC. PKC-induced phosphorylation of CPI-17 inhibits MLC phosphatase and enhances the myofilament force sensitivity to Ca²⁺. PKC-induced phosphorylation of calponin (Cap) allows more actin to bind myosin. PKC may also activate a protein kinase cascade involving Raf, MAPK kinase (MEK) and MAPK, leading to phosphorylation of the actin-binding protein caldesmon (CaD). RhoA/Rho-kinase is another signaling pathway that inhibits MLC phosphatase and further enhances the Ca²⁺ sensitivity of VSM contractile proteins. AA, arachidonic acid; G, heterotrimeric GTP-binding protein; PC, phosphatidylcholine; PE, phosphatidylethanolamine; PIP2, phosphatidylinositol 4,5-bisphosphate; PS, phosphatidylserine. Interrupted line indicates inhibition. Adapted with permission from Salamanca, Khalil 2005.

myosin filaments and VSM relaxation (Khalil, van Breemen 1995; Horowitz, Menice, Laporte et al. 1996; Somlyo, Somlyo 2003; Salamanca, Khalil 2005).

One typical example of Ca^{2+}-dependent VSM contraction occurs during depolarization of VSM cell membrane. Cell membrane depolarization in response to mechanical stretch, nerve stimuli, electrical stimulation, or in the presence of high KCl solution activates voltage-gated Ca^{2+} channels and increases the probability of the channels being open. Because of the large concentration gradient between extracellular Ca^{2+} (millimolar) and $[Ca^{2+}]_i$ (nanomolar), the opening of Ca^{2+} channels facilitates Ca^{2+} influx, which stimulates MLC phosphorylation and causes sustained contraction of VSM. The VSM response to physiological agonists such as norepinephrine, prostaglandin $F_2\alpha$ and thromboxane A_2 differs from membrane depolarization in that it involves activation of other intracellular signaling pathways in addition to voltage-gated Ca^{2+} channels. The binding of a physiological agonist to its specific receptor at the VSM plasma membrane causes activation of phospholipase C (PLC), an enzyme that promotes the hydrolysis of phosphatidylinositol 4,5-bisphosphate into inositol 1,4,5-trisphosphate (IP_3) and diacylglycerol (DAG) (Berridge, Irvine 1984; Nishizuka 1992; Kanashiro, Khalil 1998). IP_3 is water soluble and therefore diffuses in the cytosol to the sarcoplasmic reticulum where it binds to IP_3 receptors and stimulates Ca^{2+} release from the intracellular stores, and the resulting transient increase in $[Ca^{2+}]_i$ initiates VSM contraction. Agonist-induced stimulation of VSM is also coupled to activation of ligand-gated and store-operated Ca^{2+} channels, causing a sustained increase in Ca^{2+} influx, $[Ca^{2+}]_i$, MLC phosphorylation, and VSM contraction (Fig. 2.1). However, the $[Ca^{2+}]_i$/MLC-dependent theory of VSM contraction has been challenged by several observations. For instance, agonist-induced VSM contraction is not completely inhibited by Ca^{2+}-channel blockers such as nifedipine, verapamil, or diltiazem. The insensitivity of agonist-induced contraction in certain blood vessels to Ca^{2+}-channel blockers could be related in part to the differential dependence of these vessels on Ca^{2+} release from the intracellular stores versus Ca^{2+} influx from the extracellular fluid (Khalil, van Breemen 1995). However, agonist-induced dissociations between $[Ca^{2+}]_i$ and force development have been demonstrated in several vascular preparations. Also, agonist-induced sustained VSM contraction has been observed in blood vessels incubated in Ca^{2+}-free solution and in the absence of detectable increases in $[Ca^{2+}]_i$ or MLC phosphorylation. Dissociations between $[Ca^{2+}]_i$ and MLC phosphorylation have also been observed during agonist-induced VSM contraction. These observations have suggested the activation of additional signaling pathways that

cause sensitization of the contractile myofilaments to $[Ca^{2+}]_i$ and enhance VSM contraction. These $[Ca^{2+}]_i$ sensitization pathways include Rho-kinase and protein kinase C (PKC) (Horowitz, Menice, Laporte et al. 1996; Somlyo, Somlyo 2003).

PKC has been identified and characterized for almost 30 years as one of the downstream effectors of guanosine triphosphate (GTP)-binding proteins and DAG. However, the role of PKC in VSM contraction is not as widely perceived as that of Ca^{2+}. This may be related to the fact that PKC is relatively larger in size than Ca^{2+}, making it more difficult to diffuse in the cytoplasm and activate the contractile myofilaments. Also, DAG, an activator of PKC, is lipid soluble and resides in the cell membrane, and therefore may hinder the movement of PKC into the core of the cell. Additionally, PKC isoforms have differential subcellular distribution and a wide spectrum of substrates and biological functions in various systems. An important question is how the different PKC isoforms are identified among other protein kinases in VSM, and how the signal from activated PKC is transferred from the cell surface to the contractile myofilaments in the center of the cell. Also, PKC may function in concert with other pathways in the control of VSM contraction and the regulation of vascular resistance and blood pressure (BP). Studies have suggested possible interaction between PKC and inflammatory cytokines (Ramana, Chandra, Srivastava et al. 2003; Tsai, Wang, Pitcher et al. 2004; Ramana, Tammali, Reddy et al. 2007), reactive oxygen species (ROS) (Heitzer, Wenzel, Hink et al. 1999; Ungvari, Csiszar, Huang et al. 2003), and matrix metalloproteinases (MMPs) (Hussain, Assender, Bond et al. 2002; Park, Park, Lee et al. 2003; Mountain, Singh, Menon et al. 2007) in the setting of vascular reactivity, growth, and remodeling. Studies have also suggested possible association between the vascular changes observed in hypertension and coronary artery disease and the amount and activity of cytokines (Nijm, Wikby, Tompa et al. 2005; McLachlan, Chua, Wong et al. 2005; Libby 2006), ROS (Cardillo, Kilcoyne, Quyyumi et al. 1998; Heitzer, Wenzel, Hink et al. 1999; Ungvari, Csiszar, Huang et al. 2003), and MMPs in the plasma and vascular tissues (Laviades, Varo, Fernandez et al. 1998; Ergul, Portik-Dobos, Hutchinson et al. 2004; Watts, Rondelli, Thakali et al. 2007). These observations have suggested that changes in the amount and activity of PKC and related pathways such as inflammatory cytokines, ROS, and MMPs in VSM as well as in the endothelium and extracellular matrix (ECM) could contribute to the pathogenesis of hypertension.

In this chapter, we will further examine PKC as a major regulator of VSM function. The chapter will provide a description of PKC isoforms and their protein substrates, discuss the subcellular distribution of

PKC isoforms and the mechanisms that promote their translocation during VSM activation, describe the various PKC activators and inhibitors, and evaluate the usefulness of determining PKC activity in the diagnosis and prognosis of VSM hyperactivity disorders and the potential use of PKC inhibitors in the treatment of certain forms of hypertension.

PKC ISOFORMS

PKC is a ubiquitous enzyme that has been identified in many organs and tissues. PKC was originally described as a Ca^{2+}-activated, phospholipid-dependent protein kinase (Takai, Kishimoto, Iwasa et al. 1979). Biochemical analysis and molecular cloning have revealed that PKC comprises a family of different isozymes of closely related structure. Members of the PKC family are a single polypeptide, comprised of N-terminal regulatory domain and C-terminal catalytic domain (Fig. 2.2). The regulatory and the catalytic halves are separated by a hinge region that becomes proteolytically labile when the enzyme is membrane-bound (Newton 1995).

The classic PKC structure has four conserved regions (C1–C4) and five variable regions (V1–V5). The C1 domain contains a tandem repeat of the characteristic cysteine-rich zinc finger–like sequence. The sequence Cys-X2-Cys-X13(14)-Cys-X7-Cys-X7-Cys,

where X represents any amino acid, is conserved among the different PKC subspecies. Each 30-residue sequence of this type is an independently folded unit that binds a zinc ion (Klevit 1990). The Cys-rich motif is duplicated in most PKC isozymes and may also form the DAG or phorbol ester–binding site. The cysteine-rich zinc finger–like motif is immediately preceded by an autoinhibitory pseudosubstrate sequence. The C1 domain also contains the recognition site for acidic phospholipids such as phosphatidylserine (Newton 1995). In the Ca^{2+}-dependent PKC isoforms, the C2 region is rich in acidic residues and has a binding site for Ca^{2+}. The C3 and C4 regions contain the adenosine triphosphate (ATP)- and substrate-binding sites. All PKC subspecies contain the ATP-binding sequence, Gly-X-Gly-X-X-Gly-----Lys, which is observed in most protein kinases (Fig. 2.2) (Nishizuka 1992; Newton 1995).

According to their biochemical structure and specific modulators, the PKC isoforms are classified into three subgroups.

1. The conventional PKC isoforms (cPKC) include the α, βI, βII, and γ isoforms. They have the traditional four conserved regions (C1–C4) and the five variable regions (V1–V5).

   The cDNA clones for α, βI, βII, and γ PKC were isolated from bovine (Coussens, Parker, Rhee et al. 1986; Parker, Coussens, Totty et al. 1986), rat (Ono, Fujii, Ogita et al. 1989), rabbit (Ohno, Konno, Akita

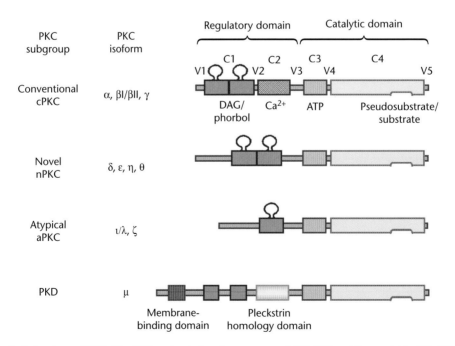

Figure 2.2 Biochemical structure of PKC. The PKC molecule has four conserved (C1–C4) and five variable (V1–V5) regions. C1 region contains binding sites for DAG, phorbol ester, and phosphatidylserine. C2 region contains Ca^{2+}-binding site. C3 and C4 regions contain binding sites for ATP and PKC substrate. Endogenous or exogenous pseudosubstrate binds to the catalytic domain and prevents PKC from phosphorylating the true substrate. Upon activation, the PKC molecule unfolds to remove the endogenous pseudosubstrate and bring ATP into proximity with the substrate. Adapted with permission from Salamanca, Khalil 2005.

Table 2.1 Vascular Tissue and Subcellular Distribution of PKC Isoforms

PKC Isoform	M.W. (kDa)	Blood Vessel	Resting State	Activated State	References
Conventional					
α	74–82	Ferret portal vein	Cytosolic	Surface membrane	Khalil et al. 1994
		Rat aorta	Cytosolic	Nuclear	Haller et al. 1994
		Carotid artery	Cytosolic	Membrane	Singer 1990
		Rat mesenteric artery	Cytosolic/membrane	Cytosolic/membrane	Ohanian et al. 1996
		Coronary artery	Cytosolic	Membrane	Kanashiro 2000
		Bovine aorta	Cytosolic	Membrane	Watanabe 1989
β	80–82	Rat aorta	Cytosolic	Nuclear	Haller et al. 1994
		Carotid artery	Cytosolic	Membrane	Singer 1990
γ	70–82	Rat mesenteric artery	Cytosolic	Cytosolic	Ohanian et al. 1996
Novel					
δ	76–82	Rat aorta	Cytoskeleton/organelle	Cytoskeleton/organelle	Liou 1994
		Rat mesenteric artery	Membrane	Membrane	Ohanian et al. 1996
ε	90–97	Ferret aorta	Cytosolic	Surface membrane	Khalil et al. 1992
		Rat mesenteric artery	Cytosolic/membrane	Cytosolic/membrane	Ohanian et al. 1996
		Coronary artery	Cytosolic	Membrane	Kanashiro 2000
η		NIH 3T3 fibroblasts	Cytosolic/membrane	Membrane	Goodnight 1995
Atypical					
ζ	64–82	Ferret aorta, portal vein	Perinuclear	Intranuclear	Khalil et al. 1992
		Rat aorta	Perinuclear	Intranuclear	Liou 1994
		Rat mesenteric artery	Cytosolic	Cytosolic	Ohanian et al. 1996
λ/ι	70	Rabbit femoral artery	Cytosolic	Cytosolic	Gailly et al. 1997
		Rabbit portal vein			

et al. 1990), and human brain libraries (Coussens, Parker, Rhee et al. 1986). Partial genomic analysis has clarified that βI and βII cDNAs are derived from a single mRNA transcript by alternative splicing, and differ from each other only in a short range of ≈50 amino acid residues in their carboxyl-terminal end in the variable region V5 (Ono, Fujii, Ogita et al. 1989; Ohno, Konno, Akita et al. 1990). α, βI, βII, and γ-PKC are downregulated by extended exposure to phorbol ester, although with different sensitivities.

2. The novel PKC isoforms (nPKC) include the δ, ε, η(L), and θ isoforms. They lack the C2 region and are therefore Ca^{2+}-independent (Ono, Fujii, Ogita et al. 1989).

The major areas of divergence of ε-PKC from α-, βI-, βII-, and γ-PKC are the regions V1 and C2 that are extended and deleted, respectively (Schaap et al. 1989. η-PKC shows phorbol ester–binding activity comparable to that observed for α-PKC. The nature of the binding activity, however, differs from that of α-PKC in that Ca^{2+} does not affect the affinity of η-PKC for [³H]PDBu (Ohno, Konno, Akita et al. 1990). η-PKC shows the highest sequence similarity to ε-PKC with 59.4% identity (Osada, Mizuno, Saido et al. 1992). PKC L is the human homologue of the mouse η-PKC (Bacher, Zisman, Berent et al. 1991). θ-PKC consists of 707 amino acid residues and shows the highest

sequence similarity to δ-PKC (67% identity) (Osada, Mizuno, Saido et al. 1992).

3. The atypical PKC isoforms (aPKC) include the ζ and λ/ι isoforms. These isoforms have only one cysteine-rich zinc finger–like motif. They are dependent on phosphatidylserine, but are not affected by DAG, phorbol esters, or Ca^{2+}. Consistent with this, the atypical PKC isoforms do not translocate or downregulate in response to phorbol esters or DAG derivatives (Fig. 2.2; Table 2.1) (Ono, Fujii, Ogita et al. 1989).

COMMON PKC SUBSTRATES

In the inactivated state, the PKC molecule is folded so that the basic autoinhibitory pseudosubstrate is tightly attached to the acidic patch in the substrate-binding site, and is therefore protected from proteolysis. The pseudosubstrate is unmasked when PKC is activated by conventional (phosphatidylserine, DAG, and Ca^{2+}), nonconventional (e.g., short chained phosphatidylcholines), or cofactor-independent substrates (e.g., protamine) (Takai, Kishimoto, Iwasa et al. 1979). Also, incubation of PKC with an antibody directed against the pseudosubstrate has been shown to activate the enzyme, presumably by removing the pseudosubstrate from the active substrate-binding site (Makowske, Rosen 1989).

Activated PKC phosphorylates protein substrates that are rich in arginine and displace the pseudosubstrate from the substrate-binding site in the catalytic domain (House, Kemp 1987; Orr, Keranen, Newton 1992; Newton 1995). These arginine-rich peptides neutralize the acidic patch that maintains the pseudosubstrate in the active site, thus releasing the basic pseudosubstrate by competing for contact (Newton 1995). The amino acid sequence in the vicinity of the substrate phosphorylation site may provide a substrate recognition guide for PKC. Although there is considerable diversity in the local phosphorylation site sequences for PKC, evidence obtained from structure–function studies with synthetic peptide substrates suggests that the enzyme has a requirement for basic residue determinants in common with other serine or threonine protein kinases (House, Kemp 1987).

Some of the common PKC substrates include lysine-rich histone and myelin basic protein (Takai, Kishimoto, Iwasa et al. 1979). PKC isoforms show some specificity for their substrates. α-, β-, γ-, and ζ-PKC are potent histone IIIS kinases. δ-, ε-, and η-PKC do not adequately phosphorylate histone IIIS, but readily phosphorylate myelin basic protein (Schaap et al. 1989; Dekker, McIntyre, Parker 1993; Kanashiro, Khalil 1998). However, removal of the regulatory domain of ε-PKC by limited proteolysis generates a catalytic fragment that can phosphorylate histone IIIS (Schaap et al. 1989).

One of the major PKC substrates is myristoylated, alanine-rich C-kinase substrate (MARCKS). MARCKS is an 87-kDa protein that binds to F-actin and may function as a crossbridge between cytoskeletal actin and the plasma membrane (Wang, Walaas, Sihra et al. 1989; Hartwig, Thelen, Rosen et al. 1992). Other membrane-bound PKC substrates include the inhibitory GTP-binding protein G_i. PKC-induced phosphorylation of G_i facilitates the dissociation of its α_i subunit from adenylyl cyclase and thereby transforms it from the inhibited to activated state (Katada, Gilman, Watanabe et al. 1985).

Plasma membrane ion channels and pumps are also known substrates for PKC. PKC inhibits the activity of Ca^{2+}-dependent large conductance K^+ channel (BK_{Ca}) in pulmonary VSM (Barman, Zhu, White 2004). Also, thromboxane A_2 may inhibit voltage-gated K^+ channels and pulmonary vasoconstriction via a pathway involving ζ-PKC (Cogolludo, Moreno, Bosca et al. 2003). PKC-induced phosphorylation of the sarcoplasmic reticulum Ca^{2+}-ATPase may promote Ca^{2+} uptake, and activation of plasmalemmal Ca^{2+}-ATPase may promote Ca^{2+} extrusion, and thereby contribute to reducing the agonist-induced increase in VSM $[Ca^{2+}]_i$ (Limas 1980). The α_1 subunit of Na/K-ATPase may also function as a PKC substrate.

Additionally, PKC may phosphorylate and activate the Na^+/H^+ exchanger and thereby increase the cytoplasmic pH and cause cell alkalinization (Rosoff, Stein, Cantley 1984; Aviv 1994).

PKC may also phosphorylate some of the structural and regulatory proteins associated with the VSM cytoskeleton and contractile myofilaments. PKC-induced phosphorylation of vinculin, a cytoskeletal protein localized at adhesion plaques, could cause significant changes in cell shape and adhesion properties. Tryptic peptide analysis revealed two major sites of PKC-mediated phosphorylation of vinculin, one containing phosphoserine and the other containing phosphothreonine. It has also been shown that while intact vinculin and its isolated head domain are only weakly phosphorylated by PKC, the isolated tail fragment is strongly phosphorylated (Schwienbacher, Jockusch, Rudiger 1996). PKC could also induce the phosphorylation of the CPI-17 regulatory protein, which in turn promotes inhibition of MLC phosphatase and thereby increases MLC phosphorylation and enhances VSM contraction (Woodsome, Eto, Everett et al. 2001). PKC could also phosphorylate the 20-kDa MLC as well as MLC kinase; however, this could counteract the Ca^{2+}-dependent actin–myosin interaction and force development (Inagaki, Yokokura, Itoh et al. 1987). Interestingly, α-PKC may cause the phosphorylation of the actin-associated regulatory protein calponin, a process that could free more actin to interact with myosin and thereby enhance VSM contraction (Parker, Takahashi, Tao et al. 1994).

DISTRIBUTION OF PKC IN VARIOUS TISSUES

PKC isoforms are expressed in different amounts in the VSM layer of various vascular beds (Table 2.1). α-PKC is a universal isoform that has been identified in almost all blood vessels examined. γ-PKC is mainly expressed in the neurons and may be found in the nerve endings of blood vessels. δ-PKC is mainly associated with the VSM cytoskeleton. ζ-PKC, another universal PKC isoform, has been found in many vascular tissues. η/L-PKC is exclusively present in the lung, skin, heart, and brain. θ-PKC has been identified in skeletal muscle. ι/λ-PKC is expressed in the testis and ovary (Kanashiro, Khalil 1998).

SUBCELLULAR DISTRIBUTION OF PKC ISOFORMS

In resting unstimulated cells, the PKC isoforms α, β and γ are mainly localized in the cytosolic fraction. Activation of PKC is generally associated with translocation of PKC isoforms to plasma membrane or specific binding domains of cells (Newton 1997; Mochly-Rosen, Gordon 1998). The Ca^{2+}-dependent α-, β-, and γ-PKC usually undergo translocation from the cytosol to the cell membrane fraction during activation (Kraft, Anderson 1983 (Table 2.1). However, exceptions to this redistribution pattern have been reported.

In normal fibroblasts, α-PKC is tightly associated with the cytoskeleton and appears to be organized into focal contacts of the plasma membrane that associates with both the cytoskeleton and the extracellular matrix. The focal contact is composed of several structural proteins (vinculin, talin, integrin, and α-actinin), which mediate the attachment of microfilament bundles to the plasma membrane (Hyat, Klauck, Jaken 1990).

In neural cells, the βI-subspecies is sometimes associated with plasma membranes, whereas the βII-subspecies is often localized in the Golgi complex (Nishizuka 1992).

In the cerebellum, γ-PKC is present in the cell bodies, dendrites, and axons of Purkinje's cells. Immunoelectron microscopic analysis has revealed that the γ-PKC is associated with most membranous structures present throughout the cell, except for the nucleus (Kose, Saito, Ito et al. 1988).

The localization of δ-PKC in the vicinity of the cytoskeleton makes it feasible to identify this isoform in the particulate fraction of both unstimulated and activated cells. In contrast, ε-PKC undergoes translocation from the cytosol to the surface membrane during activation of VSM cells. ζ-PKC has been localized in the vicinity of the nucleus of unstimulated and activated mature VSM cells (Khalil, Morgan 1996). However, ζ-PKC may have different distribution and function in the developing embryo and may play a role in pulmonary vasoconstriction during the perinatal period (Cogolludo, Moreno, Lodi et al. 2005).

TARGETING MECHANISMS FOR PKC TRANSLOCATION

What causes PKC to translocate from one cell compartment to another? Simple diffusion of PKC could be a possible driving force, while targeting mechanisms would allow tight binding of PKC when it happens to be in the vicinity of its target or substrate (Khalil, Morgan 1996). Some of the targeting mechanisms may include the following:

1. Conformation changes and altered hydrophobicity: The binding of Ca^{2+} or DAG to PKC could cause conformational change that unfolds the PKC molecule and results in exposure of the pseudosubstrate region or increases the hydrophobicity of PKC and thereby facilitates its binding to membrane lipids (Newton 1995).

2. Lipid modification: Modification in the lipid components of proteins could influence their subcellular distribution. For example, myristoylation of MARCKS is essential for its binding to actin and the plasma membrane. PKC is known to phosphorylate MARCKS and it interferes with its actin cross-linking and thereby causes its displacement from the plasma membrane. Dephosphorylation of MARCKS is associated with its re-association with the plasma membrane via its stably attached myristic acid membrane-targeting moiety (Thelen, Rosen, Nairn et al. 1991).

The architecture of the VSM plasma membrane may also be regulated by various cellular proteins. The VSM plasma membrane is composed of several domains of focal adhesions alternating with zones rich in caveolae, and both harbor a subset of membrane-associated proteins. Also, the plasma membrane lipids are segregated into domains of cholesterol-rich lipid rafts and glycerophospholipid-rich nonraft regions. The segregation of membrane lipids is critical for preserving the membrane protein architecture and for the translocation of proteins to the sarcolemma. In smooth muscle, membrane lipid segregation is supported by annexins that target membrane sites of distinct lipid composition, and each annexin requires different $[Ca^{2+}]$ for its translocation to the sarcolemma, thereby allowing a spatially confined, graded response to external stimuli and intracellular PKC (Draeger, Wray, Babiychuk 2005).

3. Phosphorylation: The phosphorylation of proteins could change their conformation or electric charge and thereby affect their affinity to lipids and their binding to surface membrane. For example, phosphorylation of MARCKS may induce an electrostatic effect that could be as important as myristoylation in determining the protein affinity to the plasma membrane. Also, phosphorylation of the PKC molecule itself may be essential for its translocation and full activation. PKC phosphorylation sites have been identified in the catalytic domain of α-, β-, and δ-PKC isoforms (Cazaubon, Parker 1993).

4. Targeting sequence: Binding sites for arginine-rich polypeptides have been identified in the PKC molecule distal to its catalytic site, allowing targeting of PKC to specific subcellular locations (Leventhal, Bertics 1993). Also, receptors for activated C-kinase (RACKs) have been suggested to target PKC to cytoskeletal elements. Additionally, a peptide inhibitor derived from the PKC-binding proteins annexin I and RACKI may interfere with translocation of the β-PKC isoform (Ron, Mochly-Rosen 1994).

PKC FUNCTIONS

The presence of PKC in many cells and tissues allows it to play a pivotal role in adjusting the cell to the environment by stimulating or inhibiting certain cellular processes. PKC has many physiological functions including secretion and exocytosis, modulation of ion channel conductance, gene expression, and cell growth and proliferation (Nishizuka 1992; Kanashiro, Khalil 1998).

One important approach to study the role of PKC in normal and deregulated growth has been through the production of cells that overexpress PKC. For example, the introduction of a vector containing the full-length cDNA encoding the βI-isozyme in rat fibroblasts led to overexpression of the isozyme and caused multiple cell growth abnormalities that mimicked the effects of tumor promoter phorbol esters. However, these cell lines did not exhibit the typical characteristics of malignantly transformed fibroblasts. Hence, the overproduction of PKC per se may not be sufficient to cause cancer, although it may facilitate the cell conversion to malignancy by genotoxic agents (Housey, Johnson, Hsiao et al. 1988).

Tumor promoters enhance tumor formation when administered after subcarcinogenic levels of initiators. However, they have little, if any, carcinogenic activity when administered alone. While the tumors formed in response to sequential application of initiators and tumor promoters are usually benign, they may spontaneously progress to a malignant phenotype. Although the most well-characterized initiation–promotion system is the mouse skin model, other studies indicate that cancers of the breast, colon, bladder, and liver also develop as a consequence of initiating and promoting events (O'Brian, Ward 1989).

PKC may exert negative-feedback control over cell signaling by downregulation of surface receptors and/or inhibition of agonist-induced activation of PLC and phosphoinositide hydrolysis (Nishizuka 1992). Also, numerous studies have suggested a prominent role of PKC in VSM contraction (Nishizuka 1992; Horowitz, Menice, Laporte et al. 1996; Kanashiro, Khalil 1998; Dallas, Khalil 2003). The most direct evidence is that DAG analogues and phorbol esters, known activators of PKC, cause significant contraction in vascular segments isolated from various blood vessels and examined ex vivo (Khalil, van Breemen 1988; Horowitz, Menice, Laporte et al. 1996; Kanashiro, Khalil 1998). Interestingly, the phorbol ester–induced vascular contraction may not be associated with detectable increases in $[Ca^{2+}]_i$, suggesting the involvement of a Ca^{2+}-independent PKC isoform such as ε-PKC (Jiang, Morgan 1987; Khalil, Lajoie, Resnick et al. 1992). Also, PKC inhibitors have been shown to cause significant inhibition of agonist-induced contraction of coronary VSM (Khalil, van Breemen 1988; Dallas, Khalil 2003). However, some studies have demonstrated that PKC-induced phosphorylation of MLC kinase may inhibit VSM contraction and may thereby promote vascular relaxation (Inagaki, Yokokura, Itoh et al. 1987).

ACTIVATORS OF PKC

PKC isoforms have different sensitivity to Ca^{2+}, phosphatidylserine, DAG, and other phospholipid degradation products. PKC-dependent isoforms bind Ca^{2+} in a phospholipid-dependent manner. The Ca^{2+} ion may form a "bridge" holding the PKC–phospholipid complex at the plasma membrane (Bazzi, Nelseusten 1990). Phosphatidylserine is essential for activation of most PKC isoforms. Phosphatidylinositol and phosphatidic acid may activate PKC, but may require high Ca^{2+} concentrations. DAG activates Ca^{2+}-independent PKC isoforms and may reduce the Ca^{2+} requirement for the activation and membrane association of Ca^{2+}-dependent PKC isoforms (Nishizuka 1992).

Lipids derived from sources other than glycerolipid hydrolysis such as cis-unsaturated free fatty acids and lysophosphatidylcholine, ceramide (a sphingomyelinase product), phosphatidylinositol 3,4,5-trisphosphate, and cholesterol sulfate may also activate PKC (Nishizuka 1995). Phorbol esters such as 12-o-tetradecanoylphorbol-13-acetate (TPA), phorbol myristate acetate (PMA), and phorbol 12,13-dibutyrate (PDBu) can substitute for DAG and activate PKC. Phorbol esters reduce the apparent K_m of PKC for Ca^{2+} and thereby stabilize its membrane association (Kanashiro, Khalil 1998).

Bryostatin, a marine natural product, is another PKC activator that binds to and activates PKC and is more potent than PMA for translocating δ- and ε-PKC, but it is not a carcinogen or a complete tumor promoter (Szallasi, Smith, Pettit et al. 1994). On the other hand, γ-rays may cause activation of the α- and ε-PKC isoforms, a process that could play a role in smooth muscle cell apoptosis in response to γ-radiation (Claro, Kanashiro, Oshiro et al. 2007). Also, oxidized low-density lipoprotein (LDL) increases the activity of α- and ε-PKC isoforms in coronary VSM, a process that could be involved in oxidized LDL–induced coronary artery vasoconstriction and atherogenesis (Giardina, Tanner, Khalil et al. 2001).

Multisite phosphorylation of PKC plays an important role in the regulation of the enzyme's function both in vitro and in vivo (Keranen, Dutil, Newton 1995; Li, Zhang, Bottaro et al. 1996; Edwards, Newton 1997). PKC activity and affinity for its substrate may be modified by protein kinase–induced phosphorylation or even its own autophosphorylation.

The α-, βI-, and βII-PKC proteins are expressed as inactive precursors that may require phosphorylation by a putative "PKC kinase" for permissive activation. For example, multiple phosphorylation of α-PKC prevents its downregulation during prolonged stimulation by phorbol ester (Keranen, Dutil, Newton 1995). Also, phosphorylation of βII-PKC at the extreme C-terminus allows the active site to bind ATP and substrate with higher affinity. Additionally, phosphorylation of structure determinants in the regulatory region of PKC increases its binding affinity with Ca^{2+} (Edwards, Newton 1997).

Autophosphorylation has also been reported for the Ca^{2+}-independent δ-PKC isoform. It has been demonstrated that the Ser-643 of δ-PKC is phosphorylated in vivo, a process that could play an important role in controlling the activity and biological function of the δ-PKC isoform (Li, Zhang, Bottaro et al. 1996).

INHIBITORS OF PKC

In the last 25 years, several PKC inhibitors with different affinities, efficacies, and specificities have been developed (Table 2.2). Some of the first PKC inhibitors appear to act on the catalytic domain and compete with ATP, and therefore may not be specific and could inhibit other protein kinases. PKC inhibitors acting on the regulatory domain by competing at the DAG- or phorbol ester-, or the phosphatidylserine-binding site may be more specific. Extended exposure to phorbol esters can downregulate α-, β-, γ-, and ε-PKC (Kanashiro, Altirkawi, Khalil et al. 2000), but the tumor promoting properties of phorbol esters significantly limit their use.

The pseudosubstrate region in the regulatory domain of PKC contains an amino acid sequence between the 19 and 36 residues that resembles the substrate phosphorylation site. Synthetic oligopeptides based on the pseudosubstrate sequence have been developed. The pseudosubstrate inhibitor peptides inhibit specific PKC isoforms because they exploit their substrate specificity and do not interfere with ATP binding. The synthetic peptide (19 to 36) inhibits not only protein substrate phosphorylation but also PKC autophosphorylation (House, Kemp 1987). Also, myr-ψPKC, a myristoylated peptide based on the substrate motif of α- and β-PKC, inhibits TPA-induced PKC activation and phosphorylation of the MARCKS protein (Eicholtz, de Bont, Widt et al. 1993).

α-Tocopherol inhibits the expression, activity, and phosphorylation of α-PKC in smooth muscles, while

Table 2.2 Examples of Inhibitors of PKC

Chemical Group	Examples	Specificity	Site of Action
1-(5-isoquinolinesulfonyl)-2-methylpiperazines	H-7	Also inhibits cyclic AMP and cyclic GMP-dependent protein kinases	Catalytic domain Compete with ATP at the ATP-binding site
Microbial alkaloids, product of *Streptomyces*	Staurosporine SCH 47112 CGP 41251 (PKC412, midostaurin)	Also inhibits MLC kinase and tyrosine kinase	Catalytic domain, ATP-binding site
Benzophenanthridine alkaloids	Chelerythrine	Competitive inhibitor with histone IIIS	Catalytic domain
Indocarbazoles	Gö6976	Ca^{2+}-dependent isoforms α and βI	Catalytic domain
Bisindolylmaleimide derivatives of staurosporine	GF109203X Ro-318220	PKC isozymes α, βI, βII, γ, δ, and ε	Catalytic domain
Others	Aminoacridine Apigenin Sangivamycin UCN-01, UCN-02		
Perylenequinone metabolites isolated from *Cladosporium cladosporioides*	Calphostin C (UCN-1028A)	Binds to the regulatory domain at DAG-/phorbol ester–binding site	Regulatory domain
Membrane lipids	Sphingosine	Competitive inhibitor with phosphatidylserine	Regulatory domain
Others	Adriamycin Cercosporin Chlorpromazine Dexniguldipine Polymixin B Tamoxifen Trifluoperazine		

β-tocopherol protects PKC from the inhibitory effects of α-tocopherol (Clement, Tasinato, Boscoboinik et al. 1997).

Short-interference RNA (siRNA) have been developed to prevent the expression of specific PKC isoforms and are becoming very useful in studying the role of PKC in various cell functions. Antisense techniques, knockout mice, and transgenic animals have also been useful in studying the effects of downregulation of specific PKC isoforms in vivo.

PKC-ACTIVATED PROTEIN KINASE CASCADES AND VSM CONTRACTION

VSM contraction may involve the activation of several protein kinases and the phosphorylation of more than one substrate. For instance, PKC-induced phosphorylation of one of its protein substrates may activate a cascade of protein kinases that ultimately stimulate or enhance VSM contraction (Khalil, Menice, Wang et al. 1995). PKC-induced phosphorylation of CPI-17 promotes the inhibition of MLC phosphatase and thereby increases the amount of MLC phosphorylation and enhances VSM contraction (Fig. 2.1) (Woodsome, Eto, Everett et al. 2001). The α-PKC may also induce the phosphorylation of the actin-binding protein calponin, a process that could reverse the calponin-mediated inhibition of the actin-activated myosin ATPase, and may thereby allow more actin to interact with myosin and enhance VSM contraction (Fig. 2.1) (Parker, Takahashi, Tao et al. 1994; Horowitz, Menice, Laporte et al. 1996).

In undifferentiated VSM cells, PKC may function in concert with MAPK and c-Raf-1 to promote cell growth and proliferation. MAPK is a Ser/Thr protein kinase that requires dual phosphorylation at both the Thr and Tyr residues for its activation. In quiescent undifferentiated VSM cells, MAPK is mainly distributed in the cytosol. On VSM cell activation by a growth factor or a mitogen, MAPK undergoes translocation from the cytosol to the nucleus where it stimulates mRNA gene expression and cell growth (Mii, Khalil, Morgan et al. 1996). Tyrosine kinase and MAPK activities have been identified in differentiated VSM, suggesting a potential role in VSM contraction (Khalil, Menice, Wang et al. 1995; Khalil, Morgan 1996). In differentiated VSM cells, contractile agonists such as the α-adrenergic agonist phenylephrine induce an initial and transient translocation of MAPK from the cytosol to the surface membrane. However, during maintained VSM activation MAPK undergoes redistribution from the surface membrane and localizes in the cytoskeleton (Khalil, Menice, Wang et al. 1995). It has been suggested that agonist-induced activation and generation of DAG at the surface membrane

promotes the translocation of the Ca^{2+}-independent ε-PKC from the cytosol to the surface membrane, where it becomes fully activated. The activated ε-PKC in the surface membrane then promotes the translocation of both MAPK kinase (MEK) and MAPK from the cytosol to the plasmalemma, where the three protein kinases form a complex at the surface membrane. PKC then induces the phosphorylation and activation of MEK, which in turn causes phosphorylation of MAPK at both Thr and Tyr residues (Adam, Gapinski, Hathaway 1992). Tyrosine phosphorylation of MAPK would then target it to the cytoskeleton, where it induces the phosphorylation of the actin-binding protein caldesmon (D'Angelo, Graceffa, Wang et al. 1999; Hedges, Oxhorn, Carty et al. 2000). The phosphorylation of caldesmon reverses its inhibition of actin-mediated MgATPase activity, and thus increases the actin–myosin crossbridge cycling and enhances VSM contraction (Fig. 2.1) (Khalil, Menice, Wang et al. 1995; Horowitz, Menice, Laporte et al. 1996; Kordowska, Hetrick, Adam et al. 2006).

ROLE OF PKC IN HYPERTENSION

Hypertension is a multifactorial disorder that involves changes in the vascular, hormonal, neural, and renal control mechanisms of BP (Cain, Khalil 2002). Increases in the amount and activity of PKC and activation of PKC-mediated pathways could cause persistent disturbance in one or more of the physiological control mechanisms, leading to significant increases in BP and hypertension. The pathophysiological mechanisms underlying the relation between PKC and hypertension could also involve potential interactions with VSM growth, proliferation and contraction pathways, vascular inflammation and inflammatory cytokines, oxidative stress and free radicals, and vascular remodeling by MMPs. The role of PKC and these related pathways has been demonstrated in some of the common forms of experimental and human hypertension.

PKC AND VSM GROWTH AND REACTIVITY IN HYPERTENSION

Increased expression/activity of PKC isoforms in VSM could promote VSM growth and proliferation (Fig. 2.3). The trophic changes in VSM cause significant increases in the vascular wall thickness and hypertrophic remodeling that lead to increased peripheral vascular resistance and hypertension. For instance, overexpression of α-PKC in A7r5 VSM cell line stimulates cell proliferation (Wang, Desai, Wright et al. 1997). Also, the localization of ζ-PKC in the

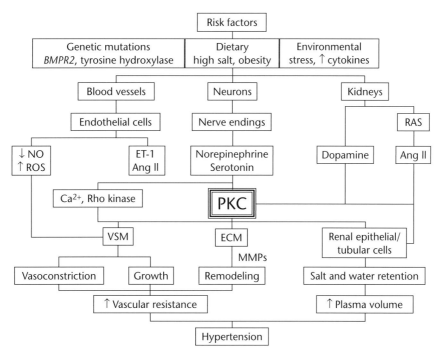

Figure 2.3 Role of PKC in hypertension. Genetic, dietary, and environmental risk factors lead to endothelial cell, neural, and renal dysfunction, and increased release of various mediators such as reactive oxygen species (ROS), ET-1, Ang II, norepinephrine, serotonin, and dopamine. Some of these mediators could stimulate VSM and activate PKC, as well as Ca^{2+} and Rho-kinase, and thereby induce vasoconstriction and VSM growth and proliferation. The interaction of PKC with matrix metalloproteinases (MMPs) in the extracellular matrix (ECM) could contribute to vascular remodeling. Ang II and dopamine could enhance PKC-mediated vasoconstriction, or induce salt and water retention and increased plasma volume. Persistent increases in vascular resistance and plasma volume lead to hypertension. RAS, renin–angiotensin system.

vicinity of the nucleus suggests that it may be involved in the VSM growth and the hypertrophic remodeling commonly observed in hypertension (Khalil, Lajoie, Resnick et al. 1992; Liou, Morgan 1994). The increased PKC activity in conjunction with elevation of $[Ca^{2+}]_i$ may exert trophic effects on the vasculature and the heart, thereby explaining the narrowing of the lumen in peripheral arteries and the cardiac hypertrophy of long-standing hypertension (Aviv 1994).

Increased expression and activity of specific PKC isoforms could also cause excessive vasoconstriction, which could contribute to the increased vascular resistance and BP (Fig. 2.3). The Ca^{2+}-dependent α-PKC has been shown to enhance VSM contraction, and its overexpression in VSM may be involved in the pathogenesis of hypertension (Khalil, Lajoie, Morgan et al. 1994; Liou, Morgan 1994). Also, the Ca^{2+}-independent ε-PKC has been suggested to play a role in enhancing the myofilament force sensitivity to $[Ca^{2+}]_i$ in VSM, a signaling pathway that could increase the vasoconstriction associated with hypertension (Khalil, Lajoie, Resnick et al. 1992; Horowitz, Menice, Laporte et al. 1996). The localization of δ-PKC in the cytoskeleton suggests that it may play a role in the vascular remodeling associated with hypertension (Kanashiro, Khalil 1998).

PKC AND INFLAMMATORY CYTOKINES IN HYPERTENSION

A growing body of evidence suggests that vascular inflammation contributes to cardiovascular disease (Young, Libby, Schonbeck U 2002; Libby 2006). Elevations in plasma tumor necrosis factor α (TNF-α), interleukin 1β (IL-1β), and IL-6 are observed in patients with hypertension and coronary disease (Waehre, Yndestad, Smith et al. 2004; Funayama, Ishikawa, Kubo et al. 2004; Lubrano, Cocci, Battaglia et al. 2005; Nijm, Wikby, Tompa et al. 2005; McLachlan, Chua, Wong et al. 2005; Sardella, Mariani, D'Alessandro et al. 2006). Also, studies have shown that infusion of angiotensin II (Ang II) fails to induce hypertension in IL-6 knockout mice, supporting a role of the cytokine in hypertension (Lee, Sturgis, Labazi et al. 2006). Interestingly, in isolated pulmonary arteries, hypoxia induces an increase in the expression of TNF-α and IL-1β, a process that is dependent on PKC activation and could promote pulmonary vasoconstriction (Tsai, Wang, Pitcher et al. 2004). TNF-α also activates PKC and mitogenic signaling in cultured VSM cells (Ramana, Chandra, Srivastava et al. 2003). Furthermore, inhibitors of PKC-δ block high glucose-induced secretion of TNF-α in rat and human aortic VSM cells in culture (Ramana, Tammali, Reddy et al. 2007).

PKC AND OXIDATIVE STRESS IN HYPERTENSION

Increased oxidative stress has been demonstrated in all forms of hypertension including essential and renovascular hypertension. Increased production of superoxide ($O_2^-\bullet$) is known to decrease the bioactivity of the major vasodilator nitric oxide (NO), thereby contributing to the increased peripheral vascular resistance associated with hypertension (Cardillo, Kilcoyne, Quyyumi et al. 1998; Heitzer, Wenzel, Hink et al. 1999; Ungvari, Csiszar, Huang et al. 2003). Evidence suggests that increased $O_2^-\bullet$ production in hypertension involves PKC. Studies have shown that high pressure induces $O_2^-\bullet$ production in isolated arteries via PKC-dependent activation of NAD(P)H oxidase (Ungvari, Csiszar, Huang et al. 2003). Other studies have shown that $O_2^-\bullet$ is elevated in sympathetic neurons in deoxycorticosterone acetate (DOCA)-salt hypertension via activation of NAD(P)H oxidase (Dai, Cao, Kreulen et al. 2006). Also, increased NAD(P)H oxidase-mediated $O_2^-\bullet$ production has been demonstrated in renovascular hypertension, and the possible involvement of PKC has been suggested (Heitzer, Wenzel, Hink et al. 1999).

PKC AND VASCULAR REMODELING BY MMPS IN HYPERTENSION

MMPs are a family of structurally related, zinc-containing enzymes that play a role in the degradation of ECM proteins (Liu, Wang, Greene et al. 1997; Galis, Khatri 2002; Visse, Nagase 2003; Raffetto, Khalil 2007). Additional effects of MMPs on the endothelium and VSM have also been suggested (Chew, Conte, Khalil et al. 2004; Raffetto, Ross, Khalil et al. 2007). The activities of MMPs are regulated at the transcription level as well as by activation of their pro-form, interaction with specific ECM components, and inhibition by endogenous tissue inhibitors of MMPs (TIMPs). Factors that upregulate MMP activities promote vascular remodeling and include chronic changes in hemodynamics, vessel injury, inflammatory cytokines, and ROS.

Hypertension is associated with vascular remodeling and rearrangement of various components of the vascular wall, including ECM proteins. Some clinical studies have shown that the plasma levels and activities of MMP-2, MMP-9, and TIMP-1 are increased in hypertensive patients (Derosa, D'Angelo, Ciccarelli et al. 2006). Other studies have reported the opposite

finding and demonstrated that the plasma levels of active MMP-2 and -9 are depressed in patients with essential hypertension. Also, treatment with amlodipine normalized MMP-9 plasma concentration (Zervoudaki, Economou, Stefanadis et al. 2003). These findings suggested a relationship between abnormal ECM metabolism and hypertension and raised the possibility that antihypertensive treatment may modulate collagen metabolism. A recent study has examined the serum concentrations of carboxy-terminal telopeptide of collagen type I (CITP) as a marker of extracellular collagen type I degradation, MMP-1 (collagenase), TIMP-1, and MMP-1–TIMP-1 complex in patients with untreated essential hypertension and normotensive controls. It was found that baseline free MMP-1 was decreased and baseline free TIMP-1 was increased in hypertensives compared with normotensives. Hypertensive patients treated with the angiotensin-converting enzyme (ACE) inhibitor lisinopril for 1 year showed an increase in free MMP-1, a decrease in free TIMP-1, and an increase in serum CITP. It was concluded that systemic extracellular degradation of collagen type I is depressed in patients with essential hypertension and may facilitate organ fibrosis, which can be normalized by treatment with lisinopril (Laviades, Varo, Fernandez et al. 1998).

Studies have also examined the expression and activity of MMPs in internal mammary artery specimens obtained from normotensive and hypertensive patients undergoing coronary artery bypass surgery. Zymographic analysis indicated a decrease in total gelatinolytic activity of MMP-2 and -9 in hypertension. MMP-1 activity was also decreased by fourfold without a significant change in protein levels. Immunoblot analysis revealed a decrease in the tissue levels of ECM inducer protein (EMMPRIN, a known stimulator of MMPs transcription), MMP activator protein (MT1-MMP), and MMP-9 in hypertension. Also, measurement of plasma markers of collagen synthesis (procollagen type I amino-terminal propeptide [PINP]) and collagen degradation (carboxy-terminal telopeptide of collagen type I [ICTP]) indicated no difference in PINP levels but suppressed the degradation of collagen in hypertension. These data demonstrate that not only MMP-1 and MMP-9 but also MMP inducer and activator proteins are downregulated in the hypertensive state, which may result in enhanced collagen deposition in hypertension (Ergul, Portik-Dobos, Hutchinson et al. 2004).

Experimental studies have shown that the wall thickness was increased in the aorta of DOCA-salt versus sham rats as was the medial area, but neither measure was altered in the vena cava. In hypertension, MMP-2 expression and activity were increased in the aorta but not the vena cava, while MMP-9 was weakly expressed in both vessels. TIMP-2 expression was increased in the aorta of DOCA rats compared to sham, but barely detectable in the vena cava of sham or DOCA-salt hypertensive rats. These data suggest that vascular remodeling in the aorta of DOCA-salt hypertensive rats, observed as an increase in wall thickness and medial area, is linked to the action of MMP-2. The increase in TIMP-2 expression observed in the aorta from DOCA-salt rats is presumably an adaptive increase to the higher-than-normal levels of MMP-2 (Watts, Rondelli, Thakali et al. 2007).

A recent study has evaluated how MMP-9 might contribute to the progression of hypertension in vivo. Wild-type and MMP-9$^{(-/-)}$ mice were treated with Ang II, 1 µg/kg per minute by minipump, and a 5% NaCl diet for 10 days. It was found that the onset of Ang II-induced hypertension was accompanied by increased MMP-9 activity in conductance vessels. The absence of MMP-9 activity results in vessel stiffness and increased pulse pressure. It was suggested that MMP-9 activation is associated with a beneficial role early on in hypertension by preserving vessel compliance and alleviating BP increase (Flamant et al. 2007).

Growth factors and cytokines such as nuclear factor κB and IL-1α stimulate VSM cells to secrete MMP-1, -3, -9. These effects appear to be dependent on activation of ζ-PKC, and may contribute to inhibition of VSM proliferation and vascular remodeling in pathological states (Hussain, Assender, Bond et al. 2002). PKC also increases MMP-2 secretion in endothelial cells (Papadimitriou, Waters, Manolopoulos et al. 2001), and PKC-α plays a critical role in MMP-9 secretion in bovine capillary endothelial cells through ERK1/2 signaling pathway (Park, Park, Lee et al. 2003). Additionally, PKC-β plays an important signaling role in the expression and activity of MMP-1 and -3 in human coronary artery endothelial cells (Li Liu, Chen et al. 2003). Furthermore, in cardiac microvascular endothelial cells, IL-1β activates PKC-α and -βI and causes upregulation in the expression and activity of MMP-2, while inhibition of PKC-α and -βI abrogates the IL-1β stimulated increase in MMP-2 (Mountain, Singh, Menon et al. 2007).

ROLE OF PKC IN AORTIC CONSTRICTION MODEL OF HYPERTENSION

Studies have demonstrated an increase in the activation and translocation of PKC in a rat model of pressure overload and left ventricular hypertrophy produced by banding or clipping of the aorta (Liou, Morgan 1994). The increased PKC activity was found to be associated with increased tritiated phorbol ester ([^{3}H]PDBu) binding and PKC concentration in both the cytosolic and membrane fractions (Gu, Bishop 1994). Immunoblot analysis has revealed

that the increased PKC activity mainly involves increases in the amount of βI-, βII- and ε-PKC in the surface membrane and nuclear-cytoskeletal fractions (Gu, Bishop 1994). Imaging of the subcellular distribution of PKC revealed that in VSM cells of normotensive rats α-PKC is mainly localized in the cytosol, while ζ-PKC is located in the perinuclear area (Khalil, Lajoie, Resnick et al. 1992; Khalil, Lajoie, Morgan et al. 1994). In VSM of hypertensive rats, α-PKC is hyperactivated and concentrated at the surface membrane, while ζ-PKC is localized in the nucleus (Liou, Morgan 1994).

ROLE OF PKC IN GENETIC MODELS OF HYPERTENSION

Genetic studies in certain families have generated important information regarding the genetic origins of hypertension. For example, mutations in *BMPR2* gene, which encodes a bone morphogenetic protein receptor II, a TGF-β super family member, have been linked to 55% of familial pulmonary arterial hypertension (Deng, Morse, Slager et al. 2000; Machado, Pauciulo, Thomson et al. 2001; Aldred, Vijayakrishnan, James et al. 2006). Mice carrying BMPR2 heterozygous alleles (BMPR2$^{+/-}$) are genetically equivalent to mutant human gene and develop pulmonary artery hypertension under stressed condition (Song, Jones, Beppu et al. 2005). Proteomics studies on murine tissues have identified β-PKC as one of the signaling components associated with BMPR2 (Hassel, Eichner, Yakymovych et al. 2004), raising the possibility that PKC contributes to the pathogenesis of genetic hypertension.

Vascular PKC may also play a role in the increased BP observed in the genetic model of spontaneously hypertensive rats (SHR). It has been demonstrated that the norepinephrine-induced contraction of isolated aortic segments is more readily inhibited by the PKC inhibitor 1-(5-isoquinolinesulfonyl)-2-methylpiperazine (H-7) in the aortas from SHR than those from Wistar-Kyoto rats (WKY). Also, treatment of the aortic segments with H-7 caused a shift to the right in the concentration–contraction curve of the PKC activator TPA in the aortas of SHR, but not in those of WKY (Shibata, Morita, Nagai et al. 1990). It has also been shown that the PKC activator PDBu produces increased contraction and greater reduction in cytosolic PKC activity in the aortas from SHR than in those from WKY, suggesting greater functional alterations of PKC in VSM of SHR (Bazan, Campbell, Rapoport 1992). In SHR, γ-interferon can restore PKC level to that in the normal control rat, suggesting an interaction between PKC and the cytokine in genetic hypertension (Sauro, Hadden 1992).

To further understand the role of PKC in genetic hypertension, studies have examined vascular contraction and PKC activity during the development of hypertension in young (5–6 weeks) SHR. It was found that contractions in response to high K⁺ depolarizing solution in intact mesenteric arteries and the Ca^{2+}-force relation in vessels permeabilized with α-toxin are not different in SHR and WKY rats. Treatment with the PKC activator PDBu augmented the high K⁺-contraction in intact vascular segments, and enhanced the Ca^{2+}-force relation in permeabilized vessels of SHR in than those of WKY. Also, the PKC inhibitors H-7 and calphostin C caused greater suppression of the contractile responses in vascular segments of SHR than in those of WKY. These data further suggest that PKC enhances the Ca^{2+} sensitivity of the contractile proteins in VSM and that the effects of PKC are greater in blood vessels of the young prehypertensive SHR than in those of WKY. The data also suggest that activation of PKC in VSM occurs before overt hypertension, and thereby provide evidence for a role of PKC as a causative factor in the development of genetic hypertension (Sasajima, Shima, Toyoda et al. 1997).

To further examine potential inborn differences in vascular PKC before the onset of hypertension, studies have compared the proliferation of VSM cells from young (1–2 weeks) SHR and WKY rats. In cultured aortic VSM from SHR and WKY rats, both Ang II and endothelin-1 (ET-1) enhanced thymidine incorporation into DNA, an indicator of DNA synthesis. Treatment of the cells with the PKC inhibitor chelerythrine caused greater suppression of Ang II– and ET-1–induced DNA synthesis and VSM growth in cells of SHR than in those of WKY, suggesting an inborn increase in PKC activity in VSM cells of SHR (Rosen, Barg, Zimlichman 1999).

Studies have also assessed the role of PKC in the changes in vascular tone associated with genetic hypertension in vivo, and examined the vascular effects of perfusing the PKC activator PDBu in the hindlimbs of anesthetized SHR and WKY rats. It was found that PDBu infusion into the hindlimb caused prolonged vasoconstriction and elevation of the perfusion pressure. The PDBu-induced vasoconstriction and elevated perfusion pressure were inhibited by the PKC inhibitor staurosporine to a greater extent in the SHR as compared to that in the WKY rats. These data provided evidence for a role of PKC in the regulation of vascular function and BP in vivo and further suggest an increase in PKC expression and activity in VSM in rat models of genetic hypertension (Bilder, Kasiewski, Perrone 1990).

Interestingly, gender differences in the expression and activity of PKC isoforms have been observed in the aortic VSM of WKY and SHR. It has been shown that the VSM contraction and the expression and activity of α-, δ- and ζ-PKC in response to the phorbol ester PDBu are reduced in intact female WKY compared with that in intact male WKY, and that the gender-related differences are greater in VSM from SHR compared with those from WKY rats (Kanashiro, Khalil 2001). The PDBu-induced contraction and PKC activity were not significantly different between castrated and intact male rats, but were greater in ovariectomized (OVX) female rats than in intact ones. Treatment of OVX females with 17β-estradiol subcutaneous implants caused a significant reduction in PDBu contraction and PKC activity, which was more prominent in SHR than WKY rats. These data suggested gender-related reduction in VSM contraction and the expression and activity of α-, δ-, and ζ-PKC in female rats compared with male rats and that these differences are possibly mediated by estrogen and are enhanced in genetic forms of hypertension (Kanashiro, Khalil 2001).

ROLE OF PKC IN ANIMAL MODELS OF SALT-SENSITIVE HYPERTENSION

Increased dietary sodium intake has been implicated in the pathogenesis of hypertension in salt-sensitive individuals (Smith, Payne, Sedeek et al. 2003; Khalil 2006). The role of vascular PKC in salt-sensitive hypertension has not been clearly established. However, evidence from cardiac tissues suggests an increase in PKC activity in this form of hypertension. Studies have demonstrated an increase in the BP and the heart-to-body weight ratio in the DOCA salt-sensitive hypertensive rats as compared to those in control rats. Also, the relative expression of α-, γ-, and ε-PKC is increased, while that of δ-PKC is not altered in cardiac extracts of DOCA-salt rats as compared to controls. Additionally, δ-PKC is increased in cardiac fibroblasts from DOCA-salt rats as compared to controls. These data suggest that the hearts of DOCA-salt hypertensive rats demonstrate cell-specific increase in the expression of α, γ, δ, or ε-PKC (Fareh, Touyz, Schiffrin et al. 2000). Interestingly, the PKC inhibitor GF109203X (2-[1-(3-dimethylaminopropyl)-1H-indol-3-yl]-3-(1H-indol-3-yl)maleimide) has been shown to decrease both basal tone and MAPK (ERK1/2) activity in DOCA-salt hypertensive rats. These studies have suggested that in DOCA-salt hypertensive rats the basal vascular tone is elevated by the altered activation of MAPK and that these effects are regulated by PKC (Kim, Lee, Lee et al. 2005).

Studies have also suggested significant changes in PKC in the hearts of Dahl salt-sensitive hypertensive rats. Marinobufagenin, an endogenous ligand of the α1 subunit of the cardiac Na/K-ATPase, is elevated in NaCl-loaded Dahl salt-sensitive rats and may contribute to the hypertension observed in this animal model (Fedorova, Talan, Agalakova et al. 2003). It has been suggested that PKC-induced phosphorylation of the $\alpha1$-Na/K-ATPase may increase its sensitivity to marinobufagenin, and thereby contribute to the elevated BP in the Dahl salt-sensitive rat (Fedorova, Talan, Agalakova et al. 2003).

ROLE OF PKC IN RENOVASCULAR HYPERTENSION

PKC could also play a role in the development of renovascular hypertension. Studies have measured vascular function in aortic segments isolated from two kidney–one clip (2K-1C) rat model of hypertension and age-matched controls. It was found that the PDBu-induced vascular contraction was enhanced, and the superoxide ($O_2^-\bullet$) production was increased in aortic segments from the 2K-1C hypertensive rats as compared to those from controls. The increased vascular contraction and $O_2^-\bullet$ production were normalized in aortic segments treated with superoxide dismutase or the PKC inhibitor calphostin C. These data suggest that the increased vascular $O_2^-\bullet$ and impaired vascular function associated with renovascular hypertension in the 2K-1C rats are possibly due to PKC-mediated activation of NADPH-dependent oxidase (Heitzer, Wenzel, Hink et al. 1999).

PKC may also affect the renin–angiotensin–aldosterone system and thereby, the renal control mechanism of BP. Studies have shown that infusion of Ang II in rats causes hypertension as well as vascular endothelial dysfunction and increased vascular $O_2^-\bullet$ production. Some of the vascular effects of Ang II appear to be mediated by increased endothelial cell release of ET-1, which is known to activate PKC (Sirous, Fleming, Khalil 2001; Cain, Tanner, Khalil 2002; Hynynen, Khalil 2006). Interestingly, Ang II–induced ET-1 production and vascular PKC activity are greater in blood vessels of SHR as compared with those of normotensive control rats (Schiffrin 1995). Other evidence for an effect of PKC on the renin–angiotensin system is derived from studies using angiotensin-converting enzyme inhibitors such as enalapril. It has been demonstrated that PKC activity is higher in the cytosolic compartment of the aortic VSM from SHR than those from WKY or enalapril-treated SHR. The changes in vascular PKC activity were closely associated with the changes in BP. Membrane-bound PKC activity was detected in aortic VSM of SHR, but not in that of the WKY or enalapril-treated SHR. Also, the expression of α-PKC mRNA and protein was higher in aortic VSM from SHR than those from WKY or enalapril-treated SHR. These data suggest that the beneficial effects of angiotensin-converting

enzyme inhibitors in hypertension may in part involve changes in expression and activity of α-PKC in VSM (Kanayama, Negoro, Okamura et al. 1994). Other studies have shown that PKC could affect the Na^+/Ca^{2+} exchange mechanism in the renal arterioles, leading to defective renal vasodilation associated with salt-sensitive hypertension (Bell, Mashburn, Unlap 2000).

PKC may also affect the renal tubular cells and the kidney function. For instance, in kidney tubular epithelial cells, δ- and ζ-PKC are localized to the plasma membrane whereas the other isoforms α- and ε-PKC are cytoplasmic. Dopamine, an important intrarenal modulator of sodium metabolism and BP, causes translocation of α- and ε-PKC to the plasma membrane (Nowicki, Kruse, Brismar et al. 2000; Ridge, Dada, Lecuona et al. 2002), supporting the role of PKC in the control of the renal sodium and water reabsorption and BP (Banday, Fazili, Lokhandwala 2007).

ROLE OF PKC IN PULMONARY HYPERTENSION

This type of hypertension involves sustained vasoconstriction of the pulmonary arteries. PKC may have specific effects on the pulmonary vessels that may contribute to the pathogenesis of pulmonary hypertension. It has been demonstrated that both insulin-like growth factor I and PKC activation stimulate the proliferation of pulmonary artery VSM cells. Activation of PKC may also be one of the signaling pathways involved in hypoxia-induced pulmonary artery VSM cell proliferation. Additionally, chronic hypoxia may act via specific PKC isozymes to enhance the growth responses in pulmonary artery adventitial fibroblasts (Das, Dempsey, Bouchey et al. 2000). Interestingly, mice deficient in ε-PKC have decreased hypoxic pulmonary vasoconstriction (Littler, Morris, Fagan et al. 2003). Also, ET-1 is one of the most potent vasoconstrictors, and the use of endothelin-receptor antagonist has yielded clinical benefits in patients with pulmonary hypertension (Ito, Ozawa, Shimada 2007; Puri, McGoon, Kushwaha 2007). The effects of ET-1 on pulmonary vessels appear to be mediated by PKC, and inhibitors of PKC isoforms have been shown to downregulate ET-1 induced pulmonary arterial contraction in several animal models (Barman 2007).

ROLE OF PKC IN ESSENTIAL HUMAN HYPERTENSION

A large body of evidence suggests that PKC may play a role in the pathogenesis of essential hypertension in humans. Studies have demonstrated an increase in oxidative stress and growth responses in VSM cells from resistant arteries of patients with essential hypertension as compared to cells from normotensive controls. It was found that Ang II caused an increase in ROS, which was enhanced in VSM from hypertensive subjects as compared to that from normotensive controls. Also, Ang II stimulated phospholipase D (PLD) activity and DNA and protein synthesis to a greater extent in VSM cells from hypertensive subjects as compared to those from normotensive controls. Treatment of the cells with the PKC inhibitors chelerythrine and calphostin C partially decreased the Ang II–induced effects. These data suggest that the increased oxidative stress and augmented growth-promoting effects of Ang II observed in VSM cells from patients with essential hypertension are associated with increased activation of PLD- and PKC-dependent pathways, and that these pathways may contribute to vascular remodeling associated with hypertension (Touyz, Schiffrin 2001).

ROLE OF PKC IN HYPERTENSION IN PREGNANCY AND PREECLAMPSIA

During normal pregnancy decreased BP, increased uterine blood flow, and decreased vascular responses to vasoconstrictors and agonists are often observed (Khalil, Granger 2002; Stennett, Khalil 2006). Studies on uterine artery from pregnant sheep and the aorta of late pregnant rats have demonstrated that decreased vascular contraction during normal pregnancy is associated with decrease in vascular PKC activity (Magness, Rosenfeld, Carr 1991; Kanashiro, Altirkawi, Khalil et al. 2000). Studies have also shown that the expression and subcellular redistribution of the Ca^{2+}-dependent α-PKC and the Ca^{2+}-independent δ- and ζ-PKC are reduced in aortic VSM isolated from late pregnant rats compared with those from nonpregnant rats (Kanashiro, Alexander, Granger et al. 1999; Kanashiro, Cockrell, Alexander 2000).

In 5% to 7% of pregnancies, women develop a condition called preeclampsia characterized by proteinuria and severe increases in peripheral vascular resistance and BP (Stennett, Khalil 2006). Because of the difficulty to perform mechanistic studies in pregnant women, animal models of hypertension in pregnancy have been developed. We have recently shown that the mean arterial pressure is greater in late pregnant rats treated with the NO synthase inhibitor L-NAME, compared with normal pregnant rats or virgin rats nontreated or treated with L-NAME (Khalil, Crews, Novak et al. 1998). Also, measurements of vascular contraction in aortic segments demonstrated an increase in phenylephrine-induced contraction in

aortas from L-NAME–treated pregnant rats as compared to tissues from normal pregnant rats or virgin rats (Khalil, Crews, Novak et al. 1998; Crews, Novak, Granger et al. 1999). Additionally, the vascular PKC activity and the expression and subcellular distribution of α- and δ-PKC isoforms were enhanced in L-NAME–treated pregnant rats compared with normal pregnant rats (Kanashiro, Alexander, Granger et al. 1999; Kanashiro, Cockrell, Alexander 2000). These data suggest that an increase in the expression and activity of α- and δ-PKC isoforms may play a role in the increased vasoconstriction and vascular resistance observed in hypertension during pregnancy (Kanashiro, Alexander, Granger et al. 1999; Kanashiro, Cockrell, Alexander 2000; Khalil, Granger 2002).

PKC may also play a role in the changes in Ang II receptor-mediated signaling associated with preeclampsia. Studies on cultured neonatal rat cardiomyocytes have shown that immunoglobulin from preeclamptic women enhances angiotensin type 1 (AT_1) receptor-mediated chronotropic response, whereas immunoglobulin from control subjects has no effect. Treatment of cardiomyocytes with the PKC inhibitor calphostin C prevented the stimulatory effect of immunoglobulin from preeclamptic women on AT_1 receptor-mediated chronotropic response. Examination of VSM cells with confocal microscopy has also shown colocalization of purified IgG from preeclamptic women and AT_1 receptor antibody. These studies concluded that preeclamptic patients develop stimulatory autoantibodies against AT_1 receptor, and this process appears to be mediated via PKC. These autoantibodies may participate in the Ang II-induced vascular lesions in patients with preeclampsia (Wallukat, Homuth, Fischer et al. 1999).

Several studies have suggested that the reduction in uteroplacental perfusion pressure and the ensuing placental ischemia or hypoxia cause an increase in the release of cytokines into the maternal circulation, which in turn leads to the generalized vascular changes and hypertension (Kupferminc, Peaceman, Wigton et al. 1994; Vince, Starkey, Austgulen et al. 1995; Conrad, Benyo 1997; Williams, Mahomed, Farrand et al. 1998; Khalil, Granger 2002; Stennett, Khalil 2006). In support of the cytokine hypothesis, it has been shown that the plasma levels of TNF-α are elevated in women with preeclampsia (Conrad, Benyo 1997; Williams, Mahomed, Farrand et al. 1998). Studies have also suggested that sources other than the placenta may contribute to the elevated concentrations of TNF-α in the circulation of preeclamptic women (Benyo Smarason, Redman et al. 2001). We and others have shown that infusion of plasma TNF-α or IL-6 in normal pregnant rats, to reach plasma levels similar to those observed in preeclampsia, are associated with significant increases in BP and systemic vasoconstriction (Davis, Giardina, Green et al. 2002; Orshal, Khalil 2004). We have also shown that treatment of vascular segments isolated from pregnant rats with cytokines enhances vascular reactivity to vasoconstrictor stimuli (Giardina, Green, Cockrell et al. 2002; Orshal, Khalil 2004). Cytokines likely increase the expression and activity of vascular PKC, leading to increase in the myofilament force sensitivity to $[Ca^{2+}]_i$ and the enhancement of VSM contraction associated with hypertension in pregnancy.

ROLE OF PKC IN ENDOTHELIUM-MEDIATED CONTROL MECHANISMS OF BP

Changes in PKC activity in the endothelium could contribute to the regulation of vascular function and BP. Studies have suggested a role of PKC in the endothelial cell dysfunction observed in blood vessels of SHR and DOCA hypertensive rats (Soloviev, Parshikov, Stefanov 1998; Fatehi-Hassanabad, Fatehi, Shahidi 2004). NO is one of the major vasodilators produced by the endothelium. Activated endothelial NO synthase (eNOS) catalyzes the transformation of L-arginine to L-citrulline and the concomitant production of NO. Mice deficient in eNOS are hypertensive and lack NO-mediated vasodilation (Huang, Huang, Mashimo et al. 1995). Studies suggest possible effects of PKC on NOS activity and NO production or bioactivity. For instance, PKC may regulate eNOS activity by phosphorylating the Thr 495 residue and dephosphorylating Ser 1175 residue of eNOS, thus inhibiting the production of NO (Michell, Chen, Tiganis et al. 2001; Fleming, Fisslthaler, Dimmeler et al. 2001). Other studies have shown that α- and δ-PKC isoforms phosphorylate eNOS at Ser 1175 and induce an increase in NO production (Partovian, Zhuang, Moodie et al. 2005; Motley, Eguchi, Patterson et al. 2007). PKC has also been suggested to play a role in eNOS "uncoupling," a process in which an attempt to get more NO to reduce the vessel tone conversely produces superoxide when eNOS is overexpressed or hyperactivated (Vasquez-Vivar, Kalyanaraman, Martásek et al. 1998; Xia, Tsai, Berka et al. 1998). In SHR, oral administration of the PKC inhibitor midostaurin, a derivative of staurosporine, has been shown to reverse aortic eNOS "uncoupling" and to cause upregulation of eNOS expression and to diminish ROS production. Also, aortic levels of (6R)-5,6,7, 8-tetrahydro-L-biopterin (BH4), a NOS cofactor, were significantly reduced in SHR compared with WKY. In addition, midostaurin lowered BP in SHR

and to a lesser extent (Li, Witte, August et al. 2006). These findings suggest potential benefits of PKC inhibitors in genetic forms of hypertension. Similarly, studies have suggested that the impaired vasodilation and increased vascular $O_2^-\bullet$ production observed in the 2K-1C rat model of renovascular hypertension are likely related to PKC-mediated activation of membrane-associated NADPH-dependent oxidase (Fedorova, Talan, Agalakova et al. 2003; Ungvari, Csiszar, Huang et al. 2003).

ROLE OF PKC IN NEURAL CONTROL MECHANISMS OF BP

PKC may also participate in the neural control mechanisms of BP. It has been demonstrated that the expression and redistribution of PKC isozymes are increased in brain tissue of SHR (Hughes-Darden, Wachira, Denaro et al. 2001). Also, sympathetic and parasympathetic nerves are known to control the contraction and dilation of VSM by releasing chemical transmitters such as norepinephrine, which in turn trigger the increase in $[Ca^{2+}]_i$ and PKC activity and thereby control the VSM contraction and vessel tone. Polymorphisms in human tyrosine hydroxylase gene have been associated with increased sympathetic activity, norepinephrine release, and hypertension (Rao, Zhang, Wessel et al. 2007), and the role of PKC in these hypertensive subjects remains to be investigated.

ROLE OF PKC IN THE METABOLIC SYNDROME

The metabolic syndrome is characterized by hyperglycemia and glucose intolerance, insulin resistance, central and overall obesity, dyslipidemia (increased triglyceride and decreased high-density lipoprotein [HDL] cholesterol levels), and different vascular manifestations and complications including hypertension. Evidence suggests a prominent role of PKC in the metabolic syndrome. For example, the glucose-induced increase in endothelial cell permeability is associated with activation of the α-PKC isoform. Also, glucose, via activation of PKC, may alter the Na^+/H^+ exchanger gene expression and activity in VSM cells. It has also been demonstrated that an antisense complementary to the mRNA initiation codon regions for the α- and β-PKC induces the downregulation of these PKC isoforms and inhibits insulin-induced glucose uptake. Furthermore, inhibitors of the β-PKC isoform have been shown to ameliorate the vascular dysfunction observed in rat models of diabetes and attenuate the progression of experimental diabetic nephropathy and hypertension (Ishii, Jirousek, Daisuke et al. 1996; Kelly, Zhang, Hepper et al. 2003).

PKC INHIBITORS AS MODULATORS OF VASCULAR FUNCTION IN HYPERTENSION

Several in vitro and ex vivo studies have suggested a role of PKC in the increased VSM contraction observed in blood vessels of animal models of hypertension. However, few studies have examined the in vivo effects of PKC inhibitors. Recent studies using the antihypertensive compound cicletanine may provide strong evidence for potential benefits of targeting vascular PKC in the treatment of hypertension. Salt-sensitive hypertension has been shown to be associated with dysregulation of the plasmalemmal sodium pump, possibly due to elevated marinobufagenin, an endogenous inhibitor of α1 Na/K-ATPase. Cicletanine appears to be effective in salt-sensitive hypertension. Dahl salt-sensitive rats on high NaCl (8%) diet exhibit an increase in BP, marinobufagenin excretion, and left ventricular mass. An increase in Na/K-ATPase and βII-PKC and δ-PKC has also been observed in the myocardium of Dahl salt-sensitive rats. In Dahl salt-sensitive rats treated with cicletanine, a reduction in BP and left ventricular weight, decreased sensitivity of Na/K-ATPase to marinobufagenin, no increase in βII-PKC, and reduced phorbol diacetate–induced Na/K-ATPase phosphorylation are observed. These data suggest that cicletanine may target PKC-induced phosphorylation of cardiac α1 Na/K-ATPase in the treatment of hypertension (Fedorova, Talan, Agalakova et al. 2003).

The in vivo effects of cicletanine in treating hypertension may involve an effect on vascular function. Studies on mesenteric arteries isolated from humans have demonstrated that marinobufagenin induces sustained vasoconstriction, possibly due to inhibition of the plasmalemmal Na/K-ATPase activity. Cicletanine causes relaxation of marinobufagenin-induced contraction of mesenteric arteries, by attenuating marinobufagenin-induced Na/K-ATPase inhibition. Treatment of the vessels with phorbol diacetate attenuates cicletanine-induced relaxation of marinobufagenin-mediated inhibition of Na/K-ATPase and vascular contraction. It has also been shown that cicletanine inhibits rat brain PKC activity, and the PKC inhibition is not observed in the presence of phorbol diacetate. These data suggest that PKC induces the phosphorylation of α1 Na/K-ATPase and thereby increases its sensitivity and susceptibility to inhibition by marinobufagenin. Cicletanine, by inhibiting PKC, reverses the marinobufagenin-induced Na/K-ATPase

and the consequent increase in vasoconstriction. Taken together, these data suggest that PKC is involved in the cardiotonic steroid–Na/K-ATPase interactions on vascular tone, and may represent a potential target for therapeutic intervention in hypertension (Bagrov, Dmitrieva, Dorofeeva et al. 2000).

We should note that PKC inhibitors alone may not be sufficient for treatment of hypertension. On the other hand, PKC inhibitors could be beneficial in attenuating the VSM growth and hyperactivity associated with hypertension, particularly when used in combination with other treatment strategies. For instance, PKC inhibitors could potentiate the inhibitory effects of Ca^{2+}-channel blockers on vasoconstriction. Targeting of Ca^{2+}-independent PKC isoforms could be specifically effective in Ca^{2+} antagonist-resistant forms of hypertension. The beneficial effects of PKC inhibitors in reducing vasoconstriction and BP could also be potentiated by inhibitors of other protein kinases such as Rho-kinase and MAPK-dependent pathways. This mechanism is supported by reports that agonist-induced activation of RhoA/Rho-kinase causes inhibition of MLC phosphatase and increases the $[Ca^{2+}]_i$ of VSM contraction, and the enhanced vascular tone contributes to the development and progress of hypertension (Seko, Ito, Kureishi et al. 2003; Lee, Webb, Jin et al. 2004).

PERSPECTIVES

The identification of at least 11 PKC isoforms in various tissues and cells has made the task of characterizing the role of PKC in vascular function and vascular disease more challenging. PKC isoforms have different tissue and subcellular distribution, cellular substrate, and cell function. Although several pieces of evidence suggest a role of PKC in the regulation of VSM contraction and the vascular control mechanisms of BP, several points remain to be investigated.

One of the interesting properties of some PKC isoforms is their translocation from the cytosol to the cell membrane during VSM activation. Such a property could be useful in the diagnosis and prognosis of the VSM hyperactivity state associated with hypertension. We should caution that the subcellular redistribution of activated PKC may vary depending on the type and abundance of membrane lipids. Studies have shown increased cholesterol/phospholipid ratio, higher levels of monounsaturated fatty acids, and lower levels of polyunsaturated fatty acids in erythrocyte membranes from elderly hypertensive subjects as compared to those from normotensive controls. However, the levels of activated membrane-associated PKC are not elevated, but rather reduced in elderly hypertensive subjects. The reduction in PKC translocation and membrane association in the erythrocytes of elderly subjects may not be related to the etiopathology of hypertension, but may represent an adaptive compensatory mechanism in response to hypertension (Escriba, Sanchez-Dominguez, Alemany et al. 2003).

Upregulation of PKC expression appears to play a pathogenic role not only in vascular disease such as hypertension and atherogenesis but also in other co-morbidities such as the metabolic syndrome and cancer promotion. The interaction between PKC and other pathways such as inflammatory cytokines, ROS, and MMPs could also be associated with many forms of vascular disease and other related disorders. The involvement of PKC in many cellular processes and diseases may be collectively termed as the "PKC syndrome" (McCarty 1996). Thus, it is important to further screen the effects of PKC inhibitors in vivo and their simultaneous effects on multiple systems. Studies of the effects of PKC inhibitors in animal models of hypertension with other comorbidities such as hypercholesterolemia and diabetes should be carried out. The development of knockout mice and transgenic animals that lack certain PKC isoforms has been useful in determining the role of specific PKC isoforms in a particular cell function or disease. These discoveries have encouraged investigators to design inhibitors of the expression and activity of the specific PKC isoforms. Although the first generation of PKC inhibitors is not very selective, the newly developed PKC inhibitors appear to be more selective. However, further experimental and specificity studies are needed before these compounds can be used safely in treatment of human disorders. Also, isoform-specific PKC inhibitors, particularly when used in combination with cytokine antagonists, antioxidants, and MMPs inhibitors, may provide new approaches for the treatment of certain forms of Ca^{2+} antagonist-insensitive forms of hypertension.

ACKNOWLEDGMENTS   This work was supported by grants from National Heart, Lung, and Blood Institute (HL-65998, HL-70659).

REFERENCES

Adam LP, Gapinski CJ, Hathaway DR. 1992. Phosphorylation sequences in h-caldesmon from phorbol ester-stimulated canine aortas. *FEBS Lett.* 302(3):223–226.

Aldred MA, Vijayakrishnan J, James V et al. 2006. BMPR2 gene rearrangements account for a significant proportion of mutations in familial and idiopathic pulmonary arterial hypertension. *Hum Mutat.* 27(2):212–213.

Aviv A. 1994. Cytosolic Ca^{2+}, Na^+/H^+ antiport, protein kinase C trio in essential hypertension. *Am J Hypertens.* 7(2):205–212.

Bacher N, Zisman Y, Berent E, Livneh E. 1991. Isolation and characterization of PKC-L, a new member of the protein kinase C-related gene family specifically expressed in lung, skin, and heart. *Mol Cell Biol.* 11:126–133.

Bagrov AY, Dmitrieva RI, Dorofeeva NA et al. 2000. Cicletanine reverses vasoconstriction induced by the endogenous sodium pump ligand, marinobufagenin, via a protein kinase C-dependent mechanism. *J Hypertens.* 18(2):209–215.

Banday AA, Fazili FR, Lokhandwala MF. 2007. Oxidative stress causes renal dopamine D1 receptor dysfunction and hypertension via mechanisms that involve nuclear factor-kappaB and protein kinase C. *J Am Soc Nephrol.* 18(5):1446–1457.

Barman SA. 2007. Vasoconstrictor effect of endothelin-1 on hypertensive pulmonary arterial smooth muscle involves Rho-kinase and protein kinase C. *Am J Physiol Lung Cell Mol Physiol.* 293(2):L472–L479.

Barman SA, Zhu S, White RE. 2004. Protein kinase C inhibits BK_{Ca} channel activity in pulmonary arterial smooth muscle. *Am J Physiol Lung Cell Mol Physiol.* 286:L149–L155.

Bazan E, Campbell AK, Rapoport RM. 1992. Protein kinase C activity in blood vessels from normotensive and spontaneously hypertensive rats. *Eur J Pharmacol.* 227(3):343–348.

Bazzi MD, Nelseusten GL. 1990. Protein kinase C interaction with calcium: a phospholipid-dependent process. *Biochemistry.* 29:7624–7630.

Bell PD, Mashburn N, Unlap MT. 2000. Renal sodium/calcium exchange; a vasodilator that is defective in salt-sensitive hypertension. *Acta Physiol Scand.* 168(1):209–214.

Benyo DF, Smarason A, Redman CW, Sims C, Conrad KP. 2001. Expression of inflammatory cytokines in placentas from women with preeclampsia. *J Clin Endocrinol Metab.* 86(6):2505–2512.

Berridge MJ, Irvine RF. 1984. Inositol trisphosphate, a novel second messenger in cellular signal transduction. *Nature.* 312:315–325.

Bilder GE, Kasiewski CJ, Perrone MH. 1990. Phorbol-12,13-dibutyrate-induced vasoconstriction in vivo: characterization of response in genetic hypertension. *J. Pharmacol Exp Ther.* 252(2):526–530.

Cain AE, Khalil RA. 2002. Pathophysiology of essential hypertension: role of the pump, the vessel, and the kidney. *Semin Nephrol.* 22(1):3–16.

Cain AE, Tanner DM, Khalil RA. 2002. Endothelin-1-induced enhancement of coronary smooth muscle contraction via MAPK-dependent and MAPK-independent $[Ca^{2+}]_i$ sensitization pathways. *Hypertension.* 39(2 Pt 2): 543–549.

Cardillo C, Kilcoyne CM, Quyyumi AA, Cannon RO 3rd, Panza JA. 1998. Selective defect in nitric oxide synthesis may explain the impaired endothelium-dependent vasodilation in patients with essential hypertension. *Circulation.* 97(9):851–856.

Cazaubon SM, Parker PJ. 1993. Identification of the phosphorylated region responsible for the permissive activation of protein kinase C. *J Biol Chem.* 268(23): 17559–17563.

Chew DK, Conte MS, Khalil RA. 2004. Matrix metalloproteinase-specific inhibition of Ca²⁺ entry mechanisms of vascular contraction. *J Vasc Surg.* 40(5):1001–1010.

Claro S, Kanashiro CA, Oshiro ME, Ferreira AT, Khalil RA. 2007. α- and ε-Protein kinase C activity during smooth muscle cell apoptosis in response to γ-radiation. *J Pharmacol Exp Ther.* 322(3):964–972.

Clement S, Tasinato A, Boscoboinik D, Azzi A. 1997. The effect of α-tocoferol on the synthesis, phosphorylation and activity of protein kinase C in smooth muscle cells after phorbol 12-myristate 13-acetate. *Eur J Biochem.* 246:745–749.

Cogolludo A, Moreno L, Bosca L, Tamargo J, Perez-Vizcaino F. 2003. Thromboxane A2-induced inhibition of voltage-gated K⁺ channels and pulmonary vasoconstriction: role of protein kinase Czeta. *Circ Res.* 93(7):656–663.

Cogolludo A, Moreno L, Lodi F, Tamargo J, Perez-Vizcaino F. 2005. Postnatal maturational shift from PKCzeta and voltage-gated K⁺ channels to RhoA/Rho kinase in pulmonary vasoconstriction. *Cardiovasc Res.* 66(1):84–93.

Comer FI, Parent CA. 2007. Phosphoinositides specify polarity during epithelial organ development. *Cell.* 128(2):239–240.

Conrad KP, Benyo DF. 1997. Placental cytokines and the pathogenesis of preeclampsia. *Am J Reprod Immunol.* 37(3):240–249.

Coussens L, Parker PJ, Rhee L et al. 1986. Multiple, distinct forms of bovine and human protein kinase C suggest diversity in cellular signaling pathways. *Science.* 233:859–866.

Crews JK, Novak J, Granger JP, Khalil RA. 1999. Stimulated mechanisms of Ca²⁺ entry into vascular smooth muscle during NO synthesis inhibition in pregnant rats. *Am J Physiol.* 276(2 Pt 2):R530–R538.

Dai X, Cao X, Kreulen DL. 2006. Superoxide anion is elevated in sympathetic neurons in DOCA-salt hypertension via activation of NADPH oxidase. *Am J Physiol Heart Circ Physiol.* 290(3):H1019–H1026.

Dallas A, Khalil RA. 2003. Ca²⁺ antagonist-insensitive coronary smooth muscle contraction involves activation of ε-protein kinase C-dependent pathway. *Am J Physiol Cell Physiol.* 285(6):C1454–C1463.

D'Angelo G, Graceffa P, Wang CA, Wrangle J, Adam LP. 1999. Mammal-specific, ERK-dependent, caldesmon phosphorylation in smooth muscle. Quantitation using novel anti-phosphopeptide antibodies. *J Biol Chem.* 274(42):30115–30121.

Das M, Dempsey EC, Bouchey D, Reyland ME, Stenmark KR. 2000. Chronic hypoxia induces exaggerated growth responses in pulmonary artery adventitial fibroblasts: potential contribution of specific protein kinase c isozymes. *Am J Respir Cell Mol Biol.* 22(1):15–25.

Davis JR, Giardina JB, Green GM, Alexander BT, Granger JP, Khalil RA. 2002. Reduced endothelial NO-cGMP vascular relaxation pathway during TNF-α-induced hypertension in pregnant rats. *Am J Physiol Regul Integr Comp Physiol.* 282(2):R390–R399.

Dekker LV, McIntyre P, Parker PJ. 1993. Mutagenesis of the regulatory domain of rat protein kinase C-η: a molecular basis for restricted histone kinase activity. *J Biol Chem.* 268:19498–19504.

Deng Z, Morse JH, Slager SL et al. 2000. Familial primary pulmonary hypertension (gene PPH1) is caused by mutations in the bone morphogenetic protein receptor-II gene. *Am J Hum Genet.* 67(3):737–744.

Derosa G, D'Angelo A, Ciccarelli L et al. 2006. Matrix metalloproteinase-2, -9, and tissue inhibitor of metalloproteinase-1 in patients with hypertension. *Endothelium.* 13(3):227–231.

Draeger A, Wray S, Babiychuk EB. 2005. Domain architecture of the smooth-muscle plasma membrane: regulation by annexins. *Biochem J.* 387(Pt 2):309–314.

Edwards AS, Newton AC. 1997. Phosphorylation at conserved carboxyl-terminal hydrophobic motif regulates the catalytic and regulatory domains of protein kinase C. *J Biol Chem.* 272:18382–18390.

Eicholtz T, de Bont DB, Widt J, Liskamp RMJ, Ploegh HL. 1993. A myristoylated pseudo substrate peptide, a novel protein kinase C inhibitor. *J Biol Chem.* 268: 1982–1986.

Ergul A, Portik-Dobos V, Hutchinson J, Franco J, Anstadt MP. 2004. Downregulation of vascular matrix metalloproteinase inducer and activator proteins in hypertensive patients. *Am J Hypertens.* 17(9):775–782.

Escriba PV, Sanchez-Dominguez JM, Alemany R, Perona JS, Ruiz-Gutierrez V. 2003. Alteration of lipids, G proteins, and PKC in cell membranes of elderly hypertensives. *Hypertension.* 41(1):176–182.

Fareh J, Touyz RM, Schiffrin EL, Thibault G. 2000. Altered cardiac endothelin receptors and protein kinase C in deoxycorticosterone-salt hypertensive rats. *J Mol Cell Cardiol.* 32(4):665–676.

Fatehi-Hassanabad Z, Fatehi M, Shahidi MI. 2004. Endothelial dysfunction in aortic rings and mesenteric beds isolated from deoxycorticosterone acetate hypertensive rats: possible involvement of protein kinase C. *Eur J Pharmacol.* 494(2–3):199–204.

Fedorova OV, Talan MI, Agalakova NI, Droy-Lefaix MT, Lakatta EG, Bagrov AY. 2003. Myocardial PKC beta2 and the sensitivity of Na/K-ATPase to marinobufagenin are reduced by cicletanine in Dahl hypertension. *Hypertension.* 41(3):505–511.

Flamant M, Placier S, Dubroca C et al. 2007. Role of matrix metalloproteinases in early hypertensive vascular remodeling. *Hypertension.* 50(1):212–218.

Fleming I, Fisslthaler B, Dimmeler S, Kemp BE, Busse R. 2001. Phosphorylation of Thr(495) regulates Ca²⁺/calmodulin-dependent endothelial nitric oxide synthase activity. *Circ Res.* 88:E68–E75.

Funayama H, Ishikawa SE, Kubo N et al. 2004. Increases in interleukin-6 and matrix metalloproteinase-9 in the infarct-related coronary artery of acute myocardial infarction. *Circ J.* 68(5):451–454.

Gailly P, Gong MC, Somlyo AV, Somlyo AP. 1997. Possible role of atypical protein kinase C activated by arachidonic acid in Ca²⁺ sensitization of rabbit smooth muscle. *J Physiol.* 500(Pt 1):95–109

Galis ZS, Khatri JJ. 2002. Matrix metalloproteinases in vascular remodeling and atherogenesis: the good, the bad, and the ugly. *Circ Res.* 90(3):251–262.

Giardina JB, Tanner DJ, Khalil RA. 2001. Oxidized-LDL enhances coronary vasoconstriction by increasing the activity of protein kinase C isoforms alpha and epsilon. *Hypertension.* 37(2 Pt 2):561–568.

Giardina JB, Green GM, Cockrell KL, Granger JP, Khalil RA. 2002. TNF-α enhances contraction and inhibits endothelial NO-cGMP relaxation in systemic vessels of pregnant rats. *Am J Physiol Regul Integr Comp Physiol.* 283(1):R130–R143.

Goodnight J, Mischak H, Kolch W, Mushinski F. 1995. Immunocytochemical localization of eight protein kinase C isozymes overexpressed in NIH 3T3 fibroblasts. *J Biol Chem.* 270:9991–10001.

Gu X, Bishop SP. 1994. Increased protein kinase C and isozyme redistribution in pressure-overload cardiac hypertrophy in the rat. *Circ Res.* 75(5):926–931.

Haller H, Quass P, Lindschau C, Luft FC, Distler A. 1994. Platelet-derived growth factor and angiotensin II induce different spatial distribution of protein kinase C-α and -β in vascular smooth muscle cells. *Hypertension.* 23:848–852.

Hartwig JH, Thelen M, Rosen A, Janmey PA, Nairn AC, Aderem A. 1992. MARCKS is an actin filament cross-linking protein regulated by protein kinase C and calcium-calmodulin. *Nature.* 356:618–622.

Hassel S, Eichner A, Yakymovych M, Hellman U, Knaus P, Souchelnytskyi S. 2004. Proteins associated with type II bone morphogenetic protein receptor (BMPR-II) and identified by two-dimensional gel electrophoresis and mass spectrometry. *Proteomics.* 4(5):1346–1358.

Hedges JC, Oxhorn BC, Carty M, Adam LP, Yamboliev IA, Gerthoffer WT. 2000. Phosphorylation of caldesmon by ERK MAP kinases in smooth muscle. *Am J Physiol Cell Physiol.* 278(4):C718–C726.

Heitzer T, Wenzel U, Hink U et al. 1999. Increased NAD(P)H oxidase-mediated superoxide production in renovascular hypertension: evidence for an involvement of protein kinase C. *Kidney Int.* 55(1):252–260.

Horowitz A, Menice CB, Laporte R, Morgan KG. 1996. Mechanisms of smooth muscle contraction. *Physiol Rev.* 76(4):967–1003.

House C, Kemp BE. 1987. Protein kinase C contains a pseudosubstrate prototope in its regulatory domain. *Science.* 238:1726–1728.

Housey GM, Johnson MD, Hsiao WLW et al. 1988. Overproduction of protein kinase C causes disordered growth control in rat fibroblasts. *Cell.* 52:343–354.

Huang PL, Huang Z, Mashimo H et al. 1995. Hypertension in mice lacking the gene for endothelial nitric oxide synthase. *Nature.* 377(6546):239–242.

Hughes-Darden CA, Wachira SJ, Denaro FJ et al. 2001. Expression and distribution of protein kinase C isozymes in brain tissue of spontaneous hypertensive rats. *Cell Mol Biol. (Noisy-le-grand).* 47(6):1077–1088.

Humbert PO, Dow LE, Russell SM. 2006. The Scribble and Par complexes in polarity and migration: friends or foes? *Trends Cell Biol.* 16(12):622–630.

Hussain S, Assender JW, Bond M, Wong LF, Murphy D, Newby AC. 2002. Activation of protein kinase Czeta is essential for cytokine-induced metalloproteinase-1, -3, and -9 secretion from rabbit smooth muscle cells and inhibits proliferation. *J Biol Chem.* 277(30):27345–27352.

Hyat SL, Klauck T, Jaken S. 1990. Protein kinase C is localized in focal contacts of normal but not transformed fibroblasts. *Mol Carcinogenesis.* 3:45–53.

Hynynen MM, Khalil RA. 2006. The vascular endothelin system in hypertension—Recent patents and discoveries. *Recent Pat Cardiovasc Drug Discov.* 1(1):95–108.

Inagaki M, Yokokura H, Itoh T, Kanmura Y, Kuriyama H, Hidaka H. 1987. Purified rabbit brain protein kinase C relaxes skinned vascular smooth muscle and phosphorylates myosin light chain. *Arch Biochem Biophys.* 254(1):136–141.

Ishii H, Jirousek MR, Daisuke K et al. 1996. Amelioration of vascular dysfunction in diabetes rats by an oral PKC β inhibitor. *Science.* 272:728–731.

Ito T, Ozawa K, Shimada K. 2007. Current drug targets and future therapy of pulmonary arterial hypertension. *Curr Med Chem.* 14(6):719–733.

Jiang MJ, Morgan KG. 1987. Intracellular calcium levels in phorbol ester-induced contractions of vascular muscle. *Am J Physiol.* 253(6 Pt 2):H1365–H1371.

Kanashiro CA, Khalil RA. 1998. Signal transduction by protein kinase C in mammalian cells. *Clin Exp Pharmacol Physiol.* 25(12):974–985.

Kanashiro CA, Alexander BT, Granger JP, Khalil RA. 1999. Ca^{2+}-insensitive vascular protein kinase C during pregnancy and NOS inhibition. *Hypertension.* 34(4 Pt 2): 924–930.

Kanashiro CA, Altirkawi KA, Khalil RA. 2000. Preconditioning of coronary artery against vasoconstriction by endothelin-1 and prostaglandin F2α during repeated downregulation of ε-protein kinase C. *J Cardiovasc Pharmacol.* 35(3):491–501.

Kanashiro CA, Cockrell KL, Alexander BT, Granger JP, Khalil RA. 2000. Pregnancy-associated reduction in vascular protein kinase C activity rebounds during inhibition of NO synthesis. *Am J Physiol Regul Integr Comp Physiol.* 278(2):R295–R303.

Kanashiro CA, Khalil RA. 2001. Gender-related distinctions in protein kinase C activity in rat vascular smooth muscle. *Am J Physiol Cell Physiol.* 280(1):C34–C45.

Kanayama Y, Negoro N, Okamura M et al. 1994. Modulation of protein kinase C in aorta of spontaneously hypertensive rats with enalapril treatment. *Osaka City Med J.* 40(2):83–97.

Katada T, Gilman AG, Watanabe Y, Bauer S, Jakobs KH. 1985. Protein kinase C phosphorylates the inhibitory guanine-nucleotide-binding regulatory component and apparently suppresses its function in hormonal inhibition of adenylate cyclase. *Eur J Biochem.* 151:431–437.

Kelly DJ, Zhang Y, Hepper C et al. 2003. Protein kinase C beta inhibition attenuates the progression of experimental diabetic nephropathy in the presence of continued hypertension. *Diabetes.* 52(2):512–518.

Keranen LM, Dutil EM, Newton AC. 1995. Protein kinase C is regulated in vivo by three functionally distinct phosphorylations. *Curr Biol.* 5:1394–1403.

Khalil RA. 2006. Dietary salt and hypertension: new molecular targets add more spice. *Am J Physiol Regul Integr Comp Physiol.* 290(3):R509–R513.

Khalil RA, van Breemen C. 1988. Sustained contraction of vascular smooth muscle: calcium influx or C-kinase activation? *J Pharmacol Exp Ther.* 244(2):537–542.

Khalil RA, Lajoie C, Resnick MS, Morgan KG. 1992. Ca^{2+}-independent isoforms of protein kinase C differentially translocate in smooth muscle. *Am J Physiol.* 263(3 Pt 1):C714–C719.

Khalil RA, Lajoie C, Morgan KG. 1994. In situ determination of $[Ca^{2+}]_i$ threshold for translocation of the α-protein kinase C isoform. *Am J Physiol.* 266:C1544–C1551.

Khalil RA, Menice CB, Wang CL, Morgan KG. 1995. Phosphotyrosine-dependent targeting of mitogen-activated protein kinase in differentiated contractile vascular cells. *Circ Res.* 76(6):1101–1108.

Khalil RA, van Breemen C. 1995. Mechanisms of calcium mobilization and homeostasis in vascular smooth muscle and their relevance to hypertension. In: Laragh JH, Brenner BM, eds. *Hypertension: Pathophysiology, Diagnosis and Management.* New York: Raven Press,. 523:40.

Khalil RA, Morgan KG. 1996. Enzyme translocations during smooth muscle activation. In: Barany M, ed. *Biochemistry of Smooth Muscle Contraction.* New York: Academic Press, 307–318.

Khalil RA, Crews JK, Novak J, Kassab S, Granger JP. 1998. Enhanced vascular reactivity during inhibition of nitric oxide synthesis in pregnant rats. *Hypertension.* 31(5):1065–1069.

Khalil RA, Granger JP. 2002. Vascular mechanisms of increased arterial pressure in preeclampsia: lessons from animal models. *Am J Physiol Regul Integr Comp Physiol.* 283(1):R29–R45.

Kim J, Lee YR, Lee CH et al. 2005. Mitogen-activated protein kinase contributes to elevated basal tone in aortic smooth muscle from hypertensive rats. *Eur J Pharmacol.* 514(2–3):209–215.

Klevit RE. 1990. Recognition of DNA by Cys2, His2 Zinc fingers. *Proteins: Struct Funct Genet.* 7:215.

Kordowska J, Hetrick T, Adam LP, Wang CL. 2006. Phosphorylated l-caldesmon is involved in disassembly of actin stress fibers and postmitotic spreading. *Exp Cell Res.* 312(2):95–110.

Kose A, Saito N, Ito H, Kikkawa U, Nishizuka Y, Tanaka C. 1988. Electron microscopic localization of type I protein kinase C in rat Purkinje cells. *J Neurosci.* 8:4262–4268.

Kraft AS, Anderson WB. 1983. Phorbol esters increase the amount of Ca^{2+}, phospholipid-dependent protein kinase associated with plasma membrane. *Nature.* 301(5901):621–623.

Kupferminc MJ, Peaceman AM, Wigton TR, Rehnberg KA, Socol ML. 1994. Tumor necrosis factor-alpha is elevated in plasma and amniotic fluid of patients with severe preeclampsia. *Am J Obstet Gynecol.* 170(6):1752–1759.

Laviades C, Varo N, Fernandez J et al. 1998. Abnormalities of the extracellular degradation of collagen type I in essential hypertension. *Circulation.* 98(6):535–540.

Lee DL, Webb RC, Jin L. 2004. Hypertension and RhoA/Rho-kinase signaling in the vasculature: highlights from the recent literature. *Hypertension.* 44(6):796–799.

Lee DL, Sturgis LC, Labazi H et al. 2006. Angiotensin II hypertension is attenuated in interleukin-6 knockout mice. *Am J Physiol Heart Circ Physiol.* 290(3):H935–H940.

Leventhal PS, Bertics PJ. 1993. Activation of protein kinase C by selective binding of arginine-rich polypeptides. *J Biol Chem.* 268:13906–13913.

Li D, Liu L, Chen H, Sawamura T, Ranganathan S, Mehta JL. 2003. LOX-1 mediates oxidized low-density lipoprotein-induced expression of matrix metalloproteinases in human coronary artery endothelial cells. *Circulation.* 107(4):612–617.

Li H, Witte K, August M et al. 2006. Reversal of endothelial nitric oxide synthase uncoupling and up-regulation of endothelial nitric oxide synthase expression lowers blood pressure in hypertensive rats. *J Am Coll Cardiol.* 47(12):2536–2544.

Li W, Zhang J, Bottaro DP, Pierce JH. 1996. Identification of serine 643 of protein kinase C-delta as an important autophosphorylation site for its enzymatic activity. *J Biol Chem.* 272:24550–24555.

Libby P. 2006. Inflammation and cardiovascular disease mechanisms. *Am J Clin Nutr.* 83(2):456S–60S.

Limas CJ. 1980. Phosphorylation of cardiac sarcoplasmic reticulum by a calcium-activated, phospholipid-dependent protein kinase. *Biochem Biophys Res Commun.* 96:1378–1383.

Liou YM, Morgan KG. 1994. Redistribution of protein kinase C isoforms in association with vascular hypertrophy of rat aorta. *Am J Physiol.* 267:C980–C989.

Littler CM, Morris KG Jr, Fagan KA, McMurtry IF, Messing RO, Dempsey EC. 2003. Protein kinase C-epsilon-null mice have decreased hypoxic pulmonary vasoconstriction. *Am J Physiol Heart Circ Physiol.* 284(4):H1321–H1331.

Liu YE, Wang M, Greene J et al. 1997. Preparation and characterization of recombinant tissue inhibitor of metalloproteinase 4 (TIMP-4). *J Biol Chem.* 272(33):20479–20483.

Lubrano V, Cocci F, Battaglia D, Papa A, Marraccini P, Zucchelli GC. 2005. Usefulness of high-sensitivity IL-6 measurement for clinical characterization of patients with coronary artery disease. *J Clin Lab Anal.* 19(3):110–114.

Machado RD, Pauciulo MW, Thomson JR et al. 2001. BMPR2 haploinsufficiency as the inherited molecular mechanism for primary pulmonary hypertension. *Am J Hum Genet.* 68(1):92–102.

Magness RR, Rosenfeld CR, Carr BR. 1991. Protein kinase C in uterine and systemic arteries during ovarian cycle and pregnancy. *Am J Physiol.* 260(3 Pt 1):E464–E470.

Makowske M, Rosen OM. 1989. Complete activation of protein kinase C by an antipeptide antibody directed against the pseudosubstrate prototope. *J Biol Chem.* 264:16155–16159.

McCarty MF. 1996. Up-regulation of intracellular signalling pathways may play a central pathogenic role in hypertension, atherogenesis, insulin resistance, and cancer promotion—the 'PKC syndrome.' *Med Hypotheses.* 46(3):191–221.

McLachlan CS, Chua WC, Wong PT, Kah TL, Chen C, El Oakley RM. 2005. Homocysteine is positively associated with cytokine IL-18 plasma levels in coronary artery bypass surgery patients. *Biofactors.* 23(2):69–73.

McNair LL, Salamanca DA, Khalil RA. 2004. Endothelin-1 promotes Ca^{2+} antagonist-insensitive coronary smooth muscle contraction via activation of ε-protein kinase C. *Hypertension*. 43(4):897–904.

Michell BJ, Chen Z, Tiganis T et al. 2001. Coordinated control of endothelial nitric-oxide synthase phosphorylation by protein kinase C and the cAMP-dependent protein kinase. *J Biol Chem*. 276:17625–17628.

Mii S, Khalil RA, Morgan KG, Ware JA, Kent KC. 1996. Mitogen-activated protein kinase and proliferation of human vascular smooth muscle cells. *Am J Physiol*. 270(1 Pt 2):H142–H150.

Mochly-Rosen D, Gordon AS. 1998. Anchoring proteins for protein kinase C: a means for isozyme selectivity. *FASEB J*. 12:35–42.

Motley ED, Eguchi K, Patterson MM, Palmer PD, Suzuki H, Eguchi S. 2007. Mechanism of endothelial nitric oxide synthase phosphorylation and activation by thrombin. *Hypertension*. 49(3):577–583.

Mountain DJ, Singh M, Menon B, Singh K. 2007. Interleukin-1beta increases expression and activity of matrix metalloproteinase-2 n cardiac microvascular endothelial cells: role of PKCalpha/bea1 and MAPKs. *Am J Physiol Cell Physiol*. 292(2):C867–C875.

Newton AC. 1995. Protein kinase C: structure, function, and regulation. *J Biol Chem*. 270:28495–28498.

Newton AC. 1997. Regulation of protein kinase C. *Curr Opin Cell Biol*. 9:161–167.

Nijm J, Wikby A, Tompa A, Olsson AG, Jonasson L. 2005. Circulating levels of proinflammatory cytokines and neutrophil-platelet aggregates in patients with coronary artery disease. *Am J Cardiol*. 95(4):452–456.

Nishizuka Y. 1992. Intracellular signaling by hydrolysis of phospholipids and activation of PKC. *Science*. 258:607–614.

Nishizuka Y. 1995. Protein kinase C and lipid signaling for sustained cellular responses. *FASEB J*. 9:484–496.

Nowicki S, Kruse MS, Brismar H, Aperia A. 2000. Dopamine-induced translocation of protein kinase C isoforms visualized in renal epithelial cells. *Am J Physiol Cell Physiol*. 279(6):C1812–C1818.

O'Brian CA, Ward NE. 1989. Biology of protein kinase family. *Cancer Metastasis Reviews*. 8:199–214.

Ohanian V, Ohanian J, Shaw L, Scarth S, Parker PJ, Heagerty AM. 1996. Identification of protein kinase C isoforms in rat mesenteric small arteries and their possible role in agonist-induced contraction. *Circ Res*. 78:806–812.

Ohno S, Konno Y, Akita Y, Yano A, Suzuki K. 1990. A point mutation at the putative ATP-binding site of protein kinase Ca abolishes the kinase activity and renders it down-regulation-insensitive. *J Biol Chem*. 265:6296–6300.

Ono Y, Fujii T, Ogita K, Kikkawa U, Igarashi K, Nishizuka Y. 1989. Protein kinase Cδ subspecies from rat brain: its structure, expression, and properties. *Proc Natl Acad Sci U S A*. 86:3099–3103.

Orr JW, Keranen LM, Newton AC. 1992. Reversible exposure of the pseudosubstrate domain of protein kinase C by phosphatidylserine and diacylglycerol. *J Biol Chem*. 267:15263–15266.

Orshal JM, Khalil RA. 2004. Reduced endothelial NO-cGMP-mediated vascular relaxation and hypertension in IL-6-infused pregnant rats. *Hypertension*. 43(2):434–444.

Orshal JM, Khalil RA. 2004. Interleukin-6 impairs endothelium-dependent NO-cGMP-mediated relaxation and enhances contraction in systemic vessels of pregnant rats. *Am. J Physiol Regul Integr Comp Physiol*. 286(6):R1013–R1023.

Osada S, Mizuno K, Saido TC, Suzuki K, Kuroki T, Ohno S. 1992. A new member of the protein kinase C family, nPKC theta, predominantly expressed in skeletal muscle. *Mol Cell Biol*.12:3930–3938.

Papadimitriou E, Waters CR, Manolopoulos VG, Unsworth BR, Maragoudakis ME, Lelkes PL. 2001. Regulation of extracellular matrix remodeling and MMP-2 activation in cultured rat adrenal medullary endothelial cells. *Endothelium*. 8(3):181–194.

Park MJ, Park IC, Lee HC et al. 2003. Protein Kinase C-alpha activation by phorbol ester induces secretion of gelatinase B/MMP-9 through ERK1/2 pathway in capillary endothelial cells. *Int J Oncol*. 22(1):137–143.

Parker CA, Takahashi K, Tao T, Morgan KG. 1994. Agonist-induced redistribution of calponin in contractile vascular smooth muscle cells. *Am J Physiol*. 267(5 Pt 1): C1262–C1270.

Parker PJ, Coussens L, Totty N et al. 1986. The complete primary structure of protein kinase C-the major phorbol ester receptor. *Science*. 233:853–859.

Partovian C, Zhuang Z, Moodie K et al. 2005. PKC-alpha activates eNOS and increases arterial blood flow in vivo. *Circ Res*. 97(5):482–487.

Puri A, McGoon MD, Kushwaha SS. 2007. Pulmonary arterial hypertension: current therapeutic strategies. *Nat Clin Pract Cardiovasc Med*. 4(6):319–329.

Raffetto JD, Khalil RA. 2007. Matrix metalloproteinases and their inhibitors in vascular remodeling and vascular disease. *Biochem Pharmacol*. [Epub ahead of print].

Raffetto JD, Ross RL, Khalil RA. 2007. Matrix metalloproteinase 2-induced venous dilation via hyperpolarization and activation of K$^+$ channels: relevance to varicose vein formation. *J Vasc Surg*. 45(2):373–380.

Ramana KV, Chandra D, Srivastava S, Bhatnagar A, Srivastava SK. 2003. Aldose reductase mediates the mitogenic signals of cytokines. *Chem Biol Interact*. 143–144:587–596

Ramana KV, Tammali R, Reddy AB, Bhatnagar A, Srivastava SK. 2007. Aldose reductase-regulated tumor necrosis factor-alpha production is essential for high glucose-induced vascular smooth muscle cell growth. *Endocrinology*. 148(9):4371–4384.

Rao F, Zhang L, Wessel J et al. 2007. Tyrosine hydroxylase, the rate-limiting enzyme in catecholamine biosynthesis: discovery of common human genetic variants governing transcription, autonomic activity, and blood pressure in vivo. *Circulation*. 116(9):993–1006.

Ridge KM, Dada L, Lecuona E et al. 2002. Dopamine-induced exocytosis of Na,K-ATPase is dependent on activation of protein kinase C-epsilon and -delta. *Mol Biol Cell*. 13(4):1381–1389.

Ron D, Mochly-Rosen D. 1994. Agonists and antagonists of protein kinase C function, derived from its binding proteins. *J Biol Chem*. 269(34):21395–21398.

Rosen B, Barg J, Zimlichman R. 1999. The effects of angiotensin II, endothelin-1, and protein kinase C inhibitor on DNA synthesis and intracellular calcium mobilization in vascular smooth muscle cells from young normotensive and spontaneously hypertensive rats. *Am J Hypertens*. 12(12 Pt 1–2):1243–1251.

Rosoff PM, Stein LF, Cantley LC. 1984. Phorbol esters induce differentiation in a pre-B-lymphocyte cell line by enhancing Na$^+$/H$^+$ exchange. *J Biol Chem*. 259:7056–7060.

Salamanca DA, Khalil RA. 2005. Protein kinase C isoforms as specific targets for modulation of vascular smooth muscle function in hypertension. *Biochem Pharmacol*. 70(11):1537–1547.

Sardella G, Mariani P, D'Alessandro M et al. 2006. Early elevation of interleukin-1beta and interleukin-6 levels after bare or drug-eluting stent implantation in patients with stable angina. *Thromb Res*. 117(6):659–664.

Sasajima H, Shima H, Toyoda Y et al. 1997. Increased Ca^{2+} sensitivity of contractile elements via protein kinase C in alpha-toxin permeabilized SMA from young spontaneously hypertensive rats. *Cardiovasc Res*. 36(1):86–91.

Sauro MD, Hadden JW. 1992. Gamma-interferon corrects aberrant protein kinase C levels and immunesuppression in the spontaneously hypertensive rat. *Int J Immunopharmacol*. 14(8):1421–1427.

Schaap D, Parker PJ, Bristol A, Kriz R, Knopf J. 1989. Unique substrate specificity and regulatory properties of PKC-epsilon: a rationale for diversity. *FEBS Lett*. 243(2):351–357.

Schiffrin EL. 1995. Endothelin: potential role in hypertension and vascular hypertrophy. *Hypertension*. 25(6): 1135–1143.

Schwienbacher C, Jockusch BM, Rudiger M. 1996. Intramolecular interactions regulate serine/threonine phosphorylation of vinculin. *FEBS Lett*. 384:71–74.

Seko T, Ito M, Kureishi Y et al. 2003. Activation of RhoA and inhibition of myosin phosphatase as important components in hypertension in vascular smooth muscle. *Circ Res*. 92(4):411–418.

Shibata R, Morita S, Nagai K, Miyata S, Iwasaki T. 1990. Effects of H-7 (protein kinase inhibitor) and phorbol ester on aortic strips from spontaneously hypertensive rats. *Eur J Pharmacol*. 175(3):261–271.

Singer HA. 1990. Phorbol ester-induced stress and myosin light chain phosphorylation in swine medial smooth muscle. *J Pharmacol Exp Ther*. 252:1068–1074.

Sirous ZN, Fleming JB, Khalil RA. 2001. Endothelin-1 enhances eicosanoids-induced coronary smooth muscle contraction by activating specific protein kinase C isoforms. *Hypertension*. 37(2 Pt 2):497–504.

Smith L, Payne JA, Sedeek MH, Granger JP, Khalil RA. 2003. Endothelin-induced increases in Ca^{2+} entry mechanisms of vascular contraction are enhanced during high-salt diet. *Hypertension*. 41(3 Pt 2):787–793.

Soloviev AI, Parshikov AV, Stefanov AV. 1998. Evidence for the involvement of protein kinase C in depression of endothelium-dependent vascular responses in spontaneously hypertensive rats. *J Vasc Res*. 35(5):325–331.

Somlyo AP, Somlyo AV. 2003. Ca^{2+} sensitivity of smooth muscle and nonmuscle myosin II: modulated by G proteins, kinases, and myosin phosphatase. *Physiol Rev*. 83(4):1325–1358.

Song Y, Jones JE, Beppu H, Keaney JF Jr, Loscalzo J, Zhang YY. 2005. Increased susceptibility to pulmonary hypertension in heterozygous BMPR2-mutant mice. *Circulation*. 112(4):553–562.

Stennett AK, Khalil RA. 2006. Neurovascular mechanisms of hypertension in pregnancy. *Curr Neurovasc Res*. 3(2):131–148.

Szallasi Z, Smith CB, Pettit GR, Blumberg PM. 1994. Differential regulation of protein kinase C isozymes by bryostatin 1 and phorbol 12-myristate 13-acetate in NIH 3T3 fibroblasts. *J Biol Chem*. 269:2118–2124.

Takai Y, Kishimoto A, Iwasa Y, Kawahara Y, Mori T, Nishizuka Y. 1979. Calcium-dependent activation of a multifunctional protein kinase by membrane phospholipids. *J Biol Chem*. 254:3692–3695.

Thelen M, Rosen A, Nairn AC, Aderem A. 1991. Regulation by phosphorylation of reversible association of a myristoylated protein kinase C substrate with the plasma membrane. *Nature*. 351(6324):320–322.

Touyz RM, Schiffrin EL. 2001. Increased generation of superoxide by angiotensin II in smooth muscle cells from resistance arteries of hypertensive patients: role of phospholipase D-dependent NAD(P)H oxidase-sensitive pathways. *J Hypertens*. 19(7):1245–1254.

Tsai BM, Wang M, Pitcher JM, Meldrum KK, Meldrum DR. 2004. Hypoxic pulmonary vasoconstriction and pulmonary artery tissue cytokine expression are mediated by protein kinase C. *Am J. Physiol Lung Cell Mol Physiol*. 287(6):L1215–L1219.

Ungvari Z, Csiszar A, Huang A, Kaminski PM, Wolin MS, Koller A. 2003. High pressure induces superoxide production in isolated arteries via protein kinase C-dependent activation of NAD(P)H oxidase. *Circulation*. 108(10):1253–1258.

Vásquez-Vivar J, Kalyanaraman B, Martásek P et al. 1998. Superoxide generation by endothelial nitric oxide synthase the influence of cofactors. *Proc Natl Acad Sci U S A*. 95(16):9220–9225.

Vince GS, Starkey PM, Austgulen R, Kwiatkowski D, Redman CW. 1995. Interleukin-6, tumour necrosis factor and soluble tumour necrosis factor receptors in women with pre-eclampsia. *Br J Obstet Gynaecol*. 102(1):20–25.

Visse R, Nagase H. 2003. Matrix metalloproteinases and tissue inhibitors of metalloproteinases: structure, function, and biochemistry. *Circ Res*. 92(8):827–839.

Waehre T, Yndestad A, Smith C et al. 2004. Increased expression of interleukin-1 in coronary artery disease with downregulatory effects of HMG-CoA reductase inhibitors. *Circulation*. 109(16):1966–1972.

Wallukat G, Homuth V, Fischer T et al. 1999. Patients with preeclampsia develop agonistic autoantibodies against the angiotensin AT1 receptor. *J Clin Invest*. 103(7):945–952.

Wang JKT, Walaas SI, Sihra TS, Aderem A, Greengard P. 1989. Phosphorylation and associated translocation of the 87-kDa protein, a major protein kinase C substrate, in isolated nerve terminals. *Proc Natl Acad Sci U S A.* 86:2253–2256.

Wang S, Desai D, Wright G, Niles RM, Wright GL. 1997. Effects of protein kinase C alpha overexpression on A7r5 smooth muscle cell proliferation and differentiation. *Exp Cell Res.* 236(1):117–126.

Watts SW, Rondelli C, Thakali K et al. 2007. Morphological and biochemical characterization of remodeling in aorta and vena cava of DOCA-salt hypertensive rats. *Am J Physiol Heart Circ Physiol.* 292:H2438–H2448.

Williams MA, Mahomed K, Farrand A et al. 1998. Plasma tumor necrosis factor-alpha soluble receptor p55 (sTNFp55) concentrations in eclamptic, preeclamptic and normotensive pregnant Zimbabwean women. *J Reprod Immunol.* 40(2):159–173.

Woodsome TP, Eto M, Everett A, Brautigan DL, Kitazawa T. 2001. Expression of CPI-17 and myosin phosphatase correlates with Ca^{2+} sensitivity of protein kinase C-induced contraction in rabbit smooth muscle. *J Physiol.* 535(Pt 2):553–564.

Xia Y, Tsai AL, Berka V, Zweier JL. 1998. Superoxide generation from endothelial nitric-oxide synthase. A Ca^{2+}/calmodulin-dependent and tetrahydrobiopterin regulatory process, *J Biol Chem.* 273:25804–25808.

Young JL, Libby P, Schonbeck U. 2002. Cytokines in the pathogenesis of atherosclerosis. *Thromb Haemost.* 88(4):554–567.

Zervoudaki A, Economou E, Stefanadis C et al. 2003. Plasma levels of active extracellular matrix metalloproteinases 2 and 9 in patients with essential hypertension before and after antihypertensive treatment. *J Hum Hypertens.* 17(2):119–124.

Chapter 3

BRAIN TEMPERATURE REGULATION DURING NORMAL NEURAL FUNCTION AND NEUROPATHOLOGY

Eugene A. Kiyatkin

ABSTRACT

This chapter is focused on brain temperature as a physiological parameter, which is determined primarily by neural metabolism, regulated by cerebral blood flow, and affected by various environmental factors and drugs. First, we consider normal fluctuations in brain temperature that are induced by salient environmental stimuli and occur during motivated behavior at stable normothermic conditions. On the basis of thermorecording data obtained in animals, we define the range of physiological fluctuations in brain temperature, their underlying mechanisms, and relations to body temperatures. Second, we discuss the temperature dependence of neural activity and the dual "functions" of temperature as a reflection of metabolic brain activity and as a factor that affects this activity. Third, we discuss pharmacological brain hyperthermia, focusing on the effects of psychomotor stimulants, highly popular drugs of abuse that increase brain metabolism, diminish heat dissipation, and may induce pathological brain overheating. We will demonstrate that the effects of these drugs are state dependent, showing strong modulation by activity states and environmental conditions that restrict heat dissipation. Finally, we discuss the adverse effects of high temperature on neural structures and functions under various pathological conditions. Particularly, we provide evidence for the role of brain hyperthermia in leakage of the blood–brain barrier, development of brain edema, acute abnormalities of neural cells, and neurotoxicity. These data are relevant for understanding the tight links between brain metabolism, temperature, and edema during various pathological processes in humans. Although most data were obtained in animals and several important aspects of brain temperature regulation in humans remain unknown, our focus is on the relevance of these data for human physiology and neuropathology.

Keywords: metabolism, cerebral blood flow, hyperthermia, metabolic brain activation, arousal, behavior, addictive drugs, blood–brain barrier, neuronal injury, neurotoxicity.

Body temperature is usually viewed as a tightly regulated homeostatic parameter that is maintained in mammals at highly stable levels during robust fluctuations in ambient temperatures (Schmidt-Nielsen 1997). A temperature increase above these "normal" levels (hyperthermia, fever) is a sensitive but nonspecific index of disease. While temperature regulation is traditionally studied within physiology (see Satinoff 1978; Gordon, Heath 1986 for review), much less is known about brain temperature, its normal and pathological fluctuations, and its role in brain functions under physiological and pathological conditions.

In contrast to electrophysiological and neurochemical parameters, which reflect brain functions, temperature is a physical property of brain tissue, one traditionally not of interest to the fields of neuroscience and clinical medicine. Interestingly, the first recordings of brain temperature in animals were performed more than 130 years ago (Schiff 1870, cited by Schiff 1894–1898), when the knowledge of brain functions was quite limited. Multipoint temperature recording from the human scalp was also used in the second part of the 19th century (Lombard 1879; Amidon 1880) as a tool to assess the selectivity of cortical activation with respect to mental functions. This can be thought of as a forerunner to the modern functional imagining techniques developed in the last two decades. Despite further sporadic work with brain temperature monitoring in animals (Feitelberg, Lampl 1935; Serota, Gerard 1938; Serota 1939; Abrams, Hammel 1964; Delgado, Hanai 1966; McElligott, Melzack 1967; Hayward, Baker 1968; Kovalzon 1972), renewed interest in this physiological parameter has derived from clinical observations that temperature strongly modulates the outcome of a stroke (Rosomoff 1957; Busto, Dietrich, Globus et al. 1987; see Maier, Steinberg 2003 for review). This work underscored the negative impact of fever on stroke-induced neural damage and attenuation of structural damage by hypothermia. Another point of interest in brain temperature arrived from the realization that extreme environmental heat has an enormous impact on human health. Many thousands of people die each year as a direct result of heatstroke, but if the negative impact of environmental heating on human diseases is taken into account the real numbers would be much higher.

The present chapter is aimed at answering the question "Why is brain temperature important for normal neural function and neuropathology?" Although most thermorecording data discussed in this chapter were obtained in rats under various physiological, pharmacological, and behavioral conditions, our focus is on the relevance of these data to human conditions.

This work is structured according to the following outline. First, we will consider physiological brain temperature fluctuations and demonstrate that brain temperature is an unstable parameter that fluctuates within relatively large limits ($\approx 3°C$), reflecting alterations in metabolic neural activity associated with environmental stimulation and/or performance of motivated behavior. Second, we will consider heat exchange between the brain and the rest of the body under different situations and discuss the source and

mechanisms of brain temperature fluctuations. Third, we will analyze the temperature dependence of neural activity and neural functions. Here our focus is on the dual "functions" of temperature: as a reflection of brain metabolic activity and as a physical factor that affects neural activity. Fourth, we will discuss pharmacological brain hyperthermia, focusing on psychomotor stimulants (methamphetamine or METH, ecstasy or MDMA), highly popular drugs of abuse that increase brain metabolism, diminish heat dissipation, and may induce pathological hyperthermia. We will demonstrate that the effects of these drugs are state dependent, showing strong modulation by environmental conditions that restrict heat dissipation. Finally, we will consider the adverse effects of high brain temperature on neural structures and functions. Here we will discuss a possible role of high brain temperature in leakage of the brain–blood barrier (BBB) and development of brain edema during acute METH intoxication. Pathological hyperthermia, coupled with rapidly developing brain edema, is the most dangerous complication of acute intoxication by psychomotor stimulant drugs and a possible contributor to latent neurotoxicity with chronic use of these drugs. These data are relevant for understanding the tight link between metabolism, temperature, and edema during various pathological processes in humans.

PHYSIOLOGICAL BRAIN TEMPERATURE FLUCTUATIONS: LIMITS AND MECHANISMS

The brain is part of the body, and brain temperature under quiet resting conditions is close to body temperature and in most cases fluctuates synchronously. However, both temperatures are, to some extent, abstractions because there are significant quantitative and qualitative differences in different body locations and brain structures. Despite the belief that brain temperature in the healthy organism is a stable, tightly regulated homeostatic parameter, our thermorecording studies in rats revealed rapid and relatively large temperature increases following exposure to quite different somatosensory stimuli (novel environment, biological smells, tail touch and tail pinch, presentation of another rat of the same or opposite sex, procedures of sc and ip injections, rectal temperature measurements).

Figure 3.1 shows typical examples of temperature fluctuations in the brain (nucleus accumbens or NAcc) and several peripheral locations (skin, temporal muscle) in male rats following two types of salient somatosensory stimulation (tail pinch and social interaction with another male rat). As can be seen, both somatosensory stimuli induced robust increases in

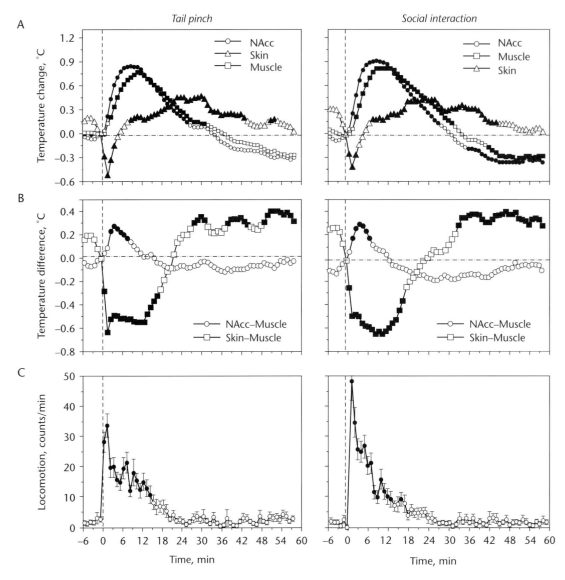

Figure 3.1 Changes in brain (nucleus accumbens or NAcc), muscle, and skin temperatures. (A) Relative change vs. baseline; (B) brain–muscle and skin–muscle temperature differentials; and (C) locomotion in male rats during one-minute tail pinch and social interaction with another male rat. Filled symbols indicate values significantly different versus baseline ($P < 0.05$).

NAcc and muscle temperatures, a biphasic, down–up fluctuation in skin temperature, and locomotor activation. Although the duration of both stimuli was 1 minute, temperature and locomotor responses were more prolonged, with different time courses for each parameter. Temperature changes in the NAcc and muscle generally paralleled each other, but increases in the NAcc were more rapid and stronger than those in muscle, resulting in a significant increase in NAcc–muscle temperature differentials during the first 4 to 6 minutes after stimulus onset (Fig. 3.1B). Since temporal muscle is a nonlocomotor head muscle that receives the same arterial blood (from common carotid artery) as the brain, this recording location provides not only a measure of body temperature but also allows one to control for the contribution of heat

inflow by arterial blood. The increase in brain–muscle differential, therefore, suggests brain activation as the primary cause for intrabrain heat production, rather than heat delivery from the periphery, and a factor that determines, via activation of effector mechanisms, subsequent body hyperthermia. Increase in brain–muscle differential correlated more tightly with locomotor activation, which increased momentarily and slowly decreased for about 20 minutes (Fig. 3.1C).

Each stimulus also induced rapid and robust decreases in skin temperature, suggesting acute vasoconstriction (Baker, Cronin, Mountjoy 1976). While changes in skin temperature are also determined by arterial blood inflow, they are modulated by changes in vessel tone. Skin hypothermia was always evident within the first 20 to 30 seconds after stimulus onset, resulting in a significant temperature fall during the first minute. In contrast to slower and more prolonged increases in brain and muscle temperature, this effect was brief, peaking at the first 2 to 4 minutes, and was followed by a rebound-like hyperthermia. This transient skin hypothermic response may be due to acute peripheral vasoconstriction, a phenomenon known to occur in humans and animals after various arousing and stressful stimuli (Altschule 1951; Solomon, Moos, Stone et al. 1964; Baker, Cronin, Mountjoy 1976), which diminishes heat dissipation. This diminished heat dissipation was especially evident in skin–muscle differential, which robustly decreased following each stimulus presentation (Fig. 3.1B). Skin–muscle differential then gradually increased, pointing at the post-stimulation increase in heat dissipation. Skin also showed an initial, opposite correlation with brain and body temperature following stimulation and inversely mirrored locomotor activation, which also peaked within the first 1 to 3 minutes after the stimulus starts.

Each recording location also had specific basal temperatures. When evaluated in habituated rats under quiet resting conditions, mean temperature was maximal in the NAcc (36.71 ± 0.04; SD = 0.51°C), lower in muscle (35.82 ± 0.05; SD = 0.57°C; $P < 0.01$ vs. NAcc), and minimal in the skin (34.80 ± 0.04; SD = 0.47°C; $P < 0.01$ vs. NAcc and muscle). These "basal" temperatures widely fluctuated in each location. The range of normal fluctuations (mean ± 3 SD, or 99% of statistical variability) were 35.2°C to 38.2°C, 34.1°C to 37.5°C, and 33.4°C to 36.2°C for NAcc, temporal muscle, and skin, respectively, that is, within ≈3°C. These three parameters also significantly correlated with each other (Fig. 3.2). NAcc and muscle temperature correlated strongly (r = 0.82, $P < 0.001$), showing a linear relationship that was parallel to the line of equality (Fig. 3.2A). Therefore, although muscle temperature was about 0.9°C lower than NAcc temperature in quiet resting conditions, both temperatures changed in parallel. Therefore, brain temperatures are higher when muscle temperatures are higher and vice versa. Although the correlation was weaker, skin temperature was also dependent upon brain and muscle temperatures (Fig. 3.2B and C). In contrast to parallel changes in brain–muscle temperatures, the temperature difference between skin and both NAcc and muscle was larger at high brain and body temperatures and progressively decreased at lower temperatures. At lower muscle temperatures, the difference between skin and muscle temperatures disappeared. This may reflect vasoconstriction that is present at higher brain and muscle temperatures (relatively decreasing skin temperature), but absent at very low basal temperatures when the rat is asleep.

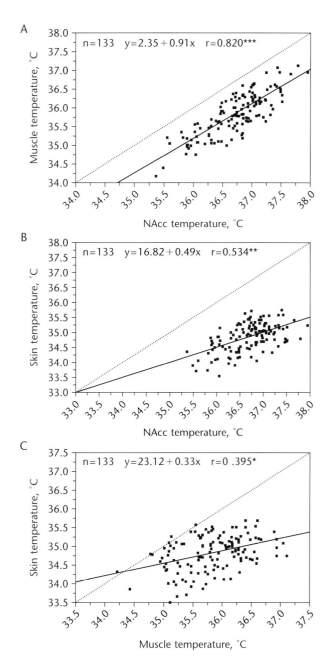

Figure 3.2 (A, B, and C) Relationships between brain (NAcc), muscle, and skin temperatures in habituated rats under quiet resting conditions. Each graph shows a coefficient of correlation, regression line, line of no effect, and regression equation.

Our work revealed that brain hyperthermic effects of all natural arousing stimuli tested were dependent on baseline brain temperatures. As shown in Figure 3.3, the temperature-increasing effects of social interaction, tail pinch, and presentation of a sexual partner were significantly stronger at low basal temperatures and became progressively weaker at higher brain temperatures [r = (−)0.61, 0.71, and 0.81 to 0.90]. Similar relationships were found for the temperature-increasing effects of other stimuli

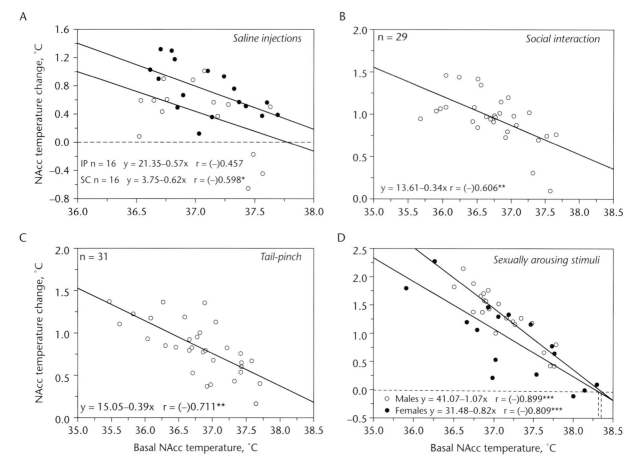

Figure 3.3 Relationships between basal brain temperature and its changes induced by various arousing stimuli. (A) Procedures of sc and ip saline injection; (B) social interaction; (C) tail pinch; and (D) sexually arousing stimuli (smell and sight of a sexual partner in male and female) in rats. Each graph shows coefficient of correlation, regression line, and regression equation. In each case, the temperature-increasing effects of arousing stimuli were inversely dependent upon basal brain temperature.

(procedure of ip and sc injections: $r = 0.46$ and 0.60, respectively; procedure of rectal temperature measurement: $r = 0.64$), as well as for several psychoactive drugs (i.e., cocaine). Therefore, this correlation appears to be valid for any arousing stimulus, reflecting some basic relationships between basal activity state (basal arousal) and its changes induced by environmental stimuli. These observations may be viewed as examples of the "law of initial values," which postulates that the magnitude and even direction of autonomic response to an "activating" stimulus is related to the pre-stimulus basal values (Wilder 1957, 1958). This relationship was evident for a number of homeostatic parameters, including arterial blood pressure, body temperature, and blood sugar levels.

This relatively tight relationship also suggests that there are upper limits of brain temperature increases (or arousal) when arousing stimuli become ineffective. As shown in Figure 3.3, these values slightly differ for each stimulus, but are close to $38.5°C$, that is, comparable to the upper limits of basal temperatures ($38.24°C$ for NAcc). These same levels were tonically

maintained during various motivated behavior (see following text).

Figure 3.4 shows examples of changes in brain and muscle temperatures during sexual behavior in male and female rats (Kiyatkin, Mitchum 2003; Mitchum, Kiyatkin 2004). As can be seen, brain temperature robustly increased following exposure to sexually arousing stimuli (A1 and A2: smell and sight of a sexual partner, respectively) and then phasically fluctuated during subsequent copulatory behavior (mounts and intromissions are shown as vertical lines), consistently peaking at ejaculation (E). While the pattern of tonic temperature elevation and their phasic fluctuations associated with copulatory cycles were similar in both males and females and in different brain structures, there were several important between-sex differences. Male rats showed larger temperature elevations following sexually arousing stimulation, stronger and more phasic increases that preceded ejaculations, and stronger temperature decreases during postejaculatory hypoactivity. Male rats also showed maximal increases in brain–muscle

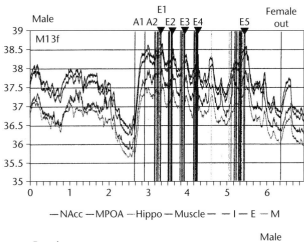

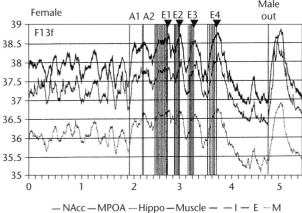

Figure 3.4 Original records of changes in brain (nucleus accumbens or NAcc, medial preoptic hypothalamus or MPOA, hippocampus or Hippo) and muscle temperatures in male and female rats during sexual behavior. Vertical lines show behavioral events: A1, placement in the cage of previous sexual interaction; A2, animals are divided by a transparent wall with holes, allowing a limited interaction; third vertical line shows the moment when animals began to interact freely; each subsequent line indicates mounts, intromissions, and ejaculations (E) The last vertical line shows the moment when sexual partner was removed from the cage (female out, male out).

differentials (i.e., maximal brain activation) immediately preceding ejaculation, but in females, these peaks occurred within the first minute after ejaculation. Importantly, sexual behavior was accompanied by robust brain and body hyperthermia with phasic, ejaculation-related temperature peaks that were similar in animals of both sexes. In males, these increases in NAcc and anterior preoptic hypothalamus were approximately 38.6°C to 38.8°C (with peaks in individual animals up to 39.8°C), obviously indicating the upper limits of physiological fluctuations in brain temperature. Although it is unknown whether such robust temperature increase may occur in humans, these data are consistent with multiple evidences, suggesting high-energy consumption during human sexual behavior and robust fluctuations of other

homeostatic parameters (Masters, Johnson 1966; Goldfarg 1970; Bohlen, Held, Sanderson et al. 1984; Stein 2002; Eardley 2005). For example, male sexual behavior was associated with maximal physiological increases in arterial blood pressure (up to doubling)—another tightly regulated homeostatic parameter.

HEAT EXCHANGE BETWEEN THE BRAIN AND THE REST OF THE BODY: BRAIN–BODY TEMPERATURE HOMEOSTASIS

The brain has a high level of metabolic activity, accounting for $\approx 20\%$ of the organism's total oxygen consumption (Siesjo 1978; Schmidt-Nielsen 1997). Most of the energy used for neuronal metabolism is spent restoring membrane potentials after electrical discharges (Hodgkin 1967; Ritchie 1973; Siesjo 1978; Laughlin, de Ruyter van Steveninck, Anderson et al. 1998; Sokoloff 1999; Shulman, Rothman, Behar et al. 2004), suggesting a relationship between metabolic and electrical neural activity. Energy is also used on other neural processes not directly related to electrical activity, particularly for synthesis of macromolecules and transport of protons across mitochondrial membranes. Since all energy used for neural metabolism is finally transformed into heat (Siesjo 1978), intense heat production appears to be an essential feature of brain metabolism.

To maintain temperature homeostasis, thermogenic activity of the brain needs to be balanced by heat dissipation from the brain to the body and then to the external environment. Because the brain is isolated from the rest of the body and protected by the skull, cerebral circulation provides the primary route for dissipation of brain-generated metabolic heat. Similar to any working, heat-producing engine, which receives a liquid coolant, the brain receives arterial blood, which is cooler than brain tissue (Feitelberg, Lampl 1935; Serota, Gerard 1938; Delgado, Hanai 1966; McElligott, Melzack 1967; Hayward, Baker 1968; Kiyatkin, Brown, Wise 2002; Nybo, Secher, Nielson 2002). Similar to a coolant, which takes heat from the engine, arterial blood removes heat from brain tissue, making venous blood warmer. After warm venous blood from the brain is transported to the heart and mixed with blood from the entire body (cooler blood from skin surfaces and warmer blood from internal organs), it travels to the lungs, where it is oxygenated and cooled by contact with air. This oxygenated, cooled blood travels to the heart again and is then rapidly transported to the brain.

While brain temperature homeostasis is determined primarily by intrabrain heat production and dissipation by cerebral blood flow, it also depends on the organism's global metabolism and the efficiency of heat dissipation to the external environment via skin and lung surfaces. Total energy consumption in humans is about 100 W at rest and may increase by 10 to 12 times (>1 kW) during intense physical activity such as running, cycling, or speed skating (Margaria, Cretelli, Aghemo et al. 1963). While this enhanced heat production is generally compensated by enhanced heat loss via skin and lung surfaces, physical exercise increases body and arterial blood temperatures (Nybo, Secher, Nielson 2002), thus affecting brain temperatures. While it is difficult to separate brain and body metabolism, it was suggested that physical activity also increases brain metabolism (Ide, Secher 2000; Ide, Schmalbruch, Quistorff et al. 2000), enhancing brain thermogenesis. In contrast, Nybo et al. (2002) explained a weak, ≈7% rise in metabolic heat production found in the brain during intense physical exercise in humans as an effect entirely dependent upon rise in brain temperature. Because heat from the body dissipates to the external environment, body temperature is also affected by the physical parameters of the external environment. Humans have efficient mechanisms for heat loss, which depend on a well-developed ability to sweat and the dynamic range of blood flow rates to the skin, which can increase from ≈0.2 to 0.5 L/min in thermally neutral conditions to 7 to 8 L/min under maximally tolerable heat stress (Rowell 1983). Under these conditions sweat rates may reach 2.0 L/h, providing a potential evaporative rate of heat loss in excess of 1 kW, that is, more than the highest possible heat production. These compensatory mechanisms, however, become less effective in hot, humid conditions, resulting in progressive heat accumulation in the organism. For example, body temperatures measured at the end of a marathon run on a warm day were found to be as high as 40°C (Schaefer 1979), and cases of fatigue during marathon running were associated with even higher temperatures (Cheuvront, Haymes 2001). While intense cycling at normal ambient temperatures increased brain temperature less than 1°C, increases of 2.0°C to 2.5°C (up to 40°C) were found when cycling was performed in water-impermeable suits that restricted heat loss via skin surfaces (Nybo, Secher, Nielson 2002). Therefore, changes in brain temperature may be determined not only by thermogenic activity of the brain but also by thermogenic activity of the body and the physical parameters of the environment.

To clarify the source of physiological brain hyperthermia, we simultaneously recorded temperatures from several brain structures and arterial blood in awake, unrestrained rats (Kiyatkin, Brown, Wise 2002). Both basal temperatures and their changes induced by various arousing and stressful stimuli were analyzed in this study. In these experiments we

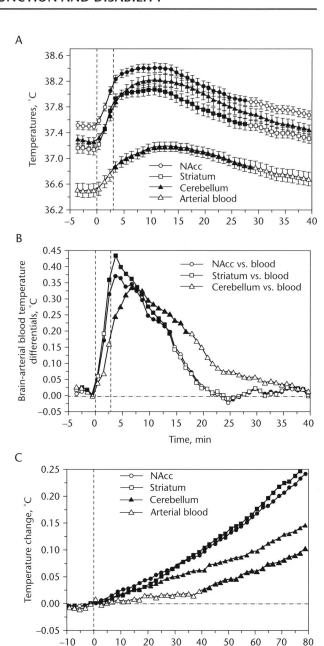

Figure 3.5 Changes in brain (nucleus accumbens or NAcc, striatum, and cerebellum) and arterial blood temperatures in male rats during three-minute tail pinch. (A) Shows mean changes (±standard errors); (B) shows temperature differentials between each brain structure and arterial blood; (C) shows rapid time-course resolution of temperature recording. Filled symbols in each graph indicate values significantly different from baseline.

confirmed previous work conducted in cats, dogs, monkeys, and humans, which demonstrated that aortal temperature during quiet rest at normal ambient temperatures (23°C, low humidity) is lower than the temperature of any brain structure (Fig. 3.5A). We also found that temperature increases occurring in brain structures following salient stimuli are more rapid and stronger than those in arterial blood

(Fig. 3.5B), suggesting intrabrain heat production rather than delivery of warm blood from the periphery as the primary cause of brain hyperthermia. This study, in combination with subsequent studies (Kiyatkin 2005), also confirmed classic observations (Serota 1939; Delgado, Hanai 1966) that brain temperature increases are qualitatively similar in different brain structures, although there are some important between-structure differences in both basal temperature and the pattern of changes with respect to different stimuli. As shown in Figure 3.5C, increases in brain temperature occurred on the second scale, consistently preceding slower and weaker increases in arterial temperature. Although the pattern of temperature changes generally paralleled in all tested structures, there were also between-structure differences, evident at rapid timescale.

Although arterial blood was consistently cooler than any brain structure under resting conditions and this difference could only increase during physiological activation, this was not true for body core temperature. Figure 3.6 shows the relationships between temperatures in medial preoptic hypothalamus (a deep brain structure), hippocampus (more dorsally located structure), and body core directly assessed in awake, habituated rats under quiet resting conditions. As can be seen, the medial preoptic hypothalamus and body core had virtually identical temperatures, while temperature in hippocampus was consistently lower than in body core. Although the fact that body core or rectal temperature may be higher than brain temperature is often considered as proof of heat inflow from the body to the brain (see Cabanac 1993 for review), heat exchange between the brain and the body is determined by the temperature gradient between brain tissue and arterial blood.

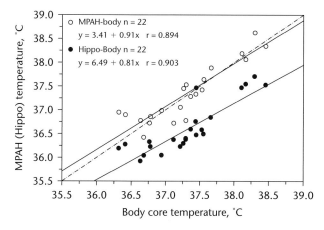

Figure 3.6 Relations between temperatures in body core, medial preoptic hypothalamus (MPAH), and hippocampus (Hippo) assessed by chronically implanted electrodes in male rats under quiet resting conditions. Each graph shows coefficient of correlation, regression line, line of no effect, and regression equation.

Although the differences between brain and body core temperatures in awake animals and humans are minimal, the brain becomes cooler than the body during general anesthesia (Kiyatkin, Brown 2005). As shown in Figure 3.7A, pentobarbital anesthesia results in powerful temperature decreases that were evident in brain structures, muscle, and skin. These decreases, however, are significantly stronger in both brain structures than in the body core (Fig. 3.7B), suggesting metabolic brain inhibition, a known feature of barbiturate drugs (Crane, Braun, Cornford et al. 1978; Michenfeider 1988), as a primary cause of brain hypothermia. In contrast, temperature decrease in skin was significantly weaker than that in body core, resulting in relative skin warming (Fig. 3.7B). This effect reflects enhanced heat dissipation that occurs because of loss of vascular tone during anesthesia. On the other hand, this enhanced heat dissipation is another contributor to body hypothermia. While the brain becomes cooler than the body core during anesthesia, it is unclear whether arterial blood arriving to the brain is warmer than the brain during anesthesia. To test this possibility, we simultaneously recorded brain (hypothalamus and hippocampus) and arterial blood temperatures during pentobarbital anesthesia (unpublished observations). As shown in Figure 3.7C, hypothalamic temperature under quiet resting conditions was about 0.5°C higher than aortal temperature, and the difference increased during activation (placement in the cage, 3-minute tail pinch, and social interaction with a female). After pentobarbital injection, the temperature difference between the hypothalamus and arterial blood decreased rapidly, reaching its minima (≈0.1°C) at ≈90 minutes after drug injection (Fig. 3.7D). The difference, however, remained positive within the entire period of anesthesia. Awakening from anesthesia was preceded by a gradual increase in hypothalamus–blood differential, which peaks at the time of the first head movement. Although changes in hippocampal temperature mirrored those in the hypothalamus, basal temperature in the hippocampus was equal to that in the abdominal aorta. During physiological activation, hippocampal temperature became higher than the temperature of arterial blood, but was lower during anesthesia.

These data complement observations suggesting selective brain cooling during anesthesia. While in awake animals and humans brain temperatures in different locations are similar to, or slightly higher than, body temperature under control conditions (Hayward, Baker 1968; Mariak, Jadeszko, Lewko et al. 1998; Mariak, Lebkowski, Lyson et al. 1999; Mariak, Lyson, Peikarski et al. 2000), these relationships become inverted during anesthesia. In cats, for example, during halothane and pentobarbital

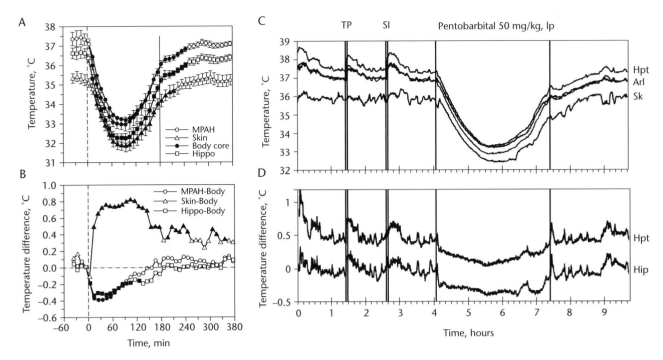

Figure 3.7 (A and B) Changes in brain (medial preoptic hypothalamus or MPAH and hippocampus or Hippo), body core, and skin temperatures assessed in rats by chronically implanted electrodes during sodium pentobarbital anesthesia (50 mg/kg). (A) shows absolute temperature changes and (B) shows temperature differentials. (C and D) shows individual record of temperature fluctuations in the same brain locations (Hpt and Hip), skin, and arterial blood.

anesthesia with body warming, cortical tissue was, respectively, 1.0°C and 1.8°C colder than body core (Erikson, Lanier 2003). Similar negative brain–body temperature differentials were found during pentobarbital anesthesia in dogs (Wass, Cable, Schaff et al. 1998), urethane anesthesia in rats (Moser, Mathiesen 1996), and anesthesia induced by α-chloralose and chloral hydrate in rats (Zhu, Nehra, Ackerman et al. 2004). In the latter study, when α-chloralose was combined with body warming, the difference between cortex and core body reached 4.3°C. In contrast to our study, these evaluations were performed in acute experiments, often with an open skull and electrodes that were not properly thermo-isolated. Although these experimental conditions would result in brain cooling and undervalued brain temperatures, especially in superficial recording sites and on small animals, these findings suggest that anesthesia may invert normal brain–body temperature homeostasis. Barbiturate anesthesia also decreases brain and rectal temperatures in humans, making the positive brain–body temperature difference smaller than that in drug-free conditions (Rumana, Gopinath, Uzura et al. 1998).

It is well known that increased brain metabolism is accompanied by increased cerebral blood flow (Fox, Raichle 1986; Raichle 2003; Trubel, Sacolick, Hyder 2006). However, the relationships between brain temperatures and interrelated changes in metabolism

and cerebral blood flow are complex and currently poorly understood. Although some consider brain temperature a passive parameter that depends entirely upon the ability of blood flow to remove metabolic heat from brain tissue (Yablonskiy, Ackerman, Raichle 2000; Sukstanskii, Yablonskiy 2006), direct relations between temperature and blood flow have been established in peripheral tissues. An increase in local temperature is accompanied by strong blood flow increases in skin (Ryan, Taylor, Bishop et al. 1997; Charkoudian 2003), muscle tissue (Oobu 1993), the intestine (Nagata, Katayama, Manivel et al. 2000), and the liver (Nakajima, Rhee, Song et al. 1992). This relationship is also observed in the brain tissue of monkeys (Moriyama 1990), rats (Uda, Tanaka 1990), and humans (Nybo, Secher, Nielson 2002). Therefore, increased local brain temperature resulting from increased neural metabolism can increase local blood flow. This factor may contribute to the blood flow increases that exceed the metabolic activity of brain tissue (Fox, Raichle 1986). As a result, the brain is able to increase blood flow more and in advance of actual metabolic demands ("anticipatory" metabolic activation), thus providing a crucial advantage for successful goal-directed behavior and the organism's adaptation to potential energetic demands. By increasing blood flow above current demand, more potentially dangerous metabolic heat is removed from intensively working brain tissue.

BRAIN TEMPERATURE AS A FACTOR AFFECTING NEURAL FUNCTIONS

Heat release is an obvious "by-product" of metabolic activity, but the changes in brain temperature it triggers may affect various neural processes and functions. While it is generally believed that most physical and chemical processes governing neuronal activity are affected by temperature with the average Van't Hoff coefficient $Q_{10} = 2.3$ (i.e., doubling with $10°C$ change (Swan 1974), experimental evaluations, using in vitro slices, revealed widely varying effects of temperature on passive membrane properties, single spike and spike bursts, as well as on the neuronal responses (i.e., excitatory postsynaptic and inhibitory postsynaptic potentials) induced by electric stimulation of tissue or its afferents (Thompson, Musakawa, Rince 1985; Volgushev, Vidyasagar, Chistiakova et al. 2000; Tryba, Ramirez 2004; Lee, Callaway, Foehring 2005). While confirming that synaptic transmission is more temperature dependent than the generation of action potentials (Katz, Miledi 1965), these studies showed that temperature dependence varies greatly for each parameter, the type of cells under study, and the nature of afferent input involved in mediating neuronal responses.

Although temperature-sensitive neurons were first described in the preoptic/anterior hypothalamus (Berner, Heller 1998; Boulant 2000; Nadel 2003) and were viewed as primary central temperature sensors, cells in many other structures (i.e., visual, motor and somatosensory cortex, hippocampus, medullary brain stem, thalamus) also show dramatic modulation of impulse activity by temperature. Many of these cells, moreover, have a Q_{10} similar to classic warmth-sensitive hypothalamic neurons. In the medial thalamus, for example, 22% of cells show a positive thermal coefficient >0.8 imp/s/°C (Travis, Bockholt, Zardetto-Smith et al. 1995), exceeding the number of temperature-modulated cells found in both anterior (8%) and posterior (11.5%) hypothalamus. About 18% of neurons in the superchiasmatic nucleus are warmth sensitive (Burgoon, Boulant 2001) while >70% of these cells decrease their activity rate with cooling below physiological baseline ($37°C$ to $25°C$) (Ruby, Heller 1996). Finally, electrophysiologically identified substantia nigra dopamine neurons in vitro are found to be highly temperature sensitive (Guatteo, Chung, Bowala et al. 2005). Within the physiological range ($34°C$ to $39°C$), their discharge rate increases with warming ($Q_{10} = 3.7$) and dramatically decreases ($Q_{10} = 8.5$) during cooling below physiological range ($34°C$ to $29°C$).

While the effects on discharge rate and evoked synaptic responses suggest that transmitter release is also strongly temperature dependent, and these data

agree with direct evaluation of stimulated release of different neuroactive substances in vivo (i.e., $Q_{10} = 3.6$ to 5.5 for K^+-induced glutamate release; $Q_{10} = 3.5$ to 6.3 for GABA release, and $Q_{10} = 11.3$ to 37.7 for K^+- and capsaicin-induced release of calcitonin gene-related peptide; Nakashima, Todd 1996; Vizi 1998), these changes in release are compensated for by increased transmitter uptake. For example, within the physiological range ($24°C$ to $40°C$), DA uptake almost doubles with a $3°C$ temperature increase ($Q_{10} = 3.5$ to 5.9 [Xie, McGann, Kim et al. 2000]), a fluctuation easily achieved in the brain under conditions of physiological activation.

The fact that temperature has strong effects on various neural parameters, ranging from the activity of single ionic channels to such integrative processes as transmitter release and uptake, has important implications. First, it suggests that naturally occurring fluctuations in brain temperature affect various parameters of neural activity and neural functions. While in vitro experiments permit individual cells to be studied and individual components of neural activity and synaptic transmission to be separated, neural cells in vivo are interrelated and interdependent. Therefore, their integral changes may be different from those of individual components assessed in in vitro experiments. For example, increased transmitter uptake should compensate for temperature-dependent increase in transmitter release, thus limiting fluctuations in synaptic transmission. By increasing both release and uptake, however, brain hyperthermia makes neurotransmission more efficient and neural functions more effective at reaching behavioral goals. Therefore, changes in temperature may play an important integrative role, involving and uniting numerous central neurons within the brain.

BRAIN HYPERTHERMIA INDUCED BY PSYCHOMOTOR STIMULANT DRUGS: STATE AND ENVIRONMENTAL MODULATION

Most psychotropic (psychoactive) drugs act on various receptor sites in both the brain and periphery to induce their behavioral, physiological, and psychoemotional effects. Most of these drugs affect brain metabolism and heat dissipation in the organism.

Our focus during the last several years was on psychomotor stimulants—METH and MDMA—widely used drugs of abuse. It is estimated that a yearly production of METH and MDMA is at 500 tons, with more than 40 million people using them in the last 12 months (United Nations Office on Drugs and Crime 2003). The prevalence of abuse among youth is higher than that in the general population, and much higher than that for heroin and cocaine. In recent years, abuse continues to spread in terms of geography, age, and income. Although METH is the most popular drug, MDMA has shown the largest increases in abuse in recent years. MDMA is usually used in pill form as part of recreational, leisure activities, thus becoming part of a "normal" lifestyle for certain groups of young people, with more than 1.4 billion tablets consumed annually. METH, in contrast, is typically injected, snorted or smoked, and is associated with heavy abuse, severe psychological problems, and addiction (United Nations Office on Drugs and Crime 2003).

Both METH and MDMA increase metabolism and induce hyperthermia (Sandoval, Hanson, Fleckenstein 2000; Mechan, O'Shea, Elliot et al. 2001; Green, Mechan, Elliott et al. 2003), which is believed to be an important contributor to pathological changes associated with both acute drug intoxication and their chronic abuse (Ali, Newport, Slikker 1996; Davidson, Gow, Lee et al. 2001; Kalant 2001; Schmued 2003). Both METH and MDMA are considered club drugs typically used under conditions of physical and emotional activation and often in a warm and humid environment. While the effects of any drug may be modulated by environmental conditions and specific activity states of the individual, these factors may be especially important for METH and MDMA because, in addition to metabolic activation, they induce peripheral vasoconstriction (Gordon, Watkinson, O'Callaghan et al. 1991; Pederson, Blessing 2001), thus diminishing heat dissipation from the body to the external environment.

To assess how these drugs affect brain temperature and how their effects are modulated by environmental conditions that mimic human use, we examined temperature changes in NAcc, hippocampus, and temporal muscle induced in male rats by METH and MDMA (1 to 9 mg/kg, sc) in quiet resting conditions at normal laboratory temperatures (23°C), during social interaction with a female, and at moderately warm ambient temperatures (29°C) (Brown, Wise, Kiyatkin 2003; Brown, Kiyatkin 2004, 2005).

Both METH and MDMA had dose-dependent hyperthermic effects. As shown in Figure 3.8, both drugs used at the same high dose (9 mg/kg, sc) increased brain and muscle temperatures (A). In both cases, the increases were stronger in brain sites than the muscle, exceeding those following natural arousing stimuli (B; compare with Fig. 3.1). Therefore, intrabrain heat production associated with metabolic brain activation appears to be the primary cause of brain hyperthermia and a factor behind more delayed and weaker body hyperthermia. While hyperthermia is stronger for METH (>3°C) than for MDMA (≈1.4°C), in both cases changes were prolonged, greatly exceeding

those seen following exposure to natural arousing stimuli. While METH induced a rapid increase in temperature immediately after the injection, there was a transient hypothermia after MDMA administration that is consistent with the robust vasoconstrictive effect of this drug (Pederson, Blessing 2001).

Hyperthermic effects of METH and MDMA were strongly dependent on the environmental conditions. As shown in Figure 3.9, the hyperthermic effect of MDMA was stronger and more prolonged when the drug was administered during social interaction with another animal. Even stronger potentiation of MDMA-induced hyperthermia was seen in animals with bilateral occlusion of jugular veins. Although this procedure did not result in evident changes in animal behavior or basal temperature of brain or muscle, drug-induced hyperthermia was about three times stronger and more prolonged than in control. Importantly, under these conditions, MDMA induced robust increases in brain–muscle differentials, greatly exceeding those seen in control. This finding once more suggests a role for metabolic brain activation and intrabrain heat production in the genesis of hyperthermia. Since jugular veins are the primary routs for blood outflow from the brain, potentiation of hyperthermia may result from inability to properly remove metabolic heat from the brain. Finally, the effects of MDMA were greatly potentiated by a slight increase in ambient temperature. Although 29°C is close to normothermy in rats (Romanovsky, Ivanov, Shimansky 2002), mean temperatures after MDMA administration increase rapidly in all animals, resulting in most animals in the clearly pathological values (>41°C to 42°C) and death in five of six animals (Fig. 3.10). Similar changes occur with METH. In this case, four of six tested animals that showed maximal temperature increases (>41°C) died within 3.5 hours after drug administration. In each case, up to the moment of death, brain–muscle differentials were maximal immediately preceding the moment of death and then rapidly inverted, with the brain becoming cooler than the body.

A similar phenomenon of selective brain cooling has been described in patients with brain death (Lyson, Jadeszko, Mariak et al. 2006). Although all temperatures decreased by 2°C to 4°C, the decrease was maximal in the brain, and brain temperature, in fact, was the lowest temperature of the body. Apparently, brain temperature lower than temperature in arterial blood appears to be incompatible with ongoing brain metabolism, and such a temperature profile might be indicative of brain death.

A powerful modulation of drug-induced toxicity by environmental conditions may explain exceptionally strong, sometimes fatal, responses of some individuals to amphetamine-like substances. Although

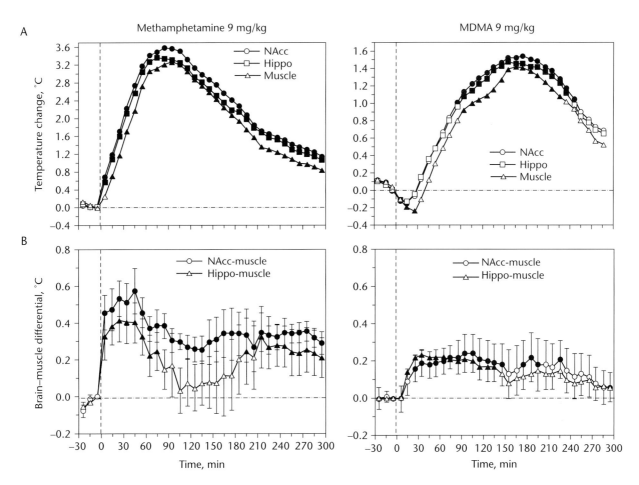

Figure 3.8 Changes in temperature induced by methamphetamine (METH) and MDMA administered at normal laboratory conditions (23°C). In contrast to natural arousing stimuli, both drugs (9 mg/kg) induced strong and prolonged increases in brain and muscle temperature (A) that were accompanied by robust increases in brain–muscle differentials (B). Mean METH-induced temperature increase exceeded 3°C, with some animals showing clearly pathological hyperthermia (>40°C).

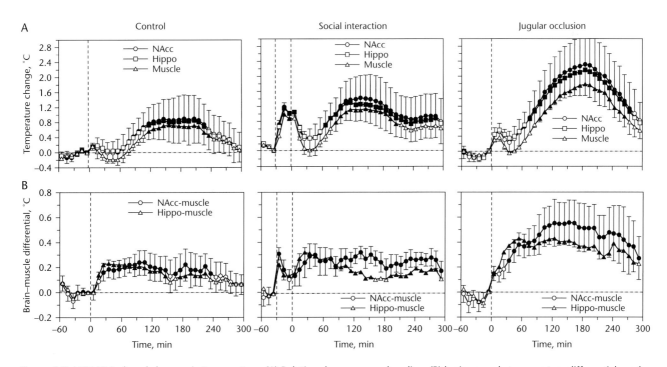

Figure 3.9 MDMA-induced changes in temperature. (A) Relative change versus baseline; (B) brain–muscle temperature differentials under control conditions (left), during social interaction (middle), and in rats with chronically occluded jugular veins (right).

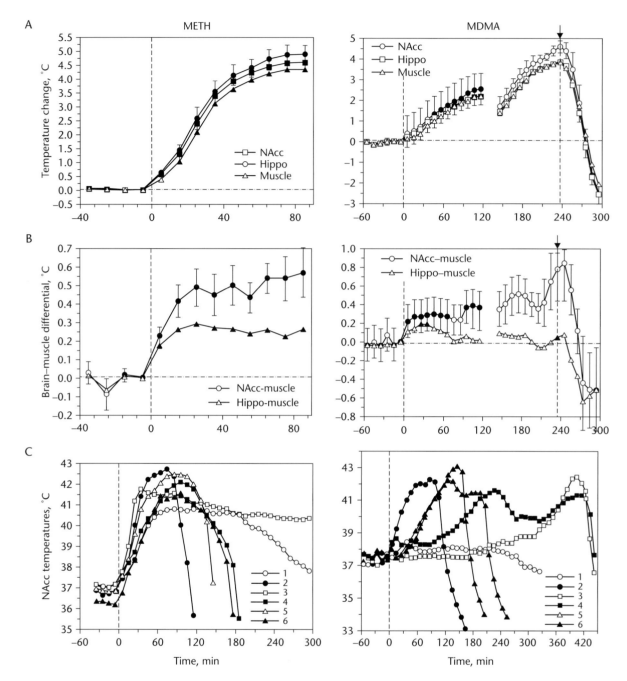

Figure 3.10 Changes in temperature. (A) Relative change vs. baseline and (B) brain–muscle differentials induced by methamphetamine (METH, 9 mg/kg) and MDMA (9 mg/kg) in rats housed at warm ambient temperatures (29°C). In contrast to normal environmental conditions (23°C, see Fig. 3.8), the temperature increase was more rapid and much stronger, resulting in pathological hyperthermia and death in most tested animals. (C) Individual animals.

9 mg/kg of MDMA is a two- threefold larger dose than that typically used by humans, it corresponds to only one-sixth of the LD_{50} in rats (Davis, Hatoum, Walters 1987) and does not result in lethality in normal environmental conditions. The same dose, however, is lethal for most animals in a moderately warm environment. Therefore, one (1.5 mg/kg) or two tablets of MDMA may be highly toxic in predisposed individuals if consumed in adverse environmental conditions.

PATHOLOGICAL BRAIN HYPERTHERMIA AND ITS RELATION TO DAMAGE OF NEURAL STRUCTURE AND FUNCTIONS

High temperature has harmful effects on any cell in the human body, and the brain is the most heat-sensitive organ (Dewhirst, Viglianti, Lora-Michiels et al. 2003). Neural cells tolerate low temperatures (at least to 30°C; Arai, Uto, Ogawa et al. 1993; Lucas,

Emery, Wang et al. 1994), but morphological and functional abnormalities start to occur at $\approx 40°C$, only about $3°C$ above baseline, and increase exponentially with slight increases above these levels (Lepock, Cheng, Al-Qysi et al. 1983; Iwagami 1996; Willis, Jackman, Bizeau et al. 2000; Lepock 2003, 2005).

While it is generally agreed that high temperature negatively affects neural cells, the exact role of this factor is difficult to discern in most in vivo experiments because other factors that may affect neural cells usually exist in most situations associated with brain hyperthermia. For example, multiple abnormalities in neural cells were described during exposure to environmental heat (Kucherenko 1970; Oifa, Kleshchnov 1985; Godlewski et al. 1986; Sharma, Cervos-Navarro, Dey 1991), a situation that is accompanied by gradual increase in body and brain temperature. However, environmental heating results in metabolic activation (oxidative stress), robust changes in systemic and cerebral blood flow, leakage of the BBB, and finally, hypoxia (Lin 1997). Each of these factors, along with high temperature, may contribute to reported neural structural abnormalities. Similar multiple contributions exist in other situations associated with robust brain hyperthermia. METH, which induces robust hyperthermia, is known to induce both acute and chronic morphological abnormalities and death of neural cells (Bowyer, Ali 2006). But, METH also induces metabolic activation (oxidative stress) with increased levels of many potentially neurotoxic substances and alterations in cerebral blood flow.

While in vitro work cannot mimic conditions of the active, fully functional brain, it allows one to exclude other contributions and examine the role of temperature per se in alterations of cellular structure and functions. Cellular abnormalities induced by high temperature were described on different cells studied in slices and cultures. The most common deficit was in mitochondrial structure and functions (Gwozdz, Dyduch, Grzybek et al. 1978; Iwagami 1996; Willis, Emery, Nonner et al. 2003; Du, Di, Wang 2007), implicating this damage in apoptotic cell death, which is common to hyperthermia (White, Emery, Nonner et al. 2003; Ren, Guo, Ye et al. 2006). While all cells were sensitive to hyperthermia, this sensitivity, and thus a harmful effect of hyperthermia, is stronger in metabolically active cells (i.e., cancer cells, epithelial and endothelial cells); the most temperature-sensitive cellular elements are mitochondrial and plasma membranes. Temperature also has direct destructive effects on protein structure, resulting in conformational changes and denaturation of some proteins at temperatures as low as $39.5°C$ to $40.0°C$ (McDuffee, Sensisterra, Huntley et al. 1997; Lepock, Cheng, Al-Qysi et al. 1983; Lepock 2003, 2005).

Although all brain cells are affected by high temperature, destruction of endothelial cells and leakage of serum proteins across the BBB (Sharma, Hoopes 2003) are important factors in determining brain edema, the most dangerous acute complication of pathological brain hyperthermia (Dewhirst, Viglianti, Lora-Michiels et al. 2003; Sharma 2006). Heat-induced damage occurs in different brain structures, but it is stronger within the edematous areas of the brain, suggesting swelling as an important cofactor of heat-induced damage of brain tissue (Sharma, Alm, Westman et al. 1998). Heat-induced brain injury is not limited to the neurons but includes glial cells and cerebral microvessels. In addition to water accumulation in the brain, hyperthermia-related leakage of the BBB results in alterations of ionic environment and travel of some potentially toxic substances (i.e., glutamate) to brain tissue.

Although high temperature and leakage of the BBB may be important for cellular damage, more often they are potentiating factors. An increase in temperature amplifies neural damage induced by experimental hypoxia, ischemia, and cerebral trauma, while hypothermia is generally neuroprotective (Busto, Dietrich, Globus et al. 1987; Maier, Steinberg 2003; Miyazawa, Tamara, Fukui et al. 2003; Olsen, Weber, Kammersgaard 2003). For example, hyperthermia potentiates the cytotoxic effects of reactive oxygen species in vitro (Lin, Quamo, Ho et al. 1991) and glutamate-induced neurotoxicity (Suehiro, Fujisawa, Ito et al. 1999). While prevention of fever and mild hypothermia may be important therapeutic tools to minimize the extent and severity of neural damage associated with these pathological conditions, it is unknown how brain temperature is changed during these conditions.

Although high temperature per se may harm brain cells, it is possible that leakage of the BBB, which appears to occur at high brain temperature, may be an important contributing factor. Although the tight link between hyperthermia and leakage of the BBB has been assumed in studies with environmental warming (Sharma, Cervos-Navarro, Dey 1991) and effects of some "hyperthermic" drugs (i.e., morphine and METH; Bowyer, Ali 2006; Sharma, Ali 2006), the relationships between these parameters were never investigated. This issue is of great importance for medicine because leakage of the BBB is the cause of brain edema, a dangerous pathological condition, which is difficult to treat and often results in lethality.

To investigate this issue, we examined the relationships between brain temperatures and several parameters that characterize the state of the BBB during acute METH intoxication (Kiyatkin, Brown, Sharma 2007). Animals were implanted with chronic thermocouple electrodes and their temperatures were monitored (in brain, muscle, and skin) after METH administration (9 mg/kg) at normal (23°C) and warm (29°C) environmental temperatures. When brain temperature peaked or reached clearly pathological values (>41.5°C), the rat was rapidly anesthetized, perfused, and brains were taken for analysis. The state of BBB permeability and edema were determined by measuring brain water content and levels of several ions (Na⁺, K⁺, and Cl⁻) as well as diffusion of Evans blue dye, an exogenous protein tracer that is normally retained by the BBB, into brain tissue. Immunohistochemistry was used to quantitatively evaluate albumin leakage, a measure of breakdown of the BBB permeability, and glial fibrillary acidic protein (GFAP), an index of astrocytic activation (see Sharma, Ali 2006; Gordh, Chu, Sharma 2006). These parameters were correlated with temperatures recorded immediately before animals were sacrificed.

As shown in Figure 3.11, animals that were administered METH showed significant and robust increases in NAcc temperature (2.3°C and 4.7°C increase vs. control), brain water accumulation (0.6% and 1.1% increase vs. control), brain levels of Evans blue (2.8- and 5-fold increase vs. control), as well as a strong immunoreactivity for albumin and GFAP (36- and 83-fold increases and 5- to 12-fold increases vs. control, respectively). While changes in all brain parameters were significantly different from those in controls, animals that received METH at 29°C and showed larger brain temperature elevation had significantly larger increases in all brain parameters.

While these data suggest that higher brain temperature elevations are associated with stronger leakage of the BBB, these relationships were clarified by correlative analysis (Fig. 3.12). As can be seen, there are exceptionally tight, liner relationships between NAcc temperatures and each brain parameter studied. Coefficient of correlation was 0.95 for brain water, 0.97 for intrabrain diffusion of Evans blue, and 0.97 to 0.98 for immunoreactivity for albumin and GFAP, respectively.

Despite a tight correlation between NAcc temperatures and albumin immunoreactivity during METH intoxication, suggesting that brain hyperthermia may play a role in regulating BBB permeability, it is unclear whether this correlation will hold with brain temperature elevations resulting from other causes. It appears that this correlation stands during environmental warming (Sharma, Zimmer, Westman et al. 1992; Cervos-Navarro, Sharma, Westman et al. 1998) and is strongly dependent on the strength of body hyperthermia as evaluated by rectal measurements. Evans blue staining, albumin immunoreactivity, and an increase in brain water content were intense when body temperature reached clearly pathological levels (>41°C). An increase in BBB permeability was also

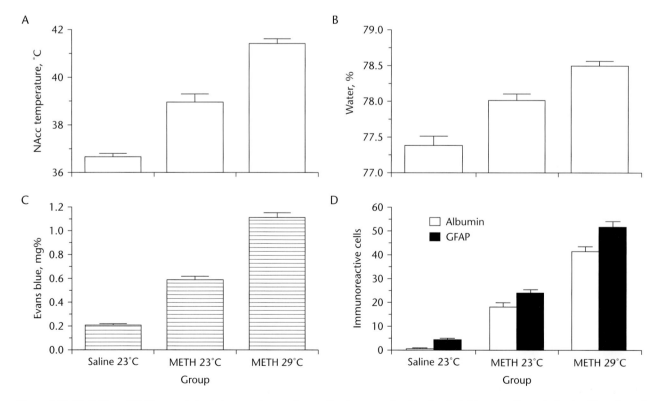

Figure 3.11 (A, B, C, and D) Changes in brain temperature and several brain parameters in rats administered methamphetamine (9 mg/kg, sc) at 23°C and 29°C. Control animals received saline at 23°C. Differences between groups were significant for each individual parameter.

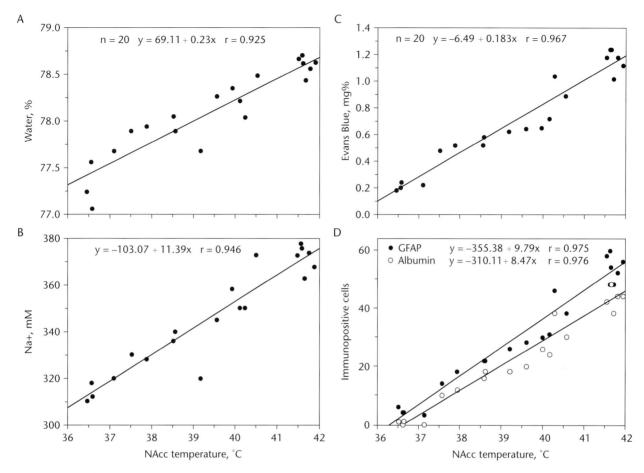

Figure 3.12 Correlative relationships between NAcc temperature and several brain parameters. (A) Brain water, %; (B) Na+, mM; (C) Evans blue concentration, mg%; (D) numbers of albumin- and GFAP-positive cells). All values (4 for control, 8 for METH—23°C, and 8 for METH—29°C, a total n = 20) were accepted for this analysis. Each graph shows regression line, regression equation, and coefficient of correlation.

found in humans during intense physical exercise at warm ambient temperatures (Watson, Shirreffs, Maughan 2005) and during restraint and forced swim stress (Sharma, Dey 1986; Esposito, Cheorghe, Kendere et al. 2001; Ovadia, Abramsky, Feldman et al. 2001), each inducing brain hyperthermia.

Although METH-induced brain temperature increases correlate tightly with several parameters of BBB permeability, it does not mean that high temperature per se is the only cause for these changes. Brain hyperthermia is not only a factor that may directly affect brain cells but is also an integral physiological index of METH-induced metabolic activation, which also manifests as an enhanced release of several neurochemicals, lipid peroxidation and the generation of free radicals, numerous changes combined as oxidative stress (Seiden, Sabol 1996; Kuhn, Geddes 2000; Cadet, Thiriet, Jayanthi 2001), as well as autonomic activation, including a robust increase in arterial blood pressure (Yoshida, Morimoto, Makisumi et al. 1993; Arora, Owens, Gentry 2001). Although all these factors may contribute to changes in BBB permeability, it is quite difficult to separate them from each

other because they are interdependent, representing various manifestations of METH-induced metabolic activation.

It is well known that increased permeability of the BBB and leakage of serum albumin will initiate a series of reactions causing alterations in brain homeostasis as well as neuronal, glial, and myelin function. It appears that BBB disruption is the main cause of vasogenic edema formation, a feature seen in this investigation by measuring water and electrolyte contents. The changes in these parameters were tightly related to brain temperature increase as well as to albumin staining in the brain, suggesting direct relationships between increased permeability of the BBB and brain edema. While brain edema results in increased intracranial pressure, tissue softening, increase in brain volume, and compression of vital centers, thus damaging brain functions, it is also responsible for secondary cell and tissue injury in the brain (Barber, Antonetti, Gardner 2000; Li, Ballinger, Nordal et al. 2001; Li, Chen, Jain et al. 2004; Sharma 2006). While many cellular changes occurring during acute METH intoxication appear to be reversible, some of them may also reflect the initial stages that will later result in irreversible cell damage—the most serious complications of chronic METH use. This issue, however, is secondary to acute METH intoxication, which may result in decompensation of vital functions and an organism's death before any evident death of neural cells. At least several rats administered METH at 29°C would naturally die if the experiment continued. Importantly, this study confirms that pathological brain hyperthermia resulting from METH intoxication under conditions of diminished heat loss results in a robust increase in brain water content (edema), which is tightly related to dramatic leakage of the BBB. Brains of rats that showed >41°C NAcc hyperthermia (6/8) had more than 1.2% higher content of water, 5.5-fold higher concentration of Evans Blue and 88-fold higher albumin immunoreactivity versus controls.

Although glial activation is usually thought to represent a late outcome of traumatic, ischemic, or hypoxic insults or a correlate of various neurodegenerative diseases (Cervos-Navarro, Sharma, Westman et al. 1998; Finch 2003; Hausmann 2003; Gordh, Chu, Sharma 2006), our data suggest that METH induces a robust increase in GFAP immunoreactivity within a surprisingly short period (up to 30 minutes). The levels of GFAP immunoreactivity, moreover, correlated tightly with the levels of albumin immunoreactivity and Evans blue concentrations, brain water, and ion content, as well as with the magnitude of drug-induced brain temperature elevation, but not with the postinjection timing per se. While rapid increase in both GFAP (30 to 60 minutes) and FOS proteins was previously described after injury to the brain and spinal cord (Lindsberg, Frericks, Siren et al. 1996; Cervos-Navarro, Sharma, Westman et al. 1998; Zhao, Ahram, Berman et al. 2003; Gordh, Chu, Sharma 2006; Sharma 2006) as well as during environmental heating (Sharma, Zimmer, Westman et al. 1992; Cervos-Navarro, Sharma, Westman et al. 1998), this study is the first to suggest that increase in GFAP immunoreactivity could be induced in the CNS by METH even within 30 to 40 minutes after drug administration. Therefore, the intensity of brain hyperthermia may play a crucial role in increased GFAP immunoreactivity. Rats administered METH at 29°C that showed robust brain hyperthermia had GFAP levels more than twice those in animals administered this drug at 23°C. The levels of GFAP in individual rats, moreover, were tightly correlated with brain temperature ($r = 0.975$) and the mean value of GFAP-positive cells in six of eight rats with pathological hyperthermia (>41°C) was ≈13-fold higher than in control.

This rapid and strong increase in GFAP immunoreactivity appears to be inconsistent with what is known about slow expression of this cytoskeleton protein (Norton, Aquino, Hozumi et al. 1992; O'Callaghan 1993; Miller, O'Callaghan 2003) and previous data suggesting later changes in expression of this protein after a series of METH injections (4 ×10 mg/kg each 2 hours) in mice (Miller, O'Callaghan 1994; O'Callaghan, Miller 1994). In this case, GFAP levels increased at 12 to 24 hours, peaked at the second day, and remained elevated for 7 days after a single series of METH exposure. These changes, moreover, were evident only in the striatum and to a lesser degree in the cortex, correlating with decreased dopamine levels in these areas. In contrast to our study, in which GFAP levels were increased at the peak of brain hyperthermia and related to robust leakage of the BBB, it is reasonable to assume that at these later intervals (several days) all subjects had temperatures and permeability of the BBB restored to normal or near-normal levels.

Since GFAP levels tightly correlate with brain temperature and albumin immunoreactivity, a strong GFAP immunoreactivity may reflect the interaction of antibodies with GFAP somehow released or made available during cellular damage. Thus, binding sites to GFAP antigens could be increased because of acute breakdown of the BBB rather than because of proliferation of astrocytes or elevated levels of GFAP proteins that require more time. This reaction could also be related to acute, possibly reversible, damage of glial cells. Damage of astrocytes and swelling of astrocytic end feet is known to increase binding of GFAP antibodies (Bekay, Lee, Lee et al. 1977; Bondarenko, Chesler 2001; Gordh, Chu, Sharma 2006). Therefore, rapid increase in GFAP immunoreactivity that occurs at peak brain temperatures and tightly correlates with robust leakage of the BBB may reflect acute abnormalities of astrocytes rather than classic astrocytic activation or astrogliosis. While this hypothesis needs to be verified morphologically, our preliminary data suggest that acute METH intoxication in fact results in multiple cellular abnormalities, especially evident in brain areas with the most pronounced changes in BBB permeability and edema (i.e., cortex, hippocampus, some areas of thalamus and hypothalamus). Although high temperature may have destructive effects on different cells (Iwagami 1996; Willis, Jackman, Bizeau et al. 2000; Du, Di, Wang 2007), multiple evidence suggests that hyperthermia-induced abnormalities might be stronger in metabolically active brain cells (Oifa, Kleshchnov 1985; Lin, Quamo, Ho et al. 1991; Lin 1997; Lee, Lee, Akuta et al. 2000; Chen, Xu, Huang et al. 2003), including glia, endothelial, and epithelial cells (Bechtold, Brown 2003; Sharma, Hoopes 2003)—the primary components of the blood–brain and blood–CSF barriers, respectively. Our preliminary data suggesting extensive cellular damage within the *plexus chorioideus* in animals showing pathological

(>41°C) brain hyperthermia during METH intoxication appears to be consistent with this view.

Therefore, although robust brain hyperthermia might have direct destructive effects on neural cells, it appears that these effects are further enhanced by the breakdown of the BBB and development of vasogenic brain edema, thus allowing numerous factors, including many blood-borne ions, neurotransmitters (i.e., glutamate, the levels of which are much higher in plasma than in CSF), and metabolic substances to enter the brain microenvironment. All these factors, alone and in combination, will further potentiate brain damage. These peripheral factors and associated alteration of the CNS microenvironment could play an important role in acute damage of brain cells following drug intoxication. While most of these changes appear to be reversible, they may contribute to neurotoxicity following chronic drug use. Because astrocytes are critical for maintaining normal functions of neurons and endothelial cells, acute astrocytic reaction may be a valuable early indicator of potential future brain pathology caused by METH.

CONCLUSIONS: NEUROBIOLOGICAL AND HUMAN IMPLICATIONS

While the brain plays an essential role in sensing fluctuations in environmental temperature and altering heat production and loss, it is unclear whether the idea of temperature regulation can be applied to the brain itself. This chapter suggests that brain temperature of the rat fluctuates within 3°C under physiological conditions. It is not known yet whether these fluctuations occur in the human brain but, based on similarities found between rats and monkeys (Hayward, Baker 1968), it appears likely.

Although recording of brain temperature in humans is possible only in patients, available data suggest that this temperature is consistently higher than in the body core (Mellergard, Nordstrom 1990; Mariak, Lewko, Luczaj et al. 1994; Mariak, Jadeszko, Lewko et al. 1998; Rumana, Gopinath, Uzura et al. 1998; Mariak, Lebkowski, Lyson et al. 1999; Mariak, Lyson, Peikarski et al. 2000; Mcilvoy 2004). These data also suggest the existence of a dorsoventral temperature gradient, with ventrally located structures being warmer than dorsally located structures. The degree of this gradient, however, varies depending on the functional state of the individual and technical aspects of temperature recording. This work also suggests that the human brain has no specific cooling mechanism (Bringelmann 1993 vs. Cabanac 1993 for an alternative point of view) and brain temperature always remains higher than that of arterial blood inflow during physiological conditions.

This chapter suggests that physiological brain hyperthermia is a part of normal brain functioning rather than an index of disease. Since arterial blood is cooler than brain tissue, metabolic neural activation, accompanied by intrabrain heat production, may be viewed as the primary cause of physiological brain hyperthermia. Cerebral blood flow, therefore, not only provides oxygen and nutrients for enhanced brain metabolism but also removes potentially dangerous metabolic heat from neural tissue. While brain heat production is an obvious by-product of cerebral metabolism, physiological fluctuations in brain temperature affect various neural parameters ranging from the activity of single ionic channels to transmitter release and uptake. Thus, brain hyperthermia may have adaptive significance, changing the dynamics of neural functions and making them more efficient for reaching behavioral goals. Brain hyperthermia may also result from impaired heat dissipation during intense physical activity in a hot, humid environment. While temperature in arterial blood remains cooler than in brain tissue under these conditions, heat is accumulated in the brain because of progressive body warming due to an inability to dissipate metabolic heat to the external environment. While this deficit remains compensated under quiet resting conditions, it may result in dramatic changes in temperature responses following exposure to various activating stimuli and pharmacological drugs.

Brain hyperthermia may also be induced by various addictive drugs, which increase brain metabolism and impair heat dissipation. Such frequently used psychomotor stimulants as METH and MDMA induce dose-dependent brain hyperthermia, which is enhanced during physiological activation and under conditions that restrict heat dissipation. Because high temperature exacerbates drug-induced toxicity and is destructive to neural cells and brain functions, pathological brain hyperthermia (>40°C) is an important contributor to both acute life-threatening complications and chronic destructive CNS changes induced by psychomotor stimulants. Although humans have more effective mechanisms for heat dissipation than rats, this drug–activity–environment interaction is important for understanding potential health hazards of these drugs of abuse, which are typically taken during high-energy activity in a hot, humid environment that prevents heat dissipation from the brain and body.

Brain hyperthermia may develop during several pathological conditions (heatstroke, head trauma, ischemic and necrotic damage), which are accompanied by neural cell damage, inflammation, and impairment of venous blood outflow from the brain, even under conditions of decreased brain metabolism and relatively normal body temperatures. These abnormalities in brain–body temperature homeostasis make these patients especially sensitive to fever and environmental overheating, both of which dramatically increase the extent of neural damage and mortality.

This chapter also indicates that monitoring of brain temperatures in animals is a valuable tool for assessment of alterations in metabolic neural activity induced by environmental stimuli or drugs and occurring during the development and performance of motivated behaviors. Although heat production is a basic feature of neural metabolism, locally released metabolic heat is continuously redistributed within brain tissue and affected by a variable inflow of cooler arterial blood, determining a similar pattern of temperature fluctuations in different brain structures. Rapid time-course temperature monitoring and determining temperature gradients between brain structures and body, muscle, or arterial blood allow one to discern between-structure differences and peaks of neural activation. Brain temperature fluctuation, however, is a different reflection of neural activity than a change in neuronal electrical discharges. While the relationships between these parameters remain unclear and need to be clarified in the future, similar to neuronal discharges, brain temperatures are affected by various salient sensory stimuli and drugs, show consistent changes during learning, and fluctuate during motivated behavior, tightly correlating with key behavioral events.

ACKNOWLEDGMENTS   I would like to thank Paul Leon Brown and David Bae for valuable comments regarding this manuscript. This research was supported by the Intramural Research Program of the NIH, NIDA.

REFERENCES

Abrams R, Hammel HT. 1964. Hypothalamic temperature in unanesthetized albino rats during feeding and sleeping. *Am J Physiol.* 206:641–646.

Ali SF, Newport GD, Slikker W. 1996. Methamphetamine-induced dopaminergic toxicity in mice: role of environmental temperature and pharmacological agents. *Ann N.Y Acad Sci.* 801:187–198.

Altschule MD. 1951. Emotion and circulation. *Circulation.* 3:444–454.

Amidon RM. 1880. Cerebral temperature. *Am J Insanity.* 37:111–112.

Arai H, Uto A, Ogawa Y, Sato K. 1993. Effect of low temperature on glutamate-induced intracellular calcium accumulation and cell death in cultured hippocampal neurons. *Neurosci Lett.* 163:132–134.

Arora H, Owens SM, Gentry WB. 2001. Intravenous (+)-methamphetamine causes complex dose-dependent physiological changes in awake rats. *Eur J Pharmacol.* 426:B1–B7.

Baker M, Cronin M, Mountjoy D. 1976. Variability of skin temperature in the waking monkey. *Am J Physiol.* 230:449–455.

Barber AJ, Antonetti DA, Gardner TW. 2000. Altered expression of retinal occluding and glial fibrillary acidic protein in experimental diabetes. *Invest Ophthalmol Vis Sci.* 41:3561–3568.

Bechtold DA, Brown IR. 2003. Induction of Hsp27 and Hsp32 stress proteins and vimentin in glial cells of the rat hippocampus following hyperthermia. *Neurochem Res.* 28:1163–1173.

Bekay L, Lee JC, Lee GC, Peng GR. 1977. Experimental cerebral concussion: an electron microscopic study. *J Neurosurg.* 47:525–531.

Berner NJ, Heller HC. 1998. Does the preoptic anterior hypothalamus receive thermoafferent information? *Am J Physiol.* 274:R9–R18.

Bohlen JG, Held JP, Sanderson MO, Patterson RP. 1984. Heart rate, rate-pressure product and oxygen uptake during four sexual activities. *Arch Intern Med.* 144:1745–1748.

Bondarenko A, Chesler M. 2001. Rapid astrocyte death induced by transient hypoxia, acidosis, and extracellular ion shifts. *Glia.* 34:134–142.

Boulant JA. 2000. The role of preoptic-anterior hypothalamus in thermoregulation and fever. *Clin Infect Dis.* 31(Suppl 5):S157–S161.

Bowyer JF, Ali S. 2006. High doses of methamphetamine that cause disruption of the blood–brain barrier in limbic regions produce extensive neuronal degeneration in mouse hippocampus. *Synapse.* 60:521–532.

Brengelmann GL. 1993. Specialized brain cooling in humans? *FASEB J.* 7:1148–1153.

Brown PL, Wise RA, Kiyatkin EA. 2003. Brain hyperthermia is induced by methamphetamine and exacerbated by social interaction. *J Neurosci.* 23:3924–3929.

Brown PL, Kiyatkin EA. 2004. Brain hyperthermia induced by MDMA ("ecstasy"): modulation by environmental conditions. *Eur J Neurosci.* 20:51–58.

Brown PL, Kiyatkin EA. 2005. Fatal intra-brain heat accumulation induced by meth-amphetamine at normothermic conditions in rats. *Int J Neurodegener Neuroregener* 1:86–90.

Burgoon PW, Boulant JA. 2001. Temperature-sensitive properties of rat suprachiasmatic nucleus neurons. *Am J Physiol.* 281:R706–R715.

Busto R, Dietrich WD, Globus MYT, Valdes I, Scheinberg R, Ginsberg MD. 1987. Small differences in intraischemic brain temperature critically determine the extent of ischemic neuronal injury. *J Cer Blood Flow Metab.* 7:729–738.

Cabanac M. 1993. Selective brain cooling in humans: "fancy" or fact? *FASEB J.* 7:1143–1147.

Cadet JL, Thiriet N, Jayanthi S. 2001. Involvement of free radicals in MDMA-induced neurotoxicity in mice. *Ann. Intern Med.* 152(Suppl 3):IS57–IS59.

Cervos-Navarro J, Sharma HS, Westman J, Bongcum-Rudloff E. 1998. Glial cell reactions in the central nervous system following heat stress. *Progr Brain Res.* 115:241–274.

Charkoudian N. 2003. Skin blood flow in adult human thermoregulation: how it works, when it does not, and why? *Mayo Clin Proc.* 78:603–612.

Chen YZ, Xu RX, Huang QJ, Xu ZJ, Jiang XD, Cai YO. 2003. Effect of hyperthermia on tight junctions between endothelial cells of the blood–brain barrier model in vitro. *Di Yi Jun Da Xue Xue Bao.* 23:21–24.

Cheuvront SN, Haymes EM. 2001. Thermoregulation and marathon running: biological and environmental influences. *Sports Med.* 31:743–762.

Crane P, Braun L, Cornford E, Cremer J, Glass J, Oldendorf M. 1978. Dose-dependent reduction of glucose utilization by pentobarbital in rat brain. *Stroke.* 9:12–18.

Davidson C, Gow AJ, Lee TH, Ellinwood EH. 2001. Methamphetamine neurotoxicity: necrotic and apoptotic mechanisms and relevance to human abuse and treatment. *Brain Res Rev.* 36:1–22.

Davis WM, Hatoum HT, Walters IW. 1987. Toxicity of MDA (2,4-methylenedioxyamphetamine) considered for relevance to hazards of MDMA (Ecstasy) abuse. *Alcohol Drug Res.* 7:123–134.

Delgado JMR, Hanai T. 1966. Intracerebral temperatures in free-moving cats. *Am J Physiol.* 211:755–769.

Dewhirst MW, Viglianti BL, Lora-Michiels M, Hanson M, Hoopes PJ. 2003. Basic principles of thermal dosimetry and thermal thresholds for tissue damage from hyperthermia. *Int J Hyperthermia.* 19:267–294.

Du J, Di HS, Wang GL. 2007. Establishment of a bovine mammary cell line and its ultrastructural changes when exposed to heat stress. *Sheng Wu Gong Cheng Xue Bao.* 23:471–476.

Eardley I. 2005. The hemodynamics of sex. *Heat Metabol.* 28:1–3.

Erikson K, Lanier W. 2003. Anesthetic technique influences brain temperature, independently of core temperature, during craniotomy in cats. *Anesth Analg.* 96:1460–1466.

Esposito P, Cheorghe D, Kendere K et al. 2001. Acute stress increases permeability of the blood–brain barrier through activation of brain must cells. *Brain Res.* 888:117–127.

Feitelberg S, Lampl H. 1935. Warmetonung der Grosshirnrinde bei Erregung und Ruhe. Functionshemmung. *Arch. Exp Path Pharmak.* 177:726–736 (in German).

Finch CE. 2003. Neurons, glia, and plasticity in normal brain aging. *Neurobiol Aging.* 24(Suppl 1):S123–127.

Fox RT, Raichle ME. 1986. Focal physiological uncoupling of cerebral blood flow and oxidative metabolism during somatosensory stimulation in human subjects. *Proc Natl Acad Sci U S A.* 83:1140–1144.

Godlewski A, Wygladalska-Jernas H, Szczech J. 1986. Effect of hyperthermia on morphology and histochemistry of spinal cord in the rat. *Folia Histochem Cytobiol.* 24:53–63.

Goldfarg AN. 1970. Energy cost of sexual activity. *Arch Intern Med.* 126:526.

Gordh T, Chu H, Sharma HS. 2006. Spinal nerve lesion alters blood–spinal cord barrier function and activates astrocytes in the rat. *Pain.* 124:211–221.

Gordon CJ, Heath JE. 1986. Integration and central processing in temperature regulation. *Ann Rev Physiol.* 48:595–612.

Gordon CJ, Watkinson WO, O'Callaghan JP, Miller DB. 1991. Effects of 3,4-methylenedioxymethamphetamine on autonomic thermoregulatory responses of the rat. *Pharmacol Biochem Behav.* 38:339–344.

Green AR, Mechan AO, Elliott JM, O'Shea E, Colado MI. 2003. The pharmacology and clinical pharmacology of 3,4-methylenedioxymethamphetamine (MDMA, "Ecstasy"). *Pharmacol Rev.* 55:463–508.

Guatteo E, Chung KK, Bowala TK, Bernardi G, Mercuri ND, Lipski J. 2005. Temperature sensitivity of dopaminergic neurons of the substantia nigra pars compacta: involvement of transient receptor potential channels. *J Neurophysiol.* 94:3069–3080.

Gwozdz B, Dyduch A, Grzybek H, Panz B. 1978. Structural changes in brain mitochodria of mice subjected to hyperthermia. *Exp Pathol. (Jena)* 15:124–126.

Hausmann ON. 2003. Post-traumatic inflammation following spinal cord injury. *Spinal Cord.* 41:369–78.

Hayward JN, Baker MA. 1968. Role of cerebral arterial blood in the regulation of brain temperature in the monkey. *Am J Physiol.* 215:389–403.

Hodgkin AL. 1967. *The Conduction of the Nervous Impulse.* Liverpool Univ. Press: Liverpool.

Ide K, Secher NH. 2000. Cerebral blood flow and metabolism during exercise. *Prog Neurobiol.* 61:397–414.

Ide K, Schmalbruch IK, Quistorff B, Horn A, Secher NH. 2000. Lactate, glucose, and oxygen uptake in human brain during recovery from maximal exercise. *J Physiol.* 522:159–164.

Iwagami Y. 1996. Changes in ultrastructure of human cell related to certain biological responses under hyperthermic culture condition. *Hum Cell.* 9:353–366.

James W. 1892. *Psychology Briefer Course.* Henry Holt: New York.

Kalant H. 2001. The pharmacology and toxicology of "ecstasy" (MDMA) and related drugs. *Can Med Assoc J.* 165:917–928.

Katz B, Miledi R. 1965. The effect of temperature on the synaptic delay at the neuromuscular junction. *J Physiol.* 181:656–670.

Kiyatkin EA. 2005. Brain hyperthermia as physiological and pathological phenomena. *Brain Res Rev.* 50:27–56.

Kiyatkin EA, Brown PL, Wise RA. 2002. Brain temperature fluctuation: a reflection of functional neural activation. *Eur J Neurosci.* 16:164–168.

Kiyatkin EA, Mitchum R. 2003. Fluctuations in brain temperatures during sexual behavior in male rats: an approach for evaluating neural activity underlying motivated behavior. *Neuroscience.* 119:1169–1183.

Kiyatkin EA, Brown PL. 2005. Brain and body temperature homeostasis during sodium pentobarbital anesthesia with and without body warming in rats. *Physiol Behav.* 84:563–570.

Kiyatkin EA, Brown PL, Sharma HS. 2007. Brain edema and breakdown of the blood–brain barrier during methamphetamine intoxication: critical role of brain temperature. *Eur J Neurosci.* 26:1242–1253.

Kovalzon VM. 1972. Brain temperature variations during natural sleep and arousal in white rats. *Physiol Behav.* 10:667–670.

Kucherenko RP. 1970. Submicroscopic changes in Purkinje cells of the cerebellum under the effects of hyperthermia. *Tsitologiia* (in Russian). 12:312–316.

Kuhn DM, Geddes TJ. 2000. Molecular footprints of neurotoxic amphetamine action. *Ann N.Y Acad Sci.* 914:92–103.

Laughlin SB, de Ruyter van Steveninck RR, Anderson JC. 1998. The metabolic cost of neural information. *Nat Neurosci.* 1:36–41.

Lee JCF, Callaway JC, Foehring RC. 2005. The effects of temperature on calcium transients and Ca^{2+}-dependent afterhyperpolarizations in neocortical pyramidal neurons. *J Physiol.* 93:2012–2020.

Lee SY, Lee SH, Akuta K, Uda M, Song CW. 2000. Acute histological effects of interstitial hyperthermia on normal rat brain. *Int J Hyperthermia.* 16:73–83.

Lepock JR. 2003. Cellular effects of hyperthermia: relevance to the minimum dose for thermal damage. *Int J Hyperthermia.* 19:252–266.

Lepock JR. 2005. How do cells respond to their thermal environment. *Int J Hyperthermia.* 21:681–687.

Lepock JR, Cheng K-H, Al-Qysi H, Kruuv J. 1983. Thermotropic lipid and protein transitions in Chinese hamster lung cell membranes: relationship to hyperthermic cell killing. *Can J Biochem Cell Biol.* 61:421–427.

Li Y-Q, Ballinger JR, Nordal RA, Su Z-H, Wong CS. 2001. Hypoxia in radiation-induced blood–spinal cord barrier breakdown. *Cancer Res.* 61:3348–3354.

Li Y-Q, Chen P, Jain V, Reilly RM, Wong CS. 2004. Early radiation-induced endothelial cell loss and blood–spinal cord barrier breakdown in the rat spinal cord. *Radiat Res.* 161:143–152.

Lin PS, Quamo S, Ho KC, Gladding J. 1991. Hyperthermia enhances the cytotoxic effects of reactive oxygen species to Chinese hamster cells and bovine endothelial cells in vitro. *Radiat Med.* 126:43–51.

Lin M-T. 1997. Heatstroke-induced cerebral ischemia and neuronal damage. Involvement of cytokines and monoamines. *Ann N.Y Acad Sci.* 813:572–580.

Lindsberg PJ, Frericks KU, Siren AL, Hallenbeck JM, Nowak TS. 1996. Heat shock protein and C-fos expression in focal microvascular brain damage. *J Cereb Blood Flow Metab.* 16:82–91.

Lombard JS. 1879. *Experimental Researches on the Regional Temperatures of the Head under Conditions of Rest, Intellectual Activity and Emotion.* London: H.K. Lewis.

Lucas JH, Emery DG, Wang G, Rosenberg-Schaffer LJ, Jordan RS, Gross GW. 1994. In vitro investigation of the effect of nonfreezing low temperatures on lesioned and uninjured mammalian spinal neurons. *J Neurotrauma.* 11:35–61.

Lyson T, Jadeszko M, Mariak Z, Kochanowicz J, Lewko J. 2006. Intracerebrain temperature measurements in brain death *Neurol Neurosurg.* Pol 40:269–275.

Maier CM, Steinberg GK. 2003. *Hypothermia and Cerebral Ischemia.* Humana Press: New York.

Margaria R, Cretelli P, Aghemo P, Sassi G. 1963. Energy cost of running. *J Appl Physiol.* 18:367–370.

Mariak Z, Lewko J, Luczaj J, Polocki B, White MD. 1994. The relationship between directly measured human cerebral and tympanic temperatures during changes in brain temperature. *Eur J Appl Physiol Occup Physiol.* 69:545–549.

Mariak Z, Jadeszko M, Lewko J, Lebkowski W, Lyson T. 1998. No specific brain protection against thermal stress in fever. *Acta Neurochir (Wien).* 140:585–590.

Mariak Z, Lebkowski W, Lyson T, Lewko J, Piekarski P. 1999. Brain temperature during craniotomy in general anesthesia. *Neurol Neurochir.* Pol 33:1325–1327.

Mariak Z, Lyson T, Peikarski P, Lewko J, Jadeszko M, Szydlik P. 2000. Brain temperature in patients with central nervous system lesions. *Neurol Neurosurg.* Pol 34:509–522.

Masters WH, Johnson VE. 1966. *Human Sexual Response.* Little, Brown and Co.: Boston.

McDuffee AT, Sensisterra G, Huntley S et al. 1997. Protein containing non-native disulfide bonds generated by oxidative stress can act as signals for the induction if heat shock response. *J Cell Physiol.* 171:143–151.

McElligott JC, Melzack R. 1967. Localized thermal changes evoked in the brain by visual and auditory stimulation. *Exp Neurol.* 17:293–312.

Mcilvoy L. 2004. Comparison of brain temperature to core temperature: a review of the literature. *J Neurosci Nurs.* 36:23–31.

Mechan AO, O'Shea E, Elliot JM, Colado MI, Green AR. 2001. A neurotoxic dose of 3,4-methylenedioxymethamphetamine (MDMA; ecstasy) to rats results in a long-term deficit in thermoregulation. *Psychopharmacology.* 155:413–418.

Mellergard P, Nordstrom CH. 1990. Epidural temperatures and possible intracerebral temperature gradients in man. *Br J Neurosurg.* 4:31–38.

Michenfelder J. 1988. *Anesthesia and the Brain: Clinical, Functional and Vascular Correlates.* New York: Churchill Livingstone.

Miller DB, O'Callaghan JP. 1994. Environment-, drug- and stress-induced alterations in body temperature affect the neurotoxicity of substituted amphetamines in the C57BL/6J mouse. *J Pharmacol Exp Ther.* 270:752–760.

Miller DB, O'Callaghan JP. 2003. Elevated environmental temperature and methamphetamine neurotoxicity. *Environ Res.* 92:48–53.

Mitchum R, Kiyatkin EA. 2004. Brain hyperthermia and temperature fluctuations during sexual interaction in female rats. *Brain Res.* 1000:110–122.

Miyazawa T, Tamara A, Fukui S, Hossmann KA. 2003. Effects of mild hypothermia on focal cerebral ischemia: review of experimental studies. *Neurol Res.* 25:457–464.

Moriyama E. 1990. Cerebral blood flow changes during localized hyperthermia. *Neurol Med Chir. (Tokyo)* 30:923–929.

Moser E, Mathiesen I, Andersen P. 1993. Association between brain temperature and dentate field potentials in exploring and swimming rats. *Science.* 259:1324–1326.

Nadel E. 2003. Regulation of body temperature. In Boron WF, Boulpaep EL, eds. *Medical Physiology* Philadelphia: Saunders, 1231–1241.

Nagata Y, Katayama K, Manivel CJ, Song CW. 2000. Changes in blood flow in locally heated intestine of rats. *Int J Hyperthermia.* 16:159–170.

Nakajima T, Rhee JG, Song CW, Onoyama Y. 1992. Effect of a second heating on rat liver blood flow. *Int J Hyperthermia.* 8:679–687.

Nakashima K, Todd MM. 1996. Effects of hypothermia on the rate of excitatory amino acid release after ischemic depolarization. *Stroke*. 27:913–918.

Norton WT, Aquino DA, Hozumi I, Chiu F-C, Brosnan CF. 1992. Quantitative aspects of reactive gliosis: a review *Neurochem Res*. 17:877–885.

Nybo L, Secher NH, Nielson B. 2002. Inadequate heat release from the human brain during prolonged exercise with hyperthermia. *J Physiol*. 545:697–704.

O'Callaghan JP. 1993. Quantitative features of reactive gliosis following toxicant-induced damage of the CNS *Ann N.Y Acad Sci*. 679:195–210.

O'Callaghan JP, Miller DB. 1994. Neurotoxicity profiles of substituted amphetamines in the C57BL/6J mouse. *J Pharmacol Exp Ther*. 270:741–751.

Oifa AI, Kleshchnov VN. 1985. Ultrastructural analysis of the phenomenon of acute neronal swelling. *Zh Nevropatol Psikhiatr Im S.S Korsakova*. 85:1016–1020.

Olsen TS, Weber UJ, Kammersgaard LP. 2003. Therapeutic hypothermia for acute stroke. *Lancet Neurol*. 2:410–416.

Oobu K. 1993. Experimental studies on the effect of heating on blood flow in the tongue of golden hamsters *Fukuoka Igaku Zasshi*. 84:497–511.

Ovadia H, Abramsky O, Feldman S, Weidenfeld J. 2001. Evaluation of the effects of stress on the blood–brain barrier: critical role of the brain perfusion time. *Brain Res*. 905:21–25.

Pederson NP, Blessing WW. 2001. Cutaneous vasoconstriction contributes to hyperthermia induced by 3,4-methylenedioxymethamphetamine (ecstasy) on conscious rabbits. *J Neurosci*. 21:8648–8654.

Raichle ME. 2003. Functional brain imaging and human brain functions. *J Neurosci*. 23:3959–3962.

Ren GX, Guo W, Ye DX et al. 2006. A study on the mechanism of inducing apoptosis of Tca8113 cells by means of ultrasound hyperthermia. *Shanghai Kou Oiang Yi Xue*. 15:507–511.

Ritchie JM. 1973. Energetic aspects of nerve conduction: the relationships between heat production, electrical activity and metabolism. *Progr Biophys Mol Biol*. 26:147–187.

Romanovsky AA, Ivanov AI, Shimansky YP. 2002. Ambient temperature for experiments in rats: a new method for determining the zone of thermal neutrality. *J Appl Physiol*. 92:2667–2679.

Rosomoff HL. 1957. Hypothermia and cerebral vascular lesions. II. Experimental interruption followed by induction of hypothermia. *Arch Neurol Psych*. 78:454–464.

Rowell LB. 1983. Cardiovascular aspects of human thermoregulation. *Circ Res*. 52:367–376.

Ruby NF, Heller HC. 1996. Temperature sensitivity of the suprachiasmatic nucleus of ground squirrels and rats in vitro. *J Biol Rhythms*. 11:126–136.

Rumana CS, Gopinath SP, Uzura M, Valadka AB, Robertson CS. 1998. Brain temperatures exceeds systemic temperatures in head-injured patients. *Clin Care Med*. 26:562–567.

Ryan KL, Taylor WF, Bishop VS. 1997. Arterial baroreflex modulation of heat-induced vasodilation in the rabbit ear. *J Appl Physiol*. 83:2091–2097.

Sandoval V, Hanson GR, Fleckenstein AE. 2000. Methamphetamine decreases mouse striatal dopamine transporter activity: roles of hyperthermia and dopamine. *Eur J Pharmacol*. 409:265–271.

Satinoff E. 1978. Neural organization and evolution of thermal regulation in mammals. *Science*. 201:16–22.

Schaefer CF. 1979. Possible teratogenic hyperthermia and marathon running. *JAMA*. 241:1892.

Schiff M. 1870. *Archives de Physiologie*, t. iii, p. 6.

Schiff M. 1894–1898. *Gesammelte Beitrage zur Physiologie*. Lausanne.

Schmidt-Nielsen K. 1997. *Animal Physiology Adaptation and Environment*. 5th edition, Cambridge Univ. Press: Cambridge.

Schmued LC. 2003. Demonstration and localization of neuronal degeneration in the rat forebrain following a single exposure to MDMA. *Brain Res*. 974:127–133.

Seiden LS, Sabol KE. 1996. Methamphetamine and methylenedioxymethamphetamine neurotoxicity: possible mechanisms of cell destruction *NIDA Res Monogr*. 163:251–276.

Serota HM. 1939. Temperature changes in the cortex and hypothalamus during sleep *J Neurophysiol*. 2:42–47.

Serota HM, Gerard RW. 1938. Localized thermal changes in cat's brain. *J Neurophysiol*. 1:115–124.

Sharma HS. 2006. Hyperthermia-induced brain edema: current status and future perspectives. *Indian J Med Res*. 123:629–652.

Sharma HS, Dey PK. 1986. Influence of long-term immobilization stress on regional blood–brain permeability, cerebral blood flow and 5-HT levels in conscious normotensive young rats. *J Neurol Sci*. 72:61–76.

Sharma HS, Cervos-Navarro J, Dey PK. 1991. Acute heat exposure causes cellular alterations in cerebral cortex of young rats. *Neuroreport*. 2:155–158.

Sharma HS, Zimmer C, Westman J, Cervos-Navarro J. 1992. Acute systemic heat stress increases glial fibrillary acidic protein immunoreactivity in brain. An experimental study in the conscious normotensive young rats. *Neuroscience*. 48:889–901.

Sharma HS, Alm P, Westman J. 1998. Nitric oxide and carbon monoxide in the pathophysiology of brain functions in heat stress. *Prog Brain Res*. 115:297–333.

Sharma HS, Hoopes PJ. 2003. Hyperthermia-induced pathophysiology of the central nervous system. *Int. J Hyperthermia*. 19:325–354.

Sharma HS, Ali SF. 2006. Alterations in blood–brain barrier function by morphine and methamphetamine. *Ann N.Y Acad Sci*. 1074:198–224.

Shulman RG, Rothman DL, Behar KL, Hyder F. 2004. Energetic basis of brain activity: implications for neuroimaging. *Trends Neurosci*. 27:489–495.

Siesjo B 1978 *Brain Energy Metabolism*. Wiley: New York.

Sokoloff L. 1999. Energetics of functional activation in neural tissues. *Neurochem Res*. 24:321–329.

Solomon GF, Moos RH, Stone GC, Fessel WJ. 1964. Peripheral vasoconstriction induced by emotional stress in rats. *Angiology*. 15:362–365.

Stein RA. (2002). Managing concomitant cardiac disease and erectile dysfunction. *Rev Urol*. 4(Suppl 3):S39–S47.

Suehiro E, Fujisawa H, Ito H, Ishikawa T, Maekawa T. 1999. Brain temperature modifies glutamate neurotoxicity in vivo. *J Neurotrauma*. 16:285–297.

Sukstanskii AL, Yablonskiy DA. 2006. Theoretical model of temperature regulation in the brain during changes in functional activity. *Proc Natl Acad Sci U S A.* 103:12144–12149.

Swan H. 1974. *Thermoregulation and Bioenergetics.* Elsevier: New York.

Thompson SM, Musakawa LM, Rince DA. 1985. Temperature dependence of intrinsic membrane properties and synaptic potentials in hippocampal CA1 neurons in vitro. *J Neurosci.* 5:817–824.

Travis KA, Bockholt HJ, Zardetto-Smith AM, Johnson AK. 1995. In vitro thermosensitivity of the midline thalamus. *Brain Res.* 686:17–22.

Trubel HKF, Sacolick LI, Hyder F. 2006. Regional temperature changes in the brain during somatosensory stimulation. *J Cereb Blood Flow Metab.* 26:68–78.

Tryba AK, Ramirez J-M. 2004. Hyperthermia modulates respiratory pacemaker bursting properties. *J Neurophysiol.* 92:2844–2852.

Uda M, Tanaka Y. 1990. Arterial blood flow changes after hyperthermia on normal liver, normal brain, and normal small intestine. *Gan No Rinsho.* 36:2362–2366.

United Nations Office on Drugs and Crime. 2003. *Ecstasy and Amphetamines: Global Survey 2003.* New York: United Nations Publication.

Vizi ES. 1998. Different temperature dependence of carrier-mediated (cytoplasmic) and stimulus-evoked (exocytotic) release of transmitter: a simple method to separate the two types of release. *Neurochem Int.* 33:359–356.

Volgushev M, Vidyasagar TR, Chistiakova M, Eysel UT. 2000. Synaptic transmission in the neocortex during reversible cooling. *Neuroscience.* 98:9–22.

Wass C, Cable D, Schaff H, Lanier W. 1998. Anesthetic technique influences brain temperature during cardiopulmonary bypass in dogs. *Ann Thorac Surg.* 65:454–460.

Watson P, Shirreffs SM, Maughan RJ. 2005. Blood–brain barrier integrity may be threatened by exercise in a warm environment. *Am J Physiol Regul Integr Comp Physiol.* 288:R1689–R1694.

White MG, Emery M, Nonner D, Barrett JN. 2003. Caspase activation contributes to delayed death of heat-stressed striatal neurons. *J Neurochem.* 87:958–968.

Wilder J. 1957. The law of initial value in neurology and psychiatry; facts and problems. *J Nerv Ment Dis.* 125:73–86.

Wilder J. 1958. Modern psychophysiology and the law of initial value. *Am J Psychother.* 12:199–221.

Willis WT, Jackman MR, Bizeau ME, Pagliassotti MJ, Hazel JR. 2000. Hyperthermia impairs liver mitochondrial functions. *Am J Physiol.* 278:R1240–R1246.

Xie T, McGann UD, Kim S, Yuan J, Ricaurte GA. 2000. Effect of temperature on dopamine transporter function and intracellular accumulation of methamphetamine: Implications for methamphetamine-induced dopaminergic neurotoxicity. *J Neurosci.* 20:7838–7845.

Yablonskiy DA, Ackerman JH, Raichle ME. 2000. Coupling between changes in human brain temperature and oxidative metabolism during prolonged visual stimulation. *Proc Natl Acad Sci U S A.* 97:7603–7608.

Yoshida K, Morimoto A, Makisumi T, Murakami N. 1993. Cardiovascular, thermal and behavioral sensitization to methamphetamine in freely moving rats. *J Pharmacol Exp Ther.* 267:1538–1543.

Zhao A, Ahram A, Berman RT, Muizelaar JP, Lyeth BG. 2003. Early loss of astrocytes after experimental traumatic brain injury. *Glia.* 44:140–152.

Zhu M, Nehra D, Ackerman J, Yablonskiy DA. 2004. On the role of anesthesia on the body/brain temperature differential in rats. *J Thermal Biol.* 29:599–603.

Chapter *4*

RETINAL CELLULAR METABOLISM AND ITS REGULATION AND CONTROL

Dao-Yi Yu, Stephen J. Cringle, Paula K. Yu, Er-Ning Su, Xinghuai Sun, Wenyi Guo, William H. Morgan, Xiao-Bo Yu, and Chandrakumar Balaratnasingam

ABSTRACT

The retina is an extension of the brain with a high functional activity and high metabolic rate but with only a limited blood supply. Consequently there is a delicate balance between high metabolic demands and limited nutrient supply. Oxygen is known to be the most supply-limited metabolite in the human retina, and intraretinal hypoxia is thought to be a major pathogenic factor in retinal diseases with a vascular component. These diseases include diabetic retinopathy, vascular occlusion, and glaucoma. The metabolic and functional properties of the retina are highly compartmentalized, and the highly layered structure of the retina provides an opportunity for investigating the properties of different subcellular components not achievable in the brain due to the complex cell architecture. In this chapter, we demonstrate the marked heterogeneity of oxygen metabolism across the retina, even in different components of the same cell, and contrast the requirements of the inner retina in vascularized and avascular retinas. We examine the influence of several models of retinal disease and describe the potent regulation and control mechanisms that exist to protect the retina from challenges posed by alterations of the extracellular environment in normal and disease conditions. Knowledge of key molecules and pathways is essential to understand such regulation and control mechanisms. If we can determine how the retina is able to cope with the constraints imposed by the fragility of the retinal circulation, then we can begin to devise therapeutic strategies to help protect the retina from the effects of retinal disease.

Keywords: oxygen metabolism, retina, oxygen, ischemia, hypoxia.

Retinal neurons have a high functional activity, yet the retina necessarily has a limited blood supply to preserve retinal transparency. The retina is therefore particularly vulnerable to ischemic/hypoxic insults, which play a major role in many retinal diseases. Oxygen is the only molecule serving as the primary biological oxidant (Vanderkooi, Erecinska, Silver et al. 1991) and is essential for the survival of cells. The retina is one of the highest oxygen-consuming tissues in the body (Anderson 1968). Since oxygen cannot be "stored" in tissue, a constant and adequate supply must be guaranteed to preserve function. Oxygen supply to the retina is arguably more vulnerable to vascular deficiencies than in any other organ. Numerous studies have demonstrated the marked heterogeneity of oxygen metabolism across the retina, even in different components of the same cell. In this chapter, we describe key aspects of retinal metabolism and vascular regulation and control, the molecules and pathways involved, and their ability to respond to changes in the internal or external environment and the response to induced retinal diseases. This is essential for conserving the stability of the intracellular environment and for maintaining cellular function in normal and diseased retinas. By building a better picture of the metabolic requirements of each subcellular component and of how they react to changes in their particular microenvironment, new avenues of therapeutic intervention in retinal diseases and glaucoma with an ischemic or hypoxic component may be developed.

NORMAL RETINAL STRUCTURE AND BLOOD SUPPLY

Across the mammalian species studied to date, there are patterns of retinal vascularization ranging from completely avascular (anangiotic), very poorly vascularized (paurangiotic), partly vascularized (merangiotic), and extensively vascularized (holangiotic). Examining the metabolic properties of retinas with such differing degrees of vascularization can shed light on the mechanisms that have evolved to cope with limited metabolic supply to the retina. Common to all mammals is the presence of a well-supplied vascular bed immediately behind the retina, the choroid. In vascularized retinas such as our own, the choroid provides the dominant oxygen supply for the outer retina, but in avascular species it is essentially the only oxygen supply for the full thickness of retina. The regulatory properties of the choroidal and retinal circulations differ markedly. The choroid has a very high blood flow and no clearly demonstrated regulatory capacity (Riva, Cranstoun, Grunwald et al. 1994), despite the presence of autonomic innervation (Beckers, Klooster, Vrensen et al. 1993; Li, Grimes 1993). In contrast, the retinal circulation is relatively sparse, presumably to minimize disruption to the light path, and exhibits a well-developed regulatory capacity (Riva, Pournaras, Tsacopoulos 1986), which is thought to be purely "local" as there is no apparent autonomic innervation (Laties 1967). It seems likely that these opposing requirements of minimal interference with the light path and provision of sustenance to the metabolizing retinal tissue have led to the development of a system that is delicately, if not

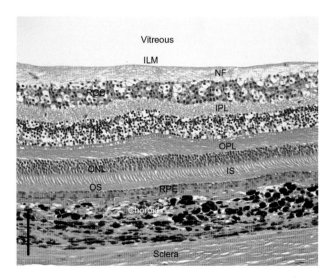

Figure 4.1 Micrograph of retina and choroid of a normal monkey in the parafoveal region. Retinal layers are as labeled: Inner limiting membrane (ILM); nerve fiber layer (NF); ganglion cell layer (RGC); inner plexiform layer (IPL); inner nuclear layer (INL); outer plexiform layer (OPL); outer nuclear layer (ONL); inner segments (IS); outer segments (OS); retinal pigment epithelium (RPE), choroid, and sclera. Haematoxylin and eosin staining; Scale bar = 100 μm.

precariously, balanced. This is borne out by the high incidence of retinal diseases with a vascular component, making it important to understand the mechanisms that regulate blood flow and oxygen metabolism in the eye in both health and disease.

As an example of retinal structure, Figure 4.1 shows a cross-section of the monkey retina. The section is from the parafoveal area. The anatomy of retinal neurons is such that the layered structure consists of sub cellular components rather than neurons alone. All retinal neurons are densely packed in a thin sheet of retina that is ≈300 μm thick. The structure is highly organized. All cell bodies are located in specific layers and other cellular components such as the synapses, axons, inner and outer segments are also constrained to specific layers.

INTRARETINAL OXYGEN DISTRIBUTION IN A VASCULAR RETINA

The highly layered structure of the retina provides an opportunity to study the oxygen metabolism of subcellular components using microelectrode-based techniques. This is the only technique currently available for measuring intraretinal oxygen distribution with such high resolution. Figure 4.2 shows an intraretinal oxygen distribution in the parafoveal area of the monkey retina (Yu, Cringle, Su 2005a). Oxygen tension is shown as a function of track distance from the retinal surface. Depth into the retina is expressed as track distance because the angle of penetration of the retina is not accurately known. The heterogeneous distribution of oxygen across different retinal layers is evident. Inner retinal oxygen levels are relatively low and show perturbations which reflect the influence of retinal vascular elements in this region. Deeper into the retina (≈250-μm track distance) the electrode enters the avascular region of the retina. The oxygen level then falls to an intraretinal minimum in the region of the photoreceptor inner segments, and then rises dramatically to high values within the outermost retina and choroid. It is evident that the high oxygen level in the choroid is barely enough to avoid anoxia in some regions of the outer retina. A recent study in monkeys demonstrated that oxygen levels in the outer retina could fall to zero during dark adaptation (Birol, Wang, Budzynski et al. 2007) when outer retinal oxygen consumption is increased (Stefansson, Wolbarsht, Landers 1983; Linsenmeier 1986). The critical point is that in terms of oxygen supply and consumption there is a very delicate balance between supply and demand. The monkey retina has a very interesting response to increased oxygen availability during systemic hyperoxia (Yu, Cringle, Su 2005a). In monkeys breathing increasing percentages of oxygen (20%, 40%, 60%, 80%, and 100%), choroidal oxygen tension closely follows the increase in systemic arterial oxygen levels (Fig. 4.3), reaching almost 400 mmHg during 100% oxygen ventilation. However, the increase in oxygen levels in the inner retina is much more constrained. Autoregulation of the retinal circulation may be partly responsible for this effect, but it has been demonstrated that a dramatic rise in inner retinal oxygen consumption is likely to be the dominant mechanism controlling inner retinal oxygen levels (Cringle, Yu 2002; Yu, Cringle, Su 2005a).

Experimental studies in primates pose difficulties both in terms of cost and ethical considerations. It is reassuring therefore to know that in terms of retinal oxygen supply and consumption, lower mammals such as rats (Yu, Cringle, Alder et al. 1994b) and mice (Yu, Cringle 2006) exhibit a similar intraretinal oxygen distribution to the primate. Additionally, the response to systemic hyperoxia in the monkey is not unlike that seen in the pig (Pournaras, Riva, Tsacopoulos et al. 1989), cat (Linsenmeier, Yancey 1989), and rat (Yu, Cringle, Alder et al. 1999; Cringle, Yu 2002). The striking similarities between the intraretinal oxygen distribution in the monkey and in these more readily available animal models is certainly encouraging in terms of the ultimate relevance of animal studies in these species to the human eye.

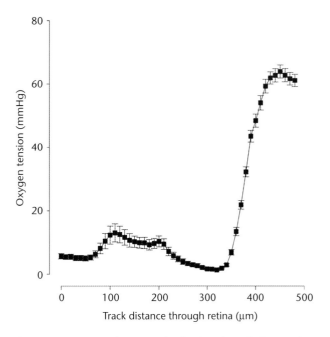

Figure 4.2 Intraretinal oxygen distribution through the monkey retina in the parafoveal region. Oxygen tension is shown as a function of track distance through the retina (Yu, Cringle, Su 2005a). Reproduced with permission from the Association for Research in Vision and Ophthalmology.

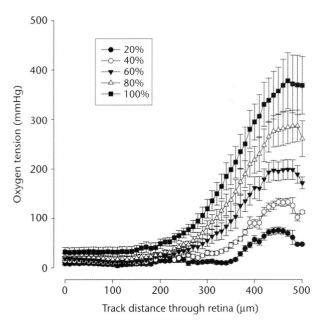

Figure 4.3 Intraretinal oxygen distributions through the monkey retina in the parafoveal region with increasing levels of oxygen in the inspired gas mixture. Oxygen tension in the choroid closely follows the increase in systemic oxygen level but the increase in oxygen level in the inner retina is muted compared to that in the choroid (Yu, Cringle, Su 2005a). Reproduced with permission from the Association for Research in Vision and Ophthalmology.

INTRARETINAL OXYGEN DISTRIBUTION IN AN AVASCULAR RETINA

It is in the mammals with avascular or partly avascular retinas that the intraretinal oxygen environment and metabolic requirements are significantly different from those in species with vascularized retinas. Studies in such species may therefore provide useful information as to how they cope without a retinal circulation, perhaps highlighting new strategies for ameliorating retinal damage in vascularized retinas in which the retinal circulation is compromised. The first such studies of intraretinal oxygen distribution were performed in the avascular retina of the guinea pig (Yu, Cringle, Alder et al. 1996). It was demonstrated that much of the inner retina in the guinea pig had oxygen levels close to zero, and, not surprisingly, very low rates of oxygen consumption in the inner retina (Cringle, Yu, Alder et al. 1996b). This contradicted well argued assumptions that the thickness of avascular retinas would correspond to the penetration depth of choroidally delivered oxygen (Chase 1982; Buttery, Haight, Bell 1990). To further explore the properties of avascular retinas, measurements were also performed in the avascular region of the rabbit retina (Yu, Cringle 2004). In the rabbit, the retinal vasculature is confined to a narrow band on either side of the optic disk as shown in Figure 4.4. Although oxygen levels in the inner retina of the rabbit did not approach zero, it was demonstrated that the inner retina of the rabbit also had a low oxygen consumption rate, even in the area of the visual streak, the region of highest visual acuity in the rabbit (Yu, Cringle 2004). Thus it has been demonstrated that the inner retina in some mammals has evolved to be able to function with minimal oxygen consumption.

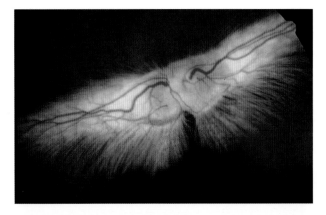

Figure 4.4 Fundus photograph of the rabbit retina. The narrow band of retinal vasculature can be seen on either side of the optic disk. The majority of the retina is avascular.

HYPOXIA AND ISCHEMIA IN HUMAN RETINAL DISEASES

In man, lack of oxygen is known to be the primary cause of visual loss following total ischemia of the intraocular vasculature (Anderson, Saltzman 1964). Since the retinal oxygen requirements must be derived from the local blood supply, it is not surprising that tissue hypoxia is thought to be an important factor in retinal diseases with a vascular component. These diseases include diabetic retinopathy, retinal vascular occlusion, and glaucoma. Such diseases account for the majority of retinal blindness in our community (Cooper 1990). The oxygen consumption of the retina on a per gram basis has been described as higher than that of the brain (Ames 1992). Given that the brain consumes a highly disproportionate share of the total body oxygen uptake (Coyle, Puttfarcken 1993), this places the retina as one of the highest oxygen-consuming tissues in the body. The requirement for a relatively unobstructed light path to the photoreceptors presumably places a constraint on the degree to which the retina can be vascularized. This results in a very limited blood oxygen supply to a highly consuming retina. It is understandable that to keep the retinal neurons in an efficient state, intracellular homeostasis must be maintained, and this requires considerable energy (Ames, Li, Heher et al. 1992; Ames 2000; Yu, Cringle, Su et al. 2005b).

There is very little direct evidence linking intraretinal hypoxia with retinal disease. This stems from the general inability to use invasive measurements in a clinical setting and the absence of noninvasive techniques with the required resolution. Indirect evidence comes from the use of supplemental oxygen therapy to treat diseases in which retinal hypoxia is suspected. Supplemental oxygen therapy has been used clinically in cases of retinal artery occlusion, but with limited success (Beiran, Reissman, Scharf et al. 1993). In diabetic retinopathy, supplemental oxygen therapy has also been suggested to have beneficial effects (Harris, Arend, Danis et al. 1996). Supplemental oxygen therapy has clear limitations in terms of treatment delivery, requiring hyperbaric chamber therapy or the patient being required to carry an oxygen supply device (Haddad, Leopold 1965; Dean, Arden, Dornhorst 1997; Nguyen, Shah, Van Anden et al. 2004). The most common therapy in which additional oxygen availability is thought to play a role is in panretinal laser photocoagulation. This therapy is commonly used in diabetic retinopathy and ischemic retinal diseases. In both instances, the underlying philosophy is that the destruction of selected regions of ischemic outer retina reduces the stimulus for retinal vascular proliferation. Intraretinal hypoxia as a result of retinal ischemia is thought to upregulate VEGF expression, which is a key factor in the proliferative process (Aiello, Avery, Arrigg et al. 1994; Takagi, King, Ferrara et al. 1996; Ozaki, Yu, Della et al. 1999). Reduced oxygen consumption of the outer retina and the presumed increase in oxygen levels in the inner retina are thought to be the mechanism relieving the hypoxic insult to the inner retina following panretinal photocoagulation (Wolbarsht, Landers III, 1980). There is some direct clinical experimental work supporting this proposal (The Diabetic Retinopathy Study Research Group 1987). In the future, other noninvasive techniques for measuring retinal oxygen levels (Wilson, Berkowitz, McCuen et al. 1992), induced changes in oxygen level (Berkowitz, Penn 1998), or oxygen saturation of the blood in the retinal vasculature (Hardarson, Harris, Karlsson et al. 2006) may give us a better picture of the retinal oxygen environment in different forms of retinal disease. There is certainly a great need for improved diagnostic techniques to determine the location and extent of intraretinal hypoxia in a clinical setting.

OXYGEN METABOLISM IN ANIMAL MODELS OF RETINAL DISEASE

Retinal Ischemia in Holangiotic and Merangiotic Retinas

Contrasting effects of total retinal ischemia have been demonstrated in holangiotic and merangiotic retinas of the rat and the rabbit. In the rat, the closure of the retinal circulation (by laser photocoagulation) results in the development of extensive anoxia in the inner retina (Yu, Cringle, Yu et al. 2007). Figure 4.5 shows the rat fundus before and after laser occlusion and Figure 4.6 shows the intraretinal oxygen distribution shortly after the induced ischemia.

Under conditions in which the retinal circulation no longer contributes any oxygen to the inner retina, mathematical analysis of the intraretinal oxygen

distribution can quantify oxygen consumption rates in specific retinal layers of the outer and inner retina. Without going into details of the mathematics, which are fully described elsewhere (Cringle, Yu, Alder et al. 1996a; Cringle, Yu, Alder et al. 1996b; Cringle, Yu, Alder et al. 1999), it is sufficient to note that the retinal layers with the highest oxygen consumption rates cause the greatest change in oxygen gradient. Thus, oxygen consumption is greatest in locations in which the oxygen profile "bends" the most. In the case of the example shown, there are two regions of high oxygen consumption corresponding to the inner segments of the photoreceptors and the outer plexiform layer. While it had long been known that the inner segments of the photoreceptor had a high oxygen uptake (Linsenmeier 1986), the discovery that the outer plexiform layer (OPL) had a high oxygen uptake was novel. Under these experimental conditions of retinal occlusion nothing could be said about the oxygen needs of other layers in the inner retina since much of the inner retina is essentially anoxic and necessarily has minimal oxygen uptake. However, when choroidal oxygen levels are increased by increasing the levels of oxygen that the rat breathes, much of the anoxic component of the ischemic insult can be overcome (Yu, Cringle, Yu et al. 2007). Figure 4.7 shows the intraretinal oxygen distribution in a rat with an occluded retinal circulation at increasing levels of inspired oxygen. Using the same mathematical analysis it was discovered that the inner plexiform layer was also a high consumer of oxygen under these ischemic, but no longer hypoxic, conditions. It was remarkable that in the acutely ischemic rat retina, it was not generally possible to raise choroidal oxygen levels to the point where all of the retina could be supplied with choroidally derived oxygen. This was somewhat surprising, given that similar studies in other species suggested that this should have been readily achieved (Landers 1978). Species differences alone cannot be the explanation since in work in pigs the relief of hypoxia has been achieved in some studies but not in other studies

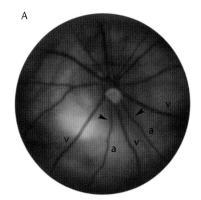 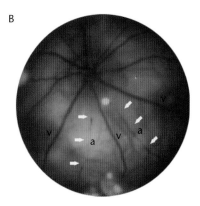

Figure 4.5 Fundus photographs of the rat retina before (A) and after (B) laser photocoagulation of the retinal arteries supplying the region subjected to intraretinal oxygen profile measurement. Cessation of blood flow in the laser treated arteries is indicated by the white arrows (Yu, Cringle, Yu et al. 2007). Reproduced with permission from the Association for Research in Vision and Ophthalmology.

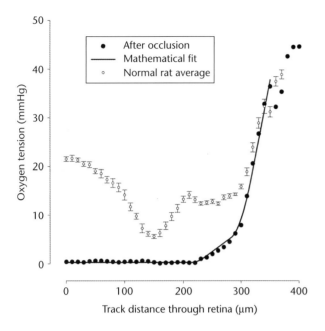

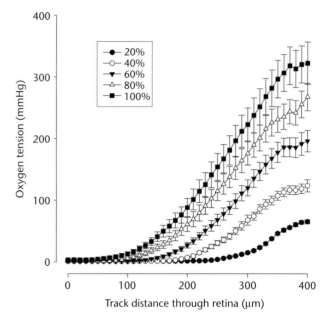

Figure 4.6 Intraretinal oxygen distribution in the rat following occlusion of the retinal circulation (full symbols). For reference, the normal oxygen profiles for these rats is shown superimposed (empty symbols). The mathematical fit of the data to a multilayer oxygen consumption model is also shown (Yu, Cringle, Yu et al. 2007).

Figure 4.7 Intraretinal oxygen distributions in the rat retina following occlusion of the retinal circulation and stepwise increments in systemic oxygen (Yu, Cringle, Yu et al. 2007). Reproduced with permission from the Association for Research in Vision and Ophthalmology.

from the same authors (Tsacopoulos, Beauchemin, Baker et al. 1976; Pournaras, Tsacopoulos, Riva et al. 1990; Pournaras, Petropoulos, Munoz et al. 2004). It may be that the duration of the ischemic insult is an important factor (which is often not well documented), with longer-term occlusion resulting in retinal damage and suppression of oxygen metabolism, thus allowing all retinal layers to be supported with oxygen from the choroid during systemic hyperoxia. This is supported by our observation of longer-term ischemia and reperfusion in the rat retina. Figure 4.8 shows the intraretinal oxygen distribution in a rat 1 month after initial treatment. The retinal circulation spontaneously reperfused on day 3 and was occluded again on the day of the final experiment. It is evident that the result is very different from that seen in short-term occlusion of the retinal circulation.

The inability to avoid some degree of hypoxia in the innermost retina of the rat with an occluded retinal circulation with an acute insult means that no conclusions regarding the oxygen requirements of retinal ganglion cells (RGCs) can be drawn, since there is very little oxygen available in this region, even under 100% oxygen ventilation conditions. It is clear, however, that in the holangiotic rat retina there are at least three retinal layers with high rates of oxygen consumption, namely, the inner segments of the photoreceptors, the outer plexiform layer, and the deeper region of the inner plexiform layer (Yu, Cringle, Alder et al. 1994b; Yu, Cringle 2001; Cringle, Yu, Yu et al. 2002). This contrasts markedly with the situation in the

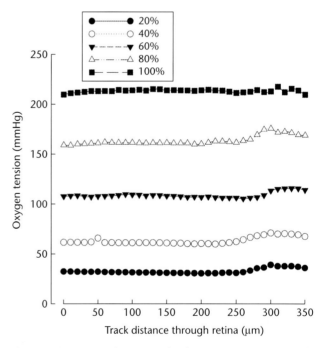

Figure 4.8 Intraretinal oxygen distribution in a rat 1 month after initial occlusion of the retinal circulation. Within 3 days the retinal circulation cleared the occlusion and the retina was reperfused. The retinal circulation was laser occluded once more just before measurement of the intraretinal oxygen distribution as a function of inspired oxygen level. It is evident that the intraretinal oxygen distribution is very different from the acute insult shown in Figure 4.7. Almost all intraretinal oxygen uptake has been lost and oxygen levels closely follow those in the choroid (Yu, Cringle 2001). Reproduced with permission from Elsevier Limited.

avascular guinea pig retina and in the avascular region of the rabbit retina in which only the inner segments of the photoreceptors have been found to have a high rate of oxygen consumption (Cringle, Yu, Alder et al. 1996b; Yu, Cringle 2004).

In the merangiotic retina of the rabbit, the consequences of loss of the retinal circulation have more localized effects. In addition to the unusual vascular distribution in the rabbit retina, the rabbit is also unusual in that the nerve fibers within the globe are myelinated. This is what gives the white background to the region underlying the retinal vasculature (Fig. 4.4). The more common myelination pattern is for the nerve fibers to become myelinated posterior to the lamina at the optic nerve head. Thus, the rabbit provides a rare opportunity to study the metabolic requirements of myelinated nerves and also provides a model in which well-controlled ischemic insults can be induced. This is difficult to achieve in the optic nerve because of a very complex vascular distribution and the relative inaccessibility of the optic nerve. In the rabbit, the intraocular nerve fibers are readily visualized and supplied from a relatively simple arrangement of easily occluded retinal vessels. Guo et al. (2006) used laser occlusion of the retinal arteries in the rabbit and conducted morphological and electrophysiological assessment of retinal function. They demonstrated that the loss of the retinal circulation impacted only on the viability of the nerve fibers underlying the previously vascularized area of retina. The remainder of the retina was unaffected and electrophysiological function was well maintained. Figure 4.9 shows the extent of damage 6 hours after the occlusion. At this point the retinal circulation remains occluded, and we are dealing with a purely ischemic insult. Retinal damage is relatively mild and confined to the nerve fiber layer. Figure 4.10 shows the extent of damage to the nerve fiber layer (NFL) following occlusion and subsequent reperfusion of the retinal circulation in the rabbit. Extensive vacuolization and necrosis of myelinated axons is evident but again the underlying retina is relatively undamaged. This mixture of ischemia and reperfusion insult appears to be more damaging than ischemia alone, an observation well supported by other ischemia-reperfusion studies. It seems that in the rabbit the retinal vasculature is primarily responsible for the metabolic support of the thick layer of myelinated nerve fibers that underlie the area of retinal vascularization.

Animal Models of Diabetic Retinopathy

Although currently there is no animal model which duplicates all the features of human diabetic retinopathy, much has been learnt from experimental work in

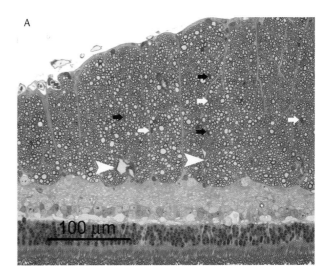

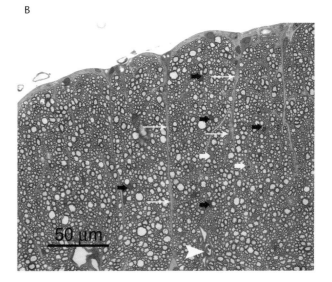

Figure 4.9 Retinal section of the vascular area of a rabbit 6 hours after laser-induced retinal arterial occlusion. In the lower power micrograph (A) diffuse swelling of the myelinated nerve fibre layer can be seen. However, changes in the body of the retinal ganglion cells and in the inner plexiform layer are not significant. Scale bar: 100 μm. At higher power (B), the nuclei of many of the oligodendrocytes are pyknotic (dark arrows); however, changes in the astrocytes (white arrows) are less obvious. Muller cell fibers (long white arrows) are more clearly evident. Scale bar: 50 μm (Guo, Cringle, Su et al. 2006). Reproduced with permission from Elsevier Limited.

animals (Gariano, Gardner 2005). In terms of oxygen effects, it has been demonstrated that the inner retina in long-term diabetic cats was hypoxic (Linsenmeier, Braun, McRipley et al. 1998) and a reduction of oxygen tension in the vicinity of retinal arteries was noted in rats after only 5 weeks of induced diabetes (Alder, Yu, Cringle et al. 1991). Impaired oxygen response to hyperoxic ventilation has also been reported in diabetic rats (Berkowitz, Ito, Kern et al. 2001).

It is very important to address retinal metabolism at the subcellular level of retinal neurons to answer some

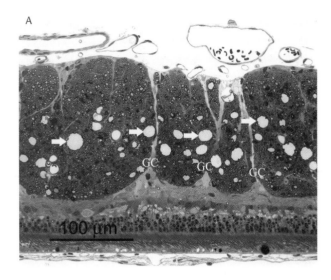

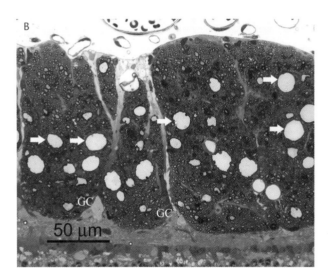

Figure 4.10 Sections through the vascularized region of the rabbit retina following laser occlusion of the retinal vasculature and subsequent reperfusion of the retinal vasculature. The eye was enucleated and fixed one day after treatment. Many large vacuoles are evident. Some retinal ganglion cells (GC) appear to have empty spaces in their cytoplasm (Guo, Cringle, Su et al. 2006). Reproduced with permission from Elsevier Limited.

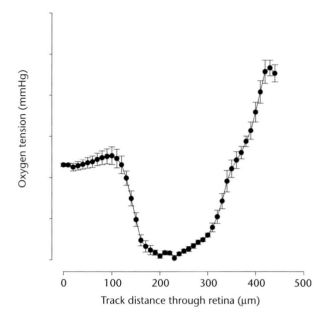

Figure 4.11 Intraretinal oxygen distribution in rats 5 weeks after STZ-induced diabetes. There is no difference in preretinal or choroidal Po_2 at this early time point, but there is a marked reduction in intraretinal oxygen levels in the middle retinal layers when compared with controls.

fundamentally important questions, such as whether the retina is really hypoxic in diabetes. Most studies have emphasized the role of hypoxia, based on clinical retinal angiography showing areas of nonperfused capillaries. However, direct empirical evidence for reduced retinal oxygen tension in human diabetic retinopathy is surprisingly limited. In fact, no studies have directly demonstrated reduction of retinal oxygen levels in humans with diabetes compared with those in controls. Therefore, while substantial indirect evidence argues for retinal hypoxia, current data does not establish a causal relationship between retinal hypoxia and retinal neovascularization in diabetes (Gariano, Gardner 2005). However, review

of evidence by Arden et al. (1998) suggests that before any change in the fundi of diabetics changes occur to blood flow, electroretinogram (ERG), and visual function and argues that hypoxia is a major factor in the development of diabetic retinopathy and recommends intervention in the early stages. Recently, we have found some solid and direct evidence of intraretinal Po_2 changes in early diabetes in rats. Figure 4.11 shows the averaged intraretinal oxygen distribution 6 weeks after inducing diabetes with streptozotocin (STZ). In comparison with normal animals, there are no significant changes of Po_2 at the surface of the retina or within the choroid. However, the intraretinal oxygen environment is markedly affected, with Po_2 in the middle layers of the retina being much lower than in controls. There were no apparent changes in the fundus and retinal microvasculature at this stage but retinal vasoactive changes and redistribution of retinal flow have been demonstrated (Cringle, Yu, Alder et al. 1993; Su, Yu, Alder et al. 1995; Su, Alder, Yu et al. 2000; Su, Alder, Yu et al. 2001; Yu, Cringle, Su et al. 2001a; Yu, Yu, Cringle et al. 2001c). Taken together, these observations suggest that diversion of blood flow away from the deep capillary layer may be a feature of this animal model of early diabetes.

Vascular changes in animal models of longer-term induced diabetes have also been reported. We performed a long-term (2.3 years) study to determine the temporal relationship between systemic glucose levels and the progression of diabetic retinopathy

Control   STZ-induced changes in the retinal vasculature

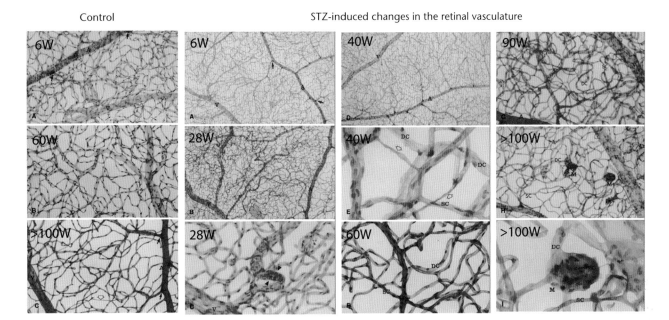

Figure 4.12 Trypsin digests of the retinal circulation of control and STZ rats as a function of time post injection.

Left panel: Control animals. (A) Six weeks (6W): Arteriole (A)–venule (V) pair and the two capillary beds providing homogeneous coverage of the retina. Darker PAS staining occurs at arterial branch points (arrows). In the capillaries endothelial cell nuclei are visible, as are pericyte nuclei. A basement membrane strand (small arrows) can also be seen. (B) Sixty weeks (60W): Retinal vascular structure is still close to normal. (C) More than 100 weeks (>100W): Sparser capillary beds are seen in this region containing an arteriole (A)–venule (V) pair. There is marked endothelial cell nuclei loss in capillary beds, leaving some as acellular vessels (empty arrow).

Right three panels: STZ animals. (A) 6W: Note darker PAS staining at arterial branch points (arrows) similar to age-matched controls. (B) 28W: Dramatic changes evident by this stage. Note enlarged tortuous venules (v) with dilated capillaries. Endothelial cell distribution heterogeneous with clusters of endothelial cells on the venous side, whereas other regions show loss of endothelial cells. (C) 28W: Region close to a venule (V) with higher magnification. Note tortuosity of smaller venule and clustered endothelial cells (arrowheads). Note also adjacent region where loss of endothelial cells is evident. (D) 40W: The retinal vasculature is clearly more quiescent than during the active stage observed at 28 weeks. (E) 40W: Higher magnification. Note the darker PAS staining in the superficial capillaries (SC) than in the deep capillaries (DC) and the narrower superficial capillaries with at least two acellular vessels (arrows). (F) 60W: Qualitatively the retina appears to have almost stabilized with some further reduction in numbers of capillaries. (G) 90W: The retina has become severely abnormal. Superficial capillaries (SC) are mainly ghost vessels, whereas the deep capillaries (DC) are dilated and still retain a few mural cells. (H) >100W: The darkly stained superficial capillaries (SC) are almost totally acellular, whereas the deeper capillaries (DC) are dilated and contain mural cells. Saccular microaneurysms (M) are present on the venous side of circulation. (I) >100W: Higher magnification. Note a saccular microaneurysm (M). Note the mural cell nuclei in the microaneurysm located in the deep capillaries (DC) which still contain mural cells, whereas the superficial capillaries (SC) are devoid of mural cells (Su, Alder, Yu et al. 2001).

during the natural course of STZ-induced diabetes in rats (Su, Alder, Yu et al. 2000). The severity of retinopathy was assessed quantitatively and qualitatively by trypsin digests of the retinal vasculature. Examples of trypsin digests of control and diabetic retinas are shown in Figure 4.12. Morphological changes were evident in the diabetic group, with late stage changes showing many of the features of clinical diabetic retinopathy. Concurrently, blood glucose, body weight, and death rate were monitored. Interestingly, in terms of glucose levels there was a general recovery from the initial hyperglycemia, with normoglycemia being restored after ≈40 weeks. The retinal microangiopathy was marked at 28 weeks during the earlier stage, and then developed more slowly but continued to worsen, with loss of capillaries in all retinas and saccular microaneurysms being present in 50% of retinas. The worsening retinopathy, despite sustained

recovery to normoglycemia, implies that good glucose control alone does not stop the progression of retinal microangiopathy in the later stages. It is notable that the pathological changes in the retinal vasculature, such as proliferation of endothelial cells, microaneurysms, loss of pericytes, and loss of endothelial cells predominantly occurred in the deep layer of the retinal capillary bed. Intracellular cytoskeleton changes and vascular leakage have been shown in the deep capillary bed in the early stage of the STZ-induced diabetes in rats (Yu, Yu, Cringle et al. 2001c; Yu, Yu, Cringle et al. 2005d). The location of these changes in the vascular endothelial cells may be associated with the alteration in the intraretinal oxygen distribution, although a cause and effect relationship cannot yet be confirmed. These findings may provide some clues to aid interpretation of the clinical data in diabetic retinopathy. Serial observations of diabetic patients before the development of proliferative diabetic retinopathy have shown that the appearance or worsening of certain intraretinal lesions is a crucial risk factor for the development of ocular neovascularization on the surface of the retina (The Diabetic Retinopathy Study Research Group 1987).

Retinal vascular endothelium changes have been further implicated by the observation of tetrahydrobiopterin improving vascular endothelium function in experimental diabetic retinopathy (Yu, Yu, Cringle et al. 2001c). The conversion of arginine to form nitric oxide by nitric oxide synthase is dependent on arginine concentration and the availability of the cofactors such as calcium, calmodulin, and tetrahydrobiopterin. It has been reported that tetrahydrobiopterin is decreased in neural tissue, such as the brain in diabetic rats (Hamom, Culter, and Blair 1989).

As mentioned previously, the current treatment of choice for the proliferative stages of diabetic retinopathy is panretinal photocoagulation. Although the role of additional oxygen supply to the ischemic inner retina due to reduced oxygen consumption in the treated areas of outer retina has long been proposed as the mechanism responsible for the therapeutic effect, only recently have such effects been quantified. We performed measurements of intraretinal oxygen distribution in the avascular region of the rabbit retina before and after graded doses of laser photocoagulation. Since only a small area of retina is treated, many measurements can be performed in the same eye, allowing a dose–response relationship to be determined. Different modes of laser delivery were assessed. The effect of pulsed or continuous wave (CW) laser delivery were compared to micropulse (MP) techniques in which the laser energy is modulated to be present for only a small portion of the duty cycle (15%, 10%, or 5%). Figure 4.13 shows the relationship between energy level and the resultant reduction in outer retinal oxygen consumption for the different modes of laser delivery. It was apparent that duty cycles of 10% or more produced an effect similar to that achieved with CW laser delivery. However, 5% MP delivery produced a significantly milder burn for the same laser power, allowing greater control of the degree of retinal damage and consequent reduction in outer retinal oxygen consumption. At the cellular level this may be explained by short pulse delivery creating less collateral damage to the cells surrounding the absorption site, the highly pigmented retinal pigment epithelium (Moorman, Hamilton 1999). Whatever the mechanism involved, it seems encouraging that such laser techniques may give the clinician better control over the extent of retinal damage and help produce the desired therapeutic effect of panretinal laser photocoagulation.

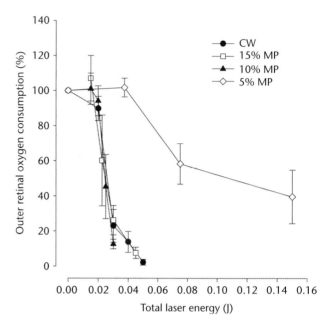

Figure 4.13 The relationship between reduction of outer retinal oxygen consumption as a function of the mode of laser delivery and laser power in a rabbit model of laser photocoagulation. The absence of inner retinal vasculature in the treated area greatly simplifies the analysis of the intraretinal oxygen distribution and allows quantification of outer retinal oxygen consumption changes. Short duration (5%) micropulse (MP) delivery gives greater control of outer retinal damage for a given laser power (Yu, Cringle, Su et al. 2005c). Reproduced with permission from the Association for Research in Vision and Ophthalmology.

Histological changes to the retinal vascular system have been studied in a wide variety of animal models of diabetes (Cogan, Toussaint, Kuwabara 1961; Su, Alder, Yu et al. 2000; Yu, Cringle, Su et al. 2001a). While many of the observed changes such as pericyte loss, capillary fallout, and vascular dysfunction reflect the clinical observations in diabetic retinopathy, the proliferation of retinal vasculature is rarely noted in animal models of diabetes (Su, Alder, Yu et al. 2000; Yu, Cringle, Su et al. 2001a), even in primates with long-term diabetes (Tso et al., 1998). Fortunately, the rat is one animal model in which retinal vascular proliferation can be achieved, although only with an almost complete lifetime of diabetic insult (Su, Alder, Yu et al. 2000).

Axonal Transport and Raised Intraocular Pressure

The importance of the RGCs and their axons in retinal and optic nerve physiology and pathology is well known. However, we have only very limited knowledge of their metabolic requirements in normal and diseased conditions. Clearly, subcellular components of RGCs such as the synapse, cell processes, cell body, and axons are located in significantly different

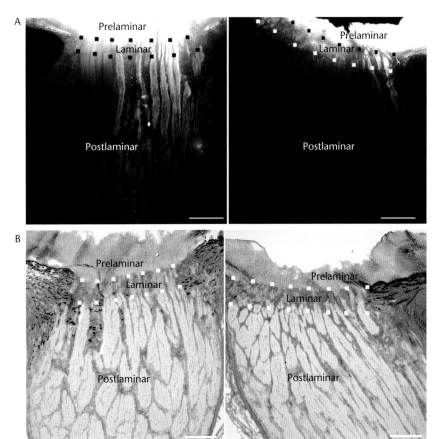

Figure 4.14 Axonal transport (A) in pig eyes in control (left) and high IOP (right) eyes. In the high-IOP eye there is very little transport of the RITC tracer beyond the lamina cribrosa. (B) Van Giesen stained sections from an adjacent region of nerve are shown for reference. Scale bar = 400 μm (Balaratnasingam, Morgan, Bass et al. 2007). Reproduced with permission from the Association for Research in Vision and Ophthalmology.

microenvironments, and most likely have different metabolic demands. The axons of the RGCs are very long (>5 cm) and thin, and usually consist of both myelinated and nonmyelinated zones. In man, approximately 1 million axons form the optic nerve and pass through a high pressure gradient at the lamina cribrosa (Morgan, Yu, Cooper et al. 1995). These unique features potentially make the axon particularly vulnerable to disease processes. In most cases, unmyelinated nerve fibers exit the eye via the lamina cribrosa, becoming myelinated at its posterior border. The pig has a strong lamina cribrosa similar to man, and steep pressure gradients have been demonstrated in this region (Morgan, Yu, Cooper et al. 1995). Mitochondria are concentrated in the prelaminar and laminar regions of the optic nerve, where the axons are unmyelinated. This distribution of mitochondria has traditionally been attributed to mechanical constriction or axoplasmic stasis at the lamina. However, mitochondrial distribution can also reflect the energy requirements to maintain conduction in the unmyelinated regions as compared to the myelinated regions of the axon. Functional roles of the cytoskeleton and mitochondria are extremely critical. The cytoskeleton not only plays a supporting role in keeping heterogeneous cellular structure but also has close intimacy with mitochondria. Interactions and linkage between mitochondria and intermediate

filaments, microtubules, and actin fibrils have been reported (Bereiter-Hahn, Voth 1994). The intensity of cytochrome oxidase staining is closely related to physiological activity (Caldwell, Roque, Solomon 1989), and mitochondrial electron transport chain complexes are directly involved in the most important function of mitochondria (Jung, Higgins, Xu 2002). Understanding the structural and functional aspects of each retinal subcomponent is fundamentally important for understanding the pathogenic cascade in ischemic/hypoxic insults in the subcellular components of retinal neurons.

The metabolic needs of the RGCs and their axons are difficult to assess directly in vivo. However, insights into the impact of ischemic insults can be obtained by assessing the efficiency of the axonal transport systems that are vital for healthy function of the axons. Such information is of direct relevance to the study of glaucoma, a common blinding disease in which both the ischemic and mechanical effects of raised intraocular pressure (IOP) are important. Figure 4.14 shows the reduction in axonal transport in pig eyes after 6 hours of raised IOP. The high-IOP eye was maintained at 40 to 45 mmHg and the control eye at 10 to 15 mmHg. The tracer rhodamine-β-isothiocyanate (RITC) was injected into the vitreous cavity at the start of the experiment. It is evident that in the high-IOP eye there is collection of RITC in the prelaminar

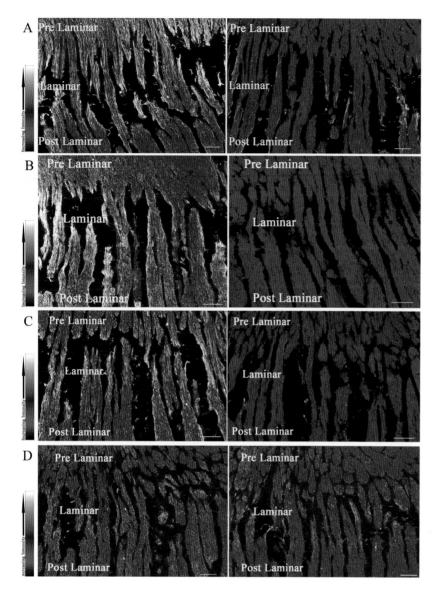

Figure 4.15 Confocal images of neurofilament stains. The left panel shows images of the control eye and the right panel those of the high-IOP eye. The prelaminar, laminar, and postlaminar regions of the nerve are labeled. (A) NFHp, (B) NFH, (C) NFM, and (D) NFL. Scale bar = 100 μm (Balaratnasingam, Morgan, Bass et al. 2007). Reproduced with permission from the Association for Research in Vision and Ophthalmology.

and laminar regions and relatively little transport to the postlaminar regions compared to the control eye. Thus, it was demonstrated that axonal transport was compromised in the high-IOP eye.

Confocal images of neurofilament-stained optic nerves (control and high-IOP eyes) are shown in Figure 4.15. Antibodies to phosphorylated neurofilament heavy (NFHp), phosphorylation-independent neurofilament heavy (NFH), neurofilament medium (NFM), and neurofilament light (NFL) were used to study the axonal cytoskeleton. Montages of confocal microscopy images were quantitatively analyzed to investigate simultaneous changes in optic nerve axonal transport and cytoskeletal proteins in the high-IOP and control eyes. The extent of neurofilament staining is reduced in the high-IOP eye, indicating that protein synthesis may have been affected. It was also demonstrated that microtubule proteins, which are necessary for mitochondrial movement,

were not substantially affected at this time point (Balaratnasingam, Morgan, Bass et al. 2007).

Given the disparate findings regarding oxygen metabolism properties and the influence of retinal ischemia in different species with varying degrees of retinal vascularization, it seemed appropriate to turn to other tools with which to study the potential for oxygen metabolism in different retinal layers. The retina is particularly amenable to histological, histochemical, and immunohistochemical studies. Morphologically the retina in a wide variety of mammals has essentially the same appearance in terms of a highly layered structure and the organization of different cell types. At the gross structural level there is little hint of the widely varying oxygen metabolism properties that have been demonstrated in vascularized and avascular retinas. Figure 4.16 shows retinal histology of a rat, mouse, guinea pig, and rabbit, and Figure 4.17 shows examples of normal intraretinal

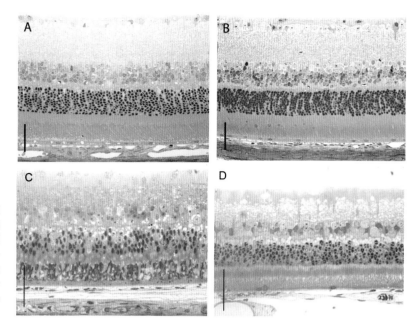

Figure 4.16 Micrographs of retina and choroid of normal rat (A), mouse (B), guinea pig (C), and rabbit (D). In the vascular retina of the rat and mouse, the layered structure of the retina is similar to that in the avascular retina of the guinea pig and in the avascular region of the rabbit retina; however, the avascular retinas are thinner. Scale bar = 50 μm.

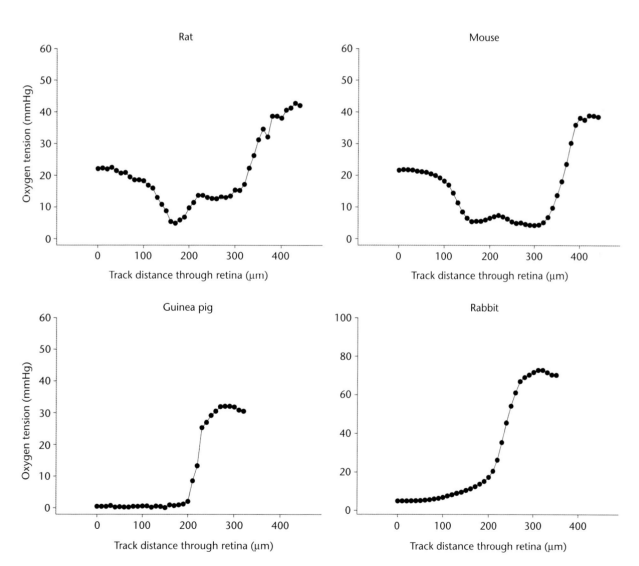

Figure 4.17 Intraretinal oxygen profiles under air-breathing conditions in four different species, rat, mouse, guinea pig, and rabbit. The influence of the retinal circulation is evident in the rat and the mouse. In the avascular retina of the guinea pig inner retinal oxygen levels fall close to zero. In the avascular region of the rabbit retina oxygen levels do not fall to zero but the choroid is the only source of retinal oxygenation.

oxygen profile in each species. Apart from a thinner retina, the avascular guinea pig and rabbit retina exhibit the same layered structure as seen in the vascularized retinas of the rat and mouse. The intraretinal oxygen distribution reflects the lack of a retinal circulation in the guinea pig and in the avascular region of the rabbit retina, and the choroid is the only source of retinal oxygenation. These special conditions can offer very simple models for studying retinal oxygen metabolism (Cringle, Yu, Alder et al. 1996a; Cringle, Yu, Alder et al. 1996b; Cringle, Yu, Su et al. 1998). Other researchers who have made intraretinal oxygen measurements in species with vascularized retinas of the cat (Linsenmeier 1986; Linsenmeier, Yancey 1989; Braun, Linsenmeier, Goldstick 1995), pig (Molnar, Poitry, Tsacopoulos et al. 1985; Pournaras, Riva, Tsacopoulos et al. 1989; Pournaras, Tsacopoulos, Riva et al. 1990) and monkey (Ahmed, Braun, Dunn et al. 1993; Birol, Wang, Budzynski et al. 2007) have reported the same general findings that we have found in the cat (Alder, Cringle, Constable 1983; Alder, Ben-nun, Cringle 1990), rat (Yu, Cringle, Alder et al. 1994b; Yu, Cringle, Alder et al. 1999; Cringle, Yu, Yu et al. 2002), mouse (Yu, Cringle 2006), and monkey (Yu, Cringle, Su 2005a).

Regulation of Intraretinal Oxygen Levels

Surprisingly little is known about the specific mechanisms that regulate the intraretinal oxygen environment. Perhaps the most striking example of regulation of intraretinal oxygen level is that seen in the avascular retina of the guinea pig. Figure 4.18 shows the result of stepwise increments in systemic oxygen levels in the guinea pig. Remarkably the oxygen level in the choroid rises very little, even in the face of 100% oxygen ventilation. Since the choroid is the only source of retinal oxygenation in the guinea pig this results in intraretinal oxygen levels being almost unchanged during systemic hyperoxia. Blood gas levels were closely monitored in those studies to observe the typical increase in systemic arterial oxygen level with stepwise increments in oxygen percentage in the ventilation gas. Figure 4.19 shows the arterial blood gas levels which increased to more than 400 mmHg with 100% oxygen ventilation. It is evident that the guinea pig has mechanisms in place to tightly regulate intraretinal oxygen levels through control of choroidal oxygen level. How this is achieved is not presently known, although it has been demonstrated that such regulation is disrupted to some extent by systemic hypercapnia (Yu, Cringle, Alder et al. 1996), so blood flow regulation may be implicated.

In contrast, the avascular retina of the rabbit shows no ability to regulate intraretinal oxygen levels

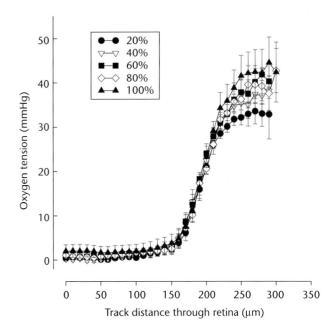

Figure 4.18 Intraretinal oxygen distribution in the avascular guinea pig retina during stepwise increments in systemic oxygen level. The choroid shows only a very small increase in oxygen tension, and intraretinal oxygen levels show almost no change (Yu, Cringle, Alder et al. 1996). Reproduced with permission from Elsevier Limited.

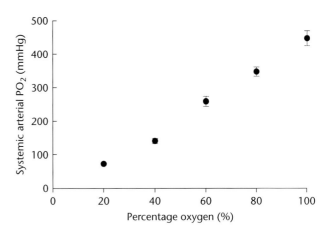

Figure 4.19 Arterial blood gas values in the guinea pig retina during stepwise increments in systemic oxygen level. The expected rise in systemic arterial oxygen level with increasing percentage of oxygen in the ventilation gases is evident (Yu, Cringle, Alder et al. 1996).

in the face of systemic hyperoxia (Cringle, Yu 2004). Figure 4.20 shows the intraretinal oxygen distribution in the avascular region of the rabbit retina during systemic hyperoxia. For each increment in inspired oxygen percentage the choroidal oxygen tension increases and this flows on to an increased oxygen level in all retinal layers. With 100% oxygen ventilation, the inner retinal oxygen levels in the rabbit far exceed

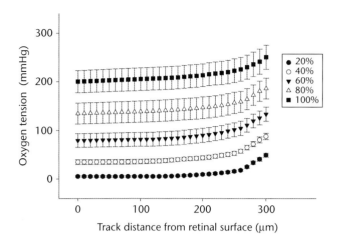

Figure 4.20 Intraretinal oxygen distribution in the avascular region of the rabbit retina during stepwise increments in systemic oxygen level. Systemic hyperoxia creates very high oxygen levels in all retinal layers (Cringle, Yu 2004). Reproduced with permission from the Association for Research in Vision and Ophthalmology.

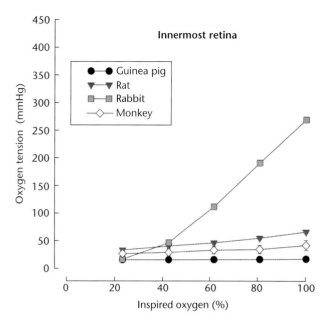

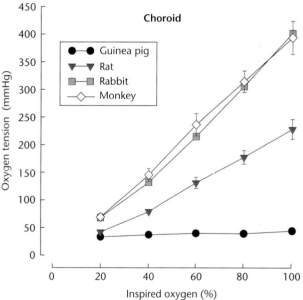

Figure 4.21 Average oxygen levels in the innermost retina and choroid in four different species as a function of inspired oxygen percentage. The oxygen level within the retina shows a high degree of variability between species.

anything seen in any other animal studied. This finding is consistent with the earlier work of Berkowitz et al. (1991a, 1991b), who showed very large changes in preretinal oxygen tension in the rabbit.

The absence of any clear oxygen regulatory ability in the rabbit may help explain the potent toxicity of systemic oxygen supplementation to the adult rabbit retina (Noell 1955; Noell 1962; Bresnick 1970) that is not seen in other species. Noell reported that more than 70% of the visual cells were degenerated after only 48 hours of oxygen exposure (Noell 1955). There is clearly scope for further studies on the effects of oxygen exposure on the adult rabbit retina.

These differing oxygen regulation properties in the retina in different species are well demonstrated by Figure 4.21, which summarizes the oxygen levels in the innermost retina and choroid as a function of inspired oxygen percentage. It is evident that as far as inner retinal oxygen level during systemic hyperoxia is concerned, the rabbit is the odd one out. In the choroid, it is the guinea pig which goes against the trend. This highlights the need to carefully consider the choice of animal model when planning studies of the effect of supplemental oxygen on the retina. It is evident from Figure 4.21 that in the avascular region of the rabbit and guinea pig retinas the change in inner retinal oxygen level during systemic hyperoxia ranges from extreme in the rabbit to essentially no change at al in the guinea pig. In their work on miniature pig retinas, Pournaras et al. (1989) showed that innermost retinal Po_2 in the pig was essentially unchanged by systemic hyperoxia, so such control mechanisms seem to be operating in a range of species.

REGULATION AND CONTROL OF RETINAL METABOLISM

Intracellular Homeostasis and Microenvironment

Intracellular homeostasis is essential for maintaining cell stability and efficient function in response to changes in the internal or external environment. All living cells have to closely communicate with their external environments via abundant signal molecules, which are interlinked and which interact forming multiple pathways. To adapt to changes in the extracellular environment, cells can control and regulate their own metabolic rate, and also interact with other cells such as glial cells and vascular endothelial and smooth muscle cells, resulting in alteration of the extracellular environment. The mechanisms and processes of cellular regulation and control are complex and must be dynamic.

The retina performs the vital task of transducing and encoding the visual input for later processing by the visual centers of the brain. Of all afferent fibers of cranial nerves, 38% are from the optic nerve. The retina has the conflicting constraints of a high metabolic requirement and transparency of the retina that cannot be compromised by an overly rich vascular network on the inner retinal side. It is now established that specific layers within the retina dominate the oxygen requirements of the retina. There is no doubt that the functionally active retina with high metabolic demands and a limited blood supply needs a considerable capacity for metabolic control and regulation to cope with alterations of supply and demand. The anatomy of retinal neurons is such that the layered structure consists of subcellular components rather than of neurons alone. All cell bodies are located in specific layers, and other cellular components such as the synapses, axons, inner and outer segments, are also constrained to specific layers. It is important to study each microenvironment as a compartment within the retina. The individual enzymes of a metabolic pathway are capable of converting a starting material to end products without accumulating elevated concentrations of the metabolic intermediates. This further compounds the problem of adequate provision of nutrients and the removal of metabolic waste products to maintain retinal homeostasis. The inner segments of the photoreceptors lie in a completely avascular region of the retina, and the relatively sparse retinal vasculature needs to supply both the inner and outer plexiform layers. This can only be achieved by precise regulation of vascular elements to match local blood flow with tissue demands.

Metabolic Regulation and Control Mechanisms in the Retina

Metabolic regulation and control mechanisms in the retina are complicated, and our knowledge in this field is very limited. Understanding regulation and control of retinal metabolism requires studies not only at the cellular and molecular levels, but also from a dynamic point of view. Many of the small metabolites and ions do not diffuse freely through the cytoplasm because they are often associated with the macromolecular structure. Concentration gradients are therefore present in most neurons (Bereiter-Hahn, Voth 1994). Restricted molecular mobility forms microcompartmentations, which are morphological and functional entities. These concentration gradients reflect the nonuniform nature of the function and metabolism within the neuron. This is also reflected in the uneven distribution of mitochondria across the retina. This distribution is dynamic. The dynamics of mitochondria have been demonstrated in single cells (Bereiter-Hahn, Voth 1994) and in supportive cells such as Muller cells (Germer, Biedermann, Wolburg et al. 1998a; Germer, Schuck, Wolburg et al. 1998b). Mitochondria are endowed with the ability to change their shape and location and play a prominent role in cellular energy production and coordinate all microcompartmentations inside a living cell to face all physiological and pathological challenges (Bereiter-Hahn, Voth 1994). Furthermore, metabolic control and regulation are interlinked, but different. Metabolic control is a response to an altered external environment by adjusting the output of a metabolic pathway while metabolic regulation maintains some variable relatively constant over time. As each cellular reaction is catalyzed by its own enzyme, every cell contains a large number of different enzymes. The amount of metabolite produced through any metabolic pathway will depend upon the activities of the individual enzymes involved. From a theoretical viewpoint, metabolic control can be categorized as two levels of alterations in response to environment changes: (1) long-term changes—the total cellular population of enzyme molecules is changed; and (2) fast changes—the activity of the preexisting enzyme molecule is modulated. However, the results from most acute experiments appear to be short-term changes. This means that the control mechanism may be based on preexisting enzyme activity changes. This can be thought of as metabolic transducers "sensing" the momentary metabolic needs of the cell and modulating flux through the various pathways accordingly (Plaxton 2004). Long-term control mechanisms were evident in our previous work in retinal degeneration models such as P23H and Royal College of Surgeons (RCS) rats (Yu, Cringle, Su et al. 2000a; Yu, Cringle 2001; Yu, Cringle, Valter et al. 2004). It has been demonstrated that the retina has control and regulation capabilities and switches mechanism between aerobic and anaerobic conditions (Winkler 1981; Ames 1983; Ames, Li 1992; Ames 1992; Winkler, Arnold, Brassell et al. 1997; Yu, Cringle, Alder et al. 1999; Yu, Cringle, Su 2005a; Yu, Cringle, Yu, et al. 2007). However, the regulatory or pacemaker enzyme(s) of a pathway such as in retinal ischemia/hypoxia have not yet been clearly defined, although such information may be useful in developing therapeutic strategies. Currently, we are working on the retinal biochemistry and mitochondria in the retina in the hope that we can identify the mechanisms behind the metabolic differences in vascular and avascular retinas. This may then open up the possibility of modification of the inner retinal oxygen uptake in vascular retinas in order to ameliorate the effects of ischemic/hypoxic insults.

As we described, hyperoxia induces increased heterogeneities in intraretinal oxygen distribution in vascular retinas, both with intact retinal circulations and under ischemic conditions induced by retinal artery occlusion and also in naturally avascular retinas (Yu, Cringle, Alder et al. 1996; Yu, Cringle, Alder et al. 1999; Yu, Cringle, Su et al. 2000b; Yu, Cringle 2001; Cringle, Yu, Yu et al. 2002; Cringle, Yu 2004; Yu, Cringle, Su 2005a; Yu, Cringle 2006; Yu, Cringle, Yu et al. 2007). Hyperoxia-induced heterogeneity changes in tissue oxygen distribution have also been found in other organs (Johnston, Steiner, Gupta et al. 2003). For example, in muscle tissue, hyperoxia increases the mean tissue oxygen tension but with increased heterogeneity, such that some regions of the tissue have lower oxygen tension than that in normoxia (Lund, Jorfeldt, Lewis 1980). Hyperoxia also induces tissue oxygen heterogeneity in the brain (Eintrei, Lund 1986).

An important question in the management of tissue ischemia/hypoxia in retina and brain is how to ensure adequate tissue oxygen delivery in the face of systemic and regional hypoxemia by modulation of blood flow and tissue oxygen uptake and increase in inspired oxygen level. It has been clearly shown that interactions between changes of blood flow and tissue oxygen uptake, and tissue oxygen level existed. There is increasing appreciation of the modulatory role of hyperoxia in vascular tone and blood circulation and a consideration of the effects of such modulation on the maintenance of tissue oxygen tension. It is expected that vascular and tissue oxygen responses to hyperoxia may change in disease. Our knowledge in these areas may provide important insights into pathophysiological mechanisms and may provide novel targets for therapy.

The mechanisms of hyperoxia-induced changes in the heterogeneities in intraretinal oxygen distribution remain unclear. The increase in heterogeneity is speculated to be a result of redistribution of blood flow, with vasoconstriction in some areas and shunting in others. The intricate relationship involved in producing an accurate matching between oxygen supply and oxygen demand in a tissue requires some feedback to allow regulation of blood flow. Oxygen is known to be a vasoactive trigger in many circulations, including the cerebral and retinal circulations.

There are some limited studies in the ocular vasculature (Hickam, Frayser 1966; Riva, Grunwald, Sinclair 1983; Brinchmann-Hansen, Myhre 1989). Various mediators and mechanisms have been suggested to play a role in ocular vessels (Alder, Su, Yu et al. 1993) and in cerebral vessels (Johnston, Steiner, Gupta et al. 2003), including increased effects of serotonin, nitric oxide synthase inhibition, inhibition of endothelial prostaglandin synthesis, and increased leukotriene production.

However, vascular responses to increased oxygen tension vary with different vasculature and species. In vascular retinas such as in rats and monkeys, there is significant difference between retinal and choroidal vasculature in response to stepwise increases in inspired oxygen levels and blood oxygen tension. The retinal vasculature generally has more regulatory capability to maintain normoxic oxygen levels than the choroid. However, the regulatory capability in the choroidal vasculature varies dramatically in different species with avascular retinas. For example, the choroidal vasculature in the guinea pig has potent response to increased blood oxygen level in the choroid, whereas the rabbit has none. It is predictable that various mediators and mechanisms must be involved but they remain to be investigated.

Control and regulation of cellular metabolism plays a major role in hyperoxia-induced increases in heterogeneity of intraretinal oxygen distribution. There is no doubt that occlusion of the retinal circulation renders the majority of the inner retina anoxic. Ventilation with 100% oxygen ventilation does not generally avoid some degree of intraretinal anoxia. Under 100% oxygen ventilation conditions the oxygen consumption of the inner retina is more than four times that of the outer retina. A marked degree of heterogeneity in oxygen uptake of different retinal layers is clearly evident. We also confirmed that the dominant oxygen consumers are the inner segments of the photoreceptors, the outer plexiform layer, and the inner plexiform layer (Yu, Cringle 2001; Yu, Cringle, Yu et al. 2007). Increased oxygen uptake in these dominant oxygen consumers during graded hyperoxia has also been found in the vascular retina with intact retinal circulation in which contraction of the retinal circulation and the relative lack of blood vessels in the inner plexiform layers allow oxygen consumption to be measured (Cringle, Yu, Yu et al. 2002).

One possible explanation for the significant increase in oxygen uptake in the plexiform layers is that there is normally a high rate of both oxidative and anaerobic metabolism in the plexiform layers in normoxia. Anaerobic metabolism is known to exist in the rat inner retina (Winkler 1995). When environmental oxygen levels are raised following total retinal ischemia, a switching to more oxidative metabolism in the plexiform layers may be responsible for this effect (Pasteur Effect). We have shown that the synaptic layers of the inner retina have a particularly high rate of oxygen metabolism, which may provide new insights into the particular vulnerability of the inner retina to ischemic or hypoxic insult. The use of hyperoxic ventilation in this acute model of arterial occlusion is able to partially overcome the intraretinal anoxia seen in the inner retina with successive increases in choroidal oxygen tension confining the anoxic zone to the more proximal retinal layers. However, even with 100% oxygen ventilation complete relief from intraretinal anoxia could not be guaranteed.

Oxygen availability is crucial for cellular metabolism. The matching of oxygen supply to metabolic demand in tissues and cells is one of the principal physiological challenges. It is interesting to know the signal molecules and pathway in response to changes in oxygen tension at tissues and cells. The exact site and mechanism of the oxygen sensor is yet to be fully elucidated. There may be more than one sensor. Research over the last few decades has provided significant insights into the molecular processes underlying this complex task, and has revealed a central role for a set of dioxygenases belonging to the Fe(II) and 20G (2-oxoglutarate)-dependent oxygenase superfamily in directing the activity of a major transcriptional regulator termed *hypoxia inducible factor* (HIF) (Schofield, Ratcliffe 2005). HIF-1 is the major oxygen homeostasis regulator and at the transcriptional level. A diverse range of genes including those encoding glycolytic enzymes (for anaerobic metabolism), VEGF (for angiogenesis), inducible nitric oxide synthase and heme oxygenase-1 (for production of vasodilators), EPO (for erythropoiesis), and possibly tyrosine hydroxylase (for dopamine production to increase breathing) are all under the control of a crucial transcription factor: hypoxia-inducible factor 1 (HIF-1) (Guillemin, Krasnow 1997). HIF-1 is rapidly degraded by the proteasome under normoxic conditions. However, under hypoxic conditions, HIF-1 is stabilized and permits the activation of genes essential to cellular adaptation to low oxygen conditions. These molecules include the vascular endothelial growth factor (VEGF), erythropoietin, inducible nitric oxide synthase and glycolytic enzymes, and glucose transporter-1. There is increasing evidence showing that HIF-1 is also implicated in biological functions requiring its activation under normoxic conditions. Among others, growth factors and vascular hormones are implicated in this normoxic activation. These enzymes catalyze the posttranslational hydroxylation of specific prolyl and asparaginyl residues, the oxidation state of which governs both the rate of degradation and transcriptional activity of HIF-a subunits.

The sensitivity of HIF hydroxylase to oxygen concentrations enables the regulation of a wide array of cellular and systemic responses to oxygen availability.

This oxygen-dependent instability may provide a means by which gene expression is controlled during changes in oxygen tension. Johnston et al. (2003) speculates that hyperoxia reduces the intracellular HIF-1 concentration, thus reducing the activity of important enzymes involved in glycolysis, such as phosphofructokinase and 6-phosphofructo-2-kinase/fructose-2,6-bisphosphatase. A reduction in glycolysis would reduce lactic acid production and intracellular buffering, and thus modulate cerebral blood flow. Unfortunately, it is unlikely that it will be possible to measure HIF-1 concentrations in vivo because of its intracellular position and instability.

Mitochondrial Subunits in Vascular and Avascular Retinas

Mitochondria play a pivotal role in cell metabolism, being the major site of adenosine triphosphate (ATP) production via oxidative phosphorylation. Defects of mitochondrial metabolism are associated with a wide spectrum of diseases (Leonard, Schapira 2000). Energy is produced by the electron transport chain. This pathway involves five multi-subunit complexes. We have studied the subunits and respiratory enzymes of retinal mitochondria to determine the differences between vascular and avascular retinas. These differences may provide some clues for possible manipulation of the nucleic acids and gene expression to modify specific subunits and respiratory enzymes. Figures 4.22, 4.23, and 4.24 are representative data from immunohistochemical studies using mitochondrial subunit antibodies in the rat, guinea pig, and rabbit retinas respectively. Mitochondrial antibodies, complex II 30 kDa, 70 kDa, complex III core II, complex IV subunit I, II, IV and IVc, and Vα as well as prohibitin were used. Prohibitin, an evolutionarily conserved protein with homologues located in cytoplasmic mitochondria, appears to be a very reliable marker of mitochondria (Ikonen, Fiedler, Parton et al. 1995). Positive staining for prohibitin is evident in the RGCs and nerve fiber layers, the inner and outer plexiform layers and the inner segment of the photoreceptor layer in all these species. This is somewhat surprising since we have shown earlier that there is very little oxidative metabolism in the inner retina in the avascular species. These results indicate that the presence of mitochondria, as implied by prohibitin staining, does not always correspond to sites of high oxygen uptake.

We have further addressed whether the differences of metabolic properties in these species are

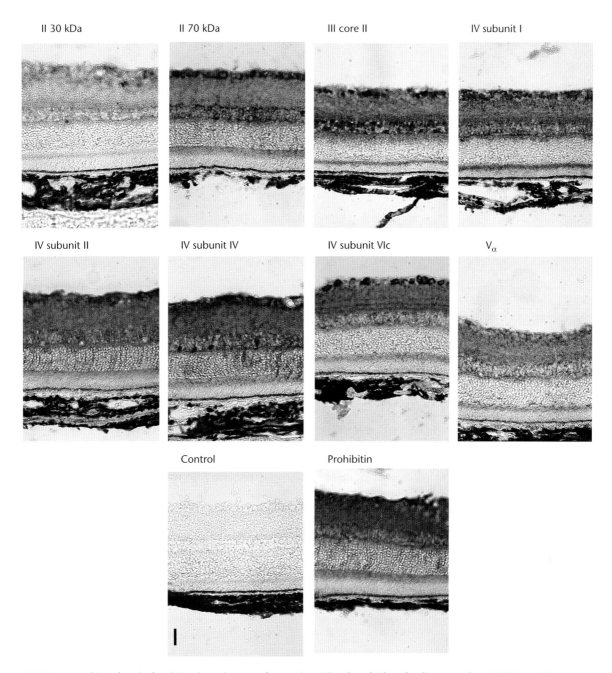

Figure 4.22 Immunohistochemical staining in a pigmented rat retina. Mitochondrial antibodies, complex II 30 kDa, 70 kDa, complex III core II, complex IV subunit I, II, IV and IVc, and Vα as well as the control are showed as labeled. Prohibitin staining is used as a marker of mitochondria. Scale bar = 50 μm.

caused by variations of mitochondrial subunits. There are remarkable differences in expression of the mitochondrial subunits in these three species. It is difficult to directly compare the degree of expression in the various layers and interpret the in vivo experimental data using microelectrode techniques within these three species. However, the best match between the immunohistochemistry and in vivo studies are the complex IV subunits, particularly subunit VIc, which is a nuclear coded subunit and may have a regulatory effect on cytochrome oxidase

(Gagnon, Kurowski, Weisner et al. 1991). Figure 4.25 shows cytochrome oxidase staining in the retinas of the rat, guinea pig, and rabbit. The distribution of cytochrome oxidase staining is completely consistent with our understanding of oxygen uptake based on the previously described oxygen profile measurements.

Recent immunohistochemical evidence from Bentmann et al. (2005) also provides supportive evidence for localized layers of high oxygen consumption in vascularized and avascular retinas (Yu, Cringle

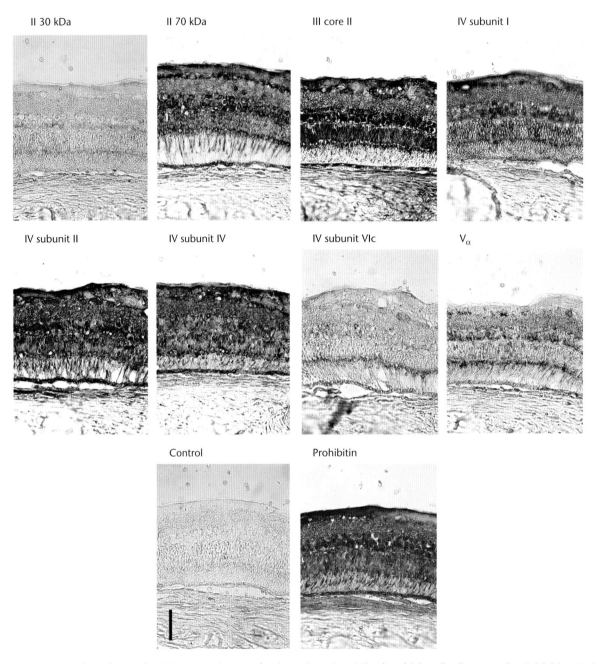

Figure 4.23 Immunohistochemical staining in a pigmented guinea pig retina. Mitochondrial antibodies, complex II 30 kDa, 70 kDa, complex III core II, complex IV subunit I, II, IV and IVc, and Vα as well as the control are shown as labeled. Prohibitin staining is used as a marker of mitochondria. Note that although the expression of complex IV subunits in the inner segment of the photoreceptor layer is similar to that in the rat retina, staining in the inner retina is much weaker than that in the rat retina, particularly in complex IV subunit VIc. Scale bar = 50 μm.

2001). Figure 4.26 shows their schematic illustration of retinal structure and vascular elements in a vascularized and an avascular retina. Figure 4.27 shows that the distribution of mitochondria and neuroglobin corresponds well with the identified layers of high oxygen uptake from the oxygen profile studies as demonstrated by Bentmann et al. Neuroglobin is a respiratory protein thought to play an essential role in oxygen homeostasis of neuronal cells. They showed that in rat and mouse retinas, mitochondria are concentrated in the inner segments of photoreceptor cells, the outer and the inner plexiform layers, and the ganglion cell layer. These are the same regions in which neuroglobin is present at high levels. They demonstrated that in the retina of guinea pigs, both neuroglobin and mitochondria are restricted to the layer containing the inner segments of the photoreceptors.

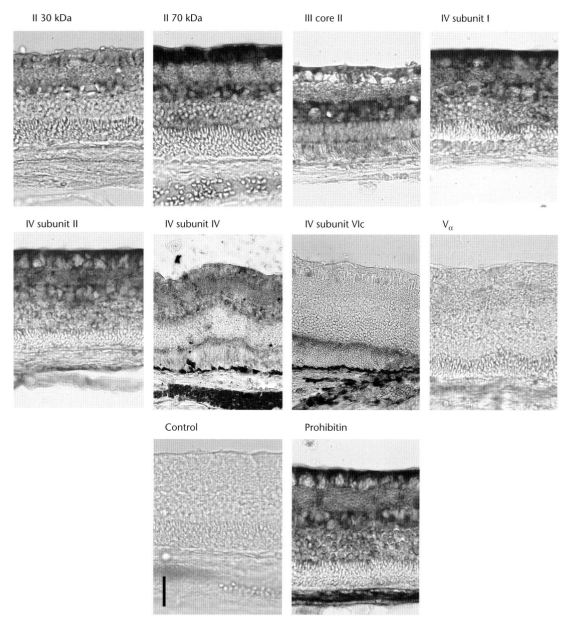

Figure 4.24 Immunohistochemical staining in a pigmented rabbit retina. Mitochondrial antibodies, complex II 30 kDa, 70 kDa, complex III core II, complex IV subunit I, II, IV and VIc, and Vα as well as the control are shown as labeled. Prohibitin staining is used as a marker of mitochondria. Note that although the expression of complex IV subunits in the inner segment of the photoreceptor layer is similar to that in the rat retina, staining in the inner retina is much weaker, particularly for complex IV subunit VIc. Scale bar = 50 μm.

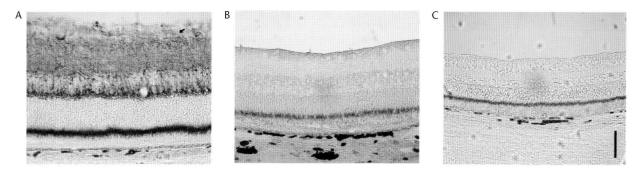

Figure 4.25 Cytochrome oxidase staining of rat retina (A), guinea pig (B), and rabbit retina (C). Note that there is a clearly defined staining of cytochrome oxidase in the inner segment of the photoreceptor layer in all three species, the staining, however, being remarkably different in the inner retina. The outer and inner plexiform layers are clearly stained in the rat retina, but not in the guinea pig or rabbit retina. Scale bar = 50 μm.

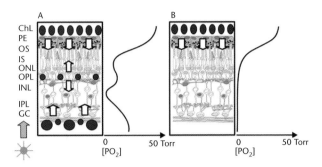

Figure 4.26 Schematic representation of intraretinal oxygen distribution, retinal structure, and vascular supplies in a vascularized and avascular retina (Bentmann, Schmidt, Reuss et al. 2005). Reproduced with permission from the American Society for Biochemistry and Molecular Biology.

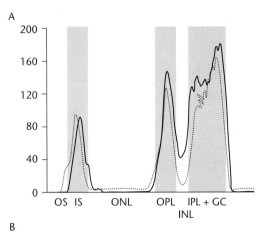

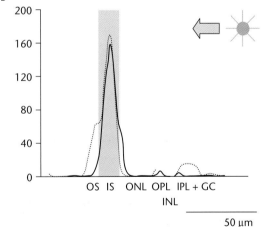

Figure 4.27 Distribution of neuroglobin (solid lines) and cytochrome C (dotted lines) in the vascularized retina of the mouse (A) and the avascular retina of the guinea pig (B) (Bentmann, Schmidt, Reuss et al. 2005). Reproduced with permission from the American Society for Biochemistry and Molecular Biology

In the future it is conceivable that we might be in a position to modulate the expression of particular enzymes in the retina. An initial target might be to increase the enzymes associated with metabolism in the inner retina of avascular species. This may

compensate in part for the presence of retinal ischemia and hypoxia in disease states in vascularized retinas. It appears that the target of metabolic engineering should perhaps begin with manipulating complex IV, particularly subunits IV and VIc. It is now possible to manipulate nucleic acids and gene expression using contemporary genetic engineering techniques, which have the potential to target subunits IV and VIc. However, with our present level of understanding we can make only strategic decisions that may not have a practical solution. Not only has the ability to manipulate the genetics far transcended our ability to predict the effects of these manipulations on metabolism, but our fundamental understanding of metabolic control in the retina also remains very poor. Major metabolic pathways are interconnected in each compartmentation and interactions are also present between these compartmentations within retina. Even if the expression of a gene encoding a particular enzyme such as cytochrome oxidase is suitably manipulated to ameliorate retinal ischemia and diabetic retinopathy, this manipulation may cause a corresponding complex change in retinal metabolism and functions through other pathways in which the enzyme works. From our perspective, metabolic engineering is a logical step for the future rather than a purposeful plan to develop therapeutic intervention, given our current level of understanding. Fortunately, we have an increasing number of tools with which to monitor intraretinal metabolism and retinal function in various animal models of retinal ischemia/hypoxia. In the future, the combination of genetic engineering with other technologies such as biochemistry and physiology will be required to ensure the long-term outcome desired. The management of retinal ischemia/hypoxia via modulation of the metabolic pathways must not be at the expense of other pathways equally important for healthy vision. We should continue to enhance our knowledge in protein/enzyme and metabolic biochemistry as a stepping stone to manipulating metabolic properties of the retina for therapeutic purposes.

CONTROL AND REGULATION OF OCULAR VASCULATURE

Control and Regulation of Ocular Blood Flow Is Crucial for Retinal Cells

The control and regulation of blood flow in the eye is a vital component in maintaining retinal microenvironment in a relatively consistent state and in keeping retinal cell homeostasis. Understanding how such control and regulation is achieved is fundamental to understanding the mechanisms in the communications between retinal neurons and microvasculature within the microcompartment, and the development of appropriate therapeutic strategies aimed at restoring adequate blood flow in disease states. However, this is no simple task, as the mechanisms and molecular pathways responsible for vascular control and regulation are complex, and within the different components that make up the ocular vasculature there is a high degree of heterogeneity in vasoactive properties.

In general, the eye is supplied through an ophthalmic artery, which leads into the ciliary arteries feeding the choroidal/uveal circulation, and a central retinal artery or cilioretinal arteries, which feed the retinal circulation. These two circulations, choroidal and retinal, possess very different properties and constraints. The outer segments of the photoreceptors are where the visual image is focused. This region is avascular to ensure optimal visual acuity with minimum optical interference from any vascular bed. As a consequence, the photoreceptors' main source of nutrients, the choroidal circulation, lies totally outside the retina and supplies the photoreceptor layer with nutrients such as oxygen by passive diffusion (Linsenmeier 1986; Pournaras, Riva, Tsacopoulos et al. 1989; Yu, Cringle 2001). It is known that the oxygen supply from the choroid is barely enough to prevent some regions of the outer retina from becoming hypoxic, which suggests that the high rate of blood flow through the choroid may be essential to maintain a high oxygen level in the choriocapillaris (Linsenmeier 1986). We have further demonstrated that the deep capillary bed also provides oxygen supply to the outer retina when oxygen demand in the inner segment of the photoreceptors is increased such as during the dark adaptation (Yu, Cringle 2002).

The choroidal circulation possesses both sympathetic and parasympathetic innervation (Laties, Jacobowitz 1966), presumably allowing systemic control of choroidal blood flow. However, there has been considerable disagreement as to whether the choroidal circulation is capable of functional regulation (Bill 1962; Friedman 1970; Alm, Bill 1970; Yu, Alder, Cringle et al. 1988; Kiel, Shepherd 1992; Hardy, Abran, Li, et al. 1994). In contrast, the retinal circulation is differently constrained in its design. Although it is responsible for feeding a high metabolic rate tissue, it must be anatomically sparse to minimize optical interference with the light path to the photoreceptors. A further unusual feature of the retinal circulation is that it has no autonomic innervation (Laties 1967), so total reliance must be placed on local vascular control mechanisms. These requirements result in a limited flow circulation, with a high arteriovenous oxygen tension difference. This circulation has in general, two capillary beds, one feeding into the nerve fiber/ganglion cell layer and the other

feeding the middle retinal layers including the inner nuclear layer and plexiform layers. There is no controversy about the regulatory ability of the retinal circulation. It has long been accepted that the retinal circulation has powerful regulatory mechanisms. Human and animal data demonstrate that flow in the major vessels is regulated (measured by laser Doppler velocimetry) and that the circulation regulates in response to changes in blood pressure and (Grunwald, Riva, Brucker et al. 1984a). Moreover, we have demonstrated that in the rat retina the oxygen level in the region supported by the superficial capillary layer is well regulated, while that of the deeper capillary layer is not (Yu, Cringle, Alder et al. 1994b). This apparent vulnerability of the deep capillary bed area is an important observation as it provides a possible explanation for the high incidence of pathological involvement of the deep capillaries in retinal vascular disease (Yanoff, Fine 1989). The feeder vessels to the eye are also involved in the regulation of ocular blood flow and it is known that their vasoactive properties can vary significantly along their length (Yu, Su, Alder et al. 1992c). This adds yet another dimension to the heterogeneity of vascular control mechanisms in the ocular vasculature.

In any particular vessel there are a number of competing or complementary mechanisms that are responsible for locally regulating the vessel tone. These local factors combine to ensure that the blood flow to the tissue is matched to the metabolic requirements. To understand the local control mechanisms, in vitro preparations have been used to study the vascular reactivity of different components of the ocular vasculature, determining their response to blood-borne factors, tissue-released factors, and factors released from the autonomic system. This integration of total blood flow is known to be achieved by the continuous and dynamic interplay between many regulatory factors, including factors emanating from the blood, the endothelial and smooth muscle cells of the vessel walls, the surrounding metabolizing tissue, and the input pressure.

Several hypotheses have been tested in an attempt to understand whole organ regulation in other organs such as the brain and kidney (Holstein-Rathlou, Marsh 1994; Defily, Chilian 1995), but no such hypothesis has yet been proposed for ocular circulations. To partially remedy this deficit, the research covered in this chapter takes the first step in unraveling control mechanisms of the individual components of the ocular circulation. The vascular endothelium is a vital component of vascular regulation. It consists of a monolayer of thin squamous cells, which line the inside surface of blood vessels. One intracellular structure implicated in sensing external changes and mediating the output of the huge array of autocoids known to change smooth muscle cell response is the cytoskeleton. The cytoskeleton gives the cell its shape as well as mediates the transmission of intracellular signaling. The response of the endothelium to shear stresses associated with local blood flow is another important mechanism for regulation of blood flow (Smiesko, Johnson 1993).

Given the complexity of all the factors involved in the regulation of vascular tone, it is perhaps not surprising that systemic diseases such as diabetes disrupt the normal control mechanisms. Of all the vascular diseases of the retina, diabetic retinopathy is the probably the most extensively studied and documented (Cogan, Toussaint, Kuwabara 1961; Davis 1992; Frank 1995). The frustrating feature of human diabetic retinopathy is that the disease follows a long, clinically silent course, during which undetectable vascular and neural damages occur, some of which are irreversible by the time the damage is revealed clinically. It is vital that the cascade of vascular changes is better understood, and in this respect the availability of rat models of induced diabetes provides a useful avenue for research (Su, Alder, Yu et al. 2000; Yu, Yu, Cringle et al. 2001c).

Vasoactivity of Ocular Vasculature Can Be Modulated

Although most ocular vessels consist of only one cell layer of endothelium and a few layers of smooth muscle cells, clear-cut definitions of the mechanisms and effects of many vasoactive substances have not yet been obtained. However, the effects of vasoactive endogenous and pharmacologic substances have been studied by our and other groups. Controversy exists concerning the responses of the retinal vasculature to catecholamines (Alm 1972; Forster, Ferrari-Dileo, Anderson 1987). However, direct vascular responsiveness must be demonstrated before concluding that any induced vasoactivity may be important.

It has been shown that noradrenaline, adrenaline, and phenylephrine induce a contractive response in the cat ophthalmociliary artery (Yu, Su, Alder et al. 1992c), and in the human long posterior ciliary artery (Yu, Alder, Su et al. 1992b). We have also shown that noradrenaline, adrenaline, and phenylephrine induce vascular contraction in intact ocular vasculature (Su, Yu, Alder et al. 1995), in isolated ophthalmic artery, and in retinal arterioles and veins (Yu, Alder, Su et al. 1992b; Yu, Su, Alder et al. 1992c; Alder, Su, Yu et al. 1993; Yu, Cringle, Alder et al. 1994b). An asymmetry in the responses to adrenergic agonists with contractions significantly larger when the drug was applied to the intraluminal surface rather than extraluminal surface has also been demonstrated (Yu, Alder, Cringle et al. 1994a).

Unlike other vasculatures, there is clear evidence that much of the ocular vasculature is relatively devoid of β-adrenergic receptors, and, as demonstrated in vitro in several species of animals and in humans, that any β-adrenergic receptors present are at best only weakly functional (Nielsen, Nyborg 1989a; Hoste, Boels, Andries et al. 1990; Yu, Alder, Su et al. 1992a; Yu, Alder, Su et al. 1992b; Yu, Su, Alder et al. 1992c; Su, Yu, Alder et al. 1995). Thus, one would anticipate a minimal β-adrenergic effect in the retinal vasculature. Our group has demonstrated that 5-hydroxytryptamine (5-HT) induces contractile responses in the long posterior ciliary artery and ophthalmic arteries (Yu, Alder, Su et al. 1992b; Yu, Su, Alder et al. 1992c) and in isolated perfused eye preparations (Su, Yu, Alder et al. 1995) as well as isolated retinal arteriole preparations. These results imply that 5-HT receptors are present in the ocular vasculature.

We have demonstrated that histamine induces potent contractile responses in the cat ophthalmociliary artery with significantly heterogenous response in the proximal and distal segments of the same artery (Yu, Su, Alder et al. 1992c). However, in the human posterior ciliary artery, histamine produced biphasic responses (Yu, Alder, Su et al. 1992b). More recently, we have compared the differences between histamine-induced responses in retinal arterioles and in the posterior ciliary artery in the pig. We demonstrated that histamine induces opposing vasoactive effects at different levels of the porcine ocular vasculature (Su, Yu, Alder et al. 2005). In examining the mechanism of action in the retinal arterioles, we found that in retinal arterioles the histamine-induced vasodilatation may be mediated by endothelial cell H_1 receptors and by H_2 receptors on the smooth muscle cells. Acetylcholine has not only been implicated as a mediator of vascular tone but also been recognized as an important pharmacological tool to assay the endothelium function (Angus, Lew 1992).

The endothelium modulates smooth muscle cell activity by releasing vasoactive substances such as endothelium-derived relaxing factor/nitric oxide, and potent vasoconstrictor endothelin-1. Damaged or dysfunctional endothelium therefore has an important role in the pathology of vascular diseases. It is known to cause endothelium-dependent vasodilatation by stimulating the release of nitric oxide from the endothelium. This endothelium-dependent dilatation function has been shown to be impaired in the vasculature of many organs in diseases such as hypertension and diabetes. Hypertension and diabetes have associated ocular pathologies, such as hypertensive or diabetic retinopathy, which have specific relevance to the vascular component of the eye. It is therefore suspected that endothelial dysfunction also occurs in the eye vasculature. Several studies (Su, Yu, Alder et al.

1994; Bakken, Vincent, Sjaavaag et al. 1995; Stowe, O'Brien, Chang et al. 1997) on normal ocular circulations have been performed using acetylcholine. The responses varied with species studied but most studies demonstrated endothelium-dependent vasodilation effects of acetylcholine administration on isolated retinal vessels, isolated eyes, and ring segments of ophthalmic arteries. In vitro studies from our laboratory on human retinal vessels (Yu, Su, Cringle et al. 1998) have also demonstrated vasodilatation with acetylcholine administration. Furthermore, we have specifically addressed the question of tone dependency in acetylcholine-induced relaxation response using isolated eye preparation (Yu, Yu, Cringle et al. 2000c). The issue of tone dependency is important in view of vascular disease situations as in systemic hypertension or glaucoma where perfusion pressure is altered. If tone dependency exists in acetylcholine-induced dilatation responses, then this has implications for the ability of vessels to dilate with acetylcholine in disease states and also for the interpretation of acetylcholine studies. Our results show that acetylcholine-induced relaxation responses are highly dependent on vascular tone in the rat ocular vasculature. Particularly, there is a strong linear relationship between acetylcholine-induced vascular relaxation and precontracted perfusion pressure at higher dosages of acetylcholine (Yu, Yu, Cringle et al. 2000c).

The dopaminergic system, like those of all other neurotransmitters, can effect alterations in ocular blood flow by a number of distinct mechanisms. Contractile response to dopamine in cat ophthalmociliary arteries is only $\approx 50\%$ of that to noradrenaline and 30% of K^+-induced contraction under the same conditions (Yu, Su, Alder et al. 1992c). Dopamine induced contraction in the human long posterior ciliary artery but these were less potent than seen in the cat ophthalmociliary artery (Yu, Alder, Su et al. 1992b).

The prostanoids and other arachidonate-mediated metabolites represent a vast family of compounds; there are at least two issues of direct interest to the ocular vasculature. A large number of diverse eicosanoids such as prostaglandin $F_2\alpha$ ($PGF_2\alpha$) and prostacyclin are known to be potent modulators of the ocular circulation. Second, a number of eicosanoids have been used as therapeutic agents for glaucoma. $PGF_2\alpha$ is known to have contractile effects on the feeder vessels to the eye (Su, Yu, Alder et al. 1994; Ohkubo, Chiba 1987; Su, Yu, Alder et al. 1995; Hoste 1997; Stjernschantz, Selen, Astin et al. 2000) and also in bovine retinal arteries (Nielsen, Nyborg 1989b; Hoste, Andries 1991). However, comparatively little is known about the vasoactive effect of $PGF_2\alpha$ and other prostanoids on retinal arterioles. We have

studied vasoactive effects of selected prostanoids on retinal arterioles (Yu, Su, Cringle et al. 2001b) and demonstrated that in normal tone arterioles without endothelin 1 (ET-1) contraction, $PGF_2\alpha$ and the thromboxane A_2 analog U46619 both produced a potent dose-dependent contraction. In ET-1 contracted retinal arterioles, U46619 produced further contraction, whereas $PGF_2\alpha$ produced a slight vasodilatation.

Endothelins are endogenous vasocontracting peptide agents. ET-1, ET-2, and ET-3 are produced in a variety of tissues, where they act as modulators of important cell processes and act through binding to two classes of transmembrane receptors, ETa and ETB, where the stimulation of several signaling pathways leads to their mitogenic, vasoconstriction, and developmental actions. ET-1 has been shown to be one of the most potent vasocontractors in the ocular vasculature. Significant reduction in blood flow in the retina, choroid, and optic nerve head by exogenously administered ET-1 has been reported in humans and in a number of animal species (Granstam, Wang, Bill 1992; Sugiyama, Haque, Onda et al. 1996; Dallinger, Dorner, Wenzel et al. 2000; Kiel 2000; Polak, Petternel, Luksch et al. 2001). Altered plasma concentration of ET-1 has been demonstrated in a variety of ocular diseases, such as retinal vein occlusion (Masaki, Yanagisawa 1992), glaucoma (Liu, Chen, Casley et al. 1990; Kaiser, Flammer, Wenk et al. 1995), diabetic microangiopathy (Ak, Buyukberber, Sevinc et al. 2001), and ocular microangiopathy syndrome in patients with acquired immune deficiency syndrome (Geier, Rolinski, Sadri et al. 1995). Normal plasma level of ET-1 is about 1 to 8 pg/mL (0.4 to 3.2×10^{-12} M) (Masaki, Yanagisawa 1992; Iannaccone, Letizia, Pazzaglia et al. 1998), and the values in these reported diseases are roughly twice those of normal subjects. However, 10^{-12} to 10^{-7} M ET-1 induced potent contraction of porcine ciliary artery with EC of 8.3 (Meyer, Lang, Flammer et al. 1995). ET-1 induced dose-dependent vasocontraction in retinal arterioles with a similar range of dosage. Extraluminal ET-1 application, 10^{-9} M, $\approx EC_{50}$ of the vasocontraction, produced a potent and stable vasocontraction in the pig and human retinal arterioles (Yu, Su, Cringle et al. 1998; Yu, Su, Cringle et al. 2001b). More recently, we have found that retinal arterioles exhibit asymmetry in their responses to ET-1, with contractions significantly larger when the drug was applied to the extraluminal surface rather than to the intraluminal surface (Yu, Su, Cringle et al. 2003). Vasoactive factors stimulate endothelial cells to release ET-1. Release of ET-1 stimulates ETA receptors on smooth muscle and ETB on endothelial cells. Two factors, prostacyclin and endothelium-derived relaxing factor (EDRF), are released and act on smooth muscle cells as vasorelaxation factors. It is likely that ET-1 levels in the vicinity of the smooth muscle cells could be more than 1 ng/mL, which is significantly higher than that seen in the plasma. As ET-1 is locally secreted, only that portion, a several-thousand-times smaller amount of ET-1, crossing back across the endothelium will enter the plasma, making plasma concentration of 1 to 2 pg/mL. Therefore, there is a diffusion barrier for ET-1 and an efficient regulatory system in the vascular wall, particularly in microvessels. In general, data on levels of circulating ET-1 in blood or plasma do not provide any valid information on local activity of this system, nor do they allow association of enhanced formation rates to particular cells or tissues. At best, levels of circulating ET-1 give some information regarding the "overall" activity of the system.

Adenosine, along with the excitatory amino acids glutamate and aspartate, is known to be released from ischemic and hypoxic neural tissue (Rudolphi, Schubert, Parkinson et al. 1992; Sciotti, Park, Berne et al. 1997). Indeed, elevation of aspartate and glutamate are both accompanied by an increase in extracellular adenosine (Sciotti, Park, Berne et al. 1997). The excitatory amino acids are damaging to neural cells, whereas the concomitant release of adenosine has been shown to ameliorate the damage. Indeed, extracellular concentrations of adenosine increase in ischemia in a graded fashion by factors of greater than 10, with extracellular adenosine concentration being related to the level of tissue ischemia, a necessary criterion if it is to function as a vasoactive signaler. In the retina, adenosine has been shown to cause retinal artery dilatation after vitreal microsuffusion onto the vessels, acting through A_2 receptors (Gidday, Park 1993a; Gidday, Park 1993b). Experimental increase of endogenous adenosine was also accompanied by dilatation. We have demonstrated an asymmetrical response to exogenous adenosine in retinal arterioles in that extraluminal administration of adenosine produces a dose-dependent dilatation, whereas intraluminal adenosine fails to produce a significant dilatation response (Alder, Su, Yu et al. 1996). In vivo, in hypoxic or ischemic situations, adenosine is released by extraluminal neural tissue and minimizes tissue damage, partially by acting as a signaler of metabolic status to the vasculature, leading to vasodilatation and increased local blood flow. Thus, adenosine is capable of both signaling metabolic needs and causing vasodilatation in the retina. Normally, extracellular levels of adenosine are about 10^{-7} M, which is close to the threshold values found in our and other studies for extraluminal application (Park, Gidday 1990; Rudolphi, Schubert, Parkinson et al. 1992; Alder, Su, Yu et al. 1996). Adenosine probably acts as a neuromodulator as well as a vascular mediator in the retina. A_1 and A_2 receptors are also present in neural tissue.

Dynamic alterations in blood insulin and glucose levels are hallmark features of both insulin-dependent and non–insulin-dependent diabetes. Within the retina, the vasculature is the prime site of diabetes-induced changes (Cogan, Toussaint, Kuwabara 1961). Insulin is known to exert diverse biological effects. Insulin has a physiological role to play in controlling vascular activity in some vessels (Baron 1994). We tested the hypothesis that insulin dilates retinal arterioles by a direct mechanism. Our results showed that extraluminal delivery of insulin alone had no significant effect on vessel diameter. Intraluminal delivery of insulin produces a dose-dependent mild dilatation, whereas combined intraluminal and extraluminal application of insulin causes remarkable dilatation at all concentrations (Su, Yu, Alder et al. 1996). These results imply that insulin is a vascular regulator in normal conditions and may have relevance to the vascular changes occurring in diabetes and hypertension in the retina.

Both plasmalemma and sarcoplasmic reticulum membranes establish a Ca^{2+} concentration gradient of about 10,000-fold. $[Ca^{2+}]_i$ in the resting smooth muscle cell lies between 120 and 270 nM and rises to 500 to 700 nM in the activated smooth muscle cell. This means that $[Ca^{2+}]_i$ of smooth muscle cells in the activated condition is only 3 to 4 times higher than that in the resting condition. The voltage-activated Ca^{2+} channels are often loosely referred to as Ca^{2+} channels although three major Ca^{2+} control pathways, voltage-activated Ca^{2+} channels, receptor-operated Ca^{2+} channels, and Na^+-Ca^{2+} exchangers, are present. The biological role of L-type Ca^{2+} channels is well established and most current calcium-channel entry blockers act on L-type Ca^{2+} channels. The three major subclasses of Ca^{2+} entry blockers have demonstrated important differences in their inhibitory potency, when their action on cerebral vessels is compared. The dihydropyridines are the most potent, with IC_{50} values usually around 10^{-8} M to 10^{-9} M, reaching even 10^{-10} M in some cases, whereas the phenylkylamines and benzothiazepines have significantly higher IC_{50} values. We have extensively studied the effects of calcium-channel entry blockers. Our data from studies on human and pig retinal arteries are comparable with similar studies on cerebral vessels (Yu, Su, Cringle et al. 1998). The relative importance of the intracellular and extracellular Ca^{2+} sources in contributing to vasodilatation has been shown to vary in different regions of the vasculature, as well as with different vasoactive agents. For example, we have demonstrated that the phasic component of an α_1-adrenergic contraction is mainly dependent on intracellular Ca^{2+} stores, whereas the tonic component relies almost exclusively on extracellular Ca^{2+} (Yu, Alder, Su et al. 1992a). It is well recognized that the selectivity of Ca^{2+} entry blockers depends on the tissue (with greater selectivity in cerebral arteries when compared with other peripheral arteries), the species, the vasoconstrictor agent used, and the chemical type of the Ca^{2+} entry blocker, which probably reflects differences not only in the quantity but also in the quality of the Ca^{2+} channels activated in the different cases.

In addition to these vasoactive substances, other factors, such as oxygen, pH, blood flow and pressure, can also modulate vessel tone. Oxygen tension in vivo is known to play an important role in regulating retinal blood flow (Grunwald, Riva, Petrig et al. 1984b). Our results (Alder, Su, Yu et al. 1993) indicated that endothelial cells modify the intrinsic smooth muscle response to a gradual reduction in Po_2 by releasing relaxing and contracting factors, causing the observed dichotomous response in noradrenaline-activated vessels. However, the KCl-induced response is only modulated by low oxygen tensions (Alder, Su, Yu et al. 1993).

We have studied the effects of changes in extracellular pH (pHe) on passive tone and agonist responses in the ophthalmociliary artery and mediator roles of the endothelial cells in any pH-induced effect to explore the ability of the ophthalmociliary artery to influence retinal and choroidal blood flow in response to metabolic stimuli (Su, Yu, Alder et al. 1994). Our results show that $PGF_2\alpha$ produces a concentration-dependent contraction that is insensitive to an alkaline shift but sensitive to acidic shifts. All pHe-induced relaxations of K^+ are endothelium independent. Passive tension is unaffected by all pHe manipulations.

We have demonstrated myogenic responses and flow-induced dilatation in the retinal artery (Yu, Alder, Cringle et al. 1994a). Pressure dependency in vasoactive substance–induced vascular responses is also present in the intact ocular vascular preparation. As mentioned, we have demonstrated perfusion pressure dependency in acetylcholine-induced relaxation response using an isolated eye preparation (Yu, Yu, Cringle et al. 2000c).

Although a vascular component in glaucoma is more controversial, there is an increasing body of evidence that blood flow changes are involved. There is also evidence that some glaucoma medications may help restore retinal blood flow in addition to their IOP-lowering effect (Drance 1997; Yu, Su, Cringle et al. 1998). There is clearly scope for investigating new therapeutic agents that may beneficially influence ocular blood flow in disease states.

SUMMARY

This chapter has briefly described retinal cellular metabolism and its regulation and control, based largely on our work in the fields of retinal oxygen metabolism and vascular biology. Retinal neurons have

a high functional activity, yet the retina necessarily has a limited blood supply, creating the need for a delicate balance between metabolic supply and demand. This renders the retina particularly vulnerable to ischemic/hypoxic insults, which play a major role in many retinal diseases. The significant heterogeneity of intraretinal oxygen distribution in the normal and diseased conditions suggests that there is a potent ability to regulate and control retinal and vascular cells. Studies of retinal cellular metabolism should include their microenvironment, including the relationship between neural and glial cells and the microvasculature. Many molecules such as neurotransmitters are not only involved in retinal neurons but also in regulation of retinal vasculature. Understanding the control and regulation mechanisms of the retinal neuron is essential for knowing how these cells are able to perform their demanding functions for our whole life and how to protect them from physiological and pathological challenges. However, the complexity and dynamic nature of retinal cellular metabolism and its control and regulation are still far beyond our current knowledge. The layered structure of the retina provides us with a golden opportunity to look into the compartments within the retina at the spatial and temporal level. Many molecules including ions and proteins have been shown to be involved and multiple pathways have been identified. These molecules and pathways are interlinked and interact in physiological conditions maintaining intracellular homeostasis. Functional activity of these molecules and pathways could be modulated to help adapt to external environmental changes and pathological challenges. Each molecule may have multiple effects such as a signaling molecule to perform a physiological role or becoming a pathogenic factor if its location or concentration is disrupted. For example, oxygen is the most important molecule for oxidative metabolism and for keeping cells viable and functional; however, "extra" oxygen may be problematic in some locations. It is critical that each key molecule has the appropriate distribution under physiological conditions and that changes in pathological conditions can be accommodated by regulatory pathways. Some important insights into retinal cellular metabolism and its control and regulation have been gained from our multidisciplinary approach. We believe that knowledge gained in this field, either from retinal cellular metabolism and its regulation and control or vascular regulation, and determination of the system's ability to respond to changes in the internal or external environment and the response to induced retinal diseases is valuable. No doubt that retina has a strong capability to stabilize the intra- and extracellular environment through various molecules and pathways. This provides us a great opportunity to further investigate and explore the pathogenesis of ocular ischemic/hypoxic diseases and ultimately assist in the development of new therapeutic strategies.

ACKNOWLEDGMENTS Funding was provided by the National Health and Medical Research Council of Australia and the ARC Centre of Excellence in Vision Science.

REFERENCES

Ahmed J, Braun RD, Dunn R, Linsenmeier RA. 1993. Oxygen distribution in the Macaque Retina. *Invest Ophthalmol Vis Sci.* 34:516–521.

Aiello LP, Avery RL, Arrigg PG et al.1994. Vascular endothelial growth factor in ocular fluid of patients with diabetic retinopathy and other retinal disorders. *N Engl J Med.* 331:1480–1487.

Ak G, Buyukberber S, Sevinc A et al. 2001. The relation between plasma endothelin-1 levels and metabolic control, risk factors, treatment modalities, and diabetic microangiopathy in patients with Type 2 diabetes mellitus. *J Diabetes Complic.* 15:150–157.

Alder VA, Cringle SJ, Constable IJ. 1983. The retinal oxygen profile in cats. *Invest Ophthalmol Vis Sci.* 24:30–36.

Alder VA, Ben-nun J, Cringle SJ. 1990. PO_2 profiles and oxygen consumption in cat retina with an occluded retinal circulation. *Invest Ophthalmol Vis Sci.* 31:1029–1034.

Alder VA, Yu D-Y, Cringle SJ, Su EN. 1991. Changes in vitreal oxygen tension distribution in the streptozotocin-diabetic rat. *Diabetologia.* 34:469–476.

Alder VA, Su EN, Yu D-Y, Cringle SJ. 1993. Oxygen reactivity of the feline isolated ophthalmociliary artery. *Invest Ophthalmol Vis Sci.* 34:1–9.

Alder VA, Su EN, Yu D-Y, Cringle SJ, Yu PK. 1996. Asymmetrical response of the intraluminal and extraluminal surfaces of the porcine retinal artery to exogenous adenosine. *Exp Eye Res.* 63:557–564.

Alm A. 1972. Effects of norepinephrine, angiotensin, dihydroergotamine, papaverine, isoproterenol, histamine, nicotinic acid, and xanthinol nicotinate on retinal oxygen tension in cats. *Acta Ophthalmol.* 50:707–719.

Alm A, Bill A. 1970. Blood flow and oxygen extraction in the cat uvea at normal and high intraocular pressure. *Acta Physiol Scand.* 80:19–28.

Ames A. 1983. Earliest irreversible changes during ischemia. *Am J Emerg Med.* 2:139–146.

Ames A. 1992. Energy requirements of CNS cells as related to their function and to their vulnerability to ischemia: a commentary based on studies on retina. *Can J Pharmacol.* 70:S158–S164.

Ames A. III 2000. CNS energy metabolism as related to function. *Brain Res. Brain Res. Rev.* 34:42–68.

Ames A, Li YY. 1992. Energy requirements of glutamatergic pathways in rabbit retina. *J Neurosci.* 12:4234–4242.

Ames A, Li YY, Heher EC, Kimble CR. 1992. Energy metabolism of rabbit retina as related to function: high cost of Na$^+$ transport. *J Neurosci.* 12:840–853.

Anderson B. 1968. Ocular effects of changes in oxygen and carbon dioxide tension. *Trans Am Ophthalmol Soc.* 66:423–474.

Anderson B, Saltzman HA. 1964. Retinal oxygen utilization measured by hyperbaric blackout. *Arch Ophthalmol.* 72:792–795.

Angus JA, Lew MJ. 1992. Interpretation of the acetylcholine test of endothelial cell dysfunction in hypertension. *J Hypertens.* 10:S179–S186.

Arden GB, Wolf JE, Tsang Y. 1998. Does dark adaption exacerbate diabetic retinopathy? Evidence and a linking hypothesis. *Vision Res.* 38:1723–1729.

Bakken IJ, Vincent MB, Sjaavaag I, White LR. 1995. Vasodilation in porcine ophthalmic artery: peptide interaction with acetylcholine and endothelial dependence. *Neuropeptides.* 29:69–75.

Balaratnasingam C, Morgan WH, Bass L, Matich G, Cringle SJ, Yu D-Y. 2007. Axonal transport and cytoskeletal changes in the laminar regions following elevated intraocular pressure. *Invest Ophthalmol Vis Sci.* 48:3632–3644.

Baron ad. 1994. Hemodynamic actions of insulin. *Am J Physiol.* 30:E187–E202.

Beckers HJM, Klooster J, Vrensen GFJM, Lamers WPMA. 1993. Facial parasympathetic innervation of the rat choroid, lacrimal glands and ciliary ganglion. *Ophthalmic Res.* 25:319–330.

Beiran I, Reissman P, Scharf J, Nahum Z, Miller B. 1993. Hyperbaric oxygenation combined with nifedipine treatment for recent-onset retinal artery occulsion. *Eur J Ophthalmol.* 3:89–94.

Bentmann A, Schmidt M, Reuss S, Wolfrum U, Hankeln T, Burmester T. 2005. Divergent distribution in vascular and avascular mammalian retinae links neuroglobin to cellular respiration. *J Biol Chem.* 280:20660–20665.

Bereiter-Hahn J, Voth M. 1994. Dynamics of mitochondria in living cells: shape changes, dislocations, fusion and fission of mitochondria. *Microsc Res Tech.* 27:198–219.

Berkowitz BA, Wilson CA, Hatchell DL. 1991a. Oxygen kinetics in the vitreous substitute perfluorotributylamine: a ^{19}F NMR study in vivo. *Invest Ophthalmol Vis Sci.* 32:2382–2387.

Berkowitz BA, Wilson CA, Hatchell DL, London RE. 1991b. Quantitative determination of the partial oxygen pressure in the vitrectomized rabbit eye in vivo using ^{19}F NMR. *Magn Reson Med.* 21:233–241.

Berkowitz BA, Penn JS. 1998. Abnormal panretinal response pattern to carbogen inhalation in experimental retinopathy of prematurity. *Invest Ophthalmol Vis Sci.* 39:840–845.

Berkowitz BA, Ito Y, Kern TS, McDonald C, Hawkins R. 2001. Correction of early subnormal superior hemiretinal DeltaPO(2) predicts therapeutic efficacy in experimental diabetic retinopathy. *Invest Ophthalmol Vis. Sci.* 42:2964–2969.

Bill A. 1962. Intraocular pressure and blood flow through the uvea. *Arch Ophthalmol.* 67:336–348.

Birol G, Wang S, Budzynski EWangsa-Wirawan ND, Linsenmeier RA. 2007. Oxygen distribution and consumption in the macaque retina. *Am J Physiol. Heart Circ Physiol.* 293:H1696–H1704.

Braun RD, Linsenmeier RA, Goldstick TK. 1995. Oxygen consumption in the inner and outer retina of the cat. *Invest Ophthalmol Vis Sci.* 36:542–554.

Bresnick GH. 1970. Oxygen-induced visual cell degeneration in the rabbit. *Invest Ophthalmol.* 9:373–387.

Brinchmann-Hansen O, Myhre K. 1989. The effect of hypoxia on the central light reflex of retinal arteries and veins. *Acta Ophthalmol. (Copenh).* 67:249–255.

Buttery RG, Haight JR, Bell K. 1990. Vascular and avascular retinae in mammals. A funduscopic and fluorescein angiographic study. *Brain Behav Evol.* 35:156–175.

Caldwell RB, Roque RS, Solomon SW. 1989. Increased vascular density and vitreo-retinal membranes accompany vascularization of the pigment epithelium in the dystrophic rat retina. *Curr Eye Res.* 8:923–937.

Chase J. 1982. The evolution of retinal vascularization in mammals. A comparison of vascular and avascular retinae. *Ophthalmology.* 89:1518–1525.

Cogan DG, Toussaint D, Kuwabara T. 1961. Retinal vascular pattern. IV Diabetic retinopathy. *Arch Ophthalmol.* 66:366–378.

Cooper RL. 1990. Blind registrations in Western Australia: a five-year study. *Aust N Z J Ophthalmol.* 18:421–426.

Coyle JT, Puttfarcken P. 1993. Oxidative stress, glutamate, and neurodegenerative disorders. *Science.* 262:689–695.

Cringle SJ, Yu D-Y, Alder VA, Su EN. 1993. Retinal blood flow by hydrogen clearance polarography in the streptozotocin-induced diabetic rat. *Invest Ophthalmol Vis Sci.* 34:1716–1721.

Cringle S, Yu D-Y, Alder V, Su EN, Yu PK. 1996a. Modelling oxygen consumption across an avascular retina. *Aust N Z J Ophthalmol Suppl.* 24:70–72.

Cringle S, Yu D-Y, Alder V, Su EN, Yu PK. 1996b. Oxygen consumption in the avascular guinea pig retina. *Am J Physiol.* 40:H1162–H1165.

Cringle SJ, Yu D-Y, Su EN, Alder VA, Yu PK. 1998. Quantification of retinal oxygen consumption changes from preretinal oxygen transients. *Aust N Z J Ophthalmol.* 26:S71–S73.

Cringle SJ, Yu D-Y, Alder VA, Su EN. 1999. Light and choroidal PO_2 modulation of intraretinal oxygen levels in an avascular retina. *Invest Ophthalmol Vis Sci.* 40:2307–2313.

Cringle SJ, Yu D-Y. 2002. A multi-layer model of retinal oxygen supply and consumption helps explain the muted rise in inner retinal PO_2 during systemic hyperoxia. *Comp Biochem Physiol.* 132:61–66.

Cringle SJ, Yu D-Y, Yu PK, Su EN. 2002. Intraretinal oxygen consumption in the rat in vivo [published erratum appears in *Invest Ophthalmol Vis Sci.* 2003 Jan;44(1)]. *Invest Ophthalmol Vis Sci.* 43:1922–1927.

Cringle SJ, Yu D-Y. 2004. Intraretinal oxygenation and oxygen consumption in the rabbit during systemic hyperoxia. *Invest Ophthalmol Vis Sci.* 45:3223–3228.

Dallinger, Dorner GT, Wenzel R et al. 2000. Endothelin-1 contributes to hypoxia-induced vasoconstriction in the human retina. *Invest Ophthalmol Vis Sci.* 41:864–869.

Davis MD. 1992. Diabetic Retinopathy. A Clinical Overview. *Diabetes Care.* 15:1844–1874.

Dean FM, Arden GB, Dornhorst A. 1997. Partial reversal of protan and tritan colour defects with inhaled oxygen in insulin-dependent diabetic subjects. *Br J Ophthalmol.* 81:27–30.

Defily DV, Chilian WM. 1995. Coronary microcirculation: autoregulation and metabolic control. *Basic Res Cardiol.* 90:112–118.

Drance SM. 1997. Glaucoma: a look beyond intraocular pressure. *Am J Ophthalmol.* 123:817–819.

Eintrei C, Lund N. 1986. Effects of increases in the inspired oxygen fraction on brain surface oxygen pressure fields in pig and man. *Acta Anaesthesiol Scand.* 30:194–198.

Forster BA, Ferrari-Dileo G, Anderson DR. 1987. Adrenergic $alpha_1$ and $alpha_2$ binding sites are present in bovine retinal blood vessels. *Invest Ophthalmol Vis Sci.* 28:1741–1746.

Frank RN. 1995. Diabetic retinopathy. *Prog Retina Eye Res.* 14:361–392.

Friedman E. 1970. Choroidal blood flow. Pressure–flow relationships. *Arch Ophthalmol.* 83:95–99.

Gagnon J, Kurowski TT, Weisner RJ, Zak R. 1991. Correlations between a nuclear and a mitochondrial mRNA of cytochrome c oxidase subunits, enzymatic activity and total mRNA content, in rat tissues. *Mol Cell Biochem.* 107:21–29.

Gariano RF, Gardner TW. 2005. Retinal angiogenesis in development and disease. *Nature.* 438:960–966.

Geier SA, Rolinski B, Sadri I et al. 1995. Ocular microangiopathy syndrome in patients with AIDS is associated with increased plasma levels of the vasoconstrictor endothelin-1. *Klin Monatsbl Augenheilkd.* 207:353–360.

Germer A, Biedermann B, Wolburg H et al. 1998a. Distribution of mitochondria within Muller cells I correlation with retinal vascularization in different mammalian species. *J Neurocytol.* 27:329–345.

Germer A, Schuck J, Wolburg H, Kuhrt H, Mack AF, Reichenbach A. 1998b. Distribution of mitochondria within Muller cells. II Post natal development of the rabbit retinal periphery in vivo and in vitro: dependence on oxygen supply. *J Neurocytol.* 27:347–359.

Gidday JM, Park TS. 1993a. Adenosine-mediated autoregulation of retinal arteriolar tone in the piglet. *Invest Ophthalmol Vis Sci.* 34:2713–2719.

Gidday JM, Park TS. 1993b. Microcirculatory responses to adenosine in the newborn pig retina. *Pediatr Res.* 33:620–627.

Granstam E, Wang L, Bill A. 1992. Ocular effects of endothelin-1 in cats. *Curr Eye Res.* 11:325–332.

Grunwald JE, Riva CE, Brucker AJ, Sinclair SH, Petrig BL. 1984a. Altered retinal vascular response to 100% oxygen breathing in diabetes mellitus. *Ophthalmology.* 91:1447–1452.

Grunwald JE, Riva CE, Petrig BL, Sinclair SH, Brucker AJ. 1984b. Effect of pure O_2-breathing on retinal blood flow in normals and in patients with background diabetic retinopathy. *Curr Eye Res.* 3:239–242.

Guillemin K, Krasnow MA. 1997. The hypoxic response: huffing and HIFing. *Cell.* 89:9–12.

Guo W, Cringle SJ, Su EN et al. 2006. Structure and function of myelinated nerve fibers in the rabbit eye following ischemia/reperfusion injury. *Curr Neurovasc Res.* 3:55–65.

Haddad HM, Leopold IH. 1965. Effect of hyperbaric oxygenation on microcirculation: use in therapy of retinal vascular disorders. *Invest Ophthalmol.* 4:1141–1149.

Hamon CG, Cutler P, Blair JA. 1989. Tetrahydrobiopterin metabolism in the streptozotocin induced diabetic state in rats. *Clin Chim Acta.* 181:249–254.

Hardarson SH, Harris A, Karlsson AR et al. 2006. Automatic retinal oximetry. *Invest Ophthalmol Vis Sci.* 47:5011–5016.

Hardy P, Abran D, Li DY, Fernandez H, Varma DR, Chemtob S. 1994. Free radicals in retinal and choroidal blood flow autoregulation in the piglet: interaction with prostaglandins. *Invest Ophthalmol Vis Sci.* 35:580–591.

Harris A, Arend O, Danis RP, Evans D, Wolf S, Martin BJ. 1996. Hyperoxia improves contrast sensitivity in early diabetic retinopathy. *Br J Ophthalmol.* 80:209–213.

Hickam JB, Frayser R. 1966. Studies of the retinal circulation in man: observations on vessel diameter, arteriovenous oxygen difference, and mean circulation time. *Circulation.* 33:302–316.

Holstein-Rathlou NH, Marsh DJ. 1994. A dynamic model of renal blood flow autoregulation. *Bull Math Biol.* 56:411–429.

Hoste am, Andries LJ. 1991. Contractile responses of isolated bovine retinal microarteries to acetylcholine. *Invest Ophthalmol Vis Sci.* 32:1996–2005.

Hoste am. 1997. Reduction of IOP with latanoprost. *Ophthalmology.* 104:895–896.

Hoste am, Boels PJ, Andries LJ, Brutsaert DL, de Laey JJ. 1990. Effects of beta-antagonists on contraction of bovine retinal microarteries in vitro. *Invest Ophthalmol Vis Sci.* 31:1231–1237.

Iannaccone A, Letizia C, Pazzaglia S, Vingolo EM, Clemente G, Pannarale MR. 1998. Plasma endothelin-1 concentrations in patients with retinal vein occlusions. *Br J Ophthalmol.* 82:498–503.

Ikonen E, Fiedler K, Parton RG, Simons K. 1995. Prohibitin, an antiproliferative protein, is localized in mitochondria. *FEBS Lett.* 358:273–277.

Johnston AJ, Steiner LA, Gupta AK, Menon DK. 2003. Cerebral oxygen vasoreactivity and cerebral tissue oxygen reactivity. *Br J Anaesth.* 90:774–786.

Jung C, Higgins CM, Xu Z. 2002. A quantitative histochemical assay for activities of mitochondrial electron transport chain complexes in mouse spinal cord sections. *J Neurosci. Methods.* 114:165–172.

Kaiser HJ, Flammer J, Wenk M, Luscher T. 1995. Endothelin-1 plasma levels in normal-tension glaucoma: abnormal response to postural changes. *Graefes Arch Clin Exp Ophthalmol.* 233:484–488.

Kiel JW. 2000. Endothelin modulation of choroidal blood flow in the rabbit. *Exp Eye Res.* 71:543–550.

Kiel JW, Shepherd AP. 1992. Autoregulation of choroidal blood flow in the rabbit. *Invest Ophthalmol Vis Sci.* 33:2399–2410.

Landers MB. 1978. Retinal oxygenation via the choroidal circulation. *Trans Am Ophthalmol Soc.* 76:528–556.

Laties am. 1967. Central retinal artery innervation. *Arch Ophthalmol.* 77:405–409.

Laties am, Jacobowitz D. 1966. A comparative study of the autonomic innervation of the eye in monkey, cat, and rabbit. *Anat Rec.* 156:383–389.

Leonard JV, Schapira AHV. 2000. Mitochondrial respiratory chain disorders I: mitochondrial DNA defects. *Lancet.* 299–304.

Li H, Grimes P. 1993. Adrenergic innervation of the choroid and iris in diabetic rats. *Curr Eye Res.* 12:89–94.

Linsenmeier RA. 1986. Effects of light and darkness on oxygen distribution and consumption in the cat retina. *J Gen Physiol.* 88:521–542.

Linsenmeier RA, Yancey CM. 1989. Effects of hyperoxia on the oxygen distribution in the intact cat retina. *Invest Ophthalmol Vis Sci.* 30:612–618.

Linsenmeier RA, Braun RD, McRipley MA et al. 1998. Retinal hypoxia in long-term diabetic cats. *Invest Ophthalmol Vis Sci.* 39:1647–1657.

Liu J, Chen R, Casley DJ, Nayler WG. 1990. Ischemia and reperfusion increase ^{125}I-labeled endothelin-1 binding in rat cardiac membranes. *Am J Physiol.* 258:H829–H835.

Lund N, Jorfeldt L, Lewis DH. 1980. Skeletal muscle oxygen pressure fields in healthy human volunteers. A study of the normal state and the effects of different arterial oxygen pressures. *Acta Anaesthesiol Scand.* 24:272–278.

Masaki T, Yanagisawa M. 1992. Physiology and pharmacology of endothelins. *Med Res Rev.* 12:391–421.

Meyer P, Lang MG, Flammer J, Luscher TF. 1995. Effects of calcium channel blockers on the response to endothelin-1, bradykinin and sodium nitroprusside in porcine ciliary arteries. *Exp Eye Res.* 60:505–510.

Molnar I, Poitry S, Tsacopoulos M, Gilodi N, Leuenberger pm. 1985. Effect of laser photocoagulation oxygenation of the retina in miniature pigs. *Invest Ophthalmol Vis Sci.* 26:1410–1414.

Moorman CM, Hamilton am. 1999. Clinical applications of the MicroPulse diode laser. *Eye.* 13 (Pt 2):145–150.

Morgan WH, Yu D-Y, Cooper RL, Alder VA, Cringle SJ, Constable IJ. 1995. The influence of cerebrospinal fluid pressure on the lamina cribrosa tissue pressure gradient. *Invest Ophthalmol Vis Sci.* 36:1163–1172.

Nguyen QD, Shah SM, Van Anden E, Sung JU, Vitale S, Campochiaro PA. 2004. Supplemental oxygen improves diabetic macular edema: a pilot study. *Invest Ophthalmol Vis Sci.* 45:617–624.

Nielsen PJ, Nyborg NCB. 1989a. Adrenergic responses in isolated bovine retinal resistance arteries. *Int Ophthalmol.* 13:103–107.

Nielsen PJ, Nyborg NCB. 1989b. Calcium antagonist-induced relaxation of the prostaglandin-F_2 response of isolated calf retinal resistance arteries. *Exp Eye Res.* 48:329–335.

Noell WK. 1955. Visual cell effects of high oxygen pressures. *American Physiological Society.* 14:107–108.

Noell WK. 1962. Effect of high and low oxygen tension on the visual system. In Schaeffer KE, eds. *Environmental Effects on Consciousness.* New York: Macmillan, 3–18.

Ohkubo H, Chiba S. 1987. Vascular reactivities of simian ophthalmic and ciliary arteries. *Curr Eye Res.* 6:1197–1203.

Ozaki H, Yu AY, Della N et al. 1999. Hypoxia inducible factor-1alpha is increased in ischemic retina: temporal and spatial correlation with VEGF expression. *Invest Ophthalmol Vis Sci.* 40:182–189.

Park TS, Gidday JM. 1990. Effect of dipyridamole on cerebral extracellular adenosine level in vitro. *J Cereb Blood Flow Metab.* 10:424–427.

Plaxton WC. 2004. Principles of metabolic control. In Storey KB, eds. *Functional Metabolism: Regulation and Adaptation.* New York: John Wiley & Sons, 1–24.

Polak K, Petternel V, Luksch A et al. 2001. Effect of endothelin and BQ123 on ocular blood flow parameters in healthy subjects. *Invest Ophthalmol Vis Sci.* 42:2949–2956.

Pournaras CJ, Riva ce, Tsacopoulos M, Strommer K. 1989. Diffusion of O$_2$ in the retina of anesthetized miniature pigs in normoxia and hyperoxia. *Exp Eye Res.* 49:347–360.

Pournaras CJ, Tsacopoulos M, Riva ce, Roth A. 1990. Diffusion of O$_2$ in normal and ischemic retinas of anesthetized miniature pigs in normoxia and hyperoxia. Graefes *Arch Clin Exp Ophthalmol.* 228:138–142.

Pournaras JC, Petropoulos IK, Munoz J-L, Pournaras CJ. 2004. Experimental retinal vein occlusion: effect of acetazolamide and carbogen (95% 02/5% C02) on preretinal P02. *Invest Ophthalmol Vis Sci.* 45:3669–3677.

Riva ce, Grunwald JE, Sinclair SH. 1983. Laser Doppler velocimetry study of the effect of pure oxygen breathing on retinal blood flow. *Invest Ophthalmol Vis Sci.* 24:47–51.

Riva ce, Pournaras CJ, Tsacopoulos M. 1986. Regulation of local oxygen tension and blood flow in the inner retina during hyperoxia. *J Appl Physiol.* 61:592–598.

Riva ce, Cranstoun SD, Grunwald JE, Petrig BL. 1994. Choroidal blood flow in the foveal region of the human ocular fundus. *Invest Ophthalmol Vis Sci.* 35:4273–4281.

Rudolphi KA, Schubert P, Parkinson FE, Fredholm BB. 1992. Adenosine and brain ischemia. *Cerebrovasc Brain Metab Rev.* 4:346–369.

Schofield CJ, Ratcliffe PJ. 2005. Signalling hypoxia by HIF hydroxylases. *Biochem Biophys Res Commun.* 338:617–626.

Sciotti VM, Park TS, Berne RM, Vanwylen DGL. 1997. Changes in extracellular adenosine during chemical or electrical brain stimulation. *Brain Res.* 613:16–20.

Smiesko V, Johnson PC. 1993. The arterial lumen is controlled by flow-related shear stress. *News Physiol Sci.* 8:34–38.

Stefansson E, Wolbarsht ML, Landers MB. 1983. In vivo O$_2$ consumption in rhesus monkeys in light and dark. *Exp Eye Res.* 37:251–256.

Stjernschantz J, Selen G, Astin M, Resul B. 2000. Microvascular effects of selective prostaglandin analogues in the eye with special reference to latanoprost and glaucoma treatment. *Prog Retina Eye Res.* 19:459–496.

Stowe DF, O'Brien WC, Chang D, Knop CS, Kampine JP. 1997. Reversal of endothelin-induced vasoconstriction by endothelium-dependent and -independent vasodilators in isolated hearts and vascular rings. *J Cardiovasc Pharmacol.* 29:747–754.

Su EN, Yu D-Y, Alder VA, Cringle SJ. 1994. Effects of extracellular pH on agonist-induced vascular tone of the cat ophthalmociliary artery. *Invest Ophthalmol Vis Sci.* 35:998–1007.

Su EN, Yu D-Y, Alder VA, Cringle SJ. 1995. Altered vasoactivity in the early diabetic eye: measured in the isolated perfused rat eye. *Exp Eye Res.* 61:699–712.

Su EN, Yu D-Y, Alder VA, Cringle SJ, Yu PK. 1996. Direct vasodilatory effect of insulin on isolated retinal arterioles. *Invest Ophthalmol Vis Sci.* 37:2634–2644.

Su EN, Alder VA, Yu D-Y, Yu PK, Cringle SJ. 2000. Continued progression of retinopathy despite spontaneous recovery to normoglycemia in a long-term study of streptozotocin-induced diabetes in rats. *Graefes Arch Clin Exp Ophthalmol.* 238:163–173.

Su EN, Alder VA, Yu D-Y, Yu PK, Cringle SJ. 2001. Continued progression of retinopathy despite spontaneous recovery to normoglycemia in a long term study of streptozotocin-induced diabetes in rats. *Focus of Diabetic Retinopathy.* 8:41–43.

Su EN, Yu D-Y, Cringle SJ. 2005. Histamine induces opposing vasoactive effects at different levels of the ocular vasculature. *Curr Eye Res.* 30:205–212.

Sugiyama K, Haque MSR, Onda E, Taniguchi T, Kitazawa Y. 1996. The effects of intravitreally injected endothelin-1 on the iris-ciliary body microvasculature in rabbits. *Curr Eye Res.* 15:633–637.

Takagi H, King GL, Ferrara N, Aiello LP. 1996. Hypoxia regulates vascular endothelial growth factor receptor KDR/Flk gene expression through adenosine A2 receptors in retinal capillary endothelial cells. *Invest Ophthalmol Vis Sci.* 37:1311–1321.

The Diabetic Retinopathy Study Research Group. 1987. Indications for photocoagulation treatment of diabetic retinopathy: diabetic retinopathy study report no. 14. *Int Ophthalmol Clin.* 27:239–253.

Tsacopoulos M, Beauchemin ML, Baker R, Babel J. 1976. Studies of experimental retinal focal ischaemia in miniature pigs. In Cant JS, eds. *Vision and Circulation.* London: Henry Kimpton Publishers, 93–103.

Tso MOM, Kurosawa A, Benhamou E, Bauman A, Jeffrey J, Jonasson O. 1988. Microangiopathic retinopathy in experimental diabetic monkeys. *Tr Am Ophth Soc.* 86:389–421.

Vanderkooi JM, Erecinska M, Silver IA. 1991. Oxygen in mammalian tissue: methods of measurement and affinities of various reactions. *Am J Physiol.* 260:C1131–C1150.

Wilson CA, Berkowitz BA, McCuen BW, Charles HC. 1992. Mcasurement of preretinal oxygen tension in the vitrectomized human eye using fluorine-19 magnetic resonance spectroscopy. *Arch Ophthalmol.* 110:1098–1100.

Winkler BS. 1981. Glycolytic and oxidative metabolism in relation to retinal function. *J Gen Physiol.* 77:667–692.

Winkler BS. 1995. A quantitative assessment of glucose metabolism in the isolated rat retina. In Christen Y, Doly M, Droy-Lefaix MT, eds. *Les Seminaires Ophtalmologiques DIPSEN: Vision Et Adaptation.* Amsterdam: Elsevier, 78–96.

Winkler BS, Arnold MJ, Brassell MA, Sliter DR. 1997. Glucose dependence of glycolysis, hexose monophosphate shunt activity, energy status, and the polyol pathway in retinas isolated from normal (nondiabetic) rats. *Invest Ophthalmol Vis Sci.* 38:62–71.

Wolbarsht ML, Landers MB III. 1980. The rationale of photocoagulation therapy for proliferative diabetic retinopathy: a review and a model. *Ophthalmic Surg.* 11:235–245.

Yanoff M, Fine BS. 1989. Chapter 11. Retina. In Cooke DB, Patterson D, Andresen W, Hallowell R, eds. *Ocular Pathology: A Text and Atlas.* Third Edition. Philadelphia: JB Lippincott Company, 377–465.

Yu D-Y, Alder VA, Cringle SJ, Brown MJ. 1988. Choroidal blood flow measured in the dog eye in vivo and in vitro by local hydrogen clearance polarography: validation of a technique and response to raised intraocular pressure. *Exp Eye Res.* 46:289–303.

Yu D-Y, Alder VA, Su EN, Cringle SJ. 1992a. Relaxation effects of diltiazem, verapamil, and tolazoline on isolated cat ophthalmociliary artery. *Exp Eye Res.* 55:757–766.

Yu D-Y, Alder VA, Su EN, Mele EM, Cringle SJ, Morgan WH. 1992b. Agonist response of human isolated posterior ciliary artery. *Invest Ophthalmol Vis Sci.* 33:48–54.

Yu D-Y, Su EN, Alder VA, Cringle SJ, Mele EM. 1992c. Pharmacological and mechanical heterogeneity of cat isolated ophthalmociliary artery. *Exp Eye Res.* 54:347–359.

Yu D-Y, Alder VA, Cringle SJ, Su EN, Yu PK. 1994a. Vasoactivity of intraluminal and extraluminal agonists in perfused retinal arteries. *Invest Ophthalmol Vis Sci.* 35:4087–4099.

Yu D-Y, Cringle SJ, Alder VA, Su EN. 1994b. Intraretinal oxygen distribution in rats as a function of systemic blood pressure. *Am J Physiol.* 36:H2498–H2507.

Yu D-Y, Cringle SJ, Alder VA, Su EN, Yu PK. 1996. Intraretinal oxygen distribution and choroidal regulation in the avascular retina of guinea pigs. *Am J Physiol.* 270:H965–H973.

Yu D-Y, Su EN, Cringle SJ, Alder VA, De Santis L. 1998. Effect of betaxolol, timolol and nimodipine on human and pig retinal arterioles. *Exp Eye Res.* 67:73–81.

Yu D-Y, Cringle SJ, Alder VA, Su EN. 1999. Intraretinal oxygen distribution in the rat with graded systemic hyperoxia and hypercapnia. *Invest Ophthalmol Vis Sci.* 40:2082–2087.

Yu D-Y, Cringle SJ, Su EN, Yu PK. 2000a. Intraretinal oxygen levels before and after photoreceptor loss in the RCS rat. *Invest Ophthalmol Vis Sci.* 41:3999–4006.

Yu D-Y, Cringle SJ, Su EN, Yu PK et al. 2000b. Retinal oxygen distribution in a rat model of retinal ischemia. *Invest Ophthalmol Vis Sci.* 41:S19

Yu PK, Yu D-Y, Cringle SJ, Su EN. 2000c. Acetylcholine-induced relaxation in rat ocular vasculature. *J Ocul Pharmacol Ther.* 16:447–454.

Yu D-Y, Cringle SJ. 2001. Oxygen distribution and consumption within the retina in vascularised and avascular retinas and in animal models of retinal disease. *Prog Retina Eye Res.* 20:175–208.

Yu D-Y, Cringle SJ, Su EN, Yu PK, Jerums G, Cooper ME. 2001a. Pathogenesis and intervention strategies in diabetic retinopathy. *Clin Experiment Ophthalmol.* 29:164–166.

Yu D-Y, Su EN, Cringle SJ, Schoch C, Percicot CP, Lambrou GN. 2001b. Comparison of the vasoactive effects of the docosaoid unoprostone and selected prostanoids on isolated perfused retinal arterioles. *Invest Ophthalmol Vis Sci.* 42:1499–1504.

Yu PK, Yu D-Y, Cringle SJ, Su EN. 2001c. Tetrahydrobiopterin reverses the impairment of acetylcholine-induced vasodilatation in diabetic ocular microvasculature. *J Ocul Pharmacol Ther.* 17:123–129.

Yu D-Y, Cringle SJ. 2002. Outer retinal anoxia during dark adaptation is not a general property of mammalian retinas. *Comp Biochem Physiol.* 132:47–52.

Yu D-Y, Su EN, Cringle SJ, Yu PK. 2003. Isolated preparations of ocular vasculature and their applications in ophthalmic research. *Prog Retina Eye Res.* 22:135–169.

Yu D-Y, Cringle SJ. 2004. Low oxygen consumption in the inner retina of the visual streak of the rabbit. *Am J Physiol Heart C.* 286:H419–H423.

Yu D-Y, Cringle SJ, Valter K, Walsh N, Lee D, Stone J. 2004. Photoreceptor death, trophic factor expression, retinal oxygen status and photoreceptor function in the P23H rat: stress and protection in a slow degeneration. *Invest Ophthalmol Vis Sci.* 45:2013–2049.

Yu D-Y, Cringle SJ, Su EN. 2005a. Intraretinal oxygen distribution in the monkey retina and the response to systemic hyperoxia. *Invest Ophthalmol Vis Sci.* 4728–4733.

Yu D-Y, Cringle SJ, Su EN, Yu PK. 2005b. Retinal degeneration and local oxygen metabolism. *Exp Eye Res.* 80:745–751.

Yu D-Y, Cringle SJ, Su EN, Yu PK, Humayun MS, Dorin G. 2005c. Laser induced changes in intraretinal oxygen distribution in pigmented rabbits. *Invest. Ophthalmol Vis Sci.* 46:988–999.

Yu PK, Yu D-Y, Cringle SJ, Su EN. 2005d. Endothelial f-actin cytoskeleton in the retinal vasculature of normal and diabetic rats. *Curr Eye Res.* 30:279–290.

Yu D-Y, Cringle SJ. 2006. Oxygen distribution in the mouse retina. *Invest Ophthalmol Vis Sci.* 47:1109–1112.

Yu D-Y, Cringle SJ, Yu PK, Su EN. 2007. Intraretinal oxygen distribution and consumption during retinal artery occlusion and hyperoxic ventilation in the rat. *Invest Ophthalmol Vis Sci.* 48:2290–2296.

Chapter **5**

CROSS TALK BETWEEN THE AUTONOMIC AND CENTRAL NERVOUS SYSTEMS: MECHANISTIC AND THERAPEUTIC CONSIDERATIONS FOR NEURONAL, IMMUNE, VASCULAR, AND SOMATIC-BASED DISEASES

Fuad Lechin and Bertha van der Dijs

ABSTRACT

In the present chapter, we summarize anatomical, physiological, pathophysiological, pharmacological, immunological, and some therapeutic information dealing with most types of diseases. We present evidence supporting our postulation that clinical symptoms (cardiovascular, gastrointestinal, respiratory, dermatological, nephrological, rheumatological, haemathological, endocrinological, and others) depend on central nervous system (CNS) disorders that project to the peripheral organs throughout the peripheral autonomic nervous system (ANS) and neuroendocrine pathways. In addition, psychological disturbances such as depression, psychosis, and so on also provoke ANS, hormonal, and immunological disorders that are responsible for different somatic symptoms. Finally, we present evidence showing that the adrenal glands are hypoactive during both childhood and senescence. This peripheral ANS profile explains why they are affected by specific pathophysiological disorders that are rarely observed in young adult subjects. This physiological profile depends on the predominance of the A5(NA) nucleus at the CNS level in the groups mentioned.

We present data emanating from the routine assessment of circulating neurotransmitters that showed that diseases are underlain by PNS or adrenal sympathetic overactivity. The former ANS profile is underlain by very high noradrenaline over adrenaline plasma ratio, whereas the latter depends on a very low noradrenaline/adrenaline ratio. Predominance of the A5(NA) is responsible for the neural sympathetic overactivity, whereas C1(Ad) medullary nuclei display overwhelming activity in the other group. The fact that both CNS nuclei interchange inhibitory axons explains the ANS peripheral dissociation.

We have quoted evidence showing that the two ANS profiles are paralleled by two different immunological profiles. The TH-1 immune profile is registered in patients affected by neural sympathetic predominance, whereas the TH-2 immunological profile is registered in patients affected by adrenal sympathetic overactivity. Furthermore, we also present evidence showing that an adequate neuropharmacological therapy, addressed to revert the neuroimmunological disorders mentioned, was able to provoke clinical, ANS, and immunological normalization.

In addition, we have described neuropharmacological manipulations addressed to revert the ANS and CNS disorders responsible for both types of diseases. We have alerted physicians about the deleterious effects triggered by the labeling of neuropharmacological drugs as "antidepressants" or "antipsychotics" or "anxiolytics," and so on. These labels, introduced by the pharmaceutical industry, interfere with the scientific information that allows adequate therapeutic approaches addressed to normalize both the CNS and peripheral ANS disturbances.

We have devoted special attention to the physiological and pathophysiological mechanisms that underlie senescence. We afford a bulk of evidence showing that the A6(NA) neurons (locus coeruleus) fade with aging. Thus, taking into account that the number of these neurons is also minimized in both children and psychotics facilitates the understanding of the similarity of the clinical profiles shared by these three groups. The aforementioned fading depends on the peripheral neural sympathetic preponderance (poor adrenal sympathetic activity). Furthermore, other psychiatric disorders such as endogenous depression and post-traumatic stress disorder are also underlain by the aforementioned CNS profile. These facts facilitate some types of speculations. For instance, psychotics and depressed subjects are able to commit suicide whereas obese subjects affected by hyperinsulinism parallel this psychological behavior because they are not able to reduce feeding, which is responsible for the progressive damage of their health. The well-demonstrated fact showing that these patients show neural sympathetic overactivity—A5(NA) predominance and A6(NA) underactivity—supports our postulation. Finally, the demonstrated fact that neuropharmacological manipulations addressed to revert the disorders mentioned earlier is addressed to enhance A6(NA) activity supports the inferences.

We devoted some limited information dealing with the physiology and pathophysiology of sleep. The routine assessment of circulating neurotransmitters throughout the polysomnographic investigation in both normal and diseased subjects led us to postulate that all diseases are underlain by one of the two types of disorders. Our findings showing that adrenaline plasma levels reach zero values at the first 10 minutes of supine resting (waking) state, whereas noradrenaline reaches minimal values (but not zero values) at the first REM sleep period support the postulation that the A5(NA) does not interrupt its activity at any period. This phenomenon explains why systolic but not diastolic blood pressure showed maximal reduction during the sleep cycle. Furthermore, the finding that neither diastolic blood pressure nor noradrenaline plasma level show significant reductions in patients affected by the obstructive sleep apnea syndrome supports the postulation that this sleep disorder is registered in patients affected by neural sympathetic activity (essential hypertension, hyperinsulinism, obesity and all types of TH-1 autoimmune diseases). Furthermore, taking into account that these patients are also affected by a short REM latency allows the inference that the A5(NA) overwhelming overactivity is annulled by the A6(NA) activity. The latter is responsible for the maintenance of the slow-wave sleep (SWS), the disappearance of which allows the abrupt appearance of the REM sleep stage.

In addition, we support our point of view with a great deal of research papers that describe the neuropharmacological therapeutic success of hundreds of patients affected by the aforementioned two types of ANS disorders.

Keywords: central nervous system, peripheral autonomic nervous system, neural immune interactions, neural system, parasympathetic system, noradrenaline, adrenaline, serotonin, stress, depression, psychosis, post-traumatic stress disorder, Alzheimer's disease, myasthenia gravis, multiple sclerosis, sleep disorders, gastrointestinal diseases, irritable bowel syndrome, pancreatitis, carcinoid, malignant diseases, thrombocytopenic purpura, polycythemia vera, thrombostasis, bronchial asthma.

Most clinicians, physiologists, and pharmacologists tend to consider the peripheral autonomic nervous system (ANS) as a two-faced structure that displays two opposite functional roles, which would underlie all clinical syndromes. Furthermore, most of them are not aware that these clinical syndromes depend on a complex cross talk among the central nervous system (CNS) nuclei, which integrate interacting circuits responsible for both central and peripheral physiological and pathophysiological oscillations. This simpleness may lead to deleterious therapeutic manipulations (Swedberg, Brislow, Cohn et al. 2002; Lechin, Lechin, van der Dijs 2002d). In addition, this lack of knowledge has also led to the inability to find adequate neuropharmacological manipulations aimed at successful therapeutic approaches. In addition, clinicians should be aware that drugs can act at both peripheral and/or CNS levels; hence, they must know that the CNS circuitry is provided by a complex diversity of circuits and receptors and, thus, that the "black versus white" (sympathetic vs. parasympathetic) concept is an anachronism that interferes with the advance of the medical sciences.

CENTRAL NERVOUS SYSTEM CIRCUITRY RESPONSIBLE FOR THE FUNCTIONING OF THE PERIPHERAL AUTONOMIC NERVOUS SYSTEM

Anatomical, Physiological, and Neuropharmacological Data

Both monoaminergic and acetylcholinergic (ACh) neurons integrate the CNS circuitry responsible for the peripheral ANS activity. Monoaminergic nuclei include the noradrenergic (NA), adrenergic (Ad), dopaminergic (DA), serotonergic (5-HT), and histaminergic (H) neurons; these nuclei are modulated by excitatory glutamatergic and inhibitory GABAergic neurons.

Noradrenergic System

Noradrenergic nuclei include the A6 (locus coeruleus), the A5, the A2, and the A1 nuclei. The A6(NA) pontine nucleus comprises some 18,000 neurons, whereas the pontomedullary A5 and the medullary A2 and A1 nuclei include progressively decreasing numbers of NA neurons. The A6(NA) nucleus sends monosynaptic and polysynaptic axons to the A5(NA) and C1(Ad) nuclei, respectively. In addition, the A6(NA) receives monosynaptic inhibitory axons from the latter nuclei (Lechin, van der Dijs, Hernandez-Adrian 2006a; Lechin, van der Dijs 2006a, 2006b).

Both A6(NA) and A5(NA) pontine and the C1(Ad) medullary nuclei are crowded by inhibitory α-2 receptors (Langer, Angel 1991). In addition, the A5(NA) and the C1(Ad) medullary nuclei interchange inhibitory axons also (Li, Wesselingh, Blessing 1992; Fenik, Marchenko, Janssen et al. 2002). According to these facts and considering that the C1(Ad) and the A5(NA)

nuclei are responsible for the adrenal and the neural sympathetic activities, respectively, the A6(NA) or locus coeruleus nucleus is able to modulate both branches of the peripheral sympathetic system. These two sympathetic branches can function in association or dissociation, according to the physiological circumstances (Young, Rosa, Landsberg 1984).

A6(NA) VERSUS A5(NA) INTERACTIONS Both nuclei interchange inhibitory axons (Byrum, Guyenet 1987; Dampney 1994). Although predominance of the former is observed during wakefulness, it diminishes during the supine resting and sleep periods. Maximal reduction of the A6(NA) activity is seen during rapid eye movement (REM) sleep (Lechin, Pardey-Maldonado, van der Dijs et al. 2004a), at which time, A5(NA) neurons display slight but significant firing activity. Predominance of the A5(NA) over the A6(NA) is also observed at the 1-minute orthostasis state. However, both types of NA neurons are excited during all types of exercise (Lechin, van der Dijs, Lechin et al. 1997a). In addition, there also exist several types of polysynaptic A6(NA) versus A5(NA) interactions. For instance, the A6(NA) sends excitatory and inhibitory polysynaptic drives to the medullary C1(Ad) nuclei, whereas the latter sends inhibitory axons to both the A6(NA) and the A5(NA) nuclei (Kostowski 1979; Levitt, Moore 1979; Young, Rosa, Landsberg 1984; Ennis, Aston-Jones 1987; Pieribone, Aston-Jones 1991; Fenik, Marchenko, Janssen, et al. 2002). This cross talk explains the black versus white—C1(Ad) versus A5(NA) activity—when the A6(NA) nucleus is exhausted (uncoping stress state) (Anisman, Irwin, Sklar 1979; Fenik, Marchenko, Janssen et al. 2002).

Adrenergic System

The adrenergic system includes the ventrolateral medullary C1(Ad), C2(Ad), and C3(Ad) nuclei, which interchange modulatory axons with cholinergic, noradrenergic, and serotonergic medullary nuclei as well as with supramedullary (pontine) and inframedullary (spinal) structures. Special mention should be made of the interconnections between C1(Ad) and the pontine nuclei A5(NA), A6(NA), and dorsal raphe nucleus DR(5-HT), and to the C1(Ad) axons, which innervate the spinal sympathetic preganglionic (ACh) neurons responsible for the adrenal gland secretion (Granata, Numao, Kumada et al. 1986; Byrum, Guyenet 1987; Pieribone, Aston-Jones 1991; Li, Wesselingh, Blessing 1992).

Dopaminergic System

The DA-A10 ventral tegmental area (VTA) neurons release dopamine at cortical levels, whereas A8(DA) and A9(DA) subcortical neurons are responsible for the mesostriatal and mesolimbic subcortical areas (Hand, Kasser, Wang 1987a; Hand, Hu, Wang 1987b; Vezina, Blanc, Glowinski et al. 1991). Dopaminergic cortical system modulates dopaminergic subcortical system through both glutamate and γ-aminobutyric acid (GABA) intermediary neurons. Cortical and subcortical dopaminergic systems are positively correlated with intellectual and emotional, and motility behaviors, respectively (Sagvolden 2006).

Serotonergic System

Six major serotonergic nuclei distributed along the midline of the CNS pontomedullary area integrate the serotonergic CNS, in addition to serotonergic neurons grouped at the hypothalamus. This system includes the pontine median raphe (MR)—B8 and B9; the dorsal raphe (DR)—B7 and the periaqueductal gray (PAG); and the medullary raphe magnus (RM)—raphe obscurus (RO) and raphe pallidus (RP). In addition, there exist several serotonergic small nuclei located at the hypothalamic level (Lechin, van der Dijs, Hernandez-Adrian 2006a).

ROLE OF THE SEROTONERGIC SYSTEM IN THE CNS CIRCUITRY RESPONSIBLE FOR THE PERIPHERAL ANS Serotonergic axons arising from the pontine and medullary nuclei modulate the DA, NA, Ad, and ACh nuclei. Serotonergic axons exert excitatory effects on the release of prolactin, growth hormone, corticotrophin releasing hormone (CRH), and adrenocorticotropic hormone (ACTH) by acting at the paraventricular hypothalamic nucleus (PVN), at which level a complex cross talk among NA, DA, and 5-HT neurons is responsible for the neuroendocrine CNS versus peripheral interactions (Herman, Ostrander, Mueller et al. 2005; Ho, Chow, Yung 2007).

These monoaminergic, acetylcholinergic, and hormonal interactions are too complex a crossroad that makes it difficult to assign a specific physiological role to each of these 5-HT nuclei. Furthermore, the fact that some of the serotonergic neurons are not protected by the blood–brain barrier (BBB) makes them accessible to both CNS and peripheral stimuli (Lechin, van der Dijs, Hernandez-Adrian 2006a; Lechin, van der Dijs 2006a, 2006b).

The DR(5-HT) axons modulate A6(NA) neurons and in addition, DR(5-HT) axons innervate cortical areas, which also receive A6(NA) axons. These phenomena are consistent with the absolute A6(NA) versus DR(5-HT) antagonism. Thus, exhaustion of DR(5-HT) neurons allows the excessive release of noradrenaline from the A6 axons. This unbalance underlies the obsessive-compulsive syndrome (during acute maniac periods). The noradrenergic over serotonergic predominance has been also demonstrated at the ventral hippocampus area, which receives both types of axons. This neurochemical unbalance is consistent with the therapeutic effects triggered in these patients by drugs that provoke serotonin release and, in addition, inhibit the uptake of 5-HT by both serotonergic dendrites and axons (Lechin, van der Dijs, Lechin 2002a).

Serotonin released from DR(5-HT) axons modulates the CNS circuitry responsible for the ANS activity. We will mention some examples for this. The DR(5-HT) axons are able to inhibit A6(NA) neurons that would redound in the A5(NA) over the A6(NA) predominance (neural sympathetic predominance). However, because A5(NA) axons excite and inhibit DR(5-HT) neurons by acting at α-1 and α-2 postsynaptic receptors, respectively any prolongation of this unbalance would be responsible for the exhaustion of DR(5-HT) neurons. These pathophysiological mechanisms have been postulated to be underlying endogenous depression (ED), essential hypertension (EH), hyperinsulinism, and all TH-1 autoimmune diseases. A great bulk of clinical and scientific evidence supports the above postulations. In summary, there exists enough evidence that allows postulating that the above psychiatric, somatic, and autoimmune diseases are caused by the predominance of both A5(NA) over A6(NA), and C1(Ad), and MR(-5-HT) over DR(5-HT). This postulation is reinforced by the successful neuropharmacological therapy addressed to normalize the CNS and neuroautonomic disorders (Lechin, van der Dijs, Lechin 2002a; Lechin, van der Dijs, Hernandez-Adrian 2006a; Lechin, van der Dijs 2006a, 2006b).

DR VERSUS MR INTERACTIONS A great bulk of evidence demonstrates that the DR(5-HT) neurons are positively correlated with the C1(Ad) medullary nuclei, whereas the MR(5-HT) neurons display the opposite physiological role and cooperate with the A5(NA) neural sympathetic activity. These DR(5-HT) and C1(Ad) versus MR(5-HT) and A5(NA) interaction constitutes two complex neuroendocrine circuitries responsible for two types of physiological mechanisms, whose disorders underlie most clinical syndromes (Lechin, van der Dijs, Hernandez-Adrian 2006a).

Noradrenergic Versus Serotonergic Interactions

The A5(NA) but not the A6(NA) modulates the DR(5-HT) nucleus (Pudovkina, Cremers, Westerink 2002). In turn, the latter sends inhibitory axons to the A6(NA) neurons (Szabo, Blier 2001). Noradrenaline released from the A5(NA) axons excites and inhibits DR(5-HT) neurons. Excitation is exerted through α-1 receptors whereas inhibition depends on α-2 receptors (Saavedra, Grobecker, Zivin 1976; Marwaha, Aghajanian 1982).

Although the MR(5-HT) neurons do not receive significant inhibitory and/or excitatory axons from other nuclei, they send inhibitory axons to both the A6(NA) (Marwaha, Aghajanian 1982) and the DR(5-HT) nuclei (Saavedra, Grobecker, Zivin 1976; Vertes, Fortin, Crane 1999). The fact that MR(5-HT) neurons are organized as a long chain of neurons and not within a compact nucleus helps understand this physiological peculiarity.

According to the physiological cross talk, the predominance of the MR(5-HT) activity triggers inhibition of the A6(NA) and DR(5-HT) nuclei and disinhibition of the A5(NA) neurons. In addition, predominance of the latter provokes inhibition of the C1(Ad) medullary nuclei. In short, the A5(NA) and MR(5-HT) binomial is the CNS circuitry responsible for the neural sympathetic (peripheral) hyperactivity, which underlies EH (Lechin, van der Dijs, Hernandez-Adrian 2006a; Lechin, van der Dijs 2006a), hyperinsulinism (Lechin, van der Dijs 2006b), ED (Lechin, van der Dijs, Orozco et al. 1995a), and TH-1 autoimmune diseases (as will be discussed in subsequent text) (Lechin, van der Dijs, Lechin 2002a).

Conversely, the C1(Ad)—DR(5-HT) circuitry is positively correlated with the adrenal sympathetic activity that underlies non–essential hypertension and all psychosomatic syndromes associated with the "uncoping stress" disorder (Lechin, van der Dijs, Lechin et al. 1993; Peyron, Luppi, Fort et al. 1996).

Both the A6(NA) and the DR(5-HT) nuclei receive excitatory (glutamic) and inhibitory (GABA) axons from the brain cortex. In turn, both nuclei innervate the frontal and other cortical areas. In addition, A6(NA) axons excite the A10(DA) neurons (DA mesocortical nucleus) (Tassin 1992). This noradrenergic and dopaminergic cortical drive is responsible for the high-level intellectual function (Lechin, van der Dijs, Lechin 1979a; Lechin, van der Dijs 1989). This latter activity is attenuated by the release of serotonin from DR(5-HT) axons (at both pre- and postsynaptic levels). Thus, any deficit of noradrenaline and dopamine at cortical areas is responsible for the neurochemical and physiological disorders that underlie both psychological and intellectual activities (psychosis, attention-deficit hyperactive disorder [ADHD], Alzheimer's disease, ED, and post-traumatic stress disorder [PTSD]) (Lechin, van der Dijs 1989). This noradrenaline and dopamine cortical deficit is also triggered by the overactivity of DR(-5-HT) neurons such as that seen in anxiety patients and subjects affected by sleep disorders (Lechin, van der Dijs,

Lechin 2002a). It should be taken into account that both A6(NA) and A10(DA) neurons become silent at the rapid eye movement (REM) sleep stage, at which period they are at absolute resting state. Thus, all types of sleep disorders, which interfere with the restoration of the above nuclei, will facilitate their exhaustion. Exhaustion of the A6(NA), A10(DA), and DR(5-HT) neurons is also seen in most types of convulsive syndromes. These syndromes are triggered by the abrupt discharge of cortical pyramidal neurons (that release glutamate). The nonmodulated glutamatergic discharge should be attributed to a deficit of the GABA bridle, which would result in the intermittent (epileptic) noradrenergic and dopaminergic discharges at cortical and other CNS levels (Lechin, van der Dijs, Lechin 2002a). These noncontinuous flowing would favor also the alternation of up- and downregulation of noradrenergic and dopaminergic postsynaptic receptors, which should potentiate all types of convulsive syndromes. The above inference receives strong support from findings showing that most anticonvulsant drugs are GABAmimetic and/or serotonin-releasing drugs.

Acetylcholinergic System

The ACh CNS includes both cortical and subcortical neurons. Cortical neurons are short axon ACh neurons (interneurons) whereas several ACh nuclei integrated by long axon neurons are located in the pontine and medullary areas. They include the pedunculopontine nucleus (PPN) or gigantotegmental field (GTF) and the medullary nuclei tractus solitarius (NTS), nucleus ambiguus, nucleus reticularis gigantocellularis, nucleus originis dorsalis vagi, and area postrema (AP). The ACh nuclei receive long axons from all monoaminergic nuclei as well as from the nucleus originis nervi hypoglossi, and the trigeminal and the phrenic nuclei. In addition, a bulk of ACh neurons is disseminated through the brain stem reticular formation. Ach neurons, which integrate the aforementioned medullary dorsal vagal complex (DVC), receive excitatory axons from the RM and RO serotonergic neurons and inhibitory axons from the A6(NA) and the A5(NA) nuclei. In addition, DVC(ACh) and C1(Ad) medullary nuclei interchange excitatory and inhibitory axons. This interchange of axons allows the fast modulation of the peripheral autonomic nervous system. Special mention should be made of the AP. This ACh nucleus is located at the floor of the IV ventricle, and hence the blood–brain barrier (BBB) does not protect these neurons; they transmit signals from the peripheral blood to the CNS fast. This mechanism allows quick responses addressed to restore homeostasis (Lechin, van der Dijs, Lechin 2002a; Lechin, van der Dijs 2006a, 2006b).

PERIPHERAL AUTONOMIC NERVOUS SYSTEM

Both the parasympathetic and the sympathetic branches of the peripheral ANS depend on the CNS circuitry that includes catecholaminergic, serotonergic, and acetyl cholinergic neuronal nuclei. In addition, the peripheral sympathetic system is integrated by two well-differentiated branches: (1) neural sympathetic and (2) adrenal sympathetic. These two branches may display independent and/or associated activities, according to the physiological and pathophysiological requirements.

CNS Circuitry Underlying Neural Sympathetic Activity

The CNS circuitry underlying neural sympathetic activity includes the A5(NA) pontomedullary nucleus, which sends glutamatergic axons to the lumbar lateral spinal area. ACh neurons located at this segment send ACh axons to lumbar sympathetic (but not thoracic sympathetic) ganglia. Acetylcholine released from these preganglionic axons excites postganglionic NA neurons, which are provided by ACh (nicotine) receptors. Axons that are emanated from these sympathetic ganglia (sympathetic nerves) release noradrenaline at the target areas (muscles, gastrointestinal, cardiovascular, endocrine, peripheral blood, etc.). In addition, noradrenaline released at the adrenal gland from the sympathetic nerves triggers inhibition of these glands by acting at α-2 receptors located at this level (Lechin, van der Dijs, Azócar et al. 1988a; Lechin, van der Dijs, Lechin et al. 1989a; Porta, Emsenhuber, Felsner et al. 1989; Engeland 1998; Lechin, van der Dijs 2006b) (Fig. 5.1). Noradrenaline released at these glands inhibits both the cortisol and adrenaline secretions.

CNS Circuitry Underlying Adrenal Sympathetic Activity

CNS circuitry underlying adrenal sympathetic activity includes the C1(Ad) medullary nuclei, which sends glutamatergic axons to the thoracic spinal segment. ACh neurons located at this segment send axons to the adrenal glands, which are modified sympathetic ganglia. These glands are also crowded by nicotine receptors whose excitation by ACh released from the thoracic sympathetic (preganglionic) axons triggers adrenal gland secretion (adrenaline 80%, dopamine 10%, and noradrenaline 10% approximately). Both sympathetic nerves and adrenal gland secretions are released to the blood; however, it should be known that sympathetic nerves are able to take up circulating noradrenaline, adrenalin, and dopamine. The catecholamines might be released further (Lechin, van der Dijs, Azócar et al. 1988a; Lechin, van der Dijs, Lechin et al. 1989a; Lechin, van der Dijs 2006b).

In addition, it should be known that sympathetic nerves are provided by a dopamine (neuronal) pool; thus, dopamine is coreleased with noradrenaline from these terminals. This dopamine pool is excited during neural sympathetic activity and exerts a modulatory role. Dopamine, which is released before noradrenaline during neural sympathetic excitation, acts at DA-2 inhibitory autoreceptors located at these nerves, to limit further noradrenaline release (Mercuro, Rossetti, Rivano et al. 1987; Mannelli, Pupilli, Fabbri et al. 1988). Pathophysiological predominance of this inhibitory mechanism is responsible for the orthostatic hypotension syndrome. This phenomenon is also observed in patients affected by the Shy Dragger syndrome as well as after the therapeutic administration of DA-2 agonists, such as bromocriptine and L-dopa.

The aforementioned branches (neural and adrenal) of the peripheral sympathetic system may act in association or dissociation, according to the physiological and/or pathophysiological circumstances (Young, Rosa, Landsberg 1984).

Neural Sympathetic Predominance

Stressor agents such as restraint, photic, acoustic, and psychological agents excite the MR(5-HT) but not the DR(5-HT) neurons. The latter are inhibited by the MR(5-HT) axons that release serotonin at postsynaptic 5-HT-1A and 5-HT-2 receptors located at the DR(5-HT) nucleus. In addition, the MR(5-HT) axons excite the CNS circuitry, which includes the central nucleus of the amygdala (CEA), A5(NA), bed nucleus of stria terminalis (BNST), and PVN. No significant participation of the C1(Ad) and the A6(NA) nuclei is seen under this circumstance because both nuclei are inhibited by the A5(NA) and MR(5-HT) axons. Glutamate neurons located at the A5(NA) nucleus send excitatory axons to the lumbar sympathetic (ACh) but not to the thoracic sympathetic (ACh) preganglionic neurons. Acetylcholine released from axons of these sympathetic neurons synapses at the lumbar sympathetic (NA) ganglia, which are provided with nicotine (excitatory) receptors. NA axons, which arise from these sympathetic ganglia, constitute the sympathetic nerves. Noradrenaline released from these nerves inhibits the adrenal gland secretion of both

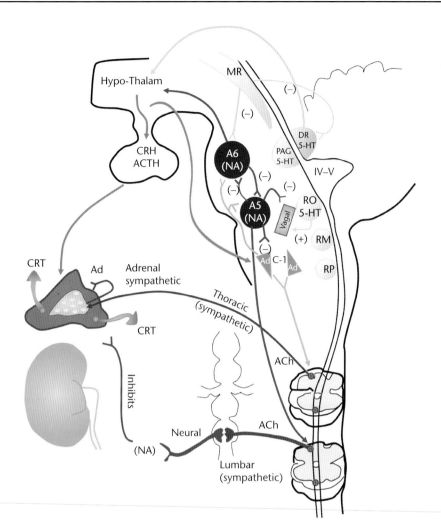

Figure 5.1 Central nervous system (CNS) plus peripheral autonomic nervous system circuitry responsible for both adrenal and neural sympathetic activity. Pontomedullary A5(NA) and C1(Ad) nuclei are responsible for neural and adrenal sympathetic activity, respectively. A5(NA) axons excite acetylcholine (ACh) spinal (preganglionic) neurons whose axons synapse at the neural sympathetic ganglia. Acetylcholine release at this level excites postsynaptic noradrenergic (NA) neurons, whose axons integrate sympathetic nerves. These postsynaptic sympathetic neurons are provided with ACh nicotine receptors; thus, ACh released from preganglionic sympathetic axons act at this level. Medullary C1(Ad) axons excite ACh-preganglionic neurons located at the thoracic lateral spinal segment. Ach axons from these neurons innervate the adrenal gland and excite ACh nicotine receptors responsible for the adrenal gland secretion. In addition to these two branches of the peripheral sympathetic system, ACTH released to the blood by hypophysis excites the release of cortisol from the adrenal cortical gland. Both the adrenaline and cortisol secretions depend on a common CNS circuitry, which includes the A6(NA), the hypothalamic paraventricular nucleus (PVN), and the C1(Ad) nuclei. Both sympathetic activities may act in association or dissociation, according to the physiological requirements. At the CNS level, dissociation depends on the interchange of inhibitory axons between the A5(NA) and C1(Ad) nuclei. Noradrenaline released from the former and Ad released from the latter nuclei act at postsynaptic α-2 inhibitory receptors, located at both type of neurons. At the peripheral level, noradrenaline released from sympathetic nerves inhibits corticoadrenal gland whereas CRT crosses the BBB and excites the DR(5-HT) and C1(Ad) nuclei and inhibits the sympathetic ganglia. These anatomical and physiological interactions allow the modulation of the peripheral sympathetic system.

catecholamines and cortisol (Engeland 1998). The CNS and peripheral interconnections mentioned are consistent with the high noradrenaline/adrenalin plasma ratio observed in these circumstances. In addition, it also explains the nonsignificant increase of cortisol in the plasma, seen during this type of stress (Lechin, van der Dijs, Lechin et al. 1994a; Lechin, van der Dijs 2006a, 2006b).

Adrenal Sympathetic Predominance

ANS unbalance is observed during most types of acute stress that can trigger the activation of the A6(NA), DR(5-HT), C1(Ad), PVN(CRH), and ACTH–cortisol cascade (Anisman 1978). The fact that the motility behavior excites the DR(5-HT) and the C1(Ad) nuclei but not the MR(5-HT) neurons explains the CNS–peripheral cascade, which provokes this type of stress (Jacobs, Heym, Trulson 1981). Prolongation of this behavior triggers the progressive inhibition of the A6(NA) neurons because both adrenalin and serotonin are coreleased at this nucleus from axons arising from the C1(Ad) and the DR(5-HT) nuclei, respectively. In addition, adrenalin released from the C1(Ad) axons limits and/or inhibits the A5(NA) neurons, responsible for neural sympathetic activity, by acting at α-2 postsynaptic receptors located at the somatodendritic area of these neurons (Li, Wesselingh, Blessing 1992; Lechin, van der Dijs, Benaim 1996a; Fenik, Marchenko, Janssen et al. 2002).

Parasympathetic Predominance

The uncoping stress disorder is caused by two alternating periods: (1) adrenal sympathetic predominance and (2) parasympathetic predominance. Neural sympathetic drive is absent in both circumstances. Raised adrenalin and plasma serotonin (f5-HT) underlie both alternating periods. The raised f5-HT depends on the maximal serotonin release from the enterochromaffin cells excited by the enhanced parasympathetic drive. In addition, the raised levels of plasma adrenalin observed during this uncoping stress syndrome triggers platelet aggregation. Serotonin arising from platelets is split to the plasma.

Carcinoid Syndrome

Carcinoid syndrome should be included among the uncoping stress disorders. Both adrenal sympathetic hyperactivity and raised cortisol plasma levels are observed in these patients (Lechin, van der Dijs, Orozco et al. 2005c). Noradrenaline plasma level does not rise at the 1-minute orthostasis challenge, and in addition, the adrenalin plasma levels show maximal increases through the exercise challenge. The facts that both f5-HT and platelet serotonin (p5-HT) reach maximal levels during relapsing periods indicate overactivation of both the enterochromaffin cells and the adrenal gland. These cells are submitted to two opposite neurological stimuli: parasympathetic (excitatory) and neural sympathetic (inhibitory) (Tobe, Izumikawa, Sano et al. 1976). The latter is absent during relapsing periods. In addition, enterochromaffin cells are also present at both hepatic and pancreatic areas. Patients affected by this type of tumor, present symptomatic and symptomless alternating periods. Gastrointestinal (diarrhea, vomit, abdominal pain, etc.) and cardiovascular (tachycardia, extrasystoles, blood pressure

fall) symptoms are seen during relapsing periods. Lung metastases are frequently observed. Worsening and death cannot be avoided because of liver, pancreatic, and lung metastases.

Circulating 5-HT arises from the enterochromaffin cells that release it in response to parasympathetic drive (Tobe 1974). Although most serotonin is secreted into the intestinal lumen, a fraction reaches portal circulation. Serotonin that escapes from uptake by the liver and lungs is trapped by platelets (Rausch, Janowsky, Risch et al. 1985). However, some fraction of serotonin always remains free in the plasma (f5-HT). The normal f5-HT/p5-HT circulating ratio is about 0.5% to 1%. This ratio increases during both platelet aggregation and deficit of platelet uptake (Larsson, Hjemdahl, Olsson et al. 1989). Both circulating acetylcholine because of hyperparasympathetic activity and circulating dopamine interfere with platelet uptake (De Keyser, De Waele, Convents et al. 1988). The increase of f5-HT observed in these circumstances may be exacerbated because indolamine excites 5-HT-3 and 5-HT-4 receptors located at the medullary AP (outside the BBB), which is connected with the motor vagal complex (Reynolds, Leslie, Grahame-Smith et al. 1989). The increased f5-HT results in a further increase of the peripheral parasympathetic discharge over the enterochromaffin cells (Bezold–Jarisch reflex). Such mechanisms explain the hyperserotonergic storm occurring in carcinoid patients frequently.

Patients affected by carcinoid tumors present alternation of clinical syndromes (parasympathetic and adrenal sympathetic predominance). This bipolar syndrome depends on the interaction between the medullary DVC and the C1(Ad) nuclei. The fact that both systems are under control of the A5(NA) nucleus (responsible for the peripheral neural sympathetic activity) (Fenik, Marchenko, Janssen et al. 2002) suggests that any neuropharmacological therapy should be addressed to restore the hierarchical supremacy of the latter nucleus.

The immunological investigation of these patients showed a TH-2 profile (raised levels of TH-2 cytokines IL-6, IL-10, and β-interferon, reduced natural killer (NK) cell cytotoxicity against the K-562 target cells, and reduced CD4/CD8 ratio (lower than 1; normal values ≈2).

An adequate neuropharmacological therapy to enhance neural sympathetic activity and to reduce adrenal sympathetic activity was able to normalize clinical, neurochemical, neuroautonomic, and immunological parameters. Up to the present, we have successfully treated nine patients affected by the carcinoid syndrome. Control periods ranged between 6 months and 7 years. No relapses have been observed. The treatment is interrupted periodically every 5 to 6 months (Lechin, van der Dijs, Orozco et al. 2005c; Lechin, van der Dijs 2005c).

Acute Pancreatitis

Acute pancreatitis is a severe and frequently uncontrollable disease, which shows an important index of mortality. Severe abdominal pain, vomits, and disorders of cardiovascular parameters are always present. Usually, these patients are treated at the intensive care units and the mortality rate is high. In 1992, we published our first clinical report showing the successful therapy of this disease with a small dose of intramuscularly injected clonidine (0.15 mg) 2 to 3 times daily (Lechin, van der Dijs, Lechin et al. 1992b). All patients recovered within the next 48 to 72 hours. The amylase plasma levels become normal after the first clonidine administration and remain normal further. Up to the present, we have successfully treated more than 100 acute pancreatitis patients, without any failure (Lechin, van der Dijs, Lechin et al. 1992b, 2002c; Lechin, van der Dijs 2004b).

We outlined this therapy because we were aware that clonidine is able to provoke dry mouth (inhibition of the salivary gland), which parallels pancreatic exocrine secretion. It is commonly accepted that both salivary and pancreatic exocrine secretion share a common CNS excitatory mechanism. In addition, it was recently demonstrated that pancreatic nerves responsible for the pancreatic exocrine secretion depend on the C1(Ad) medullary nuclei (Roze, Chariot, Appia et al. 1981), which are the CNS nuclei connected to the pancreatic exocrine gland (Loewy, Haxhiu 1993; Loewy, Franklin, Haxhiu 1994). These findings fit well with the known fact that clonidine exerts maximal CNS sympathetic inhibition by acting at the α-2 receptors located at these nuclei, which are the adrenergic medullary neurons whose excitation triggers the release of noradrenalin from sympathetic nerves at the pancreatic gland.

Clonidine is an important therapeutic tool to treat other pancreatic exocrine disorders (chronic pancreatitis, cancer of the pancreas, pancreatic cysts, and cystic fibrosis of the pancreas) (Lechin, van der Dijs, Orozco et al. 2005d). The abrupt hyposecretory effect exerted by this drug would explain the relief of acute pain and the beneficial chronic therapeutic effects (Roze, Chariot, Appia et al. 1981).

The above reports are good examples that demonstrate the relevance of coupling physiological, pathophysiological, clinical, and pharmacological information to outline therapeutic approaches. However, despite this, doctors remain in the same state and treat pancreatitis throughout stressful and dramatic harmful procedures.

Cystic Fibrosis and Pancreatic Cysts

The two syndromes, cystic fibrosis and pancreatic cysts, are caused by similar autonomic nervous system (ANS) disorder, which allows a common neuropharmacological therapy. Six patients affected by pancreatic cysts and four patients affected by cystic fibrosis have been successfully treated with neuropharmacological therapy. All of them showed an uncoping stress profile: predominance of adrenal over neural sympathetic activity. In addition, all they showed raised levels of p5-HT. This latter parameter indicated that all patients secreted higher than normal serotonin from the enterochromaffin cells (Lechin, van der Dijs, Orozco et al. 2005d).

The enterochromaffin cells release serotonin during postprandial periods and during peripheral parasympathetic activity. These cells are excited by vagal nerves. Serotonin released to the portal vein is taken up by the liver; however, some fraction of this indolamine escapes from liver uptake and reaches the blood stream. In addition, it has been demonstrated that serotonergic nerves innervate pancreatic exocrine gland.

Overexcited pancreatic exocrine glands secrete a greater than normal amount of pancreatic juice, which would enhance intraacinar pressure and provoke the degeneration of the acinos. Thus, pancreatic exocrine glands turn into pancreatic cysts.

Our therapeutic strategy was addressed the inhibition of the parasympathetic activity, which depends on both the excessive adrenal sympathetic and the neural sympathetic activities. The ANS unbalance triggered by the absence of the neural sympathetic drive would favor the parasympathetic versus adrenal sympathetic instability. In addition, these patients present positive antipancreatic (++) and antinuclear (+) antibodies when immunologically investigated. All immunoglobulins were also raised.

Doxepin (25 mg) before bed, clonidine (0, 15 mg) before meals, and propantheline (15 mg) at 10:00 AM and 4:00 PM were prescribed. Significant clinical, ANS, and immunological improvements were obtained after the first 4-week period and continue up to the present (June 2008).

It may be postulated that pancreatic cyst formation will be favored by factors that overwhelm the pancreatic duct drainage capacity by excessive acinar cell secretion.

Several ANS and hormonal factors are involved in pancreatic exocrine secretion. Sympathetic nerves terminate on intrapancreatic blood vessels. In addition, inhibition of exocrine secretion may occur in the absence of vascular effects (α-receptor blockade) (Roze, Chariot, Appia et al. 1981), suggesting that the catecholamines may act directly on the secretory cells (Holst, Schaffalitzky, Muckadell et al. 1979). Noradrenergic and serotonergic fibers end at intra-pancreatic ganglia whose stimulation abolishes vagal-induced secretion, by acting at α-2 adrenoceptors (Alm, Cegrell, Ehinger et al. 1967; Holst, Schaffalitzky, Muckadell et al. 1979). These findings are supported by the capacity of neural sympathetic enhancement to antagonize the hyperparasympathetic-induced hypersecretion, which underlies pancreatic cyst formation (Hong, Magee 1970). Considering that post-ganglionic α-2 receptors mediate sympathetic nerve effects at this level, we find an explanation for the benefits triggered by clonidine (an α-2 agonist) in both pancreatic cysts and pancreatitis (Lechin, Benshimol, van der Dijs et al. 1970; Lechin, van der Dijs, Lechin 2002c; Lechin, van der Dijs, Orozco 2002h). Roze et al. (1981) found that a small dose of intramuscular injected clonidine is able to stop pancreatic secretion from the excretory duct abruptly in experimental rats. This peripheral noradrenergic versus parasympathetic antagonism is consistent with the inhibitory effects exerted by both A5(NA) and A6(NA) axons ending at the dorsal motor nucleus of the vagus located in the medullary area (Barlow, Greenwell, Harper et al. 1971; Lechin, van der Dijs 1989).

In addition, nicotine receptor antagonists effectively block the vagal-induced pancreatic secretion. This finding fits well with the beneficial effects that we obtained by the addition of small doses of propantheline, a nicotine-antagonist that does not cross the BBB.

Not only ANS but also hormonal (cholecystokinin [CCK]-pancreozymin and secretin) mechanisms are involved in pancreatic exocrine secretion. The release of both hormones is less dependent on the ANS influence (Lechin, van der Dijs, Bentolila et al. 1978; Lechin, van der Dijs 1981e; Lechin 1992b; Lechin, van der Dijs, Orozco 2002b, 2002h). However, ANS drives are able to interfere with the secretory hormone release and/or its effects (Lechin, van der Dijs, Orozco et al. 2002h). For instance, α-adrenergic influences are able to interfere with CCK-pancreozymin effects (Lechin, van der Dijs, Bentolila et al. 1978; Lechin, van der Dijs 1981e; Lechin 1992b; Lechin, van der Dijs, Orozco 2002b). Thus, we believe that the therapeutic success we obtained with this small casuistic of pancreatic cysts and cystic fibrosis patients has enough scientific support to attempt additional neuropharmacological approaches to treat these patients.

Neuroautonomic and Immunological Interactions

The levels of both cortisol and adrenaline in the plasma are responsible for significant immunological changes. All TH-1 autoimmune diseases are caused by the disinhibition of the thymus gland from the cortisol bridling. In addition, the excitatory effect of the neural sympathetic overactivity at the spleen and sympathetic ganglia contributes to the enhancement and further predominance of the TH-1 immunological profile (Fig. 5.2). This predominance of the neural sympathetic activity triggers the enhancement of plasma TH-1 cytokines (γ-interferon, IL-2, IL-12, IL-18, TNF, etc.). On the contrary, enhanced cortisol level inhibits the thymus gland and increases the plasma values of TH-2 cytokines (IL-4, IL-6, IL-10, β-interferon, and others) whereas adrenaline provokes a cascade of hematological, metabolic, gastrointestinal, cardiovascular, and respiratory disorders. These two types of peripheral endocrine factors (Ad and cortisol) converge to the deviation of the immune system to the TH-2 profile. Overactivity of humoral immunity predominates over cellular immunity, in this circumstance (Romagnani 1996; Lechin, van der Dijs, Lechin 2002a) (Fig. 5.3).

Uncoping Stress in the Elderly

Uncoping stress in the elderly differs from that seen in young people. Both atrophy of the A6(NA) (Ishida, Shirokawa, Miyaishi et al. 2000; Grudzien, Shaw, Weintraub et al. 2007) and hyporeactivity of the adrenal gland cause the absolute predominance of neural over adrenal sympathetic activity observed in the elderly (Seals, Esler 2000). It is consistent with findings indicating that aging prolongs the stress-induced release of noradrenaline in rat hypothalamus (Perego, Vetrugno, De Simoni et al. 1993). The assessment of circulating neurotransmitters in approximately 30,000 subjects carried out in our institute demonstrated that absolute noradrenergic over adrenergic predominance was observed in the elderly. In addition, adrenaline plasma level does not increase during exercise; thus the noradrenaline/adrenaline plasma ratio does not show a decrease but an increase (Lechin, van der Dijs, Lechin 1996c). However, significant plasma dopamine rises are always noted in these circumstances. Artalejo et al. (1985) demonstrated that circulating dopamine is able to inhibit the adrenal glands secretion. The aforementioned adrenaline versus noradrenaline and dopamine dissociation, observed during the orthostasis and exercise challenge supports the postulation of the hyperresponsiveness of neural sympathetic activity versus the hyporresponsiveness of the adrenal sympathetic system seen in the elderly. This neuroautonomic response to the orthostatic and exercise challenge in old subjects when they are submitted to the aforementioned stressors fits well with the orthostatic hypotension but not with the heart rate

A6-NA = Locus coeruleus
DR-5-HT = Dorsal raphe
MR-5-HT = Median raphe
PVN = Paraventricular nucleus
⟶ Excitation
⟼ Inhibition

Figure 5.2 TH-1 autoimmune profile. Predominance of the A5(NA) neurons is responsible for the inhibition of both the C1(Ad) (adrenergic) and vagal (parasympathetic) activities. In addition, the absence of the C1(Ad) excitatory drive to the DR(5-HT) neurons is responsible for the MR(5-HT) predominance. At the peripheral level, raised noradrenaline/adrenaline plasma ratio is observed. The hypoactivity of the DR(5-HT) and the hyperactivity of the MR(5-HT) nucleus are responsible for the low plasma tryptophan as well as the high platelet serotonin levels, always seen in these circumstances. Predominance of neural sympathetic activity inhibits adrenocortical secretion, which is responsible for the disinhibition of the thymus gland. This latter provokes enhancement of cell-mediated immunity (TH-1 immunological profile). At the blood level, predominance of the cytokines IL-2, IL-12, IL-18, and γ-interferon is seen in patients affected by the TH-1 profile.

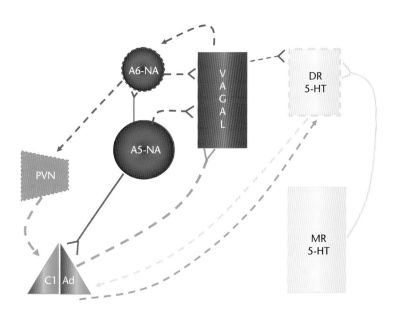

A6-NA = Locus coeruleus
DR-5-HT = Dorsal raphe
MR-5-HT = Median raphe
PVN = Paraventricular nucleus
⟶ Excitation
⟼ Inhibition

Figure 5.3 TH-2 autoimmune profile. This profile depends on the release of corticotrophin-releasing hormone (CRH) from the hypothalamic paraventricular nucleus (PVN). A positive feedback among the A6(NA), DR(5-HT), and C1(Ad) is observed at this circumstance (uncoping stress). Highest adrenaline (Ad) and cortisol plasma levels are observed during this disorder. Conversely, very low levels of plasma noradrenaline (NA) underlie this profile. Predominance of corticoadrenal sympathetic activity inhibits the thymus gland. This latter provokes predominance of humoral immunity (TH-2 immunological profile). At the blood level, cytokines IL-6, IL-10, and β-interferon predominates at this circumstance. However, the most important immunological parameter involved in this disorder should depend on the natural killer (NK) cell cytotoxicity against the K-562 target cells. This parameter is found very low in TH-2 autoimmune patients. Sastry et al. (2007) ratified our findings showing that the raised levels of plasma Ad are responsible for the inability by NK cells to destroy the K-562 target cells (Lechin et al. 1987).

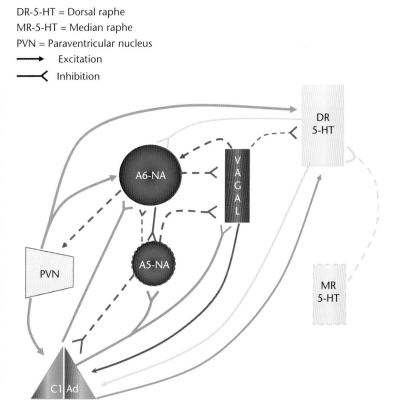

increase seen in them. Diastolic, but not systolic, blood pressure fall is always reported in old subjects during the 1-minute orthostasis test. We found a negative correlation between the diastolic blood pressure fall and the rise of dopamine plasma levels (Lechin, van der Dijs, Lechin 2004c; Lechin, van der Dijs, Lechin 2005a). This phenomenon should be attributed to the release of dopamine from sympathetic nerves, which are provided by a dopamine pool. This neurotransmitter is released before noradrenaline during sympathetic nerve excitation. Dopamine released from these terminals excites dopamine-2 inhibitory autoreceptors located at this level and modulates the further release of noradrenaline from sympathetic nerves (Mercuro, Rossetti, Rivano et al. 1987; Mannelli, Pupilli, Fabbri et al. 1988). Failure of the modulatory mechanism contributes to the EH syndrome, frequently seen in the elderly (Lechin, van der Dijs, Baez et al. 2006c). In addition, many research studies demonstrated a negative correlation between CNS-NA activity and secretion of adrenal glands (Bialik, Smythe, Sardelis et al. 1989). Furthermore, other findings by Porta et al. (1989) demonstrated that noradrenaline overactivity triggers medullar adrenaline depletion during normoglycemia. Other findings by Sato and Trzebski (1993) demonstrated that the excitatory response of the adrenal sympathetic nerve decreases in aged rats. This issue has been widely investigated and discussed by many authors, including Seals and Esler (2000). These authors summarize their research work as follows: (a) tonic whole-body sympathetic nervous system (SNS) activity increases with age; (b) skeletal muscle and the gut, but not the kidney, are some of the most important targets; and (c) the SNS tone of the heart is highly increased. In contrast to SNS activity, tonic adrenaline secretion from the adrenal medulla is markedly reduced with age. They also found that the adrenaline release in response to acute stress is substantially attenuated in older men.

It should be remembered that the pontomedullary A5(NA) nucleus is responsible for the neural sympathetic activity whereas the medullary C1(Ad) nuclei are responsible for the adrenal glands secretion (Fenik, Davies, Kubin 2002). Finally, the CNS nuclei interchange inhibitory axons, which release noradrenaline and adrenaline, respectively (Li, Wesselingh, Blessing et al. 1992). Noradrenaline and adrenaline act at postsynaptic (inhibitory) α-2 receptors located at both types of neurons.

Additional comments should be made with respect to the progressive reduction of the A6(NA) neurons with aging (Ishida, Shirokawa, Miyaishi et al. 2000; Grudzien, Shaw, Weintraub et al. 2007).It should be remembered that psychosis is caused by the congenital deficit of the A6(NA) neurons (Craven, Priddle,

Crow et al. 2005); thus, any reduction of them would explain the intellectual and psychological disturbances observed in patients affected by Alzheimer's disease, whose symptoms resembled those observed in psychotic patients (Grudzien, Shaw, Weintraub et al. 2007).

Neural Sympathetic Versus Parasympathetic Cross Talk in the Elderly

The absence or deficit of adrenal sympathetic activity in the elderly explains the sympathetic versus parasympathetic antagonism present in them. This dialog substitutes the compliance supported by the cross talk among three interacting factors. This limited ANS compliance explains why the elderly cannot prolong the exercise time. Elder people do not have enough adrenaline to maintain cardiovascular and respiratory hyperactivity required in these circumstances. These subjects have neural sympathetic and parasympathetic activity but not adrenal sympathetic activity. We found that a small dose of L-arginine (50 mg) or digitalis (both of which enhance parasympathetic activity) is enough to suppress cardiovascular, respiratory, and/or gastrointestinal symptoms triggered by any type of stressors in the elderly (Lechin, van der Dijs, Baez et al. 2006c).

The absolute neural sympathetic predominance observed in the elderly is responsible for all types of vascular thrombosis seen during aging. The absence of the β-adrenergic vasodilator mechanism facilitates all types of vasospasm. When the latter phenomenon depends on the effect of circulating noradrenaline at the α-1 receptors located at this level this mechanism would be no more attenuated by the opposite effect displayed by adrenaline at the vasodilator β-receptors.

The A5(NA) predominance over both A6(NA) and C1(Ad) nuclei is responsible for the overwhelming neural sympathetic activity. It is similar to that observed in patients with both ED (Kitayama, Nakamura, Yaga et al. 1994) and psychosis, both syndromes caused by auto-aggressive behavior. It brings to my mind the Freud's sentence: *suicide underlies all deaths.*

The predominance of noradrenaline over adrenaline observed in the peripheral sympathetic system in the elderly is also responsible for the TH-1 immunological profile, always observed in the elderly. This phenomenon fits well with the inhibitory effect exerted by sympathetic nerves on cortisol and adrenaline from the adrenal glands. Minimization of the latter redounds in the disinhibition of the thymus. This phenomenon is frequently seen despite the fact that this gland tends to involute during senescence. However, it has been demonstrated that neural sympathetic innervation of the spleen is responsible for the TH-1 immunological predominance seen in the elderly (Felten, Felten, Bellinger et al. 1988). This means that the spleen is able to substitute the thymus immunological activity.

PATHOPHYSIOLOGY OF CLINICAL SYNDROMES

Two Types of Stress Mechanisms

Type 1: Motility Behavior—Acute Stress

Both the A6(NA) and DR(5-HT) neurons receive excitatory glutamate axons, which trigger the release of noradrenaline and serotonin, respectively, at the hypothalamic PVN. CRH secreted at this level excites the ACTH—cortisol cascade and, in addition, excites the C1(Ad) medullary nuclei. Furthermore, CRH released from axons arising from the PVN at the A6(NA) and the DR(5-HT) nuclei is responsible for a positive feedback between these two CNS levels. Even more, cortisol released from the adrenal gland crosses the BBB and excites both the C1(Ad) and the DR(5-HT) nuclei. The latter nucleus, but not other serotonergic nuclei, is crowded by excitatory cortisol receptors. In addition, the overexcited C1(Ad) nuclei send excitatory and inhibitory drives to the DR(5-HT) and the A5(NA) neurons, respectively. Summarizing, the acute stress syndrome includes overactivity of the A6(NA), DR(5-HT), PVN(CRH), and C1(Ad) CNS circuitry, and the inhibition of the A5(NA) nucleus.

Type 2: Restraint, Photic, Acoustic, and Psychological Stimuli—Acute Stress

Predominance of the MR(5-HT) nucleus is responsible for this type of stress. MR(5-HT) axons inhibit both A6(NA) and DR(5-HT) nuclei. Both the A6(NA) and the MR(5-HT) but not the DR(5-HT) neurons are excited by glutamatergic axons. The MR(5-HT) axons do not innervate the hypothalamic PVN directly, but throughout polysynaptic drives which include the CEA, the BNST and the A5(NA) nuclei and finally, the hypothalamic PVN. The inhibition of the A6(NA) by the MR(5-HT) axons triggers the disinhibition of the A5(NA) neurons, which are also excited by the CEA + BNST drive. The overexcited A5(NA) nucleus triggers the inhibition of both the C1(Ad) and the A6(NA) nuclei. In addition, the CRH—ACTH—cortisol cascade is not so intense as that observed during the Type 1 acute stress, thus the plasma cortisol rise is not so high to disinhibit the DR(5-HT) neurons from the MR(5-HT) bridle. This well-known inhibitory effect exerted by MR(5-HT)

axons at the DR(5-HT) level, annuls the predominance of the DR(5-HT), PVN (CRH), hypophysis (ACTH), and corticoadrenal cascade.

According to the above there are two different and even opposite types of neuroendocrine circuits which underlie two types of stress profiles: Type 1 is caused by the DR(5-HT,) PVN(CRH), and C1(Ad) predominance, whereas Type 2 depends on the MR(5-HT), CEA, and A5(NA) overactivity. At the peripheral level, Type 1 stress would provoke corticoadrenal hypersecretion whereas Type 2 stress would provoke neural sympathetic overactivity and inhibition of the corticoadrenal activity, because sympathetic nerves, which innervate the corticoadrenal gland (Engeland 1998), inhibit the CRH–ACTH–cortisol cascade.

The aforementioned postulation is supported by the assessment of circulating neurotransmitters in approximately 30,000 normal and diseased subjects and a bulk of experimental mammals during the last 36 years. (Lechin, van der Dijs, Benaim 1996a; Lechin, van der Dijs, Lechin 2002a; Lechin, van der Dijs, Hernandez-Adrian 2006a; Lechin, van der Dijs 2006b).

Coping Stress

It should be known that the A6(NA) neurons do not display spontaneous firing activity. They should be excited by glutamatergic axons arising from the pyramidal cortical neurons. Glutamate released from these axons excites A6(NA) neurons by acting on other than *N*-methyl D-aspartate (NMDA) receptors located at these latter (Koga, Ishibashi, Shimada et al. 2005). Excitation of the A6(NA) neurons initiates all type of stress. Facts showing that MR(5-HT) rather than DR(5-HT) receives heavy glutamate innervation (Tao, Auerbach 2003) contrast with the opposite findings showing the heavy GABAergic innervation of the latter but not the former serotonergic nucleus (Lechin, van der Dijs, Lechin et al. 2002a). These findings allow the understanding why both serotonergic nuclei are included into two different anatomical and physiological circuitries. The above anatomical circuitry allows the necessary physiological independence needed for the accomplishment of two distinct behavioral activities. Serotonergic axons from these two nuclei inhibit the A6NA) neurons. The modulatory role exerted by them would depend on the type of stress stimulus. This specialization is possible because DR(5-HT) neurons are excited by the motility behavior whereas MR(5-HT) responds to restraint, photic, acoustic, fear and all types of psychological stimuli (Lechin, van der Dijs, Hernandez-Adrian et al. 2006a).

The locus coeruleus (LC) or A6(NA) axons innervate the brain cortex and the pontomedullary DVC(ACh) and the NTS cholinergic neurons. These two anti-ACh drives provoke the alerting state and diminish peripheral parasympathetic activity. The augmentation and/or prolongation of this acute stress phenomenon contributes to the excitation of the PVN hypothalamic and the C1(Ad) medullary nuclei, which are responsible for the CRH—ACTH—cortisol and the adrenal sympathetic cascades, respectively (Kvetnansky, Bodnar, Shahar et al. 1977; Burchfield 1979; Liu, Fung, Reddy et al. 1991; Sternberg, Glowa, Smith et al. 1992; Calogero, Bagdy, D'Agata 1998). The fact that CRH is also released at both the A6(NA) and the DR(5-HT) levels constitutes a positive feedback mechanism that favors the prolongation of the firing activity of these nuclei (Koob 1999). Both the A6(NA) and the C1(Ad) axons over-release noradrenaline and adrenaline, respectively, at the A5(NA) nucleus. Both catecholamines trigger inhibition of the latter, by acting at α-2 inhibitory receptors located at the A5(NA) nucleus. This cross talk is responsible for the predominance of the adrenal sympathetic over the neural sympathetic observed at the peripheral level during this acute period (Kvetnansky, Bodnar, Shahar et al. 1977; Burchfield 1979). At these circumstances, the serotonin released at the A6(NA) is not enough to be able for stop the stress cascade because of the overwhelming release of CRH at the A6(NA) neurons. However, prolongation and/or augmentation of the stressful process triggers maximal enhancement of the cortisol plasma levels. This hormone crosses the BBB and provokes additional excitation of the DR(5-HT) neurons activity because they are crowded by excitatory cortisol receptors. The over-release of serotonin from the DR(5-HT) axons at the A6(NA) neurons attenuates the stress cascade; however, prolongation of this process triggers the exhaustion of the DR(5-HT) neurons. The exhaustion and further disappearance of the activity of the serotonergic nucleus underlies the uncoping stress phenomenon. It is the "learned helplessness behavior," "uncontrollable stress," or "behavioral despair" (Kant, Mougey, Meyerhoff et al. 1989; Szabo, Blier 2001).

Uncoping Stress

Learned helplessness or inescapable (uncontrollable) stress, also known as behavioral despair constitutes the maximal expression of this syndrome and is experimentally induced in rats submitted to prolonged exercise (e.g., swimming until exhaustion). These rats do not try more to escape and lie flat on the experimental table. Hypotonic legs and neck are always seen in these circumstances. Neurochemical investigation carried out at this period demonstrated exhaustion of the DR(5-HT) neurons plus an excess of extracellular 5-HT at the spinal motor (anterior) horns. This latter depends on the release of serotonin from the disinhibited RP(5-HT) neurons, which receive inhibitory DR(5-HT) axons. According to the above, this syndrome depends on the predominance of RP(5-HT) over A6(NA) at the anterior spinal horns (Kvetnansky, Bodnar, Shahar et al. 1977; Anisman, Irwin, Sklar 1980; Desan, Silbert, Maier et al. 1988; Tanaka, Okamura, Tamada et al. 1994). This syndrome is similar to that observed in the called *akathisia syndrome* (restlessness of legs), usually observed in benzodiazepine's consumers (Lechin, van der Dijs, Vitelli-Flores et al. 1994b; Lechin, van der Dijs, Benaim 1996b); these drugs trigger the inhibition of DR(5-HT) neurons (which are crowded by inhibitory GABA neurons) and disinhibition of the RP(5-HT) neurons. Summarizing, the exhaustion of both A6(NA) and DR(5-HT) nuclei underlies this disorder. However, the fact that the disinhibition of the A5(NA) nucleus from the exhausted A6(NA) axons but not from the overactive C1(Ad) nuclei explains the prolongation of the uncoping stress disorder (Granata, Numao, Kumada et al. 1986; Peyron, Luppi, Fort et al. 1996; Koob 1999). Nevertheless, the progressive disinhibition of the A5(NA) neurons from the A6(NA) and C1(Ad) nuclei, allows that axons from the former nucleus bridle the RP(5-HT) neurons, whose hyperactivity is responsible for the restlessness syndrome (Hokfelt, Phillipson, Goldstein 1979; Byrum, Guyenet 1987; Zhang 1991; Tanaka, Okamura, Tamada et al. 1994; Laaris, Le Poul, Hamon et al. 1997; Hermann, Luppi, Peyron et al. 1997; Gerin, Privat 1998). This postulation is reinforced by findings showing that neuropharmacological and/or electrical excitation of the A5(NA) neurons and/or the DR(5-HT) neurons normalized the motility behavior in rats affected by this syndrome. With respect to this, we demonstrated that low doses (10 mg) of amitriptyline or desipramine, intramuscularly injected (which excites A5(NA) neurons), suppresses drastically the restlessness syndrome (Lechin, van der Dijs, Benaim 1996a). These findings are also consistent with the demonstration that the A5(NA) neurons send inhibitory axons to the RP(5-HT) neurons (Tanaka, Okamura, Tamada et al. 1994).

In humans, the restlessness syndrome is frequently seen in benzodiazepine's consumers and in myasthenia gravis patients (during acute periods). The fact that recovery in this last syndrome is fast with the administration of corticosterone (which excite the DR(5-HT) and/or intramuscularly injected amitriptyline or desipramine, which excites the

A5(NA) neurons, fits well with the experimental findings in rats. The failure of oral administration of both amitriptyline and desipramine to provoke results similar to that obtained after parenteral route should be attributed to interference by the liver uptake of the oral administered drugs. This liver uptake interferes with the fast and direct CNS effect triggered by the intramuscularly injection. We have successfully treated hundreds of these patients during acute as well as nonacute episodes with this neuropharmacological strategy (Lechin, van der Dijs, Jara et al. 1997b; Lechin, van der Dijs, Pardey-Maldonado 2000; Lechin, van der Dijs, Lechin 2002a).

Other monoaminergic neurons are involved in the uncoping stress versus coping stress. All types of stressor agents excite the glutamate (pyramidal) cortical neurons. Glutamate axons excite the A6(NA) + MR(5-HT) rather than DR(5-HT) neurons or the dopaminergic nuclei A10, and A8 + A9 (substantia nigra). (Olpe, Steinmann, Brugger et al. 1989; Ping, Wu, Liu 1990; Nitz, Siegel 1997; Hervas, Bel, Fernandez et al. 1998; Tao, Auerbach 2003). The above monoaminergic nuclei are located at the first or second line of the stress cascade (Calogero, Bagdy, D'Agata et al. 1988; Midzyanovskaya, Kuznetsova, van Luijtelaar et al. 2006). However, other CNS nuclei receive also glutamatergic axons, such as the A5(NA) and the C1(Ad) nuclei (Shanks, Zalcman, Zacharko et al. 1991; Fung, Reddy, Zhuo et al. 1994; Liu, Fung, Reddy et al. 1995). These glutamate axons do not arise from cortical but subcortical levels. In addition, both the A6(NA) and the DR(5-HT) nuclei receive also heavy GABA ergic innervation, which arise from cortical levels. Finally, although the MR(5-HT) neurons receive both GABA and glutamic cortical inputs, this latter predominates over the former (Tao, Auerbach 2003).

Although the A10(DA) mesocortical neurons receive also glutamate (excitatory) and GABA (inhibitory) axons, these neurons are maximal excited by the A6(NA) and inhibited by the DR(5-HT) axons. The understanding of this "cross talk" helps to outline adequate neuropharmacological therapy for several psychological and neurological disturbances (Vezina, Blanc, Glowinski et al. 1991; Pozzi, Invernizzi, Cervo et al. 1994; Matsumoto, Togashi, Mori et al. 1999; Devoto, Flore, Pani et al. 2001; Lechin, van der Dijs, Lechin et al. 2002a; Ishibashi, Shimada, Jang et al. 2005).

The rationality of the aforementioned cross talk should be understood on the basis of experimental data emanating from a bulk of research studies. For instance, DR(5-HT) neurons fire during movement and cease to fire during immobility (Trulson, Jacobs 1979; Jacobs, Heym, Trulson 1981). Conversely, MR(5-HT) neurons display the opposite physiological profile (Lechin, van der Dijs, Hernandez-Adrian 2006a). Other findings demonstrate that the A8(DA), A9(DA), and the A10(DA) nuclei display firing activities, which parallel the activities of DR(5-HT) and MR(5-HT), respectively (Ferre, Artigas 1993; Broderick, Phelix 1997; Jackson, Cunnane 2001; Yan, Zheng, Feng et al. 2005). Furthermore, the fact that cortical and subcortical DA are positively associated with thinking and motility, respectively (Bunney and Aghajanian, 1978) facilitates the understanding of why these two serotonergic nuclei are included into the two circuitries responsible for the aforementioned profiles, respectively. This knowledge allows explaining why mammals interrupt movements to think (Fuxe, Hokfelt, Agnati et al. 1977; Herve, Simon, Blanc et al. 1981; Herve, Pickel, Joh et al. 1987).

Other types of stressors (restraint, photic, sound, and psychological) excite the MR but not the DR serotonergic neurons (Tanaka, Kohno, Nakagawa et al. 1983; Dilts, Boadle-Biber 1995; Laaris, Le Poul, Hamon et al. 1997; Midzyanovskaya, Kuznetsova, van Luijtelaar et al. 2006; Rabat, Bouyer, George et al. 2006). These findings allow understanding why both stressed mammals and humans present with different clinical, biochemical, and hormonal profiles, according to the distinct types of stressful situations (Lechin, van der Dijs, Hernandez-Adrian 2006a).

The exhaustion of the DR(5-HT) neurons redounds in the disinhibition of the subordinate serotonergic nuclei: PAG, RM, RO, and RP (Byrum, Guyenet 1987; Krowicki, Hornby 1993; Vertes, Kocsis 1994; Hermann, Luppi, Peyron et al. 1997). Thus, serotonin released from the disinhibited nuclei excites all ACh medullary nuclei such as the NTS and the nucleus ambiguus (Behbehani 1982; Newberry, Watkins, Reynolds et al. 1992; Porges 1995; Thurston-Stanfield, Ranieri, Vallabhapurapu et al. 1999), which interchange modulatory axons with the C1(Ad) medullary nuclei. This cross talk at the medullary level explains the alternancy between the peripheral adrenal sympathetic and parasympathetic activities. Maximal oscillations of this binomial circuitry are observed during uncoping stress situations. Abrupt alternation of adrenal sympathetic and parasympathetic predominance is observed during these periods (Young, Rosa, Landsberg 1984; Krowicki, Hornby 1993; Porges 1995). Gastrointestinal, biliary, and cardiovascular symptoms would reflect the hyperactivity of these two opposite ANS profiles. The absence of the neural sympathetic activity under these circumstances allows the aforementioned peripheral ANS instability among the adrenal, sympathetic, and parasympathetic activities.

The progressive (chronic) exhaustion of the A6(NA) and DR(5-HT) binomial observed during the uncoping stress disorder may lead to the gradual predominance of the A5(NA) and MR(5-HT) nuclei. Both NA and 5-HT axons arising from the latter inhibit the C1(Ad) and parasympathetic binomial as well as the medullary serotonergic nuclei (Levine, Litto, Jacobs 1990; Shanks, Zalcman, Zacharko et al. 1991; Laaris, Le Poul, Hamon et al. 1997; Koob 1999; Kvetnansky, Bodnar, Shahar et al. 2006). This emergent CNS neurochemical predominance underlies the "coping stress" syndrome. At the peripheral level, the neural sympathetic overactivity would be responsible for the spastic colon, biliary hypokinesia, bradycardia, diastolic blood pressure rise, and many other physiological changes.

The uncoping versus coping stress CNS mechanism and the peripheral mechanisms that underlie them are responsible for most, if not all, the clinical syndromes seen during these circumstances, and will be illustrated with several examples. These examples will include acute pancreatitis, ulcerative colitis, Crohn's disease, nervous diarrhea, spastic colon, biliary dyskinesia, bronchial asthma, EH, vascular thrombosis, hyperinsulinism, duodenal ulcer, infertility in women, malignant diseases, thrombocytopenic purpura, polycythemia vera, cystic fibrosis, carcinoid tumor, and several autoimmune diseases.

In summary, the uncoping stress disorder would be caused by the exhaustion of the A6(NA) and A5(NA) nuclei and the absolute predominance of the C1(Ad) and ACh medullary nuclei. Adrenocortical and adrenal sympathetic predominance over neural sympathetic activity is observed at the peripheral level. This adrenocortical hyperactivity is paralleled by the absolute DR(5-HT) predominance over MR(5-HT) activity at the CNS. Finally, the absence of the A6(NA) and A5(NA) bridle is responsible for the C1(Ad) and vagal(ACh) nuclei alternancies that underlie the instability of the peripheral ANS activity, at which level frequent and maximal adrenal sympathetic versus parasympathetic oscillations are observed (Lechin, van der Dijs, Jakubowicz et al. 1987a; Lechin, van der Dijs, Lechin et al. 1989a, 1993, 1994a; Lechin, van der Dijs, Benaim 1996a; Lechin, van der Dijs, Lechin 1996c; Lechin, van der Dijs, Orozco et al. 1996d, 1996e; Lechin, van der Dijs, Lechin et al. 1997a; Lechin, van der Dijs, Hernandez-Adrian 2006a; Lechin, van der Dijs 2006a, 2006b).

Maximal accentuation of the uncoping stress disorder leads to the "inescapable" or "uncontrollable" stress. The recovery from this disorder would depend on the physiological or neuropharmacological activation of the A6(NA), A5(NA), and MR(5-HT) activities. However, overactivity of the two latter nuclei may lead to the maximal inhibition of the DR(5-HT) and

A6(NA) binomial. This excessive response (predominance) from the A5(NA) and MR(5-HT) may lead to the pathophysiological disorder that underlies the ED. Irreversibility of this disorder is responsible for PTSD. Hence, the ED syndrome depends on the absolute but reversible predominance of A5(NA) and MR(-5-HT) over the A6(NA) and DR(5-HT) binomial (Lechin, van der Dijs, Orozco et al. 1995a, 1995b; Lechin 2006a, 2006b) whereas the PTSD would be the irreversible version of the same disorder.

Endogenous Depression

We were the first to demonstrate that ED is caused by hyperneural sympathetic activity (Lechin, van der Dijs 1982; Lechin, van der Dijs, Gómez et al. 1983a; Lechin, van der Dijs, Acosta et al. 1983b; Lechin, van der Dijs 1984; Lechin, van der Dijs, Jakubowicz et al. 1985a, 1985b; Lechin, van der Dijs, Amat et al. 1986; Gomez, Lechin, Jara et al. 1988; Lechin, van der Dijs, Vitelli et al. 1990a; Lechin, van der Dijs, Lechin et al. 1991; Lechin 1992a; Lechin, van der Dijs, Orozco et al. 1995a). Additional studies carried out in our and other laboratories demonstrated that ED is also associated with severe endocrinological disorders.

Endogenously depressed patients present with a raised plasma cortisol level in the afternoons, and the level does not show reduction after dexamethasone challenge. It should be known that the MR(5-HT) and not the DR(5-HT) is responsible for the 5-HT–CRH–ACTH cascade, which triggers the endocrine disorder in these patients. This circuitry does not depend on the DR(5-HT) and PVN hypothalamic nuclei but on the MR(5-HT), CEA, BNST, A5(NA), and anterior hypothalamic area. This CNS circuitry is less accessible to the cortisol and/or dexamethasone plasma levels and would thus explain the "nonsuppression" of plasma cortisol after dexamethasone challenge, seen in ED patients (Lechin, van der Dijs, Hernandez-Adrian 2006a).

Endogenously depressed patients do not show the normal increase in plasma levels of growth hormone (GH) when they are challenged with clonidine (an α-2 agonist). This null response is explained by the downregulation of α-2 receptors at the anterior hypothalamic area, which receives heavy innervation from the overexcited A5(NA) axons. This abnormal response to clonidine, observed in ED patients is consistent with the postulation that this syndrome is caused by overactivity of the A5(NA) nucleus and hypoactivity of the A6(NA) neurons (Lechin, van der Dijs, Jakubowicz et al. 1985a, 1985b; Eriksson, Dellborg, Soderpalm et al. 1986; Lechin, van der Dijs, Jakubowicz 1987a; Lechin, van der Dijs, Vitelli et al.

1990a; Lechin, van der Dijs, Benaim 1996a; Lechin, van der Dijs, Orozco et al. 1996d, 1996e; Lechin, van der Dijs 2004a).

Raised nocturnal cortisol and prolactin plasma levels have been the most frequent hormonal findings seen in these patients (Oliveira, Pizarro, Golbert et al. 2000). Most studies associated increase in prolactin levels with an excess of serotonin and a deficit of dopamine at the median eminence hypothalamic nucleus. However, the fact that not only L-dopa (a DA precursor) but also fenfluramine (a serotonin-releasing agent) were able to counteract this hypothalamic disorder and to reduce the plasma prolactin level indicates that the CNS disorder underlying the neuroendocrine disturbance should be explained. It has been shown that enhanced and prolonged serotonin release at the median eminence depends on the MR(5-HT) neurons, which display an overwhelming activity in ED patients, which annuls DR(5-HT) functioning (Lechin, van der Dijs, Hernandez-Adrian 2006a). This chronic hyperprolactinemia is responsible for the mammary and ovarian cysts and the female infertility presented by many depressed women, who also show hyperinsulinism, obesity, and EH frequently (Lechin, van der Dijs, Jakubowicz et al. 1985a, 1985b; Lechin, van der Dijs, Hernandez-Adrian 2006a; Lechin, van der Dijs 2006a, 2006b).

A bulk of evidence supports the postulation that the raised prolactin plasma levels in ED patients depend on the MR(5-HT) overactivity. Although acute excitation of DR(5-HT) neurons triggers a peak of plasma prolactin level, only MR(5-HT) overactivity is responsible for the chronic, sustained rise in plasma prolactin level seen in ED patients. It was demonstrated that sustained (chronic) raised plasma levels of this hormone parallels the higher NA plasma levels, also observed in these patients. Indeed, we were the first to demonstrate that buspirone, a 5-HT-1A agonist, which inhibits the DR(5-HT) neurons, reduced plasma prolactin levels in normal but not in ED patients (Lechin, van der Dijs, Jara et al. 1997c, 1998a). Conversely, we found that this parameter is normalized after an adequate neuropharmacological therapy of ED patients (Lechin, van der Dijs, Lechin 2002a). This evidence reinforces the postulation that the hyperprolactinemia in ED patients would depend on the MR(5-HT), CEA, A5(NA), BNST, and median eminence circuitry. This circuitry excludes areas which are innervated by the DR(5-HT) axons.

We also demonstrated in 1979 that captivity (restraint stress) was able to provoke not only the depressive syndrome but also hyperprolactinemia and hyperinsulinism in dogs (Lechin, Coll-Garcia, van der Dijs et al. 1979b).

The MR(5-HT)-induced prolactin hypersecretion is responsible for the mammary and ovarian cysts and infertility, often observed in patients who frequently show an ED profile. With respect to this, we found that a small dose of daily L-dopa was able to revert the infertility disorder reported in a bulk of these patients (Lechin, van der Dijs 1980, 2004a). The fact that L-dopa crosses the BBB and acts at all CNS circuitries is consistent with the earlier postulation.

Finally, it should be known that this type of hyperprolactinemia is closely associated to A5(NA) hyperactivity (neural sympathetic hyperactivity). This association allows understanding why TH-1 autoimmune diseases frequently affect depressed patients. It should be remembered that this autoimmune disorder depends on the thymus gland disinhibition from the plasma cortisol, which is silenced by the over-release of NA from the sympathetic nerves, at the adrenal gland level. Furthermore, it should be known that although ED patients show cortisol levels which are not lowered by the dexamethasone challenge, these patients present with lower-than-normal cortisol values in the mornings because of the underactivity of the DR(5-HT)–CRF–ACTH–cortisol cascade at this period. This phenomenon reflects the maximal inhibition of the cortical adrenal gland triggered by the overwhelming neural sympathetic activity, which underlies this syndrome (Robertson, Johnson, Robertson et al. 1979; Young, Rosa, Landsberg 1984; Brown, Fisher 1986; Barbeito, Fernandez, Silveira et al. 1986; Porta, Emsenhuber, Felsner et al. 1989).

In Summary, it has been exhaustively demonstrated that the chronic and sustained prolactin plasma rise and the hyperactivity of the neural sympathetic (peripheral) branch seen in endogenously depressed subjects depend on the MR(5-HT) predominance over DR(5-HT), which are responsible for the CNS and endocrine disorders observed in this syndrome. The mechanisms described might explain the physiological disorders that underlie other syndromes such as EH and hyperinsulinism, which should be included into this common pathology. We will go deeply into the experimental, clinical, and therapeutic evidence underlying the pathophysiology of endogenous (major) depression, which support our point of view dealing with the postulation that a great bulk of the so-called psychosomatic disorders are the other face of the coin of the ED syndrome (Fig. 5.4).

Endogenous Depression and Some Psychosomatic Disorders

We demonstrated that major (endogenous) depressed patients presented with neural sympathetic

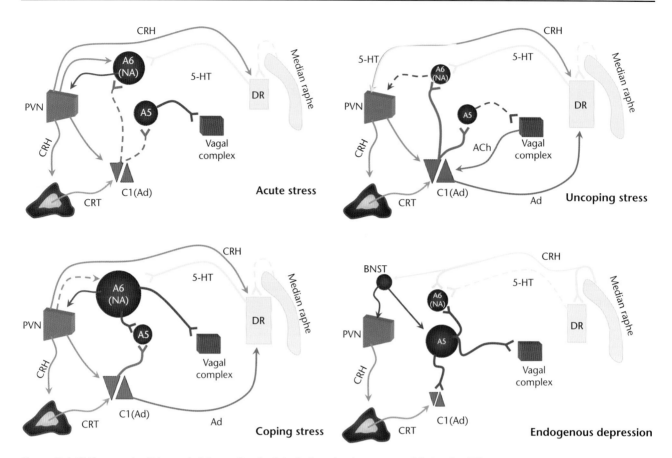

Figure 5.4 CNS neurocircuitries underlying pathophysiological mechanisms responsible for the different stress stages and depression.

Stress: Stressors excite both A6(NA) and DR(5-HT) neurons. These effects are triggered by glutamatergic axons. Both noradrenaline and serotonin released from A6 and DR axons excite the hypothalamic paraventricular nucleus (PVN). PVN axons release corticotropin-releasing hormone (CRH) at the median eminence (hypophysis) and the A6(NA) and DR(5-HT) nuclei. Thus, CRH is responsible for the hypophysis and adrenal gland excitation, which releases ACTH and cortisol (Crt), respectively. In addition, CRH axons excite the medullary Cl(Ad) nuclei that send excitatory (polysynaptic) drives to the adrenal glands, which release adrenaline (Ad) to the blood stream.

Attenuation of the A6(NA) neurons plus C1(Ad) nuclei is responsible for the disinhibition of the A5(NA) neurons, which receive direct inhibitory axons from the C1(Ad) nuclei. The progressive enhancement of the A5(NA) activity redounds in the peripheral neural sympathetic overactivity. This latter triggers the inhibition of both adrenal and cortical gland secretion.

Considering that both Cl(Ad) axons and plasma cortisol excite DR(5-HT) neurons, the attenuation of both activities redounds in the fading of both excitatory drives to the serotonergic nucleus.

Disappearance of neural sympathetic activity and overwhelming adrenal sympathetic activity underlies the "uncoping stress disorder." The plasma noradrenaline/adrenaline ratio reaches minimal levels (less than 2; normal, 3 to 5). The highest levels of adrenaline are responsible for maximal platelet aggregation, which is responsible for the maximal increase of plasma serotonin (f-5-HT).

Considering that medullary acetylcholinergic (ACh) nuclei, responsible for the peripheral parasympathetic activity, are controlled by both the A6(NA) and A5(NA) nuclei, absolute disinhibition of the former from the two latter nuclei is observed during uncoping stress. This phenomenon fits well with the lability of the peripheral autonomic nervous system (ANS), which shows frequent oscillations between parasympathetic and adrenal sympathetic periods. In addition, uncontrollable parasympathetic drives trigger overexcitation of the enterochromaffin cells, which release serotonin to the blood stream. This indolamine overexcites the medullary area postrema (outside the BBB). This parasympathetic structure is responsible for the maximal enhancement of the medullary (ACh) nuclei. It is the physiological disorder named Bezold Jarish syndrome. Lowest blood pressure, heart rate, diarrhea, vomits, and so on are seen at this period. However, overexcited parasympathetic nuclei are antagonized by the Cl(Ad) medullary nuclei that are responsible for the adrenal glands secretion. Thus, parasympathetic and adrenal sympathetic predominance are alternatively observed at peripheral level in mammals, caused by the uncoping stress disorder. Findings showing that adequate excitation of the pontine NA and 5-HT nuclei is able to normalize this disorder demonstrate that the absolute failure of these nuclei is responsible for the uncontrollable stress syndrome.

Endogenous depression: Exhaustive evidence demonstrated that this syndrome is caused by the absolute predominance of the peripheral neural sympathetic over adrenal sympathetic activity. This peripheral disorder depends on the predominance of the A5(NA) over the Cl(Ad) nucleus. In addition, considering that the A5(NA) and the A6(NA) interchange direct inhibitory axons, predominance of the former results in the inhibition of the latter.

Several mechanisms explain the overwhelming predominance of MR(5-HT) over DR(5-HT) that underlies this syndrome, namely, the exhaustion of the Cl(Ad) and DR(5-HT) axis, as demonstrated by the lower-than-normal levels of both adrenaline and cortisol plasma levels in mammals affected by this syndrome.

hyperactivity (higher than normal NA plasma levels), which was also underlying distal colon hypertonicity (spastic colon) (Lechin, van der Dijs 1982). Both psychiatric and gastrointestinal disorders were improved with the administration of some neuropharmacological agents that were able to deplete CNS serotonin stores (Lechin, van der Dijs, Gómez et al. 1982a, 1983a; Lechin, van der Dijs, Acosta et al. 1983b). These findings were further ratified and amplified in other research studies (Lechin, van der Dijs, Jakubowicz et al. 1985a, 1985b). These studies allowed us to postulate that the CNS circuitry underlying the endogenous depressive syndrome includes hyperactivity of both the MR(5-HT) and the A5(NA) nuclei and hypoactivity of the C1(Ad) medullary nuclei. In addition, we found that endogenously depressed patients also showed raised levels of plasma cortisol at night but not in the mornings. Furthermore, we also demonstrated that endogenously depressed patients had high levels of both plasma noradrenaline and p5-HT, and low levels of plasma adrenaline. Both neurochemical and endocrine disorders were associated to adrenal gland hypoactivity and neural sympathetic hyperactivity. Finally, we afforded evidence that allowed the association of the low levels of plasma tryptophan detected in ED patients to hypoactivity of the DR(5-HT) nucleus. These findings have received additional support from the routine peripheral neuroautonomic assessment of these patients as well as the therapeutic success obtained in hundreds of them. The fact that our neuropharmacological therapy normalized not only clinical but also neurochemical, endocrinological , andneuroautonomic disorders gave a definitive support to our postulation (Lechin, van der Dijs, Gómez et al. 1983a; Lechin, van der Dijs, Acosta et al. 1983b; Lechin, van der Dijs, Jakubowicz et al. 1985b; Lechin, van der Dijs, Orozco et al. 1995a; Lechin, van der Dijs, Benaim 1996a; Lechin, van der Dijs, Hernandez-Adrian 2006a; Lechin, van der Dijs 2006a, 2006b).

Other research studies carried out in our institute demonstrated that not only gastrointestinal but also biliary motility disorders should be associated with ED. For instance, patients affected by the spastic colon syndrome (hyperactivity of the rectosigmoid function) (Chowdhury, Dinoso, Lorber 1976) also presented with biliary motility disorders such as biliary dyskinesia and no gallbladder emptying after the test meal (Lechin, van der Dijs, Bentolila et al. 1977a, 1977b, 1978; Lechin, van der Dijs 1979a, 1979b, 1979c, 1981a, 1982; Lechin, van der Dijs, Gómez et al. 1982a, 1982b, 1982c, 1983a; Lechin, van der Dijs, Acosta et al. 1983b; Lechin, van der Dijs, Jakubowicz et al. 1985a, 1985b; Lechin A, Jara, Rada et al. 1988; Lechin M, Jara, Rada et al. 1988a; Lechin, van der Dijs, Gómez et al. 1988b; Lechin, van der Dijs, Lechin-Báez et al.

1994c; Lechin 1992b; Lechin, van der Dijs, Orozco et al. 1995b; Lechin, van der Dijs, Benaim 1996a; Lechin, van der Dijs, Orozco 2002b; Lechin, van der Dijs, Lechin 2002c).

Our research work allowed us to conclude that both biliary dyskinesia and the irritable bowel syndrome (IBS) should be considered as somatization syndromes (depending on ED) rather than true gastrointestinal diseases. In addition, we have exhaustively demonstrated that ED is closely associated to TH-1 autoimmune disorders. This hypothesis is reinforced by our findings showing that the therapeutic effects triggered by an adequate neuropharmacological therapy was able to suppress not only gastrointestinal and psychiatric symptoms but also the immunological disorders (Lechin, van der Dijs, Lechin et al. 1989a; Lechin, van der Dijs, Vitelli et al. 1990a; Lechin 1992a; Lechin, van der Dijs, Hernandez-Adrian 2006a; Lechin 2006b; Lechin, van der Dijs 2007a, 2007b).

The findings showing no reduction of the levels of plasma cortisol after the dexamethasone challenge may be explained because this neuro-endocrine disorder depends on the MR(5-HT) overactivity. This statement is supported by facts showing that whereas the DR(5-HT)–PVN(CRH)–ACTH–cortisol circuitry overactivity observed during acute stress is inhibited (suppressed) by dexamethasone, the disorder responsible for the nocturnal (not diurnal) hypersecretion of cortisol, observed in ED patients, would depend on another circuitry. We have quoted enough evidence showing that MR(5-HT)–CEA–BNST–PVN circuitry is less accessible to the circulating dexamethasone. Even more, the demonstrated fact that the DR(5-HT) but not MR(5-HT) neurons are crowded by both CRH and cortisol (excitatory) receptors (Kalin, Weiler, Shelton 1982; Laaris, Le Poul, Hamon et al. 1997; Gerendai, Halasz 2000; Vazquez, Bailey, Dent et al. 2006) fits well with our postulation. The above findings afford definitive explanations to the controversial facts showing that acute stress is caused by elevated cortisol plasma levels in the morning whereas ED patients show this endocrine disorder at night (Roy 1988; Yehuda, Teicher, Trestman et al. 1996; Choi, Furay, Evanson et al. 2007), at which period the DR(5-HT) but not the MR(5-HT) neurons show significant fading (Lechin, van der Dijs, Lechin et al. 2002a; Lechin, Pardey-Maldonado, van der Dijs et al. 2004a; Lechin, van der Dijs, Lechin 2004b).

The aforementioned CNS circuitry disorder, which underlies ED, might also explain the lack of increase in plasma levels of growth hormone when ED patients were challenged with a dose of oral clonidine (Lechin, van der Dijs, Jakubowicz et al. 1985a, 1985b; Lechin, van der Dijs 2004a).

Endogenous Depression and Hyperinsulinism

In 1979, we demonstrated that the depressive syndrome induced by captivity (restraint stress) in experimental dogs was caused by the increase of both noradrenaline and p5-HT in the blood (Lechin, Coll-Garcia, van der Dijs et al. 1979b). In addition, we also demonstrated that these dogs showed a rise of both insulin and glucose (insulin resistance). Furthermore, in 1991 we also published a research article, which demonstrated that ED patients showed hyperinsulinism but not hypoglycemia (Lechin, van der Dijs, Lechin et al. 1991). These patients also had higher than normal levels of noradrenaline, which were increased after the oral glucose load (3 hours). On the contrary, plasma adrenaline levels did not rise throughout the postprandial period in these patients. Thus, the noradrenaline/adrenaline plasma ratio augmented throughout the test. This neurotransmitters profile was paralleled by both diastolic blood pressure and plasma insulin rises. Conversely, systolic blood pressure and heart rate remained constant or showed slight decreases throughout the test. The finding that the therapy with doxepin (50 mg before bed) normalized clinical, neuroautonomic, metabolic, and cardiovascular parameters (within the 4 weeks of treatment), allowed us to postulate that an A5(NA) predominance over C1(Ad) was responsible for the peripheral disorder (neural sympathetic over adrenal sympathetic predominance). Eighty-three percent of these patients showed a depressive profile when they were tested with the Hamilton Depression Rating Scale.

Other patients affected by postprandial hypoglycemia and hyperinsulinism (included in this research study) showed the opposite clinical, metabolic, and neuroendocrine profiles. Namely, they presented with abrupt hypoglycemia 45 to 50 minutes after the oral glucose load, which was followed by adrenaline peaks (10 to 15 minutes later). Dramatic heart rate and systolic blood pressure but not diastolic blood pressure increases paralleled adrenaline peaks. This group of patients also improved with the doxepin therapy. However, the fact that the former but not the latter group showed both cortisol and growth hormone resistance to the dexamethasone and clonidine challenges, respectively, allowed us to postulate that ED was responsible for the postprandial hypoglycemia observed in them. On the contrary, taking into account that the second group did not show a depressive profile, when tested with the Hamilton Depression Rating scale, allowed us to assign them the uncoping stress label. Summarizing these results and many others sprouted from the neuroendocrine and neuroautonomic investigation, we concluded that neural sympathetic and adrenal sympathetic hyperactivities underlie ED and uncoping stress syndromes,

respectively. This postulation has received additional support from a great deal of other research studies carried out in our institute. The above findings led us to postulate that the ED syndrome is caused by a CNS circuitry that includes the predominance of the A5(NA) over A6(NA) + C1(Ad) nuclei as well as the MR(5-HT) over DR(5-HT) predominance (Lechin, van der Dijs, Hernandez-Adrian et al. 2006a). Conversely, the uncoping stress syndrome would be caused by the opposite profile: C1(Ad) and DR(5-HT) predominance over A5(NA) and MR(5-HT) (Lechin, van der Dijs, Lechin et al. 1992a).

Akathisia Syndrome (Restlessness)

This syndrome is frequently observed in chronic benzodiazepine's consumers (Lechin, van der Dijs, Vitelli-Flores et al. 1994b, Lechin, van der Dijs, Benaim 1996b). The well-known fact that benzodiazepines inhibit the DR(5-HT) and the A6(NA) but not the MR(5-HT) neurons would explain the pathophysiological disinhibition of the RP(5-HT) neurons responsible for this syndrome. Doctors prescribe L-dopa to these patients order to ameliorate symptoms affecting them. The improvement triggered by this dopamine precursor depends on the fact that not only NA axons but also DA axons innervate the anterior spinal horns. Both catecholamines cooperate to the enhancement of the motility behavior and the muscular tone. These DA axons arise from DA neurons (A11 nucleus) located at the hypothalamic level. In addition, it should be remembered that the anterior (motor) spinal horns also receive excitatory glutamic and inhibitory GABA axons. The latter predominate in those patients who consume GABA mimetic drugs such as benzodiazepines (Hokfelt, Phillipson, Goldstein 1979).

In summary, it is possible to understand that the inescapable or uncontrollable stress syndrome depends on the exhaustion of the A6(NA), A5(NA), and the DR(5-HT) neurons and the disinhibition of the subordinated Ad(C1) and 5-HT(RP) nuclei. This postulation receives additional support from findings which demonstrated that not only DR(5-HT) but also A5(NA) axons inhibit RP(5-HT) neurons (Speciale, Crowley, O'Donohue et al. 1978; Li, Wesselingh, Blessing 1992; Tanaka, Okamura, Tamada et al. 1994), which release serotonin at the anterior spinal horns (Zhang 1991). The opposite profile showing the recovery and predominance of the A5(NA) and the MR(5-HT) neurons would shift the uncoping stress to a coping stress profile. However, prolongation of the latter would lead to the ED profile [A5(NA) and MR(5-HT) predominance]. Furthermore, the fact that the A5(NA) interchanges inhibitory axons with the C1(Ad) medullary nuclei would explain the absolute inhibition of the adrenal sympathetic activity that has always been found in thousands of ED patients investigated (Li, Wesselingh, Blessing et al. 1992; Fenik, Marchenko, Janssen et al. 2002).

Endogenous Depression and Essential Hypertension

We demonstrated in 1993 that the EH patients but not the non–essential hypertensive patients showed the hyperinsulinism (insulin resistance) syndrome (Lechin, van der Dijs, Lechin et al. 1993). Furthermore, we also reported that these patients fulfilled the diagnostic criteria for depression when they were tested with the Hamilton Depression Rating Scale. These clinical research findings allowed us to postulate that both the EH and the depression syndromes are caused by similar CNS disorders.

Both syndromes showed enhanced neural sympathetic activity. In addition, essential hypertensive patients frequently present with the ED clinical profile. Both of them also showed diastolic blood pressure increase at the 1-minute orthostasis challenge (Lechin, van der Dijs, Lechin et al. 1997a). Finally, mammary and ovarian cysts, infertility, rheumatoid arthritis, scleroderma, multiple sclerosis, and other TH-1 autoimmune diseases are frequently associated with both ED and EH (Lechin, van der Dijs, Orozco et al. 1995a, 1996e; Elenkov, Wilder, Chrousos et al. 2000; Koutantji, Harrold, Lane et al. 2003; Lechin, van der Dijs 2004a; Lechin, van der Dijs, Lechin 2004c, 2005a; Beretta, Astori, Ferrario et al. 2006; Wallin, Wilken, Turner et al. 2006; Isik, Koca, Ozturk et al. 2007). Special attention should be devoted to our findings showing that both ED and EH patients are affected by the hyperinsulinism syndrome. This issue has been widely commented on in two recently published review articles (Lechin, van der Dijs 2006a, 2006b).

The fact that all these patients are significantly improved by a common neuropharmacological therapeutic approach to revert the neural predominance over adrenal sympatheticactivity reinforces our point of view. Special mention should be made with respect to multiple sclerosis patients who have been absolutely cured by this therapy (unpublished results).

Our therapeutic strategy is addressed at reverting the predominance of A5(NA) over A6(NA) and C1(Ad) and that of MR(5-HT) over DR(5-HT). Summarizing this issue, we prescribed the following drug therapies:

1. Noradrenaline uptake inhibitor (such as desipramine 25 mg; or maprotyline 75 mg; or reboxetine 30 mg) before both breakfast and lunch (but not before supper). These drugs would excite the inhibited A6(NA) rather than the overactive A5(NA) neurons.

2. Yohimbine (5 mg) or regitine orally, (before both breakfast and lunch). Both are α-2 antagonists that trigger the release of NA from the exhausted A6(NA), but not from the overactive A5(NA) neurons. In addition, these α-2 antagonists will excite the underactive C1(Ad) neurons that are able to antagonize the A5(NA) neurons (both nuclei interchange inhibitory axons) (Fenik, Marchenko, Janssen et al. 2002). The α-2 antagonists also excite DR(5-HT) neurons, which are crowded by α-2 presynaptic inhibitory autoreceptors (Raiteri 2001).

3. Amitriptyline or desipramine (10 mg) injected (at morning) intramuscularly. Both drugs are taken up and metabolized in the liver after oral administration. Thus, the parenteral administration enables these drugs to avoid the obstacle, cross the BBB, and directly excite the hypoactive A6(NA) but not the hyperactive (A5)NA neurons. Considering that amitriptyline is an inhibitor of not only noradrenaline uptake but also 5-HT uptake, it would additionally potentiate the underactive DR(5-HT) but not the hyperactive MR(5-HT) neurons.

4. Sibutramine (10 mg before breakfast), only if necessary. This drug inhibits the noradrenaline uptake and is, in addition, able to trigger noradrenaline and dopamine releases (amphetamine-like effects).

5. Tianeptine 3 mg (before breakfast and lunch). This serotonin uptake–enhancing agent inhibits the release of serotonin from the MR(5-HT) axons. These neurons display overwhelming firing activity in these patients.

6. Doxepin or imipramine (25 mg) before supper. These drugs inhibit the uptake of both noradrenaline (40%) and serotonin (60%) at the A6(NA) and DR(5-HT) nuclei, respectively. These two nuclei should be activated because they are responsible for the slow-wave sleep activity. Exhaustion of one or both of them underlies the short-REM latency seen in exhausted and in depressed patients. In addition, this neuropharmacological strategy would interfere with the precocious nocturnal fading of the above nuclei.

7. Mirtazapine (30 mg) before bed. This drug is a noradrenaline (α-2) as well as 5-HT-2 antagonist, which triggers the release of both types of neurotransmitters from the disinhibited A6(NA) and DR(5-HT) axons, respectively. These excitatory effects provoked by mirtazapine are further potentiated by the previous administration of doxepin or imipramine. These latter drugs interfere with both noradrenaline and serotonin uptake. This pharmacological manipulation favors the normalization of the sleep cycle because it prolongs the SWS duration and avoids the short-REM sleep latency.

Absolute disappearance of psychiatric, neurological, neuroendocrine, and immunological disorders is observed within the first 8 to 16 weeks, after which slow and progressive reduction of the doses of the drugs should be attempted. In our long experience with this issue, we have had no failures with this therapeutic approach. We have maintained this treatment during several months, if necessary. Higher doses are not required. Interruptions of this therapy would depend on the clinical assessment. We never administer cortisol or dexamethasone and/or prednisone to our patients.

Post-traumatic Stress Disorder

PTSD is caused by the absolute and irreversible exhaustion of the A6(NA) and DR(5-HT). This CNS circuitry disorder is similar to that seen in psychotics.

We have had the opportunity to investigated six subjects affected by this syndrome. All of them were diagnosed by more than one psychiatrist and all them satisfied the clinical criteria necessary to be labeled with this diagnosis.

The neurochemical assessment carried out in these patients revealed very high levels of plasma noradrenaline and p5-HT and low levels of plasma adrenaline, dopamine, and f5-HT. In addition, very low levels of plasma tryptophan were also detected. In accordance with our long experience with this type of assessment, these patients showed the same plasma neurotransmitters profile that underlies the psychotic syndrome. This syndrome depends on the A6(NA) and DR(5-HT) maximal hypoactivity and A5(NA) and MR(5-HT) hyperactivity. Owing to the fact that the A10-DA mesocortical neurons depend on the excitatory A6(NA) axons, both dopamine and noradrenaline deficits should be found at the frontal cortex level in both PTSD and psychotic patients.

The aforementioned findings reinforce our hypothesis that PTSD depends on an irreversible deficit of A6(NA) neurons, which would be accentuated after the sudden death of these neurons, which occurs during uncontrollable stress episodes. Definitive and irreversible A5(NA) and MR(5-HT) predominance would result in these circumstances.

We prescribed to the PTSD patients the same neuropharmacological therapy that is advised for psychotic patients. This therapy includes drugs that excite the A6(NA) neurons (intramuscularly injected amitriptyline (10 mg) and prostigmine (15 mg), and oral olanzapine (5 mg), yohimbine (2.5 mg), desipramine (25 mg), or any other noradrenaline-uptake inhibitor (maprotyline, reboxethine, etc). These drugs must be administered before breakfast. In addition, we prescribed doxepin or imipramine (25 mg) or any other noradrenaline and serotonin uptake inhibitor before supper. Finally, we added mirtazapine (30 mg)

before bed. This drug is an α-2 and 5-HT-2 antagonist, which favors the release of both noradrenaline and serotonin from their axons. A small dose of 5-hydroxytryptophan (a serotonin precursor) would be added before bed (25 to 50 mg). In addition to all these drugs, we also prescribed 3 mg of tianeptine (a 5-HT uptake enhancer) both before breakfast and lunch. Yohimbine is able to excite both A6(NA) and DR(5-HT) neurons but not MR(5-HT) neurons, which are not crowded by α-2 inhibitory receptors.

Psychotic Syndrome

We demonstrated in 1980 that noradrenaline antagonist drugs such as dihydroergotamine, phentolamine, and clonidine but not dopamine-blocking agents inhibit the distal colon hypermotility (phasic waves) always present in psychotic patients during relapses (Lechin, van der Dijs 1979c; Lechin, Gómez, van der Dijs et al. 1980a; Lechin, van der Dijs, Gómez et al. 1980b). This distal colon motility profile strongly suggested that both the acute clinical and physiological disorders were triggered by CNS noradrenergic overactivity. Hence, we postulated that an excess of CNS noradrenaline and not dopamine was responsible for the acute psychotic episodes (Lechin, van der Dijs, Gómez et al. 1980b; Lechin, van der Dijs 1981b, 1981c).

The fact that clonidine, an α-2 agonist that reduces CNS A5(NA) activity, but not DA antagonists, was able to suppress both gastrointestinal and acute psychotic episodes allowed us to postulate that both gastrointestinal and psychiatric symptoms in psychotic subjects would depend on CNS noradrenaline overactivity. Then, we stated that an excess of CNS noradrenaline and not dopamine underlies the psychotic syndrome (Lechin, van der Dijs 1979c, 1979d; Lechin, Gómez, van der Dijs et al. 1980a; Lechin, van der Dijs 1981b, 1981c, 1982; Lechin, van der Dijs, Gómez et al. 1983c; Lechin, van der Dijs 2005a).

These findings allowed us to successfully treat hundreds of psychotic patients during acute episodes, with clonidine, a drug that bridles hyperactive CNS-NA and/or CNS-Ad nuclei, but not CNS-DA nuclei. The fact that the peripheral physiological (gastrointestinal) parameters as well as the abnormal levels of circulating neurotransmitters showed different profiles during acute and nonacute periods led us to go deeply into both the clinical and neurochemical abnormal phenomena underlying the psychotic syndrome at these two periods. We demonstrated that whereas high phasic activity (waves) and low sigmoidal tone (lowered baseline) were observed during the acute periods, the opposite profile was observed during nonacute (depressive) periods: low phasic activity and high sigmoidal tone. In addition, the circulating neurotransmitters profile showed raised noradrenaline/adrenaline ratio and normal or low p5-HT during acute psychotic periods and lowered noradrenaline/adrenaline ratio and highest p5-HT values during nonacute (depressive) periods. This latter neurotransmitter profile is also seen in psychotic patients taking antipsychotic drugs. The findings that these patients also showed sedation and other clinical symptoms of hyperparasympathetic predominance after the clonidine administration allowed us to think that ACh and serotonergic overactivity was responsible for the clinical profile observed during nonacute psychotic (depressive) periods.

Neuroautonomic and neurophysiologic data have demonstrated that the A5(NA) and the MR(5-HT) are included into a common CNS circuitry, which is shared by the CEA and the BNST. This circuitry displays antagonistic activity to other circuitry integrated by the A6(NA), DR(5-HT), and the hypothalamic PVN nuclei (Lechin, van der Dijs, Hernandez-Adrian 2006a).

Considering that the A6(NA) is underdeveloped in psychotic subjects (Craven, Priddle, Crow et al. 2005), it cannot exert the normal modulatory role, which depends on the bridling of the A5(NA) neurons by A6(NA) axons (Cedarbaum, Aghajanian 1978; Byrum, Guyenet 1987; Ennis, Aston-Jones 1988). Conversely, the latter nucleus should inhibit the former in psychotic patients. Furthermore, taking into account that MR(5-HT) axons bridle both the A6(NA) and the DR(5-HT) neurons, the A5(NA) and MR(5-HT) binomial activity should overwhelm the A6(NA) + DR(5-HT) nuclei (Lechin, van der Dijs, Hernandez-Adrian 2006a). In addition, findings showing that the A5(NA) nucleus interchanges inhibitory axons with the medullary parasympathetic nuclei (Iwasaki, Kani, Maeda 1999; Fenik, Marchenko, Janssen et al. 2002) and furthermore, sends inhibitory axons to the C1(Ad) medullary nuclei (Li, Wesselingh, Blessing 1992) fit well with the understanding of the pathophysiological mechanisms that underlie the two clinical alternating periods seen in psychotic patients (maniac and depressive). At the peripheral level, both neural sympathetic and parasympathetic predominance would be observed, during manic and depressive periods, respectively. Increased phasic activity and low sigmoidal tone versus none or low phasic activity and high sigmoidal tone will be observed during acute and nonacute psychotic (depressive) clinical syndromes, respectively (Lechin, Gómez, van der Dijs et al. 1980a; Lechin, van der Dijs, Gómez et al. 1980b, 1982a).

The DR(5-HT) and the MR(5-HT) nuclei are involved into the CNS circuitry disorder that underlies the psychotic syndrome to a great extent. The assessment of circulating neurotransmitters in approximately 30,000 normal and diseased subjects,

not only during supine-resting state but also after different types of challenges, allowed us to conclude that whereas the p5-HT level is positively correlated with the activity of the MR(5-HT) neurons, a negative correlation exists between plasma tryptophan and DR(5-HT) activity. We discussed this issue in a review article (Lechin, van der Dijs, Hernandez-Adrian 2006a) where we quoted a great deal of data supporting this postulation. Thus, the very low levels of plasma tryptophan that we always found in psychotic patients during acute periods should be associated to the predominance of MR over DR.

Summarizing, the great bulk of data accumulated by our research group dealing with the neurochemical, neuroautonomic, and neurophysiological assessment of hundreds of psychotic patients during both acute and nonacute periods led us to postulate that this syndrome is caused, at the CNS level, by an A5(NA) and MR(5-HT) predominance over A6(NA) and DR(5-HT). In addition, a deficit of the A10(DA) activity (dopamine mesocortical neurons) should parallel the A6(NA) deficit (Knable, Hyde, Murray et al. 1996; Craven, Priddle, Crow et al. 2005). This well-demonstrated fact fits well with others showing that A6(NA) axons innervate A10(DA) neurons, which are crowded by α-1 excitatory receptors (Tassin 1992). Thus, any A6(NA) deficit should redound in the DA underactivity at the cortical level. Patients with other syndromes (hyperactive, PTSD, and Alzheimer's disease) also share this disorder.

ED patients (during relapsing periods) should also be included among the CNS (neurochemical and neuroautonomic) psychotic profile disorder. This postulation is consistent with our neurochemical research studies, which demonstrated that they present with maximal raised levels of both plasma noradrenaline and p5-HT levels and very low levels of plasma tryptophan at these periods. In our long experience with this issue, we found a positive correlation between the neurochemical disorders and the suicide attempts, which should be considered as a psychotic symptom.

Psychotic Disorder

Summarizing, psychotic syndrome is caused by anatomical and physiological deficits of the A6(NA), A10(DA), and DR(5-HT) nuclei. Hence, noradrenaline, dopamine, and serotonin are under-released at the frontocortical brain areas. These deficits would result in the predominance of the subcortical nuclei: A5(NA), MR(5-HT), A8(DA), and A9(DA).

The A5(NA) and MR(5-HT) binomial would predominate over the A6(NA) and DR(5-HT) during acute psychotic periods, whereas the MR(5-HT) and medullary parasympathetic activities would predominate during psychotic depressive periods.

Similar Common Disorders Shared by Endogenous Depression, Psychotic, Attention-Deficit Hyperactive Disorder, Post-traumatic Stress Disorder, and Alzheimer's Patients

We do not pretend to afford a long and detailed list of specific symptoms with reference to each of these syndromes; however, it is well known that all patients with these disorders show a low intellectual capability, deficit of memory, attention, and affection as well as learning disability. In addition, they also show an aggressive behavior and a low prepulse inhibition (Lechin, van der Dijs, Lechin 1979a; Lechin, van der Dijs 1989; Lechin, van der Dijs, Lechin 2002a). In addition, all of them present with a neurochemical profile characterized by raised levels of circulating noradrenaline and p5-HT. Conversely, both adrenaline and plasma tryptophan levels are found to be lower than normal in all of them (Lechin, van der Dijs, Orozco et al. 1995a). This neurochemical profile worsens during orthostasis and exercise challenges. Diastolic blood pressure, but neither systolic blood pressure nor heart rate, showed normal increases in healthy subjects. This phenomenon is consistent with the postulation of the predominance of the peripheral neural sympathetic activity over the adrenal sympathetic activity. At the CNS level, predominance of the A5(NA) over the C1(Ad) pontomedullary nucleus would be responsible for the peripheral sympathetic disorder (Lechin, van der Dijs 2006a). These findings receive support from those of many others researchers (Rotman, Zemishlany, Munitz et al. 1982; Kalin, Weiler, Shelton 1982; Rogeness, Mitchell, Custer et al. 1985; Roy, Pickar, Linnoila et al. 1985; Banki, Bissette, Arato et al. 1987; Faludi, Magyar, Tekes et al. 1988; Leake, Griffiths, Ferrier 1989; Murburg, McFall, Lewis et al. 1995; Yehuda, Teicher, Trestman et al. 1996; Roy 1999; Seals, Esler 2000).

Several neuroendocrinological disorders are also common to all the aforementioned psychiatric syndromes. These include lower-than-normal cortisol response to the dexamethasone challenge as well as lower-than-normal growth hormone response to the clonidine challenge. In addition, this α-2 agonist does not provoke the normal plasma noradrenaline level reduction when these patients are challenged with this drug. Other common neuroendocrinological disorder shared by all these patients is the chronically elevated prolactin plasma level (Lechin, van der Dijs, Jakubowicz et al. 1985a, 1985b; Lechin 1992c).

Increased p5-HT and reduced plasma tryptophan levels are always observed in these patients. A bulk of evidence supports the postulation that these abnormal findings should be associated with the absolute predominance of the MR(5-HT) activity over the DR(5-HT) activity (Lechin, van der Dijs, Hernandez-Adrian 2006a).

It has been exhaustively demonstrated that these abnormal findings support the postulation that the predominance is closely associated to the aggressive behavior, which is always present in all patients with the aforementioned psychiatric syndromes.

Our long experience dealing with the neurochemical plus neuroautonomic assessment of all types of psychiatric and/or somatic diseases allow us to postulate that the aforementioned patients share some common CNS circuitry disorders. This common profile would be integrated by a deficit of the A6(NA), A10(DA), + and DR(5-HT) neurons, all of which innervate the frontal cortical area. The neurochemical deficit at cortical level would favor the predominance of the A5(NA), A8(DA), A9(DA), and MR(5-HT) subcortical CNS circuitry. Indeed, this CNS profile underlies the psychotic syndrome schizophrenia. Our research group has investigated this issue since 1981, when we published our first reports dealing with the noradrenergic hypothesis of the schizophrenia (Lechin, van der Dijs 1981c). These preliminary studies have been further ratified by us and many other researchers (Yamamoto, Hornykiewicz 2004; Lechin, van der Dijs 2005a). In addition, we have had the opportunity to outline successfully neuropharmacological therapy for a bulk of these patients.

Our neuropharmacological therapeutic approach is aimed at the enhancement of the A6(NA) and A10(DA) activity, to restore the predominance of this binomial over the A5(NA), A8(DA), and A9(DA) (Vezina, Blanc, Glowinski et al. 1991; King, Zigmond, Finlay 1997). This target is reached by the administration of a noradrenaline-uptake inhibitor (such as desipramine or maprotyline or reboxethine), a noradrenaline-releasing agent (such as yohimbine or regitine or idaxozan), a noradrenaline precursor (phenylalanine or l-tyrosine), olanzapine, which excites A6(NA) neurons (Dawe, Huff, Vandergriff et al. 2001), and an MAO-B inhibitor (such as selegiline). The rationality of this treatment depends on findings showing that the two former drugs would act at the underactive A6(NA) and not at the hyperactive A5(NA) nucleus. Considering that A6(NA) axons excite A10(DA) mesocortical neurons, selegiline should interfere with the MAO-B enzyme, which catabolizes dopamine at this level. Finally, we add a small dose of modafinil or adrafinil after breakfast. This α-1 agonist is able to excite receptors located at the A10(DA) mesocortical neurons (Tassin 1992), which release dopamine from DA axons. It should be remembered that dopamine released at cortical levels is not taken up by DA axons (as occurs at subcortical areas). This neurotransmitter is destroyed by the MAO-B enzyme; thus, inhibition of this enzyme would interfere with the disappearance of dopamine at this level (Vezina, Blanc, Glowinski et al. 1991).

In addition, we prescribe an adequate neuropharmacological therapy addressed to normalize the sleep disorder always present in all these patients (Tandon, Shipley, Taylor et al. 1992). Considering that all of them show a short REM latency and frequent awake periods, we prescribe a noradrenaline and serotonin uptake inhibitor, such as doxepin (25 mg) or imipramine (25 mg) and a noradrenaline and serotonin–releasing agent, such as mirtazapine. This drug is an α-2 and 5-HT-2 antagonist that triggers both noradrenaline and serotonin release from NA and 5-HT axons, respectively. In our long experience with the polysomnography investigation, we found that prolongation of the SWS period parallels clinical improvement. Indeed, the short-REM latency they always present with (before treatment) should be attributed to the exhaustion of the A6(NA) and DR(5-HT) nuclei. This phenomenon is consistent with the well-known fact that both the A6(NA) and the DR(5-HT) nuclei are responsible for the SWS and both become silent at the REM sleep stage.

The sustained and progressive improvement obtained in all these patients might be monitored throughout the clinical assessment. We never observed any type of undesirable side effects. In addition, it should be mentioned that children with ADHD reach absolute and irreversible improvement in all the cases, after long-term sustained neuropharmacological therapy such as that we have outlined for psychotic patients.

In our long experience with this issue, we found that psychotic patients maximally improve with the addition of a small dose of olanzapine (Dawe, Huff, Vandergriff et al. 2001) or clozapine (Youngren, Moghaddam, Bunney et al. 1994) (before bed). These drugs excite the A6(NA) neurons (in addition to the other effects at both DA and 5-HT neurons). Clozapine also excites A6(NA) neurons and exerts an α-1 antagonistic effect, which explains the deep sleep that it provokes. This fact should be taken into account to enhance the SWS of these patients.

Neuroimmunological Profiles

Uncoping stress is associated with TH-2 immunological profile, which is caused by low CD4/CD8 ratio, low NK-cell cytotoxicity against K-562 target cells, and low plasma levels of TH-1 cytokines (IL-2, IL-12, IL-18, γ-interferon) (Kopin, Eisenhofer, Goldstein 1988; Cunnick, Lysle, Kucinski et al. 1990; Felsner, Hofer, Rinner et al. 1995; Buckingham, Loxley, Christian et al. 1996; Marotti, Gabrilovac, Rabatic et al. 1996; Leonard, Song 1996; Oya, Kawamura, Shimizu et al. 2000; Calcagni, Elenkov 2006; Shakhar, Rosenne, Loewenthal et al. 2006; Matsuda, Furukawa, Suzuki et al. 2007).

Coping stress is associated with TH-1 immunological profile, which is caused by high CD4/CD8 ratio, high NK-cell cytotoxicity against K-562 target cells, and high plasma levels of TH-1 cytokines (IL-2,

IL-12, IL-18, γ-interferon) (Madden, Felten, Felten et al. 1989; Ader, Felten, Cohen 1990; Madden, Felten, Felten et al. 1994; Amital, Blank, Shoenfeld 1996; Nicholson, Kuchroo 1996; Aulakh, Mazzola-Pomietto, Murphy 1996; Eilat, Mendlovic, Doron 1999; Schwarz, Chiang, Muller et al. 2001; Wrona 2006; Gaykema, Chen, Goehler 2007; Witek-Janusek, Gabram, Mathews 2007) (See Table 5.1). Adequate neuropharmacological therapy should be administered to reverse the aforementioned abnormal neuroautonomic and CNS disorders.

Neuroimmunological Diseases

We will refer to some diseases well investigated by our research group.

Gastrointestinal Diseases

Duodenal ulcer, type B gastritis and Crohn's disease are caused by raised levels of plasma noradrenaline, NA/Ad ratio, p5-HT, and nocturnal plasma cortisol. These findings fit well with the TH-1 immunological profile usually found in these subjects. The fact that the cortisol plasma levels do not show significant reduction after the dexamethasone challenges in these patients gives additional support to the postulations. Furthermore, clonidine does not trigger growth hormone increase in duodenal ulcer patients (Jara, Lechin, Rada et al. 1988; Lechin, van der Dijs, Rada et al. 1990b). These findings are caused by the down-regulation of α-2 receptors at the hypothalamic level, which depends on the over-release of noradrenaline from the A5 axons at this level. Other immunological evidence demonstrated that the gastrointestinal diseases these patients present with should be considered as being caused by the TH-1 autoimmune profile. Conversely, patients affected by type A gastritis, gastric ulcer, ulcerative colitis, reflux esophagitis, and gastric maltoma always showed the TH-2 immunological profile as well as the uncoping stress neuroendocrine and neuroautonomic disorder (Lechin, van der Dijs 1973; Lechin 1977; Christensen 1980; Lechin, van der Dijs, Jakubowicz et al. 1987a; Lechin 1988b; Lechin, van der Dijs, Rada et al. 1989b; Lechin, van der Dijs, Vitelli et al. 1990a; Lechin 1988b).

Both the ulcerative colitis and Crohn's disease merit some special comments. The former should be included among the TH-2 disorders whereas the latter always shows the TH-1 autoimmune disorder. These postulations are supported by the successful neuropharmacological therapies prescribed for them. Readers should be aware that patients with Crohn's disease are frequently misdiagnosed because intestinal lesions are located at the submucosal (deep) level, nonaccessible to punch biopsy, and in addition,

Table 5.1 Neuroautonomic and Immunological Profiles Underlying Some Somatic, Psychosomatic, and Psychiatric Diseases

	Adrenal/Neural Sympathetic Predominance	Neural/Adrenal Sympathetic Predominance	References
Central pathways activated	A6(NA), DR(5-HT), C1(Ad)	A5(NA), MR(5-HT)	Anisman 1978 Lechin et al. 1996a, 2006a
Peripheral pathways activated	Thoracic sympathetic chain and adrenal gland—raised plasma adrenaline and cortisol or serotonin	Lumbar sympathetic chain—raised plasma noradrenaline	Burchfield 1979 Kvetnansky et al. 1977 Jacobs et al. 1981 Engeland 1998; Lechin et al. 1996a, 2006a
	↓	↓	

Diseases associated with	Uncoping Stress (TH-2)		Endogenous Depression (TH-1)		
	Ad.S.	P.S.	N.S.	P.S.	
Cardiovascular disorders					
Bradyarrhythmia		X			Lechin et al. 2004c, 2005a
Tachyarrhythmia	X		X		Lechin et al. 2002d
Ischemic heart disease			X		Lechin et al. 2002g, 2005a
Essential hypertension					Lechin et al. 1993, 1997a Lechin, van der Dijs 2006a
Non–essential hypertension	X				Lechin et al. 1997a
Respiratory disorders					
Acute asthma				X	Lechin AE et al. 1994 Lechin et al. 1996f, 1998b; Lechin et al. 2002f, 2004h
Nonacute asthma			X		Lechin et al. 2005a
Sleep apnea			X		Lechin et al. 2004b Lechin, van der Dijs 2005b
Respiratory failure			X		Roussos, Koutsoukou 2003
Gastrointestinal disorders					
Type A gastritis		X			Lechin, van der Dijs 1973
Type B gastritis			X		Lechin M et al. 1988b
Gastric ulcer	X	X			Lechin et al. 2006c
Duodenal ulcer	X	X			Lechin et al. 1990b
Acute pancreatitis	X	X			Roze et al. 1981 Loewy, Haxhiu 1993 Lechin, van der Dijs 2004b
Biliary dyskinesia			X	X	Lechin et al. 2002b Lechin, van der Dijs 2007b
Spastic colon			X		Lechin et al. 1977b
Nervous diarrhea	X	X			Lechin et al. 1977a; Lechin et al. 1994c
Ulcerative colitis	X	X			Lechin et al. 1985c; Sandborn et al. 2001
Granulomatous colitis (Crohn's disease)			X		Lechin et al. 1988a; Lechin et al. 1989a
Carcinoid syndrome	X	X			Tobe et al. 1976; Lechin et al. 2005c; Lechin, van der Dijs 2005c
Pancreatic cyst fibrosis	X	X			Hong, Magee 1970 Lechin et al. 2005d

(Continued)

Table 5.1 Continued

Diseases associated with	Uncoping Stress (TH-2)		Endogenous Depression (TH-1)		References
	Ad.S.	P.S.	N.S.	P.S.	
Malignant diseases	X		X		Lechin et al. 2002a
Hematological disorders					
Thrombocytopenic purpura	X		X		Lechin 2006b, 2004e
Polycythemia vera			X		Lechin et al. 2005b, 2006b
Aplastic anemia	X		X		Nakao et al. 2005; Young 2006
Immune-mediated injury					
Allergies and anaphylaxis		X			Reeves, Todd 2000
Rheumatoid arthritis			X		Elenkov et al. 2000
Scleroderma			X		Vassilopoulos,
Vasculitis			X		Mantzoukis 2006
Raynaud's syndrome			X		Beretta et al. 2006
Fibromyalgia			X		Koutantji et al. 2003
Polymyositis			X		Young, Redmond 2007
Dermatomyositis			X		
Guillain Barré syndrome	X				Kuwabara 2007
Multiple sclerosis			X		Wallin et al. 2006
Myasthenia gravis			X		Lechin et al. 1996e, 1996f
Endocrinological syndromes					
Type 1 diabetes			X		Novak et al. 2007
Type 2 diabetes	X	X			O'Connor et al. 2006
Hyperinsulinism			X		Lechin et al. 1979b, 1991; Lechin, van der Dijs 2006b
Type 1 postprandial hypoglycemia	X	X			Lechin et al. 1991
Type 3 postprandial hypoglycemia			X		
Chronic hyperprolactinemia (mammary and ovarian cysts)			X		Lechin et al. 1979 Oliveira et al. 2000
Recurrent abortions			X	X	Peluso, Morrone 2007
Psychiatric diseases					
Endogenous depression			X	X	Leake et al. 1989, 1992; Lechin et al. 1995a, 1996a
Dysthymic depression	X	X			
Psychotic syndrome			X		Lechin, van der Dijs 2005a Craven et al. 2005
Anxiety, social phobia	X	X			Lechin et al. 1997c, 2006a
Post-traumatic stress disorder			X		Lechin 2006a

Uncoping stress: Adrenal gland secretion of catecholamines (adrenaline 80%, noradrenaline 10% , and dopamine 10%) predominates over sympathetic nerves release of catecholamines (noradrenaline 80 to 90% and dopamine 10 to 20%). Overactivity of the CNS C1(Ad) nuclei triggers excitation of the vagal (medullary) nuclei, which is responsible for the peripheral parasympathetic nerves activity. Thus, alternancy of these two ANS peripheral branches is frequently seen in patients affected by the uncoping stress syndrome (**Ad.S.,** Adrenal stage; **P.S.,** parasympathetic stage). Predominance of both adrenal and cortisol are responsible for the Th-2 immunological predominance.

Endogenous depression: Absolute predominance of neural over adrenal sympathetic activity underlies this CNS and ANS profile (**N.S.,** neural sympathetic stage). At CNS level, the A5(NA) nucleus exerts maximal inhibition of both the C1(Ad) and vagal (medullary) nuclei. This CNS disorder is responsible for the disappearance of both adrenal and parasympathetic peripheral activities. In addition, the inhibition of the adrenocortical glands is responsible for the disinhibition of the thymus, which redunds in the TH-1 immunological profile.

the lymphoid granulomas are located at the small bowel rather than at the colon level. That area of the intestine is not accessible to endoscopic investigation. Thus the diagnosis of Crohn's disease should be made according to radiological, immunological, and neuroautonomic procedures (Lechin, van der Dijs, Lechin et al. 1989a, 2002a). With respect to this, it should be known that patients with ulcerative colitis, but not those with Crohn's disease, present with positive ANCA test (antineutrophil cytoplasmic antibody) (Sandborn, Loftus, Colombel et al. 2001; Joossens, Reinisch, Vermeire et al. 2002). This test reflects TH-2 immune profile, which parallels the uncoping stress disorder.

Neurological Diseases

Two types of neurological diseases, the multiple sclerosis and the Guillian Barré syndrome, are caused by TH-1 and TH-2 immunological disorders, respectively (Lechin, van der Dijs, Lechin et al. 2002a; Kuwabara 2007). Both of them have been successfully treated in our institute with neuropharmacological therapies to restore the immunological TH-1 versus TH-2 balance.

Other neuroimmunological diseases such as myasthenia gravis (MG) merit some special comments. We have investigated and treated several hundreds of these patients (Lechin, van der Dijs, Orozco et al. 1996e, 1996f). The neuroimmunological investigation carried out in our institute demonstrated that this syndrome should be considered as a TH-1 immunological predominant disorder. Thus, exhausted A6(NA) and DR(5-HT) nuclei would be overwhelmed by the A5(NA) and MR(5-HT) binomial. The fact that thymectomy and/or steroid therapy is able to suppress both the thymus gland hyperactivity and the MR(5-HT) predominance fits well with the beneficial (short-term) therapeutic alleviation of symptoms seen in these patients submitted to these therapies. It should be known that steroids excite the DR(5-HT) but not the MR(5-HT) neurons, because the former, but not the latter, is crowded by cortisol (excitatory) receptors. In addition, it should be taken into account that steroids suppress neural sympathetic activity, which is enhanced in all TH-1 patients. The alleviation of symptoms triggered by pyridostigmine, a drug that does not cross the BBB in both seronegative and seropositive MG patients should be attributed to the ability of this drug to excite the adrenal gland, which is crowded by excitatory nicotine receptors rather than to the direct effect of the drug at the neuromuscular junction. These glands are underactive in all types of TH-1 disorders. This explanation fits well with the improvement of symptoms provoked by glucocorticoids in both seropositive and seronegative MG patients (these latter patients do not have anti-ACh autoantibodies that can interfere at the neuromuscular junction). Hence, the myasthenic symptoms cannot be attributed to this synaptic interference in seronegative MG patients.

The greater obstacle that we found in treating these patients should be attributed to both previous steroid therapy and thymectomy. Absolute recovery has been obtained in hundreds of MG patients who had not been taking steroids. These drugs provoke the exhaustion of both the DR(5-HT) and the adrenal gland. This disease affected Dr. Lechin (12 years ago) and, he is absolutely normalized because he rejected this type of therapy, which, in our opinion, should be forbidden.

Other TH-1 autoimmune diseases have been successfully treated in our institute. Multiple sclerosis, Sjögren disease, fibromyalgia, pemphigus, scleroderma, rheumatoid arthritis, recurrent abortions, and other TH-1 autoimmune patients are frequently referred to our institute for that purpose. Several photographical evidences have been published in some review articles and in our last published book (Lechin, van der Dijs, Lechin et al. 2002a). In addition, cases of Crohn's diseases are also presented in our book, which might be a useful reference on the absolute normalization of patients who presented with these radiological disorders at the small bowel level and/or colon or stomach. Special mention should be made with respect to multiple sclerosis. We have successfully treated 23 cases after the failure of β-interferon therapy to avoid the relapses always observed following the initial successes obtained with this drug. Two blind patients are included among these latter cases. Both of them recovered the sight that they had lost despite the β-interferon treatment.

Other TH-2 autoimmune diseases such as ulcerative colitis have been successfully treated also with an adequate neuropharmacological protocol that enhances the Th1/Th2 ratio. Details of these protocols can be found in our previous published articles (Lechin, van der Dijs, Insausti et al. 1982d, 1985c; Lechin, van der Dijs, Orozco 2004e, 2005c; Lechin, van der Dijs 2005c).

Hematological and Vascular Disorders

IDIOPATHIC THROMBOCYTOPENIC PURPURA AND POLYCYTHEMIA VERA We demonstrated that both idiopathic thrombocytopenic purpura (ITP) and polycythemia vera (PV) were caused by an ED profile (Lechin, van der Dijs, Orozco et al. 2004e, 2005b). In addition, immunological investigation demonstrated that both syndromes are caused by a TH-1 autoimmune profile.

An anti-TH-1 neuropharmacological therapy was successfully carried out in these patients. No relapses were observed over months and years among the 11 PV and the 13 ITP patients included in our protocol (Lechin, van der Dijs, Orozco et al. 2004e, 2005b).

Normalization (without relapses) of both the neuroautonomic and the immunological profiles has been obtained in all ITP and PV patients who had received the neuropharmacological therapy. In addition, normalization of the wake–sleep cycle was observed in all these patients. This latter issue merits some comments. In our long experience dealing with the neuro-immunopharmacological investigation and therapy, we learned that normalization of the wake–sleep cycle is the best index of improvement. We tested this parameter in our sleep research laboratory not only through polysomnographic assessment but also through investigation of circulating neurotransmitters (NA, Ad, DA, p5-HT, f5-HT, and tryptophan) during both the waking state and each stage of the nocturnal sleep cycle. It should be known that normalization of the sleep disorders depends on the accomplishment of the five sleep stages that integrate the sleep cycle: SWS-1, SWS-2, SWS-3, SWS-4, and REMs without awakenings interruptions.

THROMBOSTASIS DISORDERS These disorders are caused by a TH-1 autoimmunological profile. Autoantibodies against vascular endothelial cells are frequently reported to be present in their sera. These findings support the postulation that vasculitis, cardiovascular and cerebrovascular thrombostasis, and in addition, phlebothrombosis disorders are caused by the same TH-1 autoimmune profile. In addition, we have found that the p5-HT value is positively correlated with blood coagulation and thus, with all thrombotic events. We demonstrated that an adequate neuropharmacological therapy to enhance CNS serotonergic activity (with serotonin uptake inhibitors) triggers the parallel reduction of thrombogenesis. It should be remembered that p5-HT depletion interferes with thrombogenesis. Thus, this effect triggered by all types of serotonin uptake inhibitors would easily explain the interference by these drugs on all types of thrombotic events. (Lechin, van der Dijs 2004b, 2004c, 2004d; Lechin, van der Dijs, Orozco et al. 2004g; Lechin, van der Dijs, Lechin 2005a; Lechin, van der Dijs, Orozco et al. 2005b). This issue led us to treat all types of arterial and venous thrombosis by the administration of a minimal dose of serotonin uptake inhibitors, such as clomipramine, paroxetine, sertraline, etc. This therapeutic strategy impedes coronary, cerebrovascular, and any other vascular thrombosis. These patients have not needed any instrumental therapy to deobstruct vessels.We published some

short reports on this issue; however, we are aware that practitioners would not accept this type of therapeutic approaches. Thus, we will not discuss this issue in this chapter.

Malignant Diseases

STRESS, IMMUNOLOGY, AND CANCER: EFFECTS OF PSYCHOACTIVE DRUGS All malignant diseases but Hodgkin lymphoma, myeloma multiple, and myeloid leukemia present with the TH-2 immunological profile. We published a review article in 1987 (Lechin, van der Dijs, Jakubowicz et al. 1987a). We presented photographic evidence showing the beneficial results obtained with our therapeutic neuropharmacological approach aimed at normalizing the CNS and ANS neuroautonomic disorders after the administration of an adequate neuropharmacological therapy. Both neuroendocrinological and immunological disorders were also normalized through the 6 years that this protocol lasted.

We measured noradrenaline, adrenaline, dopamine, p5-HT, f5-HT, plasma cortisol, and plasma prolactin levels both before and after monthly control evaluation. The immunological investigation included the assessment of the number of peripheral lymphocytes CD3, CD4, CD8, and NK-cells. In addition, NK-cell cytotoxicity against the K-562 target cells was also assessed periodically. This therapeutic research has been carried out since 1980 up to the present (Lechin, van der Dijs, Azócar et al. 1988c; van der Dijs, Lechin, Vitelli et al. 1988a; van der Dijs, Lechin, Vitelli et al. 1988b; Vitelli, Lechin, Cabrera et al. 1988; Lechin S Vitelli, Martinez et al. 1988).

A total of 177 cancer patients participated in our first protocol. All patients had advanced cancer showing an uncoping stress profile and had previously refused chemotherapy. Of the 177 advanced cancer patients, 144 (81.4%) survived for more than 5 years after the initiation of therapy. In addition, the 33 remaining advanced cancer patients showed survival time that was significantly longer than that supposed to be the upper limit of their lifetime expectancy (Table 5.2). Normalization of neurochemical, endocrinological, and immunological parameters was observed within 2 to 3 months of the initiation of the neuropharmacological therapy (Fig. 5.5). Our initial research work was presented in international meetings and in many cancer centers in the United States and other countries. Some clinical reports were also published in several journals and in our last book (Lechin, van der Dijs 1982; Lechin, van der Dijs, Azócar et al. 1987b; Lechin, van der Dijs, Lechin et al. 1989a; Lechin, van der Dijs, Vitelli et al. 1990a; Lechin, van der Dijs, Lechin 2002a, 2004d).

Table 5.2 Follow-up of 177 Advanced Cancer Patients Submitted to Neuropharmacological Therapy

Cancer	Total	Alive	Dead	% Alive
Esophagus	03	00	03	00.0
Stomach	21	18	03	85.7
Right colon	05	05	00	100.0
Transverse colon	03	13	00	100.0
Sigmoid colon	11	09	02	81.8
Rectum	08	08	00	100.0
Gallbladder	01	01	00	100.0
Primary hepatoma	01	00	01	00.0
Pancreas	04	01	03	25.0
Choledochus	01	01	00	100.0
Kidney	09	09	00	100.0
Bladder	03	03	00	100.0
Prostatic gland	26	24	02	92.3
Testis	01	00	01	100.3
Mammary gland	15	11	04	73.3
Uterus	05	04	01	80.0
Ovary	03	02	01	66.6
Larynx	01	01	00	100.0
Lungs	22	18	04	81.8
Melanoma	13	08	05	61.5
Lymphoma	07	07	00	100.0
Sarcoma	03	03	00	100.0
Myeloma	01	01	00	100.0
Skin	07	07	00	100.0
Meningioma	02	02	00	100.0
Brain	01	00	01	00.0
Total	177	144	33	81.4

Adapted from the Archivos Venezolanos de Farmacologia Clinica y Terapeutica (Lechin et al. 1987b).

A total of 177 advanced cancer patients treated by neuropharmacological therapy: 5 patients survived after 6 years, 7 patients survived after 5 years, 13 patients survived after 4 years, 21 patients survived after 3 years, 24 patients survived after 2 years, 42 and patients survived after 1 year. All patients had metastatic tumors and began neuropharmacological therapy during exacerbation periods. All patients began neuropharmacological therapy immediately after partial or total removal of primary tumor. None them showed further exacerbation periods.

Furthermore, we recently sent a commentary to the *Journal of Biological Chemistry* (Lechin, van der Dijs 2007c), related to a research article by Sastry et al. (2007). These authors ratified our findings dealing with the positive correlation found between malignancy and adrenaline plasma levels as well as the negative correlation between the former parameters and NK-cell cytotoxicity.

Up to the present, we have successfully treated more than 1000 advanced cancer patients who rejected both chemotherapy and radiotherapy, because those patients were aware that both therapeutic procedures destroy the immune system.

Summarizing our long experience, we concluded that the worsening of cancer is positively correlated with uncoping stress. In addition, we demonstrated that an adequate neuropharmacological therapy enhances both the TH-1 immunological profile and the NK-cell cytoxicity against the K-562 target cells. Ovarian cancer, melanoma, and mammary, prostate, and gastric adenocarcinomas were the most easy to improve. In addition, non–Hodgkin's lymphoma and maltoma showed a 100% of improvement.

Psychosomatic Diseases

A bulk of experimental, clinical, and therapeutic data support the postulation that the gastrointestinal and biliary systems, along with the cardiorespiratory machinery, constitute the visceral areas that maximum reflect both the physiological and pathophysiological oscillations of the CNS structures that integrate the pontomedullary and spinal circuitry responsible for the CNS to ANS physiological cascade. The fact that those visceral areas are included into the more innervated structures and, in addition, considering that those peripheral systems are targeted by all types of peripheral agents as well as by psychological stressors might help understand why the visceral areas are the most frequently affected.

Although we have investigated a great deal of clinical, physiological, and pharmacological data dealing with the cardiovascular parameters, we will refer in this chapter to a bulk of both clinical and scientific research findings concerning to the physiological and pathophysiological interactions between gastrointestinal and biliary systems and the CNS circuitry. Peripheral assessment included biliary motility, distal colon motility, circulating neurotransmitters, clinical data, and some other parameters. In addition, we will present evidence dealing with the effects of some neuropharmacological drugs on both neuroautonomic and visceral functioning.

Finally, we will present physiological, pharmacological, and therapeutic evidence supporting the postulation that the so-called psychosomatic diseases depend on the peripheral ANS unbalance, which reflects on the CNS circuitry disorders. Although this issue is valid for all types of diseases, we will choose some examples that might be graphically demonstrated.

Irritable Bowel Syndrome and Biliary Dyskinesia

Clinical and pathophysiological research investigations carried out in our institute (Lechin, van der Dijs, Lechin-Báez et al. 1994c) demonstrated that

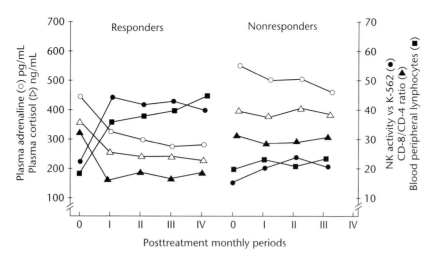

Figure 5.5 A total of 177 advanced cancer patients received neuropharmacological therapy instead of chemotherapy. They were followed up for 6 years or more. All of them showed significant improvement. Absolute disappearance of tumors was seen in 144 patients (responders), whereas significant improvement and increased survival time expectancy was seen in the other 33 patients (nonresponders). All patients showed increased levels of epinephrine, epinephrine over norepinephrine (E/NE) plasma ratio, and low levels of natural killer (NK) cell cytoxicity against the K-562 target cells. Absolute normalization of neuroimmunological parameters was seen in all responders. Adapted from Archivos Venezolanos de Farmacología Clínica y Terapéutica (Lechin, van der Dijs, Azócar et al. 1987b). This conference was lectured by invitation at the XI Congress of the Latinoamerican Association of Pharmacology and the II Congress of the Interamerican Society for Clinical Pharmacology and Therapeutics, Buenos Aires, Argentina, November 1986, and by invitation at the following centers: The University of Texas, MD Anderson Cancer Center; Arthur James Cancer Center (Iowa); National Cancer Institute (Maryland); University of South Florida (Tampa); The Ohio State University, Columbus, 1992.

there exist two types or two faces of the so-called irritable bowel syndrome (IBS): the spastic colon and the nervous diarrhea. Periodical alternation of these two clinical stages is the rule. High sigmoidal tone and low rectal activity are seen during the spastic colon periods whereas low sigmoidal tone and high rectal motility are seen during the latter period (Lechin, Jara, Rada et al. 1988a, 1988; Cabrera, van der Dijs, Jimenez et al. 1988; Lechin, van der Dijs, Lechin-Báez et al. 1994c). In addition, biliary dyskinesia is frequently seen during the spastic but not the diarrheic period. Gallbladder emptying was triggered neither by the Boyden test meal (eggs, milk, butter) nor by the intravenous administration of CCK during the spastic colon period. Furthermore, it has been also demonstrated that dihydroergotamine (an α-2 antagonist) was able to interfere with the cholecystokinetic effect of the intravenously injected CCK to both normal subjects and diarrheic patients (Lechin, van der Dijs, Bentolila et al. 1978; Lechin, van der Dijs 1979b; Lechin, van der Dijs, Orozco et al. 2002b; Lechin, van der Dijs 2007b). Finally, this drug was also able to enhance the sigmoidal tone of both normal and diarrheic subjects significantly (Lechin, van der Dijs, Bentolila et al. 1977a, 1977b; Lechin, van der Dijs 1983, 2007a). In summary, it was found that both the spastic colon syndrome and the biliary dyskinesia were frequently associated in the same patients and, furthermore, that both types of motility disorders

were experimentally triggered by the same neuropharmacological manipulation. Even more, we found that mianserine, a serotonin-releasing agent at CNS level, was able to revert both the sigmoidal hypertony and the biliary dyskinesia (Fig. 5.6).

In summary, we found that both ANS disorders (colonic and biliary) reflected a common CNS abnormality that allows us to postulate that both spastic colon and biliary dyskinesia were triggered by hyperneural sympathetic activity (at the peripheral level) and by A5(NA) and MR(5-HT) overactivity at the CNS level (Lechin, van der Dijs 1979b, 1979c, 1979d, 1979e, 1981a; Lechin, van der Dijs, Gómez et al. 1982a, 1982a, 1982c, 1982c; Lechin, van der Dijs 1983; Lechin 1992b). However, this CNS and neuroautonomic preponderance was reverted to the opposite phase during the diarrheic period: low sigmoidal tone, rectal hypermotility, and biliary hypermotility. At this period a C1(Ad) and DR(5-HT) predominance over A5(NA) and MR(5-HT) would be underlying this clinical syndrome (Lechin, van der Dijs, Bentolila et al. 1977b; Lechin, van der Dijs 1981d, 1981e; Lechin, van der Dijs, Acosta et al. 1983b; Lechin 1992b).

CNS Circuitry Involved in Distal Colon Motility and Biliary Disorders

We demonstrated that both high sigmoidal tone and gallbladder hypokinesia are frequently associated

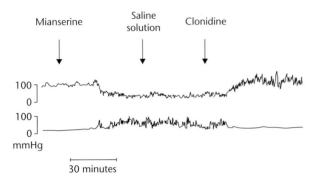

Figure 5.6 High sigmoidal tone in a patient affected by the "spastic colon" syndrome, who also showed hypokinetic gallbladder (no emptying after the Boyden test meal). Mianserine (an α-2 and serotonin-2 antagonist), which enhances the release of serotonin from CNS serotonergic neurons reduced the sigmoidal tone and eliminated abdominal pain. The enhanced rectal activity provoked by mianserine should be attributed to the α-2 antagonist activity exerted by the drug. Clonidine, an α-2 agonist suppresses rectal activity and augments sigmoidal tone. A second oral cholecystography (X-ray), performed 7 days after a therapeutic trial with mianserine (15 mg, daily), was enough to normalize the gallbladder emptying and to eliminate spastic colon symptoms.

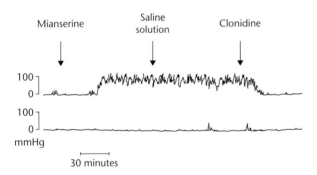

Figure 5.7 Distal colon motility carried out in a normal subject showed low sigmoidal tone and no phasic activity (waves). Mianserine (an α-2 antagonist and serotonin-2 antagonist) enhanced phasic activity at the sigmoidal but not rectal segment. Clonidine, an α-2 agonist, suppressed both the abdominal pain and the increased sigmoidal activity provoked by mianserine. These findings are consistent with the demonstrated fact that the sigmoidal segment is heavily innervated by the myenteric plexa, which includes serotonergic neurons and NA nerves. Parasympathetic nerves cooperate with the former and antagonize the latter neurological activities.

in those patients with IBS during the colon spastic phase. These patients frequently report postprandial abdominal pain at the right hypochondria and/or hypogastria, as well as constipation. No gallbladder emptying after the Boyden test meal or the intravenously injected cholecystokinin is also frequently observed in these subjects when they are submitted to these challenges. Furthermore, it has been demonstrated that both biliary and sigmoidal disorders can

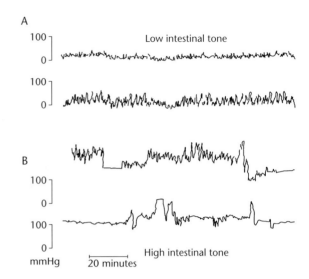

Figure 5.8 (A) Patient with irritable bowel syndrome (investigated during diarrheic period). He showed low sigmoidal tone and raised rectal activity. In addition, this patient had normal gallbladder emptying when tested with an intravenous dose of cholecystokinin (CCK). Administration of dihydroergotamine (DHE, an α-2 antagonist) (6 mg intramuscularly injected) suppresses diarrhea and increased both sigmoidal and rectal tone (more than 100 mmHg). At the same time, DHE interferes with the CCK-induced gallbladder emptying. The DHE injection also provoked abdominal pain. (B) Patient with irritable bowel syndrome (investigated during the constipation period). Abdominal pain was exacerbated during postprandial periods. High sigmoidal tone was demonstrated during the distal colon motility investigation (more than 100 mmHg). Cholecystokinin intravenously injected was not able to provoke gallbladder emptying and in addition, triggered abdominal pain at both right hypochondrium and hypogastrium. Mianserine (an α-2 and serotonin-2 antagonist) orally administered, was able to reduce sigmoidal tone and increase rectal phasic activity (waves). Gallbladder emptying was normalized by the drug. Abdominal pain was also relieved. However, further administration of intramuscular clonidine (0.15 mg), an α-2 agonist, increased sigmoidal tone and provoked abdominal pain.

be experimentally induced by the administration of centrally acting α-2 antagonists to normal subjects (such as dihydroergotamine, yohimbine, regitine, mianserine) (Figs. 5.7, 5.8, and 5.9). These findings allowed us to postulate that these drugs provoked by acting at the CNS level. Considering that both the C1(Ad) and the A5(NA) nuclei are crowded by α-2 inhibitory autoreceptors, both α-2 agonists and α-2 antagonists would act at those CNS nuclei (Li, Wesselingh, Blessing 1992; Lechin 1992b; Lechin, van der Dijs, Orozco 2002b; Lechin, van der Dijs, Lechin 2002c; Fenik, Davies, Kubin 2002; Lechin, van der Dijs 2007b). Furthermore, considering that other experimental evidence demonstrating that clonidine, an α-2 agonist, was able to antagonize the effects provoked by dihydroergotamine reinforced our postulations. Summarizing and taking into account that both

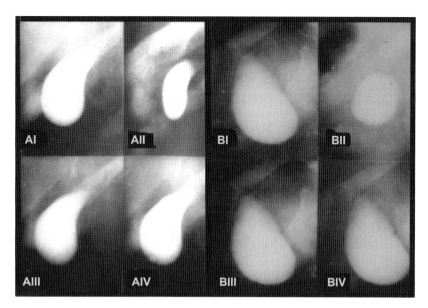

Figure 5.9 Low sigmoidal tone and normal gallbladder emptying after the Boyden test meal (AII and BII) was reverted by high sigmoidal tone and no gallbladder emptying (AIV and BIV) after 7 days of dihydroergotamine administration (an α-2 antagonist), 2.5 mg three times daily. Symptoms of spastic colon (constipation and abdominal pain) were observed at this period.

A5(NA) and C1(Ad) nuclei interchange inhibitory axons (Li, Wesselingh, Blessing 1992), both α-2 antagonists and α-2 agonists would be able to reverse both types of physiological and pathophysiological predominance by acting at those nuclei. (Lechin, van der Dijs, Bentolila et al. 1977a, 1977b, 1978; Lechin, van der Dijs 1979b, 1983; Lechin 1992b; Lechin, van der Dijs 2008; Lechin, van der Dijs, Orozco 2002b; Lechin, van der Dijs 2007b; Lechin, van der Dijs 1981d). The fact that C1(Ad) and (A5)NA predominance underlie both the uncoping stress and the ED syndromes, respectively, allowed us to think that the gastrointestinal disorders discussed should be considered as peripheral symptoms reflecting CNS pathophysiological disorders. Finally, this postulation received additional support by the demonstration that an adequate neuropharmacological therapy was able to normalize both gastrointestinal and psychological syndromes.

Patients with IBS show periodical alternation of constipation and diarrhea. Low sigmoidal tone and rectal hypermotility were found during diarrheic periods, whereas high sigmoidal tone and rectal hypoactivity was observed during spastic periods. Circulating neurotransmitter assessment demonstrated that the noradrenaline/adrenaline ratio and p5-HT levels are significant lowered during the diarrheic periods, at which time f5-HT is significantly increased (because of platelet aggregability). This last parameter always showed close positive correlation with adrenaline and cortisol plasma levels (at morning periods). In accordance with this observation, we postulated that the uncoping stress disorder was responsible for the diarrheic syndrome. The fact that significant positive correlations have been found among adrenaline, f5-HT, and cortisol at these periods reinforced our point of view (Lechin, van der Dijs, Jakubowicz et al. 1987a;

Lechin, van der Dijs, Lechin et al. 1989a, 1994a, 1996c; Lechin, van der Dijs, Orozco et al. 1996d, 1996e). Finally, tthe fact that clinical, neurochemical, and distal colon motility disorders were normalized by an adequate neuropharmacological therapy addressed to enhance neural sympathetic activity supports our postulation. This therapy included a small dose of buspirone (5 mg) before breakfast and lunch (this serotonin-1A agonist triggers the inhibition of the overactive DR(5-HT) neurons). In addition, a small dose of doxepin (25 to 50 mg) or imipramine (25 mg) before supper and a small dose of mirtazapine (15 to 30 mg) before bed should be administered to these patients. This treatment triggered normalization of both clinical and neuroautonomic parameters within the first few (3 to 4) weeks. Normalization of the sleep cycle paralleled the clinical improvement (Lechin, van der Dijs, Lechin et al. 1989a; Lechin, van der Dijs, Jara et al. 1997c, 1998a).

The findings summarized in this chapter allow one to understand why medical knowledge should not be divided into fractions, and in addition, why only an adequate integration of physiological, pathophysiological, and pharmacological knowledge is required for the right understanding of the clinical syndromes, which enables formulation of adequate therapeutic strategies.

We will offer a highly experimental and illustrative example to the readers. We demonstrated that dogs subjected to captivity (median raphe stressor agent) presented with glucose intolerance (insulin resistance) within 5 to 7 days after the restraint stress (Lechin, van der Dijs, Lechin 1979b). In addition, these dogs also showed the spastic colon syndrome when tested using distal colon motility procedure. Significant increases of p5-HT levels were observed at this period. Furthermore, dogs became apathetic, neither barked, nor showed the normal responses to the environmental stimuli. For instance, they did not react to aggression by other dogs or to children's caresses. At that time we ignored that serotonin is positively correlated with MR(5-HT) activity and that restraint stress excites MR(5-HT) but not DR(5-HT) neurons. Finally, the fact that these dogs showed also enhanced neural sympathetic and reduced adrenal sympathetic activities as revealed by the plasma noradrenaline/adrenaline ratio demonstrated that the A5(NA) and MR(5-HT) predominance underlies not only depression but also the insulin resistance and the spastic colon syndromes (Lechin, van der Dijs, Hernandez-Adrian 2006a; Lechin, van der Dijs 2006a, 2006b).

We will add some comments on the CNS and peripheral serotonergic mechanisms involved in the IBS. We have investigated hundreds of these patients during both the spastic colon and the diarrheic periods. We found that raised noradrenaline and p5-HT and lowered adrenaline levels caused the spastic phase whereas predominant adrenaline levels over noradrenaline, low p5-HT levels, raised f5-HT levels, and increased platelet aggregability were observed during the diarrheic periods. In addition, we also found that whereas plasma cortisol levels (at morning) increased in diarrheic patients (when compared with spastic patients) the opposite profile was observed with respect to prolactin plasma levels. This hormone was found to be much more increased in spastic than in diarrheic patients. Considering that this parameter is positively correlated with the MR(5-HT) activity, we assumed that the neuroendocrine disorder described, which underlies the spastic colon syndrome, should be associated to the ED syndrome. We quoted a great deal of evidence that allowed postulating that this psychological syndrome would depend on the predominance of the MR(5-HT) and A5(NA) binomial over the C1(Ad), A6(NA), and DR(5-HT) CNS circuitry. Conversely, predominance of the latter circuitry would underlie the uncoping stress disorder (Lechin, van der Dijs 2006a, 2006b, 2007a).

Additional experimental evidence that emanated from our research work allows the understanding that the sigmoidal tone depends on the serotonergic neurons located between the two muscular intestinal layers and that this neuronal system should be considered as part of the CNS rather than as a peripheral nervous system structure; thus, these serotonergic neurons should react in parallel with some CNS serotonergic circuitry. This issue should be associated also with the concept of the "brain-gut axis" that we introduced in 1977 (Lechin, van der Dijs, Bentolila et al. 1977b; Lechin, van der Dijs, Gómez et al. 1982c, 1983a). In support we demonstrated that both fenfluramine and

d-amphetamine, which are able to deplete CNS and distal colon serotonin stores, were also able to reduce both sigmoidal spasticity and depressive symptoms. Our findings ratified others by Gershon and Bursztajn (1978), who demonstrated that serotonin neurons located at the myenteric plexa level are protected, isolated from the peripheral blood by the hemato–myenteric barrier. This hemato–myenteric barrier would be similar to the BBB and thus, would interfere with the direct cross talk between the myenteric plexa and blood stream. Thus, these 5-HT neurons should be considered as belonging to the CNS. This presumption is supported by our findings showing that p5-HT values are significantly reduced during the diarrheic periods (lowered sigmoidal tone and reduced noradrenaline/adrenaline plasma ratio), which afforded definite support to our point of view.

Other studies carried out by our research group demonstrated that spastic colon patients present a depressive profile frequently. The frequent association between these clinical syndromes and EH and the TH-1 autoimmune profile, which has been reported by us and many other authors, should also be considered (Lechin, van der Dijs, Bentolila et al. 1977a, 1977b, 1978, 1981d; Lechin, van der Dijs 1979b, 1981a, 1982; Lechin, van der Dijs, Gómez et al. 1982a, 1982c; Lechin, van der Dijs 1983; Lechin, van der Dijs, Gómez et al. 1983a; Lechin, van der Dijs, Acosta et al. 1983b; Lechin, van der Dijs, Jakubowicz et al. 1985a, 1985b; Lechin, van der Dijs, Vitelli et al. 1990a; Lechin 1992b; Lechin, van der Dijs, Lechin-Báez et al. 1994c; Lechin, van der Dijs, Orozco 2002b; O'Brien, Lamb, Muller et al. 2005; Ladep, Obindo, Audu et al. 2006; Cole, Rothman, Cabral et al. 2006; Kurland, Coyle, Winkler et al. 2006; Masuko, Nakamura 2007; Radziwillowicz, Gil 2007; North, Hong, Alpers 2007; Liebregts, Adam, Bredack et al. 2007; Lechin, van der Dijs 2007a, 2007b). Thus, clinicians should try to understand that the fragmentation of the truth withdraws doctors from the right way to diagnose and treat patients.

Summarizing, we quoted evidence which demonstrates that both spastic colon and spastic biliary sphincter are caused by the same neuroautonomic disorder. Our findings showing that an α-2 and 5-HT-2 antagonist drug (mianserine) is able to antagonize both higher sigmoidal tone and rectal phasic hypoactivity, and in addition, allows the gallbladder emptying induced by CCK, indicates that both the sphincter of Oddi and the sigmoidal–rectal sphincter are positively correlated with the neural sympathetic activity. Furthermore, considering that both mianserine and fenfluramine, two serotonin releasing agents, were able to revert both the colonic and the biliary disorders allows assigning a primordial role to the serotonergic neurons located at the myenteric plexus of the Auerbach. Axons of these neurons innervate and excite the longitudinal (external) muscle layer and are responsible for the intestinal tone. Furthermore, taking into account a bulk of experimental and clinical data, it is possible to postulate the parallelism between both the CNS and the peripheral ANS.

BRONCHIAL ASTHMA

This syndrome should be considered as a two-faced coin, the symptoms of which would depend on the CNS physiological disorder period. An uncoping stress profile underlies acute asthma attacks whereas a "major depression" CNS circuitry is detected during nonacute periods. In addition, both TH-2 and TH-1 immunological profiles parallel both syndromes, respectively.

Asthma attacks are caused by raised levels of plasma adrenaline and f5-HT whereas, predominant levels of noradrenaline and p5-HT are found during nonattack periods. Increased platelet aggregability would be responsible for the f5-HT peaks, because these both disorders are closely positively correlated with plasma adrenaline values, observed during asthma attacks (Lechin, van der Dijs, Lechin et al. 1994a, 1996c; Lechin, van der Dijs, Orozco et al. 1996f; Lechin A Varon, van der Dijs et al. 1994).

Dissociation of the two ANS peripheral branches is also observed at those two periods of bronchial asthma disease. Thus, adrenal sympathetic and neural sympathetic branches are positively correlated with the acute and nonacute asthma periods, respectively (Fig. 5.10).

Considering that adrenergic activity triggers bronchial dilatation, whereas bronchial spasms depend on neural sympathetic activity (Salonen Webber SE, Widdicombe 1990) some other pathophysiological mechanisms should be invoked in order to explain this apparently contradictory phenomenon.

Acute Periods

We demonstrated (Lechin, Varon, van der Dijs et al. 1994) that both plasma catecholamines (adrenaline, noradrenaline and dopamine) and plasma indolamine (serotonin f5-HT) but not (p5-HT) were raised during asthma attacks. In addition, we also found that the f5-HT plasma levels were positively and negatively correlated with clinical severity and pulmonary function, respectively (Lechin, van der Dijs, Orozco et al. 1996f). In addition, we demonstrated that plasma cortisol was also raised during acute but not at the remission periods.

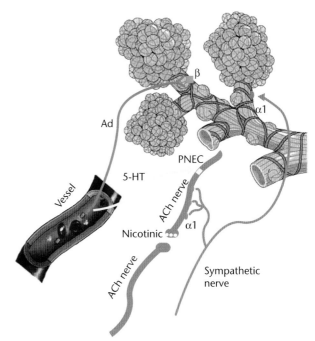

Figure 5.10 Peripheral neuroautonomic factors involved in bronchial physiological and pathophysiological mechanisms. Postsynaptic parasympathetic nerves contract muscular fibers by releasing acetylcholine (ACh) at nicotine receptors located at bronchial level. Plasma adrenaline (Ad) antagonizes this effect by acting at β-adrenergic receptors located the same muscular (bronchial) level. Plasma serotonin (f5-HT) is taken up by the pulmonary neuroendocrine cells (PNEC). These cells are excited and release serotonin during parasympathetic excitation. Both ACh and serotonin cooperate to contract the bronchial tubes during parasympathetic overactivity (sleep periods and/or over-release of histamine from excited mast cells). These bronchoconstrictor mechanisms are favored by the low adrenal glands activity seen in both asthmatic children and old subjects. Maximal noradrenaline/adrenaline plasma ratio is always observed in both types of patients (neural sympathetic over adrenal sympathetic predominance). Furthermore, sympathetic nerves excite parasympathetic nerves by acting at α-1 receptors located at the latter. At the central nervous system (CNS) level, this peripheral autonomic disorder depends on the overwhelming inhibitory effects exerted by A5(NA) axons over the Cl(Ad) medullary nuclei. These pathophysiological mechanisms are consistent with the abrupt suppression of asthma attacks triggered by a small dose of tianeptine (which enhances the serotonin uptake) during these acute periods. However, preventive therapeutic approach should be addressed to the reduction of the overwhelming neural sympathetic activity. This target is reached through neuropharmacological manipulation able to enhance the A6(NA) activity. This nucleus sends inhibitory axons to the A5(NA) neurons.

Additional findings showed that f5-HT plasma levels were negatively correlated with FEV1 (forced expiratory volume in one second). This finding led us to think that reducing the concentration of f5-HT in plasma may be useful in treating patients during acute periods.

On the basis of these findings, we might understand how and why plasma serotonin may provoke asthma attacks during both acute (diurnal) active waking periods and during (nocturnal) quiet waking and sleep periods. Adrenaline-induced platelet aggregability allows the dispersion of serotonin to the plasma during diurnal periods whereas the nocturnal enhancement of plasma ACh, which interferes with the serotonin uptake by platelets, would provoke the f5-HT rise during sleep periods (Lechin 2000; Lechin, van der Dijs, Lechin et al. 2002e; Lechin, Pardey-Maldonado, van der Dijs et al. 2004a; Lechin, van der Dijs, Lechin 2004b, 2005a, 2007; Lechin, van der Dijs 2005b).

In addition, it should be known that pulmonary vascular preparations always contract also in response to serotonin (Hechtman 1978; Webber, Salonen, Widdicombe et al. 1990). These findings allow understanding why serotonin plays also a primary role into the pathophysiological mechanisms, which underlie pulmonary hypertension (Lechin, van der Dijs 2001, 2002; Lechin, van der Dijs, Lechin et al. 2002e, 2002f, 2002g, 2005a; Eddahibi, Adnot 2006). We will refer to this subsequently.

Neuropharmacological Therapy

Tianeptine enhances the uptake of serotonin from the synaptic cleft by the serotonergic axons. Taking into account that 5-HT axons from the medullary nuclei raphe obscurus, RM, and raphe pallidus release serotonin at the medullary respiratory center, which includes the C1, C2, and C3(Ad) and other medullary nuclei (Kumaido 1988; Holtman, Marion, Speck 1990) it is understandable why this neurotransmitter plays a primary excitatory role at this CNS nuclei complex (Strum, Junod 1972; Fozard 1984; Lauweryns, van Rast 1988; Reynolds, Leslie, Grahame-Smith et al. 1989; Johnson, Georgieff 1989; Richard, Stremel 1990; Arita, Ochiishi 1991; Colebatch, Olsen, Nadel 1966; Lalley, Benacka, Bischoff et al. 1997; Pan, Copland, Post, Yeger et al. 2006). In addition, serotonin stored and further released from pulmonary neuroendocrine cells (PNEC) triggers bronchoconstriction; thus tianeptine should interfere at this circumstance, also. It suppresses sudden asthma attacks. However, it should not be administered during remission periods, because it also acts at the CNS level. It should be known that tianeptine enhances the uptake of serotonin by axons of active but not inactive serotonergic neurons (Lechin, van der Dijs, Lechin et al. 1998b; Lechin, van der Dijs, Orozco et al. 1998c; Lechin, van der Dijs, Lechin 2002f, 2004f; Lechin 2005; Lechin, van der Dijs, Hernandez 2006b).

Tianeptine may be used to improve pulmonary hypertension also (Lechin, van der Dijs 2001, 2002; Lechin, van der Dijs, Lechin et al. 2002e, 2003). This drug will reduce f5-HT plasma levels and thus, will interfere with the pulmonary vasoconstrictor effect provoked by the excess of serotonin at the vascular pulmonary area. However, this drug should be administered during acute periods only.

Other neuropharmacological strategies might be used to treat asthma patients, during nonacute periods. In our long experience obtained from the treatment of more than 10,000 asthmatic patients, we found that a small dose of doxepin (10 mg) before bed is able to prevent asthma attacks, after the first 3 weeks of administration of this drug. Other noradrenaline and serotonin uptake inhibitors, such as imipramine might be administered instead of doxepin. Absolute inhibitors of noradrenaline or serotonin uptake should not be used.

It has been shown that serotonin can induce bronchoconstriction by an effect on presynaptic neuronal 5-HT-3 receptors located at the parasympathetic ganglia (Fozard 1984). In addition, free- but not p5-HT is able to stimulate 5-HT-3 receptors, which crowd the medullary AP located outside the BBB (Reynolds, Leslie, Grahame-Smith et al. 1989). Thus, any rise of f5-HT would provoke the parasympathetic cascade (Bezold Jarisch reflex) responsible for nocturnal asthma attacks (Lechin 2000).

Other findings showed that serotonin is actively transported by the PNEC, where it is metabolized by the MAO enzyme (Strum, Junod 1972). In addition, Colebatch et al. (1966) demonstrated that serotonin causes constriction of both central and peripheral airways when given to vagotomized cats and other mammals. Thus, plasma serotonin is able to trigger asthma attacks both directly and/or mediated by parasympathetic nerves. Furthermore, in man, serotonin is concentrated in platelets and is released when platelets aggregate. This occurs during stress situation and is also observed in immunological diseases. (Hechtman, Lonergan, Staunton et al. 1978; Capron, Joseph, Ameisen et a1. 1987; Cazzola, Matera, Gusmitta et al. 1991; Freitag, Wessler, Racke 1997). Finally, in human airways, considering that serotonin is localized at nerve terminals in the so-called PNEC (Lauweryns, van Rast 1988) and may be released upon exposure to local airway under conditions such as hypoxia, hyperoxia, and hypercapnia (Keith, Will 1982; Moosavi, Smith, Heath et al. 1973), this indoleamine can exert a direct bronchoconstrictor effect (Strum, Junod 1972).

Pulmonary neuroendocrine cells are granulated epithelial cells and can be detected throughout the lung from the trachea to the alveoli (Johnson, Georgieff 1989). This PNEC is the presynaptic element and the nerve vagal ending is the postsynaptic element (Levitt, Mitzner 1989).

Bronchoconstriction evoked by serotonin involves vagal afferent nerves and is inhibited by atropine

(Islam, Melville, Ulmer 1974). These findings are consistent with other observation that inhaled serotonin induces an acute fall in lung function (greater than 20% in FEV1) in asthmatic patients but not in normals (Tonnesen 1985; Cushley, Wee, Holgate et al. 1986).

The fact that nocturnal asthma attacks are associated with increased parasympathetic activity should be added to other findings, which show that this activity releases serotonin from intestinal source and provokes an increase of blood serotonin (Tobe, Izumikawa, Sano et al. 1976). In addition, hyperparasympathetic activity (as occurs during sleep and postprandial periods) interferes with p5-HT uptake, which redounds in an increase of plasma serotonin (Rausch, Janowsky, Risch et al. 1985; Skaburskis, Shardonofsky, Milic-Emili et al. 1990).

CNS and Peripheral ANS Interactions

PERIPHERAL LEVEL Parasympathetic nerves release ACh from terminals, which contracts bronchial structures by acting at nicotine receptors located at the bronchial muscles (Haxhiu, Jansen, Cherniack et al. 1993; Hadziefendic, Haxhiu 1999; Jordan 2001). This effect is potentiated by serotonin released at this level from the PNEC. These cells are located at ACh nerves and serotonin is coreleased with acetylcholine during parasympathetic activation. These neuroendocrine structures are able to uptake serotonin from the plasma; thus, any increase of plasma 5-HT enhances PNEC stores and is further released during parasympathetic excitation (Pan, Yeger, Cutz 2004; Pan, Copland, Post et al. 2006).

NA sympathetic nerves excite parasympathetic nerves by acting at α-1 receptors located at these terminals (Haxhiu, Kc, Neziri et al. 2003; Haxhiu, Kc, Moore et al. 2005). Conversely, plasma adrenaline triggers bronchial dilatation by acting at β-adrenergic receptors located at muscular fibers, which are provided with β-adrenergic receptors (Larsson, Carlens, Bevegard et al. 1995). Thus, any predominance of parasympathetic or neural sympathetic activity would result in bronchial contraction. Both plasma serotonin and plasma histamine also trigger bronchial contraction by acting directly at the bronchial muscular layer (Larsson, Carlens, Bevegard et al. 1995; Kinkead, Belzile, Gulemetova 2002).

Asthma Attacks

Asthma attacks may be triggered by both exercise (diurnal) and sleep (nocturnal) periods. The former is associated with the rise of plasma serotonin triggered by platelet aggregation, which releases serotonin. Platelet aggregation is triggered by the increase of adrenaline from the adrenal glands during exercise. The nocturnal attack should be associated with

parasympathetic activity (Haxhiu, Rust, Brooks et al. 2006). Acetylcholine released to the plasma interferes with the platelet uptake and is responsible for the increase of f5-HT (Lechin, van der Dijs, Orozco et al. 1996f). The low levels of plasma adrenaline but not of noradrenaline observed at these periods favors the bronchoconstriction triggered by f5-HT. Predominance of the noradrenaline/adrenaline ratio is always observed in asthmatic subjects and is caused by neural sympathetic over adrenal sympathetic predominance (Lechin, van der Dijs, Lechin et al. 2004h).

CNS Level

Both the RO and the RP serotonergic nuclei excite the medullary parasympathetic (ACh) nuclei responsible for the excitation of the peripheral parasympathetic activity (Haxhiu, Jansen, Cherniack et al. 1993). Conversely, the RM-5-HT nucleus cooperates with the A5(NA) nucleus, which is responsible for the neural sympathetic activity (Richard, Stremel 1990). The A5(NA) nucleus interchanges inhibitory axons with the Cl(Ad) medullary nuclei, which send excitatory polysynaptic drive to the adrenal glands (adrenal sympathetic activity) (Lindsey, Arata, Morris et al. 1998; Lalley, Benacka, Bischoff et al. 1997). Exercise-induced asthma attacks depends on the overactivity of the latter CNS circuitry: RM(5-HT)–Cl(Ad). However, considering that the plasma level of adrenaline but not noradrenaline reaches minimal level during sleep periods, nocturnal asthma attacks should be associated with both neural and parasympathetic but not adrenal sympathetic activity (Kumaido 1988; Li, Wesselingh, Blessing 1992; Lima, Souza, Soares et al. 2007). These findings fit well with others, showing that asthma in children is always caused by neural sympathetic predominance. This predominance is the profile always seen in old patients affected by the obstructive sleep apnea syndrome (OSAS). In addition, parasympathetic predominance seen during sleep periods is responsible for the raised plasma levels of acetylcholine, which enhances f5-HT plasma levels. Finally, the overwhelming neural sympathetic over adrenal sympathetic predominance observed in both asthmatic and OSAS patients may explain the overexcitation of parasympathetic nerves, which contract bronchial structures. The β-adrenergic dilatator effect of plasma adrenaline is not enough to attenuate this bronchoconstriction.

Summarizing, both nocturnal asthma attacks and OSAS depend on the predominance of neural sympathetic over adrenal sympathetic activity (Li, Wesselingh, Blessing 1992), whereas exercise-induced asthma attacks depend on the serotonin released because of the platelet aggregation (Lechin, van der Dijs, Orozco et al. 1996f), which cooperates

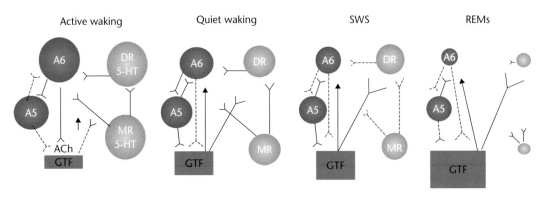

Figure 5.11 Neurophysiological changes throughout the wake sleep cycle at the CNS level. A6(NA), DR(5-HT), and MR(5-HT) neurons receive excitatory glutamatergic axons from the cortical pyramidal neurons during active waking periods. These excitatory drives are progressively substituted by cortical GABAergic inputs reaching the two former nuclei but not the MR(5-HT). Thus, the fading of the A6(NA) and DR(5-HT) redounds in the predominance of the A5(NA) and MR(5-HT) binomial. In addition to the above, the gigantotegmental field (GTF) or pedunculonpontine (PPN) acetylcholinergic (ACh) neurons become progressively disinhibited from the A6(NA) axons and reach maximal firing activity at the rapid eye movement (REM) sleep period. Acetylcholine (ACh) released from GTF(ACh) axons excite A6(NA) neurons, which re-initiate the GTF(ACh) inhibition. This latter redounds in disinhibition of DR(5-HT) from the GTF(ACh) bridle. This ACh bridle is exerted through inhibitory nicotine receptors located at the DR(5-HT) neurons. Serotonin released from DR(5-HT) axons at the A6(NA) neurons avoids maximal excitation of the latter, which would trigger sudden wakening as occurs in endogenous depressed patients [MR(5-HT) over DR(5-HT) predominance].

with plasma histamine, leukotrienes, and other factors, leading to bronchial contraction. Serotonin released from PNEC plays a primordial role, since a small dose of tianeptine is able to suppress bronchial contraction. However, our long experience obtained from the treatment of thousands of these patients (Lechin, van der Dijs, Lechin 2004h) led us to postulate that all those patients should be treated with an adequate neuropharmacological therapy to revert the overwhelming predominance of CNS A5(NA) over C1(Ad).

CNS CIRCUITRY INVOLVED IN BOTH PHYSIOLOGICAL AND PATHOPHYSIOLOGICAL MECHANISMS OF SLEEP

We will refer to the active waking period as well as to the four sleep periods: SWS I, II, III, and IV (δ-sleep) and the REM sleep period.

Both A6(NA) and DR(5-HT) activities show progressive fading throughout SWS and reach zero firing activity at the REM sleep period. The MR(5-HT) also shows progressive reduction of its firing activity, but does not reach zero firing at REM sleep stage (Lechin, van der Dijs 1984; Lechin van der Dijs, Lechin et al. 1992a, 2002a; Lechin, Pardey-Maldonado, van der Dijs et al. 2004a; Lechin, van der Dijs, Lechin 2004b; Lechin, van der Dijs 2005b).

The A5(NA) neurons show slow fading also but do not reach zero firing at REM period. The PPN(ACh)

or GTF(ACh) neurons showed progressive disinhibition from the A6(NA) and the A5(NA) bridling and became maximally excited at the REM sleep stage. The C1(Ad) medullary nuclei reach zero firing activity within the first 10 minutes after the supine-resting (wake) state (Lechin, Pardey-Maldonado, van der Dijs et al. 2004a) (Fig. 5.11).

Both the PAG(5-HT) and the RM(5-HT) nuclei also show reductions of firing activity but remain active throughout the sleep cycle. The RP(5-HT) is hyperactive at the REM sleep period and is responsible for the leg movements (jerking) observed at the REM sleep stage (Trulson, Trulson 1982). The RO(5-HT) is active throughout all sleep stages. Axons from these 5-HT neurons excite the medullary parasympathetic (ACh) nuclei (ambiguus, NTS) whose activity is responsible for the predominance of the ANS branch during the sleep cycle (Woch, Davies, Pack et al. 1996; Fenik, Davies, Kubin et al. 2005). The disinhibited pontine (ACh) neurons, which integrate the PPN, send axons that excite and inhibit the A6(NA) and the A5(NA) neurons, respectively and trigger the progressive disinhibition of the A6(NA) but not the A5(NA) nucleus (Behbehani 1982; Kubin, Reignier, Tojima et al. 1994; Lalley, Benacka, Bischoff et al. 1997; Lindsey, Arata, Morris et al. 1998; Datta, Patterson, Spoley 2001). This noradrenaline versus acetylcholine feedback avoids the prolongation of the REM sleep stage (≈10 minutes).

Axons arising from the PPN inhibit and excite DR(5-HT) and MR(5-HT), respectively. This mechanism is consistent with the absolute DR but not MR fading at the REM sleep period. The absolute A6(NA) fading at the REM sleep stage is responsible for the disinhibition of the A5(NA), whose neurons display some degree of activity at this period. However, this physiological interaction is abruptly changed in stressed and elderly subjects, whose A6(NA) neurons are exhausted in the former and diminished in the latter subjects. This pathophysiological factor is responsible for the sudden and abrupt (nonphysiological) predominance of the A5(NA) over the A6(NA) neuronal activity at this sleep period (Verdecchia, Schillaci, Gatteschi et al. 1993; van Diest, Appels 1994). Noradrenaline released from the prematurely disinhibited A5(NA) axons inhibits the hypoglossal and glossopharyngeal nuclei and provokes the peripheral dysfunction responsible for the obstructive sleep apnea syndrome (Lalley Benacka, Bischoff et al. 1997; Narkiewicz, Somers 2003). This disorder is facilitated by the A5(NA)-induced inhibition of the RO(5-HT) neurons, the axons of which are responsible for the excitation of the medullary vagal complex, which, in these circumstances, is no more able to attenuate the sudden A5(NA) disinhibition (Meredith, Eisenhofer, Lambert et al. 1993).

At the peripheral level, the above CNS physiological movements are paralleled by cardiovascular, respiratory, gastrointestinal, and other peripheral physiological oscillations. This CNS versus peripheral cross talk explains why all diseases are caused by sleep disorders. In addition, we demonstrated that the adequate assessment of the circulating neurotransmitter oscillations reflects the CNS neurochemical movements, which underlie the sleep cycle. We will try to summarize our results obtained from thousands of normal and diseases subjects, who were investigated during both wake and sleep periods.

Plasma Catecholamines: Adrenaline, Noradrenaline, Dopamine, and Plasma Indoleamines: p5-HT, f5-HT, and Tryptophan

Adrenaline plasma levels fall abruptly 10 minutes after the supine resting (waking) state. Additional decrease is observed throughout the SWS and reaches almost zero values before the first REM sleep period.

Noradrenaline plasma level decreases slowly and does not reach zero value at any period. Maximal adrenaline versus noradrenaline dissociation is observed at the REM sleep.

DA plasma values are also reduced through the sleep periods, but no parallelism with adrenaline or noradrenaline can be established.

p5-HT shows slow but progressive increase throughout the sleep cycle. f5-HT show two peaks, which correlated negatively with the maximal adrenaline fall and noradrenaline fall (at REM sleep). Considering that this parameter should be associated to the activity of the MR(5-HT) nucleus, the p5-HT rise fits well with the known fact the DR(5-HT) but not the MR(5-HT) reaches zero firing activity at the REM sleep stage.

Plasma tryptophan does not show significant change; however, progressive rise is seen before waking (at morning). The tryptophan rise should be associated to the progressive recovery of the DR(5-HT) neurons, which predominate at the active waking period.

Although this issue has been exhaustively discussed in our published articles, we will try to summarize the interpretation of these findings.

Adrenaline fall should be associated with the abrupt reduction of the C1(Ad) medullary activity, which is responsible for the adrenal gland secretion. The slow noradrenaline fall would depend on the slow fading of the A5(NA) neurons responsible for neural sympathetic activity. We observed noradrenaline peaks during the obstructive sleep apnea (OSA) episodes. Noradrenaline fading is seen neither in patients with EH and/or hyperinsulinism nor in patients affected by TH-1 autoimmune diseases. In addition, no or poor noradrenaline firing is observed in all people and/or ED and/or psychotic patients. These findings contrast with the nocturnal adrenaline peaks observed in stressed patients, and in patients affected by TH-2 autoimmune diseases or by all types of malignant diseases.

Platelet serotonin rises should be associated with the predominance of the MR(5-HT) over the DR(5-HT) activity throughout the sleep cycle. The fact that all syndromes caused by the predominance of MR(5-HT) over DR(5-HT) show greater than normal p5-HT values is consistent with the earlier finding (ED, psychoses, hyperactive and ADHD, PTSD subjects). Furthermore, we have found that a close positive correlation exists between p5-HT values and any type of aggressive behavior (Lechin, van der Dijs, Lechin 2002a).

We would like to inform that there are few subjects showing a normal sleep profile. Abnormal circulating neurotransmitter profile is a most accurate index than the electroencephalographic assessment of the sleep cycle. However, we have also found that an adequate neuropharmacological therapy is able to normalize both the sleep and wake physiology. Thus, a great bulk of evidence showing that normalization of both cycles is followed by the improvement of most diseases has been accumulated. We hope that both scientific and practitioner doctors might reach some degree of cooperation and understanding about this point of view.

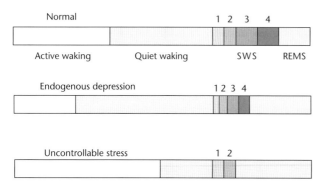

SWS (slow wave sleep) = stages 1,2,3, and 4
REMS (rapid eye movement sleep)

Figure 5.12 Short rapid eye movement (REM) sleep latency in endogenous depressed patients. This phenomenon depends on the predominance of A5(NA) over A6(NA), which triggers inhibition of the latter nucleus. Uncontrollable stress is responsible for the disappearance of the deep slow-wave sleep (stages 3 and 4 of the SWS). Exhaustion of the A6(NA) neurons is responsible for the sudden disappearance of the firing activity of these NA neurons. Frequent awakenings are always observed in these subjects.

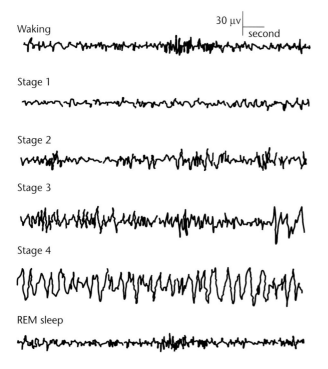

Figure 5.13 The EEG of sleep in a human adult shown for each stage of sleep, in a single-channel monopolar recording from the left parietal area, with the ears as neutral reference point.

Two Types of Sleep Disorders Underlie Both Uncoping Stress and Endogenous Depression

Uncoping Stress

Uncoping stress is caused by the exhaustion of both the A6(NA) and the A5(NA) nuclei, which are additionally annulled by the excessive release of adrenaline and serotonin from the C1(Ad) and the DR(5-HT) axons at both levels, respectively. This binomial is overactive in this circumstance and is responsible for the frequent wakening periods observed in these patients. These abrupt awakenings provoked by the sudden fall of the A6(NA) neuronal activity triggers the over-release of glutamate at these neurons; thus, the glutamate versus GABA balance is lost in these circumstances (Figs. 5.12 and 5.13).

Endogenous Depression and Obstructive Sleep Apnea Syndrome

The obstructive sleep apnea syndrome is frequently observed in both endogenously depressed and stressed elderly subjects. The absolute predominance of the A5(NA) over the A6(NA), C1(Ad), and RO(5-HT) nuclei is responsible for this disorder. Noradrenaline released from the A5(NA) axons provokes the inhibition of these nuclei and triggers both laryngeal obstruction and sudden wakening. Considering that both aging and stress are caused by the death or the inhibition of the A6(NA) neurons, this syndrome is more frequently observed in the endogenously depressed and stressed elderly subjects.

Some therapeutic neuropharmacological strategies to improve sleep disorders are listed here.

In the general population, except the elderly before supper: doxepin (25 mg) and before bed: mirtazapine (15 mg).

In elderly people, clomipramine (25 mg) before supper and clonidine (0.15 mg) before bed.

In all cases, levopromazine 1 mg before bed.

This α-1 antagonist interferes with the excitatory drive, which arises from A6(NA) axons and excites A10(DA) mesocortical neurons. Greater doses should be avoided because it triggers upregulation of α-1 receptors.

REFERENCES

Ader R, Felten D, Cohen N. 1990. Interactions between the brain and the immune system. *Annu. Rev Pharmacol Toxicol.* 30:561–602. Review.

Alm P, Cegrell L, Ehinger B, Falck B. 1967. Remarkable adrenergic nerves in the exocrine pancreas. *Z Zellforsch Mikrosk Anat.* 83:178–186.

Amital H, Blank M, Shoenfeld Y. 1996. Th1/Th2 cells and autoimmunity. *Harefuah.* 131:189–192. Review.

Anisman H. 1978. Neurochemical changes elicited by stress. In Anisman H, Bignami G, eds. *Psychopharmacology of Aversively Motivated Behavior.* New York: Plenum Press, 19–172.

Anisman H, Irwin J, Sklar LS. 1979. Deficits of escape performance following catecholamine depletion: implications for behavioral deficits induced by uncontrollable stress. *Psychopharmacology. (Berl).* 64:163–170.

Anisman H, Pizzino A, Sklar LS. 1980. Coping with stress, norepinephrine depletion and escape performance. *Brain Res.* 191:583–588.

Arita H, Ochiishi M. 1991. Opposing effects of 5-hydroxytryptamine on two types of medullary inspiratory neurons with distinct firing patterns. *J Neurophysiol.* 66:285–292.

Artalejo AR, García AG, Montiel C, Sánchez-García P. 1985. A dopaminergic receptor modulates catecholamine release from the cat adrenal gland. *J Physiol.* 362:359–368.

Aulakh CS, Mazzola-Pomietto P, Murphy DL. 1996. Long-term antidepressant treatment restores clonidine's effect on growth hormone secretion in a genetic animal model of depression. *Pharmacol Biochem Behav.* 55:265–268.

Banki CM, Bissette G, Arato M, O'Connor L, Nemeroff CB. 1987. CSF corticotropin-releasing factor-like immunoreactivity in depression and schizophrenia. *Am J Psychiatry.* 144:873–877.

Barbeito L, Fernandez C, Silveira R, Dajas F. 1986. Evidences of a sympatho-adrenal dysfunction after lesion of the central noradrenergic pathways in rats. *J Neural Transm.* 67:205–214.

Barlow TE, Greenwell JR, Harper AA, Scratcherd T. 1971. The effect of adrenaline and noradrenaline on the blood flow, electrical conductance and external secretion of the pancreas. *J Physiol.* 217:665–678.

Behbehani MM. 1982. The role of acetylcholine in the function of the nucleus raphe magnus and in the interaction of this nucleus with the periaqueductal gray. *Brain Res.* 252:299–307.

Beretta L, Astori S, Ferrario E, Caronni M, Raimondi M, Scorza R. 2006. Determinants of depression in 111 Italian patients with systemic sclerosis. *Reumatismo.* 58:219–225.

Bialik RJ, Smythe JW, Sardelis M, Roberts DC. 1989. Adrenal demedullation blocks and brain norepinephrine depletion potentiates the hyperglycemic response to a variety of stressors. *Brain Res.* 502:88–98.

Broderick PA, Phelix CF. 1997. I. Serotonin (5-HT) within dopamine reward circuits signals open-field behavior. II. Basis for 5-HT–DA interaction in cocaine dysfunctional behavior. *Neurosci Biobehav Rev.* 21:227–260. Review.

Brown MR, Fisher LA. 1986. Glucocorticoid suppression of the sympathetic nervous system and adrenal medulla. *Life Sci.* 39:1003–1012.

Buckingham JC, Loxley HD, Christian HC, Philip JG. 1996. Activation of the HPA axis by immune insults: roles and interactions of cytokines, eicosanoids, glucocorticoids. *Pharmacol Biochem Behav.* 54:285–298. Review.

Bunney BS, Aghajanian GK. 1978. Mesolimbic and mesocortical dopaminergic systems: physiology and pharmacology. In Lipton MA, DiMascio A, Killam KF, eds. *Psychopharmacology: A Generation of Progress.* New York: Raven Press, 221–234.

Burchfield SR. 1979. The stress response: a new perspective. *Psychosom Med.* 41:661–672. Review.

Byrum CE, Guyenet PG. 1987. Afferent and efferent connections of the A5 noradrenergic cell group in the rat. *J Comp Neurol.* 261:529–542.

Cabrera A, van der Dijs B, Jimenez V, Guerrero H, Lechin F. 1988. Plasma neurotransmitters profile in normal subjects III Interamerican congress of clinical pharmacology and therapeutics and XII latinoamerican congress of pharmacology. *Arch Ven Farm Clin Terap.* 7(Suppl 1) Abst 107.

Calcagni E, Elenkov I. 2006. Stress system activity, innate and T helper cytokines, and susceptibility to immune-related diseases. *Ann N Y Acad Sci.* 1069:62–76. Review.

Calogero AE, Gallucci WT, Chrousos GP, Gold PW. 1988. Catecholamine effects upon rat hypothalamic corticotropin-releasing hormone secretion in vitro. *J Clin Invest.* 82:839–846.

Calogero AE, Bagdy G, D'Agata R. 1998. Mechanisms of stress on reproduction. Evidence for a complex intra-hypothalamic circuit. *Ann N Y Acad Sci.* 851:364–370. Review.

Capron A, Joseph M, Ameisen JC, Capron M, Pancre V, Auriault C. 1987. Platelets as effectors in immune and hypersensitivity reactions. *Int Arch Allergy Appl Immunol.* 82:307–312. Review.

Cazzola M, Matera MG, Gusmitta A, Rossi F. 1991. Effect of flomoxef on human platelet aggregation. *Eur J Clin Pharmacol.* 41:503–504.

Cedarbaum JM, Aghajanian GK. 1978. Afferent projections to the rat locus coeruleus as determined by a retrograde tracing technique. *J Comp Neurol.* 178:1–16.

Choi DC, Furay AR, Evanson NK, Ostrander MM, Ulrich-Lai YM, Herman JP. 2007. Bed nucleus of the stria terminalis subregions differentially regulate hypothalamic-pituitary-adrenal axis activity: implications for the integration of limbic inputs. *J Neurosci.* 27:2025–2034.

Chowdhury AR, Dinoso VP, Lorber SH. 1976. Characterization of a hyperactive segment at the rectosigmoid junction. *Gastroenterology.* 71:584–588.

Christensen NJ. 1980. Adrenergic mechanisms in selected diseases: arterial hypertension, duodenal ulcer, primary depressive illness, malignant tumors, and ketotic hypoglycemia. *Metabolism.* 29:1190–1197.

Cole JA, Rothman KJ, Cabral HJ, Zhang Y, Farraye FA. 2006. Migraine, fibromyalgia, and depression among people with IBS: a prevalence study. *BMC Gastroenterol.* 6:26–33.

Colebatch HJ, Olsen CR, Nadel JA. 1966. Effect of histamine, serotonin, and acetylcholine on the peripheral airways. *J Appl Physiol.* 21:217–226.

Craven RM, Priddle TH, Crow TJ, Esiri MM. 2005. The locus coeruleus in schizophrenia: a postmortem study of noradrenergic neurons. *Neuropathol Appl Neurobiol.* 31:115–26.

Cunnick JE, Lysle DT, Kucinski BJ, Rabin BS. 1990. Evidence that shock-induced immune suppression is mediated by adrenal hormones and peripheral beta-adrenergic receptors. *Pharmacol Biochem Behav.* 36:645–651.

Cushley MJ, Wee LH, Holgate ST. 1986. The effect of inhaled 5-hydroxytryptamine (5-HT, serotonin) on airway calibre in man. *Br J Clin Pharmacol.* 22:487–490.

Dampney RA. 1994. Functional organization of central pathways regulating the cardiovascular system. *Physiol Rev.* 74:323–364. Review.

Datta S, Patterson EH, Spoley EE. 2001. Excitation of the pedunculopontine tegmental NMDA receptors induces wakefulness and cortical activation in the rat. *J Neurosci Res.* 66:109–116.

Dawe GS, Huff KD, Vandergriff JL, Sharp T, O'Neill MJ, Rasmussen K. 2001. Olanzapine activates the rat locus coeruleus: in vivo electrophysiology and c-Fos immunoreactivity. *Biol Psychiatry.* 50:510–520.

De Keyser J, De Waele M, Convents A, Ebinger G, Vauquelin G. 1988. Identification of D1-like dopamine receptors on human blood platelets. *Life Sci.* 42:1797–1806.

Desan PH, Silbert LH, Maier SF. 1988. Long-term effects of inescapable stress on daily running activity and antagonism by desipramine. *Pharmacol Biochem Behav.* 30:21–29.

Devoto P, Flore G, Pani L, Gessa GL. 2001. Evidence for co-release of noradrenaline and dopamine from noradrenergic neurons in the cerebral cortex. *Mol Psychiatry.* 6:657–664.

Dilts RP, Boadle-Biber MC. 1995. Differential activation of the 5-hydroxytryptamine-containing neurons of the midbrain raphe of the rat in response to randomly presented inescapable sound. *Neurosci Lett.* 199:78–80.

Eddahibi S, Adnot S. 2006. The serotonin pathway in pulmonary hypertension. *Arch Mal Coeur Vaiss.* 99:621–625. Review.

Eilat E, Mendlovic S, Doron A, Zakuth V, Spirer Z. 1999. Increased apoptosis in patients with major depression: a preliminary study. *J Immunol.* 163:533–534.

Elenkov IJ, Wilder RL, Chrousos GP, Vizi ES. 2000. The sympathetic nerve--an integrative interface between two supersystems: the brain and the immune system. *Pharmacol Rev.* 52:595–638. Review.

Engeland WC. 1998. Functional innervation of the adrenal cortex by the splanchnic nerve. *Horm Metab Res.* 30:311–314. Review.

Ennis M, Aston-Jones G. 1987. Two physiologically distinct populations of neurons in the ventrolateral medulla innervate the locus coeruleus. *Brain Res.* 425:275–282.

Ennis M, Aston-Jones G. 1988. Activation of locus coeruleus from nucleus paragigantocellularis: a new excitatory amino acid pathway in brain. *J. Neurosci.* 8:3644–3657.

Eriksson E, Dellborg M, Soderpalm B, Carlsson M, Nilsson C. 1986. Growth hormone responses to clonidine and GRF in spontaneously hypertensive rats: neuroendocrine evidence for an enhanced responsiveness of brain alpha 2-adrenoceptors in genetical hypertension. *Life Sci.* 39:2103–2109.

Faludi G, Magyar I, Tekes K, Tothfalusi L, Magyar K. 1988. Measurement of 3H-serotonin uptake in blood platelets in major depressive episodes. *Biol Psychiatry.* 23:833–836.

Felsner P, Hofer D, Rinner I, Porta S, Korsatko W, Schauenstein K. 1995. Adrenergic suppression of peripheral blood T cell reactivity in the rat is due to activation of peripheral alpha 2-receptors. *J Neuroimmunol.* 57:27–34.

Felten SY, Felten DL, Bellinger DL et al. 1988. Noradrenergic sympathetic innervation of lymphoid organs. *Prog Allergy.* 43:14–36. Review.

Fenik V, Marchenko V, Janssen P, Davies RO, Kubin L. 2002. A5 cells are silenced when REM sleep-like signs are elicited by pontine carbachol. *J Appl Physiol.* 93:1448–1456.

Fenik VB, Davies RO, Kubin L. 2005. REM sleep-like atonia of hypoglossal (XII) motoneurons is caused by loss of noradrenergic and serotonergic inputs. *Am J Respir Crit Care Med.* 172:1322–1330.

Ferre S, Artigas F. 1993. Dopamine D2 receptor-mediated regulation of serotonin extracellular concentration in the dorsal raphe nucleus of freely moving rats. *J Neurochem.* 61:772–775.

Fozard JR. 1984. Neuronal 5-HT receptors in the periphery. *Neuropharmacology.* 23:1473–1486.

Freitag A, Wessler I, Racke K. 1997. Nitric oxide, via activation of guanylyl cyclase, suppresses alpha2-adrenoceptor-mediated 5-hydroxytryptamine release from neuroendocrine epithelial cells of rabbit tracheae. *Naunyn Schmiedebergs Arch Pharmacol.* 356:856–859.

Fung SJ, Reddy VK, Zhuo H, Liu RH, Wang Z, Barnes CD. 1994. Anatomical evidence for the presence of glutamate or enkephalin in noradrenergic projection neurons of the locus coeruleus. *Microsc Res Tech.* 29:219–225.

Fuxe K, Hokfelt T, Agnati L, Johansson D, Ljangdahl A, Perez de la Mora M. 1977. Regulation of the mesocortical dopamine neurons. In Costa E, Gessa GL, eds. *Nonstriatal Dopaminergic Neurons. Advanced Biochemical Psychopharmacology.* New York: Raven Press, 47–55.

Gaykema RP, Chen CC, Goehler LE. 2007. Organization of immune-responsive medullary projections to the bed nucleus of the stria terminalis, central amygdala, and paraventricular nucleus of the hypothalamus: evidence for parallel viscerosensory pathways in the rat brain. *Brain Res.* 1130:130–145.

Gerendai I, Halasz B. 2000. Central nervous system structures connected with the endocrine gland. Findings obtained with the viral transneuronal tracing technique. *Exp Clin Endocrinol Diabetes.* 108:389–395. Review.

Gerin C, Privat A. 1998. Direct evidence for the link between monoaminergic descending pathways and motor activity: II. a study with microdialysis probes implanted in the ventral horn of the spinal cord. *Brain Res.* 794:169–173.

Gershon MD, Bursztajn S. 1978. Properties of the enteric nervous system: limitation of access of intravascular macromolecules to the myenteric plexus and muscularis externa. *J Comp Neurol.* 180:467–488.

Gomez F, Lechin AE, Jara H et al. 1988. Plasma neurotransmitters in anxiety patients. III Interamerican congress of clinical pharmacology and Therapeutics and the XII latinoamerican congress of pharmacology. *Arch Ven Farm Clin Terap.* 7(Suppl 1), Abst. 4.

Granata AR, Numao Y, Kumada M, Reis DJ. 1986. A1 noradrenergic neurons tonically inhibit sympathoexcitatory neurons of C1 area in rat brainstem. *Brain Res.* 377:127–146.

Grudzien A, Shaw P, Weintraub S, Bigio E, Mash DC, Mesulam MM. 2007. Locus coeruleus neurofibrillary degeneration in aging, mild cognitive impairment and early Alzheimer's disease. *Neurobiol Aging.* 28:327–335.

Hadziefendic S, Haxhiu MA. 1999. CNS innervation of vagal preganglionic neurons controlling peripheral airways: a transneuronal labeling study using pseudorabies virus. *J Auton Nerv Syst.* 76:135–145.

Hand TH, Kasser RJ, Wang RY. 1987a. Effects of acute thioridazine, metoclopramide and SCH 23390 on the basal activity of A9 and A10 dopamine cells. *Eur J Pharmacol.* 137:251–255.

Hand TH, Hu XT, Wang RY. 1987b. Differential effects of acute clozapine and haloperidol on the activity of ventral tegmental (A10) and nigrostriatal (A9) dopamine neurons. *Brain Res.* 41:257–269.

Haxhiu MA, Jansen AS, Cherniack NS, Loewy AD. 1993. CNS innervation of airway-related parasympathetic preganglionic neurons: a transneuronal labeling study using pseudorabies virus. *Brain Res.* 618:115–134.

Haxhiu MA, Kc P, Neziri B, Yamamoto BK, Ferguson DG, Massari VJ. 2003. Catecholaminergic microcircuitry controlling the output of airway-related vagal preganglionic neurons. *J Appl Physiol.* 94:1999–2009.

Haxhiu MA, Kc P, Moore CT et al. 2005. Brain stem excitatory and inhibitory signaling pathways regulating bronchoconstrictive responses. [appears erratum in: *J Appl Physiol.* 2005,99:2476] *J Appl Physiol.* 98:1961–1982. Review.

Haxhiu MA, Rust CF, Brooks C, Kc P. 2006. CNS determinants of sleep-related worsening of airway functions: implications for nocturnal asthma. *Respir Physiol Neurobiol.* 28:151:1–30.

Hechtman HB, Lonergan EA, Staunton HP, Dennis RC, Shepro D. 1978. Pulmonary entrapment of platelets during acute respiratory failure. *Surgery.* 83:277–283.

Hermann DM, Luppi PH, Peyron C, Hinckel P, Jouvet M. 1997. Afferent projections to the rat nuclei raphe magnus, raphe pallidus and reticularis gigantocellularis pars alpha demonstrated by iontophoretic application of choleratoxin (subunit b). *J Chem Neuroanat.* 13:1–21.

Herman JP, Ostrander MM, Mueller NK, Figueiredo H. 2005. Limbic system mechanisms of stress regulation: hypothalamo-pituitary-adrenocortical axis. *Prog Neuropsychopharmacol Biol Psychiatry.* 29:1201–1213.

Hervas I, Bel N, Fernandez AG, Palacios JM, Artigas F. 1998. In vivo control of 5-hydroxytryptamine release by terminal autoreceptors in rat brain areas differentially innervated by the dorsal and median raphe nuclei. *Naunyn Schmiedebergs Arch Pharmacol.* 358:315–322.

Herve D, Simon H, Blanc G, Lemoal M, Glowinski J, Tassin JP. 1981. Opposite changes in dopamine utilization in the nucleus accumbens and the frontal cortex after electrolytic lesion of the median raphe in the rat. *Brain Res.* 216:422–428.

Herve D, Pickel VM, Joh TH, Beaudet A. 1987. Serotonin axon terminals in the ventral tegmental area of the rat: fine structure and synaptic input to dopaminergic neurons. *Brain Res.* 435:71–83.

Ho SS, Chow BK, Yung WH. 2007. Serotonin increases the excitability of the hypothalamic paraventricular nucleus magnocellular neurons. *Eur J Neurosci.* 25:2991–3000.

Hokfelt T, Phillipson O, Goldstein M. 1979. Evidence for a dopaminergic pathway in the rat descending from the A11 cell group to the spinal cord. *Acta Physiol Scand.* 107:393–395.

Holst JJ, Schaffalitzky de Muckadell OB, Fahrenkrug J. 1979. Nervous control of pancreatic exocrine secretion in pigs. *Acta Physiol Scand.* 105:33–51.

Holtman JR Jr, Marion LJ, Speck DF. 1990. Origin of serotonin-containing projections to the ventral respiratory group in the rat. *Neuroscience.* 37:541–552.

Hong SS, Magee DF. 1970. Pharmacological studies on the regulation of pancreatic secretion in pigs. *Ann Surg.* 172:41–48.

Islam MS, Melville GN, Ulmer WT. 1974. Role of atropine in antagonizing the effect of 5-hydroxytryptamine (5-HT) on bronchial and pulmonary vascular systems. *Respiration.* 31:47–59.

Ishibashi H, Shimada H, Jang IS, Nakamura TY, Nabekura J. 2005. Activation of presynaptic GABAAA receptors increases spontaneous glutamate release onto noradrenergic neurons of the rat locus coeruleus. *Brain Res.* 1046:24–31.

Ishida Y, Shirokawa T, Miyaishi O, Komatsu Y, Isobe K. 2000. Age-dependent changes in projections from locus coeruleus to hippocampus dentate gyrus and frontal cortex. *Eur J Neurosci.* 12:1263–1270.

Isik A, Koca SS, Ozturk A, Mermi O. 2007. Anxiety and depression in patients with rheumatoid arthritis. *Clin Rheumatol.* 26:872–878.

Iwasaki H, Kani K, Maeda T. 1999. Neural connections of the pontine reticular formation, which connects reciprocally with the nucleus prepositus hypoglossi in the rat. *Neuroscience.* 93:195–208.

Jackson VM, Cunnane TC. 2001. Neurotransmitter release mechanisms in sympathetic neurons: past, present, and future perspectives. *Neurochem Res.* 26:875–889. Review.

Jacobs BL, Heym J, Trulson ME. 1981. Behavioral and physiological correlates of brain serotoninergic unit activity. *J Physiol.* 77:431–436.

Jara H, Lechin A, Rada I et al. 1988. Plama neurotransmitters profile in duodenal ulcer patients. III Interamerican congress of clinical pharmacology and therapeutics and XII latinoamerican congress of pharmacology. *Arch Ven Farm Clin Terap.* 7(suppl 1) Abst. 86.

Johnson DE, Georgieff MK. 1989. Pulmonary neuroendocrine cells. Their secretory products and their potential roles in health and chronic lung disease in infancy. *Am Rev Respir Dis.* 140:1807–1812. Review.

Joossens S, Reinisch W, Vermeire S et al. 2002. The value of serologic markers in indeterminate colitis: a prospective follow-up study. *Gastroenterology* 122:1242–1247.

Jordan D. 2001. Central nervous pathways and control of the airways. *Respir Physiol.* 125:67–81. Review.

Kalin NH, Weiler SJ, Shelton SE. 1982. Plasma ACTH and cortisol concentrations before and after dexamethasone. *Psychiatry Res.* 7:87–92.

Kant GJ, Mougey EH, Meyerhoff JL. 1989. ACTH, prolactin, corticosterone and pituitary cyclic AMP responses to repeated stress. *Pharmacol Biochem Behav.* 32:557–561.

Keith IM, Will JA. 1982. Dynamics of the neuroendocrine cell-regulatory peptide system in the lung. Specific overview and new results. *Exp Lung Res.* 3:387–402. Review.

King D, Zigmond MJ, Finlay JM. 1997. Effects of dopamine depletion in the medial prefrontal cortex on the stress-induced increase in extracellular dopamine in the nucleus accumbens core and shell. *Neuroscience.* 77:141–153.

Kinkead R, Belzile O, Gulemetova R. 2002. Serotonergic modulation of respiratory motor output during tadpole development. *J Appl Physiol.* 93:936–946.

Kitayama I, Nakamura S, Yaga T et al. 1994. Degeneration of locus coeruleus axons in stress-induced depression model. *Brain Res. Bull.* 35:573–580.

Knable MB, Hyde TM, Murray AM, Herman MM, Kleinman JE. 1996. A postmortem study of frontal cortical dopamine D1 receptors in schizophrenics, psychiatric controls, and normal controls. *Biol. Psychiatry.* 40:1191–1199.

Koga H, Ishibashi H, Shimada H, Jang IS, Nakamura TY, Nabekura J. 2005. Activation of presynaptic GABA-A receptors increases spontaneous glutamate release onto noradrenergic neurons of the rat locus coeruleus. *Brain Res.* 1046:24–31.

Koob GF. 1999. Corticotropin-releasing factor, norepinephrine, and stress. *Biol. Psychiatry.* 46:1167–1180. Review.

Kopin IJ, Eisenhofer G, Goldstein D. 1988. Sympathoadrenal medullary system and stress. In Chrousos GP, Loriaux DL, Gold PW, eds. *Mechanisms of Physical and Emotional Stress.* New York: Plenum Press, 11–23.

Kostowski W. 1979. Two noradrenergic systems in the brain and their interactions with other monoaminergic neurons. *Pol J Pharmacol Pharm.* 31:425–436. Review.

Koutantji M, Harrold E, Lane SE, Pearce S, Watts RA, Scott DG. 2003. Investigation of quality of life, mood, pain, disability, and disease status in primary systemic vasculitis. *Arthritis Rheum.* 49:826–837.

Krowicki ZK, Hornby PJ. 1993. Serotonin microinjected into the nucleus raphe obscurus increases intragastric pressure in the rat via a vagally mediated pathway. *J Pharmacol Exp Ther.* 265:468–476.

Kubin L, Reignier C, Tojima H, Taguchi O, Pack AI, Davies RO. 1994. Changes in serotonin level in the hypoglossal nucleus region during carbachol-induced atonia. *Brain Res.* 645:291–302.

Kumaido K. 1988. Studies on the respiratory control mechanism of medullary raphe nuclei and their serotonergic system. *No To Shinkei.* 40:929–938.

Kurland JE, Coyle WJ, Winkler A, Zable E. 2006. Prevalence of irritable bowel syndrome and depression in fibromyalgia. *Dig Dis Sci.* 51:454–460.

Kuwabara S. 2007. Guillain-barre syndrome. *Curr Neurol Neurosci Rep.* 7:57–62. Review.

Kvetnansky R, Palkovits M, Mitro A, Torda T, Mikulaj L. 1977. Catecholamines in individual hypothalamic nuclei of acutely and repeatedly stressed rats. *Neuroendocrinology.* 23:257–267.

Kvetnansky R, Bodnar I, Shahar T, Uhereczky G, Krizanova O, Mravec B. 2006. Effect of lesion of A5 and A7 brainstem noradrenergic areas or transection of brainstem pathways on sympathoadrenal activity in rats during immobilization stress. *Neurochem Res.* 31:267–275.

Laaris N, Le Poul E, Hamon M, Lanfumey L. 1997. Stress-induced alterations of somatodendritic 5-HT1A autoreceptor sensitivity in the rat dorsal raphe nucleus—in vitro electrophysiological evidence. *Fundam Clin Pharmacol.* 11:206–214.

Ladep NG, Obindo TJ, Audu MD, Okeke EN, Malu AO. 2006. Depression in patients with irritable bowel syndrome in Jos, Nigeria. *World J Gastroenterol.* 12:7844–7877.

Lalley PM, Benacka R, Bischoff AM, Richter DW. 1997. Nucleus raphe obscurus evokes 5-HT-1A receptor-mediated modulation of respiratory neurons. *Brain Res.* 747:156–159.

Langer SZ, Angel I. 1991. Pre- and postsynaptic alpha-2 adrenoceptors as target for drug discovery. *J Neural Transm Suppl.* 34:171–177.

Larsson K, Carlens P, Bevegard S, Hjemdahl P. 1995. Sympathoadrenal responses to bronchoconstriction in asthma: an invasive and kinetic study of plasma catecholamines. *Clin Sci.* 88:439–446.

Larsson PT, Hjemdahl P, Olsson G, Egberg N, Hornstra G. 1989. Altered platelet function during mental stress and adrenaline infusion in humans: evidence for an increased aggregability in vivo as measured by filtragometry. *Clin Sci.* 76:369–376.

Lauweryns JM, Van Ranst L. 1988. Immunocytochemical localization of aromatic L-amino acid decarboxylase in human, rat, and mouse bronchopulmonary and gastrointestinal endocrine cells. *J Histochem Cytochem.* 36:1181–1186.

Leake A, Griffiths HW, Ferrier IN. 1989. Plasma N-POMC, ACTH and cortisol following hCRH administration in major depression and dysthymia. *J Affect Disord.* 17:57–64.

Lechin A, Jara H, Rada I et al. 1988. Plasma neurotransmitters profile in irritable bowel syndrome (IBS) diarrheic patients. III Interamerican congress of clinical pharmacology and therapeutics and XII latinoamerican congress of pharmacology. *Arch Ven Farm Clin Terap.* 7(Suppl 1) Abst. 88.

Lechin AE, Varon J, van der Dijs B, Lechin F. 1994. Plasma catecholamines and indoleamines during attacks and remission on severe bronchial asthma: possible role of stress. *Am J Respir Crit Care Med.* 149:A778.

Lechin F. 1977. Autoinmunidad y patologia gastroduodenal. Editorial. *Acta Gastroenter Latinoamer.* 7:39–43.

Lechin F. 1992a. Neuropharmacological therapy approach to psychosomatic diseases associated with stress and depression. Abstract. XXIII Congress of the International Society of Psychoneuroendocrinology. Madison: Wisconsin.

Lechin F. 1992b. Adrenergic-serotonergic influences on gallbladder motility and irritable bowel syndrome. *Am J Physiol. Gastrointest Liver Physiol.* 262:G375–G376.

Lechin F. 1992c. Clonidine and prolactin secretion in humans. *Clin Neuropharmacology.* 15:155–156.

Lechin F. 2000. Central and plasma 5-HT, vagal tone and airways. *Trends Pharmacol Sci.* 21:425.

Lechin F. 2005. Treatment of bronchial asthma with tianeptine. Conference. Therapeutics. Annals of the First International Congress of Therapeutics 2005. Caracas, Venezuela.

Lechin F. 2006a. Neurocircuitries involved into the psychopathologic syndromes: anxiety, phobia, major depression, dysthymic depression, panic, bipolar, obssesive-compulsive disorder, post-traumatic stress disorder and psychotic. Therapeutical considerations. Memories of the 8th Congreso Argentino de Neuropsiquiatría y Neurociencia Cognitiva, Buenos Aires, Argentina. September.

Lechin F. 2006b. Neurophysiology, neuropathophysiology, neuroimmunology and neuroimmunepharmacology associated to stress and depression. Therapeutical approaches to the Th-1 and Th-2 autoimmune diseases. Memories of the 4th Congreso Latinoamericano de Neuropsiquiatría, Buenos Aires, Argentina. September.

Lechin F, Benshimol A, van der Dijs B. 1970. Histalog and secretin effects on serum electrolytes. Influence of pancreatectomy and gastrectomy. *Acta Gastroenter Latinoamer.* 2:9–13.

Lechin F, van der Dijs B, Bentolila A, Peña F. 1977a. Antidiarrheal effects of dihydroergotamine. *J Clin Pharmacol.* 17:339–349.

Lechin F, van der Dijs B, Bentolila A, Peña F. 1977b. The spastic colon syndrome. Therapeutic and pathophysiological considerations. *J Clin Pharmacol.* 17:431–435.

Lechin F, van der Dijs B, Bentolila A, Peña F. 1978. The adrenergic influences on the gallbladder emptying. *Am J Gastroenterol.* 69:662–668.

Lechin F, van der Dijs B, Lechin E. 1979a. eds. *The Autonomic Nervous System. Physiological Basis of Psychosomatic Therapy.* Barcelona, Spain: Editorial Científico-Médica.

Lechin F, Coll-Garcia E, van der Dijs B, Bentolila A, Peña F, Rivas C. 1979b. Effects of captivity on glucose tolerance in dogs. *Experientia.* 35:876–879.

Lechin F, Gómez F, van der Dijs B, Lechin E. 1980a. Distal colon motility in schizophrenic patients. *J Clin Pharmacol.* 20:459–464.

Lechin F, van der Dijs B, Gómez F, Valls JM, Acosta E, Arocha L. 1980b. Pharmacomanometric studies of colonic motility as a guide to the chemotherapy of schizophrenia. *J Clin Pharmacol.* 20:664–671.

Lechin F, van der Dijs B, Gómez F, Arocha L, Acosta E. 1982a. Effects of d-amphetamine, clonidine and clonazepam on distal colon motility in non-psychotic patients. *Res Commun Psychol Psychiat Behav.* 7:385–410.

Lechin F, van der Dijs B, Gómez F, Arocha L, Acosta E, Lechin E. 1982b. Distal colon motility as a predictor of antidepressant response to fenfluramine, imipramine and clomipramine. *Arch Ven Farm Clin Terap.* 1:156–161.

Lechin F, van der Dijs B, Gómez F, Acosta E, Arocha L. 1982c. Comparison between the effects of d-amphetamine and fenfluramine on distal colon motility in non-psychotic patients. *Res Commun Psychol Psychiat Behav.* 7:411–417.

Lechin F, van der Dijs B, Insausti CL, Gómez F. 1982d. Treatment of ulcerative colitis with thioproperazine. *J Clin Gastroenterol.* 4:445–449.

Lechin F, van der Dijs B, Gómez F, Arocha L, Acosta E, Lechin E. 1983a. Distal colon motility as a predictor of antidepressant response to fenfluramine, imipramine and clomipramine. *J Affect Dis.* 5:27–35.

Lechin F, van der Dijs B, Acosta E, Gómez F, Lechin E, Arocha L. 1983b. Distal colon motility and clinical parameters in depression. *J Affect Dis.* 5:19–26.

Lechin F, van der Dijs B, Gómez F, Lechin E, Oramas O, Villa S. 1983c. Positive symptoms of acute psychosis: dopaminergic or noradrenergic overactivity? *Res Commun Psychol Psychiat Behav.* 8:23–31.

Lechin F, van der Dijs B, Jakubowicz D et al. 1985a. Effects of clonidine on blood pressure, noradrenaline, cortisol, growth hormone and prolactin plasma levels in low and high intestinal tone subjects. *Neuroendocrinology.* 40:253–261.

Lechin F, van der Dijs B, Jakubowicz D et al. 1985b. Effects of clonidine on blood pressure, noradrenaline, cortisol, growth hormone, and prolactin plasma levels in high and low intestinal tone depressed patients. *Neuroendocrinology.* 41:156–162.

Lechin F, van der Dijs B, Insausti CL et al. 1985c. Treatment of ulcerative colitis with clonidine. *J Clin Pharmacol.* 25:219–226.

Lechin F, van der Dijs B, Amat J, Lechin ME. 1986. Central neuronal pathways involved in depressive syndrome. Experimental findings. *Res Commun Psychol Psychiat Behav.* 11:145–192.

Lechin F, van der Dijs B, Jakubowicz D et al. 1987a. Role of stress in the exacerbation of chronic illness. Effects of clonidine administration on blood pressure, nor-epinephrine, cortisol, growth hormone and prolactin plasma levels. *Psychoneuroendocrinology.* 12:117–129.

Lechin F, van der Dijs B, Azócar J et al. 1987b. Stress, immunology and cancer: effect of psychoactive drugs. *Arch Ven Farm Clin Terap.* 6:28–43.

Lechin F, van der Dijs B, Azócar J et al. 1988a. Definite and sustained with psychoactive drugs of three Crohn's disease patients.III Interamerican congress of clinical pharmacology and therapeutics and XII latinoamerican congress of pharmacology. *Arch Ven Farm Clin Terap.* 7(Suppl 1) Abst. 89.

Lechin F, van der Dijs B, Gómez F et al. 1988b. Plasma neurotransmitters profile in depressive syndromes. III Interamerican congress of clinical pharmacology and therapeutics and the XII latinoamerican congress of pharmacology. *Arch Ven Farm Clin Terap.* 7(Suppl 1) Abst. 7.

Lechin F, van der Dijs B, Azócar J et al. 1988c. Neurochemical and inmunological profiles of three clinical stages in 50 advanced cancer patients. III Interamerican congress of clinical pharmacology and therapeutics and XII latinoamerican congress of pharmacology. *Arch Ven Farm Clin Terap.* 7(Suppl 1) Abst. 39.

Lechin F, van der Dijs B, Lechin S, Vitelli G, Lechin ME, Cabrera A. 1989a. Neurochemical, hormonal and immunological views of stress: clinical and therapeutic implications in Crohn's disease and cancer. In Velazco M, ed. *Recent Advances in Pharmacology and Therapeutics.* International Congress Series Vol 839. Amsterdam: Excerpta Medica, 57–70.

Lechin F, van der Dijs B, Rada I et al. 1989b. Recurrent gastroesophageal symptoms and precordial pain in a gastrectomized man improved by amytriptyline. Physiologic, metabolic, endocrine, neurochemical and psychiatric findings. *J Med.* 20:407–424.

Lechin F, van der Dijs B, Vitelli G et al. 1990a. Psychoneuroendocrinological and immunological parameters in cancer patients: involvement of stress and depression. *Psychoneuroendocrinology.* 15:435–451.

Lechin F, van der Dijs B, Rada I et al. 1990b. Plasma neurotransmitters and cortisol in duodenal ulcer patients: role of stress. *Dig Dis Sci.* 35:1313–1319.

Lechin F, van der Dijs B, Lechin A et al. 1991. Doxepin therapy for postprandial symptomatic hypoglycemic patients neurochemical, hormonal and metabolic disturbances. *Clin Sci.* 80:373–384.

Lechin F, van der Dijs B, Lechin M et al. 1992a. Effects of an oral glucose load on plasma neurotransmitters in humans: involvement of REM sleep? *Neuropsychobiology.* 26:4–11.

Lechin F, van der Dijs B, Lechin M et al. 1992b. Clonidine treatment of acute pancreatitis: Report of five cases. *Acta Gastroent Latinoamer.* 22:119–124.

Lechin F, van der Dijs B, Lechin M et al. 1992c. Dramatic improvement with clonidine of acute pancreatitis showing raised catecholamines and cortisol plasma levels: case report of five patients. *J Med.* 23:339–351.

Lechin F, van der Dijs B, Lechin M et al. 1993. Plasma neurotransmitters throughout an oral glucose tolerance test in essential hypertension. *Clin Exp Hypertension.* 15:209–240.

Lechin F, van der Dijs B, Lechin AE et al. 1994a. Plasma neurotransmitters and cortisol in chronic illness: role of stress. *J Med.* 25:181–192.

Lechin F, van der Dijs B, Vitelli-Flores G et al. 1994b. Peripheral blood immunological parameters in long-term benzodiazepine users. *Clin Neuropharmacology.* 17:63–72.

Lechin F, van der Dijs B, Lechin-Báez S et al. 1994c. Two types of irritable bowel syndrome: differences in behavior, clinical signs, distal colon motility and hormonal, neurochemical, metabolic, physiological and pharmacological profiles. *Arch Ven Farmac Terap.* 12:105–114. Review.

Lechin F, van der Dijs B, Orozco B et al. 1995a. Plasma neurotransmitters, blood pressure and heart rate during supine-resting, orthostasis and moderate exercise conditions in major depressed patients. *Biol Psychiatry.* 38:166–173.

Lechin F, van der Dijs B, Orozco B et al. 1995b. Plasma neurotransmitters, blood pressure and heart rate during supine-resting, orthostasis and moderate exercise in dysthymic depressed patients. *Biol Psychiatry.* 37:884–891.

Lechin F, van der Dijs B, Benaim M. 1996a. Stress versus depression. *Prog NeuroPsychopharmacol Biol Psychiatry.* 20:899–950. Review.

Lechin F, van der Dijs B, Benaim M. 1996b. Benzodiazepines: tolerability in elderly patients. *Psychother Psychosom.* 65:171–182. Review.

Lechin F, van der Dijs B, Lechin M. 1996c. Plasma neurotransmitters and functional illness. *Psychother Psychosom.* 65:293–318. Review.

Lechin F, van der Dijs B, Orozco B et al. 1996d. Plasma neurotransmitters, blood pressure and heart during supine-resting, orthostasis and moderate exercise in severely ill patients: a model of failing to cope with stress. *Psychother Psychosom.* 65:129–136.

Lechin F, van der Dijs B, Orozco B et al. 1996e. Plasma neurotransmitters, blood pressure and heart rate during supine-resting, orthostasis and moderate exercise stress test in healthy humans before and after parasympathetic blockade with atropine. *Res Comm Biol Psychol Psychiatry.* 21:55–72.

Lechin F, van der Dijs B, Orozco B, Lechin ME, Lechin AE. 1996f. Increased levels of free-serotonin in plasma of symptomatic asthmatic patients. *Ann Allergy Asthma Immunol.* 77:245–253.

Lechin F, van der Dijs B, Lechin ME et al. 1997a. Plasma neurotransmitters, blood pressure and heart rate during supine-resting, orthostasis, and moderate exercise conditions in two types of hypertensive patients. *Res Comm Biol Psychol Psychiatry.* 22:111–145.

Lechin F, van der Dijs B, Jara H et al. 1997b. Successful neuropharmacological treatment of Myasthenia Gravis. Report of eight cases. *Res Comm Biol Psychol Psychiatry.* 22:81–94.

Lechin F, van der Dijs B, Jara H, Orozco B et al. 1997c. Plasma neurotransmitter profiles of anxiety, phobia and panic disorder patients. Acute and chronic effects of buspirone. *Res Comm Biol Psychol Psychiatry.* 22:95–110.

Lechin F, van der Dijs B, Jara H et al. 1998a. Effects of buspirone on plasma neurotransmitters in healthy subjects. *J Neural Transm.* 105:561–573.

Lechin F, van der Dijs B, Lechin A, Orozco B, Lechin ME, Lechin AE. 1998b. The serotonin uptake-enhancing drug tianeptine suppresses asthmatic symptoms in children. A double-blind crossover placebo-controlled study. *J Clin Pharmacol.* 38:918–925.

Lechin F, van der Dijs B, Orozco B et al. 1998c. Neuropharmacological treatment of bronchial asthma with an antidepressant drug: tianeptine. A dowuble-blind crossover placebo-controlled study. *Clin Pharmacol Ther.* 64:223–232.

Lechin F, van der Dijs B, Pardey-Maldonado B et al. 2000. Enhancement of noradrenergic neural transmission: an effective therapy of myastenia gravis. Report of 52 consecutive patients. *J Med.* 31:333–361.

Lechin F, van der Dijs B, Lechin ME. 2002a. eds. *Neurocircuitry and Neuroautonomic Disorders Reviews and Therapeutic Strategies.* Karger: Basel.

Lechin F, van der Dijs B, Orozco B. 2002b. Gallbladder muscle dysfunction and neuroautonomic disorders. *Gastroenterology*. 123:1407–1408.

Lechin F, van der Dijs B, Lechin ME. 2002c. Neuropharmacological factors, biliary motility and pancreatitis. *J Pancreas*. 3:152–154.

Lechin F, Lechin ME, van der Dijs B. 2002d. Plasma catecholamines and chronic congestive heart failure. *Circulation*. 106(25):222.

Lechin F, van der Dijs B, Lechin AE. 2002e. Plasma serotonin, pulmonary hypertension and bronchial asthma. *Clin. Sci*. 103:345–346.

Lechin F, van der Dijs B, Lechin AE. 2002f. Severe asthma and plasma serotonin. *Allergy*. 57:258–259.

Lechin F, van der Dijs B, Lechin AE. 2002g. Pulmonary hypertension, left ventricular dysfunction and plasma serotonin. *Br J Pharmacol*. 137:937–938.

Lechin F, van der Dijs B, Orozco B. 2002h. Cholecystokinin (CCK) and secretin and pancreatic secretion of insulin and glucagon. *Dig Dis Sci*. 47:2422–2423.

Lechin F, van der Dijs B, Lechin AE. 2003. Tianeptine, plasma serotonin and pulmonary hypertension. *Lancet*. 361(9351):87.

Lechin F, Pardey-Maldonado B, van der Dijs B et al. 2004a. Circulating neurotransmitter profiles during the different wake-sleep stages in normal subjects. *Psychoneuroendocrinology*. 29:669–685.

Lechin F, van der Dijs B, Lechin AE. 2004b. The autonomic nervous system assessment throughout the wake-sleep cycle & stress. *Psychosom Med*. 66:974–976.

Lechin F, van der Dijs B, Lechin AE. 2004c. Neural sympathetic activity in essential hypertension. *Hypertension*. 44:e3–e4.

Lechin F, van der Dijs B, Lechin AE. 2004d. Natural killer cells activity and neuroimmunological treatment of cancer. *Clin Cancer Res*. 10:8120–8121.

Lechin F, van der Dijs B, Orozco B, Jahn E, Rodriguez S, Baez S. 2004e. Neuropharmacological treatment of refractory idiopathic thrombocytopenic purpura: roles of circulating catecholamines and serotonin. *Thromb Haemost*. 91:1254–1256.

Lechin F, van der Dijs B, Lechin AE. 2004f. Tianeptine: a new exploratory therapy for asthma. *Chest*. 125:348–349.

Lechin F, van der Dijs B, Orozco B, Rodriguez S, Baez S. 2004g. Elective stenting, platelet serotonin and thrombotic events. *Platelets*. 15:462.

Lechin F, van der Dijs B, Lechin AE. 2004h. Treatment of bronchial asthma with tianeptine. *Methods Find Exp Clin Pharmacol*. 26:697–701. Review.

Lechin F, van der Dijs B, Lechin AE. 2005a. Circulating serotonin, catecholamines and CNS circuitry related to some cardiorespiratory and vascular disorders. *J Appl Res*. 5: 605–621. Review.

Lechin F, van der Dijs B, Orozco B, Rodriguez S, Baez S. 2005b. Neuropharmacological therapy of Polycythemia vera: roles of circulating catecholamines and serotonin. *Thromb Haemost*. 93:175–177.

Lechin F, van der Dijs B, Orozco B, Rodriguez S, Baez S. 2005c. Neuropharmacological therapy of the neuroendocrine carcinoid syndrome: report of two cases. *J Appl Res*. 5:109–114.

Lechin F, van der Dijs B, Orozco B, Hernandez-Adrian G, Rodriguez S, Baez S. 2005d. Similar autonomic nervous system disorders underlying cystic fibrosis and pancreatic cysts allowed common neuropharmacological therapy: report of four cases. *J Appl Res*. 5:299–304.

Lechin F, van der Dijs B, Hernandez-Adrian G. 2006a. Dorsal Raphe (DR) vs. Median Raphe (MR) serotonergic antagonism. Anatomical, physiological, behavioral, neuroendocrinological, neuropharmacological and clinical evidences: relevance for neuropharmacological therapy. *Prog Neuropsychopharmacol Biol Psychiatry*. 30:565–585. Review.

Lechin F, van der Dijs B, Hernandez G, Orozco B, Rodriguez S, Baez S. 2006b. Acute effects of tianeptine on circulating neurotransmitters and cardiovascular parameters. *Prog Neuropsychopharmacol Biol Psychiatry*. 30:214–222.

Lechin F, van der Dijs B, Baez S, Hernandez G, Orozco B, Rodriguez S. 2006c. The effects of oral arginine on neuroautonomic parameters in healthy subjects. *J Appl Res*. 6:201–213.

Lechin F, van der Dijs B, Lechin AE. 2007. Serotonin bronchial hyperresponsiveness and eosinophil-associated gastrointestinal disease. *Gastroenterology*. (Accepted for publication).

Lechin F, van der Dijs B. 1973. A study of some immunological and clinical characteristics of gastritis, gastric ulcer, and duodenal ulcer in the three racial groups of the venezuelan population. *Am J Phys Anthropology*. 39:369–374.

Lechin F, van der Dijs B. 1979a. Colecistoquinina endógena y motilidad del colon distal. *Acta Cient Venez*. 29(Suppl 1):109–113.

Lechin F, van der Dijs B. 1979b. Physiological effects of endogenous CCK on distal colon motility. *Acta Gastroenter Latinoamer*. 9:195–201.

Lechin F, van der Dijs B. 1979c. The effects of dopaminergic blocking agents on distal colon motility. *J Clin Pharmacol*. 19:617–623.

Lechin F, van der Dijs B. 1979d. Dopamine and distal colon motility. *Dig Dis Sci*. 24:86.

Lechin F, van der Dijs B. 2001. Effects of diphenylhydantoin on distal colon motility. *Acta Gastroenter Latinoamer*. 9:145–151.

Lechin F, van der Dijs B. 1980. Treatment of infertility with levodopa. *Br Med J*. 280:480.

Lechin F, van der Dijs B. 1981a. Colon motility and psychological traits in the irritable bowel syndrome. *Dig Dis Sci*. 26:474–475.

Lechin F, van der Dijs B. 1981b. Clonidine therapy for psychosis and tardive dyskinesia. *Am J Psychiatry*. 138:390.

Lechin F, van der Dijs B. 1981c. Noradrenergic or dopaminergic activity in chronic schizophrenia? *Br J Psychiat*. 139:472.

Lechin F, van der Dijs B. 1981d. Intestinal pharmacomanometry and glucose tolerance: evidence for two antagonistic dopaminergic mechanisms in the human. *Biol Psychiatry*. 16:969–976.

Lechin F, van der Dijs B. 1981e. Glucose tolerance, nonnutrient drink and gastrointestinal hormones. *Gastroenterology*. 80:216.

Lechin F, van der Dijs B. 1982. Intestinal pharmacomanometry as a guide to psychopharmacological therapy. In Velazco M, ed. *Clinical Pharmacology and Therapeutics*, International Congress Series No. 604. Amsterdam: Excerpta Medica, 166–172.

Lechin F, van der Dijs B. 1983. Opposite effects on human distal colon motility of two postulated alpha-2 antagonists (mianserin and chlorprothixene) and one alpha-2 agonist (clonidine). *J Clin Pharmacol*. 23:209–218.

Lechin F, van der Dijs B. 1984. Slow wave sleep (SWS), REM sleep (REMS) and depression. *Res Commun Psychol Psychiat Behav*. 9:227–262.

Lechin F, van der Dijs B. 1989. eds. *Neurochemistry and Clinical Disorders: Circuitry of Some Psychiatric and Psychosomatic Syndromes*. Boca Raton, FL: CRC Press.

Lechin F, van der Dijs B. 2001. Plasma serotonin, bronchial asthma and tianeptine. *Clin Physiol*. 21:723.

Lechin F, van der Dijs B. 2002. Serotonin and pulmonary vasoconstriction. *J Appl Physiol*. 92:1363–1364.

Lechin F, van der Dijs B. 2004a. Growth hormone, polycystic ovary syndrome and clonidine test. *Fertil Steril*. 82:765–767.

Lechin F, van der Dijs B. 2004b. Platelet aggregation, platelet serotonin and pancreatitis. *J Pancreas*. 5:8001–8003.

Lechin F, van der Dijs B. 2004c. Platelet serotonin and thrombostasis. *J Clin Invest*. http://www.jci.org/eletters/view/20267#sec1

Lechin F, van der Dijs B. 2004d. Platelet activation, and catheter intracoronary brachytherapy. *Heart*. July 1 (on line) http://heart.bmj.com/cgi/eletters/90/2/160.

Lechin F, van der Dijs B. 2005a. Noradrenergic hypothesis of schizophrenia. *Prog Neuropsychopharmacol Biol Psychiatry*. 29:777–778.

Lechin F, van der Dijs B. 2005b. Blood pressure and autonomic system assessment throughout the sleep cycle in normal adults. *Sleep*. 28:645–646.

Lechin F, van der Dijs B. 2005c. Neuropharmacological therapy of carcinoid syndrome. *Neuroendocrinology*. 81:137–138.

Lechin F, van der Dijs B. 2006a. Central nervous system circuitry and peripheral neural sympathetic activity responsible for essential hypertension. *Curr Neurovasc Res*. 3:307–325. Review.

Lechin F, van der Dijs B. 2006b. Central nervous system (CNS) circuitry involved in the hyperinsulinism syndrome. *Neuroendocrinology*. 84:222–234. Review.

Lechin F, van der Dijs B. 2007a. Irritable bowel syndrome, depression and TH-1 autoimmune diseases. *Dig. Dis. Sci*. 52:103–104.

Lechin F, van der Dijs B. 2007b. Pathophysiology of biliary type abdominal pain. *Dig Dis Sci*.. 52(11):3157–3158.

Lechin F, van der Dijs B. 2007c. Epinephrine, norepinephrine and cancer. *J Biol Chem*. (Accepted for publication).

Lechin F, van der Dijs B. 2008. Central nervous system plus autonomic nervous system disorders responsible for gastrointestinal and pancreatobiliary diseases. *Dig Dis Sci*. (In press).

Lechin M, Jara H, Rada I et al. 1988a. Plasma neurotransmitters profile in irritable bowel syndrome (IBS); spastic colon patients (SCP). III Interamerican congress of clinical pharmacology and therapeutics and XII latinoamerican congress of pharmacology. *Arch Ven Farm Clin Terap*. 7(Suppl 1) Abst. 87.

Lechin M, Villa S, Rada I et al. 1988b. Plasma neurotransmitters profile in reflux esophagitis. III Interamerican congress of clinical pharmacology and therapeutics and XII latinoamerican congress of pharmacology. *Arch Ven Farm Clin Terap*. 7(Suppl 1) Abst. 85.

Lechin S, Vitelli G, Martinez C et al. 1988. Plasma neurotransmitters, lymphocyte subpopulations and natural killer cell activity in terminal cancer patients. III Interamerican congress of clinical pharmacology and therapeutics and XII latinoamerican congress of pharmacology. *Arch Ven Farm Clin Terap*. 7(Suppl 1) Abst. 37.

Leonard BE, Song C. 1996. Stress and the immune system in the etiology of anxiety and depression. *Pharmacol. Biochem. Behav*. 54:299–303. Review.

Levine ES, Litto WJ, Jacobs BL. 1990. Activity of cat locus coeruleus noradrenergic neurons during the defense reaction. *Brain Res*. 531:189–195.

Levitt P, Moore RY. 1979. Origin and organization of brainstem catecholamine innervation in the rat. *J Comp Neurol*. 186:505–528.

Levitt RC, Mitzner W. 1989. Autosomal recessive inheritance of airway hyperreactivity to 5-hydroxytryptamine. *J Appl Physiol*. 67:1125–1132.

Li YW, Wesselingh SL, Blessing WW. 1992. Projections from rabbit caudal medulla to C1 and A5 sympathetic premotor neurons, demonstrated with phaseolus leucoagglutinin and herpes simplex virus. *J Comp Neurol*. 317:379–395.

Liebregts T, Adam B, Bredack C et al. 2007. Immune activation in patients with irritable bowel syndrome. *Gastroenterology*. 132:913–920.

Lima C, Souza VM, Soares AL, Macedo MS, Tavares-de-Lima W, Vargaftig BB. 2007. Interference of methysergide, a specific 5-hydroxytryptamine receptor antagonist, with airway chronic allergic inflammation and remodelling in a murine model of asthma. *Clin Exp Allergy*. 37:723–734.

Lindsey BG, Arata A, Morris KF, Hernandez YM, Shannon R. 1998. Medullary raphe neurons and baroreceptor modulation of the respiratory motor pattern in the cat. *J Physiol*. 512:863–882.

Liu JP, Clarke IJ, Funder JW, Engler D. 1991. Evidence that the central noradrenergic and adrenergic pathways activate the hypothalamic-pituitary-adrenal axis in the sheep. *Endocrinology*. 129:200–209.

Liu RH, Fung SJ, Reddy VK, Barnes CD. 1995. Localization of glutamatergic neurons in the dorsolateral pontine tegmentum projecting to the spinal cord of the cat with a proposed role of glutamate on lumbar motoneuron activity. *Neuroscience*. 64:193–208.

Loewy AD, Haxhiu MA. 1993. CNS cell groups projecting to pancreatic parasympathetic preganglionic neurons. *Brain Res*. 620:323–330.

Loewy AD, Franklin MF, Haxhiu MA. 1994. CNS monoamine cell groups projecting to pancreatic vagal motor neurons: a transneuronal labeling study using pseudo-rabies virus. *Brain Res.* 638:248–260.

Madden KS, Felten SY, Felten DL, Sundaresan PR, Livnat S. 1989. Sympathetic neural modulation of the immune system. I. Depression of T cell immunity in vivo and vitro following chemical sympathectomy. *Brain Behav Immun.* 3:72–89.

Madden KS, Felten SY, Felten DL, Hardy CA, Livnat S. 1994. Sympathetic nervous system modulation of the immune system. II. Induction of lymphocyte proliferation and migration in vivo by chemical sympathectomy. *J Neuroimmunol.* 49:67–75.

Mannelli M, Pupilli C, Fabbri G et al. 1988. Endogenous dopamine (DA) and DA2 receptors: a mechanism limiting excessive sympathetic-adrenal discharge in humans. *J Clin Endocrinol. Metab.* 66:626–631.

Marotti T, Gabrilovac J, Rabatic S, Smejkal-Jagar L, Rocic B, Haberstock H. 1996. Met-enkephalin modulates stress-induced alterations of the immune response in mice. *Pharmacol Biochem Behav.* 54:277–284.

Marwaha J, Aghajanian GK. 1982. Relative potencies of alpha-1 and alpha-2 antagonists in the locus ceruleus, dorsal raphe and dorsal lateral geniculate nuclei: an electrophysiological study. *J Pharmacol Exp Ther.* 222:287–293.

Masuko K, Nakamura H. 2007. Functional somatic syndrome: how it could be relevant to rheumatologists. *Mod Rheumatol.* 17:179–184.

Matsuda A, Furukawa K, Suzuki H et al. 2007. Does impaired TH1/TH2 balance cause postoperative infectious complications in colorectal cancer surgery? *J Surg Res.* 139:15–21.

Matsumoto M, Togashi H, Mori K, Ueno K, Miyamoto A, Yoshioka M. 1999. Characterization of endogenous serotonin-mediated regulation of dopamine release in the rat prefrontal cortex. *Eur J Pharmacol.* 383:39–48.

Mercuro G, Rossetti Z, Rivano AC et al. 1987. Peripheral presynaptic dopamine receptors control the release of norepinephrine and arterial pressure in humans. *Cardiologia.* 32:643–650.

Meredith IT, Eisenhofer G, Lambert GW, Dewar EM, Jennings GL, Esler MD. 1993. Cardiac sympathetic nervous activity in congestive heart failure. Evidence for increased neuronal norepinephrine release and preserved neuronal uptake. *Circulation.* 88:136–145.

Midzyanovskaya IS, Kuznetsova GD, van Luijtelaar EL, van Rijn CM, Tuomisto L, Macdonald E. 2006. The brain 5HTergic response to an acute sound stress in rats with generalized (absence and audiogenic) epilepsy. *Brain Res Bull.* 69:631–638.

Moosavi H, Smith P, Heath D. 1973. The Feyrter cell in hypoxia. *Thorax.* 28:729–741.

Murburg MM, McFall ME, Lewis N, Veith RC. 1995. Plasma norepinephrine kinetics in patients with post-traumatic stress disorder. *Biol Psychiatry.* 38:819–825.

Nakao S, Feng X, Sugimori C. 2005. Immune pathophysiology of aplastic anemia. *Int J Hematol.* 82:196–200. Review.

Narkiewicz K, Somers VK. 2003. Sympathetic nerve activity in obstructive sleep apnoea. *Acta Physiol Scand.* 177:385–390. Review.

Newberry NR, Watkins CJ, Reynolds DJ, Leslie RA, Grahame-Smith DG. 1992. Pharmacology of the 5-hydroxytryptamine-induced depolarization of the ferret vagus nerve in vitro. *Eur J Pharmacol.* 221:157–160.

Nicholson LB, Kuchroo VK. 1996. Manipulation of the Th1/Th2 balance in autoimmune disease. *Curr Opin Immunol.* 8:837–842. Review.

Nitz D, Siegel JM. 1997. GABA release in the locus coeruleus as a function of sleep/wake state. *Neuroscience.* 78:795–801.

North CS, Hong BA, Alpers DH. 2007. Relationship of functional gastrointestinal disorders and psychiatric disorders: implications for treatment. *World J Gastroenterol.* 13:2020–2027.

Novak J, Griseri T, Beaudoin L, Lehuen A. 2007. Regulation of type 1 diabetes by NKT cells. *Int. Rev. Immunol.* 26:49–72. Review.

O'Brien AJ, Lamb EJ, Muller AF. 2005. Renal tubular proteinuria in patients with irritable bowel syndrome. *Eur J Gastroenterol Hepatol.* 17:69–72.

O'Connor JC, Johnson DR, Freund GG. 2006. Psychoneuroimmune implications of type 2 diabetes. *Neurol Clin.* 24:539–559. Review.

Oliveira MC, Pizarro CB, Golbert L, Micheletto C. 2000. Hyperprolactinemia and psychological disturbance. *Arq Neuropsiquiatr.* 58:671–676.

Olpe HR, Steinmann MW, Brugger F, Pozza MF. 1989. Excitatory amino acid receptors in rat locus coeruleus. An extracellular in vitro study. *Naunyn Schmiedeberg's Arch Pharmacol.* 339:312–314.

Oya H, Kawamura T, Shimizu T et al. 2000. The differential effect of stress on natural killer T (NKT) and NK cell function. *Clin Exp Immunol.* 121:384–390.

Pan J, Yeger H, Cutz E. 2004. Innervation of pulmonary neuroendocrine cells and neuroepithelial bodies in developing rabbit lung. *J Histochem Cytochem.* 52:379–389.

Pan J, Copland I, Post M, Yeger H, Cutz E. 2006. Mechanical stretch-induced serotonin release from pulmonary neuroendocrine cells: implications for lung development. *Am J Physiol Lung Cell Mol Physiol.* 290:185–193.

Peluso G, Morrone G. 2007. Antiphospholipid antibodies and recurrent abortions: possible pathogenetic role of annexin A5 investigated by confocal microscopy. *Minerva Ginecol.* 59:223–229.

Perego C, Vetrugno GC, De Simoni MG, Algeri S. 1993. Aging prolongs the stress-induced release of noradrenaline in rat hypothalamus. *Neurosci Lett.* 157:127–130.

Peyron C, Luppi PH, Fort P, Rampon C, Jouvet M. 1996. Lower brainstem catecholamine afferents to the rat dorsal raphe nucleus. *J Comp Neurol.* 364:402–413.

Pieribone VA, Aston-Jones G. 1991. Adrenergic innervation of the rat nucleus locus coeruleus arises predominantly from the C1 adrenergic cell group in the rostral medulla. *Neuroscience.* 41:525–542.

Ping HX, Wu HQ, Liu GQ. 1990. Modulation of neuronal activity of locus coeruleus in rats induced by excitatory amino acids. *Zhongguo Yao Li Xue Bao.* 11:193–195.

Porges SW. 1995. Cardiac vagal tone: a physiological index of stress. *Neurosci Biobehav Rev.* 19:225–233. Review.

Porta S, Emsenhuber W, Felsner P, Schauenstein K, Supanz S. 1989. Norepinephrine triggers medullar epinephrine depletion during normoglycemia. *Life Sci.* 45:1763–1769.

Pozzi L, Invernizzi R, Cervo L, Vallebuona F, Samanin R. 1994. Evidence that extracellular concentrations of dopamine are regulated by noradrenergic neurons in the frontal cortex of rats. *J Neurochem.* 63:195–200.

Pudovkina OL, Cremers TI, Westerink BH. 2002. The interaction between the locus coeruleus and dorsal raphe nucleus studied with dual-probe microdialysis. *Eur J Pharmacol.* 445:37–42.

Rabat A, Bouyer JJ, George O, Le Moal M, Mayo W. 2006. Chronic exposure of rats to noise: relationship between long-term memory deficits and slow wave sleep disturbances. *Behav Brain Res.* 171:303–312.

Radziwillowicz P, Gil K. 2007. Psychiatric aspects of the irritable bowel syndrome. *Psychiatr Pol* 41:87–97.

Raiteri M. 2001. Presynaptic autoreceptors. *J Neurochem.* 78:673–675. Review.

Rausch JL, Janowsky DS, Risch SC, Huey LY. 1985. Physostigmine effects on serotonin uptake in human blood platelets. *Eur J Pharmacol.* 109:91–96.

Reeves G, Todd I. 2000. *Lectures Notes in Immnunology.* London: Blackwell Sciences Ltd, 181–197.

Reynolds DJM, Leslie RA, Grahame-Smith DG, Harvey JM. 1989. Localization of 5-HT$_3$ receptor binding sites in human dorsal vagal complex. *Eur J Pharmacol.* 174:127–130.

Richard CA, Stremel RW. 1990. Involvement of the raphe in the respiratory effects of gigantocellular area activation. *Brain Res Bull.* 25:19–23.

Robertson D, Johnson GA, Robertson RM, Nies AS, Shand DG, Oates JA. 1979. Comparative assessment of stimuli that release neuronal and adrenomedullary catecholamines in man. *Circulation.* 59:637–643.

Rogeness GA, Mitchell EL, Custer GJ, Harris WR. 1985. Comparison of whole blood serotonin and platelet MAO in children with schizophrenia and major depressive disorder. *Biol Psychiatry.* 20:270–275.

Romagnani S. 1996. Th1 and Th2 in human diseases. *Clin Immunol Immunopathol.* 80:225–235. Review.

Rotman A, Zemishlany Z, Munitz H, Wijsenbeek H. 1982. The active uptake of serotonin by platelets of schizophrenic patients and their families: possibility of a genetic marker. *Psychopharmacology (Berl).* 77:171–174.

Roussos C, Koutsoukou A. 2003. Respiratory failure. *Eur Respir J Suppl.* 47:3s–14s. Review.

Roy A, Pickar D, Linnoila M, Potter WZ. 1985. Plasma norepinephrine level in affective disorders. Relationship to melancholia. *Arch Gen Psychiatry.* 42:1181–1185.

Roy A. 1988. Cortisol nonsuppression in depression: relationship to clinical variables. *J Affect Disord.* 14:265–270.

Roy A. 1999. Suicidal behavior in depression: relationship to platelet serotonin transporter. *Neuropsychobiology.* 39:71–75.

Roze C, Chariot J, Appia F, Pascaud X, Vaille C. 1981. Clonidine inhibition of pancreatic secretion in rats: a possible central site of action. *Eur J Pharmacol.* 76:381–390.

Saavedra JM, Grobecker H, Zivin J. 1976. Catecholamines in the raphe nuclei of the rat. *Brain Res.* 114:337–345.

Sagvolden T. 2006. The alpha-2A adrenoceptor agonist guanfacine improves sustained attention and reduces overactivity and impulsiveness in an animal model of Attention-Deficit/Hyperactivity Disorder (ADHD). *Behav Brain Funct.* 2:41–48.

Salonen RO, Webber SE, Widdicombe JG. 1990. Effects of neurotransmitters on tracheobronchial blood flow. *Eur Respir J Suppl.* 12:630–636.

Sandborn WJ, Loftus EV Jr, Colombel JF et al. 2001. Evaluation of serologic disease markers in a population-based cohort of patients with ulcerative colitis and Crohn's disease. *Inflamm Bowel Dis.* 7:192–201.

Sastry KS, Karpova Y, Prokopovich S et al. 2007. Epinephrine protects cancer cells from apoptosis via activation of camp-dependent protein kinase and bad phosphorylation. *J Biol Chem.* 282:14094–14100.

Sato A, Trzebski A. 1993. The excitatory response of the adrenal sympathetic nerve to severe hypoxia decreases in aged rats. *Neurosci Lett.* 161:97–100.

Seals DR, Esler MD. 2000. Human ageing and the sympathoadrenal system. *J Physiol.* 528:407–417. Review.

Schwarz MJ, Chiang S, Muller N, Ackenheil M. 2001. T-helper-1 and T-helper-2 responses in psychiatric disorders. *Brain Behav Immun.* 15:340–370. Review.

Shakhar K, Rosenne E, Loewenthal R, Shakhar G, Carp H, Ben-Eliyahu S. 2006. High NK cell activity in recurrent miscarriage: what are we really measuring? *Hum Reprod.* 21:2421–2425.

Shanks N, Zalcman S, Zacharko RM, Anisman H. 1991. Alterations of central norepinephrine, dopamine and serotonin in several strains of mice following acute stressor exposure. *Pharmacol Biochem Behav.* 38:69–75.

Skaburskis M, Shardonofsky F, Milic-Emili J. 1990. Effect of serotonin on expiratory pulmonary resistance in cats. *J Appl Physiol.* 68:2419–2425.

Speciale SG, Crowley WR, O'Donohue TL, Jacobowitz DM. 1978. Forebrain catecholamine projections of the A5 cell group. *Brain Res.* 154:128–133.

Sternberg EM, Glowa JR, Smith MA et al. 1992. Corticotropin releasing hormone related behavioral and neuroendocrine responses to stress in Lewis and Fischer rats. *Brain Res.* 570:54–60.

Strum JM, Junod AF. 1972. Radioautographic demonstration of 5-hydroxytryptamine-3H uptake by pulmonary endothelial cells. *J Cell Biol.* 54:456–467.

Swedberg K, Brislow M, Cohn JN et al. 2002. The effects of moxonidine SR, and imidazoline agonists, on plasma norepinephrine in patients with chronic heart failure. *Circulation.* 105:1797–1803.

Szabo ST, Blier P. 2001. Functional and pharmacological characterization of the modulatory role of serotonin on the firing activity of locus coeruleus norepinephrine neurons. *Brain Res.* 922:9–20.

Tanaka M, Kohno Y, Nakagawa R, Nishikawa T, Tsuda A, Nagasaki N. 1983. Immobilization stress increases serotonin turnover in the extended brain regions in the rat. *Kurume Med J.* 30:35–43.

Tanaka M, Okamura H, Tamada Y, Nagatsu I, Tanaka Y, Ibata Y. 1994. Catecholaminergic input to spinally projecting serotonin neurons in the rostral ventromedial medulla oblongata of the rat. *Brain Res Bull.* 35:23–30.

Tandon R, Shipley JE, Taylor S et al. 1992. Electroencephalographic sleep abnormalities in schizophrenia. Relationship to positive/negative symptoms and prior neuroleptic treatment. *Arch Gen Psychiatry.* 49:185–194.

Tao R, Auerbach SB. 2003. Influence of inhibitory and excitatory inputs on serotonin efflux differs in the dorsal and median raphe nuclei. *Brain Res.* 961:109–120.

Tassin JP. 1992. NE/DA interactions in prefrontal cortex and their possible roles as neuromodulators in schizophrenia. *J Neural Transm Suppl.* 36:135–162. Review.

Thurston-Stanfield CL, Ranieri JT, Vallabhapurapu R, Barnes-Noble D. 1999. Role of vagal afferents and the rostral ventral medulla in intravenous serotonin-induced changes in nociception and arterial blood pressure. *Physiol Behav.* 67:753–767.

Tobe T. 1974. Enterochromaffin cells and carcinoid syndrome. *Nippon Rinsho.* 32:745–750.

Tobe T, Izumikawa F, Sano M, Tanaka C. 1976. Release mechanisms of 5-HT in mammalian gastrointestinal tract–especially vagal release of 5-HT. In Fujita T, ed. *Endocrine Gut-pancreas.* Amsterdam: Elsevier. 371–390.

Tonnesen P. 1985. Effect of topically applied atropine, methysergide and chlorpheniramine on nasal challenge with serotonin. *Allergy.* 40:616–619.

Trulson ME, Jacobs BL. 1979. Raphe unit activity in freely moving cats: correlation with level of behavioral arousal. *Brain Res.* 163:135–150.

Trulson ME, Trulson VM. 1982. Activity of nucleus raphe pallidus neurons across the sleep-waking cycle in freely moving cats. *Brain Res.* 237:232–237.

van der Dijs B, Lechin S, Vitelli G et al. 1988a. Plasma neurotransmitters, lymphocyte subpopulations and natural killer cell activity in progressive cancer patients. III Interamerican congress of clinical pharmacology and therapeutics and the XII latinoamerican congress of pharmacology. *Arch Ven Farm Clin Terap.* 7(Suppl 1) Abst. 35.

van der Dijs B, Lechin S, Vitelli G et al. 1988b. Plasma neurotransmitters, lymphocyte subpopulations and natural killer cell activity in short term symptomless cancer patients. III Interamerican congress of clinical pharmacology and therapeutics and the XII latinoamerican congress of pharmacology. *Arch Ven Farm Clin Terap.* 7(Suppl 1) Abst. 34.

van Diest R, Appels WP. 1994. Sleep physiological characteristics of exhausted men. *Psychosom Med.* 56:28–35.

Vassilopoulos D, Mantzoukis D. 2006. Dialogue between the brain and the immune system in inflammatory arthritis. *Ann N Y Acad. Sci.* 1088:132–138. Review.

Vazquez DM, Bailey C, Dent GW et al. 2006. Brain corticotropin-releasing hormone (CRH) circuits in the developing rat: effect of maternal deprivation. *Brain Res.* 1121:83–94.

Verdecchia P, Schillaci G, Gatteschi C et al. 1993. Blunted nocturnal fall in blood pressure in hypertensive women with future cardiovascular morbid events. *Circulation.* 88:986–992.

Vertes RP, Kocsis B. 1994. Projections of the dorsal raphe nucleus to the brainstem: PHA-L analysis in the rat. *J Comp Neurol.* 340:11–26.

Vertes RP, Fortin WJ, Crane AM. 1999. Projections of the median raphe nucleus in the rat. *J Comp Neurol.* 407:555–582.

Vezina P, Blanc G, Glowinski J, Tassin JP. 1991. Opposed behavioural outputs of increased dopamine transmission in prefrontocortical and subcortical areas: a role for the cortical d-1 dopamine receptor. *Eur J Neurosci.* 3:1001–1007.

Vitelli G, Lechin S, Cabrera A et al. 1988. Plasma neurotransmitters, lymphocyte subpopulations and natural killer cell activity in long-term symptomless cancer patients. III Interamerican congress of clinical pharmacology and therapeutics and the XII latinoamerican congress of pharmacology. *Arch Ven Farm Clin Terap.* 7(Suppl 1) Abst. 36.

Wallin MT, Wilken JA, Turner AP, Williams RM, Kane R. 2006. Depression and multiple sclerosis: review of a lethal combination. *J Rehabil Res Dev.* 43:45–62.

Webber SE, Salonen RO, Widdicombe JG. 1990. Receptors mediating the effects of 5-hydroxytryptamine on the tracheal vasculature and smooth muscle of sheep. *Br J Pharmacol.* 99:21–26.

Witek-Janusek L, Gabram S, Mathews HL. 2007. Psychologic stress, reduced NK cell activity, and cytokine dysregulation in women experiencing diagnostic breast biopsy. *Psychoneuroendocrinology.* 32:22–35.

Woch G, Davies RO, Pack AI, Kubin L. 1996. Behaviour of raphe cells projecting to the dorsomedial medulla during carbachol-induced atonia in the cat. *J Physiol.* 490:745–758.

Wrona D. 2006. Neural-immune interactions: an integrative view of the bidirectional relationship between the brain and immune systems. *J Neuroimmunol.* 172:38–58.

Yamamoto K, Hornykiewicz O. 2004. Proposal for a noradrenaline hypothesis of schizophrenia. *Prog Neuropsychopharmacol Biol Psychiatry.* 28:913–922. Review.

Yan QS, Zheng SZ, Feng MJ, Yan SE. 2005. Involvement of 5-HT1B receptors within the ventral tegmental area in ethanol-induced increases in mesolimbic dopaminergic transmission. *Brain Res.* 1060:126–137.

Yehuda R, Teicher MH, Trestman RL, Levengood RA, Siever LJ. 1996. Cortisol regulation in post-traumatic stress disorder and major depression: a chronobiological analysis. *Biol Psychiatry.* 40:79–88.

Young JB, Rosa RM, Landsberg L. 1984. Dissociation of sympathetic nervous system and adrenal medullary responses. *Am J Physiol.* 247:E35–E40.

Young NS. 2006. Pathophysiologic mechanisms in acquired aplastic anemia. *Hematology Am Soc Hematol Educ Program.* 72–77. Review.

Young JL, Redmond JC. 2007. Fibromylagia, chronic fatigue, and adult attention deficit hyperactivity disorder in the adult: a case study. *Psychopharmacol Bull.* 40:118

Youngren KD, Moghaddam B, Bunney BS, Roth RH. 1994. Preferential activation of dopamine overflow in prefrontal cortex produced by chronic clozapine treatment. *Neurosci Lett.* 165:41–44.

Zhang L. 1991. Effects of 5-hydroxytryptamine on cat spinal motoneurons. *Can J Physiol Pharmacol.* 69:154–163.

Chapter 6

NEUROBIOLOGY OF CHRONIC PAIN

Min Zhuo

ABSTRACT

Understanding the neurobiology of sensory synapses in the central nervous system provides us with basic knowledge of physiological and pathological pain, and has the potential to reveal possible drug targets for treating chronic pain. Pain-related synapses are found not only in the spinal cord dorsal horn, but also in many cortical areas. More importantly, recent evidence suggests that injury that causes chronic pain also triggers long-term plastic changes in sensory synapses, including those in the spinal dorsal horn and frontal cortex. Plastic changes are not just limited in excitatory glutamatergic synapses but are also found in inhibitory synapses. Here I review recent progress in these areas, in particular, integrative physiological investigations of chronic pain.

Keywords: chronic pain, synaptic plasticity, cortex, gene knockout mice, spinal cord, descending modulation.

Pain is the unpleasant experience or sensation induced by noxious stimuli. Nociceptive information enters the brain through spinal–brain projecting systems, and projects to widely different brain areas. Most of all, painful inputs enter the forebrain areas including the anterior cingulate cortex (ACC) and insular cortex (IC) and trigger unpleasant sensations or experiences. Painful inputs projected into the somatosensory cortex help determine the location and quality of painful stimuli.

Hippocampus, a structure known to be important for spatial memory, is also activated by painful stimuli, and may contribute to the formation of pain-related spatial memory. Neuronal inputs into the amygdala and its related structures play important roles in forming fear memory and pain–emotional responses. Furthermore, nociceptive inputs also activate endogenous analgesia systems including neurons in the periaqueductal gray (PAG) and brainstem rostral ventromedial medulla (RVM). Activation of endogenous analgesia systems excites descending inhibitory systems and modulates sensory transmission at the level of spinal cord and possible supraspinal structures. Through activation of descending inhibitory systems, painful information entering the central nervous system is significantly reduced. Thus, acute pain or physiological pain is bearable and does not get transferred into chronic pain or pathological pain.

Previous studies of plastic changes related to pathological pain are mainly focused on the dorsal root ganglion (DRG) and spinal cord dorsal horn. However, recent studies demonstrate that central plasticity happens within the ACC after injury. There are three major reasons why the study of central cortical plasticity is important for pathological pain. First, pain or pain-related unpleasantness is encoded in the forebrain areas such as the ACC; second, higher brain structures play important roles in many mental dysfunctions related to chronic pain and long-term use of pain medicines. Finally, central activity itself may produce pain sensation and play important roles in spontaneous pain or central pain.

Here, I will divide pain into two groups: physiological pain and pathological pain. Physiological pain is a very important physiological function for the survival. Depending on pain experience, animals and humans gain knowledge of potential dangerous stimuli in the environment, and pain-related unpleasantness helps form long-term avoidance memory to protect themselves. Although animals have the capability to enhance its sensitivity as well as its motor responses to subsequent noxious stimuli, the ability of animals to distinguish pain from other sensations is intact, at least not permanently altered. Pathological pain only happens after injury (e.g., tissue or nerve injury), and is not the result of the repetitive application of physiological pain. Long-term changes are likely to occur after injury, both peripherally and centrally. Consequently, the injury and injury-related areas undergo long-term plastic changes, and pain sensation is significantly enhanced (hyperalgesia) or non-noxious stimuli cause pain (allodynia). It should be pointed out that allodynia is one of the major problems in pathological pain. Because they are induced by non-noxious stimuli, it is mostly likely that central plastic changes play important roles.

A NEW APPROACH: PLASTIC MOLECULAR TARGETS FOR CHRONIC PAIN

As discussed so far, pathological pain is likely a result of long-term plastic changes along somatosensory pathways, from the periphery to cortex. Owing to long-term plastic changes in central regions, pain specificity is lost in the somatosensory pathway, at least from areas where allodynia is reported. Thus, drugs developed on the basis of physiological pain mechanism may not be used for treating pathological pain. Understanding pathological pain requires understanding of plastic changes in somatosensory pathways, mainly, the central nervous system. In this chapter, I will review the current understanding of the basic synaptic mechanism for pain transmission, regulation, and plasticity. I will then focus on recent new findings in the ACC, and propose a model for neuronal network mechanisms for pathological pain.

PERIPHERAL NERVES AND DRG CELLS

Peripheral noxious stimuli activate peripheral nociceptive transducer receptor and/or ion channels, and cause membrane depolarization in sensory DRG cells. Transducer proteins include a family of proteins, including TRPV1–4, TRPM8, adenosine triphosphate (ATP) receptor, and others. (McKemy 2005; Lumpkin, Caterina 2007). It becomes clear that no simple protein or gene is responsible for a specific sensory process such as heat pain or cold sensation (see Table 6.1). Recent studies using gene knockout mice lacking TRPV1 or TRPM8 have nicely demonstrated that neither heat pain nor cold pain is mediated by a single protein/ion channel. In mice lacking TRPV1, behavioral deficits in response to noxious heat applied to the tail or hind paw are only partial (Caterina, Julius 2001). Recently, in mice lacking TRPM8, behavioral responses to noxious cold are partially affected or not affected (Colburn, Lubin, Stone et al. 2007; Dhaka, Murray, Mathur et al. 2007). Thus, a peripheral sensory protein may contribute multiple sensory processes, such as heat, cold, itch, and touch.

Under physiological conditions, noxious stimuli stimulate both non-noxious and nociceptive fibers. It is almost impossible to deliver a selective noxious stimulus without activating some forms of non-nociceptive receptors. In pathological pain condition, typical allodynia triggered by non-noxious stimulation is also unlikely because of selective activation of nociceptive fibers (see Fig. 6.1). It is safe to say that each sensory modality or sensation is a function of a specially organized neuronal circuit and network, from the periphery to the cortex, with some of the key proteins playing major roles.

Synaptic Transmission at the Spinal Cord Dorsal Horn

Kainate (KA) Receptor–Mediated Responses

Neurons in the spinal cord dorsal horn and related areas receive sensory inputs, including noxious information, and convey them to supraspinal structures. Studies using pharmacological and behavioral approaches show that glutamate and neuropeptides

Table 6.1 Peripheral Sensory Transduction Channels for Sensory Transmission

Sensory Modality	Ion Channel	Primary Afferent Fibers	Physiology
Thermal warm/heat	TRPV1; TRPV2; TRPV3; TREK-1	A_δ- and C-fibers	Warm sensation—heat pain
Mechanical	TRPA1; TRPV2; ASIC1-3; TREK-1	A_β- and A_δ-fibers	Touch; pressure—mechanical pain
Cold	TRPM8	C-fiber	Cold sensation—cold pain

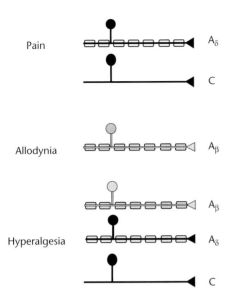

Figure 6.1 Primary afferent fibers that are likely involved in physiological pain and pathological pain. A model explaining the contribution of different groups of peripheral afferent fibers to normal pain and pathological pain. For normal or physiological pain, peripheral small myelinated A_δ-fibers and unmyelinated C-fibers contribute to the pain transmission. In pathological pain, non-noxious stimulation such as gentle touch triggers pain, and it is likely that A_β-fibers are mainly involved. For hyperalgesia, it is likely that most of the fibers are activated and contribute to the transmission.

including substance P (SP) are excitatory transmitters for pain. Electrophysiological investigation of sensory synaptic responses between primary afferent fibers and dorsal horn neurons provide evidence that glutamate is the principle fast excitatory transmitter, and synaptic responses are mediated by postsynaptic glutamate receptors. While α-amino-3-hydroxy-5-methyl-4-isoxazole propionate (AMPA) receptors mediate the largest component of postsynaptic currents, KA receptors preferentially contribute to synaptic responses induced by higher (noxious) stimulation intensities (Li, Calejesan, Zhuo 1998; Li, Wilding, Kim et al. 1999a) (Fig. 6.2). Consistent with this, antagonism of both KA and AMPA receptor yields greater analgesic effects in adult animals than AMPA receptor antagonism alone (Li, Wilding, Kim et al. 1999a). These findings suggest that sensory modality may be coded in part by different postsynaptic neurotransmitter receptors.

Pure NMDA Receptor–Mediated Responses

Silent glutamatergic synapses have been documented in spinal cord dorsal horn (Bardoni, Magherini, MacDermott 1998; Li, Zhuo 1998; Zhuo 2000). In silent synapses, no effective AMPA/KA receptors are available to detect the release of glutamate from presynaptic terminals. Consequently, these synapses do not

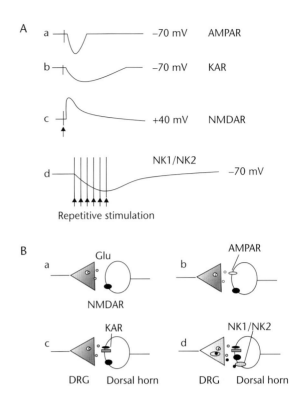

Figure 6.2 Spinal sensory synaptic transmission. (A) Synaptic currents recorded at resting membrane potentials are mostly mediated by AMPA receptors (AMPAR) (a); some synaptic currents at dorsal horn neurons receiving high-threshold inputs are mediated by KA receptors (KAR) (b). In young and adult dorsal horn neurons, some sensory synapses are "silent" and containing only functional NMDA receptors (NMDAR) (c). These pure NMDA synapses can be revealed when cells are held at +40 mV potentials. In adult dorsal horn neurons, some pure NMDA receptor synapses can be even detected at the resting membrane potentials. When a train of stimulation is applied, neuropeptide-mediated responses are recruited. Both postsynaptic NK1 and NK2 receptors contribute to substance P (SP)- and neurokinin A (NKA)–mediated excitatory postsynaptic currents (d). (B) Models for glutamate-containing and glutamate- and neuropeptide-mixed sensory synapses in the spinal cord dorsal horn. At least four different synapses are found: (a) synapses receiving low-threshold sensory inputs contain only postsynaptic NMDA receptors; (b) synapses receiving low-threshold sensory inputs contain both AMPA and NMDA receptors; (c) synapses receiving both low- and high-threshold sensory inputs contain postsynaptic AMPA, KAR, and NMDA receptors; (d) synapses receiving low- and high-threshold sensory inputs contain AMPA, KA, and NMDA receptors as well as peptidergic NK1 and NK2 receptors.

conduct any synaptic transmission at the resting membrane potential. It is important to point out that silent synapses should not be confused with potential "silent synaptic transmission." The definition of "silent synapses" is related to the condition when the postsynaptic cell is clamped at –70 mV. As *defined* by silent synapses, there are abundant *N*-methyl-D-aspartate (NMDA) receptors located in these "silent" synapses. In an unclamped cell, these NMDA receptors may conduct sensory synaptic transmission, for example, in the case of high-intensity sensory fiber activity induced by tissue injury. These results consistently suggest that different types of glutamatergic synapses exist in spinal sensory connections between primary afferent fibers and dorsal horn neurons. These silent synapses provide a key synaptic mechanism for explaining the recruitment of ineffective synapses as measured by neuronal spikes after injury.

To study synaptic regulation by serotonin (5-HT), we performed intracellular recordings in adult mouse spinal cord slices. We found that in sensory synapses of adult mouse, some synaptic responses (26.3% of a total of 38 experiments) between primary afferent fibers and dorsal horn neurons were almost completely mediated by NMDA receptors (Wang, Zhuo 2002). Dorsal root stimulation did not elicit any detectable AMPA/KA receptor–mediated responses in these synapses. These findings indicate that in adult spinal dorsal horn neurons, some of sensory synaptic transmission is mediated by pure NMDA receptors.

Neuropeptide-Mediated Response

Several neuropeptides including SP are thought to act as sensory transmitters. For many years, there has been a lack of electrophysiological evidence that SP can mediate monosynaptic responses since SP-mediated responses had a very slow onset. Recent studies using whole-cell patch-clamp recordings reveal relatively faster SP and neurokinin A–mediated synaptic currents in synapses between primary afferent fibers, and excitatory postsynaptic currents (EPSCs) in the case of burst activity allow SP-mediated responses to affect the excitability of spinal dorsal horn neurons (Li, Zhuo 2001) (Fig. 6.2). Together with glutamate-mediated synaptic responses, these neuropeptide-mediated EPSCs may cause dorsal horn neurons to fire action potentials at a high frequency for a long period. The combination of glutamate- and neuropeptide-mediated EPSCs allow nociceptive information to be conveyed from the periphery to the central nervous system.

Gastrin-Releasing Peptide (GRP) and Itching

Recently, it has been reported that GRP may act as a transmitter for behavioral itch (Sun, Chen 2007). The evidence for GRP being an "itching" transmitter is mainly from anatomic studies; GRP is expressed in some DRG cells, and GRP receptor (GRPR) is mainly expressed in spinal lamina I cells (presumably ascending projection cells). However, previous electrophysiological studies failed to observe any residual currents that may be mediated non-SP/neurokinin A (NKA)–mediated currents (Li, Zhuo 2001).

For any spinal transmitter to be qualified as one, the critical criterion is to demonstrate the involvement of this transmitter in spinal synaptic transmission. If this proves to be true, spinal synaptic transmission may be a novel pathway for G protein–related signaling transduction in these itch-related specific pathways. Alternatively, GRP may serve as a neuromodulator that affects spinal itch transmission. Recent studies have shown that GRP is highly expressed in the lateral nucleus of the amygdala (Shumyatsky, Tsvetkov, Malleret et al. 2002). Furthermore, GRP receptor (GRPR) is expressed in γ-amino butyric acid (GABA) ergic interneurons of the lateral nucleus. Mice lacking GRPR show enhanced LTP, and greater fear/anxiety responses (Shumyatsky, Tsvetkov, Malleret et al. 2002). It remains to be determined whether GRP receptor may also be expressed in inhibitory neurons in the spinal cord, and thus contribute to disinhibition of spinal sensory transmission or itch.

Regulation of Spinal Sensory Transmission

Although the dorsal horn of the spinal cord is often regarded as a simple relay for sensory transmission, recent studies reveal that synaptic transmission in the dorsal horn of the spinal cord undergoes complicated, biphasic and activity-dependent regulation. By doing so, sensory inputs from the periphery are appropriately coded and conveyed into the brain.

Postsynaptic Regulation: DRG-Dorsal Horn Synapses

Neurotransmitters or neuromodulators bind to their receptors postsynaptically at spinal dorsal horn neurons. Activation of these postsynaptic receptors leads to changes in AMPA/KA receptor–mediated synaptic responses. These neurotransmitters/neuromodulators include acetylcholine, serotonin, opioids, norepinephrine, oxytocin (Yoshimura, North 1983; Li, Zhuo 2001; Robinson, Calejesan, Zhuo et al. 2002). Recent studies using mice lacking subtype of neuromedin U receptors revealed that spinal excitatory transmission may be under the modulation by neuromedin U (Zeng, Gragerov, Hohmann et al. 2006). It is likely that spinal dorsal horn neurons are regulated by multiple members of G protein-coupled receptor family (Fig. 6.3).

Presynaptic Regulation: DRG-Dorsal Horn Synapses

Sensory transmitters or neuromodulators bind to their target receptors on the central terminals of DRG cells in the spinal cord dorsal horn. Activation of these presynaptic receptors will lead to changes

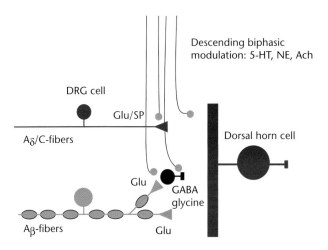

Figure 6.3 Pain control in the spinal cord integrating local modulation and descending modulation. Spinal dorsal horn neurons receive sensory inputs from nociceptive A_δ-/C-fibers and non-nociceptive A_β-fibers. Glutamate (Glu) is the principal fast excitatory transmitter at synapses between afferent fibers and dorsal horn neurons, regardless of the type of afferent fibers. In addition to glutamate, SP and neurokinin A are also released from nociceptive afferent fibers. Large diameter, non-nociceptive A_β fibers can also activate spinal inhibitory neurons. These inhibitory neurons then form inhibitory synapses with dorsal horn neurons as well. Activation of non-nociceptive afferent fibers may thus inhibit spinal nociceptive transmission by activating local spinal inhibitory influences. Glutamate release from primary afferent fibers can also act on presynaptic kainate receptors on inhibitory terminals and modulate spinal inhibitory transmission. Both projection and local neurons receive descending modulation from the supraspinal structures. Many neurotransmitters contribute to biphasic modulation at the spinal cord, including facilitatory and inhibitory modulation.

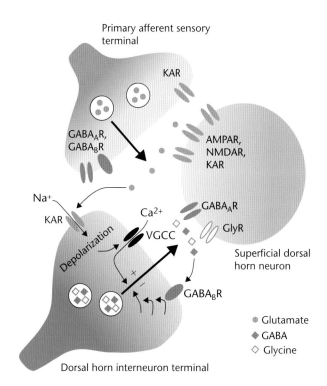

Figure 6.4 KA-mediated presynaptic regulation of spinal inhibitory transmission. Presynaptic KAR regulate spinal inhibitory transmission. A model of a synaptic glomerulus depicts the proposed function of presynaptic KA receptors at dorsal horn inhibitory synapses. These receptors, which can be activated by glutamate released from primary afferent sensory fibers, mediate Na^+ entry and terminal depolarization, triggering the opening of voltage-gated Ca^{2+} channels (VGCC) and Ca^{2+}-dependent vesicle fusion. GABA released in this manner may activate presynaptic $GABA_B$ autoreceptors, reducing action potential–dependent transmitter release. Previous work has shown that sensory neuron terminals contain $GABA_A$ and $GABA_B$ receptors (Malcangio, Bowery 1996), indicating that sensory neurons and dorsal horn interneurons engage in reciprocal heterosynaptic regulation of transmitter release. Other studies have documented additional roles for KA receptors in spinal sensory transmission: Along with AMPAR and NMDA receptors (NMDAR), KA receptors mediate a component of the postsynaptic response of dorsal horn neurons to high-threshold sensory fiber stimulation (Li et al. 1999a). In addition, sensory fibers themselves express presynaptic KA receptors that regulate glutamate release (Kerchner, Wei, Wang et al. 2001).

in the release of sensory transmitters in response to peripheral sensory stimulation. Many neurotransmitters and peptides, such as ATP, serotonin and opioids, have been reported to produce presynaptic regulatory effects in the DRG-dorsal horn synapses (Li, Calejesan, Zhuo 1998; Kohno, Kumamoto, Higashi et al. 1999; Nakatsuka, Gu 2001; Nakatsuka, Furue, Yoshimura et al. 2002) (Fig. 6.3).

Heterosynaptic Regulation: DRG-Spinal Inhibitory Neurons

In the spinal cord dorsal horn, glutamate-containing sensory fiber terminals come into close proximity with the GABA- and glycine-containing boutons of local interneurons at synaptic glomeruli (Ribeiro-da-Silva, Coimbra 1982; Todd 1996). In a recent study, we provide evidence that glutamate released from primary afferent sensory fibers can regulate spinal inhibitory transmission by activating KA receptors. These data suggest that heterosynaptic regulation of transmitter release by presynaptic ligand-gated ionic channels may be reciprocal between sensory fibers and dorsal

horn interneurons. The suppression of evoked inhibitory transmission by synaptically released glutamate suggests that with sufficiently high levels of sensory input, inhibitory tone may be reduced, possibly facilitating the relay of sensory information to higher brain centers (Kerchner, Wang, Qiu et al. 2001a; Kerchner, Wilding, Li et al. 2001b) (Fig. 6.4). Most of these observations are collected from cultured spinal neurons. Recently, Xu et al. (2006) confirmed in mouse spinal cord slice studies that presynaptic GluR5-containing kainate receptors regulates the release of the inhibitory transmission in spinal substantia gelatinosa.

Autoregulation

Neurotransmitters can act on their target receptors, also expressed in the presynaptic terminals. These can be either excitatory glutamate or inhibitory GABA synapses. In case of glutamatergic synapses, glutamate may act on presynaptic KA receptor expressed on the central terminals of primary afferent fibers, and may regulate releases of glutamate (Kerchner, Wilding, Li et al. 2001b; Kerchner, Wilding, Huettner et al. 2002). Similar autoregulation of GABA releases are also reported in the spinal cord (Kerchner et al. 2001a; Kerchner, Wilding, Huettner et al. 2002).

Retrograde Messengers

In central synapses, activation of postsynaptic receptors often leads to production of diffusible messengers, such as nitric oxide and carbon monoxide (Zhuo, Small, Kandel et al. 1993; Zhuo, Hu, Schultz et al. 1994). In the spinal cord dorsal horn, enzymes that produce retrograde messengers are found in dorsal horn neurons. It is very likely that diffusible retrograde messengers affect presynaptic release of glutamate and/or neuropeptides.

Long-Term Plasticity of Spinal Sensory Synapses

Long-Term Potentiation

Studies of LTP in spinal dorsal horn neurons draw much attention because it is believed that potentiation of sensory responses after injury may explain chronic pain (Woolf, Salter 2000; Willis 2002; Ji, Kohno, Moore et al. 2003). While it has been consistently demonstrated that spike responses of dorsal horn neurons to peripheral stimulation are enhanced after the injury (see Willis 2002), it remains to be investigated if enhanced spike responses are simply due to enhanced synaptic transmission between the DRG cells and dorsal horn neurons. Unlike synapses in other areas such as hippocampus, synaptic potentiation in the spinal dorsal horn neurons is not induced by strong tetanic stimulation (Zhuo 2003). Recent studies further show that LTP only happens in some of the spinal projecting cells (Ikeda, Heinke, Ruscheweyh et al. 2003). In the spinal cord, dorsal horn neurons that did not express SP receptors did not undergo potentiation. Furthermore, activation of NK1 receptors or NMDA receptors is required for LTP (Ikeda, Heinke, Ruscheweyh et al. 2003). Using the classic pairing protocol, Wei et al. (2006) reported that LTP can be induced in dorsal horn neurons in adult mouse dorsal horn neurons. One key experiment in future studies is needed to directly demonstrate that neurons receiving nociceptive inputs undergo LTP in the spinal cord.

Silent Synapse and Long-Term Facilitation

Spinal dorsal neurons receive innervations from descending serotonin systems from the brainstem. Application of 5-HT or 5-HT receptor agonist induced long-term facilitation of synaptic response (Hori, Endo, Takahashi 1996; Li, Kerchner, Sala et al. 1999b). One mechanism for the facilitation is the recruitment of silent synapses through interaction of glutamate AMPA receptors with proteins containing postsynaptic density-95/Discs large/zona occludens-1 (PDZ) domains. GluR2 and -3 are widely expressed in sensory neurons in the superficial dorsal horn of the spinal cord (Tachibana, Wenthold, Morioka et al. 1994; Popratiloff, Weinberg, Rustioni 1996; Li, Kerchner, Sala et al. 1999b). Glutamate receptor–interacting protein (GRIP), a protein with 7 PDZ domains that binds specifically to the C-terminus of GluR2/3, is expressed in spinal dorsal horn neurons (Dong, O'Brien, Fung et al. 1997; Li, Kerchner, Sala et al. 1999b). In many dorsal horn neurons, GluR2/3 and GRIP coexist (Li, Kerchner, Sala et al. 1999b). Long-term overexpression of the C-terminus of GluR2 in hippocampal neurons reduced the number of synaptic AMPA receptor clusters (Dong, O'Brien, Fung et al. 1997), suggesting that an interaction between GluR2/3 and PDZ proteins is involved in the postsynaptic targeting of AMPA receptors. To examine the functional significance of GluR2/3-PDZ interactions in sensory synaptic transmission, we made a synthetic peptide corresponding to the last 10 amino acids of GluR2 ("GluR2-SVKI": NVYGIESVKI) that disrupts binding of GluR2 to GRIP (Li, Kerchner, Sala et al. 1999b). As expected, GluR2-SVKI peptide blocked the facilitatory effect of 5-HT. The effect of GluR2-SVKI on synaptic facilitation is rather selective because baseline EPSCs and currents evoked by glutamate application did not change over time in these neurons (Li, Kerchner, Sala et al. 1999b). Experiments with different control peptides consistently indicate that the interaction between the C-terminus of GluR2/3 and GRIP/ABP (or called GRIP1 and GRIP2) (Dong, Zhang, Song et al. 1999) is important for 5-HT-induced facilitation. Furthermore, synaptic facilitation induced by PDBu is also blocked by GluR2-SVKI, suggesting that synaptic facilitation mediated by protein kinase C (PKC) activation is similar to that produced by 5-HT in its dependence on GluR2/3 C-terminal interactions (Li, Kerchner, Sala et al. 1999b). Figure 6.5 is a model explaining 5-HT mediated recruitment of AMPA receptors in spinal dorsal horn neurons.

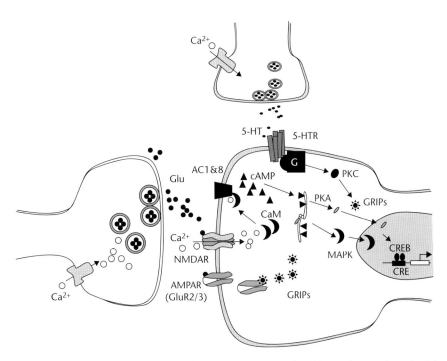

Figure 6.5 Silent glutamatergic synapses and long-term facilitation. Neurons in the RVM project to the spinal dorsal horn and modulate sensory synaptic transmission in the spinal cord. Serotonin is the most likely transmitter for mediating this facilitatory effect. The facilitation induced by serotonin likely requires activation of specific subtypes of serotonin receptors and coactivation of cAMP signaling pathways to induce facilitation in adult spinal dorsal horn neurons. 5-HT activates postsynaptic PKC through G-protein receptors. PKC activation and subsequent AMPA receptor (AMPAR) and GRIP interactions cause the recruitment of AMPA receptors to the synapse. Due to enhanced synaptic efficacy between primary afferent fibers and dorsal horn neurons, spike (action potential) responses to stimulation of afferent fibers were enhanced, as were behavioral nociceptive responses (e.g., decrease in response latencies).

Pure NMDA Receptor–Mediated Sensory Responses in Adult Spinal Cord Dorsal Horn

Cyclic adenosine monophosphate (cAMP) signal pathways have been implicated in the function of spinal dorsal horn neurons. Activation of several receptors for sensory transmitters such as glutamate and calcitonin gene–related peptide (CGRP) has been reported to raise cAMP levels. In a recent study, application of forskolin did not significantly affect synaptic responses induced by dorsal root stimulation in slices of adult mice. However, co-application of 5-HT and forskolin produced long-lasting facilitation of synaptic responses. Possible contributors to the increase in the cAMP levels are calcium-sensitive adenylyl cyclases (AC). We found that the facilitatory effect induced by 5-HT and forskolin was completely blocked in mice lacking AC1 or AC8, indicating that calcium-sensitive ACs are important. Our results demonstrate that in adult sensory synapses, cAMP signaling pathways determine whether activation of 5-HT receptors causes facilitatory or inhibitory effects on synaptic responses (Wang, Zhuo 2002). This finding provides a possible explanation for regulation of two different signaling pathways under physiological or pathological conditions. Postsynaptic increases in cAMP levels by sensory transmitters may favor 5-HT-induced facilitation. The interaction between cAMP and 5-HT may provide an associative heterosynaptic form of central plasticity in the spinal dorsal horn to allow sensory inputs from the periphery to act synergistically with central modulatory influences descending from the brainstem RVM.

CORTICAL REGIONS IN PAIN PERCEPTION: SUMMARY OF RECENT HUMAN IMAGING STUDIES

Human brain imaging techniques have provided powerful tools for mapping cortical brain activities before and during noxious stimuli or pain. Unlike animals, human subjects report the pain sensation as well as the unpleasantness related to painful stimuli in these experiments. Despite the differences in experimental subjects, and other conditions, it has been consistently reported that several cortical areas are activated during different kinds of pain stimuli, including heat pain, cold pain, and mechanical pain. There are five major areas found to be activated: ACC, insular cortex (IC), prefrontal cortex (PFC), primary somatsensory cortex (S1), and secondary somatosensory cortex (S2) (see Table 6.2).

Table 6.2 Five Major Cortical Areas that Are Activated during Pain

Cortical Region	Pain Stimulus
ACC: anterior cingulate cortex	Heat; cold; mechanical; capsaicin; acid; rectal distension; electric shock; warm–cold grill
IC: insular cortex	Heat; cold; mechanical; capsaicin; electric shock; rectal distension; warm–cold grill
PFC: prefrontal cortex	Heat; cold; mechanical; capsaicin; rectal distension; rectal distension
S1: primary somatosensory cortex	Heat; cold; mechanical; capsaicin; electric shock; rectal distension; warm–cold grill
S2: secondary somatosensory cortex	Heat; cold; mechanical; capsaicin; electric shock; rectal distension; warm–cold grill

ACC

Animal and human studies consistently suggest that forebrain neurons play important roles in nociception and pain perception. In animal studies, lesions of the medial frontal cortex including the ACC significantly increased acute nociceptive responses, and formalin injection induced aversive memory behaviors (Lee, Kim, Zhuo 1999; Johansen, Fields, Manning 2002). In patients with frontal lobotomies or cingulotomies, the unpleasantness of pain is abolished (see Zhuo 2002 for review). Electrophysiological recordings from the ACC neurons found that neurons within the ACC respond to noxious stimuli, including nociception-specific neurons (Sikes, Vogt 1992; Hutchison, Davis, Lozano et al. 1999). Neuroimaging studies further confirm these observations and show that the ACC, together with other cortical structures, are activated by acute noxious stimuli (Talbot, Marrett, Evans et al. 1991; Rainville, Duncan, Price et al. 1997; Casey 1999; Rainville, Bushnell, Duncan 2001). Thus, understanding the synaptic mechanism within the ACC will greatly help us gain insights into plastic changes in the brain related to central pain. It is important to point out here that in addition to pain, the ACC has been proposed as a neurobiological substrate for executive control of cognitive and motor processes. Human imaging studies demonstrate that the ACC region is activated by different factors including motivational drive, reward, gain or loss, conflict monitoring or error prediction, and attention or anticipation. The neuronal mechanisms for these different functions within the ACC remain mostly unknown because of the limitation of human studies. These "side-effect" or nonselective roles of the ACC further support the critical role of ACC in chronic pain-related mental disorders. It is unlikely that the contribution of ACC in humans is limited to pain, and it may also include pain-related depression, drug addiction, suicide, and loss of interests.

IC

Similar to the ACC, the IC has been also reported to play roles in pain, although most of data are imaging data in human patients (Talbot, Marrett, Evans et al. 1991; Rainville, Duncan, Price et al. 1997; Casey 1999; Rainville, Bushnell, Duncan 2001; Jasmin, Rabkin, Granato et al. 2003). Local manipulations that enhance GABA functions in the IC produced long-lasting analgesic effects (Jasmin, Rabkin, Granato et al. 2003). In the IC, it has been reported that θ-burst stimulation induces LTP, and the activity of the Ca^{2+}/CaM-dependent protein kinase CaMKIV is required for the potentiation (Wei, Qiu, Kim et al. 2002). By using whole-cell patch recording, we recently found that spike-time paring protocol also induced LTP in insular neurons (Zhuo, unpublished data).

Long-Term Potentiation in the ACC

Induction Mechanism

Glutamate is the major fast excitatory transmitter in the ACC (Wei, Li, Zhuo 1999). Different types of glutamate receptors, including AMPA, KA, NMDA, and metabotropic receptors (mGluRs) are found in the ACC. Fast synaptic responses induced by local stimulation or stimulation of thalamocortical projection pathways are mediated by AMPA/KA receptors, since both applications of CNQX completely block fast synaptic responses. In addition to fast synaptic responses, in adult ACC slices at physiological temperatures, NMDA receptor–mediated slow synaptic responses were also recorded from the ACC (Liauw, Wang, Zhuo 2003), suggesting that NMDA receptors are tonically active in this region.

Glutamatergic synapses in the ACC can undergo long-lasting potentiation in response to θ-burst stimulation, a paradigm more close to the activity of ACC neurons. The potentiation lasted for at least 40 minutes (Zhao, Toyoda, Lee et al. 2005). cAMP signaling pathways are required for the induction of ACC LTP; studies using gene knockout mice and pharmacological activators/inhibitors found that calcium-stimulated AC1 and AC8 contribute to the induction of LTP in the ACC (Liauw et al. 2005). In addition, CaMKIV, another protein kinase responding to calcium-calmodulin (CaM), is also required for the induction of LTP (Wei, Qiu, Liauw et al. 2002b).

Expression Mechanisms

At least four possible mechanisms may contribute to the expression of LTP:

1. Presynaptic enhancement of glutamate release

2. Postsynaptic enhancement of glutamate receptor–mediated responses
3. Recruitment of previously "silent" synapses or synaptic trafficking or insertion of AMPA receptors
4. Structural changes

Under in vitro brain slice conditions, it appears that LTP mechanism may depend on the induction protocol in certain cases. Paired-pulse facilitation (PPF) was not altered after the induction of cingulate LTP (Zhao, Toyoda, Lee et al. 2005). However, we do not rule out the possibility of presynaptic changes in the ACC during other physiological or pathological conditions. Among these possibilities, we have recently investigated the roles of GluR1 and GluR2/3 using genetic and pharmacological approaches. We found that GluR1 subunit C-terminal peptide analog, Pep1-TGL, blocked the induction of cingulate LTP (Toyoda, Wu, Zhao et al. 2007a). Thus, in the ACC, the interaction between the C-terminus of GluR1 and PDZ domain proteins is required for the induction of LTP. Synaptic delivery of the GluR1 subunit from extrasynaptic sites is the key mechanism underlying synaptic plasticity (Passafaro, Piech, Sheng 2001) and GluR1–PDZ interactions play a critical intermediate in this plasticity. Our pharmacological experiments show that the application of philanthotoxin (PhTx) 5 minutes after paired training reduced synaptic potentiation, while PhTx had no effect on basal responses. Therefore, we believe that Ca^{2+}-permeable GluR2-lacking receptors contribute to the maintenance of LTP and are necessary for subsequent LTP stabilization. Although our data did not provide direct evidence for the synaptic trafficking or insertion of GluR1 receptors at postsynaptic membrane, the present findings suggest selective contribution of AMPA subtype receptors to cingulate LTP.

GluR2/3 subunits may continually replace synaptic GluR2/3 subunits in an activity-independent manner that maintains constant synaptic transmission (Carroll, Beattie, von Zastrow et al. 2001; Malinow, Malenka 2002; Song, Huganir 2002; Bredt, Nicoll 2003). We also examined the role of these peptides in synaptic potentiation in the ACC and found that the GluR2/3-PDZ interaction had no effect on cingulate LTP.

Long-Term Depression in the ACC

Long-term depression (LTD) has been thought to be a reversed form of plasticity for LTP. It has been well investigated in the hippocampus. Two forms of LTD have been reported in the hippocampus: NMDA receptor–dependent and mGluR-dependent forms. In the ACC neurons of adult rats and mice, two forms of LTD can be observed, depending on the induction protocols. In ACC slices, repetitive stimulation for a long period (15 minutes) induced mGluR-dependent LTD (Wei, Li, Zhuo 1999). LTD is input specific, and unstimulated pathways remain unchanged. The induction of LTD requires activation of mGluRs and L-type voltage-gated calcium channels (L-VDCCs) (Wei, Li, Zhuo 1999). NMDA receptor–dependent LTD is recently found by using whole-cell patch-clamp recordings (Toyoda, Wu, Zhao et al. 2007b). Pairing the synaptic activity with modest postsynaptic depolarization in cingulated pyramidal cells induced LTD in the EPSCs. The induction of LTD requires activation of postsynaptic NMDA receptor and postsynaptic calcium influx. Activation of NR2A- and NR2B-containing NMDA receptors contributes the LTD. Using GluR2-interfering peptide, we found that the interfering peptides inhibited cingulated LTD (Toyoda, Wu, Zhao et al. 2007b). These findings suggest that AMPA GluR1 and GluR2/3 play different roles in cingulate LTP versus LTD (Fig. 6.6). Future studies are clearly needed to investigate signaling pathways that link activation of NMDA receptor or mGluRs to synaptic depression.

Alternations of ACC Plasticity after Injury

Long-Term Enhancement of Synaptic Responses in the ACC after Injury

One important question related to AC plasticity is whether injury causes prolonged or long-term changes in synaptic transmission in the ACC in whole animals. To test this question, we first measure synaptic responses to peripheral electrical shocks. We placed a recording electrode in the ACC of anesthetized rats (Wei, Zhuo 2001). At high intensities of stimulation sufficient to activate A_δ- and C-fibers, evoked field excitatory postsynaptic potentials (EPSPs) were found in the ACC. To detect central plastic changes, we performed amputation at the hindpaw contralateral to the one to which stimulation was delivered. Interestingly, after amputation of a central digit of the hindpaw, we observed a rapid enhancement of sensory responses to peripheral electrical shocks delivered to the normal hindpaw (Fig. 6.7). The potentiation was long-lasting; evoked responses remained enhanced for at least 120 minutes (Wei, Zhuo 2001). Synaptic changes likely happen locally within the ACC; we also observed a long-lasting potentiation of field EPSPs induced by focal stimulation in the ACC after amputation that lasted for at least 90 minutes (Wei, Zhuo 2001). The amount of potentiation is not significantly different from that in field recordings evoked by hindpaw stimulation. We hypothesize that LTP within the ACC is likely due to abnormal activity during and

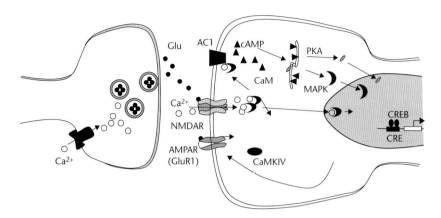

Figure 6.6 Model for the cingulate LTP. Neural activity triggered the release of excitatory neurotransmitter glutamate (Glu: filled circles) in the ACC synapses. Activation of glutamate NMDA receptors (NMDAR) leads to an increase in postsynaptic Ca^{2+} in dendritic spines. Both NMDA NR2B and NR2A subunits are important for NMDA receptor functions. Ca^{2+} serves as an important intracellular signal for triggering a series of biochemical events that contribute to the expression of LTP. Ca^{2+} binds to CaM and leads to activation of calcium-stimulated ACs, mainly AC1 and Ca^{2+}/CaM-dependent protein kinases. Through various protein kinase–related intracellular signaling pathways, the trafficking of postsynaptic AMPA receptor as well as other synaptic modifications contributes to enhanced synaptic responses. Activation of CaMKIV, a kinase predominantly expressed in the nuclei, will trigger CREB signaling pathways. In addition, activation of AC1 and AC8 lead to activation of PKA, and subsequently CREB as well. MAPK/ERK could translocate from the cytosol to the nucleus and then regulate CREB activity. Considering the upstream promoter region of the *Egr1* gene contains CRE sites, it is possible that Egr1 may contribute to CREB-related signaling targets in the ACC neurons. Considering the fact that many late signaling molecules (e.g., FMRP, Egr1, and CaMKIV) also contribute to early enhancement of responses, more works are needed to reveal the signaling pathways for the LTP in the ACC neurons.

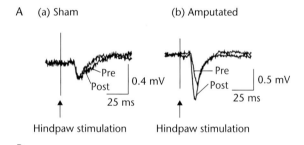

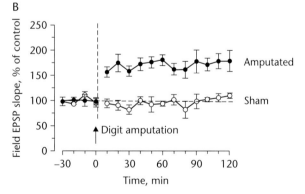

Figure 6.7 In vivo long-term potentiation triggered by digit amputation. Long-lasting enhancement following amputation of a single hindpaw digit. (A) Representative traces of EPSPs 5 minutes before amputation and 115 to 120 minutes after sham treatment (a) or amputation (b). In (b), the latency of sensory responses was not changed after the amputation, while the EPSP slope was increased. (B) Amputation of a single digit of the contralateral hindpaw (indicated in Fig. 6.1 by an arrow) caused long-lasting enhancement of sensory responses (filled circles). Sensory responses were not significantly changed in sham-treated animals (open circles). The testing frequency was 0.01 Hz.

after amputation. One important question is whether potentiated sensory responses required persistent activity from the injured hindpaw. To test this, we locally injected a local anesthetic, QX-314, into the hindpaw (5%, 50 μL) at 120 minutes after amputation. We found that QX-314 injection did not significantly affect the synaptic potentiation induced by amputation (Wei, Zhuo 2001).

Enhanced Hippocampal LTP by Amputation

Hippocampal neurons are thought to be important for spatial learning and memory. For example, hippocampal neurons fire spikes when an animal is at a particular location or performs certain behaviors in a particular place. In a natural environment, spatial memory is often associated with potentially dangerous sensory experiences such as noxious or painful stimuli. The central sites for such pain-associated memory or plasticity have been investigated in rats and mice. We found that excitatory glutamatergic synapses within the CA1 region of the hippocampus may play a role in storing pain-related information. By performing intracellular recordings from anesthetized rats, we found that peripheral noxious stimulation induced EPSPs in CA1 pyramidal cells. Tissue or nerve injury caused a rapid increase in the level of the immediate-early gene product *Egr1* (also called NGFI-A, Krox24, or zif/268) in hippocampal CA1 neurons. In parallel, synaptic potentiation induced by a single tetanic stimulation (100 Hz for 1 s) was enhanced after the injury.

This enhancement of synaptic potentiation was absent in mice lacking Egr1 (Fig. 6.8). We suggest that Egr1 may act as an important regulator of pain-related synaptic plasticity within the hippocampus.

Loss of Long-Term Depression

In support of plastic changes in the ACC after injury, activity-dependent immediate-early genes, such as *c-fos*, *Egr1*, and cyclic adenosine 3',5'-monophosphate response element binding protein (*CREB*) are activated in the ACC neurons after tissue inflammation or amputation (Wei, Li, Zhuo 1999; Wei, Wang, Kerchner et al. 2001). Furthermore, these plastic changes persist for a long period, from hours to days. Studies using AC1 and AC8 double knockout or NR2B

overexpression mice show that NMDA receptors, AC1 and AC8 contribute to activation of immediate-early genes by injury (Wei, Wang, Kerchner et al. 2001; Wei, Qiu, Kim et al. 2002a). In parallel with these dramatic changes in gene expression, synaptic plasticity recorded from in vitro ACC slices is also altered. In ACC slices of animals with amputation, the same repetitive stimulation produced less or no LTD (Fig. 6.9). The loss of LTD is regionally selective, and no change was found in other cortical areas (Wei, Li, Zhuo 1999). One possible physiological mechanism for LTD in the ACC is to serve as an autoregulatory mechanism. LTD induced during low-frequency repetitive stimulation may help maintain appropriate neuronal activity within the ACC by reducing synaptic transmission. In amputated or injured animals,

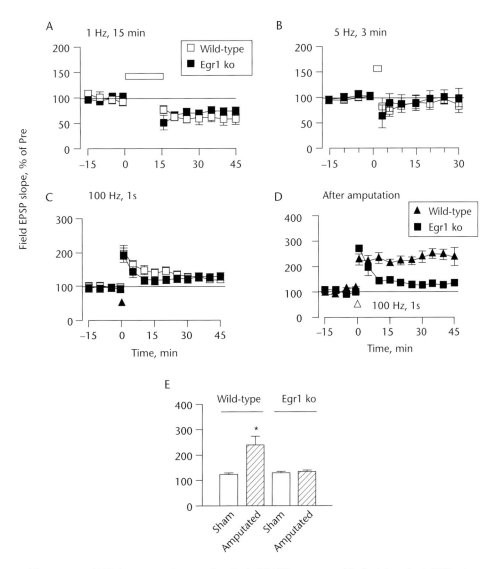

Figure 6.8 Enhanced hippocampal LTP by amputation requires Egr1. (A) LTD was normal in Egr1 knockout (KO) mice as compared with wild-type mice. (B) Synaptic responses to 5 Hz stimulation were also normal. (C) Synaptic potentiation induced by a single tetanic stimulation was similar. (D) Amputation caused enhanced LTP in wild-type mice while there was no synaptic enhancement of LTP in Egr1 knockout mice. (E) Summarized data of different treatments on the enhancement of LTP caused by amputation.

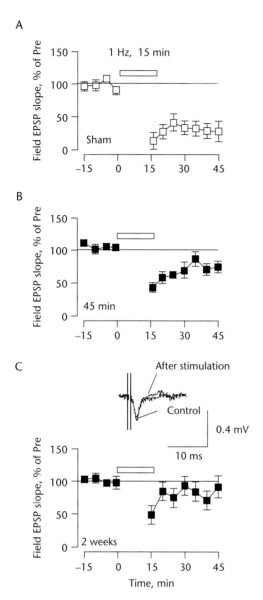

Figure 6.9 Loss of cortical LTD after amputation. Long-lasting loss of LTD in the ACC after the amputation. LTD recorded from ACC slices in sham animals (A) and rats at 45 minutes (B) and 2 weeks (C) after the amputation. (Inset in C): representative records of the EPSP recorded before and 30 minutes after 1 Hz stimulation.

the loss of autoregulation of synaptic tone may lead to overexcitation in the ACC neurons and contribute to enhancement of pain or unpleasantness related to the injury.

FOREBRAIN NMDA NR2B RECEPTORS: SMART MICE, MORE PAIN

In order to investigate molecular and cellular mechanisms for pain-related plasticity in the ACC, we decided to use genetic approaches together with integrative neuroscience techniques to investigate synaptic mechanisms in the ACC. First, we want to

test if persistent pain may be enhanced by genetically enhanced NMDA receptor functions, a key mechanism for triggering central plasticity in the brain (Zhuo 2002). Functional NMDA receptors contain heteromeric combinations of the NR1 subunit and one or more of NR2A-D. While NR1 shows a widespread distribution in the brains, NR2 subunits exhibit regional distribution. In humans and rodents, NR2A and NR2B subunits predominate in forebrain structures. NR2A and NR2B subunits confer distinct properties to NMDA receptors; heteromers containing NR1 and NR2B mediate a current that decays three to four times more slowly than receptors composed of NR1 and NR2A. Unlike other ionotropic channels, NMDA receptors are 5 to 10 times more permeable to calcium, a critical intracellular signaling molecule, than to Na+ or K+. NMDA receptor–mediated currents are long-lasting compared with the rapidly desensitizing kinetics of AMPA and kainate receptor channels. In transgenic mice with forebrain-targeted NR2B overexpression, the normal developmental change in NMDA receptor kinetics was reversed (Tang, Xhimizu, Dube et al. 1999). NR2B subunit expression was observed extensively throughout the cerebral cortex, striatum, amygdala, and hippocampus, but not in the thalamus, brainstem, or cerebellum. In both the ACC and insular cortex, NR2B expression was significantly increased, and NMDA receptor-mediated responses were enhanced (Wei, Wang, Kerchner et al. 2001). NMDA receptor-mediated responses in the spinal cord, however, were not affected. NR2B transgenic and wild-type mice were indistinguishable in tests of acute nociception; however, NR2B transgenic mice exhibited enhanced behavioral responses after peripheral injection of formalin. Late-phase nociceptive responses, but not early responses, were enhanced. Furthermore, mechanical allodynia measured in the complete Freund's adjuvant (CFA) model were significantly enhanced in NR2B transgenic mice. These findings provide the first genetic evidence that forebrain NMDA receptors play a critical role in chronic pain.

Transgenic overexpression of NMDA NR2B receptors in forebrain regions increased behavioral responses to persistent inflammatory pain. However, it is not known whether inflammation leads to the upregulation of NR2B receptors in these regions. To further investigate if the upregulation of NMDA NR2B receptors may occur in pathological conditions, we performed experiments in animals with chronic inflammation at the hindpaws (Wu, Toyoda, Zhao et al. 2005). We found that peripheral inflammation increased the expression of NMDA NR2B receptors within the ACC. The changes in NMDA receptor protein expression are subtype selective, since other NMDA receptor subunits did not show

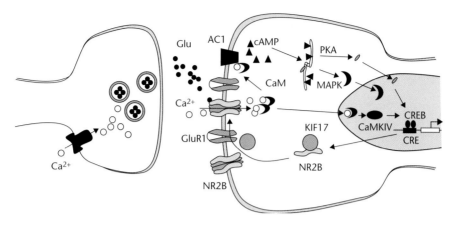

Figure 6.10 Model for upregulation of NR2B after chronic pain. Activation of postsynaptic glutamate NMDA receptors leads to an increase in postsynaptic Ca²⁺ in dendritic spines. Ca²⁺ binds to CaM and leads to activation of calcium-stimulated ACs, mainly AC1 and other Ca²⁺/CaM-dependent protein kinases (PKC, CaMKII, and CaMKIV). Activation of CaMKIV, a kinase predominantly expressed in the nuclei, will trigger CREB signaling pathways. In addition, activation of AC1 and AC8 leads to activation of PKA, and subsequently CREB as well. MAPK/ERK could translocate from the cytosol to the nucleus and then regulate CREB activity. Subsequently, postsynaptic synthesis of NMDA NR2B receptor is increased, and together with endogenous motor protein KIF17, these new NR2B subunits are added to post-synaptic NMDA receptors. Such possible positive feedback may further enhance neuronal excitability within the ACC and contribute to chronic pain. In addition to the upregulation of NMDA NR2B receptors, it is likely that AMPA receptor will undergo plastic upregulation. The enhanced AMPA and NMDA receptor–mediated responses thus likely to lead to positive enforcement of excitatory transmission within the ACC, and contribute to chronic, severe pain as well as pain-related mental disorders.

significant increases. The increased NMDA NR2B receptors are likely to be within synapses, and single-shock focal stimulation–induced NMDA NRR2B receptor–mediated synaptic currents were also enhanced in the ACC pyramidal neurons (Wu, Toyoda, Zhao et al. 2005) (Fig. 6.10).

The upregulation of NMDA NR2B receptors in the ACC can also be detected in freely moving mice. NMDA receptor-mediated evoked responses in the ACC were increased after hindpaw inflammation by CFA (Wu, Toyoda, Zhao et al. 2005). Pharmacological and behavioral studies provide further evidence supporting the roles of NMDA NR2B receptors in mediating persistent pain caused by peripheral CFA inflammation. Inhibition of NR2B receptors in the ACC selectively reduced behavioral sensitization related to inflammation. These results demonstrate that the upregulation of NR2B receptors in the ACC contributes to behavioral sensitization caused by inflammation.

Environmental Enrichment and Chronic Pain

Environmental enrichment is known to increase cortical plasticity and is one of the most reliable and well-characterized paradigms of experience-dependent plasticity in rodents. This experimental paradigm has been repeatedly shown to trigger widespread morphological changes in the mammalian brain. A vast amount of studies have focused on the positive effects of environmental enrichment

in brain regions involved in learning and memory such as the hippocampus and neocortex (van Praag et al. 1999). For example, enriched animals exhibit enhanced hippocampal LTP (Duffy, Craddock, Abel et al. 2001), enhanced performance in hippocampus-dependent behavioral task in the Morris water maze (Kempermann, Kuhn, Gage 1997; Williams, Luo, Ward et al. 2001) and in fear conditioning (Duffy, Craddock, Abel et al. 2001). Furthermore, exposure to enriched environments (EEs) has been shown to enhance plasticity and functional recovery associated with cerebral insult (Dahlqvist, Zhao, Johansson et al. 1999; Rampon, Tang, Goodhouse et al. 2000), suggesting that EE triggers cortical reorganization leading to functional recovery after injury. Recently, we examined the effects of EE on synaptic plasticity changes in the ACC and the extent to which enhanced sensory experience affects behavioral sensitization to injury. We induced cortical plasticity by placing mice in an EE for 1 month and measured the effects of EE in the ACC. EE enhanced the expression of the plasticity gene, *Egr1*, in the ACC of EE animals accompanied by enhanced cingulated LTP and decreased cingulated LTD. The increased NMDA receptor NR2B/NR2A subunits' current ratio is associated with the plasticity seen in the ACC while total protein levels remain unchanged. Furthermore, behavioral experiments show that these mice exposed to EE demonstrate enhanced responses to acute and long-term inflammation (Fig. 6.11). Thus, exposure to EE alters physiological properties within the ACC, which results in enhanced responses to inflammation.

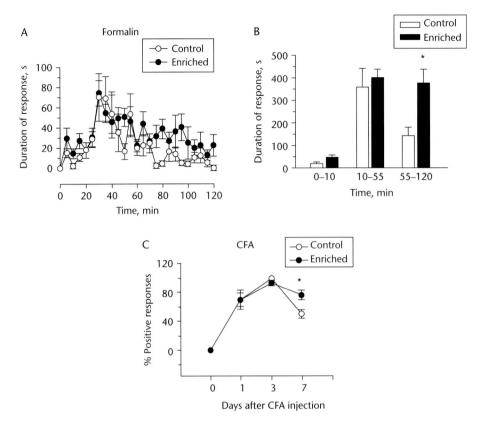

Figure 6.11 Enrichment enhanced persistent pain. (A) Enriched and control animals were injected with 10 μL of formalin (5%) in the right hindpaw and were monitored over a time course of 2 hours corresponding to the three phases of formalin-induced response. Enriched animals showed significantly enhanced licking response during the third phase. (B) Comparison with control animals. (C) Timeline showing that 10 μL CFA (50%) injection into the hindpaw of enriched animals enhanced chronic injury response on the 7th day in the ipsilateral paw.

Cortical Reorganization and Phantom Pain

Cortical reorganization acts as an adaptive mechanism during development and learning; it could also play a detrimental role in traumatic events, such as the loss of a limb (Kaas, Florence, Jain 1999; Flor, Nikolajsen, Jensen 2006). It has been demonstrated that cortical reorganization occurs after limb or digit amputation (Merzenich, Nelson, Stryker et al. 1984; Pons, Garraghty, Ommaya et al. 1991; Ramachandran, Rogers-Ramachandran, Stewart 1992; Ramachandran, Rogers-Ramachandran, Cobb 1995; Florence, Taub, Kaas 1998; Jones, Pons 1998; Kaas 1998; Merzenich 1998). After amputation of digits, neuronal terminals invade into adjacent cortical area representing deafferented fingers (see Fig. 6.12 for a model). Similarly, human amputees experience phantom limb sensation or phantom pain, and the amount of cortical reorganization correlates with the extent of phantom pain (Flor, Elbert, Knetcht et al. 1995; Birbaumer, Lutzenberger, Montoya et al. 1997; Lorenz, Kohlhoff, Hansen et al. 1998). Molecular and cellular mechanisms for cortical reorganization are still largely unknown. Here I would like to propose that cortical reorganization may also contribute to chronic pain due to peripheral injury. Recent studies in human brain imaging indeed reported brain structural changes in patients with chronic pain (Flor, Elbert, Knetcht et al. 1995; Flor, Nikolajsen, Jensen 2006).

Calcium-Stimualted ACs Are Critical for Chronic Pain

AC1 and AC8, the two major CaM-stimulated ACs in the brain, couple NMDA receptor activation to cAMP signaling pathways. In the ACC, strong and homogeneous patterns of AC1 and AC8 expression was observed in all cell layers (Wei, Qiu, Kim et al. 2002a). Behavioral studies found that wild-type, AC1, AC8, or AC1 and AC8 double knockout mice were indistinguishable in tests of acute pain including the tail flick (TF) test and hot plate test, and the mechanical withdrawal responses. However, behavioral responses to peripheral injection of two inflammatory stimuli, formalin and CFA, were reduced in AC1 or AC8 single knockout mice. Deletion of both AC1 and AC8 in AC1 and AC8 double knockout mice produced greater reduction in persistent pain (Wei, Qiu, Kim et al. 2002a). More importantly, microinjection of an AC

ENDOGENOUS ANALGESIA SYSTEM AND FACILITATORY SYSTEM: TOP-DOWN MODULATION

Endogenous Analgesic and Antinociceptive Systems

Spinal nociceptive transmission is modulated by an endogenous antinociceptive or analgesic system, consisting of the midbrain PAG and the RVM (Basbaum, Fields 1984; Gebhart 1986; Willis 1988; Gebhart, Randich 1990). The RVM serves as an important relay for descending influences from the PAG to the spinal cord. Activation of neurons in the RVM inhibits spinal nociceptive transmission and behavioral nociceptive reflexes. The inhibitory effect is mediated directly by descending pathways projecting bilaterally in the dorsolateral funiculi, and indirectly by descending activation of local spinal inhibitory neurons (Zhuo, Gebhart 1990a, 1990b, 1992, 1997).

In the spinal cord, muscarinic, noradrenergic and serotonergic receptors are important for descending inhibition of behavioral nociceptive reflexes. Electrophysiological studies using intracellular or whole-cell patch-clamp recordings of dorsal horn neurons allow investigation into the cellular mechanisms for the antinociceptive or analgesic effects induced by these transmitters. In anesthetized whole animals, electrical stimulation applied to sites within the nucleus raphe magnus or PAG produced IPSPs in dorsal horn neurons including ascending projection spinothalamic tract cells. More detailed pharmacological analysis came from studies using an in vitro brain or spinal cord slice preparation. In trigeminal nuclei, all three major transmitters, acetylcholine, serotonin, and norepinephrine are reported to inhibit glutamatergic transmission (Grudt, Williams, Travagli 1995; Travagli, Williams 1996). In the lumbar spinal cord, activation of postsynaptic muscarinic receptors inhibits excitatory sensory transmission. Unlike carbachol, the effect of which was completely attenuated by postsynaptic G-protein inhibition, agonists of serotonin and α_2-adrenergic receptors could produce inhibitory modulatory effects through both presynaptic and postsynaptic receptors, since postsynaptic G-protein blockade provided only partial attenuation of their effects (Li, Zhuo 2001). These findings are consistent with anatomic evidence that both presynaptic and postsynaptic receptors are found in these sensory synapses. Future studies are clearly needed to explore the molecular mechanism of inhibition of postsynaptic glutamate-mediated responses.

Endogenous Facilitatory Systems

In addition to descending inhibition, descending excitatory or facilitatory influences from the brainstem or

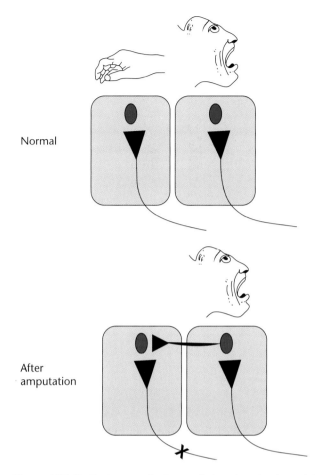

Figure 6.12 Cortical reorganization and chronic pain. A model for the possible roles of cortical reorganization in phantom pain. In normal conditions, the connections between different somatosensory cortical areas are limited. However, after amputation (a long period of time after surgery), the neurons form new intracortical connections by sprouting into adjacent cortical area. In this case, the neurons in cortical region representing the face form connections with those representing the hand fingers. Consequently, stimulation of facial area may trigger phantom sensation of amputated hand or pain in amputated hand. Early LTP after amputation may represent early changes that initiate long-term structures in patients with cortical reorganization.

activator, forskolin, can rescue defects in chronic pain in AC1 and AC8 double knockout mice. Consistently, pharmacological interventions of NMDA receptors as well as cAMP signaling pathways within the ACC also produced inhibitory effects on persistent pain in normal or wild-type animals, supporting the roles of ACC in persistent pain. Microinjection of NMDA receptor antagonists or cAMP-dependent protein kinase (PKA) inhibitors reduced or blocked mechanical allodynia related to inflammation (Wei, Qiu, Kim et al. 2002a). A recent study showed that persistent pain induced by tissue inflammation or nerve injury was significantly reduced in PDZ-93 knockout mice, in part due to the lower level of NR2B expression at the spinal and cortical levels of knockout mice (Tao, Rumbaugh, Wang et al. 2003).

forebrains have been characterized (Zhuo, Gebhart 1990a, 1990b, 1991, 1992, 1997; Calejesan, Kim, Zhuo 2000). Biphasic modulation of spinal nociceptive transmission from the RVM, perhaps reflecting the different types of neurons identified in this area, offer fine regulation of spinal sensory thresholds and responses. While descending inhibition is primarily involved in regulating suprathreshold responses to noxious stimuli, descending facilitation reduces the neuronal threshold to nociceptive stimulation (Zhuo, Gebhart 1990a, 1990b, 1991, 1992, 1997). Descending facilitation has a general impact on spinal sensory transmission, inducing sensory inputs from cutaneous and visceral organs (Zhuo, Sengupta, Gebhart 2002; Zhuo, Gebhart 2002; Zhuo 2007) (Fig. 6.13). Descending facilitation can be activated under physiological conditions, and one physiological function of descending facilitation is to enhance the ability of animals to detect potential dangerous signals in the environment. Indeed, neurons in the RVM not only respond to noxious stimuli, but also show "learning"-type changes during repetitive noxious stimuli. More importantly, RVM neurons can undergo plastic changes during and after tissue injury and inflammation.

ACC-Induced Facilitation

It is well documented that the descending endogenous analgesia system, including the PAG and RVM, plays an important role in modulation of nociceptive transmission and morphine- and cannabinoid-produced analgesia. Neurons in the PAG receive inputs from different nuclei of higher structures, including the cingulated ACC. Electrical stimulation of ACC at high intensities (up to 500 µA) of electrical stimulation did not produce any antinociceptive effect. Instead, at most sites within the ACC, electrical stimulation produced significant facilitation of the TF reflex (i.e. decreases in TF latency). Activation of mGluRs within the ACC also produced facilitatory effects in both anesthetized rats or freely moving mice (Calejesan, Kim, Zhuo 2000; Tang et al. 2006). Descending facilitation from the ACC apparently relays at the RVM (Calejesan, Kim, Zhuo 2000) (see Fig. 6.14).

Descending Facilitation Maintains Chronic Pain

Descending facilitation is likely activated after the injury, contributing to secondary hyperalgesia (Calejesan, Ch'ang, Zhuo 1998; Robinson et al. 2002b). Blocking descending facilitation by lesion of the RVM or spinal blockade of serotonin receptors is antinociceptive (Urban, Gebhart 1999; Porreca, Ossipov, Gebhart 2002; Robinson et al. 2004). The descending facilitatory system therefore serves as a

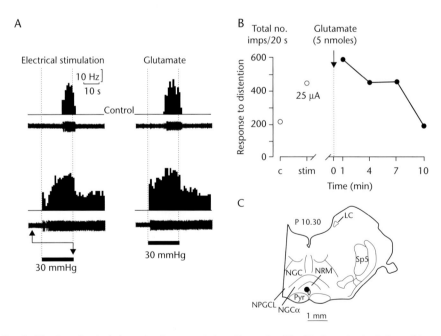

Figure 6.13 Descending facilitation of spinal visceral pain transmission. Example of facilitation of spinal visceral transmission produced by electrical stimulation and glutamate in the nucleus raphe magnus (NRM). (A) Peristimulus time histograms (1-second binwidth) and corresponding ocillographic records in the absence (top histograms) and presence (bottom histograms) of electrical stimulation (25 µA) and glutamate (5 nmoles) given in the same site in NRM. The intensity and duration of colorectal distension is illustrated below; the period of electrical stimulation (25 seconds) is indicated by the arrows. (B) Summary of the data illustrated in (A) and time course of effect of glutamate given in NRM. The point above c represents the response to 30-mmHg colorectal distension; the point above stimulation represents the response to the same intensity of distension during stimulation in NRM. (C) Site of stimulation and injection of glutamate.

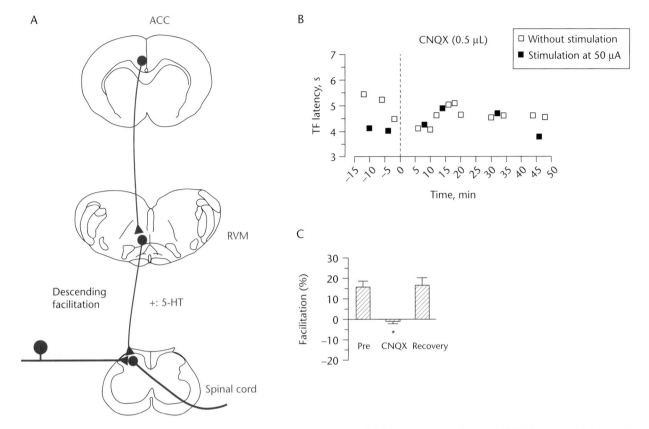

Figure 6.14 ACC controls RVM-generated descending facilitation. (A) A model shows supraspinal control of RVM-generated descending facilitation of spinal nociception by ACC) neurons. (B) An example illustrates that CNQX microinjection into the RVM reversibly blocks facilitation of the TF reflex produced by electrical stimulation at a site within the ACC; TF response latencies measured without stimulation were represented by open squares. TF latencies measured with stimulation were represented by filled squares; (C) Summary data showing mean facilitation (% of control) before CNQX injection into the RVM (Pre); after (within 10 minutes); and 30 minutes after (30 min post).

double-edged blade in the central nervous system. On one hand, it allows neurons in different parts of the brain to communicate with each other and enhances sensitivity to potentially dangerous signals; on the other hand, prolonged facilitation of spinal nociceptive transmission after injury speeds up central plastic changes related to chronic pain (Table 6.3).

CONCLUSIONS AND FUTURE DIRECTIONS

Finally, I would like to review and propose three key cellular models for future investigations of chronic pain. I would like to emphasize that integrative experimental approaches are essential for future studies to avoid the misleading discoveries; work at different sensory synapses are equally critical such as spinal cord synapses, cortical synapse, and brainstem synapses that dictate descending facilitatory and inhibitory modulations. Table 6.4 summarizes likely key mechanisms for chronic pain. They include

1. Plasticity of sensory synaptic transmission: excitatory (glutamate) and inhibitory (GABA, Gly) transmission
2. Anatomic structural changes: synaptic reorganization (e.g. changes in spines), cortical reorganization, neuronal phenotype switch, cortical gray matter loss
3. Long-term alteration in descending modulation: enhanced descending facilitation or loss of tonic descending inhibitory influences

In summary, progress made in basic neurobiology investigations has significantly helped us understand the fundamental mechanism for pain or physiological pain processes, both at the peripheral spinal cord level and at the cortical level. Studies of central plasticity, including LTP/LTD in sensory synapses, start to provide useful cellular models for our understanding of chronic pain. Novel mechanisms revealed at molecular and cellular levels will significantly affect our future approaches to search and design novel drugs for treating chronic pain in patients.

ACKNOWLEDGMENT I thank funding supports from the EJLB-CIHR Michael Smith Chair in Neurosciences

Table 6.3 Comparison of Endogenous Facilitation and Analgesia Systems

	Descending Facilitation	Descending Analgesia
Central origin	ACC; RVM	PAG; RVM
Neurotransmitter	Glutamate; neurotensin	Glutamate; opioids
Stimulation intensity	5–25 µA	50–100 µA
Stimulation–response Function (SRF)	Reduced threshold	Reduced peak response without affecting threshold
Response latency	200 ms	90 ms
Laterality	Bilateral	Bilateral
Spinal pathways	Ventrolateral funiculi (VLF)/ventral funiculi (VF)	Dorsolateral funiculi (DLF)
Spinal neurotransmitter	5-HT	Ach; NE; 5-HT
Synaptic mechanism	AMPA receptor trafficking Enhanced AMPA receptor–mediated EPSCs	Inhibit presynaptic transmitter release; reduced AMPA receptor–mediated EPSCs
Sensory modality	Non-nociceptive Nociceptive Mechanical Thermal	Non-nociceptive Nociceptive Mechanical Thermal
Origin of sensory inputs	Somatosensory Visceral	Somatosensory Visceral

Table 6.4 Proposed Key Neurobiological Mechanisms for Chronic Pain

Proposed Model	Synaptic Consequences	Key References
Plasticity of synaptic transmission		
Silent synapse	Recruit AMPA responses into NS specific cells	Li, Zhuo 1998
LTP	Enhanced existing AMPA responses GluR1 mediated LTP Enhanced glutamate release	Ikeda et al. 2003 Zhao et al. 2005 Zhao et al. 2006
Loss of LTD	Fail to depotentiate enhanced responses	Wei et al. 1999
Microglia disinhibition	Switching GABA currents	Coull et al. 2003
Structural reorganization		
Phenotype switch	Neurons making new transmitters such as SP	Woolf et al. 1992
Structural sprouting	Sprouting fibers	Neumann et al. 1996
Cortical reorganization	Growth of new cortical connections	Flor et al. 1995
Neuronal cell death	Loss of neurons due to cell death	Apkarian et al. 2004
Altered descending modulation		
Loss of descending inhibition	Activity in the PAG, RVM neuron failed to produce analgesic effects in the spinal cord	Wei et al. 1999 Robinson et al. 2002 Urban et al. 1999
Enhanced descending facilitation	Enhanced facilitatory influences from the ACC and RVM	Calejesan et al. 2000 Zhuo, Gebhart 1997

and Mental Health in Canada, CIHR operating grants, Canada Research Chair, and NeuroCanada Brain repair program.

REFERENCES

Apkarian AV, Sosa Y, Sonty S et al. 2004. Chronic back pain is associated with decreased prefrontal and thalamic gray matter density. *J Neurosci.* 24:10410–10415.

Bardoni R, Magherini PC, MacDermott AB. 1998. NMDA EPSCs at glutamatergic synapses in the spinal cord dorsal horn of the postnatal rat. *J Neurosci.* 18:6558–6567.

Basbaum AI, Fields HL. 1984. Endogenous pain control system: brainstem spinal pathways and endorphin circuitry. *Annu Rev Neurosci.* 7:309–338.

Birbaumer N, Lutzenberger W, Montoya P et al. 1997. Effects of regional anesthesia on phantom limb pain are mirrored in changes in cortical reorganization. *J Neurosci.* 17:5503–5508.

Bredt DS, Nicoll RA. 2003. AMPA receptor trafficking at excitatory synapses. *Neuron.* 40:361–379.

Calejesan AA, Ch'ang MH-C, Zhuo M. 1998. Spinal serotonergic receptors mediate facilitation of a nociceptive reflex by subcutaneous formalin injection into the hindpaw in rats. *Brain Res.* 798:46–54.

Calejesan AA, Kim SJ, Zhuo M. 2000. Descending facilitatory modulation of a behavioral nociceptive response by stimulation in the adult rat anterior cingulate cortex. *Eur J Pain.* 4:83–96.

Carroll RC, Beattie EC, von Zastrow M, Malenka RC. 2001. Role of AMPA receptor endocytosis in synaptic plasticity. *Nat Rev Neurosci.* 2(5):315–324.

Casey KL. 1999. Forebrain mechanisms of nociception and pain: analysis through imaging. *Proc Natl Acad Sci U S A.* 96:7668–7674.

Caterina MJ, Julius D. 2001. The vanilloid receptor: a molecular gateway to the pain pathway. *Annu Rev Neurosci.* 24:487–517.

Colburn RW, Lubin ML, Stone DJ Jr et al. 2007. Attenuated cold sensitivity in TRPM8 null mice. *Neuron.* 54:379–386.

Coull JA, Boudreau D, Bachand K et al. 2003. Transsynaptic shift in anion gradient in spinal lamina I neurons as a mechanism of neuropathic pain. *Nature.* 424:938–942.

Dahlqvist P, Zhao L, Johansson IM et al. 1999. Environmental enrichment alters nerve growth factor-induced gene A and glucocorticoid receptor messenger RNA expression after middle cerebral artery occlusion in rats. *Neuroscience.* 93:527–535.

Dhaka A, Murray AN, Mathur J, Earley TJ, Petrus MJ, Patapoutian A. 2007. TRPM8 is required for cold sensation in mice. *Neuron.* 54:371–378.

Dong H, O'Brien RJ, Fung ET, Lanahan AA, Worley PF, Huganir RL. 1997. GRIP: a synaptic PDZ domain-containing protein that interacts with AMPA receptors. *Nature.* 386:279–284.

Dong H, Zhang P, Song I, Petralia RS, Liao D, Huganir RL. 1999. Characterization of the glutamate receptor-interacting proteins GRIP1 and GRIP2. *J Neurosci.* 19:6930–6941.

Duffy SN, Craddock KJ, Abel T, Nguyen PV. 2001. Environmental enrichment modifies the PKA-dependence of hippocampal LTP and improves hippocampus-dependent memory. *Learn Mem.* 8:26–34

Flor H, Elbert T, Knetcht S et al. 1995. Phantom-limb pain as a perceptual correlate of cortical reorganization following arm amputation. *Nature.* 375:482–484.

Flor H, Nikolajsen L, Jensen TS. 2006. Phantom limb pain: a case of maladaptive CNS plasticity? *Nat Rev Neurosci.* 7(11):873–81.

Florence SL, Taub HB, Kaas JH. 1998. Large-scale sprouting of cortical connections after peripheral injury in adult macaque monkeys. *Science.* 282:1117–1121

Gebhart GF. 1986. Modulatory effects of descending systems on spinal dorsal horn neurons, In TL. Yaksh, ed. *Spinal Afferent Processing.* New York: Plenum Press, 391–426.

Gebhart GF, Randich A. 1990. Brainstem modulation of nociception, In WR. Klemm and RP. Vettes, eds. *Brainstem Mechanisms of Behavior.* Wiley and Sons: New York, 315–352.

Grudt TJ, Williams JT, Travagli RA. 1995. Inhibition by 5-hydroxytryptamine and noradrenaline in substantia gelatinosa of guinea-pig spinal trigeminal nucleus. *J Physiol.* 485:113–120.

Hori Y, Endo K, Takahashi T. 1996. Long-lasting synaptic facilitation induced by serotonin in superficial dorsal horn neurones of the rat spinal cord. *J Physiol.* 492:867–876.

Hutchison WD, Davis KD, Lozano AM, Tasker RR, Dostrovsky JO. 1999. Pain-related neurons in the human cingulate cortex. *Nat Neurosci.* 2:403–405.

Ikeda H, Heinke B, Ruscheweyh R, Sandkuhler J. 2003. Synaptic plasticity in spinal lamina I projection neurons that mediate hyperalgesia. *Science.* 299:1237–1240.

Jasmin L, Rabkin S, Granato A, Boudah A, Ohara P. 2003. Analgesia and hyperalgesia from GABA-mediated modulation of the cerebral cortex. *Nature.* 424(6946): 316–320

Ji RR, Kohno T, Moore KA, Woolf CJ. 2003. Central sensitization and LTP: do pain and memory share similar mechanisms? *Trends Neurosci.* 26:696–705.

Johansen JP, Fields HL, Manning BH. 2002. The affective component of pain in rodents: direct evidence for a contribution of the anterior cingulated cortex. *Proc Natl Acad Sci U S A.* 98:8077–8082.

Jones EG, Pons TP. 1998. Thalamic and brainstem contributions to large-scale plasticity of primate somatosensory cortex. *Science.* 282:1121–1125.

Kaas JH. 1998. Phantoms of the brain. *Nature.* 391:331–333

Kaas JH, Florence SL, Jain N. 1999. Subcortical contributions to massive cortical reorganizations. *Neuron.* 22:657–660.

Kempermann G, Kuhn HG, Gage FH. 1997. More hippocampal neurons in adult mice living in an enriched environment. *Nature.* 386:493–495

Kerchner GA, Wei F, Wang G-D et al. 2001. 'smart' mice feel more pain, or are they just better learners? *Nat Neurosci.* 4:453–454.

Kerchner GA, Wang GD, Qiu C-S, Huettner JE, Zhuo M. 2001a. Direct presynaptic regulation of GABA/Glycine release by kainate receptors in the dorsal horn: an ionotropic mechanism. *Neuron.* 32:477–488.

Kerchner GA, Wilding TJ, Li P, Zhuo M, Huettner JE. 2001b. Presynaptic kainate receptors regulate spinal sensory transmission. *J Neuroscience.* 21:59–66.

Kerchner GA, Wilding TJ, Huettner JE, Zhuo M. 2002. Kainate receptor subunits underlying presynaptic regulation of transmission release in the dorsal horn. *J Neuroscience.* 22:8010–8017.

Kohno T, Kumamoto E, Higashi H, Shimoji K, Yoshimura M. 1999. Actions of opioids on excitatory and inhibitory transmission in substantia gelatinosa of adult at spinal cord. *J Physiol.* 518:803–813.

Lee DE, Kim SJ, Zhuo M. 1999. Comparison of behavioral responses to noxious cold and heat in mice. *Brain Res.* 845:117–121.

Li P, Calejesan AA, Zhuo M. 1998. ATP P_{2X} receptors and sensory transmission between primary afferent fibers and spinal dorsal horn neurons in rats. *J Neurophysiol.* 80:3356–3360.

Li P, Zhuo M. 1998. Silent glutamatergic synapses and nociception in mammalian spinal cord. *Nature.* 393:695–698.

Li P, Wilding TJ, Kim SJ, Calejesan AA, Huettner JE, Zhuo M. 1999a. Kainate-receptor-mediated sensory synaptic transmission in mammalian spinal cord. *Nature.* 397:161–164.

Li P, Kerchner GA, Sala C et al. 1999b. AMPA receptor-PDZ protein interaction mediate synaptic plasticity in spinal cord. *Nat Neurosci.* 2:972–977.

Li P, Zhuo M. 2001. Substance P and neurokinin A mediate sensory synaptic transmission in young rat dorsal horn neurons. *Brain Res Bull.* 55:521–531.

Liauw J, Wang GD, Zhuo M. 2003. NMDA receptors contribute to synaptic transmission in anterior cingulate cortex of adult mice. *Sheng Li Xue Bao.* 55:373–380.

Liauw J, Wu LJ, Zhuo M. 2005. Calcium-stimulated adenylyl cyclases required for long-term potentiation in the anterior cingulate cortex. *J Neurophysiol.* 94:878–882.

Lorenz J, Kohlhoff H, Hansen HC, Kunze K, Bromm B. 1998. Abeta-fiber mediated activation of cingulate cortex as correlate of central post-stroke pain. *Neuroreport.* 9:659–663.

Lumpkin EA, Caterina MJ. 2007. Mechanisms of sensory transduction in the skin. *Nature.* 445:858–865.

Malcangio M, Bowery NG. 1996. GABA and its receptors in the spinal cord. *Trends Pharmacol Sci.* 17, 457–462.

Malinow R, Malenka RC. 2002. AMPA receptor trafficking and synaptic plasticity. *Annu Rev Neurosci.* 25:103–126.

McKemy DD. 2005. How cold is it? TRPM8 and TRPA1 in the molecular logic of cold sensation. *Mol Pain.* 1:16.

Merzenich MM, Nelson RJ, Stryker MP, Cynader MS, Schoppmann A, Zook JM. 1984. Somatosensory cortical map changes following digit amputation in adult monkeys. *J Comp Neurol.* 224:591–605.

Merzenich M. 1998. Long-term change of mind. *Science.* 282:1062–1063.

Nakatsuka T, Gu JG. 2001. ATP P2X receptor-mediated enhancement of glutamate release and evoked EPSCs in dorsal horn neurons of the rat spinal cord. *J Neurosci.* 21:6522–6531.

Nakatsuka T, Furue H, Yoshimura M, Gu JG. 2002. Activation of central terminal vanilloid receptor-1 receptors and alpha beta-methylene-ATP-sensitive P2X receptors reveals a converged synaptic activity onto the deep dorsal horn neurons of the spinal cord. *J Neurosci.* 22:1228–1237.

Neumann S, Doubell TP, Leslie T, Woolf CJ. 1996. Inflammatory pain hypersensitivity mediated by phenotypic switch in myelinated primary sensory neurons. *Nature.* 384:360–364.

Passafaro M, Piech V, Sheng M. 2001. Subunit-specific temporal and spatial patterns of AMPA receptor exocytosis in hippocampal neurons. *Nat Neurosci.* 4:917–926.

Pons TP, Garraghty PE, Ommaya AK, Kaas JH, Taub E, Mishkin M. 1991. Massive cortical reorganization after sensory deafferentation in adult macaques. *Science.* 252:1857–1860.

Popratiloff A, Weinberg RJ, Rustioni A. 1996. AMPA receptor subunits underlying terminals of fine-caliber primary afferent fibers. *J Neurosci.* 16:3363–3372.

Porreca F, Ossipov MH, Gebhart GF. 2002. Chronic pain and medullary descending facilitation. *Trends Neurosci.* 25:319–325.

Rainville P, Duncan GH, Price DD, Carrier B, Bushnell MC. 1997. Pain affect encoded in human anterior cingulate but not somatosensory cortex. *Science.* 277:968–971.

Rainville P, Bushnell MC, Duncan GH. 2001. Representation of acute and persistent pain in the human CNS: potential implications for chemical intolerance. *Ann N Y Acad Sci.* 933:130–141.

Ramachandran VS, Rogers-Ramachandran DC, Stewart M. 1992. Perceptual correlates of massive cortical reorganization. *Science.* 258:1159–1160.

Ramachandran VS, Rogers-Ramachandran DC, Cobb S. 1995. Touching the phantom limb. *Nature.* 377:489–490

Rampon C, Tang YP, Goodhouse J, Shimizu E, Kyin M, Tsien JZ. 2000. Enrichment induces structural changes and recovery from nonspatial memory deficits in CA1 NMDAR1-knockout mice. *Nat Neurosci.* 3:238–244

Ribeiro-da-Silva A, Coimbra A. 1982. Two types of synaptic glomeruli and their distribution in laminae I–III of the rat spinal cord. *J Comp Neurol.* 209:176–186.

Robinson DA, Wei F, Wang GD et al. 2002a. Oxytocin mediates stress-induced analgesia. *J Physiol. (Lond).* 540:593–606.

Robinson D, Calejesan AA, Zhuo M. 2002b. Long-lasting changes in rostral ventral medulla neuronal activity following inflammation. *J Pain.* 3:292–300.

Robinson DA, Calejesan AA, Wei F, Gebhart GF, Zhuo M. 2004. Endogenous facilitation: from molecular mechanisms to persistent pain. *Curr Neurovasc Res.* 1:11–20.

Shumyatsky GP, Tsvetkov E, Malleret G et al. 2002. Identification of a signaling network in lateral nucleus of amygdala important for inhibiting memory specifically related to learned fear. *Cell.* 111:905–918

Sikes RW, Vogt BA. 1992. Nociceptive neurons in area 24 of rabbit cingulate cortex. *J Neurophysiol.* 68:1720–1732.

Song I, Huganir RL. 2002. Regulation of AMPA receptors during synaptic plasticity. *Trends Neurosci.* 25:578–588.

Sun YG, Chen ZF. 2007. A gastrin-releasing peptide receptor mediates the itch sensation in the spinal cord. *Nature.* 448:700–703.

Tachibana M, Wenthold RJ, Morioka H, Petralia RS. 1994. Light and electron microscopic immunocytochemical localization of AMPA-selective glutamate receptors in the rat spinal cord. *J Comp Neurol.* 344:431–454.

Talbot JD, Marrett S, Evans AC, Meyer E, Bushnell MC, Duncan GH. 1991. Multiple representations of pain in human cerebral cortex. *Science.* 251:1355–1358.

Tang YP, Xhimizu E, Dube GR et al. 1999. Genetic enhancement of learning and memory in mice. *Nature.* 401:63–69.

Tang J, Ko S, Ding HK, Qiu CS, Calejesan AA, and Zhuo, M. 2005. Pavlovian fear memory induced by activation in the anterior cingulate cortex. *Mol Pain.* 1, 6.

Tao YX, Rumbaugh G, Wang GD et al. 2003. Impaired NMDA receptor-mediated postsynaptic function and blunted NMDA receptor-dependent persistent pain in mice lacking postsynaptic density-93 protein. *J Neurosci.* 23:6703–6712.

Todd AJ. 1996. GABA and glycine in synaptic glomeruli of the rat spinal dorsal horn. *Eur J Neurosci.* 8:2492–2498.

Toyoda H, Wu LJ, Zhao MG, Xu H, Zhuo M. 2007a. Time-dependent postsynaptic AMPA GluR1 receptor recruitment in the cingulate synaptic potentiation. *Dev Neurobiol.* 67:498–509.

Toyoda H, Wu LJ, Zhao MG, Xu H, Jia Z, Zhuo M. 2007b. Long-term depression requires postsynaptic AMPA GluR2 receptor in adult mouse cingulate cortex. *J Cell Physiol.* 211:336–343.

Travagli RA, Williams JT. 1996. Endogenous monoamines inhibit glutamate transmission in the spinal trigeminal nucleus of the guinea-pig. *J Physiol.* 491:177–185.

Urban MO, Gebhart GF. 1999. Supraspinal contributions to hyperalgesia. *Proc Natl Acad Sci U S A.* 96:7687–7692.

van Praag H, Christie BR, Sejnowski TJ, Gage FH. 1999. Running enhances neurogenesis, learning, and long-term potentiation in mice. *Proc Natl Acad Sci U S A.* 96:13427–13431.

Wei F, Li P, Zhuo M. 1999. Loss of synaptic depression in mammalian anterior cingulate cortex after amputation. *J Neurosci.* 19:9346–9354.

Wei F, Dubner R, Ren K. 1999. Dorsolateral funiculus-lesions unmask inhibitory or disfacilitatory mechanisms which modulate the effects of innocuous mechanical stimulation on spinal Fos expression after inflammation. *Brain Res.* 820:112–116.

Wei F, Wang GD, Kerchner GA et al. 2001. Genetic enhancement of inflammatory pain by forebrain NR2B over-expression. *Nat Neurosci.* 4:164–169.

Wei F, Zhuo M. 2001. Potentiation of synaptic responses in the anterior cingulate cortex following digital amputation in rat. *J Physiol. (Lond.).* 532:823–833.

Wang GD, Zhuo M. 2002. Synergistic enhancement of glutamate-mediated responses by serotonin and forskolin in adult mouse spinal dorsal horn neurons. *J Neurophysiol.* 87:732–739.

Wei F, Qiu CS, Kim SJ et al. 2002a. Genetic elimination of behavioral sensitization in mice lacking calmodulin-stimulated adenylyl cyclases. *Neuron.* 36:713–726.

Wei F, Qiu CS, Liauw J et al. 2002b. Calcium calmodulin-dependent protein kinase IV is required for fear memory. *Nat Neurosci.* 6:573–579.

Wei F, Vadakkan KI, Toyoda H et al. 2006. Calcium calmodulin-stimulated adenylyl cyclases contribute to activation of extracellular signal-regulated kinase in spinal dorsal horn neurons in adult rats and mice. *J Neurosci.* 26:851–861.

Williams BM, Luo Y, Ward C et al. 2001. Environmental enrichment: effects on spatial memory and hippocampal CREB immunoreactivity. *Physiol Behav.* 73:649–658.

Willis WD Jr. 1988. Anatomy and physiology of descending control of nociceptive responses of dorsal horn neurons: comprehensive review. *Prog Brain Res.* 77:1–29.

Willis WD. 2002. Long-term potentiation in spinothalamic neurons. *Brain Res Brain Res Rev.* 40:202–214.

Woolf CJ, Shortland P, Coggeshall RE. 1992. Peripheral nerve injury triggers central sprouting of myelinated afferents. *Nature.* 355:75–78.

Woolf CJ, Salter MW. 2000. Neuronal plasticity: increasing the gain in pain. *Science.* 288:1765–1769.

Wu LJ, Toyoda H, Zhao MG et al. 2005. Upregulation of forebrain NMDA NR2B receptors contributes to behavioral sensitization after inflammation. *J Neurosci.* 25:11107–11116.

Xu H, Wu LJ, Zhao MG et al. 2006. Presynaptic regulation of the inhibitory transmission by GluR5-containing kainate receptors in spinal substantia gelatinosa. *Mol Pain.* 2:29.

Yoshimura M, North RA. 1983. Substantia gelatinosa neurones hyperpolarized in vitro by enkephalin. *Nature.* 305:529–530.

Zeng H, Gragerov A, Hohmann JG et al. 2006. Neuromedin U receptor 2-deficient mice display differential responses in sensory perception, stress, and feeding. *Mol Cell Biol.* 26:9352–9363.

Zhao MG, Toyoda H, Lee YS et al. 2005. Roles of NMDA NR2B subtype receptor in prefrontal long-term potentiation and contextual fear memory. *Neuron.* 47:859–872.

Zhao MG, Ko SW, Wu LJ et al. 2006. Enhanced presynaptic neurotransmitter release in the anterior cingulate cortex of mice with chronic pain. *J Neurosci.* 26:8923–8930.

Zhuo M. 2000. Silent glutamatergic synapses and long-term facilitation in spinal dorsal horn neurons. *Prog. Brain Res.* 129:101–113.

Zhuo M. 2002. Glutamate receptors and persistent pain: targeting forebrain NR2B subunits. *Drug Discov Today.* 7:259–267.

Zhuo M. 2003. Synaptic and molecular mechanisms for pain and memory. *Acta Physiologica Sinica.* 55:1–8.

Zhuo M. 2007. *"Descending Facilitation," Encyclopedia of Pain.* CD-ROM, Springer Reference: Springer.

Zhuo M, Gebhart GF. 1990a. Characterization of descending inhibition and facilitation from the nuclei reticularis gigantocellularis and gigantocellularis pars alpha in the rat. *Pain.* 42:337–350.

Zhuo M, Gebhart GF. 1990b. Spinal cholinergic and monoaminergic receptors mediate descending inhibition from the nuclei reticularis gigantocellularis and gigantocellularis pars alpha in the rat. *Brain Res.* 535:67–78.

Zhuo M, Gebhart GF. 1991. Spinal serotonin receptors mediate descending inhibition and facilitation from the nuclei reticularis gigantocellularis and gigantocellularis pars alpha in the rat. *Brain Res.* 550:35–48.

Zhuo M, Gebhart GF. 1992. Characterization of descending facilitation and inhibition of spinal nociceptive transmission from the nuclei reticularis gigantocellularis and gigantocellularis pars alpha in the rat. *J Neurophysiol.* 67:1599–1614.

Zhuo M, Gebhart GF. 1997. Biphasic modulation of spinal nociceptive transmission from the medullary raphe nuclei in the rat. *J Neurophysiol.* 78:746–758.

Zhuo M, Small SA, Kandel ER, Hawkins RD. 1993. Nitric oxide and carbon monoxide produce activity-dependent long-term synaptic enhancement in hippocampus. *Science.* 260:1946–1950.

Zhuo M, Hu Y, Schultz C, Kandel ER, Hawkins RD. 1994. Role of guanylyl cyclase and cGMP-dependent protein kinase in long-term potentiation in hippocampus. *Nature.* 368:635–639.

Zhuo M, Gebhart GF. 1997. Biphasic modulation of spinal nociceptive transmission from the medullary raphe nuclei in the rat. *J Neurophysiol.* 78:746–758.

Zhuo M, Sengupta, JN, Gebhart GF. 2002. Biphasic modulation of spinal visceral nociceptive transmission from the rostroventral medial medulla in the rat. *J Neurophysiol.* 87:2225–2236.

Zhuo M, Gebhart GF. 2002. Modulation of noxious and non-noxious spinal mechanical transmission from the rostral medial medulla in the rat. *J Neurophysiol.* 88:2928–2941.

Chapter 7

PHYSIOLOGICAL EFFECTS AND DISEASE MANIFESTATIONS OF PERFORMANCE-ENHANCING ANDROGENIC–ANABOLIC STEROIDS, GROWTH HORMONE, AND INSULIN

Michael R. Graham, Julien S. Baker, Peter Evans, and Bruce Davies

ABSTRACT

Anabolic–androgenic steroids (AASs) were the first identified doping agents and can be used to increase muscle mass and strength in adult males. Despite successful detection and convictions by sporting antidoping agencies, they are still being used to increase physical performance and improve appearance. Their use does not appear to be diminishing. The adverse side effects and potential dangers of AAS use have been well documented. Recent epidemiological research has identified that the designer drugs, growth hormone (GH) and insulin, are also being used because of the belief that they improve sporting performance. GH and insulin are currently undetectable by urinalysis. The objective of this chapter is to summarize the classification of these drugs, their prevalence, and patterns of use. The physiology of GH and its pathophysiology in the disease states of deficiency and excess and in catabolic states has been discussed and a distinction made on the different effects between therapeutic use in replacement and abuse in a sporting context. The history, physiology, and pathophysiology of insulin in therapeutic replacement and its abuse in a sporting context have also been identified. A suggestion has been made on potential mechanisms of the effects of the designer drugs GH and insulin.

Keywords: abuse, drugs, GH, insulin, steroids.

WHAT ARE ANABOLIC–ANDROGENIC STEROIDS?

Anabolic–androgenic steroids (AASs) are a group of synthetic compounds similar in chemical structure to the natural anabolic steroid testosterone (T) (Fig. 7.1) (Haupt, Rovere 1984). T, the predominant circulating testicular androgen, is both an active hormone and a prohormone for the formation of a more active androgen, the 5α-reduced steroid dihydrotestosterone (DHT). Physiological studies of steroid hormone metabolism in the postnatal state demonstrated that DHT is formed in target tissues from circulating T and is a more potent androgen than T in several bioassay systems (Wilson, Leihy, Shaw et al. 2002).

Genetic evidence indicates that these two androgens work via a common intracellular receptor. The androgen receptor (AR) is an intracellular ligand-dependent protein that modulates the expression of genes and mediates biological actions of physiological androgens (T and 5α-DHT) in a cell-specific manner (Janne, Palvimo, Kallio et al. 1993).

During embryonic life, androgens cause the formation of the male urogenital tract and hence are responsible for development of the tissues that serve as the major sites of androgen action in postnatal life.

It has been generally assumed that androgens virilize the male fetus by the same mechanisms as in the adult, namely, by the conversion of circulating T to DHT in target tissues.

A role for steroid 5α-reduction in androgen action became apparent with the findings in 1968 that DHT, the 5α-reduced derivative of T, is formed in many androgen target tissues where it binds to the AR (Bruchovsky, Wilson 1968).

DHT binds to the AR more tightly than T, primarily as a result of stabilization of the AR complex and at low concentrations is as effective as T is at high concentrations in enhancing the transcription of one response element (Deslypere, Young, Wilson et al. 1992). This finding clearly indicated that some effects of DHT are the result of amplification of the T signal.

Loss of function mutations of the *steroid 5α-reductase 2* gene impairs virilization of the urogenital sinus and external genitalia in males (Wilson, Griffin, Russell et al. 1993).

In summary, DHT formation both acts as a general amplifier of androgen action and conveys specific function to the androgen–AR complex. The mechanism by which the specific function is mediated is unknown.

The enzyme aromatase controls the androgen/estrogen ratio by catalyzing the conversion of T into estradiol (E2). Therefore, the regulation of E2 synthesis by aromatase is thought to be critical in sexual development and differentiation (Kroon, Munday, Westcott et al. 2005).

Synthetic T was first synthesized from cholesterol in 1935 (Ruckzika, Wettstein, Kaegi 1935). T is synthesized by the interstitial Leydig cells of the testes, which are primarily under the control of the gonadotrophins secreted by the pituitary gland.

Approximately 95% of circulating T originates directly from testicular secretion (Ruckzika, Wettstein, Kaegi 1935). Following secretion, T is then transported via the blood to target organs and specific receptor sites. The bodily functions which are under

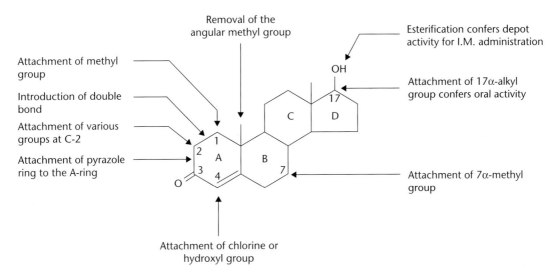

Figure 7.1 The structure of testosterone. The structural modifications to the A- and B-rings of this steroid increase the anabolic activity; substitution at carbon atom position 17 (C-17) confers oral activity. I.M., intramuscular. Reproduced with kind permission from Annals of Clinical Biochemistry 2003; 40:321–356.

direct control of T that have relevance to the athlete can be divided into two broad classifications:

1. Androgenic functions—male hormonal effects (male-characteristic determining)
2. Anabolic functions—constructive or muscle building

The clinical advantages of a pure anabolic agent were recognized many years ago and work was undertaken by a number of drug companies to modify the T molecule with a view to maximizing the anabolic effect and minimizing the androgenic activity (Hershberger, Shipley, Meyer 1953). Some of the structural modifications to testosterone to dissociate the anabolic from the androgenic effects are shown in Figure 7.1. The extent of the dissociation differs depending on the modification but there is no AAS that has an anabolic effect in an athlete without an androgenic effect (Di Pasquale 1990).

DOPING IN SPORT

AASs were the first identified doping agents to be banned in sport by the International Olympic Committee (IOC) Medical Commission in Athens in 1961. Evidence suggests that they increase muscle mass and strength and are abused to increase physical performance and improve appearance (Bhasin et al. 1996). The adverse side effects and potential dangers of AAS abuse are well documented (Ferenchick, Hirokawa, Mammen et al. 1995).

The prevalence of AAS use has risen dramatically over the last two decades and has filtered into all aspects of society. Subsequent published work indicated the concomitant abuse of recombinant human growth hormone (rhGH) and insulin (Grace, Baker, Davies 2001). Sportspersons are taking rhGH and insulin, separately or in combination, as doping agents to increase skeletal muscle mass and improve performance (Ehrnborg, Bengtsson, Rosen 2000; Jenkins 2001; Sonksen 2001).

Contemporary research has assessed the effects of taking supraphysiological levels of rhGH, but has not assessed the effects of taking rhGH and insulin in combination in a sporting context. Recent research suggests that rhGH administration in AAS abstinence may indeed improve sporting performance (Graham, Davies, Hullin et al. 2007b; Graham, Baker, Evans et al. 2008).

THE PREVALENCE OF ANABOLIC–ANDROGENIC STEROID ABUSE

A questionnaire study conducted by Perry and Littlepage (1992) found that 39% of 160 respondents were regular AAS abusers.

In 1993, a report investigating abuse of AASs in 21 gymnasia in England, Scotland, and Wales found that 119 (9.1%) of the 1310 male respondents to the questionnaire and 8 (2.3%) of the 349 female respondents had taken AASs. The youngest abuser was aged 16. The prevalence of abuse of AASs in the gymnasia ranged from 0% (in three gymnasia) to 46% (28 of 61 respondents). The response rate to the questionnaire was 59% (1677/2834) (Korkia, Stimson 1993).

In 1997, 100 AAS-using athletes were surveyed and high rates of polypharmacy (80%) with a wide array of drug abuse were reported among this sample group (Evans 1997).

Another study in 1996 examined AAS abuse among 176 abusers (171 men and 5 women) and highlighted that 37% of respondents indicated a need for more knowledge of drug effects among drug workers and a less prejudiced attitude against drug dependency from general practitioners (Pates, Barry 1996).

In 2001, 69% of 107 respondents of hardcore weight lifters were identified as abusing AASs, highlighting that AAS abuse was certainly not on the decline (Grace, Baker, Davies 2001). Recent surveys conducted by Baker et al. (2006) and Parkinson and Evans (2006) have estimated that AASs are being abused by more than 1 million UK citizens and more than 3 million Americans.

PREVALENCE AND PATTERNS OF GROWTH HORMONE AND INSULIN ABUSE

GH appeared in the underground doping literature in 1981 (Duchaine 1983). Insulin-dependent diabetics are selling insulin pen-fills on the black market to bodybuilders. Unused aliquots are being resold, with the added risk of needle sharing and potential HIV and hepatitis C infection.

Extensive literature research identifies very few cases of rhGH or insulin abuse by athletes. The few cases of rhGH abuse that have been published are case histories of individuals who have been arrested in possession at international tournaments. The possession of rhGH by the Chinese swimmers bound for the 1998 World Swimming Championships and similar problems at the Tour de France cycling event in 1998 suggested abuse at an elite level (Wallace, Cuneo, Baxter et al. 1999). Approximately 1500 vials were stolen from an Australian wholesale chemist 6 months before the Sydney Olympics in 2000 (Sonksen 2001). The few cases of insulin abuse that have been highlighted are those that have been admitted to hospital following accidental overdose (Konrad, Schupfer, Wietlisbach et al. 1998; Evans, Lynch 2003). Dawson (2001) reports that 10% of 450 patients attending his needle-exchange programme self-prescribe insulin for nontherapeutic purposes. The covert nature of its abuse precludes exact figures.

A recent questionnaire survey by Baker et al. (2006) has shown an increase in the abuse of insulin from 8% to 14% and an increase in the abuse of growth hormone (GH) from 6% to 24% in comparison to a survey conducted by Grace et al. (2001).

HISTORY OF GROWTH HORMONE

Physiological Aspects

A cascade of interacting transcription factors and genetic elements normally determines the ability of the somatotroph cells in the anterior pituitary to synthesize and secrete the polypeptide human growth hormone (hGH). The development and proliferation of somatotrophs are largely determined by a gene called the *Prophet of Pit-1 (PROP1)*, which controls the embryonic development of cells of the Pit-1 (POU1F1) transcription factor lineage. Pit-1 binds to the GH promoter within the cell nucleus, a step that leads to the development and proliferation of somatotrophs and GH transcription. Once translated, GH is secreted as a 191–amino acid, 4-helix bundle protein (70% to 80%) and a less abundant 176–amino acid form (20% to 30%), (Baumann 1991; Wu, Bidlingmaier, Dall et al. 1999) entering the circulation in a pulsatile manner under dual hypothalamic control through hypothalamic-releasing and hypothalamic-inhibiting hormones that traverse the hypophysial portal system and act directly on specific somatotroph surface receptors (Melmed 2006).

Growth hormone–releasing hormone (GHRH) induces the synthesis and secretion of GH, and somatostatin suppresses the secretion of GH. GH is also regulated by ghrelin, a GH secretagogue–receptor ligand (Kojima, Hosoda, Date et al. 1999) that is synthesized mainly in the gastrointestinal tract (GIT).

In healthy persons, the GH level is usually undetectable (<0.2 µg/L) throughout most of the day. There are approximately 10 intermittent pulses of GH per 24 hours, most often at night, when the level can be as high as 30 µg/L (Melmed 2006).

Fasting increases the secretion of GH, whereas aging and obesity are associated with suppressed secretory bursts of the hormone (Iranmanesh, Lizarralde, Velduis et al. 1991).

The action of GH is mediated by a GH receptor, which is expressed mainly in the liver and in cartilage and is composed of preformed dimers that undergo conformational change when occupied by a GH ligand, promoting signaling (Brown, Adams, Pelekanos et al. 2005).

Cleavage of the GH receptor also yields a circulating GH-binding protein (GHBP), which prolongs the half-life and mediates the cellular transport of GH. GH activates the GH receptor, to which the intracellular Janus kinase 2 (JAK2) tyrosine kinase binds. Both the receptor and JAK2 protein are phosphorylated, and signal transducers and activators of transcription (STAT) proteins bind to this complex. STAT proteins are then phosphorylated and translocated to the nucleus, which initiates transcription of GH target proteins (Argetsinger, Campbell, Yang et al. 1993).

Intracellular GH signaling is suppressed by several proteins, especially the suppressors of cytokine signaling (SOCS). GH induces the synthesis of peripheral insulin-like growth factor 1 (IGF-1) (Le Roith, Scavo, Butler 2001) and both circulating (endocrine) and local (autocrine and paracrine) IGF-1 induce cell proliferation and inhibit apoptosis (O'Reilly, Rojo, She et al. 2006).

IGF-binding proteins (IGFBP) and their proteases regulate the access of ligands to the IGF-1 receptor, either enhancing or attenuating the action of IGF-1. Levels of IGF-1 are at the highest during late adolescence and decline throughout adulthood; these levels are determined by sex and genetic factors (Milani, Carmichael, Welkowitz et al. 2004). The production of IGF-1 is suppressed in malnourished patients as well as in patients with liver disease, hypothyroidism, or poorly controlled diabetes. IGF-1 levels usually reflect the secretory activity of GH and IGF-1 is one of a number of potential markers for identification of rhGH administration in sport (Powrie, Bassett, Rosen et al. 2007).

In conjunction with GH, IGF-1 has varying differential effects on protein, glucose, lipid, and calcium metabolism (Mauras, Attie, Reiter et al. 2000), and therefore, on body composition. Direct effects result from the interaction of GH with its specific receptors on target cells. In the adipocyte, GH stimulates the cell to break down triglyceride (TG) and suppresses its ability to uptake and accumulate circulating lipids. Indirect effects are mediated primarily by IGF-1. Many of the growth-promoting effects of GH are due to the action of IGF-1 on its target cells. In most tissues, IGF-1 has local autocrine and paracrine actions, but the liver actively secretes IGF-1 and its binding proteins into the circulation (Mauras, Attie, Reiter et al. 2000). Little is known about the expression of skeletal muscle–specific isoforms of *IGF-1* gene in response to exercise in humans or about the influence of age and physical training status. Greig et al. (2006) reported that a single bout of isometric exercise stimulated the expression of mRNA for the IGF-1 splice variants IGF-1Ea and IGF-1Ec (mechano growth factor [MGF]) within 2.5 hours, which lasts for at least 2 days after exercise.

GROWTH HORMONE DEFICIENCY

The therapeutic indications for rhGH in the United Kingdom are controlled by the National Institute for Clinical Excellence guidelines (May 2002), which has recommended treatment with rhGH for children with

- Growth disturbance in short children born small for gestational age
- Proven growth hormone deficiency (GHD)
- Gonadal dysgenesis (Turner's syndrome)
- Prader–Willi syndrome
- Chronic renal insufficiency before puberty (renal function decreased to less than 50%)

NICE (2003) has recommended rhGH in adults only if the following three criteria are fulfilled:

1. Severe GHD established by an appropriate method
2. Impaired quality of life (QoL) measured by means of a specific questionnaire
3. Already receiving treatment for another pituitary hormone deficiency

Adult-onset growth hormone (A-OGH)–deficient individuals are overweight, with reduced lean body mass (LBM) (Salomon, Cuneo, Hesp et al. 1989; Amato, Carella, Fazio et al. 1993; Beshyah, Freemantle, Shahi et al. 1995) and increased fat mass (FM), especially abdominal adiposity (Salomon, Cuneo, Hesp et al. 1989; Bengtsson, Eden, Lonn et al. 1993; Amato, Carella, Fazio et al. 1993; Beshyah, Freemantle, Shahi et al. 1995; Snel, Doerga, Brummer et al. 1995). They have reduced total body water (Black 1972) and reduced bone mass (Kaufman, Taelman, Vermeuelen et al. 1992; O'Halloran, Tsatsoulis, Whitehouse et al. 1993; Holmes, Economou, Whitehouse et al. 1994). There is also reduced strength and exercise capacity (Cuneo, Salomon, Wiles et al. 1990; Cuneo, Salomon, Wiles et al. 1991a; Cuneo, Salomon, Wiles et al. 1991b), reduced cardiac performance, and an altered substrate metabolism (Binnerts, Swart, Wilson et al. 1992; Fowelin, Attvall, Lager et al. 1993; Russell-Jones, Weissberger, Bowes et al. 1993; O'Neal, Kalfas, Dunning et al. 1994; Hew, Koschmann, Christopher et al. 1996). This leads to an abnormal lipid profile (Cuneo, Salomon, Wiles et al. 1993; Rosen, Edén S, Larson et al. 1993; De Boer, Blok, Voerman et al. 1994; Attanasio, Lamberts, Matranga et al. 1997) that can predispose to the development of cardiovascular disease (CVD). A-OGH deficiency reduces psychological well-being and QoL (Stabler, Turner, Girdler et al. 1992; Rosen, Wiren, Wilhelmsen et al. 1994). The prescription of rhGH is currently being used successfully to treat this deficiency.

GROWTH HORMONE EXCESS

GH excess results in the clinical condition known as acromegaly. This condition is presented as a consequence of a pituitary tumor (Table 7.1) characterized by a multitude of signs and symptoms (Table 7.2). Pituitary tumors account for approximately 15% of primary intracranial tumors (Melmed 2006). Acromegalics have an increased risk of diabetes mellitus (DM), hypertension, and premature mortality due to CVD (Bengtsson, Eden, Lonn et al. 1993). The nontherapeutic abuse of rhGH by bodybuilders and sportspersons can predispose an individual to the same side effects as are seen in acromegaly, which would appear to be dose dependent. Bodybuilders are known to take supraphysiological doses of as much as 30 IU of rhGH per day (personal communications), though the average doses abused are much less (Graham, Baker, Evans et al. 2007a; Graham, Davies, Hullin et al. 2007b; Graham, Davies, Hullin et al. 2007c).

The most common side effects following administration arise from sodium and water retention. Weight gain, dependent edema, a sensation of tightness in the hands and feet, or carpal tunnel syndrome can frequently occur within days (Hoffman, Crampton, Sernia 1996).

Arthralgia (joint pain), involving small or large joints can occur, but there is usually no evidence of effusion, inflammation, or X-ray changes (Salomon, Cuneo, Hesp et al. 1989). Muscle pains can also occur. GH administration is documented to result in hyperinsulinemia (Hussain, Schmitz, Mengel et al. 1993), which may increase the risk of cardiovascular complications. GH-induced hypertension (Salomon, Cuneo, Hesp et al. 1989) and atrial fibrillation (Bengtsson, Eden, Lonn et al. 1993) have both been reported but are rare. There have also been reports of cerebral side effects, such as encephalocele (Salomon, Cuneo, Hesp et al. 1989) and headache with tinnitus (Bengtsson,

Table 7.1 Growth Hormone Excess (Acromegaly)

Primary Growth Hormone Excess	Extra-Pituitary Growth Hormone Excess	Growth Hormone-Releasing Hormone Excess
Pituitary adenoma	Pancreatic islet cell tumor	**Central** Hypothalamic tumor
Pituitary carcinoma	Lymphoma	**Peripheral** Bronchial Pancreatic Lung Adrenal Thyroid
Extra-pituitary tumor	Iatrogenic	
Familial syndromes		

Table 7.2 Clinical Features of Acromegaly

Local Tumor Effects	Somatic Systems	Skin	Cardiovascular System	Pulmonary System	Gastrointestinal System	Visceromegaly	Endocrine and Metabolic Systems
Enlarged Pituitary	Acral enlargement (thickness of soft tissue of hands and feet) Musculoskeletal system	Hyper-hydrosis	Left ventricular hypertrophy	Enlarged pituitary	Colon polyps	Tongue	Reproduction
Visual field defects	Gigantism	Oily texture	Asymmetric septal hypertrophy	Visual field defects		Thyroid gland	Multiple endocrine neoplasia type 1
Cranial-nerve palsy	Prognathism/Jaw malocclusion	Skin tags	Cardiomyopathy	Cranial nerve palsy		Salivary glands	Carbohydrate tolerance Insulin resistance and hyperinsulinemia Diabetes mellitus
Headache	Arthralgias and arthritis		Hypertension	Headache		Liver	Lipid hypertriglyceridemia
	Carpal tunnel syndrome/ acroparesthesia		Congestive heart failure			Spleen	Mineral hypercalciuria, increased levels of 25-hydroxyvitamin D3 and urinary hydroxyproline
	Hypertrophy of frontal bones					Kidney	Electrolyte Low renin levels Increased aldosterone levels
	Proximal myopathy					Prostate	Thyroid Low thyroxine binding–globulin levels Goiter

Eden, Lonn et al. 1993) and benign intracranial hypertension (Malozowski, Tanner, Wysowski et al. 1993). Cessation of GH therapy is associated with regression of side effects in most cases (Malozowski, Tanner, Wysowski et al. 1993).

THE EFFECTS OF GROWTH HORMONE ON THE HOSPITAL ANXIETY AND DEPRESSION SCALE QUESTIONNAIRE

More than 200 published studies worldwide have reported experiences with the Hospital Anxiety and Depression Scale (HADS) questionnaire, which was specifically developed by Zigmond and Snaith (1983) for use with physically ill patients. The questionnaire consists of 14 questions: 7 questions are related to anxiety and 7 questions are related to depression. Each item is rated from a score of 0 to 3, depending on the severity of the problem described in each question, giving a maximum subscale score of 21 for anxiety and depression, respectively. Zigmond and Snaith (1983) recommended that scores of greater than or equal to 8 on a subscale should be taken as an indication of possible psychological morbidity. The anxiety and depression scores are categorized in Table 7.3.

The HADS gives clinically meaningful results as a psychological screening tool, in clinical group comparisons and in correlational studies with several aspects of disease and QoL. It is sensitive to changes both during the course of diseases and in response to psychotherapeutic and psychopharmacological intervention. HADS scores predict psychosocial and possibly physical outcome (Herrmann 1997).

This self-assessment scale was originally developed and found to be a reliable instrument for detecting states of depression and anxiety in the setting of a hospital medical outpatient clinic. The anxiety and depressive subscales are also valid measures of severity of emotional disorders. It was suggested that the introduction of the scales into general hospital practice would facilitate the large task of detection and

management of emotional disorder in patients under investigation and treatment in medical and surgical departments (Zigmond, Snaith 1983).

There is a need to assess the contribution of mood disorder, especially anxiety and depression, in order to understand the experience of suffering in the setting of medical practice. Many physicians are aware of this aspect of illness of patients but many feel incompetent to provide the patient with reliable information. The HADS was designed to provide a simple yet reliable tool for use in medical practice. The term "hospital" in its title suggests that it is only valid in such a setting but many studies conducted throughout the world have confirmed that it is valid when used in community settings and primary care medical practice (Snaith 2003). It should be emphasized that self-assessment scales are only valid for screening purposes; definitive diagnosis must rest on the process of clinical and psychiatric examination.

HADS has also been shown to be a useful instrument for medical patients for screening and examining the disturbed emotion in groups of psychosomatic patients (Karakula, Grzywa, Spila et al. 1996). Bodybuilders have been described as suffering with an altered perception of body image, leading to psychiatric morbidity and psychopathology (Pope, Katz 1992; Pope, Phillips, Olivardia 2000).

Bulimia nervosa (characterized by eating binges) and anorexia nervosa (characterized by starvation) have both been linked with bodybuilding, in respect of the perception of body image. Binges are frequently followed by self-induced vomiting, laxative and/or diuretic abuse, prolonged fasting, or excessive exercise. Some patients with anorexia nervosa also manifest bulimia. Unrealistic, overly muscular male body ideals put individuals at risk for negative body images, unhealthy eating and exercise habits, and low self-esteem. Some individuals resort to drug taking to counteract their altered body images.

Using the Nottingham Health Profile (NHP) and the Psychological Well-being Schedule (PGWS), McGauley (1989) showed that the QoL improved after GH administration for 6 months in adults with GHD. Decreased psychological well-being has been reported in hypopituitary patients despite pituitary replacement with all hormones but GH (Stabler, Turner, Girdler et al. 1992).

There has subsequently been an increasing interest in GH-replacement therapy to improve health and QoL of older men with age-related decline in hormone levels. A new 21-item age-related hormonal decline (A-RHDQoL) is an individualized questionnaire measuring the perceived impact of age-related hormonal decline on the QoL of older men. The internal consistency reliability and content validity of the A-RHDQoL are established, but the measure is

Table 7.3 Hospital Anxiety and Depression Scale Questionnaire Scores

Aggregate Score	Interpretation
0–7	Normal
8–10	Mild
11–14	Moderate
15–21	Severe

HADS consists of 14 questions: 7 questions are related to anxiety and 7 questions are related to depression. Each item is rate with a score of 0 to 3, depending on the severity of the problem described in each question, giving a maximum subscale score of 21 for anxiety and depression, respectively.

at an early stage of its development and its sensitivity to change and other psychometric properties needs to be evaluated in clinical trials of hormone replacement (McMillan, Bradley, Giannoulis et al. 2003).

The self-reported HADS questionnaire has been used extensively to screen psychiatric morbidity (Janson, Bjornsson, Hetta et al. 1994) and has high validity when it is used as a screening instrument for this psychiatric condition in outpatients. On the basis of data from a large population, the basic psychometric properties of the HAD scale as a self-rating instrument should be considered as quite good in terms of factor structure, intercorrelation, homogeneity, and internal consistency (Wilkinson, Barczak 1988; Mykletun, Stordal, Dahl 2001; Martin, Lewin, Thompson 2003). Current research would suggest that rhGH may have a beneficial effect on psychological profile in AAS abuse on withdrawal from AASs (Graham, Davies, Hullin et al. 2007c).

THE EFFECTS OF GROWTH HORMONE ON ANTHROPOMETRY AND EXERCISE PERFORMANCE

The administration of rhGH has therapeutic value as a replacement therapy for GHD adults (Cuneo, Salomon, Wiles et al. 1991a; Cuneo, Salomon, Wiles et al. 1991b; Johannsson, Grimby, Sunnerhagen et al. 1997; Carroll, Christ, Bengtsson et al. 1998), increasing LBM and reducing total and visceral fat, which may be delayed by up to 12 months. $\dot{V}O_2$peak increased in A-OGHD after 6 months of replacement therapy (Cuneo, Salomon, Wiles et al. 1990; Cuneo, Salomon, Wiles et al. 1991b; Gullestad, Birkeland, Bjonerheim et al. 1998), 12 months therapy (Borson-Chazot, Serusclat, Kalfallah et al. 1999), and 36 months therapy, which reversed following cessation (Gullestad, Birkeland, Bjonerheim et al. 1998).

The stimulation of erythropoiesis may contribute as much to the increased exercise performance and $\dot{V}O_2$peak (Christ, Cummings, Westwood et al. 1997b) as increased cardiac output (Cuneo, Salomon, Wiles et al. 1991b).

RhGH treatment significantly increased LBM and bone mineral density (BMD), significantly decreased total cholesterol (TC) and low-density lipoprotein cholesterol (LDL-C), and significantly increased high-density lipoprotein cholesterol (HDL-C), and results were sustained after 5 and 10 years in A-OGHD (Gotherstrom, Svensson, Koranyi et al. 2001, Gotherstrom, Bengtsson, Bosaeus et al. 2007b).

The consequences of GHD differ if the disease is of childhood onset (C-OGHD) or of adulthood onset (Koranyi, Svensson, Götherstrom et al. 2001). However, after 5 years of rhGH replacement therapy, there

was no difference between C-OGHD and A-OGHD groups in any variable body composition or isometric or concentric knee extensor strength, knee flexor strength, left-hand grip strength, or in BMD (Koranyi, Svensson, Götherstrom et al. 2001).

Five years of rhGH replacement therapy in elderly adults with A-OGHD significantly normalized knee flexor strength (98% to 106% of that predicted) and significantly increased, but did not fully normalize, knee extensor strength (90% to 100% of that predicted) and handgrip strength (80% to 87%) (Gotherstrom, Bengtsson, Sunnerhagen et al. 2005).

GH-resistant states: When rhGH was given in conjunction with prednisone, it counteracted the protein catabolic effects of prednisone in eight healthy volunteers and resulted in increased whole body protein synthesis rates, with no effect on proteolysis (Horber, Haymond 1990). Bowes et al. (1997) demonstrated that the clearance of leucine into protein was increased after 2 and 7 days of GH treatment in Cushing's syndrome. This was consistent with GH stimulating the availability of amino acid transporters. However, when large therapeutic doses of rhGH are used in the treatment of cachexia and in HIV wasting syndrome, diabetic symptoms occur relatively more quickly than development of LBM (Schauster, Geletko, Mikolich 2000; Lo, Mulligan, Noor et al. 2001).

The infusion of rhGH over 24 hours causes a net glutamine release from skeletal muscle into the circulation and increased glutamine synthetase mRNA levels. This possibly compensates for reduced glutamine precursor availability after trauma in hypercatabolic trauma patients, which can account for its anticatabolic effects (Biolo, Iscra, Bosutti et al. 2000).

Hutler et al. (2002), demonstrated that GH treatment (0.037 to 0.047 mg/kg/day[1 mg = 3 IU]) improved absolute $\dot{V}O_2$peak during exercise tolerance tests in children with cystic fibrosis (CF), improving exercise tolerance, presumably resulting from the combined effects of GH on the muscular, cardiovascular, and pulmonary capacity.

RhGH treatment reverses the LBM loss allegedly responsible for diminished aerobic capacity and symptoms of increased fatigue in patients with HIV-associated wasting. It induced LBM gains and improved submaximal measurements but not maximum oxygen uptake in HIV-wasted patients (Esposito, Thomas, Kingdon et al. 2005).

Mechanisms of action: The use of acipimox (an antilipolytic) with rhGH administration in a 37-hour fasting state eliminated the ability of GH to restrict fasting protein loss, indicating that stimulation of lipolysis by GH is its principle protein-conserving mechanism (Norrelund, Nair, Nielson et al. 2003). Muscle protein breakdown increased by 50% (assessed by labeled phenylalanine). Liu et al. (2003) examined the effects of GH on myostatin (a growth inhibitory protein) regulation in A-OGHD. Skeletal muscle biopsies from the vastus lateralis were performed at 6-monthly intervals during 18 months of treatment. Myostatin mRNA expression was significantly inhibited to 31% of control by GH. The inhibitory effect of GH on myostatin was sustained after 12 and 18 months of GH treatment. These effects were associated with significantly increased LBM at 6 months, 12 months, and 18 months and translated into significantly increased aerobic performance, determined by $\dot{V}O_2$peak at 6 months and 12 months.

Effects in apparently healthy individuals: GH secretion and IGF-1 availability diminish with age, 14% per decade (Iranmanesh, Lizarralde, Velduis et al. 1991). The first researchers experimented on athletes using biosynthetic methionyl hGH (met-hGH), consisting of 192 amino acids, as opposed to recombinant (r)hGH (191 amino acids).

The administration of met-hGH (2.67 mg 3 days per week) for 6 weeks in eight well-trained exercising adults (22 to 33 years of age) who trained with progressive resistance exercise and maintained a high-protein diet significantly decreased body fat and significantly increased fat-free weight (FFW). Five subjects had a suppressed GH response to stimulation from either L-dopa or arginine or submaximal exercise (Crist, Peake, Egan et al. 1988).

It was postulated that rhGH administration would benefit elderly men, decreasing adiposity and increasing LBM (principally muscle). Rudman et al. (1990); Rudman et al. (1991) demonstrated such evidence.

Acute administration of rhGH or IGF-1 in normal healthy humans in the postabsorptive state significantly increased forearm net balance of amino acids (Fryburg, Gelfand, Barrett 1991). The effects are claimed to occur through the stimulation of protein synthesis rather than through decreased protein breakdown.

However, increased LBM has not been translated into increased strength or power in healthy individuals. For example, administration of rhGH appeared to cause no further increase in muscle mass or strength than provided by resistance training (RT) in any healthy young athletes aged 23 ± 2 years (Crist, Peake, Egan et al. 1988; Yarasheki, Campbell, Smith 1992; Yarasheki, Zachwieja, Angelopoulos 1993; Deyssig, Frisch, Blum et al. 1993) or indeed in healthy elderly men aged 70.2 ± 1.3 or 67 ± 1 years respectively (Taaffe, Pruitt, Reim et al. 1994; Yarasheki, Zachwieja, Campbell et al. 1995). There was no substantial evidence that rhGH could increase strength in healthy men and women older than 60 years (Zachwieja, Yarasheki 1999).

Muscle protein turnover and increases in muscle mass can occur over short periods of time (days) and can be measured indirectly using static techniques such as hydrostatic weighing or dual X-ray absorptiometry.

Measuring the rate of protein synthesis as the rate of incorporation of amino acids labeled with stable isotopes into the muscle rather than simply the changes in muscle mass between two time points is a more sensitive method for determining the response of muscle, but is not freely available (Rennie 2003).

RhGH administration did not enhance the muscle anabolism associated with heavy-resistance exercise in 16 men aged 21 to 34 years, with a mean weight of 70.6 kg (Yarasheki, Campbell, Smith 1992). The resistance training plus rhGH group (0.04 mg/kg/day; $n = 7$) did not differ from a resistance training plus placebo group ($n = 9$) for 12 weeks (Yarasheki, Campbell, Smith 1992).

The fractional rate of skeletal muscle protein synthesis and the whole body rate of protein breakdown did not increase during a constant intravenous infusion of [^{13}C]leucine in seven young (mean age: 23 ± 2 years; mean weight: 86.2 kg) healthy experienced male weight lifters before and at the end of 14 days of subcutaneous rhGH administration, in a dosage of 0.04 mg/kg/day (Yarasheki, Zachwieja, Angelopoulos 1993).

The administration of rhGH in 8 and 10 healthy, nonobese males (mean age: 23.4 ± 0.5 years; mean weight: 122 kg, mean body fat: 10.1%) at a dose of 0.03 mg/kg/day for a period of 6 weeks had no effect on maximal strength during concentric contraction of the biceps and quadriceps muscles (Deyssig, Frisch, Blum et al. 1993). In such highly trained power athletes with low fat mass there were no effects of rhGH treatment on strength or body composition.

RhGH administration at a dose of 0.0125 to 0.024 mg/kg/day ($n = 8$) versus placebo administration ($n = 15$) for 16-weeks did not increase muscle strength over resistance exercise training (75% to 90% maximum strength, 4 days/week) in 23 healthy, sedentary men (mean age: 67 ± 1 years, mean weight: 78.5 kg) with low serum IGF-1 levels (Yarasheki, Zachwieja, Campbell et al. 1995).

These results may be consequential to the different dosages of rhGH used, because of side effects (0.013 to 0.024 mg/kg/day). The dosages for the first two subjects were equivalent to 1.66 mg/day, but the second two subjects had 1.33 mg/day and the last four subjects had the equivalent of 1.0 mg/day.

RhGH administration (0.03 mg/kg of body weight × 3/week) for 6 months in 52 healthy men (mean age: 75 years, mean weight: 80 kg) with well-preserved functional ability but low baseline IGF-1 levels significantly increased LBM (on average by 4.3%). There were no statistically or clinically significant differences seen between the groups in knee or hand grip strength or in systemic endurance (Papadakis, Grady, Black et al. 1996).

Wallace et al. (1999) demonstrated that there was no improvement in morphological or performance characteristics, assessed by cycle ergometry and $\dot{V}O_2$peak assessment, following rhGH administration (0.05 mg/kg/day; $n = 8$) versus placebo ($n = 8$) for 7 days.

RhGH administration for 1 month significantly improved performance in "stair climb time" in 10 healthy older men (Brill, Weltman, Gentili et al. 2002).

A single rhGH dose (2.5 mg) in seven highly trained men (mean age: 26 ± 1 years; mean weight: 77 kg; mean $\dot{V}O_2$peak: 65 mL/kg/min) who performed 90 minutes of bicycling 4 hours after taking the rhGH prevented two subjects from completing the exercise protocol. It significantly increased plasma levels of lactate and glycerol as well as serum nonesterified fatty acid (NEFA) levels. This may compromise exercise performance. $\dot{V}O_2$peak remained unaltered by drug effect until exhaustion (Lange, Larsson, Flyvbjerg et al. 2002b). Plasma glucose was, on average, significantly higher (9%) during exercise after GH administration compared with placebo. This would suggest that any benefits of exercise in terms of increased glucose tolerance appeared to be negated by rhGH in the subjects.

RhGH significantly increased the myosin heavy chain (MHC) 2X isoforms (Lange, Andersen, Beyer et al. 2002a). This has been regarded as a change into a more youthful MHC composition, possibly induced by the rejuvenation of systemic IGF-1 levels. RhGH, however, had no effect on isokinetic quadriceps muscle strength, power, cross-sectional area (CSA), or fiber size. RT and placebo caused substantial increases in the isokinetic strength, power, and CSA of quadriceps; but these RT-induced improvements were not further augmented by additional rhGH administration. In the RT and GH group, there was a significant decrease in MHC 1 and 2X isoforms, whereas MHC 2A increased.

RT, therefore, seems to overrule the changes in MHC composition induced by GH administration alone.

Blackman et al. (2002) administered GH at a dose of 0.03 to 0.02 mg/kg/day and gender-related sex steroids to healthy men and women, aged 65 to 88 for 26 weeks. GH with or without sex steroids in healthy, aged women and men increased LBM and decreased fat mass. GH with testosterone increased $\dot{V}O_2$peak in men, but GH with transdermal oestradiol, 100 µg/day, plus oral medroxyprogesterone acetate, 10 mg/day did not increase $\dot{V}O_2$peak in women. The effects on strength and endurance exercise could be attributed to the effects of testosterone.

Healy et al. (2003) has shown that rhGH does exert an anabolic effect both at rest and during exercise in endurance-trained athletes, measuring whole body leucine turnover.

Healy et al. (2003) showed that plasma levels of glycerol and free fatty acids (FFA) and rate of appearance (Ra) of glycerol at rest and during and after exercise increased during treatment with rhGH as compared with placebo. Glucose Ra and its rate of disappearance (Rd) were greater after exercise during rhGH treatment as compared with placebo. Resting energy expenditure and fat oxidation were greater under resting conditions during rhGH treatment compared with placebo.

Nine males (mean age: 23.7 ± 1.9 years, mean weight: 77.3 kg, mean body fat: 17.7%, mean $\dot{V}O_2$peak: 37.9 mL/kg/min) completed six, 30-minute randomly assigned Monark cycle ergometer exercise trials at a power output midway between the lactate threshold and $\dot{V}O_2$peak consumption. Subjects received an rhGH infusion (0.01 mg/kg) at 0800 h, followed by a 30-minute exercise trial. There were no significant condition effects for total work, caloric expenditure, heart rate response, blood lactate response, or ratings of perceived exertion response (RPE). However, acute GH administration resulted in lower $\dot{V}O_2$peak without a drop-off in power output (Irving, Patrie, Anderson et al. 2004). The reduced $\dot{V}O_2$peak could not be explained but suggested that GH administration can improve exercise economy. This may have been a consequence of production of FFA by GH's lipolytic effect, providing the substrates for the maintenance of energy metabolism, despite the lower $\dot{V}O_2$.

There was no increase in strength in 30 physically active and healthy individuals of both genders (15 men and 15 women) of mean age 25.9 years (range 18 to 35) who received rhGH in a dose of 0.033 mg/kg/day ($n = 10$) and a dose of 0.067 mg/kg/day ($n = 10$) versus placebo ($n = 10$) for 1 month. IGF-1 significantly increased by 134% (baseline vs. 1 month), body weight significantly increased by 2.7%, fat-free mass significantly increased by 5.3%, total body water (TBW) significantly increased by 6.5%, and extracellular water (ECW) significantly increased by 9.6%. Body fat significantly decreased significantly by 6.6% (Ehrnborg, Ellegard, Bosaeus et al. 2005).

There was no increase in power or oxygen uptake in 30 physically active and healthy individuals of both genders (15 men and 15 women) of mean age 25.9 years (range 18 to 35) who received rhGH in a dose of 0.033 mg/kg/day ($n = 10$) and a dose of 0.067 mg/kg/day ($n = 10$) versus placebo ($n = 10$) for 1 month (Berggren, Ehrnborg, Rosen et al. 2005).

The interaction of GH and 11βhydroxysteroid dehydrogenase (11βHSD1 and 11βHSD2) has been suggested in the pathogenesis of central obesity. After 6 weeks of rhGH, the level of 11βHSD1 significantly decreased. After 9 months of rhGH, 11βHSD2 level significantly increased. Between 6 weeks to 9 months glucose disposal rate increased and visceral fat mass decreased. Changes in 11βHSD1 activity correlated with body composition and insulin sensitivity in 30 men (age range: 48 to 66 years) with abdominal obesity. However, it was considered that the data could not support the hypothesis that long-term (9 months) metabolic effects of GH are mediated through its action on 11βHSD 1 and 2 (Sigurjonsdottir, Koranyi, Axelson et al. 2006).

Plasma levels of glycerol and FFA increased at rest and during exercise during rhGH administration at a dosage of 0.066 mg/kg/day for 4 weeks in 6 trained male athletes compared to those treated with placebo. This had the effect of significantly increasing resting energy expenditure and fat oxidation and significantly increasing glucose production and uptake after exercise (Healy, Gibney, Pentecost et al. 2006). The relevance of these effects for athletic performance is as yet unknown, but one cannot exclude the postulate that enhancement is possible.

The effects of different dosages of rhGH: Professional bodybuilders and power lifters administer supraphysiological dosages of the hormone, up to 0.066 mg/kg/day (Powrie, Bassett, Rosen et al. 2007). Despite the knowledge that athletes are abusing these very high dosages, current data has identified an increase in strength and power (Graham, Baker, Evans et al. 2008) in a cohort of 24 abstinent AAS-using males taking 0.019 mg/kg/day rhGH, a comparatively small supraphysiological dose, versus 24 controls.

It is possible that the cohort sizes used by researchers have been too low to achieve the results that are still anecdotally claimed to be as a result of self-administration. However, effects of rhGH have also been studied at greater than physiological dosages, and although these may well have been below the dosages abused by bodybuilders, they have still resulted in serum concentrations of IGF-1 that are at least twice the normal values (Yarasheki, Zachwieja, Angelopoulos 1993; Yarasheki, Zachwieja, Campbell et al. 1995). There have been significant physiological effects: increased lipolysis, altered carbohydrate metabolism, activation of the renin–angiotensin system, and water retention. Mauras et al. (2000) demonstrated that when rhGH was given to severely GHD subjects, both protein synthesis and protein degradation increased with a net anabolic effect. Another explanation for the lack of evidence of increased strength in apparently healthy individuals is that rhGH has been reported to have anabolic effects on bone and collagen metabolism (Bollerslev, Moller, Thomas et al. 1996; Lissett, Shalet 2000) and the collagenous components of skeletal muscle and connective tissue elements of skin may also show up as new LBM. A small increase in visceral protein and collagen would equate to an increased positive nitrogen balance. This effect on connective tissue would not necessarily make the muscle generate greater strength or power, but may enhance resistance to injury or faster repair, which would be advantageous to athletes. This could explain why bodybuilders and power lifters self-administer AASs and rhGH together. The supraphysiological effect of GH on muscle in patients with acromegaly initiates a GH-resistant state. Therefore, true muscle hypertrophy cannot be evaluated since acromegaly is only identified when the pathology becomes fulminant. Contemporary evidence would appear to contradict an anabolic effect of rhGH, increasing strength in healthy human muscle in previously non–drug-using subjects. The difficulty lies in targeting an appropriate dose range, given the cardiovascular and metabolic hazards involved.

THE EFFECTS OF GROWTH HORMONE ON BLOOD PRESSURE

The majority of research on the effects of GH on blood pressure (BP) has involved its replacement in GHD. Reports regarding BP in GHD adults have been conflicting. In a large cohort of GHD adults, the prevalence of treated hypertension was found to have increased (Rosen, Edén S, Larson et al. 1993), but in case–control studies the BP in cases was similar to that in healthy controls (Markussis, Beshyah, Fisher et al. 1992; Valcavi, Gaddi O, Zini et al. 1995). In younger GHD adults, the systolic BP (SBP) has been found to be lower (Thuesen, Jørgensen, Müller et al. 1994), but was increased by GH replacement (Theusen, Jørgensen, Müller et al. 1994). Short-term, placebo-controlled GH-replacement trials for 4 to 12 months in GHD have demonstrated anabolic effects of GH on cardiac structure (Amato, Carella, Fazio et al. 1993; Valcavi, Gaddi O, Zini et al. 1995) and beneficial effects on SBP (Cuneo et al. 1991c). There was no change in diastolic BP (DBP) (Beshyah, Thomas, Kyd et al. 1994; Valcavi, Gaddi O, Zini et al. 1995). Hoffman et al. (1996) have shown a significant increase in body sodium, but not in plasma volume or BP in GHD adults ($n = 7$) during GH replacement at a physiological dosage of 0.013/mg/kg/day and a supraphysiological dosage of 0.027 mg/kg/day for 7 days. Other studies have shown no change in BP between GHD patients and controls before or after replacement therapy (Amato, Carella, Fazio et al. 1993; Moller, Fisker, Rosenfalck et al. 1999; Pfeifer, Verhovec, Zizek et al. 1999) despite the fact that the renin–angiotensin–aldosterone system has been demonstrated to be one of the systems responsible for the antinatriuretic effects of GH increasing plasma volume and extracellular fluid (Moller, Fisker, Rosenfalck et al. 1999). A decrease in DBP but not in SBP was demonstrated in female GHD (Bengtsson, Johannsson 1999). Studies have also demonstrated a reduced DBP in men and women as an effect of reduced peripheral vascular resistance (Caidahl, Eden, Bengtsson 1994).

Further studies have found a significant increase in SBP and DBP after 12 months, but not after 6 months, of rhGH administration (0.024 mg/kg/day), but only to the level of the controls. Such data would suggest that among other reasons, the BP response has a dosage-related action over different time intervals (Johannsson, Bengtsson, Andersson et al. 1996a). An improvement in systolic cardiac function during exercise has also been demonstrated during rhGH administration in GHD, suggesting a direct inotropic and chronotropic action by GH on the heart muscle (Cittadini, Cuocolo, Merola et al. 1994).

GH exerts direct effects on myocardial growth and function. Evidence from laboratory models shows that GH (or IGF-1) induces mRNA expression for specific contractile proteins and myocyte hypertrophy. GH increases the force of contraction and determines myosin conversion toward the low adenosine triphosphatase (ATPase) activity V3 isoform. This provides plausible explanations for the cardiac abnormalities observed in clinical settings of excessive or defective GH production. In acromegaly, the functional consequences of GH excess initially prevail, causing the hyperkinetic syndrome (high heart rate and increased systolic output). This is followed by alterations of cardiac function when myocardial hypertrophy develops. This involves both ventricles and is purposeless because it occurs without increased wall stress. Hypertrophy also entails proliferation of the myocardial fibrous tissue that leads to interstitial remodeling (Amato, Carella, Fazio et al. 1993; Sacca, Cittadini, Fazio 1994; Valcavi, Gaddi O, Zini et al. 1995). The functional consequence is an impaired ventricular relaxation that causes a diastolic dysfunction, followed by impairment of systolic function. In untreated disease, cardiac performance slowly deteriorates and heart failure eventually develops. Several lines of evidence support the specificity of heart disease in acromegaly. Particularly demonstrative are recent studies in which GH production was suppressed by octreotide, with a consequent significant regression of hypertrophy and improvement of cardiac dysfunction (Sacca, Cittadini, Fazio 1994). It is not yet established whether full recovery of normal cardiac morphology and function is possible after correction of GH excess. GHD leads to a reduced mass of both ventricles and to impaired cardiac performance with low heart rate (hypokinetic syndrome). These alterations are particularly evident during physical exercise and might provide an important contribution to the reduced exercise capacity of GHD patients, in addition to the reduced muscle mass and strength. This demonstrates a role of GH in the maintenance of a normal cardiac structure and performance. The hypokinetic syndrome is well documented in young patients in whom GHD began very early in their childhood (Sacca, Cittadini, Fazio 1994). In contrast, the data in adult-onset GHD are less consistent. This suggests that the consequences of GHD are more relevant if the disorder starts during early heart development.

As observed with other abnormalities associated with GHD, cardiac dysfunction is also susceptible to marked improvement by rhGH (Sacca, Cittadini, Fazio 1994). Attempts have been made by research enthusiasts to extrapolate the anabolic effects of GH in GHD to individuals in a state of senescence (Blackman, Sorkin, Münzer et al. 2002) and also to the exercising athlete. However, few, if any, significant effects have been recorded on BP in athletes, who were either aggressive users of AASs (Karila, Koistinen, Seppala et al. 1998) or previously non–substance users (Healy, Gibney, Russell-Jones et al. 2003).

THE EFFECTS OF GROWTH HORMONE ON HEART RATE

Amato et al. (1993) demonstrated no alteration in the heart rate in subjects with GHD, administering 0.01 mg/kg/day, three times per week for 6 months. Hoffman et al. (1996) and Johannsson et al. (1996a) have shown an increase in heart rate at rest in GHD following replacement therapy with rhGH. Hoffman et al. (1996) demonstrated that the mean 24-hour heart rate was significantly higher during low-dose (0.013 mg/kg/day) and high-dose (0.027 mg/kg/day) rhGH treatment versus placebo for 7 days (Table 7.4).

Cardiovascular morbidity and mortality are increased in the GH excess condition of acromegaly. Both GH and IGF-1 excess induce the hyperkinetic syndrome. The resultant concentric biventricular hypertrophy and diastolic dysfunction occurring in such individuals can cause heart failure if untreated (Vitale, Pivonello, Lombardi et al. 2004). Recent research has been performed in assessing both the resting and maximal heart rate response to peak exercise in early-onset GH excess following treatment. Resting, but not maximal, heart rate was significantly higher pretreatment. Following treatment with the GH antagonist octreotide, a significant reduction in the resting and maximal heart rate was demonstrated, with no amelioration of the elevated peak BP (Colao, Spinelli, Cuocolo et al. 2002).

Many researchers have not recorded maximal heart rate differences in healthy athletes who have self-administered rhGH nor demonstrated any adverse effects on the maximal heart rate (Irving, Patrie, Anderson et al. 2004). Lange, Lorentsen, Isaksson et al. (2001) demonstrated a significant lowering of heart rate after 12 weeks of rhGH administration and exercise training in females. This contrasted with a significant increase in heart rate with an acute single dose of rhGH at 65% $\dot{V}O_2$peak compared to that with placebo in males (Lange, Larsson, Flyvbjerg et al. 2002b).

Research by Ronconi et al. (2005) in excess GH disease states has shown an inverse correlation of nitric

Table 7.4 Growth Hormone Effects on Blood Pressure and Heart Rate

Effect of GH Replacement on Blood Pressure	Effect of GH Replacement on Heart Rate	Effect of GH Replacement on Hemoglobin	Effect of GH Replacement on Glucose	Effect of GH Replacement on Lipid Profile
Replacement increases BP in treated hypertension in GHD (Rosen et al. 1993)	GH deficiency results in hypokinetic syndrome (low HR and low SBP) (Sacca et al. 1994)	Low Hb present in GHD children (Eugster et al. 2002) Increases on replacement (Vihervuori et al. 1996)	Replacement increases liver glycogenolysis (Mauras, Haymond 2005)	GHD results in: Increased TC; Increased TGs; Increased LDL-C; Increased ApoB; Decreased HDL-C (Rosen et al. 1993)
Replacement increases BP to normal in hypotension in GHD (Theusen et al. 1994)	Excess GH in acromegaly results in hyperkinetic syndrome (increased HR and increased SBP) (Valcavi et al. 1995)	GHD adults have low hematopoietic precursor cells (Kotzmann et al. 1996)	GH excess induces β-cell exhaustion and DM (Sonksen et al. 1967)	Replacement: decreases TC; decreases LDL-C; decreases ApoB (Russell-Jones et al. 1994); Increases HDL-C (Attanasio et al. 1997); Increases Lp(a) (Angelin, Rudling 1994)
Replacement decreases BP in female GHD (Bengtsson, Johannsson 1999)				
Positive inotropic and chronotropic action on heart muscle (Cittadini et al. 1994)				
Excess GH in acromegaly results in concentric biventricular hypertrophy (Vitale et al. 2004)				

ApoB, Apolipoprotein B; BP, blood pressure; DM, diabetes mellitus; GH, growth hormone; GHD, growth hormone deficiency; Hb, hemoglobin; HR, heart rate; HDL-C, high-density lipoprotein cholesterol; Lp(a), lipoprotein(a); LDL-C, low-density lipoprotein cholesterol; SBP, systolic blood pressure; TC, total cholesterol; TG, triglyceride.

oxide (NO) levels (i.e., a decreased level) with GH and IGF-1. This suggests that reduced levels of platelet NO linked to GH excess may contribute to vascular alterations affecting not only heart rate but also endothelial dysfunction.

Current research has shown that supraphysiological doses of rhGH administration in apparently healthy individuals; over a short period of 6 days, there is a significant elevation of heart rate and corresponding elevation of rate–pressure product (Graham, Baker, Evans et al. 2007a).

THE EFFECTS OF GROWTH HORMONE ON HEMOGLOBIN AND PACKED CELL VOLUME (HEMATOCRIT)

Erythropoietin (Epo) is the primary regulator of erythropoiesis and promotes the survival, proliferation, and differentiation of erythroid progenitor cells. The Epo receptor belongs to the same family of receptors as growth hormone, granulocyte colony-stimulating factor, granulocyte macrophage colony-stimulating

factor, and some interleukins (ILs). In the erythropoietic process, Epo induces homodimerization of the Epo receptor, which is located on the surface of erythroid progenitor cells. Dimerization activates the receptor-associated JAK2 via transphosphorylation. Specific tyrosines in the intracellular portion of the receptor are phosphorylated and serve as a docking site for intracellular proteins, including one of STAT5. This results in activating various cascades of signal transduction. STAT5 enters the nucleus on phosphorylation, inducing the transcription of erythroid genes. The dephosphorylation of JAK2 and downregulation of the Epo receptor are performed by phosphatases. Erythropoietin receptor activation seems to exert its effect by inhibiting apoptosis rather than by affecting the commitment of erythroid lineage (Mulcahy 2001). Kotzmann et al. (1996) demonstrated that patients with GHD do not necessarily have anemia but have hematopoietic precursor cells in the lower normal range. RhGH replacement therapy over a period of 24 months has a marked effect on erythroid and myeloid progenitor precursor cells but negligible effects on peripheral blood cells in GHD.

Vihervuori et al. (1996) investigated erythropoiesis in 32 children with short stature and showed that Hb concentration was positively correlated with relative body height and with serum IGF-1 and IGFBP-3 levels but not with the concentrations of Epo. Treatment with rhGH accelerated growth significantly and elevated Hb, serum IGF-1, and IGFBP-3 significantly. When GHD is associated with multiple pituitary hormone deficiencies there are pathological influences on erythropoiesis that are not corrected until rhGH treatment is started (Valerio, Di Maio, Salerno et al. 1997).

Fetal and early postnatal erythropoiesis are dependent on factors in addition to Epo and the likely candidates are GH and IGF-1 (Halvorsen et al. 2002). Hb levels have been shown to be decreased in children with GHD compared with age-corrected norms (Eugster, Fisch, Walvoord et al. 2002).

THE EFFECTS OF GROWTH HORMONE ON GLUCOSE AND LIPID PROFILE

GH stimulates glycogenolysis in the liver in the maintenance of a homeostatic level of serum glucose. It decreases glucose uptake by the cell and thereby decreases glucose use as a substrate for ATP production, allowing neurons to continue using glucose for ATP production in glucose scarcity (Mauras, Haymond 2005).

Houssay (1936) described the diabetogenic properties of anterior pituitary hormones initially in classic animal studies. High-dose GH administration reduced forearm muscle uptake of glucose in normal adults in the postabsorptive state (Rabinowitz et al. 1965). Luft et al. (1968) demonstrated that glycemic control deteriorated following a single supraphysiological (10 mg) dose of GH in hypophysectomized adults with type 1 DM. The metabolic effects of a physiological bolus of rhGH has been studied by Moller et al. (1990) in the postabsorptive state, which demonstrated stimulation of lipolysis following a lag time of 2 to 3 hours. Plasma glucose demonstrated little fluctuation, and serum insulin and C-peptide levels remained stable. There was associated subtle reduction in glucose uptake and oxidation and substrate competition between glucose and fatty acids (glucose–fatty acid cycle). However, high GH levels induced hepatic and peripheral (muscular) resistance to insulin action on glucose metabolism, with associated increase in lipid oxidation.

GH-induced insulin resistance (IR) was associated with diminished glucose-dependent glucose disposal (Orskov, Schmitz, Jørgensen et al. 1989) and reduced muscle glycogen synthase activity (Bak, Moller, Schmitz 1991).

Active acromegaly unmasks the diabetogenic effect of GH. In its basal state, plasma glucose is elevated despite compensatory hyperinsulinemia. In both the basal and insulin-stimulated states (a euglycemic glucose clamp) hepatic and peripheral IR is associated with increased lipid oxidation and energy expenditure (Moller, Schmitz, Jørgensen et al. 1992). If untreated, this hypermetabolic state will cause pancreatic β-cell exhaustion and DM (Sonksen et al. 1967). However, if successfully treated this is reversible (Moller, Schmitz, Jørgensen et al. 1992). Only 2 weeks of supraphysiological dosages of GH (2.67 mg/day), can induce abnormalities in substrate metabolism and insulin sensitivity (Moller, Moller, Jørgensen et al. 1993).

Rizza et al. (1982) assessed the mechanisms responsible for GH-IR in man. He infused GH (2 μgm/kg/h), which increased plasma GH threefold ($\approx$9 ng/mL) within the range observed during sleep and exercise. This significantly increased plasma insulin concentrations (14 vs. 8 μU/mL) without altering plasma glucose concentrations or basal rates of glucose production and utilization. Insulin dose–response curves for both significant suppression of glucose production (half-maximal response at 37 vs. 20 μU/mL) and significant stimulation of glucose utilization (half-maximal response at 98 vs. 52 μU/mL) were shifted to the right with preservation of normal maximal responses to insulin. Monocyte insulin binding was unaffected. Thus, except at near maximal insulin receptor occupancy, the action of insulin on glucose production and utilization per number of monocyte insulin receptors occupied was decreased. These results indicate that increases in plasma GH within the physiological range can cause IR in man, which is due to decreases in both hepatic and extrahepatic effects of insulin. Assuming that insulin binding to monocytes reflects insulin binding in insulin-sensitive tissues, this decrease in insulin action can be explained on the basis of a post-receptor defect.

The GH excess (the acromegalic model) can be used to demonstrate excessive GH states to determine perturbations in metabolism, which may be precipitated by rhGH abuse.

Johnson and Rennie (1973) demonstrated that exercise in acromegalics caused marked differences in metabolites as compared with controls. Concentrations of glycerol, FFA, and ketone bodies rose rapidly to a maximum during exercise and then decreased during the period of constant exercise. However, it was shown that even in GH excess, insulin retains its effect on re-esterification of fat in spite of resistance to its effect on carbohydrate metabolism.

The known effect of increased serum glucose concentrations as a consequence of excess rhGH administration is reversible (Moller, Jørgensen, Møller et al. 1995). Its effects on glucose metabolism include suppression of glucose oxidation as a consequence of increased lipolysis and ketogenesis resulting in IR in skeletal muscles. GH increases the rate of total basal glucose turnover whereas oxidative glucose disposal is significantly decreased (Jorgensen, Pedersen, Børglum et al. 1994).

GH enhances lipolysis in adipose tissue and FFA use for ATP production. GHD patients have been shown to have elevated concentrations of TC, LDL-C, and apolipoprotein B (ApoB). HDL-C levels tend to be low and TG levels high when compared with age- and sex-matched healthy controls (Rosen, Edén S, Larson et al. 1993). GHD patients appear to have a lipid profile associated with premature atherosclerosis and CVD.

GH replacement results in a significant decrease in TC (Salomon, Cuneo, Hesp et al. 1989; Cuneo, Salomon, Wiles et al. 1993; Attanasio, Lamberts, Matranga et al. 1997) and significant decreases in LDL-C and ApoB (Russell-Jones, Watts, Weissberger et al. 1994). In addition, there is a significant increase in HDL-C (Eden, Wiklund, Oscarsson et al. 1993; Attanasio, Lamberts, Matranga et al. 1997). The plasma concentrations of TGs and apolipoprotein A do not change significantly with replacement (Salomon, Cuneo, Hesp et al. 1989; Weaver, Monson, Noonan et al. 1995; Garry, Collins, Devlin 1996).

Nine months of GH administration in apparently healthy, abdominally obese men significantly reduced TC, LDL-C, and apoB levels, but lipoprotein(a) [Lp(a)] levels significantly increased (Svensson, Bengtsson, Taskinen 2000). Lucidi et al. (2002) demonstrated that short-term treatment (1 week) with low-dose (0.0025 or 0.0033 mg/kg/day) rhGH stimulates lipolysis in apparently healthy viscerally obese men, but did not modify glucose and protein turnover rates.

These favorable effects of GH replacement on the plasma lipid and lipoprotein profile are sustained for up to 3 years after commencement (Garry, Collins, Devlin 1996; Attanasio, Lamberts, Matranga et al. 1997).

An exception following GH replacement is the elevation of Lp(a) concentration. There is a strong relationship between Lp(a) and coronary heart disease (Angelin, Rudling 1994). GH has elevated Lp(a) in four out of five studies with no change in one (Russell-Jones, Watts, Weissberger et al. 1994). There is some evidence that GH replacement upregulates the hepatic expression of the LDL receptor (Angelin, Rudling 1994) and may regulate ApoB metabolism (Christ, Carroll, Russell-Jones et al. 1997a).

There is an enhanced fat oxidation rate after prolonged GH administration (Lange, Lorentsen, Isaksson et al. 2001), supporting the idea that lipid availability upregulates lipid oxidation, in line with the Randle Cycle (Randle, Priestman, Mistry et al. 1994). This supports the concept that the metabolic processes in GH administration are akin to those in fasting or starvation, which stipulates that glucose is

essential for the energy metabolism of some cells and that conservation of glucose is obligatory for survival in starvation. The overall impact of rhGH treatment on lipoproteins may have important effects on the cardiovascular mortality in adults with GH deficiency. A reduction in TC and LDL cholesterol concentrations reduces the incidence of CVD in both men and women (Levine, Keaney, Vita 1995).

In contrast to rhGH as a treatment for the somatopause (Savinc, Sönksen 2000; Simpson, Savine, Sönksen et al. 2002; Lanfranco, Gianotti, Giordano et al. 2003), a recent review (Liu, Bravata, Olkin et al. 2007) has highlighted a mean TC decrease by 0.29 mmol/L. The clinical significance of these results has been called into question, but a limitation of the study was the mean body mass index (BMI) of 28 kg/m^2, which is associated with a blunted response to rhGH (Scacchi, Pincelli, Cavagnini 1999).

THE EFFECTS OF GROWTH HORMONE ON RESPIRATORY FUNCTION

Physical activity and exercise play a very important part in maintenance of the integrity of the respiratory system. Significantly greater diaphragmatic thickness and maximum inspiratory pressure (MIP) values in resistance trainers compared with non–weight-training adults have been reported (McCool, Conomos, Benditt et al. 1997). Insight into the physiology of a forced expiration is an important prerequisite for interpreting spirometry and recording a maximum expiratory flow-volume curve (Zach 2000).

Pathological disease states—anabolic state; GH excess: It would appear that if acromegaly exceeds 8 years duration, patients develop abnormalities of lung function from the effects of excess GH causing small airways and upper airway narrowing (Harrison, Millhouse, Harrington et al. 1978). With current identification and treatment regimes, these progressive conditions are rarely seen today. There is an association between the sleep apnoea syndrome (SAS) and acromegaly, which resolves on treatment of the active condition (Hart, Radow, Blackard et al. 1985).

At the opposite end of the scale, increased total lung capacity in acromegaly is reversed after suppression of GH hypersecretion without modifying diffusion capacity (Garcia-Rio, Pino, Diez et al. 2001). This suggests that lung growth in acromegaly may result from an increase in alveolar size, and not from increased alveolar number or inspiratory muscle strength.

A narrow window for GH/IGF-1 levels is required to maintain optimal respiratory function, as demonstrated by low $\dot{V}O_2$peak and ventilation threshold in acromegaly, which improves following treatment with the GH antagonist, octreotide (Thomas, Woodhouse, Pagura et al. 2002).

Catabolic states; GHD: There is an impairment of respiratory function in adult patients with C-OGHD, as a consequence of a reduction of lung volumes and a decrease of respiratory pressures, probably due to a reduction of respiratory muscle strength. The impairment in A-OGHD is consequential to a reduction of respiratory muscle strength. Both respond to replacement therapy with physiological dosages after 12 months (Merola, Longobardi, Sofia et al. 1996). Respiratory function does not improve in C-OGHD, with low-dose rhGH (Meineri, Andreani, Sanna et al. 1998).

Prader–Willi syndrome (a genetic abnormality of chromosome 15 with GHD) has demonstrated significant increases of carbon dioxide (CO_2) response, ventilation, and central inspiratory drive in children following GH replacement (Lindgren, Hellstrom, Ritzen et al. 1999).

Chronic obstructive pulmonary disease (COPD): Thirty percent to 60% of patients with COPD are malnourished, which adversely affects ventilatory muscle function and prognosis for survival.

Treatment of malnourished COPD patients with rhGH has been shown to significantly increase MIP within 1 week by 27% when provided with controlled high-protein diets (Pape, Friedman, Underwood et al. 1991). The same effect was not observed after 3 months of high-dose rhGH therapy (Burdet, de Muralt, Schutz et al. 1997) or 6 months of AAS administration in malnourished COPD patients (Ferreira, Verreschi, Nery et al. 1998).

Cystic Fibrosis: Exercise tolerance has been shown to improve clinically, but not statistically, on administration of biosynthetic rhGH (Huseman, Colombo, Brooks et al. 1996) and also improves significantly in CF, with rhGH replacement therapy (Hardin, Ellis, Dyson et al. 2001a; Hardin, Ellis, Dyson et al. 2001b; Hutler, Schnabel, Staab et al. 2002; Hardin, Ferkol, Ahn et al. 2005). Hutler et al. (2002) showed that the improved effect of rhGH (0.037 to 0.047 mg/kg/day) on exercise tolerance in children with CF could be explained by a significant increase in FEV1.

Surgical conditions: Respiratory function improved significantly on rhGH administration in major surgery, a catabolic condition, and was more beneficial when given pre- and postoperatively than when given postoperatively alone (Barry, Mealy, O'Neill et al. 1999).

Heart failure: Twice daily administration of Ghrelin (a GH-releasing peptide secretagogue) improved exercise capacity and left ventricular function in patients with chronic heart failure (Nagaya, Moriya, Yasumura et al. 2004).

In sport: $\dot{V}O_2$peak did not improve during exercise in healthy, young males and females with normal GH–IGF-1 axes with low- or high-dose rhGH (Berggren, Ehrnborg, Rosen et al. 2005). Current data has identified an improvement in $\dot{V}O_2$peak in abstinent AAS abuse (Graham, Davies, Hullin et al. 2007b) in a dosage of 0.017 mg/kg/day.

High-dose rhGH (0.066 mg/kg/day) has not demonstrated an improvement in $\dot{V}O_2$peak or athletic performance in endurance-trained athletes (Healey, Gibney, Pentecost et al. 2006).

ENDOTHELIAL DYSFUNCTION IN PATHOLOGICAL GROWTH HORMONE STATES

The potential mechanisms accounting for this abnormality may result from a direct IGF-1 mediated effect via increased production of NO. Qualitative alterations in lipoproteins have been described in GHD adults (O'Neal, Hew, Sikaris et al. 1996), resulting in the generation of an atherogenic lipoprotein phenotype, which would contribute to endothelial dysfunction.

GHD: Increased oxidative stress exists in GHD adults, which may be a factor in atherogenesis, and is reduced by the effects of GH therapy on oxidative stress (Evans, Davies, Anderson et al. 2000). Endothelial dysfunction exists in GHD adults (Evans, Davies, Goodfellow et al. 1999), which is reversible with GH replacement (Pfeifer, Verhovec, Zizek et al. 1999). An impaired endothelial-dependent dilatation (EDD) response was documented in GHD adults, which significantly improved after GH treatment.

Patients with GHD, with increased risk of vascular disease, have impaired endothelial function and increased augmentation index (AI^x) compared with controls. Replacement of GH resulted in improvement of both endothelial function and AI^x, without changing BP (Smith, Evans, Wilkinson et al. 2002). Administration of rhGH for 3 months corrected endothelial dysfunction in patents with chronic heart failure (Napoli, Guardasole, Matarazzo et al. 2002). Lilien et al. (2004) showed that endothelial dysfunction in renal failure and GHD is reversed by rhGH therapy. Renal failure induces GH resistance at the receptor and post-receptor level, which can be overcome by rhGH therapy.

Growth hormone excess: Acromegaly is associated with changes in the central arterial pressure waveform, suggesting large artery stiffening. This may have important implications for cardiac morphology and performance as well as in increasing the susceptibility to atheromatous disease.

Smith et al. (2003) showed that large artery stiffness is reduced in "cured" acromegaly (GH <2.5 mU/L) and partially reversed after pharmacological treatment of active disease.

THE EFFECTS OF GROWTH HORMONE ON INFLAMMATORY MARKERS OF CARDIOVASCULAR DISEASE

There have been suggestions of an association between certain inflammatory markers of CVD and GHD. Human peripheral blood T cells, B cells, natural killer (NK) cells and monocytes express IGF-1 receptors (Wit, Kooijman, Rijkers et al. 1993). Animal studies suggest a role for GH and IGF-1 in the modulation of both cell-mediated and humoral immunity. Administration of either can reverse the immunodeficiency of Snell dwarf mice (Van Buul-Offers, Ujeda, Van den Brande 1986). Crist and Kraner (1990) demonstrated that met-hGH induced a significant overall increase in the percent specific lysis of K562 tumor target cells in healthy adults. NK activity was significantly increased within the first week and this level was maintained throughout the remaining period of administration (6 weeks). In vitro studies using human lymphocytes indicate that GH is important for the development of the immune system (Wit, Kooijman, Rijkers et al. 1993). Mealy et al. (1998) showed that preoperative administration of rhGH does not alter C-reactive protein (CRP, an acute-phase protein, secreted by hepatocytes in response to in vivo inflammatory events), serum amyloid A (SAA), or interleukin-6 (IL-6, an inflammatory cytokine) release. Several studies have established homocysteine (HCY) concentration as an independent risk factor for atherosclerosis (Eichinger, Stumpflen, Hirschl et al. 1998; Stehouwer, Jacobs 1998). CRP and IL-6 levels and central fat decreased significantly in GH recipients as compared with placebo recipients in GHD after 18 months of rhGH. However, Lp(a) and glucose levels significantly increased, without affecting lipid levels (Sesmilo, Biller, Llevadot et al. 2000). HCY impairs vascular endothelial function through significant reduction of NO production. This appears to potentiate oxidative stress and atherogenic development (van Guldener, Stehouwer 2000). Acute hyperhomocysteinemia has been identified in bodybuilders regularly self-administering supraphysiological doses of various AASs (Ebenbinchler, Kaser, Bodner et al. 2001). Abdu et al. (2001) demonstrated that HCY levels are not significantly elevated in GHD adults and are unlikely to be a major risk factor for vascular disease if there are no other risk factors present. Muller et al. (2001) demonstrated that pegvisomant (GH receptor antagonist) induced no significant acute changes in the major risk markers for CVD in apparently healthy, abdominally obese men. This suggested that the secondary metabolic changes, for example, inflammatory factors, which develop as a result of long-standing GHD, are of primary importance in the pathogenesis of atherosclerosis in patients with GHD. Sesmilo et al. (2002) demonstrated that patients with active acromegaly have significantly lower CRP and significantly higher insulin levels than healthy controls. Administration of pegvisomant significantly increased CRP to normal levels. GH secretory status may be an important determinant of serum CRP levels, but the mechanism and significance of this finding is as yet unknown. Recent work of others has also demonstrated that inflammatory markers are predictive of atherosclerosis and cardiovascular events (Ridker, Rifai, Rose et al. 2002; Danesh, Wheeler, Hirschfield et al. 2004; Grace, Davies 2004). Metabolic syndrome (MS) is correlated with elevated CRP and is a predictor of coronary heart disease and DM (Sattar, Gaw, Scherbakova et al. 2003). Leonsson et al. (2003) demonstrated that IL-6 concentrations were significantly increased (208% and 248%) in GHD compared to BMI-matched and nonobese controls, respectively. CRP significantly increased (237%) in patients compared to nonobese controls, but not significantly different compared to BMI-matched controls. Age, LDL-C, and IL-6 were positively correlated, and IGF-1 was negatively correlated to arterial intima-media thickness (IMT) in the patient group, but only age and IL-6 were independently related to IMT. A recent study identified an association between raised HCY levels in long-term AAS users and sudden death (Graham, Grace, Boobier et al. 2006). Both HCY and other risk markers have been shown to decrease in AAS withdrawal and rhGH administration over a 6-day period (Graham, Davies, Hullin et al. 2007b).

THE EFFECTS OF GROWTH HORMONE ON BONE MINERAL DENSITY AND BONE METABOLISM

The effects of endocrine dysfunction on BMD are complex and are both disease and site specific, having different effects on the axial and the appendicular skeleton (Seeman et al. 1982). Both deficiency and excess of GH are related to disturbances in calcium metabolism. Bone γ-carboxyglutamic acid (Gla) protein (BGP [osteocalcin]) is a specific marker of bone turnover identified in peripheral blood.

A-OGHD patients have normal initial plasma osteocalcin concentrations. Acromegalic patients have significantly increased concentrations of osteocalcin. Treatment with rhGH, significantly increases plasma osteocalcin. One week after surgery, plasma osteocalcin concentrations are significantly decreased in acromegalic patients (Johansen, Pedersen, Jørgensen et al. 1990). GHD is associated with reduced bone mass, as assessed by BMD measurements. GH acts as an osteo-anabolic hormone when given to GHD adults. The findings in most of the trials suggest that GH has a biphasic effect; after an initial predominance of bone resorption, stimulation of bone formation leads to a net gain in bone mass after 12 to 24 months of treatment. Whether these changes in bone metabolism will result in less osteopenia and a reduced fracture rate in adults with GHD requires long-term studies. Adults with GHD are at increased risk of osteoporotic fractures. Studies have demonstrated reduced bone mass at different skeletal sites in patients with C-OGHD (Kaufman, Taelman, Vermeuelen et al. 1992; Hyer, Rodin, Tobias et al. 1992; Amato, Carella, Fazio et al. 1993; O'Halloran, Tsatsoulis, Whitehouse et al. 1993), A-OGHD (Bing-You, Denis, Rosen 1993; Holmes, Economou, Whitehouse et al. 1994), and mixed onset GHD as compared with that in healthy control subjects (Thoren, Soop, Degerblad et al. 1993; Beshyah, Freemantle, Shahi et al. 1995; Degerblad, Bengtsson, Bramnert et al. 1995). Studies investigating bone formation (osteocalcin) and resorption markers (urinary pyridinolines) have yielded conflicting results. Osteocalcin levels have been shown to be higher (Hyer, Rodin , Tobias et al. 1992), lower (Nielsen, Jørgensen, Brixen et al. 1991), or equal (Johansen, Pedersen, Jørgensen et al. 1990) in patients with A-OGH deficiency compared with those in normal controls. A radiological study of adults with long-standing GHD demonstrated that 17% had reduced vertebral height, consistent with vertebral fracture, and a further 19% had features of osteopenia (Wuster, Slenczka, Ziegler 1991). The fracture rate in adult patients with GHD, given replacement therapy other than rhGH, was significantly higher than that in a control population (24.1% vs. 8.7%) (Rosen, Wilhelmsen, Landin-Wilhelmsen et al. 1997). Markers of bone resorption increase in children with GHD and multiple pituitary deficiency but not in adults with isolated GHD (Schlemmer, Johansen, Pedersen et al. 1991; Sartorio, Conti, Monzani 1993). It was thought that the presence of other hormones partially counteracted the negative consequence of GH–IGF-1 deficiency. However, other studies have not demonstrated any difference between isolated GH deficiency and multiple deficiency (Holmes, Economou, Whitehouse et al. 1994). Bone histology of patients with mainly A-OGH deficiency showed normal trabecular bone volume, high bone volume and increased bone erosion, increased osteoid thickness, and increased mineralization lag time, indicating a delayed bone mineralization (Bravenboer, Holzmann, de Boer et al. 1996).

Significantly reduced BMD has been recorded after 6 or 12 months of rhGH therapy (Holmes, Whitehouse, Swindell et al. 1995). RhGH replacement has not been shown to increase bone mass in the short term (3 to 6 months) (Hansen, Brixen, Vahl et al. 1996). An open study of the effects of 24 months of rhGH replacement in patients with A-OGHD demonstrated a significant increase in BMD (4% to 10% above baseline) after 2 years of GH treatment, with a sustained significant increase in bone remodeling. Serum bone formation (osteocalcin, bone alkaline phophatase, and carboxyl-terminal propeptide of type I procollagen) and urinary resorption markers (deoxypyridinoline, pyridinoline, and cross-linked telopeptide of type I collagen) all significantly increased (Johannsson, Rosen, Bosaeus et al. 1996b). In patients with A-OGHD, bone formation appears to be increased at 6 months, with no further change throughout treatment (Attanasio, Lamberts, Matranga et al. 1997).

In contrast, patients with C-OGHD show a steep increase up to 12 months of rhGH therapy, followed by a sharp decrease to baseline value after 18 months of rhGH therapy (Attanasio, Lamberts, Matranga et al. 1997). 1,25-Dihydroxyvitamin D level increased in one study after 6 months (Binnerts, Swart, Wilson et al. 1992) but was unchanged after 12 months in another (Hansen, Brixen, Vahl et al. 1996). Hansen reported significant increases in serum phosphate and calcium levels and significant decreases in Parathormone (PTH) after 6 to 12 months of treatment. PTH did not change after 6 months replacement with rhGH in A-OGHD (Beshyah, Thomas, Kyd et al. 1994).

Transiliac bone biopsies of patients with A-OGHD after 6 to 12 months of rhGH treatment showed an increase in cortical thickness, increased bone formation, and decreased bone resorption. Trabecular bone volume remained unchanged (Bravenboer, Holzmann, de Boer et al. 1997).

RhGH treatment in A-OGHD for 10 years induced a sustained increase in total, lumbar (L2-L4), and femur neck BMD and bone mineral content, as measured by dual energy X-ray absorptiometry (DEXA). Females had an enhanced increase in BMD with estrogen replacement (Gotherstrom, Bengtsson, Bosaeus et al. 2007a).

GH and IGF-1 excess both stimulate osteoblast proliferation. At diagnosis GH excess has usually been present for several years. Impaired gonadotrophin secretion with hypogonadism is frequent and may account for decreased BMD. Proximal femoral and lumbar spine BMD is normal in most patients with active acromegaly, including those who have hypogonadism. Successful treatment of acromegaly does not result in major short-term changes in BMD (Ho, Fig, Barkan et al. 1992).

Fracture risk was demonstrated to be significantly decreased in patients with acromegaly compared to controls, probably because of the anabolic effect of GH on bone (Vestergaard, Mosekilde 2004).

A disadvantageous effect of acromegaly is decreased BMD. This is thought to be due to associated hypogonadism. It has been shown to occur in the distal radius (in women), the proximal femur (in men), and the total body, in both sexes (Bolanowski, Daroszewski, Medras et al. 2006). An anabolic effect of GH during active acromegaly has also been shown in the proximal femur in eugonadal men (Bolanowski, Daroszewski, Medras et al. 2006).

THE EFFECTS OF GROWTH HORMONE ON THYROID FUNCTION

GH influences thyroid function and anatomy. Goiter is frequent in acromegalic patients. The effects of GHD are difficult to assess because hypopituitary subjects who lack GH often also have a partial or complete deficit of thyroid-stimulating hormone (TSH).

The occurrence of central hypothyroidism in previously euthyroid children during GH therapy has been reported with widely varying incidence. The actual incidence is controversial, however, with some studies showing a high occurrence (Goodman, Grumbach, Kaplan 1968; Lippe, Van Herle, LaFranchi et al. 1975; Stahnke, Koehn 1990) and others little (Cacciari, Cicognani, Pirazzoli et al. 1979).

RhGH is known to increase the metabolism of thyroxin (tetra-iodothyronine [T_4]), enhancing the conversion of T_4 to triiodothyronine (T_3) (Sato, Suzukui, Taketani et al. 1977). The lowering of serum free T_4 supported the work of Grunfeld et al. (1988) where T_4 was significantly lowered by 8%, T_3 was significantly increased by 21%, and TSH was significantly decreased by 54% after 4 days of low-dose rhGH administration (0.125 mg/day). The work of Moller et al. (1992), Jorgensen et al. (1994), and Wyatt et al. (1998) demonstrated that T_4 was unaltered after 12 months of rhGH replacement therapy.

Wyatt et al. (1998) showed that shifts in thyroid hormone levels are very common during the first year of GH therapy in children who are initially euthyroid. Baseline TSH, T_4, free T_4, reverse (r)T_3, and T_3 levels were normal with negative antithyroid antibodies. By 1 month, there were significant decreases in T_4, free T_4 index, and rT_3, and significant increases in T_3 and the T_3/T_4 ratio. The changes from baseline values were greatest at 1 month, but showed a gradual return to baseline from 3 to 12 months. There were no clinical signs of hypothyroidism. T_4 supplementation is seldom needed in such patients.

Ito et al. (1998) demonstrated a significant increase in serum thyroid hormone during and after a 5-day administration of human GH in healthy male adults.

Portes et al. (2000) demonstrated that long-term rhGH replacement therapy in A-OGHD significantly decreases serum free T_4 and rT_3 levels and increases serum T_3 levels. These changes are independent of TSH and result from increased peripheral conversion of T_4 to T_3. A-OGHD does not induce hypothyroidism but simply reveals previously unrecognized cases whose serum free T_4 values fall in the low range during rhGH replacement.

Porretti et al. (2002) showed that GHD masks a state of central hypothyroidism in a consistent number of adult patients. Therefore, during rhGH treatment monitoring of thyroid function is mandatory to start or adjust T_4 substitutive therapy. Work by Kalina-Faska et al. (2004) did not support the use of thyroid hormone therapy during the first year of rhGH therapy in patients who were initially euthyroid.

Seminara et al. (2005) demonstrated that changes in thyroid function are present in C-OGHD during long-term rhGH therapy. However, these changes probably resulted from the effect of rhGH on the peripheral metabolism of thyroid hormones and appear to be transitory, disappearing during the second year of rhGH treatment.

Alcantara et al. (2006) demonstrated untreated GHD due to a homozygous GH-releasing hormone receptor (GHRHR) mutation and that heterozygous carriers of the same mutation have smaller thyroid volume than normal subjects, suggesting that GH has a permissive role in the growth of the thyroid gland. In addition, GHD subjects have reduced serum total T_3 and increased serum free T_4, suggesting a reduction in the function of the deiodinase system.

HISTORY OF INSULIN

Sir Edward Schafer, Professor of Physiology in Edinburgh, appears to have been the first to name insulin and describe its actions. He did so in a book, *The Endocrine Organs*, based on a lecture series he gave in California in 1913. In his book (Schafer 1916), he gave the hypothetical substance a name and also described its likely formation from activation of an inert precursor "pro-insuline." Insulin was subsequently discovered by Banting and Best in 1921. The first patient was treated a year later in 1922 and pro-insulin was discovered (and renamed) more than 50 years later by George Steiner of the University of Chicago in 1967. Schafer deliberately avoided using the word "hormone" and used his preferred terms "autacoid" (excitatory) and "chalonic" (inhibitory). This was as a result of long-standing academic rivalry with his contemporaries Professors Baylis and Starling at University College, London. They had previously described "secretin" as the first hormone to be isolated and characterized. They had coined the term "hormones" to describe the class of substance produced in one part of the body and acting elsewhere. Schafer preferred his own terms, which were based on terms used at the time to describe actions of drugs, autacoid being a substance with excitatory action and chalone being one with inhibitory action. Schafer went on to describe how insuline had both excitatory and inhibitory actions. His description of how he thought the hypothetical substance insuline acted in the body is remarkable because the passage of time has shown him to be correct almost word for word.

PHYSIOLOGY OF INSULIN

Insulin is a two-chain (30 and 21 amino acids) polypeptide hormone (51 amino acids; molecular weight, 5808) synthesized and secreted by the β-cells of the islets of Langerhans in the pancreas gland. Insulin acts in a stimulatory and an inhibitory manner (Schafer 1916). It stimulates the translocation of "Glut 4" glucose transporters from the cytoplasm of muscle and adipose tissue to the cell membrane. This stimulation increases the rate of glucose uptake to values greater than those in the basal state without insulin shown in isolated adipocytes from rats, as illustrated in Figure 7.2.

Insulin exhibits both inhibitory (chalonic) and excitatory (autacoid) actions via the same receptor. In these experiments carried out on rat adipose tissue, in vitro insulin simultaneously inhibits lipolysis (the release of glycerol from stored TG) and stimulates lipogenesis (formation of stored TG from glucose) (Table 7.5). Thus its anabolic action is due to two mechanisms working synergistically (Thomas, Wisher, Brandenburg et al. 1979).

There are sufficient numbers of glucose transporters in all cell membranes at all times to ensure enough glucose uptake to satisfy the cell's respiration, even in the absence of insulin. Insulin increases the number of these transporters in some cells but glucose uptake is never truly insulin dependent (Sonksen 2001). Even in uncontrolled diabetic hyperglycemia, whole body glucose uptake is increased (unless there is severe ketosis). Even under conditions of severe ketoacidosis there is no membrane barrier to glucose uptake. The block occurs where the excess ketone concentration competitively blocks the metabolites of glucose entering the Krebs cycle (Sonksen 2001). Glucose is therefore freely transported into the cell, but the pathway of metabolism is blocked at the entry point to the Krebs cycle by the excess of metabolites arising from fat and protein breakdown. As a result of this competitive block at the entry point to the Krebs cycle, intracellular glucose metabolites increase throughout the glycolytic pathway, leading to accumulation of free intracellular glucose and inhibiting initial glucose phosphorylation.

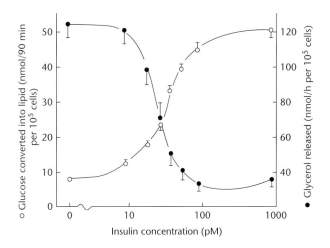

Figure 7.2 The anabolic actions of insulin. Insulin increases the rate of glucose uptake to values greater than that in the basal state without insulin; shown in isolated adipocytes from rats and is illustrated in Figure 7.2. Key: ○ = Glucose converted into Lipid; ● = Glycerol released (Thomas, Wisher, Brandenburg et al. 1979; Sonksen 2001).

Much of the "free" intracellular glucose transported into the cell is transported back out of the cell into the extracellular fluid. Under conditions of ketoacidosis, glucose metabolism (but not glucose uptake) is impaired as a direct consequence of the metabolism of fat, the "glucose–fatty acid" or Randle cycle (Randle, Priestman, Mistry et al. 1994).

In Figure 7.2 it can be seen that simultaneously with the excitatory effect in stimulating lipogenesis insulin also exhibits an inhibitory effect in preventing glycerol release. It is this inhibitory effect on lipolysis (and also glycolysis, gluconeogenesis, ketogenesis and proteolysis) that accounts for most of insulin's physiological effects in vivo in man. The inhibitory effects are also responsible for insulin's net anabolic actions.

The introduction of dynamic tracer studies enabled the identification of insulin's action in vivo in man (Sonksen, Sonksen 2000). Glucose infusion labeled with either radioactive or stable isotopes allowed the accurate measure of the rates of glucose production (rate of appearance, Ra) and rates of glucose utilization (rate of disappearance, Rd) in the circulating blood. Uncontrolled diabetics demonstrated that fasting hyperglycemia was associated with rates of glucose appearance that were increased several fold above normal (Sonksen, Sonksen 2000). Fasting glucose uptake was also increased. Since the fasting hyperglycemia in diabetes is sustained and there is a "dynamic steady state" where Ra = Rd; thus, both Ra and Rd are elevated.

In diabetes fasting blood glucose is an accurate measure of the severity of insulin deficiency. There is a linear correlation between the fasting blood glucose and the rate of hepatic glucose production (Ra)

Table 7.5 Physiological and Pathological Effects of Insulin

Physiological Effects of Insulin					
Insulin inhibits lipolysis & stimulates lipogenesis (Thomas et al. 1979)					
Pathological Effects of Insulin					
Insulin Resistance	*Hyperinsulinemia*				
Increases visceral obesity (Nyholm et al. 2004)	Increases athero sclerosis (Meissner, Legg 1973)	Increases heart rate (O' Hare et al. 1989)	Increases blood pressure (Scott et al. 1988)	Increases Hb and PCV (Facchini et al. 1998)	Decreases respiratory function (Lazarus et al. 1998a)
		Increases sympathetic nervous system activity (Landsberg 1986)			
		Increases renal sodium reabsorption (DeFronzo 1981)			

Hb, hemoglobin; PCV, packed cell volume.

and the rate of glucose disappearance (Rd) (Sonksen, Sonksen 2000). The fasting blood glucose exceeds the renal threshold; not all glucose leaving the circulation is actually being metabolized. By collecting the urine and quantifying the urinary glucose losses it is easy to measure the true rate of glucose utilization and the rate of urinary glucose loss. Glycosuria can account for as much as 30% of glucose turnover. After correcting whole body glucose turnover for urinary glucose losses, tissue glucose utilization is increased in diabetes compared with normal (Sonksen, Sonksen 2000). Insulin is not needed for glucose uptake and utilization in man, that is, glucose uptake is not totally insulin dependent.

When insulin is administered to people with diabetes who are fasting, blood glucose concentration falls. Insulin, at concentrations that are within the normal physiological range, lowers blood glucose by inhibiting hepatic glucose production (Ra) without stimulating peripheral glucose uptake (Brown, Tomkins, Juul et al. 1978). As hepatic glucose output is "switched off" by the inhibitory action of insulin, glucose concentration falls and glucose uptake actually decreases. Glucose uptake is actually increased in uncontrolled diabetes and decreased by insulin administration (Sonksen 2001). Even in insulin deficiency, there are sufficient glucose transporters in the cell membranes. The factor determining glucose uptake under these conditions is the concentration gradient across the cell membrane; this is highest in uncontrolled diabetes and falls as insulin lowers blood glucose concentration primarily (at physiological insulin concentrations) by reducing hepatic glucose production. When insulin is given to patients with uncontrolled diabetes, it switches off a number of metabolic processes (lipolysis, proteolysis, ketogenesis, and gluconeogenesis) by a similar inhibitory action. The result is that FFA concentrations fall effectively to zero within minutes and ketogenesis inevitably stops through lack of substrate. It takes some time for the ketones to clear from the circulation, as they are water

and fat soluble and distribute within body water and body fat. Both ketones and FFA compete with glucose as energy substrate at the point of entry into the Krebs cycle. Glucose metabolism increases inevitably as FFA and ketone levels fall (despite the concomitant fall in plasma glucose concentration) (Sonksen 2001).

As a consequence, insulin increases glucose metabolism more through reducing FFA and ketone levels than it does through recruiting more glucose transporters into the muscle cell membrane. Insulin does have a direct action recruiting more glucose transporters into muscle cell membranes. This facilitates glucose uptake, which is reflected as an increase in the metabolic clearance rate (MCR) of glucose. The MCR measured with tracer technology is a very important physiological measurement. It is defined as "the amount of blood irreversibly cleared of glucose in unit time." It is expressed normally in mL/kg/min and is a nonlinear function of blood glucose concentration (increasing as glucose concentration falls) and is highly sensitive to insulin (increasing with increasing insulin levels) (Sonksen, Sonksen 2000). It is measured relatively noninvasively in vivo using nonradioactive tracers or stable isotopes. All polar (water-soluble) substrates, as "transporters" are the mechanism by which they are transported across the highly nonpolar (lipid) cell membranes. The entry of a water-soluble substrate such as glucose across an impermeable lipid bilayer into a cell requires a specific transport mechanism. These protein carriers are the glucose "transporters" (GLUTs). In the case of glucose, there are at least six types and they tend to be tissue specific. In the case of muscle, the transporter is called *Glut 4*. It is normally present in excess in the cell membrane even in the absence of insulin and is not rate limiting for glucose entry into the cell (Sonksen 2001). Glucose transport into the cell is mainly determined by the concentration gradient between the extracellular fluid and the intracellular "free" glucose. Free glucose is very low inside the cell as it is immediately phosphorylated. In uncontrolled diabetes, particularly where there is a high concentration of FFA and ketones, glycolysis is inhibited, phosphorylation of free glucose stops, and intracellular free glucose rises. Insulin recruits more transporters into the cell membrane from an intracellular pool. This increases the rate of glucose entry for a given glucose concentration and this is reflected in vivo by an increase in the MCR of glucose. Thus MCR is an in vivo measure of substrate transporter activity (Boroujerdi, Umpleby, Jones et al. 1995). Experiments in normal subjects using hyperglycemic and hyperinsulinemic "clamps" have shown the importance of both glucose and insulin concentrations in determining glucose uptake. Studies illustrating these points are shown in Figure 7.3 (Gottesman, Mandarino, Verdonk et al. 1982). Subjects were studied in the overnight-fasted state with fasting insulin, averaging 18 mU/L and on two other occasions when they were infused with insulin at rates that resulted in mean plasma insulin concentrations of 80 and 150 mU/L. They were also

studied at the same insulin concentrations, but with plasma glucose increased and maintained at a steady level by an exogenous glucose infusion. Four glucose concentrations ranging from 5 to 10 mmol/L were studied with insulin levels maintained at normal fasting values. During the insulin infusions, subjects were studied at three glucose concentrations spanning the same range. Using tracer methodology, the authors were able to calculate Ra, Rd, and MCR at each glucose and insulin concentration (Fig. 7.3) (Gottesman, Mandarino, Verdonk et al. 1982; Sonksen 2001). The important points of note are as follows:

1. Total glucose uptake (Rd) is a nonlinear function of blood glucose concentration. Initially, uptake increases as blood glucose concentration rises but plateaus at higher glucose concentration. Although detectable within the range of glucose concentrations studied, it is made more obvious through extrapolation to higher glucose concentrations by use of the model. These high glucose values are unobtainable in normal subjects with existing

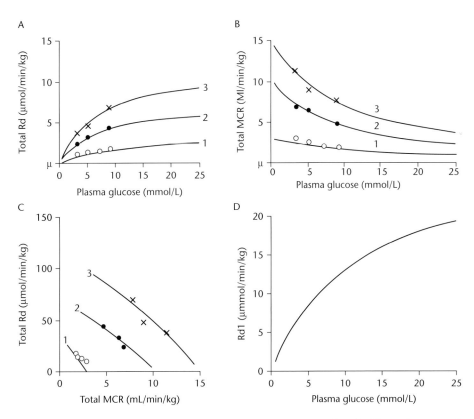

Figure 7.3 The model regulation of glucose metabolism. Graphs A, B, C, D. Data used in this illustration were obtained from normal subjects using a series of euglycemic and hyperglycemic clamps at basal or increased insulin concentrations (Sonksen 2001) (A) Total RD (increasing plasma insulin concentration) increases as blood glucose concentration rises but plateaus at higher glucose concentration. (B) Total MCR falls with increasing plasma irrespective of the plasma insulin concentration. (C, D) Total MCR increases with total RD (increasing plasma insulin concentration) irrespective of the plasma glucose concentration. This indicates that increasing insulin concentrations are associated with increasing numbers of glusoce transporters (see text for explanation). Rd, Rate of utilization; Rd1, insulin independent glucose uptake; MCR, metabolic clearance rate. Key: x, ○, ● = different concentrations.

technology. The shape of the curve suggests simple "saturation" kinetics obeying Michaelis–Menten laws.

2. Glucose MCR falls with increasing plasma glucose, independent of the plasma insulin concentration, in keeping with saturation of the glucose transporter system as plasma glucose rises.

3. MCR increases with increasing plasma insulin concentration, independent of the plasma glucose concentration. This is in keeping with translocation of more glucose transporters into the cell membrane under the influence of increasing insulin concentrations.

4. The parallel nature of the plots shown in Figure 7.3C indicates that increasing insulin concentrations are associated with increasing number of "receptors"—in this case, glucose transporters. There is no sign of a change in "affnity" of the transporters under the influence of insulin, just the number present to facilitate glucose entry into cells (Sonksen 2001).

A cohort of patients referred to a deliberate self-harm team was asked to complete the HADS questionnaire. The HADS performed well as a screening instrument; a threshold score of eight gave a sensitivity of 88% and a positive predictive value of 80%. Its use by non-psychiatrists to detect depressive disorder in patients presenting with deliberate self-harm has been recommended (Hamer 1991).

Hart and Frier (1998) retrospectively surveyed 56 admissions, to an urban teaching hospital, of hypoglycemic patients in a 12-month period and showed that 80% were diabetics receiving insulin. Of these cases, 20% was a consequence of excessive alcohol consumption or deliberate self-poisoning with insulin and had a history of psychiatric disorder. Konrad et al. (1998) discussed the hospital admission of a bodybuilder taking 70 IU insulin for its anabolic effect but suffering hypoglycemic convulsions. The HADS questionnaire was therefore considered as an appropriate tool to delineate any psychopathology in this cohort of drug users and to exclude any possibility of physical disease.

THE EFFECTS OF INSULIN ON ANTHROPOMETRY AND EXERCISE PERFORMANCE

Insulin inhibits lipolysis and stimulates lipogenesis over the same concentration range and is mediated by the same receptor (Thomas, Wisher, Brandenburg et al. 1979). Hill and Milner (1985) have shown that insulin is a potent mitogen for many cell types in vitro. They concluded that insulin promotes the growth of selected tissues by a direct action. However, in the musculoskeletal system, the action is indirect, via the regulation of IGF-1 release.

Sato et al. (1986) demonstrated that an increase in glucose metabolism to exogenous insulin in athletes (determined by euglycemic insulin-clamp technique) was significantly higher than in controls. $\dot{V}O_2$peak was also significantly increased after 1 month's physical training. His data showed that tissue sensitivity to physiological hyper-insulinemia was 46% higher in trained athletes and that physical training improved insulin sensitivity and lipid metabolism.

The IR of aging is reversible in older persons (60- to 80-year-olds). It can be decreased by increasing the level of physical training, independent of changes in weight or body composition (Tonino 1989).

Insulin has effects on protein synthesis and breakdown in muscle, at concentrations seen after meals (Bennet, Connacher, Scrimgeour et al. 1989). Protein synthesis is not performed by insulin but by its regulation of IGF-1 and GH (Bennet, Connacher, Scrimgeour et al. 1990).

Its anabolic actions are believed to improve performance by increasing protein synthesis (Bonadonna, Saccomani, Cobelli et al. 1993; Kimball et al. 1994) and inhibiting protein catabolism and enhancing transport of selected amino acids in human skeletal muscle (Biolo, Fleming, Wolfe et al. 1995). Bonadonna et al. (1993) demonstrated that physiological hyperinsulinemia stimulates the activity of amino acid transport in human skeletal muscle, thereby stimulating protein synthesis.

Seven consecutive days of exercise blunted the hyperinsulinemia associated with aging, independent of any changes in body composition (Cononie, Goldberg, Rogus et al. 1994).

Hyperaminoacidemia specifically stimulates muscle protein synthesis and even in the presence of hyperaminoacidemia insulin improves muscle protein balance, solely by inhibiting proteolysis. Hyperaminoacidemia combined with IGF-1 enhances protein synthesis more than either alone (Fryburg et al. 1995).

Impaired early insulin response and late hyperinsulinemia were predictors of type 2 DM in middle-aged Swedish men (Eriksson, Lindgarde 1996). IR preceded glucose intolerance and poor physical fitness, as measured by significantly lower $\dot{V}O_2$peak (16%), significantly lower mean vital capacity (10%), and significantly higher BMI (10%).

Healthy first-degree relatives (FDR) of patients with type 2 DM have a significantly diminished physical work capacity (determined by $\dot{V}O_2$peak), supporting the argument of a genetic predisposition (Nyholm, Mengel, Nielsen et al. 1996). Insulin-treated diabetics are known to have increased LBM versus controls (Sinha, Formica, Tsalamandris et al. 1996).

Insulin induces body weight gain by protecting lean mass, but also leads to fat accumulation in type

2 DM (Rigalleau, Delafaye, Baillet et al. 1999). In addition to its role in regulating glucose metabolism, insulin increases amino acid transport into cells. Its stimulation of lipogenesis and diminished lipolysis, are reasons why body builders and athletes will take rhGH in conjunction with insulin, to counteract this adverse effect while optimizing protein synthesis (Sonksen, Sonksen 2000; Sonksen 2001).

Insulin modulates transcription, altering the cell content of numerous mRNAs. It stimulates growth, DNA synthesis, and cell replication. Insulin administration to uncontrolled diabetics switches off certain metabolic processes (lipolysis, proteolysis, ketogenesis, and gluconeogenesis) (Sonksen 2001). It is the inhibition of proteolysis that the athlete is interested in and the physiology of the diabetic patient has been extrapolated by the "intelligent" athlete to the sporting arena. Insulin increases glucose metabolism by reducing FFA and ketone levels and recruits more glucose transporters to the muscle cell membranes, which facilitates glucose uptake and is reflected in an increase of the MCR of glucose (the amount of glucose cleared from the blood in unit time [mL/kg]).

Insulin may enhance performance. Primarily, it stimulates glycogen formation. The administration of exogenous insulin establishes an in vivo hyperinsulinemic clamp, increasing muscle glycogen before and in the recovery stages of strenuous exercise. This increase is believed by the athlete to increase power, strength, and stamina and assist recovery.

Second, by inhibiting muscle protein breakdown and in conjunction with a high-protein/high-carbohydrate diet, insulin will have the action of increasing muscle bulk, potentially improving performance.

Insulin administration is protein anabolic in the insulin-resistant state of chronic renal failure (uremia). It inhibits proteolysis and when administered with amino acids increases net protein synthesis (Lim, Yarasheki, Crowley et al. 2003).

Skeletal muscle glucose uptake is higher in trained men than in untrained men at high relative exercise intensity, although at lower relative exercise intensities no differences are observed (Fujimoto, Kemppainen, Kalliokoski et al. 2003).

Elite power athletes appear to be more insulin resistant than elite endurance athletes (Chou, Lai, Hsu et al. 2005). Chou postulated that such an individual may actually benefit from the effects of exogenous insulin. Healthy, insulin-resistant false discovery rate (FDR) of type 2 DM patients have significantly enhanced visceral obesity and significantly reduced $\dot{V}O_2$peak, compared with people without a family history of diabetes, despite similar BMI and overall fat mass (Nyholm, Nielsen, Kristensen et al. 2004).

$\dot{V}O_2$peak is significantly increased in hyperinsulinemic insulin-resistant (IR) subjects, as a consequence of exercise training. This was not associated with improvement of the inflammatory markers CRP and adiponectin (Marcell, McAuley, Traustadottir et al. 2005).

Independent of body fat, BMI, lean mass, and $\dot{V}O_2$peak, IR spares muscle glycogen and shifts substrate oxidation toward less carbohydrate use (50% lower in the IR vs. insulin sensitive [IS] group) and more lipid (28% higher in the IR vs. IS group) during exercise (Braun, Sharoff, Chipkin et al. 2004). This may contribute to the decreased $\dot{V}O_2$peak of hyperinsulinemia and the increased cardiovascular risk.

Age-related diminution in the composition of skeletal muscle (SM) mass (sarcopenia), if left untreated, may lead to functional impairment and physical disability. The accumulation of lipids within SM fibers may lead to metabolic disorders such as IR. This would appear to correlate with diminution in physical exercise, which accompanies aging (Janssen, Ross 2005).

Muscular strength is inversely associated with MS incidence, independent of age and body size in 3233 men over a 23-year period (Jurca, Lamonte, Barlow et al. 2005).

In obese subjects, dynamic strength training improves whole body and adipose tissue responsiveness. It increases responsiveness to the adrenergic β-receptor stimulation of lipolysis and to the antilipolytic action of catecholamines mediated by antilipolytic adrenergic α-2A receptors. However, there were no training-induced changes in mRNA levels of key genes of the lipolytic pathway in the subcutaneous abdominal adipose tissue (Polak, Moro, Klimcakova et al. 2005).

Strength training is more effective than endurance training over a 4-month period in improving glycemic control and lipid profile and may therefore play a very important role in the treatment of type 2 DM (Cauza, Hanusch-Enserer, Strasser et al. 2005).

As a consequence of this and similar information being available, bodybuilders and athletes are buying insulin from insulin-dependent diabetics, who get free "pen-fills" paid for by the United Kingdom national health service (NHS) (personal communications). It is possible that the sports individual, who is self-administering exogenous insulin, can be extrapolated to the hyperinsulinemic state with its concomitant metabolic risks. It is believed that sportspersons who take insulin may be counseled by physiologists within the scientific community, who are not averse to advising their protégés on the "emperor's new clothes."

THE EFFECTS OF INSULIN ON BLOOD PRESSURE

Hyperinsulinemia is a major risk factor for atherosclerosis and the changes in the vessel wall begin earlier and advance more rapidly in diabetics, than in non-diabetics (Meissner, Legg 1973). Many hyperinsuline-mic populations also have hypertension, which is not related to age or therapy for hypertension, and insulin and BP are closely related in both normotensive and hypertensive populations (Welborn, Breckenridge, Rubinstein et al. 1966; Modan, Halkin, Almog et al. 1985; Ferranini, Buzzigoli, Bonadonna et al. 1987). The work of Pfeifle and Ditschuneit (1981), has shown that insulin stimulates human arterial smooth mus-cle cell proliferation and migration in all concentra-tions in vitro, but does not appear to have an effect on endothelial cells cultured from large vessels (Stout 1990). There are several possible mechanisms by which insulin might be causally related to hyperten-sion (Reaven, Hoffman 1987). These include effects of insulin on renal sodium reabsorption (DeFronzo 1981) and enhanced sympathetic nervous system activ-ity in hyperinsulinemic states (Rowe, Young, Minaker et al. 1981; Landsberg 1986). This does not explain the full picture of hypertension in obesity. The work of O'Hare et al. (1989) has shown that at baseline, obese men displayed higher glucose and insulin lev-els and faster pulse rates and elevated mean arterial pressures (MAP) than lean controls. O'Hare infused insulin into both sets of subjects and showed only an increased sodium excretory rate in the obese subjects. He concluded that it was unlikely for the insulin to have an effect on sympathetic activity as a cause for resting tachycardia and borderline hypertension. More recent research has shown that serum glucocor-ticoid–regulated kinase 1 (SGK-1) risk carriers are at increased risk of hypertension and are more sensitive to the BP-elevating effects associated with hyperinsu-linemia. Insulin stimulation of the SGK-1 prolongs the half-life of the epithelial sodium channel, a chan-nel which is essential for BP regulation (von Wowern, Berglund, Carlson et al. 2005).

THE EFFECTS OF INSULIN ON HEART RATE

Previous research has shown enhanced sympathetic nervous system activity in hyperinsulinemic states (Rowe, Young, Minaker et al. 1981; Landsberg 1986; O' Hare, Minaker, Meneilly et al. 1989). Scott et al. (1988) have shown that during hyperinsulinemia, resting SBP rises significantly and is accompanied by forearm vasodilatation. Forearm blood flow (FABF) and heart rate (HR) are significantly higher at lower body subatmospheric pressure (LBSP) during hyperinsulinemia.

Insulin causes sympathetic excitation via the modification of baroreflex, noradrenaline release, or central sympathetic outflow.

Kohno et al. (2000) examined the effect of exer-cise training on insulin sensitivity in conjunction with the inhibition of sympathetic tone in hypertensive patients. Plasma insulin levels and arterial baroreflex function before and after 3 weeks of exercise train-ing (75% $\dot{V}O_2$peak, 6 minutes, four times daily) were evaluated. Twenty-four hour BP recordings, arterial baroreflex function testing, and 75 g glucose tolerance tests were conducted. Area under the curve of insulin (sigma insulin) to glucose load was calculated as an index of hyperinsulinemia. Heart rate significantly decreased and sigma insulin significantly decreased, and baroreflex function significantly improved. These results suggested that the improvement of neurometa-bolic factors may be involved in the depressor effect caused by exercise training.

THE EFFECTS OF INSULIN ON HEMOGLOBIN AND PACKED CELL VOLUME (HEMATOCRIT)

The work of Catalano et al. (1997) has shown that insulin sensitivity is inversely related to the packed cell volume (PCV) independently of the glucose tol-erance status. The association does not result from acute hemodynamic effects on insulin sensitivity, and may therefore reflect an action of IR/hyperinsuline-mia on blood viscosity, or the presence of a common determinant. It has also been reported that increased PCV and hemoglobin values often accompany IR and compensatory hyperinsulinemia in humans (Facchini et al. 1998). Moan et al. (1994) and Hoieggen et al. (1998) demonstrated that significant negative correla-tions between the glucose disposal rate (GDR, a mea-sure of insulin sensitivity) and calculated whole-blood viscosity at both high and low shear rates. He observed negative associations between GDR and PCV, which highlights that elevated blood viscosity is linked to the IR syndrome.

Barbieri et al. (2001) provided in vivo evidence of a relation between hyperinsulinemia/IR and eryth-ropoiesis. He demonstrated a significant correla-tion between IR and red blood cell count (r = 0.14), plasma Hb (r = 0.16), PCV (r = 0.15), and plasma iron concentrations (r = 0.1). Red blood cell count was also associated with the other biological markers of insu-lin-resistance syndrome. IR and BMI were significant and independent predictors of red blood cell count even when the analysis was adjusted for age, sex, waist-to-hip ratio, plasma iron, and any drug intake.

Brand et al. (2003) demonstrated that male and female carriers of the T allele at position 825 of the *G-protein β-(3)-subunit* gene have a significantly higher PCV and erythrocyte count. Male TT homozygotes have a significantly higher BP and are significantly more obese and IR than C allele carriers. He speculated that the higher BP in TT homozygous men might arise via a metabolic pathway characterized by obesity and IR as well as via increased peripheral resistance secondary to the higher PCV.

Taniguchi et al. (2003) showed that the IR index of homeostasis model assessment (HOMA-IR) was positively correlated to BMI, glycosylated Hb (HbA$_{1C}$), platelet count, TGs, white blood cell count, red blood cell count, PCV, TC, and SBP and DBP, and inversely correlated to HDL-C level in diabetic patients.

A proposed mechanism for the action of insulin is based on the growing evidence that increases in both PCV and body iron stores are components of the IR syndrome. The ability of insulin and of IGF-1, whose effective activity is increased in the context of IR to boost activity of the transcription factor hypoxia-inducible factor-1-α (HIF-1-α), may be at least partially responsible for this association. HIF-1-α, which functions physiologically as a detector of both hypoxia and iron deficiency, promotes synthesis of erythropoietin, and may also mediate the upregulatory impact of hypoxia on intestinal iron absorption. Insulin/IGF-1 may also influence erythropoiesis more directly as they are growth factors for developing reticulocytes. Conversely, the activation of HIF-1-α associated with iron deficiency may be responsible for the increased glucose tolerance noted in iron-deficient animals; HIF-1-α promotes efficient glucose uptake and glycolysis, a sensible adaptation to hypoxia, by inducing increased synthesis of glucose transporters and glycolytic enzymes (McCarty 2003).

An association has been noted in individuals with the MS, who in addition to IR, harbor a chronic low-grade inflammation. One postulate is that chronic inflammation might have a suppressive effect on erythropoiesis. A significant correlation between the numbers of the components of the MS and the inflammatory biomarkers including the white blood cell count, high-sensitivity CRP, fibrinogen concentrations, and the erythrocyte sedimentation rate was made. In addition, a significant correlation was noted between the number of components of the MS and the number of red blood cells in the peripheral blood in men (r = 0.192) and women (r = 0.157). Erythropoiesis may be a new component of the MS. The enhanced erythropoiesis could give an erroneous impression of general "good" health in these individuals (Mardi, Toker, Melmed et al. 2005).

THE EFFECTS OF INSULIN ON RESPIRATORY FUNCTION

Research has shown inverse correlations with lung function and IR and hyperinsulinemia. Tissue sensitivity (measurement of glucose metabolism by euglycemic insulin-clamp technique) and $\dot{V}O_2$peak were significantly increased by exogenous insulin in athletes compared with controls after 1 month's physical training (Sato, Hayamizu, Yamamoto et al. 1986). Tissue sensitivity to supraphysiological hyperinsulinemia was 46% higher in trained athletes and physical training improved IS, glucose metabolism, and lipid metabolism. Rigorous exercise, which is known to sensitize the insulin receptor, appears to counteract the adverse effect of such a hyperinsulinemic state.

Tonino (1989) demonstrated that peripheral IR in older persons (60- to 80-year-olds) can be significantly decreased by increasing the level of physical training, independent of changes in weight or body composition. This suggests that the IR of aging is reversible and that the level of physical training should be considered in its management.

Cononie et al. (1994) also showed that seven consecutive days of exercise significantly decreased the hyperinsulinemia associated with aging, independent of any changes in body composition. Fasting plasma insulin levels and plasma insulin responses to an oral glucose challenge were significantly reduced by 15% and 20% in nine men and nine women, respectively.

IR precedes glucose intolerance, type 2 DM, and poor physical fitness (as measured by significantly lower $\dot{V}O_2$peak (16%), significantly lower mean vital capacity (10%), and significantly higher BMI (11%)) (Eriksson, Lindgarde 1996). The impaired early insulin response but late hyperinsulinemia were predictors of type 2 DM in middle-aged Swedish men (Eriksson, Lindgarde 1996).

Nyholm et al. (1996) showed that healthy FDR of patients with type 2 DM had a diminished physical work capacity (determined by $\dot{V}O_2$peak). This suggested an argument for a genetic predisposition.

Lazarus et al. (1998a) demonstrated a significantly impaired ventilatory function (forced vital capacity [FVC], forced expiratory volume in 1 second [FEV$_1$], maximal midexpiratory flow rate [MMEF]), risk of cardiovascular mortality, and IR in 1050 nondiabetic males over a 20-year period.

Males in the top quintile of fasting insulin and the fasting IR index (FIRI) were defined as IR. Fasting insulin and FIRI are negatively correlated with FVC, FEV$_1$, MMEF. Baseline ventilatory function predicts the development of higher levels of fasting insulin and FIRI (Lazarus, Sparrow, Weiss 1998b).

Engstrom et al. (2003) demonstrated that subjects with a significantly reduced FVC had an increased risk of developing IR and diabetes. This relationship also contributed to an association between reduced lung function and increased incidence of CVD.

Lawlor et al. (2004) demonstrated that FEV_1 and FVC were inversely associated with IR and prevalence of type 2 DM in 3911 women aged 60 to 79 years from 23 British towns.

Nyholm et al. (2004) demonstrated that healthy but IR FDR of type 2 DM have enhanced visceral obesity and significantly reduced $\dot{V}O_2$peak compared with people without a family history of diabetes, despite similar BMI and overall fat mass.

IR, independent of body fat, BMI, lean mass, and $\dot{V}O_2$peak, shifts substrate oxidation toward less carbohydrate and more lipid use during exercise (Braun, Sharoff, Chipkin et al. 2004). This may contribute to the decreased $\dot{V}O_2$peak of hyperinsulinemia and the increased CV risk.

In the CF model, Tofe et al. (2005) demonstrated that in impaired glucose tolerance (CF-IGT) and in CF-related diabetes (CFRD), there is a significant lowering of FEV_1 and FVC.

Exercise training significantly increases $\dot{V}O_2$peak in hyperinsulinemic (IR) subjects, but is not associated with improvement of the inflammatory markers CRP and adiponectin (Marcell, McAuley, Traustadottir et al. 2005).

ENDOTHELIAL DYSFUNCTION IN PATHOLOGICAL INSULIN STATES

Increased arterial stiffness is a risk factor for CVD and is a feature associated with DM. type 1 DM patients develop alterations in the arterial connective tissue independent of the presence of atherosclerosis. These primary alterations in the vessel wall may play a role in the pathogenesis of large vessel disease among such patients (Oxlund, Rasmussen, Andreassen et al. 1989).

Kool et al. (1995) showed that in uncomplicated type 1 DM distensibility of the femoral artery was significantly lower compared with that in controls. Early atherosclerotic changes in type 1 DM frequently occur at this site. CVD is the most common cause of disability and death among subjects with type 2 DM. The atherosclerotic process begins during the prediabetic phase characterized by IGT, hyperinsulinemia, and IR. Salomaa et al. (1995) demonstrated that persons with type 2 DM or borderline glucose intolerance have significantly stiffer arteries than healthy controls with normal glucose tolerance.

Goodfellow et al. (1996) provided evidence of vascular dysfunction in non–insulin dependent diabetes before the appearance of microalbuminuria, previously regarded as its earliest marker.

Patients with DM, followed up for 9 years, have shown significantly stiffer aortas at baseline (pulse wave velocity [PWV] 12.0 m/s) who subsequently died (censored in 1996/1997) than in those who remained alive (PWV 9.9 m/s) (Lehmann, Riley, Clarkson et al. 1997).

Vehkavaara et al. (2000) demonstrated that insulin therapy significantly improves endothelium-dependent and endothelium-independent vasodilatation in type 2 DM. These data supported the idea that insulin therapy has beneficial rather than harmful effects on vascular function.

Increased arterial stiffness is associated with risk variables of the MS in middle-aged and older adults. Hedblad et al. (2002) found that age and IMT were significantly higher in MS patients than in controls and is associated with a significantly increased incidence of coronary events and deaths.

Diabetic arteries age at an accelerated rate at an earlier age and then reach a functional plateau compared with controls (Cameron, Bulpitt, Pinto et al. 2003).

Impaired glucose metabolism (IGM) and type 2 DM are associated with significantly increased central artery stiffness, more pronounced in type 2 DM. Deteriorating glucose tolerance is associated with significantly increased central and peripheral arterial stiffness, which may partly explain why both type 2 DM and IGM are associated with increased cardiovascular risk (Schram, Henry, van Dijk et al. 2004).

Lacy et al. (2004) demonstrated that pulse pressure (PP) and PWV are significantly increased in people with DM, but not associated with increased AI^x. AI^x is not an absolute measure of arterial stiffness in people with DM.

Scuteri et al. (2004) showed that the clustering of at least three of the components of the MS is independently associated with increased IMT and stiffness. The main findings were as follows:

1. MS significantly increased carotid arterial thickness (+6%) and stiffness (+32%) across all age groups.
2. MS exerts its effects on carotid structure and function independent of its individual components and other cardiovascular risk factors.

The deleterious effects of the MS on arterial stiffness underscore the importance of this syndrome in cardiovascular risk assessment even in a younger population (Li, Chen, Srinivasan et al. 2005).

Potential mechanisms: MS exerts its deleterious effects by adversely affecting the structural and functional properties of the vasculature (thickness and stiffness). It is possible that a common pathogenic factor could underlie both the arterial structural changes and the alterations in the components that comprise MS. Circumferential wall stress and flow-mediated shear stress are considered to be important determinants of arterial wall structure and function during development and their remodeling during aging or in response to disease in adults (Rubanyi, Freany,

Kauser 1990; Glagov, Giddens, Zarins 1992; Laurent 1995; Mulvany, Baumbach, Aalkjaer et al. 1996). BP and blood flow are major determinants of these mechanical stresses that act on the arterial wall and lumen. Specific alterations in carotid geometry are associated with differing levels of flow-mediated shear stress and result in specific patterns of alterations in carotid function (Scuteri, Chen, Yin et al. 2001).

Another potential mechanism by which MS can alter the structure and function of large arteries might be the glycation of matrix proteins. Alterations in matrix proteins within the vessel wall can be derived from non-enzymatic cross-links between glucose (or other reducing sugars) and amino groups that generate advanced glycation end products (AGEPs) (Lee, Cerami 1992; Airaksinen, Salmela, Linnaluoto et al. 1993). The AGEPs accumulate slowly on long-lived proteins, such as collagen and elastin, and lead to increased stiffening of both arteries and the heart (Lee, Cerami 1992).

Medication-induced cleavage of the AGEPs cross-links favorably improves measures of vascular stiffness in older human subjects (Kass, Shapiro, Kawaguchi et al. 2001). In end-stage renal disease (ESRD), the calculation of a PWV index provides information about cardiovascular and overall mortality risk with high predictive power, showing that PWV measurements provide prognostic power over and above conventional cardiovascular risk factors (Blacher, Safar, Guerin et al. 2003).

It is suspected that low-grade inflammation as represented by increased CRP plays an important role in the progression of atherosclerosis and is associated with PWV. CRP correlates significantly with age, mean arterial pressure (MAP), brachial and aortic PWV, and PPs in healthy individuals (Yasmin, McEniery, Wallace et al. 2004).

A cross-sectional study has demonstrated in the general population that arterial stiffness is independently significantly correlated with serum CRP levels after adjustment for other established cardiovascular risk factors (age, SBP, HR, BMI) (Nagano, Nakamura, Sato et al. 2005).

HCY has been implicated in a variety of cardiovascular-related diseases. Total HCY (tHCY), a byproduct of methionine metabolism, however, has been shown not to be associated with arterial PWV in a healthy young population (Woodside, McMahon, Gallagher et al. 2004).

THE EFFECTS OF GROWTH HORMONE AND INSULIN ON BLOOD PRESSURE AND HEART RATE

The combined effects of GH and insulin administration have not been studied in sport, but they have been used in bodybuilding and similar groups for more than 15 years (personal communications). To date no research has been conducted to establish the effects of such administration on the cardiovascular system. We are aware that bodybuilders are abusing these drugs in combination in an attempt to enhance the bulking effects of insulin, with the lipolytic effect of GH (Sonksen 2001).

Such a model may mimic the hyperinsulinemic state of acromegaly, induced both by insulin and rhGH administration. IR and therefore a hyperinsulinemic state are a cardinal feature of excess GH states, but the underlying mechanisms are enigmatic. Barbour et al. (2005) have shown the importance of increased p85 regulatory subunit of phosphatidylinositol kinase (PI 3-kinase) and decrease in IRS-1-associated PI 3-kinase activity in the skeletal muscle of transgenic animals overexpressing human placental growth hormone. Their findings have demonstrated the importance of increased p85α in mediating skeletal muscle IR in response to GH and suggested a potential role for reducing p85α as a therapeutic strategy for enhancing IS in skeletal muscle.

Hypertension is an important complication of excess GH as is seen in acromegaly, contributing to the increased morbidity and mortality of this condition. Prevalence of hypertension in acromegalic patients is about 35%, ranging from 18% to 60% in different clinical series, and the incidence is higher than in the general population. The lowering of BP observed concomitantly with the reduction in GH levels after successful therapy for acromegaly suggests a relationship between GH and IGF-1 excess and hypertension. The exact mechanisms underlying the development of hypertension in acromegaly are still not clear but may include several factors depending on the chronic exposure to GH and IGF-1 excess. Experimental and clinical studies suggest that the antinatriuretic action of GH (due to direct renal action of GH or IGF-1 and to indirect, systemic GH- or IGF-1-mediated mechanisms) may play a role in the pathogenesis of hypertension. Acromegaly is frequently associated with IR and hyperinsulinemia, which may induce hypertension by stimulating renal sodium absorption and sympathetic nervous activity. Whether sympathetic tone is altered in acromegalic hypertensive patients remains a matter of debate. Recent studies indicate that an increased sympathetic tone or abnormalities in the circadian activity of the sympathetic system could play an important role in development or maintenance of elevated BP in acromegaly, and may partially account for the increased risk of cardiovascular complications. Acromegalic cardiomyopathy may also elevate BP and can be aggravated by the coexistence of hypertension. Finally, a role of GH and IGF-1 as vascular growth factors cannot be excluded. In conclusion, acromegaly is associated with hypertension, but there is still no real consensus in the literature on the mechanisms behind the development of hypertension (Bondanelli, Ambrosio, degli Uberti 2001).

Colao et al. (2002) demonstrated a reduction in the resting and maximal heart rate following treatment with the GH antagonist, octreotide, in early-onset GH excess. There was also a corresponding lowering of insulin levels, demonstrating the coexistence of a hyperinsulinemic state in acromegaly, with its enhanced stimulation of the sympathetic system.

SUMMARY

AASs and insulin abuse both have overt adverse effects. GH abuse appears to offer some degree of protection in the short term; however, it is not without inherent risks as demonstrated by the significant increase in RPP. Longer studies are required to determine whether it has a place as a therapeutic replacement in AAS withdrawal or even as a hormonal therapy for replacement in the somatopause.

ACKNOWLEDGMENTS   We acknowledge the contribution and assistance of Dr Andrew Kicman, from The Drug Control Centre, King's College, London.

REFERENCES

Abdu TA, Elhadd TA, Akber M, Hartland A, Neary R, Clayton RN. 2001. Plasma homocysteine is not a major risk factor for vascular disease in growth hormone deficient adults. *Clin Endocrinol. (Oxf).* 55:635–638.

Airaksinen KE, Salmela PI, Linnaluoto MK, Ikaheimo MJ, Ahola K, Ryhanen LJ. 1993. Diminished arterial elasticity in diabetes: association with fluorescent advanced glycosylation end products in collagen. *Cardiovasc Res.* 27:942–945.

Alcantara MR, Salvatori R, Alcantara PR et al. 2006. Thyroid morphology and function in adults with untreated isolated growth hormone deficiency. *J Clin Endocrinol Metab.* 91:860–864.

Amato G, Carella C, Fazio S et al. 1993. Body composition, bone metabolism, and heart structure and function in growth hormone (GH)-deficient adults before and after GH replacement therapy at low doses. *J Clin Endocrinol Metab.* 77:1671–1676.

Angelin B, Rudling M. 1994. Growth hormone and hepatic lipoprotein metabolism. *Curr Opin Lipidol.* 5:160–165.

Argetsinger LS, Campbell GS, Yang X et al. 1993. Identification of JAK2 as a growth hormone receptor-associated tyrosine kinase. *Cell.* 237–244.

Attanasio AF, Lamberts SW, Matranga AM et al. 1997. Adult growth hormone-deficient patients demonstrate heterogeneity between childhood onset and adult onset before and during human GH treatment. *J Clin Endocrinol Metab.* 82:82–88.

Bak JF, Moller N, Schmitz O. 1991. Effects of growth hormone on fuel utilization and muscle glycogen synthase activity in normal humans. *Am J Physiol.* 260:36–42.

Baker JS, Graham MR, Davies B. 2006. "Steroid" and prescription medicine abuse in the health and fitness community: a regional study. *Eur J Intern Med.* 17:479–484.

Barbieri M, Ragno E, Benvenuti E et al. 2001. New aspects of the insulin resistance syndrome: impact on haematological parameters. *Diabetologia.* 44:1232–1237.

Barbour LA, Mizanoor Rahman S, Gurevich I et al. 2005. Increased P85alpha is a potent negative regulator of skeletal muscle insulin signalling and induces in vivo insulin resistance associated with growth hormone excess. *J Biol Chem.* 280:37489–37494.

Barry MC, Mealy K, O'Neill S et al. 1999. Nutritional, respiratory, and psychological effects of recombinant human growth hormone in patients undergoing abdominal aortic aneurysm repair. *J Parenter Enteral Nutr.* 23:128–135.

Baumann G. 1991. Growth hormone heterogeneity: genes, isohormones, variants, and binding proteins. *Endocr Rev.* 12:424–449.

Bengtsson BA, Eden S, Lonn L et al. 1993. Treatment of adults with growth hormone (GH) deficiency with recombinant human GH. *J Clin Endocrinol Metab.* 76:309–317.

Bengtsson BA, Johannsson G. 1999. Effect of growth-hormone therapy on early atherosclerotic changes in GH-deficient adults. *Lancet.* 353:1898–1899.

Bennet WM, Connacher AA, Scrimgeour CM, Smith K, Rennie MJ. 1989. Increase in anterior tibialis muscle protein synthesis in healthy man during mixed amino acid infusion: studies of incorporation of [1–^{13}C] leucine. *Clin Sci. (Lond).* 76:447–454.

Bennet WM, Connacher AA, Scrimgeour CM. 1990. Euglycaemic hyperinsulinaemia augments amino acid uptake by human leg tissues during hyperaminoacidaemia. *Am J Physiol.* 259:185–194.

Berggren A, Ehrnborg C, Rosen T et al. 2005. Short-term administration of supraphysiological recombinant human growth hormone (GH) does not increase maximum endurance exercise capacity in healthy, active young men and women with normal GH-insulin-like growth factor I axes. *J Clin Endocrinol Metab.* 90:3268–3273.

Beshyah SA, Thomas E, Kyd P, Sharp P, Fairney A, Johnston DG. 1994. The effect of growth hormone replacement therapy in hypopituitary adults on calcium and bone metabolism. *Clin Endocrinol. (Oxf).* 40:383–391.

Beshyah SA, Freemantle C, Shahi M et al. 1995. Replacement treatment with biosynthetic human growth hormone in growth hormone-deficient hypopituitary adults. *Clin Endocrinol. (Oxf).* 42:73–84.

Bhasin S, Storer TW, Berman N et al. 1996. The effects of supraphysiologic doses of testosterone on muscle size and strength in normal men. *N Engl J Med.* 335:1–7.

Bing-You RG, Denis MC, Rosen CJ. 1993. Low bone mineral density in adults with previous hypothalamic-pituitary tumours: correlations with serum growth hormone responses to GH-releasing hormone, insulin-like growth factor I, and IGF binding protein 3. *Calcif Tissue Int.* 52:183–187.

Binnerts A, Swart GR, Wilson JH et al. 1992. The effect of growth hormone administration in growth hormone-deficient adults on bone, protein, carbohydrate and lipid homeostasis, as well as body composition. *Clin Endocrinol. (Oxf).* 37:79–87.

Biolo G, Fleming RYD, Wolfe RD. 1995. Physiologic hyperinsulinaemia stimulates protein synthesis and enhances transport of selected amino acids in human skeletal Muscle. *J Clin Invest.* 95:811–819.

Biolo G, Iscra F, Bosutti A et al. 2000. Growth hormone decreases muscle glutamine production and stimulates protein synthesis in hypercatabolic patients. *Am J Physiol Endocrinol Metab.* 279:323–332.

Blacher J, Safar ME, Guerin AP, Pannier B, Marchais SJ, London GM. 2003. Aortic pulse wave velocity index and mortality in end-stage renal disease. *Kidney Int.* 63:1852–1860.

Black MM, Shuster S, and Bottoms E. 1972. Skin collagen and thickness in acromegaly and hypopituitarism. *Clin Endocrinol.* 1: 259–263.

Blackman MR, Sorkin JD, Münzer T et al. 2002. Growth hormone and sex steroid administration in healthy aged women and men. *JAMA.* 288:2282–2292.

Bolanowski M, Daroszewski J, Medras M, Zadrozna-Sliwka B. 2006. Bone mineral density and turnover in patients with acromegaly in relation to sex, disease activity, and gonadal function. *J Bone Miner Metab.* 24:72–78.

Bollerslev J, Moller J, Thomas S, Djoseland O, Christiansen JS. 1996. Dose-dependent effects of recombinant human growth hormone on biochemical markers of bone and collagen metabolism in adult growth hormone deficiency. *Eur J Endocrinol.* 135:666–6671.

Bonadonna RC, Saccomani MP, Cobelli C, Defronzo RA. 1993. Effect of insulin on system A amino acid transport in human skeletal muscle. *J Clin Invest.* 91:514–521.

Bondanelli M, Ambrosio MR, degli Uberti EC. 2001. Pathogenesis and prevalence of hypertension in acromegaly. *Pituitary.* 4:239–249.

Boroujerdi MA, Umpleby AM, Jones RH, Sonksen PH. 1995. A simulation model for glucose kinetics and estimates of glucose utilization rate in type I diabetic patients. *Am J Physiol.* 268:766–774.

Borson-Chazot F, Serusclat A, Kalfallah Y et al. 1999. Decrease in carotid intima-media thickness after one year growth hormone (GH) treatment in adults with GH deficiency. *J Clin Endocrinol Metab.* 84:1329–1333.

Bowes SB, Umpleby M, Cummings MH et al. 1997. The effect of recombinant human growth hormone on glucose and leucine metabolism in Cushing's syndrome. *J Clin Endocrinol Metab.* 84:1329–1333.

Bowes SB, Umpleby M, Cummings MH et al. 1997. The effect of recombinant human growth hormone on glucose and leucine metabolism in Cushing's syndrome. *J Clin Endocrinol Metab.* 82:243–246.

Brand E, Wang JG, Herrmann SM, Staessen JA. 2003. An epidemiological study of blood pressure and metabolic phenotypes in relation to the Gbeta3 C825T polymorphism. *J Hypertens.* 21:729–737.

Braun B, Sharoff C, Chipkin SR, Beaudoin F. 2004. Effects of insulin resistance on substrate utilization during exercise in overweight women. *J Appl Physiol.* 97:991–997.

Bravenboer N, Holzmann P, de Boer H, Blok GJ, Lips P. 1996. Histomorphometric analysis of bone mass and bone metabolism in growth hormone deficient adult men. *Bone.* 18: 551–557.

Bravenboer N, Holzmann P, de Boer H, Roos JC, van der Veen EA, Lips P. 1997. The effect of growth hormone (GH) on histomorphometric indices of bone structure and bone turnover in GH-deficient men. *J Clin Endocrinol Metab.* 82:1818–1822.

Brill KT, Weltman AL, Gentili A et al. 2002. Single and combined effects of growth hormone and testosterone administration on measures of body composition, physical performance, mood, sexual function, bone turnover, and muscle gene expression in healthy older men. *J Clin Endocrinol Metab.* 87:5649–5657.

Brown P, Tomkins C, Juul S, Sonksen PH. 1978. Mechanism of action of insulin in diabetic patients: a dose related effect on glucose production and utilisation. *Br Med J.* 1:1239–1242.

Brown RJ, Adams JJ, Pelekanos RA et al. 2005. Model for growth hormone receptor activation based on subunit rotation within a receptor dimer. *Nat Struct Mol Biol.* 12:814–821.

Bruchovsky N, Wilson JD. 1968. The conversion of testosterone to 5-alpha-androstan-17-beta-ol-3-one by rat prostate in vivo and in vitro. *J Biol Chem.* 243:2012–2021.

Burdet L, de Muralt B, Schutz Y, Pichard C, Fitting JW. 1997. Administration of growth hormone to underweight patients with chronic obstructive pulmonary disease. A prospective, randomized, controlled study. *Am J Respir Crit Care Med.* 156:1800–1806.

Cacciari E, Cicognani A, Pirazzoli P et al. 1979. Effect of long-term growth hormone administration on pituitary-thyroid function in idiopathic hypopituitarism. *Acta Pediatr Scand.* 68:405–409.

Caidahl K, Eden S, Bengtsson BA. 1994. Cardiovascular and renal effects of growth hormone. *Clin Endocrinol. (Oxf).* 40:393–400.

Cameron JD, Bulpitt CJ, Pinto ES, Rajkumar C. 2003. The ageing of elastic and muscular arteries: a comparison of diabetic and non-diabetic subjects. *Diabetes Care.* 26:2133–2138.

Carroll PV, Christ ER, Bengtsson BA et al. 1998. Growth hormone deficiency in adulthood and the effects of growth hormone replacement: a review. Growth Hormone Research Society Scientific Committee. *J Clin Endocrinol Metab.* 83:382–395.

Catalano C, Muscelli E, Natali A et al. 1997. Reciprocal association between insulin sensitivity and the haematocrit in man. *Eur J Clin Invest.* 27:634–637.

Cauza E, Hanusch-Enserer U, Strasser B et al. 2005. The relative benefits of endurance and strength training on the metabolic factors and muscle function of people with type II diabetes mellitus. *Arch Phys Med Rehabil.* 86:1527–1533.

Chou SW, Lai CH, Hsu TH et al. 2005. Characteristics of glycaemic control in elite power and endurance athletes. *Prev Med.* 40:564–9.

Christ ER, Carroll PV, Russell-Jones DL, Sonksen PH. 1997a. The consequences of growth hormone deficiency in adulthood, and the effects of growth hormone replacement. *Schweiz Med Wonchenschr.* 127:1440–1449.

Christ ER, Cummings MH, Westwood NB et al. 1997b. The importance of growth hormone in the regulation of erythropoiesis, red cell mass, and plasma volume in adults with growth hormone deficiency. *J Clin Endocrinol Metab.* 82:2985–2990.

Cittadini A, Cuocolo A, Merola B et al. 1994. Impaired cardiac performance in GH-deficient adults and its improvement after GH replacement. *Am J Physiol.* 267:219–225.

Colao A, Spinelli L, Cuocolo A et al. 2002. Cardiovascular consequences of early-onset growth hormone excess. *J Clin Endocrinol Metab.* 87:3097–3104.

Cononie CC, Goldberg AP, Rogus E, Hagberg JM. 1994. Seven consecutive days of exercise lowers plasma insulin responses to an oral glucose challenge in sedentary elderly. *J Am Geriatr Soc.* 42:394–398.

Crist DM, Peake GT, Egan PA, Waters DL. 1988. Body composition response to exogenous GH during training in highly conditioned adults. *J Appl Physiol.* 65:579–584.

Crist DM, Kraner JC. 1990. Supplemental growth hormone increases the tumor cytotoxic activity of natural killer cells in healthy adults with normal growth hormone secretion. *Metabolism.* 39:1320–1324.

Cuneo RC, Salomon F, Wiles CM, Sonksen PH. 1990. Skeletal muscle performance in adults with growth hormone-deficiency. *Horm Res.* 33:55–60.

Cuneo RC, Salomon F, Wiles CM, Hesp R, Sonksen PH. 1991a. Growth hormone treatment in growth hormone-deficient adults. I. Effects on muscle mass and strength. *J Appl Physiol.* 70:688–694.

Cuneo RC, Salomon F, Wiles CM, Hesp R, Sonksen PH. 1991b. Growth hormone treatment in growth hormone-deficient adults. II. Effects on exercise performance. *J Appl Physiol.* 70:695–700.

Cuneo RC, Salomon F, Wilmshurst P, et al. 1991c. Cardiovascular effects of growth hormone treatment in growth-hormone-deficient adults: stimulation of the renin-aldosterone system. *Clin Sci (Lond).* 81: 587–592.

Cuneo RC, Salomon F, Wiles CM, Hesp R, Sonksen PH. 1993. Growth hormone treatment improves serum lipids and lipoproteins in adults with growth hormone-deficiency. *J Clin Endocrinol Metab.* 42:1519–1523.

Danesh J, Wheeler JG, Hirschfield GM et al. 2004. C-reactive protein and other circulating markers of inflammation in the prediction of coronary heart disease. *N Engl J Med.* 350:1387–1397.

Dawson RT. 2001. Drugs in Sport. The role of the physician. *J Endocrinol.* 170:55–61.

De Boer H, Blok GJ, Voerman HJ, Phillips M, Schouten JA. 1994. Serum lipid levels in growth hormone-deficient men. *J Clin Endocrinol Metab.* 43:199–203.

DeFronzo RA. 1981. The effect of insulin on renal sodium metabolism: a review with clinical implications. *Diabetologia.* 21:165–171.

Degerblad M, Bengtsson BA, Bramnert M et al. 1995. Reduced bone mineral density in adults with growth hormone (GH) deficiency: increased bone turnover during 12 months of GH substitution therapy. *Eur J Endocrinol.* 133:180–188.

Deslypere JP, Young M, Wilson JD, McPhaul MJ. 1992. Testosterone and 5 alpha-dihydrotestosterone interact differently with the androgen receptor to enhance transcription of the MMTV-CAT reporter gene. *Mol Cell Endocrinol.* 88:15–22.

Deyssig R, Frisch H, Blum WF, Waldhor T. 1993. Effect of growth hormone treatment on hormonal parameters, body composition and strength in athletes. *Acta Endocrinol. (Copenh).* 128:313–318.

Di Pasquale MG. 1990. *Anabolic Steroid Side Effects—Facts, Fiction and Treatment.* Ontario: MGD Press. 63.

Duchaine D. 1983. *Underground Steroid Handbook*, 1st edition. California: HLR Technical Books, 84.

Ebenbichler CF, Kaser S, Bodner J et al. 2001. Hyperhomocysteinemia in anabolic steroid users. *Eur J Intern Med.* 12:43–47.

Eden S, Wiklund O, Oscarsson J, Rosén T, Bengtsson BA. 1993. Growth hormone treatment of growth hormone-deficient adults results in a marked increase in Lp(a) and HDL cholesterol concentrations. *Arterioscler Thromb.* 13:296–301.

Ehrnborg C, Bengtsson BA, Rosen T. 2000. Growth hormone abuse. *Bailleres Best Pract Res Clin Endocrinol Metab.* 14:71–77.

Ehrnborg C, Ellegard L, Bosaeus I, Bengtsson BA, Rosen T. 2005. Supraphysiological growth hormone: less fat, more extracellular fluid but uncertain effects on muscles in healthy, active young adults. *Clin Endocrinol. (Oxf).* 62:449–457.

Eichinger S, Stumpflen A, Hirschl M et al. 1998. Hyperhomocysteinemia is a risk factor of recurrent venous thromboembolism. *Thromb Haemost.* 80:566–569.

Engstrom G, Hedblad B, Nilsson P, Wollmer P, Berglund G, Janzon L. 2003. Lung function, insulin resistance and incidence of cardiovascular disease: a longitudinal cohort study. *J Intern Med.* 253:574–581.

Eriksson KF, Lindgarde F. 1996. Poor physical fitness, and impaired early insulin response but late hyperinsulinaemia, as predictors of NIDDM in middle-aged Swedish men. *Diabetologia.* 39:573–579.

Esposito JG, Thomas SG, Kingdon L, Ezzat S. 2005. Anabolic growth hormone action improves submaximal measures of physical performance in patients with HIV-associated wasting. *Am J Physiol Endocrinol Metab.* 289:494–503.

Eugster EA, Fisch M, Walvoord EC, DiMeglio LA, Pescovitz OH. 2002. Low haemoglobin levels in children with in idiopathic growth hormone deficiency. *Endocrine.* 18:135–136.

Evans LM, Davies JS, Goodfellow J, Rees JA, Scanlon MF. 1999. Endothelial dysfunction in hypopituitary adults with growth hormone deficiency. *Clin Endocrinol. (Oxf).* 50:457–464.

Evans LM, Davies JS, Anderson RA et al. 2000. The effect of GH replacement on endothelial function and oxidative stress in adult growth hormone deficiency. *Eur J Endocrinol.* 142:254–262.

Evans N. 1997. Gym and tonic: a profile of 100 male steroid users. *Br J Sports Med.* 31:54–58.

Evans PJ, Lynch RM. 2003. Insulin as a drug of abuse in body building. *Br J Sports Med.* 37:356–357.

Facchini FS, Carantoni M, Jeppesen J, Reaven GM. 1998. Haematocrit and haemoglobin are independently related to insulin resistance and compensatory hyper-insulinaemia in healthy, non-obese men and women. *Metabolism.* 47:831–835.

Ferenchick GS, Hirokawa S, Mammen EF, Schwartz KA. 1995. Anabolic-androgenic steroid abuse in weight lifters: evidence for activation of the hemostatic system. *Am J Hematol.* 49:282–288.

Ferranini E, Buzzigoli G, Bonadonna R et al. 1987. Insulin resistance in essential hypertension. *N Engl J Med.* 317:350–357.

Ferreira IM, Verreschi IT, Nery LE et al. 1998. The influence of 6 months of oral anabolic steroids on body mass and respiratory muscles in undernourished COPD patients. *Chest.* 114:19–28.

Fowelin J, Attvall S, Lager I, Bengtsson BA. 1993. Effects of treatment with recombinant human growth hormone on insulin sensitivity and glucose metabolism in adults with growth hormone deficiency. *Metab Clin Exp.* 42:1443–1447.

Fryburg DA, Gelfand RA, Barrett EJ. 1991. Growth hormone acutely stimulates forearm muscle protein synthesis in normal humans. *Am J Physiol.* 260:499–504.

Fryburg DA, Jahn LA, Hill SA, Oliveras DM, Barrett EJ. 1995. Insulin and Insulin-like Growth Factor-I enhance human skeletal muscle protein anabolism during hyperaminoacidaemia by different mechanisms. *J Clin Invest.* 96:1722–1729.

Fujimoto T, Kemppainen J, Kalliokoski KK, Nuutila P, Ito M, Knuuti J. 2003. Skeletal muscle glucose uptake in response to exercise in trained and untrained men. *Med Sci Sports Exerc.* 35:777–783.

Garcia-Rio F, Pino JM, Diez JJ, Ruíz A, Villasante C, Villamor J. 2001. Reduction of lung distensibility in acromegaly after suppression of growth hormone hypersecretion. *Am J Respir Crit Care Med.* 164:852–857.

Garry P, Collins P, Devlin JG. 1996. An open 36 month study of lipid changes with growth hormone in adults: lipid changes following replacement of growth hormone in adult acquired growth hormone deficiency. *Eur J Endocrinol.* 134:61–66.

Glagov S, Giddens DP, Zarins CK. 1992. Micro-architecture and composition of artery walls: relationship to location, diameter and the distribution of mechanical stress. *J Hypertens.* 10:101–104.

Goodfellow J, Ramsey MW, Luddington LA et al. 1996. Endothelium and inelastic arteries: an early marker of vascular dysfunction in non-insulin dependent diabetes. *BMJ.* 312:744–745.

Goodman HG, Grumbach MM, Kaplan SL. 1968. Growth and growth hormone. II. A comparison of isolated growth hormone deficiency and multiple pituitary hormone deficiencies in 35 patients with idiopathic hypopituitary dwarfism. *N Engl J Med.* 278:57–68.

Gotherstrom G, Svensson J, Koranyi J et al. 2001. A prospective study of 5 years of GH replacement therapy in GH-deficient adults: sustained effects on body composition, bone mass and metabolic indices. *J Clin Endocrinol Metab.* 86:4657–4665.

Gotherstrom G, Bengtsson BA, Sunnerhagen KS, Johannsson G, Svensson J. 2005. The effects of five-year growth hormone replacement therapy on muscle strength in elderly hypopituitary patients. *Clin Endocrinol. (Oxf).* 62:105–113.

Gotherstrom G, Bengtsson BA, Bosaeus I, Johannsson G, Svensson J. 2007a. Ten-year GH replacement increases bone mineral density in hypopituitary patients with adult onset GH deficiency. *Eur J Endocrinol.* 156:55–64.

Gotherstrom G, Bengtsson BA, Bosaeus I, Johannsson G, Svensson J. 2007b. A 10-year, prospective study of the metabolic effects of growth hormone replacement in adults. *J Clin Endocrinol Metab.* 92:1442–1445.

Gottesman I, Mandarino L, Verdonk C, Rizza R, Gerich J. 1982. Insulin increases the maximum velocity of glucose uptake without altering the Michaelis constant in man. *J Clin Invest.* 70:1310–1314.

Grace FM, Baker JS, Davies B. 2001. Anabolic androgenic steroid (AAS) use in recreational gym users—a regional sample of the Mid-Glamorgan area. *J Subst Use.* 12:45–153.

Grace FM, Davies B. 2004. Raised concentrations of C reactive protein in anabolic steroid using bodybuilders. *Br. J. Sports Med.* 38:97–98.

Graham MR, Grace FM, Boobier W et al. 2006. Homocysteine induced cardiovascular events: a consequence of long term anabolic-androgenic steroid (AAS) abuse. *Br J Sports Med.* 40:644–648.

Graham MR, Baker JS, Evans P et al. 2007a. Evidence for a decrease in cardiovascular risk factors following recombinant growth hormone administration in abstinent anabolic-androgenic steroid users. *Growth Horm. IGF Res.* 17:201–209.

Graham MR, Davies B, Hullin D et al. 2007b. The Short-term recombinant human growth hormone administration improves respiratory function in abstinent anabolic-androgenic steroid users. *Growth Horm. IGF Res.* 17:328–335.

Graham MR, Davies B, Hullin D, Kicman A, Cowan D, Baker JS. 2007c. Recombinant human growth hormone in abstinent androgenic-anabolic steroid use: psychological, endocrine, and trophic factor effects. *Curr Neurovasc Res.* 4:9–18.

Graham MR, Baker JS, Evans P et al. 2008. Physical effects of short term rhGH administration in abstinent steroid dependency. *Horm. Res.* 69:343–354.

Greig CA, Hameed M, Young A, Goldspink G, Noble B. 2006. Skeletal muscle IGF-I isoform expression in healthy women after isometric exercise. *Growth Horm. IGF Res.* 16:373–376.

Grunfeld C, Sherman BM, Cavalieri RR. 1988. The acute effects of human growth hormone administration on thyroid function in normal men. *J Clin Endocrinol Metab.* 67:1111–1114.

Gullestad L, Birkeland K, Bjonerheim R, Djøseland O, Trygstad O, Simonsen S. 1998. Exercise capacity and hormonal response in adults with childhood onset growth hormone deficiency during long-term somatropin treatment. *Growth Horm. IGF Res.* 8:377–384.

Halvorsen S, Bechensteen AG. 2002. Physiology of erythropoietin during mammalian development. *Acta. Paediatr.* 91:17–26.

Hamer D, Sanjeev D, Butterworth E, Barczak P. 1991. Using the Hospital Anxiety and Depression Scale to screen for psychiatric disorders in people presenting with deliberate self-harm. *Br J Psychiatry.* 158:782–784.

Hansen TB, Brixen K, Vahl N et al. 1996. Effects of 12 months of growth hormone (GH) treatment on calciotropic hormones, calcium homeostasis, and bone metabolism in adults with acquired GH deficiency: a double blind, randomized, placebo-controlled study. *J Clin Endocrinol Metab.* 81:3352–3359.

Hardin DS, Ellis KJ, Dyson M, Rice J, McConnell R, Seilheimer DK. 2001a. Growth hormone decreases protein catabolism in children with cystic fibrosis. *J Clin Endocrinol Metab.* 9:4424–4428.

Hardin DS, Ellis KJ, Dyson M, Rice J, McConnell R, Seilheimer DK. 2001b. Growth hormone improves clinical status in prepubertal children with cystic fibrosis: results of a randomized controlled trial. *J Pediatr.* 139:636–642.

Hardin DS, Ferkol T, Ahn C et al. 2005. A retrospective study of growth hormone use in adolescents with cystic fibrosis. *Clin Endocrinol. (Oxf).* 62:560–566.

Harrison BD, Millhouse KA, Harrington M, Nabarro JD. 1978. Lung function in acromegaly. *Q J Med.* 47:517–532.

Hart TB, Radow SK, Blackard WG, Tucker HS, Cooper KR. 1985. Sleep apnea in active acromegaly. *Arch Intern Med.* 145:865–866.

Hart SP, Frier BM. 1998. Causes, management and morbidity of acute hypoglycaemia in adults requiring a hospital admission. *Q J Med.* 91:505–510.

Haupt HA, Rovere GD. 1984. Anabolic steroids: a review of the literature. *Am J Sports Med.* 12:469–484.

Healy ML, Gibney J, Russell-Jones DL et al. 2003. High dose growth hormone exerts an anabolic effect at rest and during exercise in endurance-trained athletes. *J Clin Endocrinol Metab.* 11:5221–5226.

Healy ML, Gibney J Pentecost C, Croos P, Russell-Jones DL, Sönksen PH, Umpleby AM. 2006. Effects of high-dose growth hormone on glucose and glycerol metabolism at rest and during exercise in endurance-trained athletes. *J Clin Endocrinol Metab.* 9:320–327.

Hedblad B, Nilsson P, Engstrom G, Berglund G, Janzon L. 2002. Insulin resistance in non-diabetic subjects is associated with increased incidence of myocardial infarction and death. *Diabet Med.* 19:470–475.

Herrmann C. 1997. International experiences with the Hospital Anxiety and Depression Scale, a review of validation data and clinical results. *J Psychosom Res.* 42:17–41.

Hershberger LG, Shipley EG, Meyer RK. 1953. Myotrophic activity of 19-nortestosterone and other steroids determined by modified levator ani muscle method. *Proc Soc Exp Biol Med.* 83:175–180.

Hew FL, Koschmann M, Christopher M et al. 1996. Insulin resistance in growth hormone-deficient adults: defects in glucose utililization and glycogen synthase activity. *J Clin Endocrinol Metab.* 81:555–564.

Hill DJ, Milner RDG. 1985. Insulin as a Growth Factor. *Paediatr Res.* 19:879–886.

Ho PJ, Fig LM, Barkan AL, Shapiro B. 1992. Bone mineral density of the axial skeleton in acromegaly. *J Nucl Med.* 33:1608–1612.

Hoffman DM, Crampton I, Sernia C. 1996. Short term growth hormone (GH) treatment of GH deficient adults increases body sodium and extracellular water, but not blood pressure. *J Clin Endocrinol Metab.* 81:1123–1128.

Hoieggen A, Fossum E, Moan A, Enger E, Kjeldsen SE. 1998. Whole-blood viscosity and the insulin-resistance syndrome. *J Hypertens.* 16:203–210.

Holmes SJ, Economou G, Whitehouse RW, Adams JE, Shalet SM. 1994. Reduced bone mineral density in patients with growth hormone deficiency. *J Clin Endocrinol Metab.* 78:669–674.

Holmes SJ, Whitehouse RW, Swindell R, Economou G, Adams JE, Shalet SM. 1995. Effect of growth hormone replacement on bone mass in adults with adult onset growth hormone deficiency. *Clin Endocrinol. (Oxf).* 42:627–633.

Horber FF, Haymond MW. 1990. Human growth hormone prevents the protein catabolic side effects of prednisone in humans. *J Clin Invest.* 86: 265–272.

Houssay BA. 1936. The hypophysis and metabolism. *N Engl J Med.* 214:961–985.

Huseman CA, Colombo JL, Brooks MA et al. 1996. Anabolic effect of biosynthetic growth hormone in cystic fibrosis patients. *Pediatr Pulmonol.* 22:90–95.

Hussain MA, Schmitz O, Mengel A et al. 1993. Insulin-like growth factor I stimulates lipid oxidation, reduces protein oxidation, and enhances insulin sensitivity in humans. *J Clin Invest.* 92:2249–2256.

Hutler M, Schnabel D, Staab D et al. 2002. Effect of growth hormone on exercise tolerance in children with cystic fibrosis. *Med Sci Sports Exerc.* 34:567–572.

Hyer SL, Rodin DA, Tobias JH, Leiper A, Nussey SS. 1992. Growth hormone deficiency during puberty reduces adult bone mineral density. *Arch Dis Child.* 67:1472–1474.

Iranmanesh A, Lizarralde G, Velduis JD. 1991. Age and relative adiposity are specific negative determinants of the frequency and amplitude of growth hormone secretory bursts and the half-life of endogenous GH in healthy men. *J Clin Endocrinol Metab.* 73:1081–1088.

Irving BA, Patrie JT, Anderson SM et al. 2004. The effects of time following acute growth hormone administration on metabolic and power output measures during acute exercise. *J Clin Endocrinol Metab.* 89:4298–4305.

Ito Y, Urae A, Okuno A. 1998. Mild serum thyroid hormone increase during and after five-day administration of human growth hormone in healthy male adults. *Endocr J.* 45:125–127.

Janne OA, Palvimo JJ, Kallio P, Mehto M. 1993. Androgen receptor and mechanism of androgen action. *Ann Med.* 25:83–89.

Janson C, Bjornsson E, Hetta J, Boman G. 1994. Anxiety and depression in relation to respiratory symptoms and asthma. *Am J Respir Crit Care Med.* 149:930–934.

Janssen I, Ross R. 2005. Linking age-related changes in skeletal muscle mass and composition with metabolism and disease. *J Nutr Health Aging.* 9:408–419.

Jenkins PJ. 2001. Growth hormone and exercise: physiology, use and abuse. *Growth Horm IGF Res.* 11:71–77.

Johannsson G, Bengtsson BA, Andersson B, Isgaard J, Caidahl K. 1996a. Long-term cardiovascular effects of growth hormone treatment in GH-deficient adults: preliminary data in a small group of patients. *Clin Endocrinol. (Oxf).* 45:305–314.

Johannsson G, Rosen T, Bosaeus I, Sjostrom L, Bengtsson BA. 1996b. Two years of growth hormone (GH) treatment increases bone mineral content and density in hypopituitary patients with adult-onset GH deficiency. *J Clin.Endocrinol Metab.* 81:2865–2873.

Johannsson G, Grimby G, Sunnerhagen KS, Bengtsson BA. 1997. Two years of growth hormone (GH) treatment increases isometric and isokinetic muscle strength in GH-deficient adults. *J Clin Endocrinol Metab.* 82:2877–2884.

Johansen JS, Pedersen SA, Jørgensen JO et al. 1990. Effects of growth hormone (GH) on plasma bone Gla protein in GH-deficient adults. *J Clin Endocrinol Metab.* 70:916–919.

Johnson RH, Rennie MJ. 1973. Changes in Fat and Carbohydrate metabolism caused by moderate exercise in patients with Acromegaly. *Clinical Science.* 44:63–71.

Jorgensen JO, Pedersen SB, Børglum J et al. 1994. Fuel metabolism, energy expenditure, and thyroid function in growth hormone-treated obese women: a double-blind placebo-controlled study. *Metabolism.* 43:872–877.

Jurca R, Lamonte MJ, Barlow CE, Kampert JB, Church TS, Blair SN. 2005. Association of muscular strength with incidence of metabolic syndrome in men. *Med Sci Sports Exerc.* 37:1849–1855.

Kalina-Faska B, Kalina M, Koehler B. 2004. Effects of recombinant growth hormone therapy on thyroid hormone concentrations. *Int J Clin Pharmacol Ther.* 42:30–34.

Karakula H, Grzywa A, Spila B et al. 1996. Use of Hospital Anxiety and Depression Scale in psychosomatic disorders. *Psychiatr Pol.* 30:653–667.

Karila T, Koistinen H, Seppala M, Koistinen R, Seppala T. 1998. Growth hormone induced increase in serum IGFBP-3 level is reversed by anabolic steroids in substance abusing power athletes. *Clin Endocrinol. (Oxf).* 4:459–463.

Kass DA, Shapiro EP, Kawaguchi M et al. 2001. Improved arterial compliance by a novel advanced glycation end-product crosslink breaker. *Circulation.* 104:1464–1470.

Kaufman JM, Taelman P, Vermeuelen A, Vandeweghe M. 1992. Bone mineral status in growth hormone-deficient males with isolated and multiple pituitary insufficiencies of childhood onset. *J Clin Endocrinol Metab.* 74:118–123.

Kimball SR, Vary TC, Jefferson LS. 1994. Regulation of protein synthesis by insulin. *Ann Rev Physiol.* 56: 321–348.

Kohno K, Matsuoka H, Takenaka K et al. 2000. Depressor effect by exercise training is associated with amelioration of hyperinsulinaemia and sympathetic overactivity. *Intern Med.* 39:1013–1019.

Kojima M, Hosoda H, Date Y, Nakazato M, Matsuo H, Kangawa K 1999. Ghrelin is a growth-hormone-releasing acylated peptide from stomach. *Nature.* 9:656–660.

Konrad C, Schupfer G, Wietlisbach M, Gerber H. 1998. Insulin as an anabolic: hypoglycaemia in the body-building world. *Anaesthesiol Intensivmed Notfallmed Schmerzther.* 33:461–463.

Kool MJ, Lambert J, Stehouwer CD, Hoeks AP, Struijker Boudier HA, Van Bortel LM. 1995. Vessel wall properties of large arteries in uncomplicated IDDM. *Diabetes Care.* 18:618–624.

Koranyi J, Svensson J, Götherstrom G, Sunnerhagen KS, Bengtsson B, Johannsson G. 2001. Baseline characteristics and the effects of five years of GH replacement therapy in adults with GH deficiency of childhood or adulthood onset: a comparative, prospective study. *J Clin Endocrinol Metab.* 86:4693–4699.

Korkia P, Stimson GV. 1993. *Anabolic Steroid Use In Great Britain: An exploratory investigation.* London: The Centre for Research on Drugs and Health Behaviour.

Kotzmann H, Riedl M, Clodi M et al. 1996. The influence of growth hormone substitution therapy on erythroid and myeloid progenitor cells and on peripheral blood cells in adult patients with growth hormone deficiency. *Eur J Clin Invest.* 26:1175–1181.

Kroon FJ, Munday PL, Westcott DA, Hobbs JP, Liley NR. 2005. Aromatase pathway mediates sex change in each direction. *Proc Biol Sci.* 272:1399–1405.

Lacy PS, O'Brien DG, Stanley AG, Dewar MM, Swales PP, Williams B. 2004. Increased pulse wave velocity is not associated with elevated augmentation index in patients with diabetes. *J Hypertens.* 22:1863–1865.

Landsberg L. 1986. Diet, obesity and hypertension: an hypothesis involving insulin, the sympathetic nervous system and adaptive thermogenesis. *Q J Med.* 61:1081–1090.

Lanfranco F, Gianotti L, Giordano R, Pellegrino M, Maccario M, Arvat E. 2003. Ageing, growth hormone and physical performance. *J Endocrinol Invest.* 26:861–872.

Lange KH, Lorentsen J, Isaksson F et al. 2001. Endurance training and GH administration in elderly women: effects on abdominal adipose tissue lipolysis. *Am J Phys End Metab.* 280:886–897.

Lange KH, Andersen JL, Beyer N et al. 2002a. GH admin changes myosin heavy chain isoforms in skeletal muscle but does not augment muscle strength or hypertrophy, either alone or combined with resistance exercise training in healthy elderly men. *J Clin Endocrinol Metab.* 87:513–523.

Lange KH, Larsson B, Flyvbjerg A et al. 2002b. Acute growth hormone administration causes exaggerated increases in plasma lactate and glycerol during moderate to high intensity bicycling in trained young men. *J Clin Endocrinol Metab.* 87:4966–4975.

Laurent S. 1995. Arterial wall hypertrophy and stiffness in essential hypertensive patients. *Hypertension.* 26:355–362.

Lawlor DA, Ebrahim S, Smith GD. 2004. Associations of measures of lung function with insulin resistance and type II diabetes: findings from the British Women's Heart and Health Study. *Diabetologia.* 47:195–203.

Lazarus R, Sparrow D, Weiss ST. 1998a. Impaired ventilatory function and elevated insulin levels in non-diabetic males: the Normative Ageing Study. *Eur Respir J.* 12(3):635–640.

Lazarus R, Sparrow D, Weiss ST. 1998b. Baseline ventilatory function predicts the development of higher levels of fasting insulin and fasting insulin resistance index: the Normative Ageing Study. *Eur Respir J.* 12:641–645.

Lee AT, Cerami A. 1992. Role of glycation in ageing. *Ann N Y Acad Sci.* 663:63–70.

Lehmann ED, Riley WA, Clarkson P, Gosling RG. 1997. Non-invasive assessment of cardiovascular disease in diabetes mellitus. *Lancet.* 350:14–19.

Leonsson M, Hulthe J, Johannsson G et al. 2003. Increased Interleukin-6 levels in pituitary-deficient patients are independently related to their carotid intima-media thickness. *Clin Endocrinol. (Oxf)*. 59:242–250.

Le Roith D, Scavo L, Butler A. 2001. What is the role of circulating IGF-I? *Trends Endocrinol Metab*. 12:48–52.

Levine GN, Keaney JF Jr, Vita JA. 1995. Cholesterol reduction in cardiovascular disease. Clinical benefits and possible mechanisms. *N Engl J Med*. 332:512–521.

Li S, Chen W, Srinivasan SR, Berenson GS. 2005. Influence of metabolic syndrome on arterial stiffness and its age-related change in young adults: the Bogalusa Heart Study. *Atherosclerosis*. 180:349–354.

Lilien MR, Schroder CH, Levtchenko EN, Koomans HA. 2004. Growth hormone therapy influences endothelial function in children with renal failure. *Pediatr Nephrol*. 19:785–789.

Lim VS, Yarasheki KE, Crowley JR, Fangman J, Flanigan M. 2003. Insulin Is Protein-Anabolic in Chronic Renal Failure Patients. *J Am Soc Nephrol*. 14:2297–2304.

Lindgren AC, Hellstrom LG, Ritzen EM, Milerad J. 1999. Growth hormone treatment increases CO_2 response, ventilation and central inspiratory drive in children with Prader-Willi syndrome. *Eur J Pediatr*. 158:936–940.

Lippe BM, Van Herle AJ, LaFranchi SH, Uller RP, Lavin N, Kaplan SA. 1975. Reversible hypothyroidism in growth hormone-deficient children treated with human growth hormone. *J Clin Endocrinol Metab*. 40:612–618.

Lissett CA, Shalet SM. 2000. Effects of growth hormone on bone and muscle. *Growth Horm IGF Res*. 95–101.

Liu H, Bravata DM, Olkin I et al. 2007. Systematic review: the safety and efficacy of growth hormone in the healthy elderly. *Ann Intern Med*. 16:104–115.

Liu W, Thomas SG, Asa SL, Gonzalez-Cadavid N, Bhasin S, Ezzat S. 2003. Myostatin Is a Skeletal Muscle Target of Growth Hormone Anabolic Action. *J Clin Endocrinol Metab*. 88:5490–5496.

Lo JC, Mulligan K, Noor MA et al. 2001. The effects of recombinant human growth hormone on body composition and glucose metabolism in HIV-infected patients with fat accumulation. *J Clin Endocrinol Metab*. 86:3480–3487.

Lucidi P, Natascia N, Piccioni F, Santeusanio F, de Feo P. 2002. Short-Term Treatment with Low Doses of Recombinant Human GH Stimulates Lipolysis in Visceral Obese Men. *J Clin Endocrinol Metab*. 87:3105–3109.

Luft R, Ikkos D, Gemzell CA. 1968. Diabetogenic effects of a single supraphysiological dose of GH. *Lancet*. 721–722.

Malozowski S, Tanner LA, Wysowski D, Fleming GA. 1993. Growth hormone, insulin-like growth factor I, and benign intracranial hypertension. *N Engl J Med*. 329:665–666.

Marcell TJ, McAuley KA, Traustadottir T, Reaven PD. 2005. Exercise training is not associated with improved levels of C-reactive protein or adiponectin. *Metabolism*. 54:533–541.

Mardi T, Toker S, Melmed S et al. 2005. Increased erythropoiesis and subclinical inflammation as part of the metabolic syndrome. *Diabetes Res Clin Pract*. 69:249–255.

Markussis V, Beshyah SA, Fisher C, Sharp P, Nicolaides AN, Johnston DG. 1992. Detection of premature atherosclerosis by high-resolution ultrasonography in symptom-free hypopituitary adults. *Lancet*. 340:1188–1192.

Martin CR, Lewin RJ, Thompson DR. 2003. A confirmatory factor analysis of the Hospital Anxiety and Depression Scale in coronary care patients following acute myocardial infarction. *Psychiatry Res*. 120:85–94.

Mauras N, Attie KM, Reiter EO, Saenger P, Baptista J. 2000. High dose recombinant human growth hormone (GH) treatment of GH-deficient patients in puberty increases near-final height: a randomized, multicenter trial. Genentech, Inc., Cooperative Study Group. *J Clin Endocrinol Metab*. 85:3653–3660.

Mauras N, Haymond MW. 2005. Are the metabolic effects of GH and IGF-I separable. *Growth Horm IGF Res*. 15:19–27.

McCarty MF. 2003. Hyperinsulinaemia may boost both hematocrit and iron absorption by up-regulating activity of hypoxia-inducible factor-1alpha. *Med Hypotheses*. 61:567–573.

McCool FD, Conomos P, Benditt JO, Cohn D, Sherman CB, Hoppin FG Jr. 1997. Maximal inspiratory pressures and dimensions of the diaphragm. *Am J Respir Crit Care Med*. 155:1329–1334.

McGauley GA. 1989. Quality of Life Assessment Before and After Growth Hormone Treatment in Adults with Growth Hormone Deficiency. *Acta Paediatr Scand*. 356:70–72.

McMillan CV, Bradley C, Giannoulis M, Martin F, Sonksen PH. 2003. Preliminary development of a new individualised questionnaire measuring quality of life in older men with age-related hormonal decline: the A-RHDQoL. *Health Qual Life Outcomes*. 1:51.

Mcaly K, Barry M, O'Mahony L et al. 1998. Effects of human recombinant growth hormone (rhGH) on inflammatory responses in patients undergoing abdominal aortic aneurysm repair. *Intensive Care Med*. 24:128–131.

Meineri I, Andreani O, Sanna R, Aglialoro A, Bottino G, Giusti M. 1998. Effect of low-dosage recombinant human growth hormone therapy on pulmonary function in hypopituitary patients with adult-onset growth hormone deficiency. *J Endocrinol Invest*. 21:423–427.

Meissner WA, Legg MA. 1973. *The pathology of diabetes*. Lea, Febiger Philad. 157–190.

Melmed S. 2006. Medical progress: acromegaly. *N Engl J Med*. 14:2558–2573.

Merola B, Longobardi S, Sofia M et al. 1996. Lung volumes and respiratory muscle strength in adult patients with childhood- or adult-onset growth hormone deficiency: effect of 12 months' growth hormone replacement therapy. *Eur J Endocrinol*. 135:553–558.

Milani D, Carmichael JD, Welkowitz J et al. 2004. Variability and reliability of single serum IGF-I measurements: impact on determining predictability of risk ratios in disease development. *J Clin Endocrinol Metab*. 89:2271–2274.

Moan A, Nordby G, Os I, Birkeland KI, Kjeldsen SE. 1994. Relationship between hemorrheologic factors and insulin sensitivity in healthy young men. *Metabolism*. 43:423–427.

Modan M, Halkin H, Almog S et al. 1985. Hyperinsulinaemia: a link between hypertension, obesity and glucose intolerance. *J Clin Invest*. 75:809–817.

Moller J, Jørgensen JO, Schmitz O et al. 1990. Effects of a growth hormone pulse on total and forearm substrate fluxes in humans. *Am J Physiol.* 258:86–91.

Moller J, Schmitz O, Jørgensen JO et al. 1992. Basal- and insulin-stimulated substrate metabolism in patients with active acromegaly before and after adenomectomy. *J Clin Endocrinol Metab.* 74:1012–1019.

Moller J, Fisker S, Rosenfalck AM et al. 1999. Long-term effects of growth hormone (GH) on body fluid distribution in GH deficient adults: a four months double blind placebo controlled trial. *Eur J Endocrinol.* 140:11–16.

Moller N, Møller J, Jørgensen JO et al. 1993. Impact of 2 weeks growth hormone treatment on basal- and insulin- stimulated substrate metabolism in humans. *Clin Endocrinol. (Oxf).* 39:577–581.

Moller N, Jørgensen JO, Møller J et al. 1995. Metabolic effects of growth hormone in humans. *Metabolism.* 4:33–36.

Mulcahy L. 2001. The erythropoietin receptor *Semin Oncol.* 28:19–23.

Muller AF, Leebeek FW, Janssen JA, Lamberts SW, Hofland L, van der Lely AJ. 2001. Acute effect of pegvisomant on cardiovascular risk markers in healthy men: implications for the pathogenesis of atherosclerosis in GH deficiency. *J Clin Endocrinol Metab.* 86:5165–5171.

Mulvany JM, Baumbach GL, Aalkjaer C et al. 1996. Vascular remodelling. *Hypertension.* 28:505–506.

Mykletun A, Stordal E, Dahl AA. 2001. Hospital Anxiety and Depression (HAD) scale: factor structure, item analyses and internal consistency in a large population. *Br J Psychol.* 179:540–544.

Nagano M, Nakamura M, Sato K, Tanaka F, Segawa T, Hiramori K. 2005. Association between serum C-reactive protein levels and pulse wave velocity: a population-based cross-sectional study in a general population. *Atherosclerosis.* 180:189–195.

Nagaya N, Moriya J, Yasumura Y et al. 2004. Effects of ghrelin on left ventricular function, exercise capacity, muscle wasting in patients with chronic heart failure. *Circulation.* 110:3674–3679.

Napoli R, Guardasole V, Matarazzo M et al. 2002. Growth hormone corrects vascular dysfunction in patients with chronic heart failure. *J Am Coll Cardiol.* 39:90–95.

Nielsen HK, Jørgensen JO, Brixen K, Møller N, Charles P, Christensen JS. 1991. 24-h profile of serum osteocalcin in growth hormone (GH) deficient patients with and without GH treatment. *Growth Regul.* 1:153–159.

Norrelund H, Nair KS, Nielsen S et al. 2003. The decisive role of free fatty acids for protein conservation during fasting in humans with and without growth hormone. *J Clin Endocrinol Metab.* 88:4371–4378.

Nyholm B, Mengel A, Nielsen S et al. 1996. Insulin resistance in relatives of NIDDM patients: the role of physical fitness and muscle metabolism. *Diabetologia.* 39:813–822.

Nyholm B, Nielsen MF, Kristensen K et al. 2004. Evidence of increased visceral obesity and reduced physical fitness in healthy insulin-resistant first-degree relatives of type II diabetic patients. *Eur J Endocrinol.* 150:207–214.

O'Halloran DJ, Tsatsoulis A, Whitehouse RW, Holmes SJ, Adams JE, Shalet SM. 1993. Increased bone density after recombinant human growth hormone therapy in adults with isolated GH deficiency. *J Clin Endocrinol Metab.* 76:1344–1348.

O'Hare JA, Minaker KL, Meneilly GS, Rowe JW, Pallotta JA, Young JB. 1989. Effect of insulin on plasma nor-epinephrine and 3,4-dihydroxyphenylalanine in obese men. *Metabolism.* 38:322–329.

O'Neal D, Hew FL, Sikaris K, Ward G, Alford F, Best JD. 1996. Low density lipoprotein particle size in hypopituitary adults receiving conventional growth hormone replacement therapy. *J Clin Endocrinol Metab.* 81:2448–2454.

O'Neal DN, Kalfas A, Dunning PL et al. 1994. The effect of 3 months of recombinant human growth hormone (GH) therapy on insulin and glucose-mediated glucose disposal and insulin secretion in GH-deficient adults: a minimal model analysis. *J Clin Endocrinol Metab.* 79:975–983.

O'Reilly KE, Rojo F, She QB et al. 2006. mTOR inhibition induces upstream receptor tyrosine kinase signaling and activates Akt. *Cancer Res.* 66:1500–1508.

Orskov L, Schmitz O, Jørgensen JO et al. 1989. Influence of growth hormone on glucose-induced glucose uptake in healthy man as assessed by the hyperglycaemic clamp technique. *J Clin Endocrinol Metab.* 68:276–282.

Oxlund H, Rasmussen LM, Andreassen TT, Heickendorff L. 1989. Increased aortic stiffness in patients with type I (insulin-dependent) diabetes mellitus. *Diabetologia.* 32:748–752.

Papadakis MA, Grady D, Black D et al. 1996. Growth hormone replacement in healthy older men improves body composition but not functional ability. *Ann Intern Med.* 124:708–716.

Pape GS, Friedman M, Underwood LE, Clemmons DR. 1991. The effect of growth hormone on weight gain and pulmonary function in patients with chronic obstructive lung disease. *Chest.* 99:1495–1500.

Parkinson AB, Evans NA. 2006. Anabolic androgenic steroids: a survey of 500 users. *Med Sci Sports Exerc.* 38:644–651.

Pates R, Barry C. 1996. Steroid use in Cardiff: a problem for whom? *Perform Enhanc Drugs.* 1:92–97.

Perry H, Littlepage B. 1992. Dying to be big: a review of anabolic steroid use. *Br J Sports Med.* 4:259–261.

Pfeifer M, Verhovec M, Zizek B, Prezelj J, Poredos P, Clayton RN. 1999. Growth hormone (GH) treatment reverses early atherosclerotic changes in GH-deficient adults. *J Clin Endocrinol Metab.* 84:453–457.

Pfeifle B, Ditschuneit H. 1981. Effect of Insulin on growth of cultured human arterial smooth muscle cells. *Diabetologia.* 20:155–158.

Polak J, Moro C, Klimcakova E et al. 2005. Dynamic strength training improves insulin sensitivity and functional balance between adrenergic alpha 2A and beta pathways in subcutaneous adipose tissue of obese subjects. *Diabetologia.* 48:2631–2640.

Pope H, Phillips K, Olivardia R. 2000. *The Adonis Complex: The Secret Crisis of Male Body Obsession.* New York: The Free Press, 11.

Pope HG Jr, Katz DL. 1992. Psychiatric effects of anabolic steroids. *Psych Annals.* 22:24–29.

Porretti S, Giavoli C, Ronchi C et al. 2002. Recombinant human GH replacement therapy and thyroid function in a large group of adult GH-deficient patients: when does L-T(4) therapy become mandatory? *J Clin Endocrinol Metab.* 87:2042–2045.

Portes ES, Oliveira JH, MacCagnan P, Abucham J. 2000. Changes in serum thyroid hormones levels and their mechanisms during long-term growth hormone (GH) replacement therapy in GH deficient children. *Clin Endocrinol. (Oxf).* 53:183–189.

Powrie JK, Bassett EE, Rosen T et al. 2007. Detection of growth hormone abuse in sport. On behalf of the GH-2000 Project study group. *Growth Horm IGF Res.* 17:220–226.

Rabinowitz D, Klassen GA, Zierler KL. 1965. Effects of human growth hormone on muscle and adipose tissue metabolism in the forearm of man. *J Clin Invest.* 44:51–61.

Randle PJ, Priestman DA, Mistry SC, Halsall A. 1994. Glucose fatty acid interactions and the regulation of glucose disposal. *J Cell Biochem.* 55:1–11.

Reaven GM, Hoffman BB. 1987. A role for insulin in the aetiology and course of hypertension? *Lancet.* 2:435–437.

Ridker PM, Rifai N, Rose L, Buring JE, Cook NR. 2002. Comparison of C-reactive protein and low-density lipoprotein cholesterol levels in the prediction of first cardiovascular events. *N Engl J Med.* 347:1557–1565.

Rigalleau V, Delafaye C, Baillet L et al. 1999. Composition of insulin-induced body weight gain in diabetic patients: a bio-impedance study. *Diabetes Metab.* 4:321–328.

Rizza RA, Mandarino LJ, Gerich JE. 1982. Effects of growth hormone on insulin action in man. Mechanisms of insulin resistance, impaired suppression of glucose production, and impaired stimulation of glucose utilization. *Diabetes.* 31:663–669.

Ronconi V, Giacchetti G, Mariniello B et al. 2005. Reduced nitric oxide levels in acromegaly: cardiovascular implications. *Blood Press.* 14:227–232.

Rosen T, Edén S, Larson G, Wilhelmsen L, Bengtsson BA. 1993. Cardiovascular risk factors in adult patients with growth hormone deficiency. *Acta Endocrinol.* 129:195–200.

Rosen T, Wiren L, Wilhelmsen L, Wiklund I, Bengtsson BA. 1994. Decreased psychological well-being in adult patients with growth hormone deficiency. *Clin Endocrinol (Oxf).* 40:111–116.

Rosen T, Wilhelmsen L, Landin-Wilhelmsen K, Lappas G, Bengtsson BA 1997. Increased fracture frequency in adult patients with GH deficiency. *Eur J Endocrinol.* 137:240–245.

Rowe JW, Young JB, Minaker KL, Stevens AL, Pallotta J, Landsberg L. 1981. Effect of insulin and glucose infusions on sympathetic nervous system activity in normal man. *Diabetes.* 30:219–225.

Rubanyi GM, Freany ADK, Kauser K, Johns A, Harder DR. 1990. Mechanoreception by the endothelium: mediators and mechanisms of pressure and flow-induced vascular response. *Blood Vessels.* 27:246–257.

Ruckzika L, Wettstein A, Kaegi H. 1935. Sexual hormone VIII Darstellung von Testosterone unter Anwendung gemischter Ester. *Helv Chim Acta.* 18:1478.

Rudman D, Feller AG, Nagraj HS et al. 1990. Effect of human growth hormone in men over 60 years old. *N Engl J Med.* 323:1–6.

Rudman D, Feller AG, Cohn L, Shetty KR, Rudman IW, Draper MW. 1991. Effect of human growth hormone on Body Composition in Elderly Men. *Horm Res.* 36:73–81.

Russell-Jones DL, Weissberger AJ, Bowes SB et al. 1993. The effects of growth hormone on protein metabolism in adult growth hormone-deficient patients. *Clin Endocrinol. (Oxf).* 38:427–431.

Russell-Jones DL, Watts GF, Weissberger A et al. 1994. The effect of growth hormone replacement on serum lipids, lipoproteins, apolipoproteins and cholesterol precursors in adult growth hormone-deficient patients. *Clin Endocrinol. (Oxf).* 41:345–350.

Sacca L, Cittadini A, Fazio S. 1994. Growth hormone and the heart. *Endocr Rev.* 15:555–573.

Salomaa V, Riley W, Kark JD, Nardo C, Folsom AR. 1995. Non-insulin-dependent diabetes mellitus and fasting glucose and insulin concentrations are associated with arterial stiffness indexes. The ARIC Study. Atherosclerosis Risk in Communities Study. *Circulation.* 91:1432–1443.

Salomon F, Cuneo RC, Hesp R, Sonksen PH. 1989. The effects of treatment with recombinant human growth hormone on body composition and metabolism in adults with growth hormone deficiency. *N Engl J Med.* 321:1797–1803.

Sartorio A, Conti A, Monzani M. 1993. New markers of bone and collagen turnover in children and adults with growth hormone deficiency. *Postgrad Med J.* 69:846–850.

Sato T, Suzukui Y, Taketani T, Ishiguro K, Masuyama T. 1977. Enhanced peripheral conversion of thyroxine to triiodothyronine during hGH therapy in GH deficient children. *J Clin Endocrinol Metab.* 45:324–329.

Sato Y, Hayamizu S, Yamamoto C, Ohkuwa Y, Yamanouchi K, Sakamoto N. 1986. Improved insulin sensitivity in carbohydrate and lipid metabolism after physical training. *Int J Sports Med.* 7:307–310.

Sattar N, Gaw A, Scherbakova O et al. 2003. Metabolic syndrome with and without C-reactive protein as a predictor of coronary heart disease and diabetes in the West of Scotland Coronary Prevention Study. *Circulation.* 108:414–419.

Savine R, Sönksen P. 2000. Growth hormone—hormone replacement for the somatopause? *Horm Res.* 53:37–41.

Scacchi M, Pincelli AI, Cavagnini F. 1999. Growth hormone in obesity. *Int J Obes Relat Metab Disord.* 23:260–271.

Schafer E. 1916. *The Endocrine Organs.* London: Longman, Green & Co.

Schauster AC, Geletko SM, Mikolich DJ. 2000. Diabetes mellitus associated with recombinant human growth hormone for HIV wasting syndrome. *Pharmacotherapy.* 20:1129–1134.

Schlemmer A, Johansen JS, Pedersen SA, Jørgensen JO, Hassager C, Christiansen C. 1991. The effect of growth hormone (GH) therapy on urinary pyridinoline cross-links in GH-deficient adults. *Clin Endocrinol (Oxf).* 35:471–476.

Schram MT, Henry RM, van Dijk RA et al. 2004. Increased central artery stiffness in impaired glucose metabolism and type II diabetes: the Hoorn Study. *Hypertension*. 43:176–181.

Scott AR, Bennett T, MacDonald IA. 1988. Effects of hyperinsulinaemia on the cardiovascular responses to graded hypovolaemia in normal and diabetic subjects. *Clin Sci (Lond)*. 75:85–92.

Scuteri A, Chen CH, Yin FC, Chih-Tai T, Spurgeon HA, Lakatta EG. 2001. Functional correlates of central arterial geometric phenotypes. *Hypertension*. 38:1471–1475.

Scuteri A, Najjar SS, Muller DC et al. 2004. Metabolic syndrome amplifies the age-associated increases in vascular thickness and stiffness. *J Am Coll Cardiol*. 43:1388–1395.

Seeman E, Wahner HW, Offord KP, et al. 1982. Differential effects of endocrine dysfunction on the axial and the appendicular skeleton. *J Clin Invest*. 69:1302–1309.

Seminara S, Stagi S, Candura L et al. (2005). Changes of thyroid function during long-term hGH therapy in GHD children. A possible relationship with catch-up growth? *Horm Metab Res*. 37:751–756.

Sesmilo G, Biller BM, Llevadot J et al. 2000. Effects of growth hormone administration on inflammatory and other cardiovascular risk markers in men with growth hormone deficiency. A randomized, controlled clinical trial. *Ann Intern Med*. 133:111–122.

Sesmilo G, Fairfield WP, Katznelson L et al. 2002. Cardiovascular risk factors in acromegaly before and after normalization of serum IGF-I levels with the GH antagonist pegvisomant. *J Clin Endocrinol Metab*. 87:1692–1699.

Sigurjonsdottir HA, Koranyi J, Axelson M, Bengtsson BA, Johannsson G. 2006. GH effect on enzyme activity of 11betaHSD in abdominal obesity is dependent on treatment duration. *Eur J Endocrinol*. 154:69–74.

Simpson H, Savine R, Sönksen P et al. 2002. Growth hormone replacement therapy for adults: into the new millennium. *Growth Horm IGF Res*. 12:1–33.

Sinha A, Formica C, Tsalamandris C et al. 1996. Effects of insulin on body composition in patients with insulin-dependent and non-insulin-dependent diabetes. *Diabetic Medicine*. 13:40–46.

Smith JC, Evans LM, Wilkinson I et al. 2002. Effects of GH replacement on endothelial function and large-artery stiffness in GH-deficient adults: a randomized, double-blind, placebo-controlled study. *Clin Endocrinol (Oxf)*. 56:493–501.

Smith JC, Lane H, Davies N, et al. 2003. The effects of depot long-acting somatostatin analog on central aortic pressure and arterial stiffness in acromegaly. *J Clin Endocrinol Metab*. 88:2556–2561.

Snaith RP. 2003. The Hospital Anxiety and Depression Scale. *Health Qual Life Outcomes*. 1:29.

Snel YE, Doerga ME, Brummer RM, Zelissen PM, Koppeschaar HP. 1995. Magnetic resonance imaging-assessed adipose tissue and serum lipid and insulin concentrations in GHD adults. Effect of growth hormone replacement. *Arterioscler Thromb Vasc Biol*. 15:1543–1548.

Sonksen PH. 2001. Insulin, growth hormone and sport. *J Endocrinol*. 170:13–25.

Sonksen PH, Greenwood FC, Ellis JP, et al. 1967. Changes of carbohydrate tolerance in acromegaly with progress of the disease and in response to treatment. *J Clin Endocrinol Metab*. 27:1418–1430.

Sonksen PH, Sonksen J. 2000. Insulin: understanding its action in health and disease. *Br J Anaesth*. 85:69–79.

Stabler B, Turner JR, Girdler SS, Light KC, Underwood LE. 1992. Reactivity to stress and psychological adjustment in adults with pituitary insufficiency. *Clin Endocrinol (Oxf)*. 6:467–473.

Stahnke N, Koehn H. 1990. Replacement therapy in hypothalamus-pituitary insufficiency: management in the adolescent. *Horm Res*. 33:38–44.

Stehouwer CD, Jakobs C. 1998. Abnormalities of vascular function in hyperhomocysteinaemia: relationship to atherothrombotic disease. *Eur J Pediatr*. 157:107–111.

Stout RW. 1990. Insulin and Atheroma. 20 yr. perspective. *Diabetes Care*. 13:631–654.

Svensson J, Bengtsson BA, Taskinen MR. 2000. A nine-month, placebo-controlled study of the effects of GH treatment on lipoproteins and LDL size in abdominally obese men. *Growth Horm IGF Res*. 10:118–126.

Taaffe DR, Pruitt L, Reim J et al. 1994. Effects of recombinant human growth hormone on the muscle strength response to resistance exercise in elderly men. *J Clin Endocrinol Metab*. 79:1361–1366.

Taniguchi A, Fukushima M, Seino Y et al. 2003. Platelet count is independently associated with insulin resistance in non-obese Japanese type II diabetic patients. *Metabolism*. 52:1246–1249.

Thomas SG, Woodhouse LJ, Pagura SM, Ezzat S. 2002. Ventilation threshold as a measure of impaired physical performance in adults with growth hormone excess. *Clin Endocrinol (Oxf)*. 56:351–358.

Thomas SHL, Wisher MH, Brandenburg D, Sonksen PH. 1979. Insulin action on Adipocytes. Evidence that the anti-lipolytic and lipogenic effects of insulin are medicated by the same receptor. *Biochem J*. 184:355–360.

Thoren M, Soop M, Degerblad M, Saaf M. 1993. Preliminary study of the effects of growth hormone substitution therapy on bone mineral density and serum osteocalcin levels in adults with growth hormone deficiency. *Acta Endocrinol (Copenh)*. 128:41–43.

Thuesen L, Jørgensen JO, Müller JR et al. 1994. Short and long-term cardiovascular effects of growth hormone therapy in growth hormone deficient adults. *Clin Endocrinol (Oxf)*. 41:615–620.

Tofe S, Moreno JC, Maiz L, et al. 2005. Insulin-secretion abnormalities and clinical deterioration related to impaired glucose tolerance in cystic fibrosis. *Eur J Endocrinol*. 152:241–247.

Tonino RP. 1989. Effect of physical training on the insulin resistance of ageing. *Am J Physiol*. 256:352–256.

Valcavi R, Gaddi O, Zini M, Iavicoli M, Mellino U, Portioli I. 1995. Cardiac performance and mass in adults with hypopituitarism: effects of one year of growth hormone treatment. *J Clin Endocrinol Metab*. 80:659–666.

Valerio G, Di Maio S, Salerno M, Argenziano A, Badolato R, Tenore A. 1997. Assessment of red blood cell indices in growth-hormone-treated children. *Horm Res*. 47:62–66.

Van Buul-Offers S, Ujeda I, Van den Brande JL. 1986. Biosynthetic somatomedin C increases the length and weight of Snell dwarf mice. *Paediatric Res.* 20:825–877.

Van Guldener C, Stehouwer CD. 2000. Hyperhomocysteinemia, vascular pathology, and endothelial dysfunction. *Semin Thromb Hemost.* 26:281–289.

Vehkavaara S, Mäkimattila S, Schlenzka A, Vakkilainen J, Westerbacka J, Yki-Järvinen H. 2000. Insulin therapy improves endothelial function in type II diabetes. *Arterioscler Thromb Vasc Biol.* 20:545–550.

Vestergaard P, Mosekilde L. 2004. Fracture risk is decreased in acromegaly--a potential beneficial effect of growth hormone. *Osteoporos Int.* 15:155–159.

Vihervuori E, Virtanen M, Koistinen H, Koistinen R, Seppälä M, Siimes MA. 1996. Haemoglobin level is linked to growth hormone-dependent proteins in short children. *Blood.* 87:2075–2081.

Vitale G, Pivonello R, Lombardi G, Colao A. 2004. Cardiovascular complications in acromegaly. *Minerva Endocrinol.* 29:77–88.

von Wowern F, Berglund G, Carlson J et al. 2005. Genetic variance of SGK-1 is associated with blood pressure, blood pressure change over time and strength of the insulin-diastolic blood pressure relationship. *Kidney Int.* 68:2164–2172.

Wallace JD, Cuneo RC, Baxter R et al. 1999. Responses of the growth hormone (GH) and insulin-like growth factor axis to exercise, GH administration and GH withdrawal in trained adult males: a potential test for GH abuse in sport. *J Clin Endocrinol Metab.* 84:3591–3601.

Weaver JU, Monson JP, Noonan K et al. 1995. The effect of low dose recombinant human growth hormone replacement on regional fat distribution, insulin sensitivity and cardiovascular risk factors in hypopituitary adults. *J Clin Endocrinol Metab.* 80:153–159.

Welborn TA, Breckenridge A, Rubinstein AH, Dollery CT, Fraser TR. 1966. Serum-insulin in essential hypertension and in peripheral vascular disease. *Lancet.* 1:1336–1337.

Wilkinson MJ, Barczak P. 1988. Psychiatric screening in general practice: comparison of the general health questionnaire and the hospital anxiety depression scale. *J R Coll Gen Pract.* 38:311–313.

Wilson JD, Griffin JE, Russell DW. 1993. Steroid 5 alpha-reductase 2 deficiency. 14:577–93.

Wilson JD, Leihy MW, Shaw G, Renfree MB. 2002. Androgen physiology: unsolved problems at the millennium. *Mol Cell Endocrinol.* 198:1–5.

Wit JM, Kooijman R, Rijkers GT, Zegers BJM. 1993. Immunological findings in growth hormone treated patients. *Horm Res.* 39:107–110.

Woodside JV, McMahon R, Gallagher AM et al. 2004. Total homocysteine is not a determinant of arterial pulse wave velocity in young healthy adults. *Atherosclerosis.* 177:337–344.

Wu Z, Bidlingmaier M, Dall R, Strasburger CJ. 1999. Detection of doping with human growth hormone. *Lancet.* 353:895.

Wuster C, Slenczka E, Ziegler R. 1991. Increased prevalence of osteoporosis and arteriosclerosis in conventionally substituted anterior pituitary insufficiency: need for additional growth hormone substitution? *Klin Wochenschr.* 69:769–773.

Wyatt DT, Gesundheit N, Sherman B. 1998. Changes in thyroid hormone levels during growth hormone therapy in initially euthyroid patients: lack of need for thyroxine supplementation. *J Clin Endocrinol Metab.* 83:3493–3497.

Yarasheki KE, Campbell JA, Smith K. 1992. Effect of growth hormone and resistance exercise on muscle growth and strength in young men. *Am J Physiol.* 262:261–267.

Yarasheki KE, Zachwieja JJ, Angelopoulos TJ. 1993. Short-term growth hormone treatment does not increase muscle protein synthesis in experienced weight lifters. *J Appl Physiol.* 74:3073–3076.

Yarasheki KE, Zachwieja JJ, Campbell JA, Bier DM. 1995. Effect of growth hormone and resistance exercise on muscle growth and strength in older men. *Am J Physiol.* 268:268–276.

Yasmin, McEniery CM, Wallace S et al. 2004. C-reactive protein is associated with arterial stiffness in apparently healthy individuals. *Arterioscler Thromb Vasc Biol.* 24:969.

Zach MS. 2000. The physiology of forced expiration. *Paediatr Respir Rev.* 1:36–39.

Zachwieja JJ, Yarasheki KE. 1999. Does growth hormone therapy in conjunction with resistance exercise increase muscle force production and muscle mass in men and women aged 60 years or older? *Phys Ther.* 79:76–82.

Zigmond AS, Snaith RP. 1983. The hospital anxiety and depression scale. *Acta Psychiatr Scand.* 67:361–370.

PART II

The Potential of Stem and Progenitor Cell Applications for Degenerative Disorders

Chapter **8**

MESENCHYMAL STEM CELLS AND TRANSDIFFERENTIATED NEURONS IN CROSS TALK WITH THE TISSUE MICROENVIRONMENT: IMPLICATIONS FOR TRANSLATIONAL SCIENCE

Katarzyna A. Trzaska,* Steven J. Greco,*
Lisamarie Moore,* and Pranela Rameshwar

ABSTRACT

Stem cells hold vast therapeutic potential in facilitating the treatment of many diseases with high mortality. Stem cells are hoped to increase the quality of life for patients and also to reduce healthcare cost. Central to the advancement in stem cell therapy is a fundamental understanding of the basic biology. Currently, the rapidly growing field of stem cell research sees a dividing line between proponents of embryonic (ESC) and those of adult stem cells (ASC). While ESCs offer a tremendous potential to generate any tissue within the body, there are questions regarding their stability, with the fear of tumorigenesis and ethical concerns. ASCs are found within most organs. The harvesting of a few cells within an organ does not affect the functions of the organ, thereby circumventing the ethical qualms associated with ESCs. However, ASCs raise questions regarding their potential to form varied tissues and their isolation from living organs. Recent reports have shown the ability of ASCs to generate tissues of germ layers other than their own. This cellular plasticity has wrought excitement, as well as skepticism, within the field. In particular, the generation of specific types of neurons from adult bone marrow mesenchymal stem cells (MSCs) underscores the plasticity observed in these cells. In-depth analysis of MSCs has shown transcriptional regulatory mechanisms similar to ESCs,

*These authors contributed equally.
Grant Support: This work was supported by FM Kirby Foundation.

which may provide clues to their observed plasticity. Additionally, in vitro models have been developed to mimic the microenvironment of an injured tissue. These models have provided insights into and predictions of the behavior of implanted stem cells and/or the generated specialized cells. The field of stem cell biology will benefit from principles of biomedical engineering in controlling cellular behavior. Ultimately, the goal is to prevent untoward effects on patients as stem cell therapy is applied for tissue regeneration or organogenesis.

Keywords: stem cells, mesenchymal stem cells, bone marrow, embryonic stem cells, microenvironment, cytokines, tissue engineering.

PLASTICITY

Stem cell biology involves the study of various stem cells that could be categorized as embryonic stem cells (ESCs), fetal stem cells, umbilical cord blood cells, and adult stem cells (ASCs). ESCs are pluripotent cells from the inner cell mass of the blastocyst that have the capacity to form all the cells in the body. Typical ESC markers include OCT4, NANOG, and SOX2, which are early embryonic transcription factors that inhibit lineage-specific differentiation and maintain pluripotency (Fig. 8.1). ASCs are multipotent stem cells that reside in various tissues where they form differentiated cells resident to their tissue. A summary of the biological properties of ESCs and some ASCs can been seen in Table 8.1.

Regardless of where the stem cells reside, the fundamental paradigm of stem cell biology is that these cells are rare in occurrence, with immense self-renewal ability and the capacity to divide by symmetry or asymmetry. The hematopoietic stem cells, which reside in

the bone marrow, are classical examples of ASCs that have been studied for more than 50 years. These stem cells generate blood and immune cells while maintaining their numbers through self-renewal. Despite the long-standing view of stem cells maintaining tissue-specific lineage commitment, considerable evidence has challenged this belief, demonstrating that some ASCs are not lineage restricted, suggesting vast cellular plasticity (Krause, Theise, Collector et al. 2001).

The concept of stem cell plasticity originated in the 19th century (Cohnheim 1867; Driesch 1893). While this term has been used in several contexts, *cellular plasticity* is defined as the ability of an ASC to differentiate to cells outside of its tissue of origin. It can also be referred to as *transdifferentiation*, which is the conversion of a cell from one germ layer to another, as seen in stem cells of mesodermal origin generating cells of ectodermal origin. The immense interest in stem cells for translation in the area of regenerative medicine have caused a surge in research, which has led to the validation of plasticity among ASCs with questions on lineage determination (Wagers, Weissman 2004). The first demonstration that ASCs own a considerable plasticity was described in 2001 by Krause and colleagues. The group showed multiorgan, multilineage engraftment after transplantation of a single bone marrow–derived hematopoietic stem cell. Many laboratories support this study; however, hematopoietic stem cell plasticity remains controversial. Research by the Weissman laboratory showed that hematopoietic stem cells only reconstituted the blood and immune systems, and not any other organs or tissues, thereby refuting ASC plasticity (Wagers, Sherwood, Christensen et al. 2002).

The bone marrow also contains another type of stem cell, identified by Friedenstein in 1974, now known as the *mesenchymal stem cells* (MSCs). MSCs can generate bone, cartilage, fat, and hematopoiesis-supporting

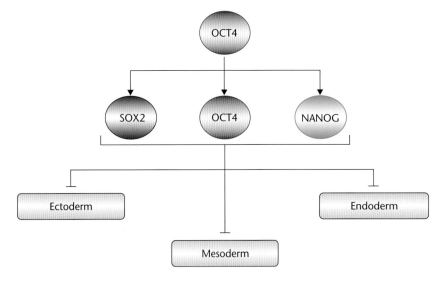

Figure 8.1 Cartoon depicting the inhibition of tissue-specific genes by OCT4, SOX2, and NANOG. OCT4 regulates expression of SOX2 and NANOG. Differentiation of ESCs leads to suppression of these transcription factors and concomitant expression of germ layer–specific genes.

Table 8.1 Characteristics of Embryonic Stem Cells and Selected Adult Stem Cells

Stem Cell	Organ/Source	Markers	Cells Generated	References
Embryonic stem cell	Inner cell mass of a blastocyst	Oct4, Nanog, Sox2, SSEA	All cells of the organism	Biswas, Hutchins 2007
Hematopoietic stem cell	Bone marrow (close to endosteum)	CD34, CD45, Sca-1, c-kit, Thy-1	Blood and immune cells; *cells exhibiting plasticity: endothelial, hepatic, muscle, neural, cardiac*	Sata et al. 2002; Chan et al. 2004
Mesenchymal stem cell	Bone marrow (close to central sinus), cord blood	CD105, CD44, CD29	Bone, cartilage, adipose, muscle, marrow stroma; *cells exhibiting plasticity: kidney, hepatocytes, muscle, neural, cardiac, pancreatic islet cells*	Bianco et al. 2001; Phinney, Isakova 2005; Zipori 2004
Neural stem cell	Brain (subventricular zone)	Nestin, vimentin, CD133	Neurons, astrocytes, oligodendrocytes; *cells exhibiting plasticity: blood and immune cells, muscle*	Sugaya 2005
Epidermal stem cell	Skin (bulge region of hair follicle, interfollicular epidermis, sebaceous gland)	Cytokeratins 14, 15, and 19; β-catenin, CD71	Keratinocytes; *cells exhibiting plasticity: connective tissue, hepatocytes, neurons, blood cells*	Liang, Bickenbach 2002
Gut stem cell	Gut (stomach, large and small intestines)	Msi-1, Hes-1	Goblet cells, columnar cells, endocrine cells, Paneth cells	Kayahara et al. 2003
Lung stem cell	Lung	GATA 1/2, CD45, FLT-1, Tie-2	Airway epithelial cells, Clara cells; *cells exhibiting plasticity: muscle and blood cells*	Summer et al. 2005
Cardiac stem cell	Heart	c-kit, Sca-1, MDR1	Cardiomyocytes, smooth muscle cells, and endothelial cells of the heart	Beltrami et al. 2003

The table summarizes selected characteristics of embryonic stem cells and selected adult stem cells. It focuses on adult stem cells showing plasticity by generating cells of other germ layers (italics).

stroma (Bianco, Riminucci, Gronthos et al. 2001). MSCs have been found to own a broad differentiation capacity, outside of their mesodermal origin (Phinney, Isakova 2005). Many recent studies have challenged the belief that they are lineage restricted, exploiting their cellular plasticity for regenerative medicine (Kashofer, Bonnet 2005). MSCs have extensive plasticity and pluripotent differentiation potential, allowing them to respond to various extracellular signals, and subsequently various differentiation pathways can be activated (Bedada, Gunther, Kubin et al. 2006). The mechanisms that facilitate the plastic nature of MSCs are a subject of intensive research. It has been suggested that MSCs are in a "stand-by" state, enabling them to shift from one position to another completely different phenotype, depending on the environmental cues (Zipori 2004). It is also proposed that their plasticity is due to the fact that they express a variety of genes, but they are not silenced, only expressed at low levels, so when necessary, the cells could respond to extracellular signals (Zipori 2004). Another possibility is that there is a genetic reprogramming on stimulation with certain growth factors (Grove, Bruscia, Krause et al. 2004).

While the plastic nature of MSCs emphasizes their potential for cellular therapy, other properties of MSCs are equally relevant. MSCs can be easily isolated from bone marrow aspirates, expanded in culture, and have a low incidence of tumor formation (Bianco, Riminucci, Gronthos et al. 2001). The unique immune properties that allow them to be transplanted across allogeneic barriers also make MSCs desirable for cell therapy (Potian, Aviv, Ponzio et al. 2003).

Several studies have shown that MSCs not only differentiate into cells of their tissue of origin but they can also generate neurons (Cho, Trzaska, Greco et al. 2005; Greco, Zhou, Ye et al. 2007), cardiomyocytes (Miyahara, Nagaya, Kataoka et al. 2006; Mazhari, Hare 2007), hepatocytes (Sato, Araki, Kato et al. 2005; Aurich, Mueller, Aurich et al. 2007), and pancreatic islet cells (Chen, Jiang, Yang et al. 2004). Thus, the immensely plastic nature of these cells is a major focus of current research studies to extrapolate the interesting biology of the cells as well as to utilize them for cellular therapy for a number of disorders. Of particular interest is the generation of neurons for several incurable nervous system disorders, such as Alzheimer's and Parkinson's diseases, spinal cord and brain injury, and multiple sclerosis, just to name a few. The destruction or dysfunction of certain limited neuronal cell types is observed in these diseases, which can all be treated theoretically by cell transplantation therapy to replace the damaged cells. Several studies have demonstrated the development of various types of neurons from both ESCs and neural stem cells (NSCs) (Wernig, Brustle 2002; Sonntag, Sanchez-Pernaute 2006; Trzaska, Rameshwar 2007).

The potential of MSCs in tissue regeneration could be discussed by revisiting the biology of ESCs. ESCs are not plastic cells because their original intent is to make all the different cells types of the body. Similarly, the normal biology of NSCs, which reside in the brain, is to generate any type of brain cell. MSCs, on the other hand, are plastic because they can generate ectodermal neurons outside of their mesodermal origin. Owing to significant problems when using ESCs, such as teratoma formation and immune rejection (Sonntag, Simantov, Isacson et al. 2005), and expansion issues with NSCs (Snyder, Olanow 2005), many researchers have focused on the use of MSCs because of their plastic nature and ease of isolation and expansion in culture.

MSC-DERIVED DOPAMINERGIC NEURONS

Research interests in our laboratory not only include the basic biology of MSCs but also utilize their plasticity to generate dopaminergic and peptidergic neurons and examine their responses to microenvironmental factors. The latter is important as MSCs or any other stem cells get closer to clinical applications. Among reports of transdifferentiation of MSCs to functional neurons (de Hemptinne, Vermeiren, Maloteaux et al. 2004; Qian, Saltzman 2004; Cho, Trzaska, Greco et al. 2005; Kondo, Johnson, Yoder et al. 2005; Wislet-Gendebien, Hans, Leprince et al. 2005; Tropel, Platet, Platel et al. 2006) are the production of dopamine (DA) neurons (Table 8.2). This generation of DA neurons is of great interest for the treatment of Parkinson's disease (PD), a movement disorder pathologically characterized by the selective degeneration of DA neurons in the nigrostriatal region of the brain (Schapira, Olanow 2004). Research studies to efficiently generate large numbers of DA neurons from MSCs are still in infancy; however, many recent studies report the transdifferentiation of MSCs to DA neurons using various induction methods and animal models (Jiang, Henderson, Blackstad et al. 2003; Dezawa, Kanno, Hoshino et al. 2004; Guo, Yin, Meng et al. 2005; Fu, Cheng, Lin et al. 2006; Tatard, D'Ippolito, Diabira et al. 2006; Suon, Yang, Iacovitti et al. 2006) (Table 8.2).

Several protocols have been described, with each utilizing the various agents linked to DA development. The common factors employed in the induction protocols are sonic hedgehog (SHH) and fibroblast growth factor 8 (FGF8). The synergistic action of SHH and FGF8 has been shown to contribute to the formation of the DA phenotype during embryogenesis (Ye, Shimamura, Rubenstein et al. 1998). Conversely, other differentiation agents have also been shown to promote the transdifferentiation of MSCs to DA neurons (Smidt, Burbach 2007). The DA cells are often identified by expression of the rate-limiting enzyme in DA synthesis, tyrosine hydroxylase (TH), and the dopamine transporter (DAT), which reuptakes DA. Additionally, secretion of DA, its electrical properties, and its function in an animal model are also used to show the function of these transdifferentiated cells. In the following sections, we describe studies that demonstrate the plastic potential of MSCs in generating neurons of DA phenotype.

Preliminary studies in this field showed that a subpopulation of MSCs, termed *mouse multipotent adult progenitor cells* (MAPC), could expand by >120 population doublings and contribute to the generation of most somatic cell lineages, including those of the nervous system (Jiang, Henderson, Blackstad et al. 2003). The MAPCs were found to generate different neuronal types, and 25% of cells were found to express DA markers after 21 days of sequential induction with SHH, FGF8, and other neurotrophic factors and chemical reagents (Jiang, Henderson, Blackstad et al. 2003). This work remains controversial, particularly with regard to whether such a cell (MAPC) exists within the bone marrow. However, many recent studies have given way to the fact that MSCs could actually transdifferentiate to cells of the nervous system, especially DA cells. An eloquent study showed that transfection of MSCs with Notch intracellular domain followed by exposure to trophic factors (forskolin, basic fibroblast growth factor (bFGF), ciliary neurotrophic factor) and addition of glial cell–derived neurotrophic factor (GDNF) generated 41% of TH+ and DA-producing cells (Dezawa, Kanno, Hoshino et al. 2004). Transplantation of the cells into a rat PD model demonstrated a significant improvement in behavioral recovery as compared to control rats. Conversely, another study reported that poor survival was observed in a PD rat model after transplantation of transdifferentiated MSCs (Suon, Yang, Iacovitti et al. 2006). While another group acquired 35% of TH+ cells from rat MSCs by adding GDNF and the cytokine, interleukin (IL)-1β, in glial cell–conditioned media with mesencephalic membrane fragments, they failed to report on DA release and the excitability of their cells (Guo, Yin, Meng et al. 2005). A similar study demonstrated 31% of TH-expressing cells, utilizing a vector with red fluorescent protein under the human TH promoter, which allows for efficient evaluation and quantification of the transdifferentiated cells

Table 8.2 Selected Reports on the Generation of Dopaminergic Neurons from Mesenchymal Stem Cells

MSC	Induction	Advantages	Disadvantages	References
Adult human BM-derived MSC	SHH, FGF8, bFGF, neurobasal medium with B27	Express DA-specific markers, 67% TH+, and secrete DA	DA progenitors by functional analysis; other inductive factors necessary	Trzaska et al. 2007
Adult human BM-derived MSC	Supplement I: bFGF, EGF, N2 supplement II: N2 supplement, BHA, dbcAMP, IBMX, RA, GDNF	31% TH+, secrete DA, generation of bioassay to evaluate induction	Optimization of protocol to obtain increased TH+ cells, electro-physiological studies necessary	Kan et al. 2007
Human BM-isolated adult multilineage inducible cells	bFGF, βME, BHA, KCL, valproic acid, forskolin, hydrocortisone, insulin, NT-3, NGF, BDNF, SHH, FGF8, RA, GDNF	62% TH+, express DA markers, inward and outward currents (20%)	Not clear whether the cells secrete DA	Tatard et al. 2006
Human BM-derived MSC cell line hMPC 32F	Sphere formation: EGF, bFGF; differentiation: TPA, IBMX, forskolin, dbcAMP	Express DA markers: Nurr1, Pitx3, TH, AADC, GIRK2	Mainly, GABA neurons with only a subset of DA neurons (15%); poor survival in PD rat model	Suon et al. 2006
Human umbilical cord–derived MSC	Neuronal conditioned media, SHH, FGF8	12.7% TH+; DA secretion, improvement in PD rat model	Low efficiency to retrieve TH+ cells; number of cells transplanted was not adequate	Fu et al. 2006
Mouse BM-derived MSC	BHA, IBMX, dbcAMP, N2 solution, RA, AA	Migration and increased survival in PD mouse model	Did not evaluate whether the cells express DA markers	Hellman et al. 2006
Rat BM-derived MSC	IBMX, glial cell–conditioned media with mesencephalic membrane fragments, GDNF, IL-1β	35% TH+	No report on DA release or electrical activity	Guo et al. 2005
Human and rat BM-derived MSC	Transfection with Notch intracellular domain, forskolin, bFGF, CNTF, GDNF	41% TH+; express DA markers, behavioral recovery in PD rat model	Behavioral recovery may simply be due to trophic support	Dezawa et al. 2004
Mouse multipotent adult progenitor cells	Linoleic acid, BSA, DMSO, AA, bFGF, SHH, FGF8, BDNF, N2 medium	25% TH and DA expressing cells	Cells are also GABAergic (18%) and serotonergic (52%), protocol needs optimization	Jiang et al. 2003
Human and rat BM-derived MSC	Genetically engineered to synthesize L-DOPA (precursor to DA)	Integrate and promote functional recovery in PD rat model	Expression of transgene ceased after 9 days in vivo	Schwarz et al. 1999

The table summarizes reported protocols to generate DA neurons from mesenchymal stem cells.

AA, amino acid; BDNF, brain-derived neurotrophic factor; bFGF, basal fibroblast growth factor; βME, β-mercaptoethanol; BM, bone marrow; CNTF, ciliary neurotrophic factor; DA, dopamine; dbcAMP, dibutyryl cyclic AMP; EGF, epidermal growth factor; FGF8, fibroblast growth factor; GABA, γ-aminobutyric acid; GDNF, glial cell line–derived neurotrophic factor; IL-1β, interleukin 1β; MSC, mesenchymal stem cells; NGF, nerve growth factor; RA, retinoic acid; SHH, sonic hedgehog; BHA, butylated hydroxyanisole; IBMX, 3-isobutyl-1-methyl-xanthine; KCL, potassium chloride; NT-3, neurotrophin-3, TPA, 4β-12-O-tetradecanoylphorbol 13-acetate; BSA, bovine serum albumin.

(Kan, Ben-Zur, Barhum et al. 2007). Our laboratory has shown an efficient 67% generation of TH+ cells in 12 days from human bone marrow (BM)–derived MSCs, which also express DA-specific markers, DAT and vesicular monoamine transporter (VMAT2), and constitutively secrete DA (Trzaska, Kuzhikandathil, Rameshwar et al. 2007). Shown in Figure 8.2 is an image of the TH+ cells generated from MSCs in our laboratory.

DA neurons have also been derived from MSCs isolated from the Wharton's jelly of the human umbilical cord blood using neuronal conditioned media, SHH, and FGF8 (Fu, Cheng, Lin et al. 2006). Even though the group only generated 12.7% TH+ cells, the studies were supported by significant behavioral recovery in a PD rat model after transplantation, but not back to the normal level as an intact rat. It is important to note that MSCs derived from the umbilical cord have been reported to have different characteristics than bone marrow–derived adult MSC (Kern, Eichler, Stoeve et al. 2006), which may have accounted for the low efficiency achieved by Fu and colleagues. Another recent study reported on a subpopulation of MSCs, termed *marrow isolated adult multilineage inducible* (MIAMI) *cells* that are plastic and characteristic of ESC (Tatard, D'Ippolito, Diabira et al. 2007). After

Days induced

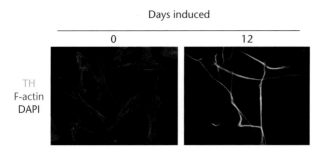

Figure 8.2 Representative images from our laboratory of MSCs induced with SHH, FGF8, and bFGF for 0 and 12 days. The panel shows just the nuclear stain, DAPI, and the cytoskeletal stain Texas Red phalloidin (F-actin) on Day 0 MSCs. In contrast, strong expression of TH) (FITC, green) is visible by 12 days of induction as indicated by the green and yellow fluorescence.

treatment with a several inductive agents, including SHH, FGF8, and retinoic acid (RA), the group generated an efficient 62% TH+ cells.

MSCs have been shown to integrate into the central nervous system (Schwarz, Alexander, Prockop et al. 1999; Li, Chen, Wang et al. 2001; Hellmann, Panet, Barhum et al. 2006; Deng, Petersen, Steindler et al. 2006). Whether the cells transdifferentiate in vivo or secrete neurotrophic factors to support damaged neurons is still in question. Regardless, transplantation of undifferentiated MSCs has shown promise for central nervous system disorders. A recent report has shown migration of contralaterally engrafted MSCs through the corpus callosum into the damaged side of the PD mouse model (Hellmann, Panet, Barhum et al. 2006). The authors suggest the presence of chemotactic agents in the lesioned area that may provide a stimulus for the MSCs to migrate and repair the injured tissue (Hellmann, Panet, Barhum et al. 2006). Since MSCs have demonstrated successful integration in the CNS, they hold promise as vehicles for gene therapy in PD. MSCs engineered to express L-DOPA successfully integrate in the CNS and promote behavioral recovery in the rat PD model (Schwarz, Alexander, Prockop et al. 1999).

Undifferentiated MSCs from human umbilical cord matrix (Weiss, Medicetty, Bledsoe et al. 2006) could be transplanted into the PD rat model without evidence of immunosuppression. Interestingly, the animals displayed considerable improvement in behavior; however, the transplanted cells could not be recovered postmortem. The authors speculate that the umbilical cord–derived MSCs dampened the immune response similar to adult MSCs, restricting secondary damage and allowing neuronal recovery. The stem cells could also secrete trophic factors that enhance functional recovery by rescuing the degenerating DA neurons (Weiss, Medicetty, Bledsoe et al.

2006). Similarly, a study reported the transplantation of human adult MSCs into a rat spinal cord injury model without immunosuppression (Cizkova, Rosocha, Vanicky et al. 2006). In comparison to the study by Weiss et al. the donor MSCs survived in the xenogenic model until the endpoint. The incorporation and survival of the human MSCs in the rat model was likely due to their immunomodulatory nature, which will be discussed in a later section (Cizkova, Rosocha, Vanicky et al. 2006).

MSC-DERIVED PEPTIDERGIC NEURONS

The derivation of different types of neurons from MSCs is desired to customize stem cell therapies for varied neural disorders. MSCs have been shown to transdifferentiate into neurons that produce the neuropeptide, SP (Cho, Trzaska, Greco et al. 2005). These results are not surprising since the anatomical location of MSCs within bone marrow suggests that they can form synapse-like structures with the innervating peptidergic fibers, and might therefore be important in the neural–hematopoietic link (Bianco, Riminucci, Gronthos et al. 2001).

SP is a 10–amino acid peptide encoded by the evolutionary conserved *Tac1* gene (Greco, Corcoran, Cho et al. 2004). *Tac1* is ubiquitously expressed, including in cells of the nervous, hematopoietic, and immune systems (Greco, Corcoran, Cho et al. 2004). SP has been linked to perception of pain, progression of cancer, and regulation of bone marrow function (Greco, Corcoran, Cho et al. 2004). In bone marrow, the functions of SP are partly mediated through the production of cytokines in bone marrow resident cells (Greco, Corcoran, Cho et al. 2004). These properties of SP make it an interesting neurotransmitter to study when considering its release by implanted stem cell–derived neurons and their interaction with the host microenvironment, which is discussed in the subsequent text.

SP-producing neurons are found within the brain and spinal cord as well as within peripheral nerve fibers such as those innervating immune organs (Greco, Corcoran, Cho et al. 2004). In addition to the generation of central DA neurons by MSCs, it would be advantageous to be able to also generate peripheral neurons, since regenerative therapies for peripheral neuropathies are needed. Future research is necessary to develop customized protocols for the development of neurons suited for many different neurological conditions.

SP-producing neurons have been derived from human MSCs by a customized induction protocol with RA as the inducing agent (Cho, Trzaska, Greco

Table 8.3 Induction Protocols for the Generation of Peptidergic Neurons from Human Mesenchymal Stem Cells

	Original Induction Protocol (Cho et al. 2005)	*Modified Induction Protocol (Greco et al. 2007)*
Efficiency	≈50%	80%–90%
Media	DMEM	DMEM/F12 Ham
Sera	10%	2%
Retinoic acid	30 μM	20 μM
Growth factors	None	bFGF
Supplement	None	1x B27

Summary of two induction protocols with varied efficiency (Cho, Trzaska, Greco et al. 2005; Greco, Liu, Rameshwar et al. 2007).

bFGF, basic fibroblast growth factor.

et al. 2005). RA is released by the neuroepithelium surrounding the developing neural tube to specify the dorsal axis, that is, the hindbrain and spinal cord. Many induction protocols use similar approaches that mimic the embryological cellular microenvironment. A recent report from our laboratory has optimized the protocol for producing mature SP-producing neurons through the inclusion of basic bFGF within the induction media (Greco, Zhou, Ye et al. 2007). bFGF is a potent mitogen, which is believed to increase the efficiency of neuronal transdifferentiation by expanding the initial development of neural progenitors, while maintaining cell survival for further lineage progression. The results from this study definitively show increased transdifferentiation efficiency by molecular, cellular, and functional approaches (Greco, Zhou, Ye et al. 2007) (Table 8.3).

Although there have been reports demonstrating the derivation of different classes of neurotransmitter-producing neurons from MSCs, little is known whether these stem cells first take on the phenotype of a neural stem/progenitor cell before undergoing lineage-specific commitment. The ability to generate and maintain a pool of neural stem/progenitor cells derived from MSCs will aid in the formation of other neural tissues, such as astrocytes and oligodendrocytes. MSCs induced with RA and bFGF appear to demonstrate a phenotype consistent with neural progenitor cells following 6 days of induction (Greco, Zhou, Ye et al. 2007). This was determined through the expression of immature neuronal markers (Nestin, Pax6, NeuroD) as well as of glial markers (GFAP) at this time point. However, further studies are needed to demonstrate that these cells behave as true neural progenitor cells in that they can form other neuronal lineages. Even so, one challenge faced is to determine how to maintain and expand this limited number of cells for further investigation.

OCT4 IN MSC FUNCTIONS

Pluripotency in ESCs and plasticity in ASCs seem to be mediated by developmental "switches," which control the fate of the cell. These switches help a stem cell decide whether to produce clones of itself, through a process known as *self-renewal*, or whether to differentiate into tissue-specific cells. Oftentimes these developmental switches are master transcriptional regulators such as transcription factors (Boiani, Scholer 2002). Three transcription factors known to mediate pluripotency in ESCs, while inhibiting tissue-specific gene expression, are OCT4, NANOG, and SOX2 (Pan, Chang, Scholer et al. 2002) (Fig. 8.1). The plasticity of MSCs suggests a level of functional similarities with ESCs. One commonality between the two stem cells comes from recent reports showing expression of OCT4 in MSCs (Tondreau, Meuleman, Delforge et al. 2005). Whether OCT4 demonstrates similar functions and regulatory circuitries in MSCs is an active area of research in our laboratory. We have shown similar regulatory circuitries by OCT4 in human MSCs and ESCs by scanning the genes that bind OCT4. These studies, as well as functional analyses, have determined similar genes expressed by OCT4 and also have similar target genes in MSCs and ESCs (Greco, Zhou, Ye et al. 2007).

One difference between MSCs and ESCs is the level of heterogeneity. While ESCs are relatively homogenous, rapidly dividing cells, MSCs appear to possess specific subpopulations of cells with different expression profiles and growth properties. However, it is unknown whether this apparent heterogeneity in vitro is indicative of MSCs within the bone marrow, since extended culture of MSCs induces some degree of lineage-specific differentiation. As a result, within a given population of MSCs there may be some cells that are self-renewing, while others undergo lineage commitment. Optimization of culture conditions is necessary to ensure efficient expansion of MSCs with minimal unwarranted differentiation.

To demonstrate the inconsistencies observed between laboratories culturing MSCs, we have compared freshly isolated MSCs and those that had been extensively passaged. The majority of early-passage MSCs expressed the embryonic transcription factors OCT4, NANOG, and SOX2, while these transcription factors were undetectable after extended passages (Greco et al. in press). In addition, significant decreases in telomerase expression and telomere length were observed in the late-passage MSCs (Greco et al. in press). Thus, despite optimal conditions in MSC expansion, the ability of these cells to continuously self-renew in culture is limited, as is their plasticity. This underscores the need to develop more efficient reagents and surfaces for MSC expansion, differentiation, and transdifferentiation as the science moves toward translational studies.

IMMUNE PROPERTIES OF MSCs

Perhaps one of the most intriguing properties of MSCs is their ability to act as antigen-presenting cells (APCs) and as immune-suppressor cells. This bimodal immune property could be partly due to their plastic nature, since it is the microenvironmental factors that will contour their functions. Their immunoprivileged and immunosuppressive functions are under intense investigation for a wide array of clinical applications, from drug or gene delivery to tissue repair (Castillo, Liu, Bonilla et al. 2007).

Their immunosuppressive function carries immense potential for transplantation, because allogeneic MSCs could be transplanted without overt fear of rejection. While the ability to veto an immune response makes MSC sufficient for immune rejection, it may not be useful when MSCs generate specialized tissue, because the veto property may be lost (Castillo, Liu, Bonilla et al. 2007). Whether transdifferentiated MSCs still carry this immunosuppressive function and how they will behave after transplantation into the damaged tissue is not clear at this time. This area of research is being pursued by our research team.

The mechanisms of MSC immunosuppression have not been completely elucidated. However, their effects are partly mediated through the release of soluble factors and secondary effects on immune cells (Groh, Maitra, Szekely et al. 2005). It has been clearly demonstrated that MSCs can inhibit the proliferation of T cells (Di Nicola, Carlo-Stella, Magni et al. 2002). Little is known about the mechanism, but it appears to depend on cross talk between the MSCs and T cells, which leads to the production of anti-inflammatory cytokines (Groh, Maitra, Szekely et al. 2005; Krampera, Cosmi, Angeli et al. 2006). Once T-cell proliferation is inhibited, the production of effector cytokines is reduced (Aggarwal, Pittenger 2005). Allogeneic MSCs can also inhibit B-cell activation, proliferation, differentiation, and immunoglobulin (Ig)G secretion (Deng, Han, Liao et al. 2005, Corcione, Benvenuto, Ferretti et al. 2006). MSCs have been reported to downregulate the expression of chemokine receptors on B cells, suggesting a blunting effect on B-cell migration to inflammatory sites (Corcione, Benvenuto, Ferretti et al. 2006). Of particular interest is the effect of MSC on dendritic cells (DCs), which are APCs. In the presence of MSCs, DC differentiation from CD14+ monocytes is inhibited, thus providing another mechanism of MSC immunosuppression (Jiang, Zhang, Liu et al. 2005). MSCs

also interact with natural killer (NK) cells; however, the studies need further research. MSC were unable to suppress the activity of IL-2–activated NK cells but could suppress NK activity in the presence of interferon (IFN)-γ (Spagiarri, Capobianco, Becchetti et al. 2006). Tumor growth factor (TGF)-β1 has also been shown to suppress NK proliferation by MSC (Sotiropoulou, Capobianco, Becchetti et al. 2006).

The immunosuppressive property of MSCs has been studied in vivo to facilitate engraftment of transplanted cells and to reduce the risk of rejection. The capability of MSCs to assist in the engraftment of hematopoietic stem cells and treat graft-versus-host disease (GVHD) during clinical bone marrow transplantation has been investigated in much detail (Le Blanc, Rasmusson, Sundberg et al. 2004; Lazarus, Koc, Devine et al. 2005; Ringden, Uzunel, Rasmusson et al. 2006). In fact, MSCs are currently under clinical trials for the treatment of GVHD in allogeneic transplantation (Giordano, Galderisi, Marino 2007). Shown in Table 8.4 are the ongoing clinical trials with MSCs. Their immunosuppressive property has also shown promise in multiple sclerosis, an autoimmune disorder. Injection of MSCs into an animal model of multiple sclerosis resulted in T-cell tolerance against the pathogenic antigen (Zappia, Casazza, Pedemonte et al. 2006). Transplantation of MSCs have also led to encouraging outcomes for a number of disorders, including osteogenesis imperfecta, breast cancer, stroke, and hematological malignancy (Koc, Gerson, Cooper et al. 2000; Horwitz, Gordon, Koo et al. 2002; Lazarus, Koc, Devine et al. 2005; Tang, Yasuhara, Hara et al. 2007). However, additional conclusive studies are warranted, since it has been reported that in some cases transplantation of allogeneic MSCs can lead to rejection (Eliopoulos, Stagg, Lejeune et al. 2005).

Despite their immense potential for clinical transplantation, MSCs express major histocompatibility complex (MHC) II, which could deter their use in cellular therapy, since they could potentially stimulate an inflammatory reaction (Potian, Aviv, Ponzio et al. 2003). The APC properties of MSCs are heightened during low levels of IFN-γ, but as levels increase, MHC II is downregulated (Chan, Tang, Patel et al. 2006) Thus, APC function is decreased and the cells switch roles to immune suppressor cells (Chan, Tang, Patel et al. 2006).

The biology of MHC II in MSCs and their differentiated cells are relevant to transplantation. At present, it is uncertain at what differentiation stages MSCs should be transplanted into patients, that is, undifferentiated versus partly transdifferentiated versus fully transdifferentiated. This issue might depend on the effects of inflammatory mediators and the expression of MHC II. Our unpublished studies indicate that MSC-derived neurons could express MHC II in the

Table 8.4 Clinical Trials with Mesenchymal Stem Cells

Pathological Condition	Treatment	Function of MSC
Graft-versus-host disease (GVHD)	Intravenous administration of autologous BM-derived MSCs	Immunosuppression
Liver failure	Injection of MSC-derived hepatocyte progenitors	Liver regeneration
Liver cirrhosis	Injection of autologous BM-derived MSCs	Regression of liver fibrosis
Tibia fractures	Implantation of autologous MSCs on a carrier at the fracture site	Fracture healing, bone regeneration
Leukemia, myelodysplastic syndrome	Transplantation of cord blood with MSC after high-dose chemotherapy	Hematopoietic reconstitution and immunosuppression
Familial hypercholesterolemia	Transplantation of hepatocytes transdifferentiated from MSC	Liver regeneration
Crohn's disease	Intravenous administration of BM-derived MSC	Immunosuppression
Heart failure	Intramyocardial BM-derived MSC transplantation	Myocardial regeneration

The information shown in the table has been obtained from the NIH clinical trials database (www.clinicaltrials.gov).

BM, bone marrow; MSC, mesenchymal stem cell.

presence of low levels of IFN-γ. This has been supported by other studies showing MHC II expression during neuronal differentiation (Liu et al. 2006). To evaluate the effect of an inflammatory environment, similar to transplantation, the authors demonstrated that addition of IFN-γ enhanced MHC II expression. Despite this, the neuronal differentiated MSCs showed some immunosuppression in the presence of T lymphocytes (Liu et al. 2007).

MICROENVIRONMENTAL CROSS TALK

In vitro, the MSC microenvironment can be determined to favor the desired outcome such as growth or differentiation. In vivo, the transplanted MSCs are exposed to immune cells and mediators that could influence the cells' behavior. MSC plasticity has principally been demonstrated in vitro, under a controlled environment. However, what if implanting the stem cells into an injured tissue alters this observed plasticity? How clinically relevant are these in vitro studies if the MSCs have untoward effects once implanted? These are important issues that need to be addressed in order to assure patient safety. Avenues of research addressing these issues will aid in the transition of stem cells from "bench to bedside."

Central to the effects of microenvironment in MSC functions are the changes in tissue-specific gene expression. This question is significant because the genes expressed in the transplanted cells could also affect the functions of cells within the microenvironment and establish a cross talk with the implanted stem cells. This type of communication could be harmful and/or beneficial. Regardless, an understanding of the mechanism by which genes are regulated by microenvironmental factors will lead to insights on communication between stem cells and their surrounding microenvironment (Moore, Lemischka 2006).

Predicting how the recipient tissue will guide stem cell implantation and behavior is challenging. To confidently make this assessment, in vitro models to study how an inflammatory microenvironment, expected in chronic and acute tissue insults, such as multiple sclerosis and spinal cord injury, need to be developed. Regardless of the stage at which stem cells are implanted, the cells will be placed in a milieu of inflammatory mediators. This issue is relevant even though particular diseases might have a special protocol for stem cell therapy. For this reason, the studies by our laboratory have examined the entire period of transdifferentiation to better predict the periods of differentiation that hold the greatest clinical significance.

To properly examine the effect of the microenvironment on the transplantable cell requires extensive experiments under a variety of conditions. Moreover, the problem becomes more complex when one considers the dynamic nature of the microenvironment and the differentiation potential of the implanted cell. Implantation of the stem cell alone will generate a local immune response and exposure to infiltrating immune cells that synthesize cytokines, chemokines, and matrix metalloproteases.

Our laboratory has investigated the effects of the ubiquitous proinflammatory cytokine, IL-1α, on

MSCs undifferentiated or transdifferentiated to neurons (Greco, Rameshwar 2007). Undifferentiated and transdifferentiated cells were found to produce the neurotransmitter, SP upon exposure to IL-1α. These results are significant because SP is also a proinflammatory peptide (Greco, Corcoran, Cho et al. 2004). Excessive production of SP by transplanted MSCs might lead to immune cell infiltration with the risk of immune rejection. In most tissues, including brain and spinal cord, exacerbated immune responses could lead to damaging outcomes.

Another surprising observation from our studies was the overall effect of IL-1α on the transdifferentiation of MSCs into neurons (Greco, Rameshwar 2007). Inclusion of IL-1α within the neuronal induction medium facilitated the neurogenic program of differentiation. These results have clinical relevance regarding the stage of differentiation at which to implant the MSCs. This is an example of the inflammatory microenvironment having a positive effect on the desired behavior of the implanted cells. Much further work is necessary to better mimic the complex tissue environment through inclusion of immune cells and other pro- and anti-inflammatory mediators.

The phenotypic effects resulting from exposure of MSCs or their transdifferentiated counterparts to an inflammatory microenvironment are due to stem cell–microenvironmental cross talk. Specifically, the host microenvironment influences the transcriptional and translational machinery of the stem cell. One example of an inflammatory microenvironment altering MSC gene regulation is the effects of IL-1α on RE-1 silencer of transcription (REST). REST, also known as neural restrictive silencing factor, is a transcription factor that represses target gene transcription by binding regulatory elements containing a consensus 21 bp RE-1 sequence (Chong, Tapia-Ramirez, Kim et al. 1995). REST expression has been demonstrated in non-neuronal cells, NSCs, and neural progenitor cells, where its function has been ascribed to repressing the expression of pan-neuronal genes in non-neuronal or immature neuronal tissues (Lunyak, Rosenfeld 2005).

Stimulation of undifferentiated MSCs with IL-1α resulted in rapid downregulation of REST (Greco, Smirnov, Murthy et al. 2007). Since REST targets many mature neuronal genes, this downregulation may be seen as conducive to neuronal transdifferentiation; however, REST also acts as both a tumor suppressor gene and an oncogene (Coulson 2005; Majumder 2006). As a result, IL-1α could predispose the implanted MSCs to tumorigenesis.

IL-1α was also observed to exert translational effects on neurons transdifferentiated from MSCs as well (Greco, Rameshwar 2007). Specifically, IL-1α caused degradation of Tac1-specific microRNAs (miRNAs) to allow synthesis of SP. miRNAs are a novel class of 19 to 23 nucleotide, small, and noncoding RNA molecules encoded in the genomes of plants and animals (as reviewed in Novina and Sharp 2004). In animals, miRNAs bind to the 3′ untranslated region (UTR) of target mRNAs to primarily mediate transient translational repression (as reviewed in Novina and Sharp 2004).

Microenvironmental influence on stem cell–specific miRNAs could lead to the premature synthesis of translationally blocked mRNAs with either beneficial or untoward effects. In either case, cross talk between a stem cell and its surrounding microenvironment can have effects at the phenotypic, transcriptional, and translational levels. Future stem cell therapies will need to take this level of regulation into consideration to prevent unforeseen harm to the patient. Through the development of in vitro models which mimic the host microenvironment, we can gain a better understanding of stem cell behavior.

BIOMEDICAL ENGINEERING APPLICATIONS

Cell therapy is a promising method for the treatment of neurodegenerative diseases and other tissue injuries. At this time, the potential for MSCs as a cell therapy for clinical disorders is irrefutable, mainly because of their plasticity and unique immune functions. However, in order to translate stem cell therapy to patients, other areas of science need to be considered. For example, combinations of matrix, growth factor, and cell adhesion cues that distinguish the microenvironment of injury are critically important for the control of cell differentiation and their proliferation (Picinich, Mishra, Glod et al. 2007) (Table 8.5).

Many in vitro studies have investigated neurons derived from transdifferentiated MSCs (Kashofer, Bonnet 2005), but have failed to significantly display the efficacy by in vivo methods (Suon, Yang, Iacovitti 2006). Overall, the current experimental evidence supports continuation for further scientific investigation. However, effective translation can only be achieved by innovative collaboration. This is where science meets engineering, commonly referred to as tissue engineering, which combines cellular and developmental biology and bioengineering designs to facilitate clinical implementations. The reports have shown that encompassing bioengineered materials that mimic the natural microenvironment produce greater accuracy in data collected in vitro and also improve in vivo capabilities of MSCs (Jager, Feser, Denck et al. 2005; Wang, Li, Zuo et al. 2007).

The recent influx of knowledge in stem cell biology has lead to a rapid increase in stem cell–based tissue

Table 8.5 Summary of Biomaterials in Stem Cell Therapy

Stem Cell	Scaffold	Biological Effect	Potential Applications and Treatments	References
In vitro				
Mouse neural stem cells (NSCs)	3D calcium alginate beads	Expression of nestin; Capacity to differentiate into neurons and glial cells	Shows feasibility of the scaffold to expand NSCs.	Li et al. 2006
Hippocampal progenitor cells (HiB5)	Films PLGA, PLCL, and PLLA	PLGA performed best and displayed maximum neurite growth. PLLA showed negative results in all categories evaluated	PLGA displayed biocompatibility for NSC transplantation and for nerve regeneration	Bhang et al. 2007
Human BM-derived MSC	PLLA, collagen I/III, and PLGA	DAG-enriched media resulted in cell proliferation on PLLA, slightly on PLGA, and inhibited on collagen	All polymers showed increases in Ca(2+) production but had significant differences in proliferation, differentiation, and adherence	Jager et al. 2005
Human BM-derived MSC	2D cultures on PDL, PLL, collagen, laminin, fibronectin and Matrigel	Expansion and differentiation were impacted due to substrates surface properties	Different in vitro substrates provide different culture results therefore optimization for each cell type is needed	Qian, Saltzman 2004
Human BM-derived MSC	PLGA beads	Shows retention of pluripotency; remained adherent and viable in the 3D electrospun nanofibrous environment.	Nanofibers may serve as a 3D vehicle for lineage-specific cells	Xin et al. 2007
Human BM-derived MSC	Chitosan conduit membrane	Induced MSCs expressed Schwann cell phenotype	Artificial peripheral nerve fields will promote nerve regeneration	Zhang et al. 2006
In vivo				
Optic tract of hamster midbrain	Peptide nanofiber scaffold	Increased axonal regeneration after injury to optic nerve	Permissive environment aided in the regeneration of axons and closed lesion gap in brain	Ellis-Behnke et al. 2006
MSCs implanted in rabbit model	3D zein porous scaffold	MSCs and scaffold were biocompatible in rabbit model	Stem/Scaffold is biocompatible therefore has potential for osteogenic procedures	Wang et al. 2007
MSCs derived neuron-like cells implanted in Rhesus monkey	methoxy polyethylene glycol-polylactic acid with controlled-release GDNF	implantation in an acute rhesus signal cord injury model showed an increase in proliferation and cellular infiltration, higher density of nerve fibers, and higher absorbance	Demonstrated optimization and benefits of combination therapy versus cellular therapy alone. Animal healing was advanced when a biomaterial was used to deliver the MSCs to the injury site.	Liu et al. 2005

Reports on the different biomaterials used with stem cells for optimizing in vitro conditions and increasing positive clinical prognosis.
GDNF, glial cell line–derived neurotrophic factor.

engineered composites. Many of these approaches are comprised of manufactured scaffolds that are seeded with stem cells and delivered as a collection to build "to the" existing tissues (Fig. 8.3). Some biomaterials such as silk, collagen, and gelatin are naturally derived and some are synthetically derived: polylactic acid, polycaprolactone, and nylon. During the healing process the construct degrades, is adsorbed, and metabolized, leaving behind newly reconstructed tissue (Stock, Vacanti 2001). Many of these materials are biodegradable and biocompatible with no adverse effect, offering a durable template for guided tissue regeneration while allowing robust stem cells, such as MSCs, to differentiate and proliferate (Wang, Li, Zuo et al. 2007; Zhang, Xu, Zhang et al. 2006; Bianco, Robey 2001). Some tissues that have been reported to

respond positively to this therapy include blood vessels, bone, cartilage, cornea, dentin, heart muscle, liver, pancreas, nervous tissue, skeletal muscle, and skin thus far.

Scientists have applied this combinatory approach to MSC research in vitro and continually strive to produce optimal microenvironments. Since MSCs are extrapolated from a 3D environment it seems applicable to provide an artificial environment that is 3D versus the planar environment where most in vitro analyses are conducted. Therefore, in vitro models that mimic the microenvironment of an injured tissue have been developed to better understand how stem cells will behave once implanted and answer many of the questions regarding the stage at which implantation should occur.

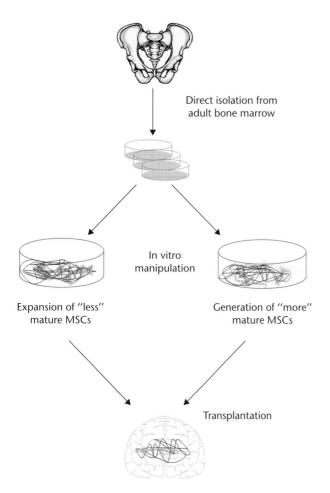

Direct isolation from adult bone marrow

In vitro manipulation

Expansion of "less" mature MSCs

Generation of "more" mature MSCs

Transplantation

Figure 8.3 MSCs are expanded from aspirated samples of the iliac crest. Shown are co-cultures of MSCs with biomaterials, such as polymeric nanofibrous scaffold. The MSCs adhere to the scaffold, then proliferate and/or differentiate into neuron-like cells. Depending on the optimal differentiation stage, MSCs and the controlled-release biodegradable scaffold are implanted in the area of damaged tissue. This approach delivers the stem cells and biomaterial as a collection to build into the existing tissue, control the microenvironment, and restrict migration of the stem cells.

Many scaffolds that can virtually mimic any tissue have been successfully developed. For example, a ceramic that is adherently brittle is being used as the construct for damaged bone or polymeric fibers to biomimic the fibrosis extracellular matrix in cartilage (Xin, Hussain, Mao 2007). In one study, poly-D-lysine, poly-L-lysine, collagen, laminin, and fibronectin coated with Matrigel were used to compare the impact on expansion and neuronal differentiation to that of standard polystyrene (Qian, Saltzman 2004). It was concluded that the surface properties of the 3D culture substrates with higher coating densities of Matrigel enhanced differentiation and significantly improved cell expansion to that of standard polystyrene.

The stem cell/scaffold constructs also yield far better in vivo results than when transdifferentiated MSCs are used alone. The construct's biomimicry properties serve as an applicable implantable device that can be used as a restricted area for implanted MSCs. It also serves as a barrier against the host immune system and a delivery vehicle for drugs and other factors. When MSCs are implanted alone at the injection site or in the blood, they may not remain in the damaged area or may have a low homing yield (Suon, Yang, Iacovitti 2006; Coronel, Musolino, Villar 2006). A recent experiment addressed this issue by using a controlled-release biodegradable biomaterial consisting of a block copolymer, methoxypolyethylene glycol-polylactic acid (mPEG-b-PLA), combined with GDNF, and seeded with "neuron-like" cells derived from MSCs (Liu, Deng, Liu et al. 2005). The construct was implanted in the posterior funiculus of Rhesus monkeys to explore the tissue regeneration of an acute spinal cord injury. The control group was injected with the biomaterial excluding the neuron-like cells and GDNF but with enough phosphate buffer saline to bring it to the same volume. The cortical somatosensory-evoked potential (CSEP) was measured and the histomorphological changes were observed. Four to 5 months after implantation, the measured amplitude of the CSEP was significantly higher in the control group. In contrast, the treatment group displayed slightly more cell proliferation, increased cellular infiltration, higher density of nerve fibers, and higher integral absorbance. The construct with neuron-like cells and controlled-release GDNF kept the CSEP at normal and decreased amplitudes, indicating an alteration in the host's judgment of the spinal cord injury, possibly controlling the immune response. Additionally, the increased number of neurons in the damaged area should accelerate the repair of the injury. This is another example of a biomaterial positively influencing regeneration and providing increased restoration of the tissue.

In the United States, there are only few approved clinical therapies available that use tissue engineered biomaterials and MSCs to regenerate and reconstruct damaged tissue. These therapies are limited to repair of skin, bone, and cartilage. There is much known about these lineages and less about neurons derived from MSCs; however, the science is advancing and new approaches to this very unique and diverse system are ongoing (Ellis-Behnke, Liang, You et al. 2006).

The ultimate goal of tissue engineers is to produce "off the shelf tissues and organs." Transplantation and tissue reconstruction are among the most expensive treatments and are needed by millions of people. "Off the shelf tissues and organs" would improve medical care immensely by lowering costs, shortening waiting periods, providing ample amounts of organs and tissues, no longer requiring donor matches and immune suppression drugs, and eliminating disease transmission. The benefits are enormous but the ultimate goal requires intensive interdisciplinary studies. Meanwhile, the products currently approved along with the products still in clinical trials offer some immediate therapies to patients. However, cell therapy in neurodegenerative diseases and disorders is still in its infancy and will be most challenging because of the complexity of the organ. Fortunately biological science and engineering collaborations are progressing onward to achieve more efficient and efficacious therapies.

SUMMARY

The application of stem cells in models of regenerative medicine is an area of intense research with great public interest. MSCs are particularly attractive, given their reduced propensity to form tumors, ease in isolation, expansion potential, and cellular plasticity. However, before extensive clinical trials using these stem cells can progress, consideration must be given to understand their basic biology and assess how they will behave once implanted. Through the development of in vitro models that mimic the characteristic microenvironment unique to each disease or disorder, and by applying principles of biomedical engineering to cell therapy, the clinical utilization of stem cells can progress with increased confidence.

REFERENCES

Aggarwal S, Pittenger MF. 2005. Human mesenchymal stem cells modulate allogeneic immune cell responses. *Blood*. 105:1815–1822.

Aurich I, Mueller LP, Aurich H et al. 2007. Functional integration of hepatocytes derived from human mesenchymal stem cells into mouse livers. *Gut*. 56:405–415.

Bedada FB, Gunther S, Kubin T, Braun T. 2006. Differentiation versus plasticity: fixing the fate of undetermined adult stem cells. *Cell Cycle*. 5:223–226.

Beltrami AP, Bariucchi L, Torella D et al. 2003. Adult cardiac stem cells are multipotent and support myocardial regeneration. *Cell*. 114:763–76.

Bhang SH, Lim JS, Choi CY, Kwon YK, Kim BS. 2007. The behavior of neural stem cells on biodegradable synthetic polymers. *J Biomater Sci Polym*. Ed 18(2):223–239.

Bianco P, Riminucci M, Gronthos S, Robey PG. 2001. Bone marrow stromal stem cells: nature, biology, and potential applications. *Stem Cells*. 19:180–192.

Bianco P, Robey P. 2001. Stem cells in tissue engineering. *Nature*. 414:118–121.

Biswas A, Hutchins R. 2007. Embryonic stem cells. *Stem Cells Dev*. 16:213–222.

Boiani M, Scholer HR. 2005. Regulatory networks in embryo-derived pluripotent stem cells. *Nat Rev Mol Cell Biol*. 6:872–884.

Castillo M, Liu K, Bonilla L, Rameshwar P. 2007. The immune properties of mesenchymal stem cells. *Intl J Biomed Sci*. 3:100–104.

Chan RJ, Yoder MC. 2004. The multiple facets of hematopoietic stem cells. *Curr Neurovas Res*. 1:197–206.

Chan JL, Tang KC, Patel AP et al. 2006. Antigen-presenting property of mesenchymal stem cells occurs during a narrow window at low levels of interferon-gamma. *Blood*. 107:4817–4824.

Chen LB, Jiang XB, Yang L. 2004. Differentiation of rat marrow mesenchymal stem cells into pancreatic islet beta-cells. *World J Gastroenterol*. 10:3016–3020.

Cho KJ, Trzaska KA, Greco SJ et al. 2005. Neurons derived from human mesenchymal stem cells show synaptic transmission and can be induced to produce the neurotransmitter substance P by interleukin-1 alpha. *Stem Cells*. 23:383–391.

Chong JA, Tapia-Ramirez J, Kim S et al. 1995. REST: a mammalian silencer protein that restricts sodium channel gene expression to neurons. *Cell*. 80:949–957.

Cizkova D, Rosocha J, Vanicky I, Jergova S, Cizek M. 2006. Transplants of human mesenchymal stem cells improve functional recovery after spinal cord injury in the rat. *Cell Mol Neurobiol*. 26:1167–1180.

Cohnheim J. 1867. Ueber entzündung und eiterung. *Path Anat Physiol Klin Med*. 40:1.

Corcione A, Benvenuto F, Ferretti E et al. 2006. Human mesenchymal stem cells modulate B-cell functions. *Blood*. 107:367–372.

Coronel MF, Musolino PL, Villar MJ. 2006. Selective migration and engraftment of bone marrow mesenchymal stem cells in rat lumbar dorsal root ganglia after sciatic nerve construction. *Neurosci Lett*. 405:5–9.

Coulson JM. 2005. Transcriptional regulation: cancer, neurons and the REST. *Curr Biol*. 15:R665–R668.

de Hemptinne I, Vermeiren C, Maloteaux JM, Hermans E. 2004. Induction of glial glutamate transporters in adult mesenchymal stem cells. *J Neurochem*. 91:155–166.

Deng W, Han Q, Liao L, You S, Deng H, Zhao RC. 2005. Effects of allogeneic bone marrow-derived mesenchymal stem cells on T and B lymphocytes from BXSB mice. *DNA Cell Biol*. 24:458–463.

Deng J, Petersen BE, Steindler DA, Jorgensen ML, Laywell ED. 2006. Mesenchymal stem cells spontaneously express neural proteins in culture and are neurogenic after transplantation. *Stem Cells*. 24:1054–1064.

Dezawa M, Kanno H, Hoshino M et al. 2004. Specific induction of neuronal cells from bone marrow stromal cells and application for autologous transplantation. *J Clin Invest*. 113:1701–1710.

Di Nicola M, Carlo-Stella C, Magni M et al. 2002. Human bone marrow stromal cells suppress T-lymphocyte proliferation induced by cellular or nonspecific mitogenic stimuli. *Blood*. 99:3838–3843.

Driesch H. 1893. Zur verlagerung der blastomeren des echinideneies. *Anat Anz*. 8:348–357.

Eliopoulos N, Stagg J, Lejeune L, Pommey S, Galipeau J. 2005. Allogeneic marrow stromal cells are immune rejected by MHC class I- and class II-mismatched recipient mice. *Blood.* 106:4057–4065.

Ellis-Behnke RG, Liang Y, You S et al. 2006. Nano neuro knitting: peptide nanofiber scaffold for brain repair and axon regeneration with functional return of vision. *Proc Nat Acad Sci U S A.* 103:5054–5059.

Friedenstein AJ, Deriglasova UF, Kulagina et al. 1974. Precursors for fibroblasts in different populations of hematopoietic cells as detected by the in vitro colony assay method. *Exp Hematol.* 2:83–92.

Fu YS, Cheng YC, Lin MY et al. 2006. Conversion of human umbilical cord mesenchymal stem cells in Wharton's jelly to dopaminergic neurons in vitro - potential therapeutic application for Parkinsonism. *Stem Cells.* 24:115–124.

Giordano A, Galderisi U, Marino IR. 2007. From the laboratory bench to the patient's bedside: an update on clinical trials with mesenchymal stem cells. *J Cell Physiol.* 211:27–35.

Greco SJ, Corcoran KE, Cho KJ, Rameshwar P. 2004. Tachykinins in the emerging immune system: relevance to bone marrow homeostasis and maintenance of hematopoietic stem cells. *Front Biosci.* 9:1782–1793.

Greco SJ, Rameshwar P. 2007. Enhancing effect of IL-1α on neurogenesis from adult human mesenchymal stem cells: implication for inflammatory mediators in regenerative medicine *J Immunol.* 179:3342–3350.

Greco SJ, Zhou C, Ye JH, Rameshwar P. 2007. An interdisciplinary approach and characterization of neuronal cells transdifferentiated from human mesenchymal stem cells. *Stem Cells Dev.* 16(5):811–826.

Greco SJ, Smirnov S, Murthy R, Rameshwar P. 2007. Synergy between RE-1 silencer of transcription (REST) and NFκB in the repression of the neurotransmitter gene *Tac1* in human mesenchymal stem cells: implication for micro-environmental influence on stem cell therapies. *J Biol Chem.* 182(41):3342–3350.

Greco SJ, Rameshwar P. 2007. miRNAs regulate synthesis of the neurotransmitter substance P in human mesenchymal stem cell-derived neuronal cells. *Proc Nat Acad. Sci U S A.* 104(39):15484–15489.

Greco SJ, Liu K, Rameshwar P. 2007. Functional similarities among genes regulated by OCT4 in human mesenchymal and embryonic stem cells. *Stem Cells.* 25(12):3143–3154.

Groh ME, Maitra B, Szekely E, Koc ON. 2005. Human mesenchymal stem cells require monocyte-mediated activation to suppress alloreactive T cells. *Exp Hematol.* 33:928–934.

Grove JE, Bruscia E, Krause DS. 2004. Plasticity of bone marrow-derived stem cells. *Stem Cells.* 22:487–500.

Guo L, Yin F, Meng HQ et al. 2005. Differentiation of mesenchymal stem cells into dopaminergic neuron-like cells in vitro. *Biomed Environ Sci.* 18:36–42.

Hellmann MA, Panet H, Barhum Y, Melamed E, Offen D. 2006. Increased survival and migration of engrafted mesenchymal bone marrow stem cells in 6-hydroxydopamine-lesioned rodents. *Neurosci Lett.* 395:124–128.

Horwitz EM, Gordon PL, Koo WK et al. 2002. Isolated allogeneic bone marrow-derived mesenchymal cells engraft and stimulate growth in children with osteogenesis imperfecta: implications for cell therapy of bone. *Proc Natl Acad Sci U S A.* 99:8932–8937.

Jager M, Feser T, Denck H, Krauspe R. 2005. Proliferation and osteogenic differentiation of mesenchymal stem cells cultured onto three different polymers in vitro. *Ann Biomed Eng.* 33:1319–1332.

Jiang Y, Henderson D, Blackstad M, Chen A, Miller RF, Verfaillie CM. 2003. Neuroectodermal differentiation from mouse multipotent adult progenitor cells. *Proc. Natl Acad Sci U S A.* 100 (Suppl 1): 11854–11860.

Jiang XX, Zhang Y, Liu B et al. 2005. Human mesenchymal stem cells inhibit differentiation and function of monocyte-derived dendritic cells. *Blood.* 105:4120–4126.

Kan I, Ben-Zur T, Barhum Y et al. 2007. Dopaminergic differentiation of human mesenchymal stem cells—utilization of bioassay for tyrosine hydroxylase expression. *Neurosci Lett.* 419:28–33.

Kashofer K, Bonnet D. 2005. Gene therapy progress and prospects: stem cell plasticity. *Gene Ther.* 12:1229–1234.

Kayahara T, Sawada M, Takaishi S et al. 2003. Candidate markers for stem and progenitor cells, Muasashi-1 and Hes1, are expressed in crypt base columnar cells of mouse and small intestine. *FEBS Lett.* 535:131–5.

Kern S, Eichler H, Stoeve J, Kluter H, Bieback K. 2006. Comparative analysis of mesenchymal stem cells from bone marrow, umbilical cord blood, or adipose tissue. *Stem Cells.* 24:1294–1301.

Koc ON, Gerson SL, Cooper BW et al. 2000. Rapid hematopoietic recovery after coinfusion of autologous-blood stem cells and culture-expanded marrow mesenchymal stem cells in advanced breast cancer patients receiving high-dose chemotherapy. *J Clin Oncol.* 18:307–316.

Kondo T, Johnson SA, Yoder MC, Romand R, Hashino E. 2005. Sonic hedgehog and retinoic acid synergistically promote sensory fate specification from bone marrow-derived pluripotent stem cells. *Proc Natl Acad Sci U S A.* 102:4789–4794.

Krampera M, Cosmi L, Angeli R et al. 2006. Role for interferon-gamma in the immunomodulatory activity of human bone marrow mesenchymal stem cells. *Stem Cells.* 24:386–398.

Krause DS, Theise ND, Collector MI et al. 2001. Multiorgan, multi-lineage engraftment by a single bone marrow-derived stem cell. *Cell.* 105:369–377.

Lazarus HM, Koc ON, Devine SM et al. 2005. Cotransplantation of HLA-identical sibling culture-expanded mesenchymal stem cells and hematopoietic stem cells in hematologic malignancy patients. *Biol Blood Marrow Transplant.* 11:389–398.

Le Blanc K, Rasmusson I, Sundberg B et al. 2004. Treatment of severe acute graft-versus-host disease with third party haploidentical mesenchymal stem cells. *Lancet.* 363:1439–1441.

Li Y, Chen J, Wang L, Zhang L, Lu M, Chopp M. 2001. Intracerebral transplantation of bone marrow stromal cells in a 1-methyl-4-phenyl-1,2,3,6-tetrahydropyridine mouse model of Parkinson's disease. *Neurosci Lett.* 316:67–70.

Li X, Liu T, Song K et al. 2006. Culture of neural stem cells in calcium alginate beads. *Biotechnol Prog.* 22:1683–1689.

Liang L, Birckenbach J. 2002. Somatic epidermal stem cells can produce multiple cell lineages during development. *Stem Cells*. 20:20–31.

Liu XG, Deng YB, Liu ZG, Zhu WB, Wang JY, Zhang C. 2005. Role of combined transplantation of neuron-like cells and controlled-release neurotrophic factor in the structural repair and functional restoration of macaca mulatta posterior funiculus following spinal cord injury. *Chinese J Clin Rehab*. 9:6–99.

Liu CT, Yang YJ, Yin F et al. 2006. The immunobiological development of human bone marrow mesenchymal stem cells in the course of neuronal differentiation. *Cell Immunol*. 244:19–32.

Lunyak VV, Rosenfeld MG. 2005. No rest for REST: REST/NRSF regulation of neurogenesis. *Cell*. 121:499–501.

Majumder S. 2006. REST in good times and bad: roles in tumor suppressor and oncogenic activities. *Cell Cycle*. 5:1929–1935.

Mazhari R, Hare JM. 2007. Mechanisms of action of mesenchymal stem cells in cardiac repair: potential influences on the cardiac stem cell niche. *Nat Clin Pract Cardiovasc Med*. 4(Suppl 1):S21–26.

Miyahara Y, Nagaya N, Kataoka M et al. 2006. Monolayered mesenchymal stem cells repair scarred myocardium after myocardial infarction. *Nat Med*. 12:459–465.

Moore KA, Lemischka IR. 2006. Stem cells and their niches. *Science*. 31:1880–1885.

Novina CD, Sharp PA. 2004. The RNAi revolution. *Nature*. 430:161–164.

Pan GJ, Chang ZY, Scholer HR, Pei D. 2002. Stem cell pluripotency and transcription factor Oct4 *Cell Res*. 12:32132–32139.

Phinney DG, Isakova I. 2005. Plasticity and therapeutic potential of mesenchymal stem cells in the nervous system. *Curr Pharm Des*. 11(10):1255–1265.

Picinich SC, Mishra PJ, Glod J, Banerjee D. 2007. The therapeutic potential of mesenchymal stem cells. Cell- & tissue-based therapy. *Expert Opin Biol Ther*. 7:965–973.

Potian JA, Aviv H, Ponzio NM, Harrison JS, Rameshwar P. 2003. Veto-like activity of mesenchymal stem cells: functional discrimination between cellular responses to alloantigens and recall antigens. *J Immunol*. 171:3426–3434.

Qian L, Saltzman WM. 2004. Improving the expansion and neuronal differentiation of mesenchymal stem cells through culture surface modification. *Biomaterials*. 25:1331–1337.

Ringden O, Uzunel M, Rasmusson I et al. 2006. Mesenchymal stem cells for treatment of therapy-resistant graft-versus-host disease. *Transplantation*. 81:1390–1397.

Sata M, Saiura A, Kunisato A et al. 2002. Hematopoietic stem cells differentiate into vascular cells that participate in the pathogenesis of atherosclerosis. *Nat Med*. 8:403–409.

Sato Y, Araki H, Kato J et al. 2005. Human mesenchymal stem cells xenografted directly to rat liver are differentiated into human hepatocytes without fusion. *Blood*. 106:756–763.

Schapira AH, Olanow CW. 2004. Neuroprotection in Parkinson disease: mysteries, myths, and misconceptions. *JAMA*. 291:358–364.

Schwarz EJ, Alexander GM, Prockop DJ, Azizi SA. 1999. Multipotential marrow stromal cells transduced to produce L-DOPA: engraftment in a rat model of Parkinson disease. *Hum Gene Ther*. 10:2539–2549.

Smidt MP, Burbach JP. 2007. How to make a mesodiencephalic dopaminergic neuron. *Nat Rev Neurosci*. 8:21–32.

Snyder BJ, Olanow CW. 2005. Stem cell treatment for Parkinson's disease: an update for 2005. *Curr Opin Neurol*. 18:376–385.

Sonntag KC, Simantov R, Isacson O. 2005. Stem cells may reshape the prospect of Parkinson's disease therapy. *Brain Res Mol Brain Res*. 134:34–51.

Sonntag KC, Sanchez-Pernaute R. 2006. Tailoring human embryonic stem cells for neurodegenerative disease therapy. *Curr Opin Investig Drugs*. 7:614–618.

Sotiropoulou PA, Perez SA, Gritzapis AD, Baxevanis CN, Papamichail M. 2006. Interactions between human mesenchymal stem cells and natural killer cells. *Stem Cells*. 24:74–85.

Spaggiari GM, Capobianco A, Becchetti S, Mingari MC, Moretta L. 2006. Mesenchymal stem cell-natural killer cell interactions: evidence that activated NK cells are capable of killing MSCs, whereas MSCs can inhibit IL-2-induced NK-cell proliferation. *Blood*. 107:1484–1490.

Stock UA, Vacanti JP. 2001. Tissue engineering: current state and prospects. *Annu Rev Med*. 53:443–451.

Sugaya K. 2005. Possible use of autologous stem cell therapies for Alzheimer's disease. *Curr Alzheimer Res*. 2:367–76.

Summer R, Kotton D, Liang S, Fitzsimmons K, Sun X, Fine A. 2005. Embryonic lung side population cells are hematopoietic and vascular precursors. *Am J Respir Cell Mol Biol*. 33:32–40.

Suon S, Yang M, Iacovitti L. 2006. Adult human bone marrow stromal spheres express neuronal traits in vitro and in a rat model of Parkinson's disease. *Brain Res*. 1106:46–51.

Tang Y, Yasuhara T, Hara K et al. 2007. Transplantation of bone marrow-derived stem cells: a promising therapy for stroke. *Cell Transplant*. 16:159–169.

Tatard VM, D'Ippolito G, Diabira S et al. 2007. Neurotrophin-directed differentiation of human adult marrow stromal cells to dopaminergic-like neurons. *Bone*. 40:360–373.

Tondreau T, Meuleman N, Delforge A et al. 2005. Mesenchymal stem cells derived from CD133-positive cells in mobilized peripheral blood and cord blood: proliferation, Oct4 expression, and plasticity. *Stem Cells*. 23:1105–1112.

Tropel P, Platet N, Platel JC et al. 2006. Functional neuronal differentiation of bone marrow-derived mesenchymal stem cells. *Stem Cells*. 24:2868–2876.

Trzaska KA, Rameshwar P. 2007. Current advances in the treatment of Parkinson's disease with stem cells. *Curr Neurovasc Res*. 4:99–109.

Trzaska KA, Kuzhikandathil EV, Rameshwar P. 2007. Specification of a dopaminergic phenotype from adult human mesenchymal stem cells. *Stem Cells*. 25(11):2797–2808.

Wagers AJ, Sherwood RI, Christensen JL, Weissman IL. 2002. Little evidence for developmental plasticity of adult hematopoietic stem cells. *Science*. 297:2256–2259.

Wagers AJ, Weissman IL. 2004. Plasticity of adult stem cells. *Cell.* 116:639–648.

Wang H, Li Y, Zuo Y, Li J, Ma S, Cheng L. 2007. Biocompatibility and osteogenesis of biomimetic nano-hydroxyapatite/polyamide composite scaffold for bone tissue engineering. *Biomaterials.* 28:3338–3348.

Wang HJ, Gong SJ, Lin ZX, Xue ST, Huang JC, Wang JY. 2007. In vivo biocompatibility and mechanical proerties of porous zein scaffolds. *Biomaterials.* 28:3962–3964.

Weiss ML, Medicetty S, Bledsoe AR et al. 2006. Human umbilical cord matrix stem cells: preliminary characterization and effect of transplantation in a rodent model of Parkinson's disease. *Stem Cells.* 24:781–792.

Wernig M, Brustle O. 2002. Fifty ways to make a neuron: shifts in stem cell hierarchy and their implications for neuropathology and CNS repair. *J Neuropathol Exp Neurol.* 61:101–110.

Wislet-Gendebien S, Hans G, Leprince P, Rigo JM, Moonen G, Rogister B. 2005. Plasticity of cultured mesenchymal stem cells: switch from nestin-positive to excitable neuron-like phenotype. *Stem Cells.* 23:392–402.

Xin X, Hussain M, Mao JJ. 2007. Continuing differentiation of human mesenchymal stem cells and induced chondrogenic and osteogenic lineages in electrospun PLGA nanofiber scaffold. *Biomaterials.* 28:316–325.

Ye W, Shimamura K, Rubenstein JL, Hynes MA, Rosenthal A. 1998. FGF and Shh signals control dopaminergic and serotonergic cell fate in the anterior neural plate. *Cell.* 93:755–766.

Zappia E, Casazza S, Pedemonte E et al. 2005. Mesenchymal stem cells ameliorate experimental autoimmune encephalomyelitis inducing T-cell anergy. *Blood.* 106:1755–1761.

Zhang P, Xu H, Zhang D, Fu Z, Zhang H, Jiang B. 2006. The biocompatibility research of functional Schwann cells induced from bone mesenchymal cells with chitosan conduit membrane. *Artif Cells Blood Substit Immobil Biotechnol.* 34:89–97.

Zipori D. 2004. Mesenchymal stem cells: harnessing cell plasticity to tissue and organ repair. *Blood Cells Mol Dis.* 33:211–215.

Chapter **9**

MOTONEURONS FROM HUMAN EMBRYONIC STEM CELLS: PRESENT STATUS AND FUTURE STRATEGIES FOR THEIR USE IN REGENERATIVE MEDICINE

K. S. Sidhu

ABSTRACT

Human embryonic stem (ES) cells are pluripotent and can produce the entire range of major somatic cell lineage of the central nervous system (CNS) and thus form an important source for cell-based therapy of various neurological diseases. Despite their potential use in regenerative medicine, the progress is hampered by difficulty in their use because of safety issues and lack of proper protocols to obtain purified populations of specified neuronal cells. Most neurological conditions such as spinal cord injury and Parkinson's disease involve damages to projection neurons. Similarly, certain cell populations may be depleted after repeated episodes of attacks such as the myelinating oligodendrocytes in multiple sclerosis. Motoneurons are the key effector cell type for control of motor function, and loss of motoneurons is associated with a number of debilitating diseases such as amyotrophic lateral sclerosis (ALS) and spinal muscular atrophy; hence, repair of such neurological conditions may require transplantation with exogenous cells. Transplantation of neural progenitor cells in animal models of neurological disorders and in patients from some clinical trial cases has shown survival of grafted cells and contribution to functional recovery. Recently a considerable progress has been made in understanding the biochemical, molecular, and developmental biology of stem cells. But translation of these in vitro studies to the clinic has been slow. Major hurdles are the lack of effective donor cells, their in vivo survival, and difficulty in remodeling the non-neurogenic adult CNS environment. Several factors play a role in maintaining their functions as stem cells. It is becoming increasingly apparent that the role of developmental signaling molecules is not over when embryogenesis has been completed. In the adult, such molecules might function in the maintenance of stem cell proliferation, the regeneration of tissues and organs, and even in the maintenance of their differentiated state. A major challenge is to teach the naïve ES cells to choose a neural fate, especially the subclasses of neurons and glial cells that are lost in neurological conditions. I review the progress that has been achieved with ES cells to obtain motoneurons and discuss how close we are to translating this research to the clinics.

Keywords: central nervous system, neuroectoderm, motoneurons, cell replacement therapy, growth factors, neural induction.

The development of CNS involves spatial distribution and networking (circuitry) of neuronal and glial cells. These anatomical developments undergo modifications during functional maturation. Insults, injury, or disease causes damage or loss of certain elements in the CNS circuitry that disrupts the neural network. Repair of these circuits would require sequential reactivation of the developmental signals in a particular spatial order, for which the adult mammalian brain and spinal cord have limited capacity (Steiner, Wolf, Kempermann 2006). Consequently, the adult brain often fails to repair the neural framework assembled by projection neurons despite the presence of stem cells or progenitors. These stem/progenitor cells in adult life appear to be designed for replenishing other parts of the CNS, because they differentiate primarily into interneurons and glial cells (Steigner, Wolf, Kempermann 2006). Most neurological conditions such as spinal cord injury and Parkinson's disease involve damages to projection neurons. In other circumstances, certain cell populations may be depleted after repeated episodes of attacks such as the myelinating oligodendrocytes in multiple sclerosis. Motoneurons are the key effector cell type for control of motor function, and loss of motoneurons is associated with a number of debilitating diseases such as ALS and spinal muscular atrophy (Lefebvre, Burglen, Reboullet et al. 1995; Cleveland, Rothstein 2001). Hence, repair of such neurological conditions may require transplantation with exogenous cells. Transplantation of neural progenitor cells in animal models of neurological disorders and in patients from some clinical trial cases has shown survival of grafted cells and contribution to functional recovery. Laboratory investigation into understanding the biochemical, molecular, and developmental biology of stem cells has progressed rapidly in the last few years. However, until relatively recently, translation of these in vitro studies to the clinic has been slow. Neural replacement as a therapy still needs further laboratory investigations. Major hurdles are the lack of effective donor cells, their in vivo survival, and difficulty in remodeling the non-neurogenic adult CNS environment. Several factors play a role in maintaining their functions as stem cells. It is becoming increasingly apparent that the role of developmental signaling molecules is not over when embryogenesis has been completed. In the adult, such molecules might function in the maintenance of stem cell proliferation, the regeneration of tissues and organs, and even in the maintenance of their differentiated state (Maden 2007).

Derivation of functional neurons from human embryonic stem cells (hESCs) as surrogate in regenerating medicine for treating various neurodegenerative diseases is the subject of intensive investigation. Three basic features of hESCs, that is, self-renewal, proliferation, and pluripotency, make them immortal, capable of unlimited expansion and differentiation into all 230 different type of cells in the body, and thus hold great potential for regenerative medicine (Hardikar, Lees, Sidhu et al. 2006; Valenzuela, Sidhu, Dean et al. 2007). Most published protocols for guiding the differentiation of these cells result in heterogeneous cultures that comprise neurons, glia, and progenitor cells, which makes the assessment of neuronal function problematic. However, many recent studies including from our laboratory (Lim, Sidhu, Tuch 2006) have demonstrated that enough purified neurons could be generated from hESCs and used for carrying out gene expression and protein analyses and for examining whether they can form functional networks in culture (Benninger, Beck, Wernig et al. 2003; Zhang 2003; Keirstead, Nistor, Bernal et al. 2005; Muotri, Nakashima, Toni et al. 2005; Ben-Hur 2006; Soundararajan, Miles, Rubin et al. 2006; Lee, Shamy, Elkabetz et al. 2007; Soundararajan, Lindsey, Leopold et al. 2007; Wu, Xu, Pang et al. 2007; Zeng, Rao 2007). This review will discuss how recent advancement in stem cell technology offers hope for generating potential effective donor cells for replacement therapy with a special emphasis on developmental potentials of ES cells.

POTENTIAL USE OF HUMAN EMBRYONIC STEM CELLS

Adult stem cells are restricted during development to a particular fate of the tissue in which they are found. Brain-derived neural stem cells may generate neurons and glia. However, the subclasses of neurons and glia differentiated from neural stem cells depend on the regions and developmental stages in which the progenitor cells are isolated and expanded. Thus, the ideal stem cell population would be those that can generate most or all subtypes of neurons and glial cells. Presently, the best known cells that possess such traits are ES cells. ES cells are able to differentiate into all cell and tissue types of the body. Technology has been developed to selectively maintain and expand mouse and human ES cells in a synchronized, undifferentiated state. Compared to adult stem cells, ES cells can be expanded in vitro with current technology for a prolonged period, and yet they retain the genetic normality. Hence, ES cells can provide a large number of normal cells for deriving the desired cells for transplant therapy. A major challenge is to teach the naïve ES cells to choose a neural fate, especially the subclasses of neurons and glial cells that are lost in neurological conditions.

hESCs are pluripotent cells derived from the inner cell mass of preimplantation embryos (Thomson 1998). Like mouse embryonic stem (ES) cells, theoretically they can differentiate into various somatic cell types (Fig. 9.1) with a stable genetic background (Thomson 1998; Amit, Carpenter, Inokuma et al. 2000; Reubinoff, Pera, Fong et al. 2000; Thomson, Odorico 2000; Sidhu, Ryan, Tuch 2008). These unique features make hESCs a favorable tool for biomedical research as well as a potential source for therapeutic application in a wide range of diseases such as Parkinson's disease, Alzheimer's disease, and spinal cord injuries. Directing ES cells to differentiate to cells of interest, such as neural lineages, depends on strategies based on the understanding of mammalian neural development (Lee Lumelsky, Studer et al. 2000; Tropepe, Hitoshi, Sirard et al. 2001; Billon, Jolicoeur, Ying et al. 2002; Wichterle, Lieberam, Porter et al. 2002; Ying, Stavridis, Griffiths et al. 2003).

Mass-scale production of functional neurons from hESCs for treating neurodegenerative diseases is the subject of intensive investigation. Most published protocols for guiding the differentiation of these cells result in heterogeneous cultures that comprise neurons, glia, and progenitor cells, which makes the assessment of neuronal function problematic. However,

recently some of the studies have been successful in purifying enough hESC-derived neurons to carry out gene expression and protein analyses and examine whether they can form functional networks in culture (Lim, Sidhu, Tuch 2006; Lee, Shamy, Elkabetz et al. 2007; Soundararajan, Lindsey, Leopold et al. 2007). However, different hESC lines behave very differently in cultures and have variable potential to produce neurons (Lim, Sidhu, Tuch 2006; Wu, Xu, Pang et al. 2007).

NEUROECTODERMAL INDUCTION

Neuroectodermal Induction and Neuronal Specification

The production of neurons involves several sequential steps precisely orchestrated by signaling events (Wilson, Edlund 2001). The initial step is the specification of neuroepithelia from ectoderm cells, the process known as *neural induction*, which is accomplished by inductive interaction with nascent mesoderm and definitive endoderm. Despite being a topic of intensive study, there is still no consensus on the mechanisms and signals involved in neural induction. Bone morphogenetic protein (BMP) antagonism has been viewed as the central and initiating event in neural induction. According to this concept, neuroepithelial specification occurs as a default pathway (Munoz-Sanjuan, Brivanlou 2002). However, recent findings challenge this neural default model and indicate some positive instructive factors, such as fibroblast growth factors (FGFs) and Wnt. For example, interference

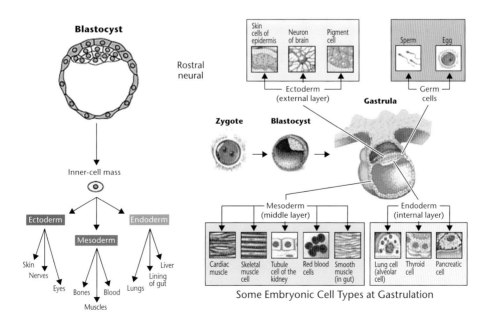

Figure 9.1 Pluripotency in embryonic stem cells and the potential derivation of various lineage-specified cells.

with FGF and Wnt signaling abolishes neural induction at an early stage in the chick (Wilson, Graziano, Harland et al. 2000; Wilson, Rydstrom, Trimborn et al. 2001). FGF might act by antagonizing the BMP signal pathway indirectly or by directly inducing specific transcription factors, which determine neuroectoderm induction and inhibit mesoderm differentiation (Bertrand, Hudson, Caillol et al. 2003; Sheng, Dos, Stern et al. 2003). Hence, a balanced view of neural induction most likely needs to include both instructive and inhibitory factors. FGF may induce a neural state at an early stage, and BMP antagonists may subsequently stabilize the neural identity. Once a neuroectodermal fate is specified, the neural plate folds to form the neural tube, from which cells differentiate into various neurons and glia. However, this process does not occur homogenously and simultaneously throughout the neural tube. Instead, the neural tube is patterned along its rostrocaudal and dorsoventral axes to establish a grid-like set of positional cues (Altmann, Brivanlou 2001). The neural plate initially acquires a rostral character, and it is then gradually caudalized by exposure to Wnt, FGF, BMP, and retinoic acid (RA) signals (Munoz-Sanjuan, Brivanlou 2001; Agathon, Thisse, Thisse et al. 2003) to establish the main subdivisions of the CNS: the forebrain, midbrain, hindbrain, and spinal cord. Along the dorsoventral axis, the neural tube is patterned into more subdivisions by the two opposing signals: sonic hedgehog (SHH) ventrally from the notochord and BMP dorsally from the roof plate (Jessell 2000; Lee, Pfaff 2001). Precursor cells in each subdivision along the rostrocaudal and dorsoventral axes, by exposure to a unique set of morphogens at specific concentrations, are fated to subtypes of neurons and glial cells (Osterfield, Kirschner, Flanagan 2003). It is this unique positional code that endows a neuron with a specific target. Thus, it will be crucial to imprint the positional information into the neurons that are generated in vitro to achieve their potential for cell replacement.

Roles of Growth Factors in Neural Tube Formation

The transition from neuroectoderm to neural plate and then to the neural tube sets up a platform from which cells differentiate into various neurons and glia (O'Rahilly, Muller 1994; O'Rahilly, Muller 2007). The neural tube is patterned along its rostrocaudal and dorsoventral axes to establish a grid-like set of positional cues (Altmann, Brivanlou 2001). Figure 9.2 depicts the central dogma of motor neuron development, where primitive ectodermal cells are converted to motor neurons through the caudalizing action of RA and the ventralizing action of SHH. Similarly,

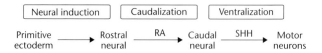

Figure 9.2 Central dogma of motor neuron development. Neural inductive signals convert primitive ectodermal cells to a rostral neural fate. Signals including retinoic acid (RA) convert rostral neural cells to more caudal identities. Spinal progenitors are converted to motor neurons by sonic hedgehog (SHH) signaling. Adapted from Wichterle, Lieberam, Porter et al. 2002.

the neural plate acquires a rostral character and is subsequently caudalized by exposure to Wnt, FGF, BMP, and RA signals (Jessell 2000; Lee, Pfaff 2001; Munoz-Sanjuan, Brivanlou 2001; Panchision, Mckay 2002; Gunhaga, Marklund, Sjodal et al. 2003) to establish the main subdivisions of the CNS: the forebrain, midbrain, hindbrain, and spinal cord. Furthermore, along the dorsoventral axis, the neural tube is patterned into more subdivisions by three signals, SHH ventrally from the notochord and BMP and Wnt dorsally from the roof plate (Jessell 2000; Lee, Pfaff 2001; Panchision, Mckay 2002; Gunhaga, Marklund, Sjodal et al. 2003). Therefore, the precursor cells in each subdivision along the rostrocaudal axes are fated to subtypes of neurons and glia, depending on its exposure to unique sets of morphogens at specific concentrations.

NEURAL DIFFERENTIATION FROM ES CELLS: METHODOLOGY

Enrichment of neural progenitors from differentiating hESCs has been achieved by exploiting the observation that cells of neural morphology form spontaneously within hESC colonies after prolonged culture. Reubinoff et al. (2001) demonstrated the mechanical isolation of these neural progenitors, and repeating the culture in chemically defined medium supplemented with B27, human epidermal growth factor (hEGF), and basic fibroblast growth factor 2 (bFGF-2) (Fig. 9.3) resulted in the formation of spherical structures called *neurospheres*. These neurospheres have highly enriched neural progenitor cells, with 99% of cells expressing neural cell adhesion molecule (N-CAM), 97% expressing nestin, and 90.5% expressing A2B5 (Reubinoff, Itsykson, Turetsky et al. 2001). According to Zhang et al. (2001), hESC-generated neuroectodermal cells usually do not form typical neurospheres. Instead, they from aggregates of columnar cells in the form of neural tube–like rosettes, where only after the long-term expansion of the neural rosette clusters will they form the morphology of neurospheres. Therefore, neurospheres formed in the spontaneous differentiation cultures may represent neural precursors at a much later developmental stage.

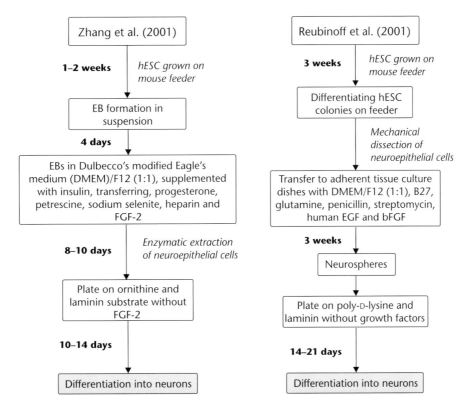

Figure 9.3 Schematic procedures for neural differentiation. Comparative analysis of methodologies by Zhang et al. (2001) and Reubinoff et al. (2001) indicate some similarities and differences. Zhang et al. utilizes the EB pathway but not Reubinoff, et al. Both isolate neuroepithelial cells by mechanical dissection or enzymatic treatment. bFGF, basic fibroblast growth factor; EB, embryoid body; FGF-2, fibroblast growth factor 2; hEGF, human epidermal growth factor.

Selection of neural cells was also used by Zhang's group as a method of enriching for neural progenitors (Zhang, Wernig, Duncan et al. 2001). hESCs were initially differentiated as EBs in chemically defined medium supplemented with FGF-2 before culturing in adherent culture for a further 8 to 10 days (Fig. 9.3). Prominent outgrowths of neural progenitors, representing 72% to 84% of the total cells, were seen in the cultures and could be isolated by limited enzymatic digestion. Culture in medium supplemented with FGF-2, but not epidermal growth factor or leukemia-inhibitory factor, was shown to promote proliferation of the isolated aggregates in suspension. Although the authors did not characterize the composition of these neurosphere-like aggregates, they demonstrated the presence of neural progenitors by differentiation potential, with the ability to form neurons, astrocytes, and oligodendrocytes on plating and withdrawal of FGF-2.

The major difference between Zhang's and Reubinoff's method is that Zhang utilizes the embryoid body (EB) pathway whereas Reubinoff spontaneously differentiates hESC colonies for a prolonged time of 3 weeks (Fig. 9.3) (Reubinoff, Itsykson, Turetsky et al. 2001; Zhang, Wernig, Duncan et al. 2001). Both protocols require the isolation of neuroepithelial cells from other non-neural cells, and propagation of these neurospheres in culture. Isolation of these neural rosettes is done either by enzymatic treatment or by mechanical dissection. Both groups utilize serum-free media (DMEM/F12) (1:1) supplemented with different types of nutrients for neural induction. The neurospheres are then plated on laminin- or ornithin-coated plates for further neural differentiation.

Another commonly used technique for the neural differentiation from ES cells is the aggregation of ES cells into so-called embryoid bodies (EBs) in suspension cultures and treatment of these EBs with RA after withdrawing pluripotent growth factors such as bFGF. The EB structure recapitulates certain aspects of early embryogenesis with the appearance of lineage-specific regions similar to that found in the embryo (Doetschman et al. 1985). After 2 to 4 days in suspension culture, primitive endoderm cells form on the surface of EBs and epiblast-like cells form inside. These EBs are termed *simple EBs*. With further culturing, differentiation of a columnar epithelium with a basal lamina and the formation of a central cavity occur, at which point the EBs are termed *cystic EBs*. Cystic EBs are similar to egg cylinder–stage embryos, consisting of a double-layered structure with an inner ectodermal layer and outer layer of endoderm enclosing a cavity. Continued culture of EBs results in the appearance of mesodermal and endodermal cell types. Hence, the differentiation of ES cells in the form of EBs in vitro obeys general rules of development that prevail in an embryo. However, EBs exhibit stochastic differentiation into a variety of cell lineages. Treatment with morphogens/growth factors and/or use of particular culture systems is necessary to achieve a directed differentiation and/or selective expansion of a specific lineage. For neural differentiation, which occurs during early embryonic development, ES cell aggregates are usually treated with morphogens at an early stage in which these aggregates do not display the structure of embryonic germ layers. Hence, the name EBs in neural differentiation paradigms is rather misleading. Spontaneous differentiation of EBs yields only a small fraction of neural lineage cells. To promote neural differentiation, ES cell aggregates, cultured in the regular ES cell medium for 4 days, are exposed to RA (0.51 mM) for another 4 days. Hence, this method is often regarded as a 42/41 protocol (Bain, Kitchens, Yao et al. 1995). This method was optimized by Gotlieb and colleagues based on neuronal differentiation from teratocarcinoma cells (Jones-Villeneuve, McBurney, Rogers et al. 1982). Other RA-triggered neural differentiation protocols are variations of the 42/41 protocol (Wobus, Grosse, Schoneich 1988; Strubing, Ahnert-Hilger, Shan et al. 1995; Fraichard, Chassande, Bilbaut et al. 1995; Dinsmore, Ratliff, Deacon et al. 1996; Renoncourt, Carroll, Filippi et al. 1998). Mouse ES cells treated with this protocol yield a good proportion (38%) of neuronal cells upon differentiation. The predominant population of neuronal cells is glutaminergic and γ-aminobutyric acid (GABAergic) neurons (Jones-Villeneuve, McBurney, Rogers et al. 1982). These neuronal cells express voltage-gated Ca^{2+}, Na^+, K^+ ion channels and form functional synapses with neighboring neurons. They generate action potentials and are functionally coupled by inhibitory (GABAergic) and excitatory (glutamatergic) synapses, as revealed by measurement of postsynaptic currents (Strubing, Ahnert-Hilger, Shan et al. 1995). Signaling through RA is important during development, particularly in rostral/caudal patterning of the neural tube (Maden 2002). However, there is little evidence to suggest that RA in these protocols acts to induce neural specifications.

DIRECTED DIFFERENTIATION: USE OF SIGNALING MOLECULES/GROWTH FACTORS

EBs treated with RA differentiate into neuronal cell types characteristic of ventral CNS: somatic motoneurons (islet1/2, Lim3, HB9), cranial motoneurons (islet1/2 and phox2b), and interneurons (lim1/2 or En1) (Renoncourt, Ahnert-Hilger, Shan et al. 1998).

The absence of several rostral neural markers, such as BF-1 and Otx2 suggests that RA may selectively promote the differentiation of caudal neuronal types. RA is required for differentiation of spinal motoneurons (Billon, Jolicoeur, Ying et al. 2002). RA is a strong morphogen that appears to push ES cells toward postmitotic neurons and results in robust neuronal differentiation in a reproducible way. Hence, it is most widely used for neuronal differentiation from ES cells, including human ES cells. FGF-2 is a survival and proliferation factor used for early neural precursor cells. On the basis of this fact, McKay and colleagues developed a method to promote the proliferation of a neural precursor population selectively with FGF-2 (Okabe, Forsberg-Nilsson, Spiro et al. 1996). ES cell aggregates are cultured in suspension for 4 days and then plated on an adhesive substrate in the presence of FGF-2 in a serum-free ITSFn medium (DMEM/F12 supplemented with insulin, transferrin, selenium, and fibronectin). Under this condition, the majority of cells die, but neural precursors survive and proliferate in the presence of FGF-2. After 6 to 8 days of selection and expansion, the nestin-positive neural precursor cells are enriched to approximately 80%. Withdrawal of FGF-2 induces spontaneous differentiation into various neurons and glia (Okabe, Forsberg-Nilsson, Spiro et al. 1996; Brustle, Jones, Learish et al. 1999), and the neuronal cells generated in this way fulfill the criteria of functional postmitotic neurons with both excitatory and inhibitory synaptic connections. In contrast to the RA approach, neural precursor cells expanded with FGF-2 are generally developmentally synchronized. They appear to be further induced to neuronal types with representatives of mid- and hindbrain, such as dopaminergic neurons (Lee, Lumelsky, Studer et al. 2000). Because FGF-2 also possesses caudalizing effects, it is reasonable to believe that FGF-2–induced neural precursors may give rise to neuronal types of a more caudal neuraxis.

In addition to methods involving formation of ES cell aggregates, direct differentiation of individual or monolayer ES cells has been developed by several groups with the use of feeder cells or media conditioned from mesoderm-derived cell lines. The rationale behind these protocols is that signals from mesodermal cells are required to induce neural specification from the ectoderm in vivo. Sasai and colleagues first established this method to derive dopaminergic neurons (Kawasaki, Mizuseki, Nishikawa et al. 2000). Mouse ES cells are dissociated into single cells and plated on PA6 stromal feeder cells at a low density. After co-culturing in a serum-free medium for 6 days, 92% of the ES cell colonies contain nestin-positive cells. The authors name the inductive factor *stromal cell–derived inducing activity* (SDIA). SDIA induces co-cultured ES cells to differentiate into rostral CNS precursor cells with both a ventral and dorsal character. Early exposure of SDIA-treated ES cells to bone morphogenetic protein 4 (BMP4) suppresses neural differentiation and promotes epidermal differentiation, whereas late BMP4 exposure (after day 4 of co-culture) causes differentiation of neural crest cells and the dorsal-most CNS cells. In contrast, SHH promotes differentiation of ventral CNS cells such as motor neurons, and SHH at a high concentration efficiently promotes differentiation of the ventral-most floor plate cells. Thus, SDIA-treated ES cells generate precursors that have the competence to differentiate into the full dorsal–ventral range of neuroectodermal derivatives in response to patterning signals (Mizuseki, Sakamoto, Watanabe et al. 2003). The neural inducing factor(s) does not appear to be restricted to PA6 cells. Studer and colleagues demonstrate that several mesoderm-derived cell lines promote the differentiation of mouse ES cells to different neuronal subtypes, astrocytes, and oligodendrocytes, in combination with morphogens at different concentrations and at different times (Barberi, Klivenyi, Calingasan, et al. 2003). Thus, neural precursor cells induced by stromal signals appear to be naive and are responsive to versatile signals for further differentiation into neurons and glia with specific regional identities, although the phenotypes of these neural precursors are not characterized. Alternatively, the stromal signals can induce a wide range of neural precursors that can be selectively promoted by different morphogens. The identity of the SDIA remains unknown, which introduces an unknown component into the experimental paradigm. This co-culture system can be combined with ES cell aggregation to yield a more homogeneous neuroectodermal differentiation (Rathjen, Haines, Hudson et al. 2002).

The aforementioned neural differentiation protocols are designed on the basis of our understanding of neural development. However, introduction of unknown factors, empirically devised steps, and selective culture systems make them irrelevant to normal neural development. In recent years, more sophisticated and chemically defined culture systems have been developed. Anti-BMP signaling is thought to play a crucial role in neural induction. Gratsch and O'Shea (2002) examined the role of BMP antagonists, noggin and chordin, in neural differentiation from mouse ES cells. Exposure of mouse ES cells to noggin in defined medium or transfection with a noggin expression plasmid promotes widespread neural differentiation. After 72 hours of noggin treatment, about 90% cells become nestin positive neural precursor cells, which are strongly inhibited by BMP4. Interestingly, exposure to chordin produces a more complex pattern of neural cell differentiation as well as mesenchymal cell

differentiation. The high efficiency of neural induction with noggin treatment is consistent with its role in the default model of neural induction.

Selection by FGF-2/bFGF

FGF-2, also known as basic fibroblast growth factor (bFGF), is a survival and proliferation factor for early neural precursor cells from mouse and human. As described previously, McKay and colleagues developed a method to promote the proliferation of neural precursor populations selectively with bFGF (Okabe, Forsberg-Nilsson, Spiro et al. 1996). Withdrawal of bFGF after 6 to 8 days of selection and expansion induces spontaneous differentiation into various neurons and glia (Okabe, Forsberg-Nilsson, Spiro et al. 1996; Brustle, Jones, Learish et al. 1999).

Another role of bFGF is its ability to direct differentiation of ES cells to neural cell types, particularly motor neurons. A study by Shin et al. (2005) demonstrated that by using bFGF alone, there was a 2.64-fold increase of motor neurons differentiated from hESCs when compared to the control treatment, suggesting that bFGF may be an effective growth factor for in vitro differentiation to human motor neurons.

FGF-2 is routinely used to expand central nervous system stem cells (CNS-SCs) in serum-free media (Ray et al. 1993; Kilpatrick, Bartlett 1995; Palmer et al. 1995; Gritti et al. 1996; Johe et al. 1996). This growth factor is considered to act simply as a neutral mitogen. Gabay et al. (2003), however, have demonstrated that contrary to this assumption, the spinal cord progenitor cells change their dorsoventral identity in FGF, even at concentrations two orders of magnitude lower than those used to grow the cells (0.2 ng/mL). In the case of dorsally derived cells, FGF causes an extinction of dorsal progenitor domain markers such as Pax3 and Pax7 and an induction of ventral markers such as Olig2 and Nkx2.2. FGF probably induces SHH signaling for ventralization in these cells. The evidence that FGF induces ventralization through SHH is based on induction of SHH mRNA and SHH antagonist (Frank-Kamenetsky et al. 2002; Williams, Guicherit, Zaharian et al. 2003), which attenuate the effect of FGF (Fig. 9.4). However, an SHH-independent mechanism does exist in telencephalon (Kuschel, Rüther, Theil 2003).

Grb2-associated binder 1 (Gab1) has been identified as an adaptor molecule downstream of many growth factors, including epidermal growth factor (EGF), fibroblast growth factor, and platelet-derived growth factor, which have been shown to play crucial roles as mitotic signals for a variety of neural progenitor cells, including stem cells, both in vitro and in vivo (Hayakawa-Yano, Nishida, Fukami et al. 2007).

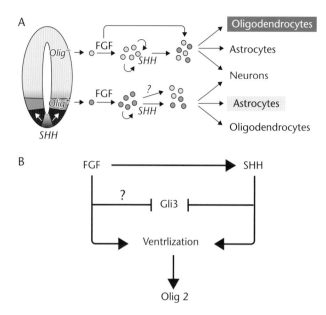

Figure 9.4 Schematic summarizing effects of FGF and SHH. (A) Dorsal (Olig2⁻; orange) and ventral (Olig2⁺; green) progenitors normally generate neurons and astrocytes, or neurons and oligodendrocytes, respectively, in vivo (black lettering). In culture, the induction and extinction of Olig2 expression by the progeny of individual founder cells from these dorsal and ventral regions, respectively, leads to competence to generate both classes of glia: oligodendrocytes (in the case of Olig2⁻ cells; blue) and astrocytes (in the case of Olig2⁺; red). (B) FGF ventralizes dorsal progenitors via both SHH-dependent and possibly SHH-independent mechanisms. The SHH-independent mechanism may involve an inhibition of Gli3 function. Adapted from Gabay, Lowell, Rubin et al. 2003.

In the developing spinal cord, after the cessation of motoneuron generation, Gab1 deficiency resulted in a reduction in the number of Olig2⁻ progenitors in the motor neuron domain (pMN), followed subsequently by a reduction in the subpopulation of Pax7⁻ dorsal progenitors expressing epidermal growth factor receptor (EGFR), without any detectable increase of apoptosis (Hayakawa-Yano, Nishida, Fukami et al. 2007). It has been shown that FGF-receptor substrate 2 (FRS2), another adaptor protein belonging to the common insulin receptor substrate family, functions as a key mediator in FGF signaling in other types of cells, including cortical progenitor cells (Kouhara, Hadari, Spivak-Kroizman et al. 1997; Yamamoto, Yoshino, Shimazaki et al. 2005). Moreover, Gab2 mediates Akt activation by FGF-2 during retinoic acid–induced neural differentiation of P19 embryonal carcinoma cells (EC) (Korhonen, Said, Wong et al. 1999). Hayakawa-Yano et al. (2007) provided evidence suggesting that Gab1 contributes to the proliferation of Olig2-expressing neural progenitors downstream of EGF signaling in a spatiotemporally regulated manner in the developing spinal cord. It is further demonstrated that a context-dependent

change in the utilization of Akt1 acts as a downstream target of Gab1 in the EGF-dependent proliferation of Olig2⁻-expressing progenitors. These findings suggest that, in addition to the differential expression of ligands and receptors, differential utilization of intercellular signaling components is integrated into the regulation of progenitor proliferation to complete the CNS histogenesis by growth factor signals.

Use of RA

The formation of neural lineages from pluripotent cells in response to RA was obtained using EC cells (Jones-Villeneuve, McBurney, Rogers et al. 1982) and subsequently from ES cells cultured as EB in 10⁻⁶ to 10⁻⁷ M RA (Bain, Kitchens, Yao et al. 1995; Fraichard, Chassande, Bilbaut et al. 1995; Strubing, Ahnert-Hilger, Shan et al. 1995; Wichterle, Lieberam, Porter et al. 2002; Soundararajan, Miles, Rubin et al. 2006; Lim, Sidhu, Tuch 2006; Lee, Shamy, Elkabetz et al. 2007). Although the efficiency of RA-induced differentiation is hard to establish because of cytotoxicity of the RA treatment, the formation of neural precursor cells, identified by the expression of markers, such as, SOX1 and SOX2, was increased 5- to 10-fold (Bain, Kitchens, Yao et al. 1995), and 50% to 70% of surviving cells exhibited properties of neural and glial cell populations, including expression of neuron-specific nuclear protein (NeuN), Tuj1, and glial fibrillary acidic protein (GFAP) (Fraichard, Chassande, Bilbaut et al. 1995; Strubing, Ahnert-Hilger, Shan et al. 1995; Wichterle, Lieberam, Porter et al. 2002). When the RA-treated neural progenitors were characterized, they showed the expression of early spinal chord markers Hoxc5, Hoxc6, but not of midbrain markers (Wichterle, Lieberam, Porter et al. 2002). This coincides with the theory of posteriorization of the neural tube in the embryo by RA (Rathjen, Rathjen 2002), where the RA-treated EBs differentiate into neural populations possessing a rostrocervical character.

Vitamin A is the source of RA. In the absence of ability to synthesize vitamin A, animals derive it from diet as carotenoids (plants) and retinyl esters (animals). These are stored as retinyl esters (also known as retinoids) in the liver and in several extrahepatic sites, including the lungs, bone marrow, and the kidneys. Transport of retinoids from these storage sites to the cells that require them is performed by retinol, and the latter circulates as bound to plasma retinol-binding protein 4 (RBP4). Retinol is taken up by target cells through an interaction with a membrane receptor for RBP4, STRA6 (Kawaguchi, Yu, Honda et al. 2007); it then enters the cytoplasm, where it binds to retinol-binding protein 1 cellular (RBP1) and is metabolized in a two-step process to all-*trans* RA3.

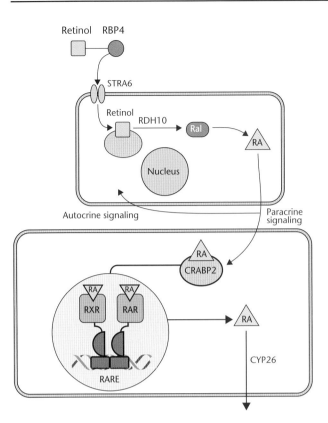

Figure 9.5 Pathways that are involved in the generation, action, and catabolism of retinoic acid (RA). Retinol, bound to retinol-binding protein 4, plasma (RBP4), is taken up by cells through a membrane receptor (STRA6) that interacts with the RBP4. In embryos, retinol dehydrogenase 10 (RDH10) metabolizes retinol to retinaldehyde (Ral), which is then metabolized to RA by retinaldehyde dehydrogenases (RALDHs). RA can be released from the cytoplasm and taken up by the receiving cell (paracrine signaling) or can act back on its own nucleus (autocrine signaling). Cellular retinoic acid–binding protein 2 (CRABP2) assists RA entry into the nucleus. In the nucleus, RA binds to RA receptors (RARs) and retinoid X receptors (RXRs), which themselves heterodimerize and bind to a sequence of DNA that is known as the retinoic acid–response element (RARE). This binding activates the transcription of target genes. RA is catabolized in the cytoplasm by the CYP26 class of P450 enzymes. From Maden 2007.

In many cell types, two cytoplasmic proteins—cellular retinoic acid–binding proteins 1 and 2 (CRABP1 and CRABP2)—bind to the newly synthesized RA. When signaling in a paracrine manner, RA must be released from the cytoplasm (by unknown mechanisms) and taken up by receiving cells; however, RA can also act in an autocrine manner (Fig. 9.5). RA enters the nucleus, assisted by CRABP2 and binds to a transcription complex that includes a pair of ligand-activated transcription factors comprising the RA receptor (RAR)–retinoic X receptor (RXR) heterodimer. There are three *RAR* genes (*RARA*, *RARB* and *RARG*) and three *RXR* genes (*RXRA*, *RXRB* and *RXRG*), and together, the heterodimeric pair binds

to a DNA sequence called a *retinoic acid–response element* (RARE). In addition to ligand binding, phosphorylation of these receptors and recruitment of a range of coactivators or co-repressors is required for the induction or repression of gene transcription. More than 500 genes have been observed to be RA-responsive, although not all are necessarily acted on directly through a RARE. Non-RARE actions on RA are known to exist but they are poorly understood. So far, the presence of a RARE has been identified unequivocally in 27 genes. Once all-*trans* RA has activated the RARs, it exits the nucleus and is catabolized in the cytoplasm by the CYP26 class of P450 enzymes (Fig. 9.5).

Signaling through RA is important during development, especially in rostral/caudal patterning of the neural tube, neural differentiation, and axon outgrowth (Maden 2002, 2007). In the anteroposterior axis of the neural plate, RA, along with Wnts and FGFs, is specifically responsible for the organization of the posterior hindbrain and the anterior spinal cord (Liu, Laufer, Jessell 2001; Maden 2002; Melton, Iulianella, Trainor et al. 2004). Impaired RA signaling leads to abnormal development of the posterior hindbrain and the anterior spinal cord (Wilson, Gale, Chambers et al. 2004). It is considered that an ascending gradient of RA from anterior to posterior mesoderm because of relative spatial distribution of the RA-synthesizing retinaldehyde dehydrogenase (RALDH2) and catabolizing enzymes (CYP26C1) causes patterning (Fig. 9.6A) in the presumptive hindbrain (Glover, Renaud, Rijli 2006). In the dorsoventral axis of the developing neural tube, RA is generated by the newly formed somites along with SHH, which is expressed ventrally; bone morphogenetic proteins (BMPs), which are expressed dorsally; and FGFs, which are expressed at the posterior end of the extending neural tube. Together, these molecules determine the fate of subsets of sensory neurons, interneurons, and motor neurons that are found in precise regions of the chick spinal cord (Fig. 9.6B) (Novitch, Wichterle, Jessell et al. 2003; Diez, Corral, Storey 2004; Wilson, Maden 2005).

RA plays a significant role in neuronal differentiation. This has been studied extensively in in vitro models, such as EC cells, neuroblastoma cells, and recently in ES cells. RA induces both neurogenesis and gliogenesis by activating various transcription factors, cell signaling molecules, structural proteins, enzymes, and cell surface receptors (Maden 2001) such as transcription factors BRN2, nuclear factor κB (NF-κB), STRA13, SOX1, SOX6, and neurogenin 1; the cytoplasmic signaling molecules protein kinase C (PKC), ceramide, presenilin 1 (PSEN 1), and microtubule-associated protein 2 (MAP2); the extracellular molecule thrombospondin; and components of the

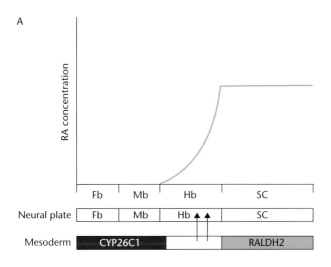

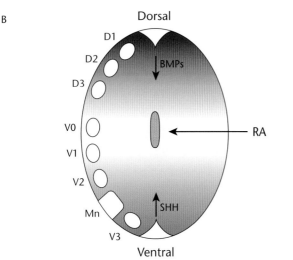

Figure 9.6 The effects of retinoic acid (RA) on patterning in the early embryo. (A) Experiments suggest that a gradient of RA in the mesoderm that is generated by retinaldehyde dehydrogenase 2 (RALDH2) (which is expressed posteriorly) and an RA-catabolizing enzyme CYP26C1 (that is expressed anteriorly) pattern the amniote hindbrain (Hb). (B) Bone morphogenetic proteins (BMPs), which are released from the dorsal region; RA, which is released from the adjacent somites; and sonic hedgehog (SHH), which is released from the ventral region, have a role in patterning the dorsoventral specification of neural cell types (D1, D2, D3, V0, V1, V2, Mn, V3) in the spinal cord. D, dorsal; Fb, forebrain; Mb, midbrain; Mn, motor neurons; SC; spinal cord; V, ventral. From Maden 2007.

canonical Wnt pathway. Some genes or pathways need to be repressed for differentiation to occur, although there has not been much research in this area and few candidates have emerged (Maden 2007). One that has is the protein tyrosine phosphatase SHP-1 (Mizuno, Katagiri, Maruyama et al. 1997), which regulates the level of phosphorylation on tyrosine residues of several intracellular proteins. Another is the Wnt inhibitor Dickkopf homologue 1 (DKK1), which

is induced by RA and is necessary for RA's effect on mouse ES cell differentiation (Verani, Cappuccio, Spinsanti et al. 2007).

The ability of RA to induce neuronal differentiation can be harnessed to produce specific neural cell types that can then be used for therapeutic transplantation (assuming that there is a high yield of a pure population of the cell type that is required). Embryonic stem cells, hematopoietic stem cells, and neural stem cells can be diverted down the neural differentiation route using combinations of RA and growth factors or neurotrophins (Table 9.1). Some of these combinations have been tested in vivo for their ability to replace lost neurons. Various embryonic neural progenitor cells and bone marrow cells, differentiated with RA, have survived and become neurons or glia when grafted into a range of locations in the adult brain, including the striatum, as a treatment for Parkinson's disease (Okada, Shimazaki, Sobue et al. 2004) or Huntington's disease (Richardson, Holloway, Bullock, et al. 2006); the lateral ventricle or subventricular zone (SVZ), as a treatment for stroke (Fraichard, Chassande, Bilbaut et al. 1995; Dinsmore, Ratliff, Deacon et al. 1996; Renoncourt, Carroll, Filippi et al. 1998); the sciatic nerve, as a treatment to induce peripheral nerve regeneration (Kilpatrick, Bartlett 1993); and the cortex, as a treatment for brain injury (Billon, Jolicoeur, Ying et al. 2002; Lee, Lumelsky, Studer et al. 2000). The potential of such differentiated cells might thus be remarkable. The role of RA in differentiation in vivo can best be exemplified in two aspects: the regulation of primary neuron number and the regulation of motor neuron differentiation.

In the chick embryo, the development of somatic motor neurons (SMN) in the caudal hindbrain and the lateral motor columns in the spinal cord is regulated by RA. SMN are found in rhombomeres 5 to 8, and grafting somites into the preotic region beneath the neuroepithelium generates ectopic SMNs in rhombomere 4 (Boillee, Cadusseau, Coulpier et al. 2001). Somites strongly express retinaldehyde dehydrogenase 2 (RALDH2) (Gard, Pfeiffer 1990; Calver, Hall, Yu et al. 1998; Stapf, Luck, Shakibaei et al. 1997) and release high levels of RA (Gabay, Lowell, Rubin et al. 2003), suggesting that RA is involved in specifying SMNs. Indeed, these effects can be mimicked with beads soaked in RA (Boillee, Cadusseau, Coulpier et al. 2001; Represa, Shimazaki, Simmonds et al. 2001; Liu, Rao 2004) and inhibited by disulphiram, an inhibitor of RA synthesis. When these experiments were performed in cultured early hindbrain neuroepithelium without adjacent cranial mesoderm, exposure to RA induced up to nine times more SMNs throughout the hindbrain than controls. This is a result strikingly similar to that observed in *Xenopus* primary neurons. When the

Table 9.1 Neuronal Types Induced by RA with or without Other Stem Cell Factors

Cell Type	Inducers	Neuronal Type
Human and mouse embryonic stem cells	RA + SHH	Cholinergic, dopaminergic
Mouse embryonic stem cells	RA + CNTF	Dopaminergic
Human embryonic stem cells	RA + BDNF, RA + TGF-α	Dopaminergic
Mouse embryonic stem cells	RA	Glutaminergic
Adult neural stem cells	RA + NT-3 RA + KCl	Mixed GABAergic
Human olfactory neural cells	RA + SHH	Dopaminergic
Bone marrow hematopoietic cells	RA, RA + NT-3, RA + BDNF, RA + FGFRA + SHH	NS Glutaminergic

From Maden 2007.

BDNF, brain-derived neurotrophic factor; CNTF, ciliary neurotrophic factor; FGF, fibroblast growth factor; KCl, potassium chloride; NS, not specified; NT-3, neurotrophin-3; RA, retinoic acid; SHH, sonic hedgehog; TGF-α, transforming growth factor α.

neuroepithelium is cultured with its adjacent cranial mesoderm, the effect of RA is markedly attenuated by the induction of CYP26 enzymes within the mesoderm. Thus, the mesoderm has an important role in precisely regulating RA levels in the normal embryo, and hence in patterning hindbrain SMNs (Fig. 9.6A). Similar effects are seen in the developing chick spinal cord. In the absence of RA, there is a reduced number of islet-1-positive motor neurons in the spinal cord, and neurites do not extend into the periphery (Sun, Echelard, Lu et al. 2001; Vallstedt, Klos, Ericson 2005; Zhou, Anderson 2002). This lack of axon outgrowth is mediated by RA that is generated in the adjacent paraxial mesoderm and that signals in a paracrine manner. RA also has a role in specifying motor neuron subtype. When brachial somites are placed at thoracic levels in the spinal cord, the types of motor neuron that are generated change from a thoracic type to a brachial type (Kuschel, Rüther, Theil 2003). These brachial motor neuron types are known as lateral motor column neurons (LMCs); they project to the dorsal and ventral limb muscles and are also found at the hindlimb level of the spinal cord. When the supply of RA from somites is reduced by 50%, there is a 20% reduction in the number of lateral LMCs (Stallcup, Beasley 1987). Later in development, however, another source of RA that supplements or replaces the somitic supply appears as the brachial and lumbar motor neurons themselves begin to express RALDH2 (Fruttiger, Karlsson, Hall et al. 1999; Nagai, Ibata, Park et al.

2002) (Fig. 9.6A). Virally induced expression of the gene encoding RALDH2 in neurons at thoracic spinal cord levels generates ectopic LMCs, demonstrating the importance of this source of RA; however, these LMCs arise not from the cells that are expressing RALHD2, but from adjacent cells that are acted on in a paracrine fashion. Conversely, reducing or eliminating RALDH2 expression (Stallcup, Beasley 1987; Kouhara, Hadari, Spivak-Kroizman et al. 1997; Lamothe, Yamada, Schaeper et al. 2004) in motor neurons reduces the number of both lateral and medial LMCs, although they are never eliminated altogether. Thus, it seems that the paraxial somitic source of RA contributes to the specification of lateral LMC numbers, whereas the neuronal source of RA contributes to the maintenance of both medial and lateral LMC populations. The role of RA in the maintenance of motor neurons is conserved in the adult, as described subsequently.

Recent data indicate that RA has a role in generating specific neuronal cell types for therapeutic transplantation and in regenerating axon after injury. Its role in maintaining the differentiated status of adult neurons and neural stem cells is also highlighted. Thus RA may have a role in both induction of nervous system regeneration and the treatment of neurodegeneration.

ES cells differentiate into motoneurons, establish functional synapses with muscle fibers, and acquire physiological properties characteristic of embryonic motoneurons when cultured with a SHH agonist and RA (Wichterle, Lieberam, Porter et al. 2002; Harper, Krishnan, Darman et al. 2004; Miles, Yohn, Wichterle et al. 2004; Lim, Sidhu, Tuch 2006; Soundararajan, Miles, Rubin et al. 2006; Lee, Shamy, Elkabetz et al. 2007). Interestingly, the vast majority of the Hb9 cells coexpressed Lhx3 when treated for 5 days with RA and the SHH agonist (Wichterle, Lieberam, Porter et al. 2002), suggesting that this treatment paradigm produces motoneurons specific to the medial aspect of the medial motor column (MMCm). Motoneurons in the MMCm innervate epaxial muscles (Tosney, Landmesser 1985a, 1985b). However, because all developing motoneurons transiently express Lhx3 (Sharma, Sheng, Lettieri et al. 1998), it is not known whether other motoneuron phenotypes would develop if the treated cells were cultured for longer periods. More importantly, the functional consequence of specific *LIM-homeobox* gene expression patterns in ES cell–derived motoneurons is not understood. It was therefore sought to determine whether SHH agonist- and RA-treated ES cell–derived motoneurons acquire phenotypic traits specific for individual motoneuron subtypes. We found that ES cell–derived motoneurons transplanted into the developing chick neural tube expressed Lhx3, migrated to the MMCm, projected axons toward epaxial muscles, received synaptic input, and developed electrophysiological properties similar to endogenous MMCm motoneurons. These results indicate that SHH and RA treatment of ES cells leads to the differentiation of functional motoneurons specific to the MMCm.

Renoncourt et al. (1998) demonstrated that EBs treated with RA can differentiate into neuronal cell types characteristic of ventral CNS: somatic motor neurons (Islet 1/2, LIM 3, HB9), cranial motor neurons (Islet 1/2 and Phox2b), and interneurons (LIM 1/2, or EN1). Similarly, another study by Gottlieb and Huettner (1999) showed that RA is required for the differentiation of spinal motor neurons where RA is a strong morphogen that appears to push ES cells toward postmitotic neurons. Therefore, neurons generated with RA treatment are likely subgroups of cells representing those in caudal and ventral part of the CNS.

Carpenter et al. (2001) utilized a complex mixture of growth factors supplemented with RA to increase the yield of neural progenitors from differentiating populations of hESC. After initial differentiation within EBs with or without RA, cells were seeded onto a poly-L-lysine/fibronectin matrix in a chemically defined medium containing neural supplements (B27 and N2) and human epidermal growth factor (hEGF), human fibroblast growth factor 2 (hFGF-2), human platelet-derived growth factor AA (hPDGF-AA), and human insulin-like growth factor 1 (hIGF-1), although the role(s) of these individual growth factors in this protocol were not defined. In these cultures, many cells exhibited a neuronal morphology and expressed the ectodermal marker, nestin. Moreover, without initial culture in RA, approximately 56% and 65% of the cells expressed neuroectodermal markers, PSA-N-CAM and A2B5, respectively. Initial EB culture in a medium supplemented with RA resulted in 87% of cells expressing PSA-N-CAM or A2B5, a 30% increase in marker expression. Although it is difficult to determine from this report if this represents enrichment for neural progenitors, other reports have shown RA to induce neuronal differentiation from hESC (Schuldiner, Eiges, Eden et al. 2001). Unlike mouse ES cell differentiation, higher concentrations of RA (10^{-6} M) promoted the formation of mature neurons, suggesting an involvement in further differentiation.

We reported a modified procedure (Lim, Sidhu, Tuch 2006) to produce motor neurons from three clonal hESC lines, hES3.1, 3.2, and 3.3 more efficiently by using a combination of growth factors such as FGF, RA, SHH compared to that reported earlier (Li, Du, Zarnowska et al. 2005; Shin, Dalton, Stice 2005; Singh, Nakano, Xuing et al. 2005). Lee et al. (2007) described a strategy to generate human motoneurons.

Based on very conservative calculations, a single hESC plated at day 0 on MS5 for neural induction yields approximately 100 HB9⁻ motoneurons at day 50 of differentiation. These numbers suggest that therapeutically relevant numbers of motoneurons can be readily achieved. Although spinal motoneurons are derived from a single ventral pMN domain (Ericson, Briscoe, Rashbass et al. 1997; Briscoe, Pierani, Jessell et al. 2000), they further acquire many different subtype identities based on positional identity, axonal projections, and gene expression. For translational applications of ES cell-derived motoneurons, it will be essential to develop motoneuron subtype–specific protocols that match the diseased population. There is evidence that most motoneurons derived from mouse ES cells using the RA/SHH protocol correspond to cervical or brachial level motoneurons based on Hoxc5 and Hoxc6 expression (Helms, Johnson 2003). Similarly, many hES cell-derived motoneurons in our protocol exhibit characteristics of brachial motoneurons. However, there is a slight caudal shift as compared with mouse ES cell-derived motoneuron progeny toward HoxC6 and HoxC8 expression.

Use of Sonic Hedgehog (SHH), Bone Morphogenetic Protein (BMP), and Wnt3A

The addition of signaling molecules to RA-treated EBs can alter the specification of neural fate. For instance, culture of RA-induced EBs in serum-free conditions, containing ITSFn and bFGF, improved the proportion of nestin-positive neuroectodermal precursors (Zhao et al. 2002). Further treatment with SHH, a determinant of ventral neural tube, induced a dorsal-to-ventral shift in gene expression, with increased expression of Nkx6.1 and Olig2, and downregulation of dorsal markers Dbx1, Irx3, and Pax6. Differentiation of RA-treated EBs resulted in inefficient formation (seven HB9 neurons/section) of motor neurons, as determined by expression of the motor neuron–specific protein, HB9. Addition of SHH (300 nM) resulted in a marked increase in the number of motor neurons produced (509 HB9 neurons/section), indicating that both posteriorization by RA and ventralization by SHH are required for the generation of motor neurons from neural progenitors. The relative formation of ventral interneurons or spinal motor neurons was dependent on the concentration of SHH in the medium, consistent with specification of these subpopulations in the embryo in response to a gradient of SHH (Wichterle, Lieberam, Porter et al. 2002).

Li et al. (2005) showed that hESC generated early neuroectodermal cells, which organized into neural rosettes and expressed Pax6 but not Sox1, and then

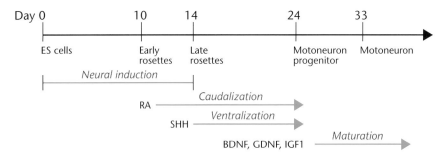

Figure 9.7 Schematic procedures for motor neuron differentiation. hESCs were differentiated to early neuroectodermal cells in the form of early rosettes in 10 days. They were then treated with retinoic acid (RA) for 1 week, and the neural tube–like rosettes were isolated through 3 to 5 days of differential adhesion and then adhered to the laminin substrate (around day 20) in the presence of RA and sonic hedgehog (SHH) for neuronal differentiation. BDNF, brain-derived neurotrophic factor; GDNF, glial cell line–derived neurotrophic factor and IGF-1, insulin-like growth factor 1. Adapted from Li, Du, Zarnowska et al. 2005.

late neuroectodermal cells, which formed neural tube–like structures and expressed both Pax6 and Sox1. Only the early (10 days of hESC aggregation), but not the late (14 days), neuroectodermal cells were efficiently posteriorized by RA, and in the presence of SHH, differentiated into spinal motor neurons (Fig. 9.7). Their findings indicate that the timing of treatments of RA and SHH is essential for motor neuron specification.

Murashov et al. (2004) demonstrated that dorsal interneurons and motor neurons specific for the spinal cord can be generated from mouse ES cells using combinations of inductive signals such as RA, SHH, BMP2, and Wnt3A. The EBs were treated with all four growth factors and showed a higher yield of interneurons (55%) and motor neurons (40%). In addition, they introduced the concept that Wnt3A morphogenic action relies on cross talk with both SHH and BMP2 signaling pathways. The roles of dorsal factors Wnt3A and BMP2 on motor neuron differentiation still remains unclear; however, this report suggests that they could play fundamental roles in motor neuron development.

The specification of neuronal subtypes in the spinal cord becomes evident with the appearance of distinct cell types at defined positions along the dorsoventral axis of the neural tube (Fig. 9.8). At early stages of ventral neural tube development, three main classes of cells are generated: floor plate cells—a specialized class of glial cells—differentiate at the ventral midline soon after neural plate formation (Figs. 9.8A and B), whereas motor neurons and interneurons are generated at more dorsal positions (Fig. 9.8D). The differentiation of these ventral cell types is triggered by signals provided initially by an axial mesodermal cell group, the notochord, and later by floor plate cells themselves (Placzek 1995) (Fig. 9.8D). As the floor plate serves as a secondary source of ventral inductive signals and is generated before any neuronal cell type, there has been interest in whether

the mechanisms that underlie floor plate differentiation are distinct from those of other ventral cell types. Many studies support the view that floor plate differentiation is mediated by inductive signaling from the notochord (Placzek 1995). An alternative view, however, argues that the floor plate emerges not by induction, but through insertion into the neural plate of a group of floor plate precursors that are set aside in the axial mesoderm before neural plate formation (Teillet, Lapointe, Le Douarin 1998; Le Douarin, Halpern 2000; Placzek, Dodd, Jessell et al. 2000). The main signaling activities of the notochord and floor plate are mediated by a secreted protein, sonic hedgehog (SHH). Ectopic expression of *SHH* in vivo and in vitro can induce the differentiation of floor plate cells, motor neurons, and ventral interneurons. Conversely, elimination of SHH signaling from the notochord by antibody blockade in vitro, or through gene targeting in mice, prevents the differentiation of floor plate cells, motor neurons, and most classes of ventral interneurons. Even though SHH can induce all ventral cell types, the generation of certain sets of interneurons in the dorsal-most region of the ventral neural tube does not depend on SHH signaling. These interneuron subtypes can be induced by a parallel signaling pathway that is mediated by retinoids derived from the paraxial mesoderm and possibly also from neural plate cells (Marti, Bumcrot, Takada et al. 1995; Roelink, Porter, Chiang 1995; Chiang, Ying, Eric et al. 1996; Ericson, Morton, Kawakami et al. 1996; Pierani, Brenner-Morton, Chiang et al. 1999). So retinoid signaling seems to have sequential roles in spinal cord development, initially imposing spinal cord identity and later specifying the identity of some of its component neurons. Progressive two- to threefold change in SHH concentration (*Graded SHH signaling*) generates five molecularly distinct classes of ventral neurons from neural progenitor cells in vitro (Ericson, Briscoe, Rashbass et al. 1997). Moreover, the position of generation of each of these neuronal classes in vivo is predicted by

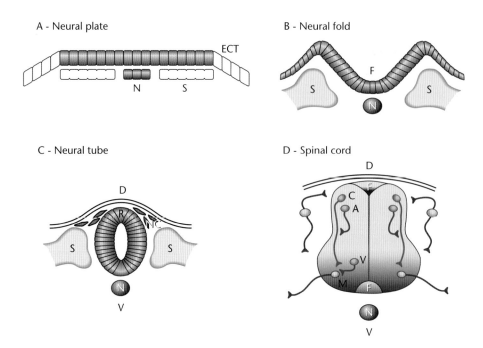

A - Neural plate

B - Neural fold

C - Neural tube

D - Spinal cord

Figure 9.8 Four stages of spinal cord development. Four successive stages in the development of the spinal cord are shown. (A) At the neural plate stage, newly formed neural cells are flanked laterally by the epidermal ectoderm (ECT). Notochord cells (N) underlie themidline of the neural plate, and segmental plate mesoderm (S) underlies the lateral region of the neural plate. (B) At the neural fold stage, floor plate cells (F) are evident at the ventral midline and the somitic mesoderm begins to develop. (C) At the neural tube stage, roof plate cells (R) begin to differentiate at the dorsal midline, and neural crest cells (NC) start to delaminate from the dorsal neural tube. (D) During the embryonic development of the spinal cord, distinct sets of commissural (C) and association (A) neurons differentiate in the dorsal half of the spinal cord, and motor neurons (M) and ventral interneurons (V) develop in the ventral half of the neural tube. Dorsal root ganglion (DRG) neurons differentiate from neural crest progenitors. The dorsal (D) and ventral (V) axes are shown in bold. From Jessell 2000.

the concentration of SHH required for their induction in vitro. Neurons generated in progressively more ventral region of the neural tube require corresponding higher concentrations of SHH for their induction. The neural progenitors interpret graded SHH signal probably through selective cross-repressive interactions between the complementary pairs of class I and class II homeodomain proteins that abut the same progenitor domain boundary (Briscoe, Pierani, Jessell et al. 2000) (Fig. 9.9B). Such interactions seem to have three main roles. First, they establish the initial dorsoventral domains of expression of class I and class II proteins. Second, they ensure the existence of sharp boundaries between progenitor domains. Third, they help relieve progenitor cells of a requirement for ongoing SHH signaling, consolidating progenitor domain identity (Briscoe, Pierani, Jessell et al. 2000). The central role of cross-repression between transcription factors in ventral neural patterning has parallels other neural and non-neural tissues. In the developing brain, cross-repressive interactions between the homeodomain proteins Pax6 and Pax2 help delineate the diencephalic–midbrain boundary, and interactions between Otx2 and Gbx2 define the midbrain–hindbrain boundary (Matsunaga, Araki, Nakamura et al. 2000; Simeone 2000). Many

studies have also provided an initial framework for defining SHH-regulated transcriptional cascades that direct neural progenitor cells along specific pathways of neurogenesis. For example, SHH-regulated homeodomain proteins can be ordered into a pathway that helps explain how motor neurons acquire an identity distinct from that of adjacent interneurons (Tanabe et al. 1998; Briscoe, Pierani, Jessell et al. 2000) (Fig. 9.10). The combinatorial actions of three homeodomain proteins—Nkx6.1, Nkx2.2, and Irx3—restrict the generation of motor neurons to a single (pMN) progenitor domain. Within this domain, Nkx6.1 activity directs the domain-restricted expression of downstream factors, such as the homeodomain protein MNR2. MNR2 is first expressed during the final division cycle of motor neuron progenitors and functions as a dedicated determinant of motor neuron identity (Fig. 9.10). Ectopic dorsal expression of MNR2 does not change the pattern of expression of class I and class II proteins, but is sufficient to subvert their activity and elicit a coherent program of postmitotic motor neuron differentiation. Moreover, once induced, MNR2 positively regulates its own expression, further consolidating the progression of progenitor cells to a motor neuron fate (Fig. 9.10). Ectopic expression of other progenitor transcription

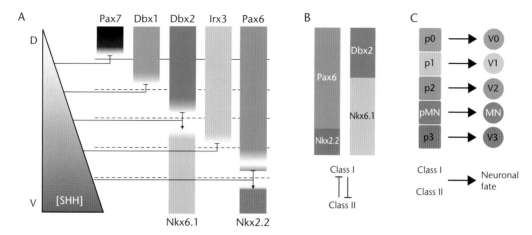

Figure 9.9 Three phases of sonic hedgehog (SHH)–mediated ventral neural patterning. (A) SHH mediates the repression of class I homeodomain proteins (Pax7, Dbx1, Dbx2, Irx3, and Pax6) at different threshold concentrations and the induction of expression of class II proteins (Nkx6.1 and Nkx2.2) at different threshold concentrations. Class I and class II proteins that abut a common progenitor domain boundary have similar SHH concentration thresholds for repression and activation of protein expression, respectively. SHH signaling defines five progenitor domains in the ventral neural tube. (B) The pairs of homeodomain proteins that abut a common progenitor domain boundary (Pax6 and Nkx2.2; Dbx2 and Nkx6.1) repress each other's expression. (C) shows the relationship between neural progenitor (p) domains and the positions at which postmitotic neurons are generated along the dorsoventral axis of the ventral spinal cord (v). From Jessell 2000.

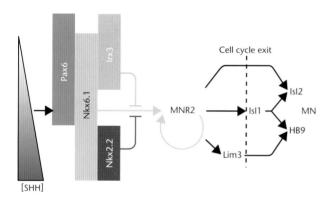

Figure 9.10 A molecular pathway for motor neuron generation. Homeodomain proteins that function downstream of SHH in the pathway of motor neuron (MN) generation in the chick embryo. Graded SHH signaling establishes an initial progenitor domain profile in which Nkx6.1 expression, in the absence of Nkx2.2 and Irx3 expression, delineates the domain from which motor neurons are generated. The activity of Nkx6.1, when unconstrained by the inhibitory effects of Irx3 and Nkx2.2, is sufficient to induce the expression of the homeodomain protein MNR2. MNR2 induces the expression of downstream transcription factors, including Lim3, Isl1, Isl2, and HB9. MNR2 also positively autoactivates its own expression, consolidating the decision of progenitor cells to select a motor neuron fate. The timing of onset of homeodomain protein expression with respect to cell cycle exit is indicated. From Jessell 2000.

determined through the actions of neuronal subtype–dedicated transcription factors. Defining such factors may aid studies that aim to direct neural stem cells along specific pathways of neuronal differentiation.

Although studies of SHH signaling have provided many insights into mechanisms of neuronal specification and patterning, it is evident that further signaling pathways are necessary to enhance the diversity of cell types that populate the ventral spinal cord. In some instances, a single progenitor domain is known to generate distinct cell types at different developmental stages (Sun, Pringle, Hardy et al. 1998), implying a temporal control of cell fate that is still poorly understood. The same progenitor domain can also generate distinct classes of neurons at spinal cord and hindbrain levels, emphasizing the idea that rostrocaudal positional cues function in concert with dorsoventral patterning mechanisms to specify individual neuronal fates. Moreover, there is evidence that more than one class of neuron can be generated from a single progenitor domain over the same developmental period. Each of these points can be illustrated through the analysis of motor neuron diversity in the spinal cord.

Role of BMP Signaling: Use of Noggin and Chordin

It has been reported that the maintenance of BMP4 signaling during early ES cell differentiation inhibits neurogenesis in vitro and in vivo, suggesting that BMP4 may either antagonize neural induction

factors that function downstream of the class I and class II proteins can similarly direct ventral cell fates in the spinal cord independently of the prior developmental history of the progenitor cell (Sasaki, Hogan 1994; Ruiz, Altaba, Jessell et al. 1995). The fates of neurons in other regions of the CNS may therefore be or direct differentiation to an alternative cell fate (Mabie, Mehler, Kessler 1999; Li, LoTurco 2000; Lim, Tramontin, Trevejo et al. 2000). Differentiation of ES cells in a medium supplemented with noggin resulted in rapid formation of neurofilament-expressing populations, with neurons comprising >91% of surviving cells after 72 hours (Gratsch, O'Shea 2002). Likewise, chordin, a second BMP4 antagonist, increased neural differentiation from ES cells but with lower (55%) efficiency (Gratsch, O'Shea 2002). These results were supported by Itsykson et al. (2005) who found that when BMP signaling is repressed by noggin in hESC aggregates, it suppresses non-neural differentiation and the aggregates develop into spheres highly enriched for proliferating neural precursors. Therefore, BMP antagonism might play a role in further differentiation of precursor cells to a neuronal cell fate rather than in directed formation of the precursor population.

Role of Wnt Signaling

During the early development of the vertebrate central nervous system, the position of generation of postmitotic neurons depends on the patterning of progenitor cells along the dorsoventral and rostrocaudal axes of the neural tube (Lumsden, Krumlauf 1996; Jessell 2000; Guthrie 2004). At many levels of the neuraxis, the dorsoventral pattern of progenitor cells, which later gives rise to motor, sensory, and local circuit neurons, is initiated by the opponent signaling activities of SHH and bone morphogenetic proteins (Briscoe, Ericson 1999; Jessell 2000; Helms, Johnson 2003). In contrast, the rostrocaudal pattern of neural progenitor cells that differentiate into distinct neuronal subtypes is imposed, in part, by opponent retinoid and FGF signals (Liu, Laufer, Jessell 2001; Bel-Vialar, Itasaki, Krumlauf 2002; Dasen, Liu, Jessell 2003; Sockanathan, Perlmann, Jessell 2003). Within the hindbrain and spinal cord, the rostrocaudal positional identity of neurons is reflected most clearly by the generation of different motor neuron (MN) subtypes. One fundamental distinction in MN subtype identity is the emergence of two major classes of MNs that exhibit distinctive axonal trajectories, ventral exiting motor neurons (VMNs), and dorsal exiting motor neurons (DMNs) (Sharma, Sheng, Lettieri et al. 1998). VMNs include most spinal MNs as well as hypoglossal and abducens MNs of the caudal hindbrain, whereas DMNs are found throughout the hindbrain and at cervical levels of the spinal cord. Each of the many subsequent distinctions in MN subtype identity emerges through the diversification of these two basic neuronal classes. Despite many advances in defining the mechanisms of MN diversification, it remains unclear how neural progenitors in the hindbrain and spinal cord acquire a rostrocaudal positional character that results in the generation of DMN and VMN classes. At both hindbrain and spinal levels, *Hox* genes are informative markers of the rostrocaudal positional identity of progenitor cells. Within the hindbrain, distinct rhombomeres are delineated by the nested expression of *3′ Hox* genes (Trainor, Krumlauf 2001), whereas the spinal expression of *5′ Hox* genes distinguishes progenitor cells and postmitotic neurons at cervical, brachial, thoracic, and lumbar levels (Shah, Drill, Lance-Jones 2004). Moreover, *Hox* genes are determinants of MN subtype identity in both hindbrain and spinal cord. In the hindbrain, for example, the restricted expression of Hoxb1 helps to determine the identity of facial MNs, and in the spinal cord the restricted expression of Hox6, Hox9, and Hox10 proteins establishes MN columnar subtype (Bell, Wingate, Lumsden 1999; Jungbluth, Bell, Lumsden 1999; McClintock, Kheirbek, Prince, 2002; Briscoe, Wilkinson 2004; Shah, Drill, Lance-Jones 2004). In addition, a more complex Hox transcriptional regulatory network specifies spinal MN pool identity and connectivity (Dasen, Tice, Brenner-Morton et al. 2005). The neural pattern of Hox expression is, in turn, regulated by members of the *Cdx homeobox* gene family (Marom, Shapira, Fainsod 1997; Charite, de Graaff, Consten et al. 1998; Isaacs, Pownall, Slack 1998; Ehrman, Yutzey 2001; van den Akker, Forlani, Chawengsaksophak et al. 2002). *Cdx* genes are transiently expressed in the caudal-most region of the neural plate prior to the onset of *5′ Hox* gene expressions and appear to be direct regulators of the expression of *5′ Hoxb* genes. Thus, analysis of spatial profiles of *Cdx* and *Hox* gene expression may provide clues about the identity of signals that pattern MN subtypes in the hindbrain and spinal cord. Several recent studies have provided insight into the signals that impose rostrocaudally restricted patterns of neural Cdx and Hox expression. RA and FGF signals appear to have opponent roles in the rostrocaudal patterning of *Hox* gene expression in the caudal hindbrain (Chb) and spinal cord. Mesodermal-derived RA signals promote the expression of *Hox* genes characteristic of the Chb and rostral spinal cord (Rsc) (Niederreither, Subbarayan, Dolle et al. 1999; Dupe, Lumsden 2001), whereas FGF signals pattern the expression of *Hox* genes at more caudal levels of the spinal cord. At an earlier developmental stage, neural progenitors have been shown to acquire caudal forebrain, midbrain, and rostral hindbrain positional identities in response to graded Wnt signaling at the gastrula stage (Muhr, Graziano, Wilson et al. 1999; Nordstrom, Jessell, Edlund 2002). It is unclear, however, whether an early phase of Wnt signaling is also required to establish *Cdx* and *Hox* gene expression profiles characteristic of the Chb and spinal cord, in turn specifying the generation of DMN and VMN subtypes. Nordstrom et al. (2006) suggest

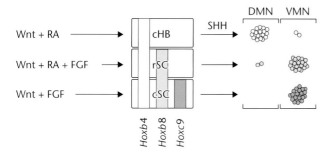

Figure 9.11 Combinatorial Wnt, RA, and FGF signals specify progenitor cell identity that prefigures MN subtype in the developing hindbrain and spinal cord. Combinatorial actions of Wnt, FGF, and RA signals specify neural progenitor cells expressing *Hox* gene profiles characteristic of the cHB, rSC, and cSC that generate patterns of differentiated MNs, with DMN or VMN exit points, characteristic of hindbrain and spinal cord, in response to SHH signaling. From Nordstrom, Jessell, Edlund 2006.

a model of how hindbrain and spinal cord cells of early rostrocaudal regional identity are generated (Fig. 9.11).

IMPLICATIONS FOR CELL REPLACEMENT THERAPY

Several studies have shown that ES cells can be directed to differentiate into electrically excitable glutamatergic (Plachta, Bibel, Tucker et al. 2004), serotonergic (Lee, Lumelsky, Studer et al. 2000), dopaminergic (Kim, Auerbach, Rodríguez-Gómez et al. 2002), or cholinergic motor (Wichterle, Lieberam, Porter et al. 2002; Harper, Krishnan, Darman et al. 2004; Miles, Yohn, Wichterle et al. 2004; Li, Du, Zarnowska et al. 2005) neurons. However, differentiated ES cells will ultimately have to be classified by other means, because subpopulations of neurons that express a given transmitter can differ dramatically with respect to size, ion channels, receptors, projection patterns, and, most importantly, function. Furthermore, several neurodegenerative disorders result in the selective loss of specific neuronal subtypes. For example, dopamine neurons expressing the G protein–coupled inward rectifying current potassium channel (Girk2) preferentially degenerate in patients with Parkinson's disease (Yamada, McGeer, Baimbridge et al. 1990; Fearnley, Lees 1991; Gibb 1992; Mendez, Sanchez-Pernaute, Cooper et al. 2005). Enkephalin-containing GABAergic neurons projecting from the striatum to the external segment of the globus pallidus are the first to degenerate in patients with Huntington's disease (Reiner, Albin, Anderson et al. 1988; Sapp, Ge, Aizawa et al. 1995). The fastest conducting, and presumably largest, motor neurons preferentially die in patients with ALS (Theys, Peeters, Robberecht 1999). One of the

guiding assumptions underlying cell replacement therapy is that the transplanted neurons will form selective connections with the appropriate target tissue. Whether this assumption is correct is not known. However, there are now several lines of evidence to suggest that specific connections do occur between transplant and host neurons. For example, fetal ventral mesencephalic tissue, used in the treatment of animal models of Parkinson's disease, contains a mixture of two dopamine neuron subtypes: A9 (Girk2$^-$) neurons of the substantia nigra that project to the striatum and A10 neurons of the ventral tegmental area. Interestingly, only A9 neurons extend axons out of the graft when the tissue is transplanted into the striatum of animal models of Parkinson's disease (Thompson, Barraud, Andersson et al. 2005) and in humans with the disease (Mendez, Sanchez-Pernaute, Cooper et al. 2005). These results suggest that many of the guidance molecules and/or trophic factors expressed during development exist in the adult CNS. They also underscore the fact that neuronal specificity is required for optimal growth and synapse formation (Thompson, Barraud, Andersson et al. 2005; for review, see Bjorklund, Isacson 2002). Thus, it may not be sufficient to simply generate generic neurons from ES cells, or even neurons of a particular transmitter phenotype, when treating diseases or trauma. Specific neuronal subpopulations that provide for the particular needs of the affected CNS will ultimately have to be developed. With respect to cell replacement therapy and the treatment of spinal cord pathologies, various studies indicate that limb innervation will be greater if ES cells are differentiated into LMC motoneurons. Although it is not known how to differentiate ES cells into LMC neurons, this process will likely require additional instructive signals that normally emanate from the developing spinal cord (Sockanathan, Jessell 1998).

PROSPECTS AND CHALLENGES

Motoneurons are the key effector cell type for control of motor function, and loss of motoneurons is associated with a number of debilitating diseases such as ALS and spinal muscular atrophy. Motoneurons are also regarded as a great model for probing mechanisms of vertebrate CNS development, and the transcriptional pathways that guide motoneuronal specification are well characterized. Recent studies have demonstrated the in vitro derivation of motoneurons from mouse and hESCs. Current hESC-derived motoneuron differentiation protocols are based on embryoid body–mediated neural induction followed by exposure to defined morphogens such as SHH and RA acting as ventralizing and caudalizing factors, respectively. It has been suggested that the ability to undergo motoneuron specification under these conditions is temporally restricted to the earliest stages of neural induction. Characterization of these cells in vitro and in vivo has been limited. Furthermore, there are currently no published data on the ability of hESC-derived motoneurons to secrete acetylcholine, the key neurotransmitter of spinal motoneurons, and to survive and maintain motoneuron characteristics in the developing or adult cord. In vivo survival and the ability for orthotopic integration are key requirements for future applications in animal models of motoneuron disease. Although the road to the clinical application of hESC-derived motoneurons remains extremely challenging, the ability to generate unlimited numbers of motoneuron progeny and the capacity for in vivo survival and integration in the developing and adult spinal cord are important first steps on this journey. Given the extensive experience in transplantation of embryonic and adult brain–derived neural precursors, one may wonder what the specific role of ESC will be in future cell therapy. A major advantage of ESC is in their potential to generate an endless supply of specific neural populations. For example, the ability to generate highly enriched oligodendroglial lineage cultures from ESC provides them with an advantage over other sources of transplantable oligodendrocyte lineage cells. The myelinogenic potential of mouse embryonic stem–derived oligodendrocyte progenitors, which were expanded in vitro, was demonstrated in embryonic rat brains, when these cells extensively myelinated the brain and spinal cord. When transplanted in a rodent model of chemically induced demyelination and in the spinal cords of *shi* mice, mouse embryonic stem–derived progenitor cells were also able to differentiate into glial cells and remyelinate demyelinated axons in vivo. A great deal of basic research should be done before persons with ALS can be considered for clinical trials. Cells with characteristics of cholinergic neurons have been generated from stem cells of various sources (Fig. 9.12), but their functional properties and ability to repair the spinal cord in ALS models are unknown. In the shorter term, strategies to retard disease progression seem to be a more realistic clinical approach as compared with neuronal replacement. Safety is the chief concern for clinical application of hES cell derivatives. The safety issue derives mainly from the pluripotency of hES cells, which could lead to potential generation of undesirable cells or tissues or even formation of teratomas. Hence, hES cells need to be instructed to become a particular cell type. For example, hES cells need to be restricted to at least a neural fate for them to be applied in neurological conditions. Because most current approaches for directed neural differentiation yield a mixture of cells, isolation of the desirable cell population appears necessary to avoid unpredictable

outcomes. It may not be sufficient merely to remove undifferentiated stem cells, because partially differentiated nontarget cells could still contribute to aberrant tissue generation. Therefore, positive selection of target cells is mostly desirable for clinical application. Selection of the versatile neurons and glial cells based on expression of specific cell surface molecules is not readily available at present. However, we know a sufficient number of transcription factors that are specifically expressed by various neuronal and glial cell types. Knock-in of a selectable marker into a cell type–specific gene using homologous recombination, as described by Zwaka, Thomson (2003), should allow the positive selection of differentiated, postmitotic cells of choice and/or removal of remaining undifferentiated stem cells, thereby minimizing the risk of teratoma formation. While genetically manipulated cells may still be a concern for clinical application, the purified target cell population using this approach will likely significantly facilitate the discovery of cell surface molecules specifically expressed by the target cells. This will, in turn, lead to the development of epigenetic approach for purifying target cells. Thus, it is reasonable to be optimistic that safe strategy can be devised to apply hES cells in clinics.

The development of stem cell–based therapies for neurodegenerative disorders is still at an early stage. Several fundamental issues remain to be resolved, and we need to move forward with caution. One challenge now is to identify molecular determinants of stem cell proliferation so as to control undesired growth and genetic alterations of ESCs, as well as to better manage the expansion of NSCs. We also need to know how to pattern stem cells to obtain a more complete repertoire of various types of cells for replacement, and how to induce effective functional integration of stem cell–derived neurons into existing neural and synaptic networks. Technological advances will be needed to make precise genetic modifications of stem cells or their progeny that will enhance their capacity for migration, integration, and pathway reconstruction. We need to develop technologies for genetic labeling of stem cell progeny so that we can firmly establish where neurogenesis occurs and which cell types are generated following damage. The functional properties of the new neurons and their ability to form appropriate afferent and efferent connections should be determined. We also need to identify, with the aid of genomic and proteomic approaches, the cellular and molecular players that, in a concerted action, regulate different steps of neurogenesis. On the basis of this knowledge, we should design strategies to deliver molecules that improve the yield of new functional neurons and other cells in the damaged area. To aid in further progress toward the clinic, we also need to develop animal models that closely mimic the human

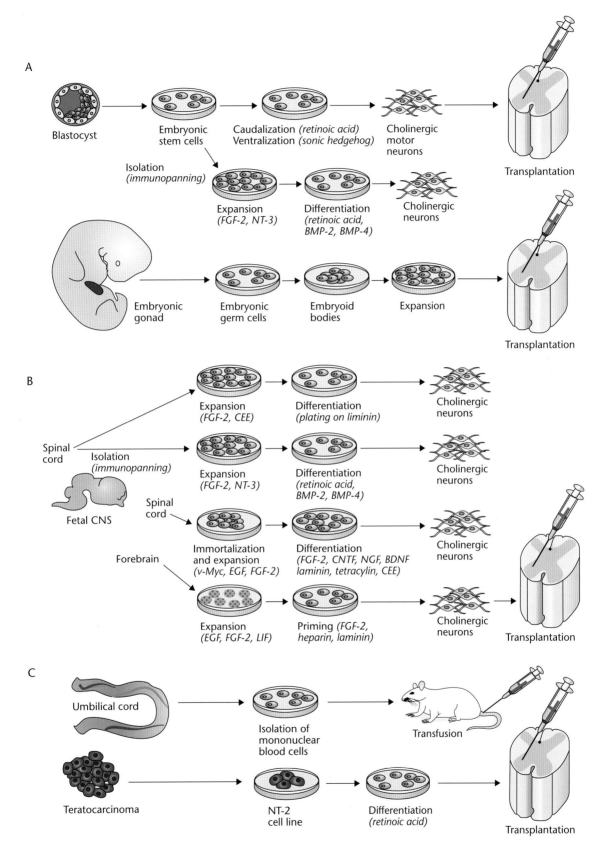

Figure 9.12 (A, B, and C) Generation of cholinergic motor neurons from various sources. BMP, bone morphogenetic protein; CEE, chicken embryo extract. From Lindvall, Zaal Kokaia, Martinez-Serrano 2004.

disease. Such models will allow us to assess and balance potential risks and benefits of stem cell therapies before their application in humans. Likewise, we need to improve noninvasive imaging technologies so that we can monitor regenerative processes subsequent to stem cell–based approaches in animals and humans. The time and the scientific effort required should not dampen our enthusiasm for developing stem cell therapies. For the first time, there is real hope that in the future we will be able to offer persons with currently intractable neurodegenerative diseases effective cell-based treatments to restore brain function.

ACKNOWLEDGMENTS   Funding was from NHMRC Program Grant of The Neuropsychiatry Institute of UNSW. Thanks to Marcus Cremonese of Medical Illustration unit of UNSW for artwork.

REFERENCES

Agathon A, Thisse C, Thisse B. 2003. The molecular nature of the zebrafish tail organizer. *Nature.* 424:448–452.

Altmann CR, Brivanlou AH. 2001. Neural patterning in the vertebrate embryo. *Int Rev Cytol.* 203:447–482.

Amit M, Carpenter MK, Inokuma MS et al. 2000. Clonally derived human embryonic stem cell lines maintain pluripotency and proliferative potential for prolonged period of culture. *Dev Biol.* 227:271–278.

Bain G, Kitchens D, Yao M, Huettner JE, Gottlieb DI. 1995. Embryonic stem cells express neuronal properties *in vitro Dev Biol.* 168:342–357.

Barberi T, Klivenyi P, Calingasan NY et al. 2003. Neural subtype specification of fertilization and nuclear transfer embryonic stem cells and application in parkinsonian mice. *Nat Biotechnol.* 21:1200–1207.

Bell E, Wingate RJ, Lumsden A. 1999. Homeotic transformation of rhombomere identity after localized Hoxbl misexpression. *Science.* 284:2168–2171.

Bel-Vialar S, Itasaki N, Krumlauf R. 2002. Initiating Hox gene expression: in the early chick neural tube differential sensitivity to FGF and RA signalling subdivides the HoxB genes in two distinct groups. *Development.* 129:5103–5115.

Ben-Hur T. 2006. Human embryonic stem cells for neural repair. *IMAJ.* 8:122–126.

Benninger F, Beck H, Wernig M, Tucker KL, Brustle O, Scheffler B. 2003. Functional integration of embryonic stem cell-derived neurons in hippocampal slice cultures. *J Neurosci.* 23:7075–7083.

Bertrand V, Hudson C, Caillol D, Popovici C, Lemaire P. 2003. Neural tissue in ascidian embryos is induced by FGF9/16/20, acting via a combination of maternal GATA and Ets transcription factors. *Cell.* 115:615–627.

Billon N, Jolicoeur C, Ying QL, Smith A, Raff M. 2002. Normal timing of oligodendrocyte development from genetically engineered, lineage-selectable mouse ES cells. *J Cell Sci.* 15:3657–3665.

Bjorklund LM, Isacson O. 2002. Regulation of dopamine cell type and transmitter function in fetal and stem cell

transplantation for Parkinson's disease. *Prog Brain Res.* 138:411–420.

Boillee S, Cadusseau J, Coulpier M, Grannec G, Junier MP. 2001. Transforming growth factor alpha: a promoter of motoneuron survival of potential biological relevance. *J Neurosci.* 21:7079–7088.

Briscoe J, Ericson J. 1999. The specification of neuronal identity by graded Sonic Hedgehog signaling. *Semin Cell Dev Biol.* 10:353–362.

Briscoe J, Pierani A, Jessell TM, Ericson J. 2000. A homeodomain protein code specifies progenitor cell identity and neuronal fate in the ventral neural tube. *Cell.* 101:435–445.

Briscoe J, Wilkinson DG. 2004. Establishing neuronal circuitry: Hox genes make the connection. *Genes Dev.* 18:1643–1648.

Brustle O, Jones KN, Learish RD et al. 1999. Embryonic stem cell-derived glial precursors: a source of myelinating transplants. *Science.* 285:754–756.

Calver AR, Hall AC, Yu WP et al. 1998. Oligodendrocyte population dynamics and the role of PDGF in vivo. *Neuron.* 20:869–882.

Carpenter MK, Inokuma MS, Denham J, Mujtaba T, Chiu CP, Rao MS. 2001. Enrichment of neurons and neural precursors from human embryonic stem cells. *Exp Neurol.* 172:383–397.

Charite J, de Graaff W, Consten D, Reijnen MJ, Korving J, Deschamps J. 1998. Transducing positional information to the Hox genes: critical interaction of cdx gene products with position-sensitive regulatory elements. *Development.* 125:4349–4358.

Chiang C, Litingtung Y, Lee Y. 1996. Cyclopia and defective axial patterning in mice lacking Sonic Hedgehog gene function. *Nature.* 383:407–413.

Cleveland DW, Rothstein JD. 2001. From Charcot to Lou Gehrig: deciphering selective motor neuron death in ALS. *Nat Rev Neurosci.* 2:806–819.

Dasen JS, Liu JP, Jessell TM. 2003. Motor neuron columnar fate imposed by sequential phases of Hox-c activity. *Nature.* 425:926–933.

Dasen JS, Tice BC, Brenner-Morton S, Jessell TM. 2005. A Hox regulatory network establishes motor neuron pool identity and target-muscle connectivity. *Cell.* 123:477–491.

Diez del Corral R, Storey KG. 2004. Opposing FGF and retinoid pathways: a signalling switch that controls differentiation and patterning onset in the extending vertebrate body axis. *Bioessays.* 26:857–869. Review.

Dinsmore J, Ratliff J, Deacon T et al. 1996. Embryonic stem cells differentiated in vitro as a novel source of cells for transplantation. *Cell Transplant.* 5:131–143.

Doetschman TC, H Eistetter, M Katz, et al. 1985. The in vitro development of blastocyst-derived embryonic stem cell lines: formation of visceral yolk sac, blood islands and myocardium. *J Embryol Exp Morphol.* 87:27–45.

Dupe V, Lumsden A. 2001. Hindbrain patterning involves graded responses to retinoic acid signaling. *Development.* 128:2199–2208.

Ehrman LA, Yutzey KE. 2001. Anterior expression of the caudal homolog cCdx-B activates a posterior genetic program in avian embryos. *Dev Dyn.* 221:412–421.

Ericson J, Morton S, Kawakami A, Roelink H, Jessell TM. 1996. Two critical periods of Sonic Hedgehog signaling required for the specification of motor neuron identity. *Cell.* 87:661–673.

Ericson J, Briscoe J, Rashbass P, van Heyningen V, Jessell TM. 1997. Graded sonic hedgehog signalling and the specification of cell fate in the ventral neural tube. *Cold Spring Harb Symp Quant Biol.* 62:451–466.

Fearnley JM, Lees AJ. 1991. Ageing and Parkinson's disease: substantia nigra regional selectivity. *Brain.* 114:2283–2301.

Fraichard A, Chassande O, Bilbaut G, Dehay C, Savatier P, Samarut J. 1995. In vitro differentiation of embryonic stem cells into glial cells and functional neurons. *J Cell Sci.* 108:3181–3188.

Frank-Kamenetsky M, Zhang XM, Bottega S et al. 2002. Small-molecule modulators of Hedgehog signaling: identification and characterization of Smoothened agonists and antagonists. *J Biol.* 1:10.

Fruttiger M, Karlsson L, Hall AC et al. 1999. Defective oligodendrocyte development and severe hypomyelination in PDGF-A knockout mice. *Development.* 126:457–467.

Gabay L, Lowell S, Rubin LL, Andeson DJ. 2003. Deregulation of dorsoventral patterning by FGF confers trilineage differentiation capacity on CNS stem cells in vitro. *Neuron.* 40:485–499.

Gard AL, Pfeiffer SE. 1990. Two proliferative stages of the oligodendrocyte lineage (a2b5_04- and 04_galc-) under different mitogenic control. *Neuron.* 5:615–625.

Gibb WR. 1992. Melanin, tyrosine hydroxylase, calbindin and substance P in the human midbrain and substantia nigra in relation to nigrostriatal projections and differential neuronal susceptibility in Parkinson's disease. *Brain Res.* 581:283–291.

Gottlieb DI, Huettner JE. 1999. An in vitro pathway from embryonic stem cells to neurons and glia. *Cells Tissues Organs.* 165:165–172.

Gratsch TE, O'Shea KS. 2002. Noggin and chordin have distinct activities in promoting lineage commitment of mouse embryonic stem (ES) cells. *Dev Biol.* 245:83–94.

Glover JC, Renaud JS, Rijli FM. 2006. Retinoic acid and hindbrain patterning. *J Neurobiol.* 66:705–725. Review.

Gunhaga L, Marklund M, Sjodal M, Hsieh JC, Jessell TM, Edlund T. 2003. Specification of dorsal telencephalic character by sequential Wnt and FGF signaling. *Nat Neurosci.* 6:701–707.

Guthrie S. 2004. Neuronal development: putting motor neurons in their place. *Curr Biol.* 14:R166–R168.

Hardikar A, Lees JG, Sidhu KS, Colvin E, Tuch BE. 2006. Stem-Cell therapy for diabetes cure: how close are we? *Curr Stem Cell Res Ther.* 1:425–436.

Harper JM, Krishnan C, Darman JS et al. 2004. Axonal growth of embryonic stem cell derived motoneurons in vitro and in motoneuron-injured adult rats. *Proc Natl. Acad Sci U S A.* 101:7123–7128.

Hayakawa-Yano Y, Nishida K, Fukami S et al. 2007. Progenitors in the embryonic spinal cord required for the spatiotemporally regulated proliferation of Olig2-expressing epidermal growth factor signaling mediated by Grb2 associated binder 1 is. *Stem Cells.* 25:1410–1422.

Helms AW, Johnson JE. 2003. Specification of dorsal spinal cord interneurons. *Curr Opin Neurobiol.* 13:42–49.

Isaacs HV, Pownall ME, Slack JM. 1998. Regulation of Hox gene expression and posterior development by the Xenopus caudal homolog Xcad3. *EMBO J.* 17:3413–3427.

Itsykson P, Ilouz N, Turetsky T et al. 2005. Derivation of neural precursors from human embryonic stem cells in the presence of noggin. *Mol Cell Neurosci.* 30(1):24–36.

Jessell TM. 2000. Neuronal specification in the spinal cord: inductive signals and transcriptional codes. *Nat Rev Genet.* 1:20–29.

Jones-Villeneuve EM, McBurney MW, Rogers KA, Kalnins VI. 1982. Retinoic acid induces embryonal carcinoma cells to differentiate into neurons and glial cells. *J Cell Biol.* 94:253–262.

Jungbluth S, Bell E, Lumsden A. 1999. Specification of distinct motor neuron identities by the singular activities of individual Hox genes. *Development.* 126:2751–2758.

Kawaguchi R, Yu J, Honda J et al. 2007. A membrane receptor for retinol binding protein mediates cellular uptake of vitamin A. *Science.* 315:820–825.

Kawasaki H, Mizuseki K, Nishikawa S et al. 2000. Induction of midbrain dopaminergic neurons from ES cells by stromal cell-derived inducing activity. *Neuron.* 28:31–40.

Keirstead HS, Nistor G, Bernal G, Totoiu M, Cloutier F, Steward O. 2005. Human embryonic stem cell-derived oligodendrocyte progenitor cell transplants remyelinate and restore locomotion after spinal cord injury. *J Neurosci.* 25:4694–4705.

Kilpatrick TJ, Bartlett PF. 1993. Cloning and growth of multipotential neural precursors: requirements for proliferation and differentiation. *Neuron.* 10:255–265.

Kim JH, Auerbach LM, Rodriguez-Gomez JA et al. 2002. Dopamine neurons derived from embryonic stem cells function in an animal model of Parkinson's disease. *Nature.* 418:50–56.

Korhonen JM, Said FA, Wong AJ, Kaplan DR. 1999. Gab1 mediates neurite outgrowth, DNA synthesis, and survival in PC12 cells. *J Biol Chem.* 274:37307–37314.

Kouhara H, Hadari YR, Spivak-Kroizman T et al. 1997. A lipid-anchored Grb2-binding protein that links FGF-receptor activation to the Ras/MAPK signaling pathway. *Cell.* 89:693–702.

Kuschel S, Rüther U, Theil T. 2003. A disrupted balance between Bmp/Wnt and Fgf signaling underlies the ventralization of the *Gli3* mutant telencephalon. *Dev Biol.* 260:484–495.

Lamothe B, Yamada M, Schaeper U, Birchmeier W. 2004. The docking protein gab1 is an essential component of an indirect mechanism for fibroblast growth factor stimulation of the phosphatidylinositol 3-kinase/akt antiapoptotic pathway. *Mol Cell Biol.* 24:5657–5666.

Lee SH, Lumelsky N, Studer L, Auerbach JM, McKay RD. 2000. Efficient generation of midbrain and hindbrain neurons from mouse embryonic stem cells. *Nat Biotech.* 18:675–679.

Lee SK, Pfaff SL. 2001. Transcriptional networks regulating neuronal identity in the developing spinal cord. *Nat Neurosci.* (Suppl 4):1183–1191.

Lee H, Shamy GA, Elkabetz Y et al. 2007. Direct differentiation and transplantation of human embryonic stem cell-derived motoneurons. *Stem Cells.* 25:1931–1939.

Lefebvre S, Burglen L, Reboullet S et al. 1995. Identification and characterization of a spinal muscular atrophy-determining gene. *Cell.* 80:155–165.

Li W, LoTurco JJ. 2000. Noggin is a negative regulator of neuronal differentiation in developing neocortex. *Dev Neurosci*. 22:68–73.

Li XJ, Du ZW, Zarnowska ED et al. 2005. Specification of motoneurons from human embryonic stem cells. *Nat Biotechnol*. 23:215–221.

Lim DA, Tramontin AD, Trevejo JM, Herrera DG, Garcia-Verdugo JM, Alvarez-Buylla A. 2000. Noggin antagonizes BMP signaling to create a niche for adult neurogenesis. *Neuron*. 28:713–726.

Lim UM, Sidhu KS, Tuch BE. 2006. Derivation of motor neurons from three clonal human embryonic stem cell lines. *Curr Neurovasc Res*. 3:281–288.

Lindvall O, Zaal Kokaia Z, Martinez Serrano A. 2004. Stem cell therapy for human neurodegenerative disorders–how to make it work. *Nat Med*. 10:S42–S50.

Liu Y, Rao MS. 2004. Olig genes are expressed in a heterogeneous population of precursor cells in the developing spinal cord. *Glia*. 45:67–74.

Liu JP, Laufer E, Jessell TM. 2001. Assigning the positional identity of spinal motor neurons: rostrocaudal patterning of Hox-c expression by Fgfs, Gdf11, and retinoids. *Neuron*. 32:997–1012.

Lumsden A, Krumlauf R. 1996. Patterning the vertebrate neuraxis. *Science*. 274:1109–1115.

Mabie PC, Mehler MF, Kessler JA. 1999. Multiple roles of bone morphogenetic protein signaling in the regulation of cortical cell number and phenotype. *J Neurosci*. 19:7077–7088.

Maden M. 2002. Retinoid signalling in the development of the central nervous system. *Nat Rev Neurosci*. 3:843–853.

Maden M. 2007. Retinoic acid in the development, regeneration and maintenance of the nervous system. *Nat Rev Neurosci*. 8:755–765.

Marom K, Shapira E, Fainsod A. 1997. The chicken caudal genes establish an anterior-posterior gradient by partially overlapping temporal and spatial patterns of expression. *Mech Dev*. 64:41–52.

Marti E, Bumcrot DA, Takada R, McMahon AP. 1995. Requirement of 19K form of Sonic hedgehog for induction of distinct ventral cell types in CNS explants. *Nature*. 375:322–325.

Matsunaga E, Araki I, Nakamura H. 2000. Pax6 defines the di-mesencephalic boundary by repressing En1 and pax2. *Development*. 127:2357–2365.

McClintock JM, Kheirbek MA, Prince VE. 2002. Knockdown of duplicated zebrafish hoxb1 genes reveals distinct roles in hindbrain patterning and a novel mechanism of duplicate gene retention. *Development*. 129:2339–2354.

Melton KR, Iulianella A, Trainor PA. 2004. Gene expression and regulation of hindbrain and spinal cord development. *Front Biosci*. 9:117–138. Review.

Mendez I, Sanchez-Pernaute R, Cooper O et al. 2005. Cell type analysis of functional fetal dopamine cell suspension transplants in the striatum and substantia nigra of patients with Parkinson's disease. *Brain*. 128:1498–1510.

Miles GB, Yohn DC, Wichterle H, Jessell TM, Rafuse VF, Brownstone RM. 2004. Functional properties of motoneurons derived from mouse embryonic stem cells. *J Neurosci*. 24:7848–7858.

Mizuno K, Katagiri T, Maruyama E, Hasegawa K, Ogimoto M, Yakura H. 1997. SHP-1 is involved in neuronal differentiation of P19 embryonic carcinoma cells. *FEBS Lett*. 417:6–12.

Mizuseki K, Sakamoto T, Watanabe K et al. 2003. Generation of neural crest-derived peripheral neurons and floor plate cells from mouse and primate embryonic stem cells. *Proc Natl Acad Sci U S A*. 100:5828–5833.

Muhr J, Graziano E, Wilson S, Jessell TM, Edlund T. 1999. Convergent inductive signals specify midbrain, hindbrain, and spinal cord identity in gastrula stage chick embryos. *Neuron*. 23:689–702.

Munoz-Sanjuan I, Brivanlou A. 2001. Early posterior/ventral fate specification in the vertebrate embryo. *Dev Biol*. 237:1–17.

Munoz-Sanjuan I, Brivanlou AH. 2002. Neural induction, the default model and embryonic stem cells. *Nat Rev Neurosci*. 3:271–380.

Muotri AR, Nakashima K, Toni N, Sandler VM, Gage FH. 2005. Development of functional human embryonic stem cell-derived neurons in mouse brain. *Proc Natl Acad Sci U S A*. 20:18644–18648.

Murashov AK, Pak ES, Hendricks WA et al. 2004. Directed differentiation of embryonic stem cells into dorsal interneurons. *FASEB J*. 19:252–254.

Nagai T, Ibata K, Park ES, Kubota M, Mikoshiba K, Miyawaki A. 2002. A variant of yellow fluorescent protein with fast and efficient maturation for cell-biological applications. *Nat Biotechnol*. 20:87–90.

Niederreither K, Subbarayan V, Dolle P, Chambon P. 1999. Embryonic retinoic acid synthesis is essential for early mouse post-implantation development. *Nat Genet*. 21:444–448.

Nordstrom U, Jessell TM, Edlund T. 2002. Progressive induction of caudal neural character by graded Wnt signaling. *Nat Neurosci*. 5:525–532.

Nordstrom U, Maier E, Jessell TM, Edlund T. 2006. An early role for Wnt signaling in specifying neural patterns of Cdx and Hox gene expression and motor neuron subtype identity. *PloS Biol*. 4:1438–1452.

Novitch BG, Wichterle H, Jessell TM, Sockanathan S. 2003. A requirement for retinoic acid-mediated transcriptional activation in ventral neural patterning and motor neuron specification. *Neuron*. 40(1):81–95.

Okabe S, Forsberg-Nilsson K, Spiro AC, Segal M, McKay RD. 1996. Development of neuronal precursor cells and functional postmitotic neurons from embryonic stem cells in vitro. *Mech Dev*. 59:89–102.

Okada Y, Shimazaki T, Sobue G, Okano H. 2004. Retinoic-acid-concentration dependent acquisition of neural cell identity during in vitro differentiation of mouse embryonic stem cells. *Dev Biol*. 275:124–142.

O'Rahilly R, Muller F. 1994. Neurulation in the normal human embryo. *Ciba Found Symp*. 181:70–82.

O'Rahilly R, Muller F. 2007. The development of the neural crest in the human. *J Anat*. 211:335–351.

Osterfield M, Kirschner MW, JG Flanagan. 2003. Graded positional information: interpretation for both fate and guidance. *Cell*. 113:425–428.

Panchision DM, McKay RD. 2002. The control of neural stem cells by morphogenic signals. *Curr Opin Genet Dev.* 12:478–487. Review.

Pierani A, Brenner-Morton S, Chiang C, Jessell TM. 1999. A sonic hedgehog-independent, retinoid-activated pathway of neurogenesis in the ventral spinal cord. *Cell.* 97:903–915.

Plachta N, Bibel M, Tucker KL, Barde YA. 2004. Developmental potential of defined neural progenitors derived from mouse embryonic stem cells. *Development.* 131:5449–5456.

Placzek M. 1995. The role of the notochord and floor plate in inductive interactions. *Curr Opin Genet Dev.* 5:499–506.

Placzek M, Dodd J, Jessell TM. 2000. The case for floor plate induction by the notochord. *Curr Opin Neurobiol.* 10:15–22.

Rathjen J, Haines BP, Hudson KM, Nesci A, Dunn S, Rathjen PD. 2002. Directed differentiation of pluripotent cells to neural lineages: homogeneous formation and differentiation of a neurectoderm population. *Development.* 129:2649–2661.

Rathjen J, Rathjen PD. 2002. Formation of neural precursor cell populations by differentiation of embryonic stem cells in vitro. *Scientific World J.* 2:690–700. Review.

Reiner A, Albin RL, Anderson KD, D'Amato CJ, Penney JB, Young AB. 1988. Differential loss of striatal projection neurons in Huntington disease. *Proc Natl Acad Sci U S A.* 85:5733–5737.

Renoncourt Y, Carroll P, Filippi P, Arce V, Alonso S. 1998. Neurons derived in vitro from ES cells express homeoproteins characteristic of motoneurons and interneurons. *Mech Dev.* 79:185–197.

Represa A, Shimazaki T, Simmonds M, Weiss S. 2001. EGF-responsive neural stem cells are a transient population in the developing mouse spinal cord. *Eur J Neurosci.* 14:452–462.

Reubinoff BE, Pera MF, Fong CY, Trounson A, Bongso A. 2000. Embryonic stem cell lines from human blastocysts: somatic differentiation in vitro. *Nat Biotechnol.* 18:399–404.

Reubinoff BE, Itsykson P, Turetsky T et al. 2001. Neural progenitors from human embryonic stem cells. *Nat Biotechnol.* 19:1134–1140.

Richardson RM, Holloway KL, Bullock MR, et al. 2006. Isolation of neuronal progenitor cells from the adult human neocortex. *Acta Neurochir (Wien).* 148:773–777.

Roelink H, Porter JA, Chiang C et al. 1995. Floor plate and motor neuron induction by different concentrations of the amino-terminal cleavage product of sonic hedgehog autoproteolysis. *Cell.* 81:445–455.

Ruiz I Altaba A, Jessell TM, Roelink H. 1995. Restrictions to floor plate induction by hedgehog and winged-helix genes in the neural tube of frog embryos. *Mol Cell Neurosci.* 6:106–121.

Sapp E, Ge P, Aizawa H et al. 1995. Evidence for a preferential loss of enkephalin immunoreactivity in the external globus pallidus in low grade Huntington's disease using high resolution image analysis. *Neuroscience.* 64:397–404.

Sasaki H, Hogan BL. 1994. HNF-3 beta as a regulator of floor plate development. *Cell.* 76:103–115.

Schuldiner M, Eiges R, Eden A et al. 2001. Induced neuronal differentiation of human embryonic stem cells. *Brain Res.* 913:201–205.

Shah V, Drill E, Lance-Jones C. 2004. Ectopic expression of Hoxd10 in thoracic spinal segments induces motoneurons with a lumbosacral molecular profile and axon projections to the limb. *Dev Dyn.* 231:43–56.

Sharma K, Sheng HZ, Lettieri K et al. 1998. LIM homeodomain factors Lhx3 and Lhx4 assign subtype identities for motor neurons. *Cell.* 95:817–828.

Sheng G, Dos RM, Stern CD. 2003. Churchill, a zinc finger transcriptional activator, regulates the transition between gastrulation and neurulation. *Cell.* 115:603–613.

Shin SJ, Dalton S, Stice SL. 2005. Human motor neuron differentiation form human embryonic stem cells. *Stem Cells Dev.* 14:1–4.

Sidhu KS, Ryan JP, Tuch BE. 2008. Derivation of a new hESC line, endeavour-1 and its clonal propagation. *Stem Cells Dev.* 17:41–51.

Simeone A. 2000. Positioning the isthmic organizer: where otx2 and gbx2 meet. *Trends Genet.* 16:237–240.

Singh RN, Nakano T, Xuing I, Kang J, Nedergaard M, Goldman SA. 2005. Enhancer specified GFP-based FACS purification of human spinal motor neurons from embryonic stem cells. *Exp Neurol.* 196:224–234.

Sockanathan S, Jessell TM. 1998. Motor neuron-derived retinoid signalling specifies the subtype identity of spinal motor neurons. *Cell.* 94:503–514.

Sockanathan S, Perlmann T, Jessell TM. 2003. Retinoid receptor signalling in post-mitotic motor neurons regulates rostrocaudal positional identity and axonal projection pattern. *Neuron.* 40:97–111.

Soundararajan P, Miles GB, Rubin LL, Brownstone RM, Rafuse VF. 2006. Motoneurons derived from embryonic stem cells express transcription factors and develop phenotypes characteristic of medial motor column neurons. *J Neurosci.* 26:3256–3268.

Soundararajan P, Lindsey BW, Leopold C, Rafuse VF. 2007. Easy and rapid differentiation of embryonic stem cells into functional motoneurons using sonic hedgehog-producing cells. *Stem Cells.* 25:1697–1706.

Stallcup WB, Beasley L. 1987. Bipotential glial precursor cells of the optic nerve express the ng2 proteoglycan. *J Neurosci.* 7:2737–2744.

Stapf C, Luck G, Shakibaei M, Blotter D. 1997. Fibroblast growth factor-2 (FGF-2) and FGF-receptor (FGFR-1) immunoreactivity in embryonic spinal autonomic neurons. *Cell Tissue Res.* 287:471–480.

Steiner B, Wolf SA, Kempermann G. 2006. Adult neurogenesis and neurodegenerative disease. *Regenerative Med.* 1:15–28.

Strubing C, Ahnert-Hilger G, Shan J, Wiedenmann B, Hescheler J, Wobus AM. 1995. Differentiation of pluripotent embryonic stem cells into the neuronal lineage in vitro gives rise to mature inhibitory and excitatory neurons. *Mech Dev.* 53:275–287.

Sun T, Pringle NP, Hardy AP, Richardson WD, Smith HK. 1998. Pax6 influences the time and site of origin of glial precursors in the ventral neural tube. *Mol Cell Neurosci.* 12:228–239.

Sun T, Echelard Y, Lu R et al. 2001. Olig bHLH proteins interact with homeodomain proteins to regulate cell fate acquisition in progenitors of the ventral neural tube. *Curr Biol.* 11:1413–1420.

Tanabe Y, William C, Jessell TM. 1998. Specification of motor neuron identity by the MNR2 homeodomain protein. *Cell.* 95:67–80

Teillet MA, Lapointe F, Le Douarin NM. 1998. The relationships between notochord and floor plate in vertebrate development revisited. *Proc Natl Acad Sci U S A.* 95:11733–11738.

Theys PA, Peeters E, Robberecht W. 1999. Evolution of motor and sensory deficits in amyotrophic lateral sclerosis estimated by neurophysiological techniques. *J Neurol.* 246:438–442.

Thompson L, Barraud P, Andersson E, Kirik D, Bjorklund A. 2005. Identification of dopaminergic neurons of nigral and ventral tegmental area subtypes in grafts of fetal ventral mesencephalon based on cell morphology, protein expression, and efferent projections. *J Neurosci.* 25:6467–6477.

Thomson JA, Itskovitz-Eldor J, Shapiro SS, Swiergiergiel JJ, Marshall VS, Jones JM. 1998. Embryonic stem cell lines derived from human blastocysts. *Science.* 282:1145–1147.

Thomson JA, Odorico JS. 2000. Human embryonic stem cell and embryonic germ cell lines. *Trends Biotechnol.* 18:53–57.

Tosney KW, Landmesser LT. 1985a. Growth cone morphology and trajectory in the lumbosacral region of the chick embryo. *J Neurosci.* 5:2345–2358.

Tosney KW, Landmesser LT. 1985b. Specificity of early motoneuron growth cone outgrowth in the chick embryo. *J Neurosci.* 5:2336–2344.

Trainor PA, Krumlauf R. 2001. Hox genes, neural crest cells, and branchial arch patterning. *Curr Opin Cell Biol.* 13:698–705.

Tropepe V, Hitoshi S, Sirard C, Mak TW, Rossant J, van der Kooy D. 2001. Direct neural fate specification from embryonic stem cells: a primitive mammalian neural stem cell stage acquired through a default mechanism. *Neuron.* 30:65–78.

Valenzuela M, Sidhu K, Dean S, Sachdev P. 2007. Neural stem cell therapy for neuropsychiatric disorders (Invited Review). *Acta Neuropsychiatrica.* 19:11–26.

Vallstedt A, Klos JM, Ericson J. 2005. Multiple dorsoventral origins of oligodendrocyte. *Neuron.* 45:1–3.

van den Akker E, Forlani S, Chawengsaksophak K et al. 2002. Cdx1 and Cdx2 have overlapping functions in anteroposterior patterning and posterior axis elongation. *Development.* 129:2181–2193.

Verani R, Cappuccio I, Spinsanti P et al. 2007. Expression of the Wnt inhibitor Dickkopf-1 is required for the induction of neural markers in mouse embryonic stem cells differentiating in response to retinoic acid. *J Neurochem.* 100:242–250.

Wichterle H, Lieberam I, Porter JA, Jessell TM. 2002. Directed differentiation of embryonic stem cells into motor neurons. *Cell.* 110:385–397.

Williams JA, Guicherit OM, Zaharian BI et al. 2003. Identification of a small molecule inhibitor of the hog signaling pathway: effects on basal cell carcinoma-like lesions. *Proc Natl Acad Sci U S A.* 100:4616–4621.

Wilson L, Gale E, Chambers D, Maden M. 2004. Retinoic acid and the control of dorsoventral patterning in the avian spinal cord. *Dev Biol.* 269:433–446.

Wilson L, Maden M. 2005. The mechanisms of dorsoventral patterning in the vertebrate neural tube. *Dev Biol.* 282:1–13.

Wilson SI, Edlund T. 2001. Neural induction: toward a unifying mechanism. *Nat Neurosci.* (Suppl 4):1161–1168.

Wilson SI, Rydstrom A, Trimborn T et al. 2001. The status of Wnt signalling regulates neural and epidermal fates in the chick embryo. *Nature.* 411:325–330.

Wilson SI, Graziano E, Harland R, Jessell TM, Edlund T. 2000. An early requirement for FGF signalling in the acquisition of neural cell fate in the chick embryo. *Curr Biol.* 10:421–429.

Wobus AM, Grosse R, Schoneich J. 1988. Specific effects of nerve growth factor on the differentiation pattern of mouse embryonic stem cells in vitro. *Biomed Biochim Acta.* 47:965–973.

Wu H, Xu J, Pang ZP et al. 2007. Integrative genomic and functional analyses reveal neuronal subtype differentiation bias in human embryonic stem cell lines. *Proc Natl Acad Sci U S A.* 21:13821–13826.

Yamada T, McGeer PL, Baimbridge KG, McGeer EG. 1990. Relative sparing in Parkinson's disease of substantia nigra dopamine neurons containing calbindin-D28K. *Brain Res.* 526:303–307.

Yamamoto S, Yoshino I, Shimazaki T et al. 2005. Essential role of Shp2-binding sites on FRS2alpha for corticogenesis and for FGF2-dependent proliferation of neural progenitor cells. *Proc Natl Acad Sci U S A.* 102:15983–15988.

Ying QL, Stavridis M, Griffiths D, Li M, Smith A. 2003. Conversion of embryonic stem cells into neuroectodermal precursors in adherent monoculture. *Nat Biotechnol.* 21:183–186.

Zeng X, Rao M. 2007. Human embryonic stem cells: long term stability, absence of senescence and a potential cell source for neural replacement. *Neuroscience.* 145:1348–1358.

Zhang SC, Wernig M, Duncan ID, Brustle O, Thomson JA. 2001. In vitro differentiation of transplantable neural precursors from human embryonic stem cells. *Nat Biotechnol.* 19:1129–1133.

Zhang SC. 2003. Embryonic stem cells for neural replacement therapy: prospects and challenges. *J Hematother Stem Cell Res.* 12:625–634.

Zhao X, Liu J, Ahmad I. 2002. Differentiation of embryonic stem cells into retinal neurons. *Biochem Biophys Res Comm.* 297:177–184.

Zhou Q, Anderson DJ. 2002. The bHLH transcription factors olig2 and olig1 couple neuronal and glial subtype specification. *Cell.* 109:61–73.

Chapter **10**

ADULT NEUROGENESIS, NEUROINFLAMMATION, AND THERAPEUTIC POTENTIAL OF ADULT NEURAL STEM CELLS

Philippe Taupin*

ABSTRACT

Contrary to a long-held dogma, neurogenesis occurs throughout adulthood in mammals, including humans. Neurogenesis occurs primarily in two regions of the adult brain, the hippocampus and the subventricular zone (SVZ), along the ventricles. Neural progenitor and stem cells have been isolated from various regions of the adult central nervous system (CNS) and characterized in vitro, providing evidence that neural stem cells (NSCs) reside in the adult CNS and are potential sources of tissue for therapy. Adult neurogenesis is modulated in animal models and patients with neurological diseases and disorders, such as Alzheimer's disease, depression, and epilepsy. The contribution of adult neurogenesis to neurological diseases and disorders, and its significance, remains to be elucidated. The confirmation that neurogenesis occurs in the adult brain and that NSCs reside in the adult CNS is as important for our understanding of the development, physiology, and pathology of the nervous system as it is for therapy. Cellular therapy may involve the stimulation of endogenous neural progenitor or stem cells and the grafting of neural progenitor and stem cells to restore the degenerated or injured pathways. Mounting evidence suggests that neuroinflammation is involved in the pathogenesis of neurological diseases and disorders. Neural progenitor and stem cells express receptors involved in neuroinflammation, and neuroinflammation modulates neurogenesis in the adult brain. Hence, neuroinflammation may underlie the contribution of adult neurogenesis to the pathologies of the nervous system and the therapeutic potential of adult NSCs.

Keywords: bromodeoxyuridine, cell cycle, cellular therapy, neurodegenerative diseases, neurological diseases.

Most nerve cells in the adult mammalian central nervous system (CNS) are post-mitotic and differentiated cells (Cajal 1928). They are born from primordial stem cells during development. It was believed that the adult brain was devoid of stem cells, and hence lacked the capacity to generate new nerve cells and regenerate after injury. Studies in the 1960s and,

*Current address: Scientific Director, Fighting Blindness Vision Research Institute, Dublin City University, Dublin, Ireland.

mostly, in the 1980s and 1990s (Taupin, Gage 2002) have reported and confirmed that, contrary to this long-held dogma, neurogenesis occurs in the adult brain of mammals (Gross 2000; Kaplan 2001). The confirmation that neurogenesis occurs in the adult mammalian brain has tremendous consequences for our understanding of brain development and functioning, as well as for therapy.

NEUROGENESIS AND NEURAL STEM CELLS IN THE ADULT CNS

Neurogenesis occurs primarily in two discrete regions of the adult brain, the dentate gyrus (DG) of the hippocampus and the anterior part of the subventricular zone (SVZ), in various species (Taupin, Gage 2002), including humans (Eriksson, Perfilieva, Bjork-Eriksson et al. 1998; Curtis, Kam, Nannmark et al. 2007). Newborn neuronal cells in the anterior part of the SVZ migrate to the olfactory bulb (OB) through the rostromigratory stream (RMS) (Luskin 1993; Lois, Alvarez-Buylla 1994). They differentiate in the OB into functional interneurons (Belluzzi, Benedusi, Ackman et al. 2003). In humans, the RMS is organized differently than in other species, around a lateral ventricular extension reaching the OB (Curtis, Kam, Nannmark et al. 2007). In the DG, newborn neuronal cells in the subgranular zone (SGZ) migrate to the granule cell layer, where they differentiate into granule-like cells (Cameron, Woolley, McEwen et al. 1993). They establish functional connections with neighboring cells (van Praag, Schinder, Christie et al. 2002; Toni, Teng, Bushong et al. 2007) and extend axonal projections to the CA3 region of Ammon's horn (Stanfield, Trice 1988; Markakis, Gage 1999). Newborn granule-like cells in the DG survive for an extended period of time—at least 2 years in humans (Eriksson, Perfilieva, Bjork-Eriksson et al. 1998). Neurogenesis may also occur in other areas of the adult brain, such as the neocortex (Gould, Reeves, Graziano et al. 1999), CA1 area (Rietze, Poulin, Weiss et al. 2000), and substantia nigra (SN) (Zhao, Momma, Delfani et al. 2003). However, some of these data have been the source of debates and controversies (Kornack, Rakic 2001; Frielingsdorf, Schwarz, Brundin et al. 2004), and remain to be further confirmed.

In rodents, 65.3% to 76.9% of bulbar neurons are replaced during a 6-week period (Kato, Yokouchi, Fukushima et al. 2001). In the DG, as many as 9000 new neuronal cells are generated per day in young adult rodents, contributing to about 3.3% per month or about 0.1% per day of the granule cell population (Kempermann, Kuhn, Gage et al. 1997; Cameron, McKay 2001). In the adult macaque monkey, at least 0.004% of the neuronal population in the granule cell layer consists of new neurons generated per day

(Kornack, Rakic 1999). The rate of neurogenesis in the human DG was also reported to be low (Eriksson, Perfilieva, Bjork-Eriksson et al. 1998). The reasons for the apparent decline of adult neurogenesis in primates are unclear. The decline of adult neurogenesis during vertebrate evolution could be an adaptive strategy to maintain stable neuronal populations throughout life (Rakic 1985).

It is hypothesized that newborn neuronal cells in the adult brain originate from residual stem cells. Neural stem cells (NSCs) are the self-renewing multipotent cells that generate the main phenotypes of the nervous system (Gage 2000) (Fig. 10.1). Neural progenitor cells are multipotent cells with limited proliferative capabilities. Self-renewing multipotent neural progenitor and stem cells have been isolated and characterized in vitro from various regions of the adult CNS, including the spinal cord (Reynolds, Weiss 1992; Gage, Coates, Palmer et al. 1995; Gritti, Parati, Cova et al. 1996; Palmer, Takahashi, Gage 1997; Shihabuddin, Horner, Ray et al. 2000). In the adult brain, populations of ependymocytes and astrocytes have been identified and proposed as candidates for stem cells in the DG and SVZ (Chiasson, Tropepe, Morshead et al. 1999; Doetsch, Caille, Lim et al. 1999; Johansson, Momma, Clarke et al. 1999; Seri, Garcia-Verdugo, McEwen et al. 2001). Despite being

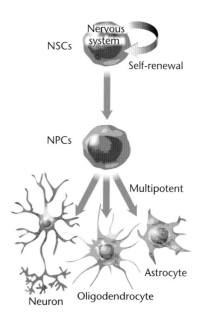

Figure 10.1 Neural stem cells. Neural stem cells (NSCs) are the self-renewing multipotent cells that generate the main phenotypes of the nervous system. Neural progenitor cells (NPCs) are multipotent cells, with limited proliferative capabilities. In the adult brain, populations of ependymocytes and astrocytes have been identified and proposed as candidates for stem cells. Self-renewing multipotent neural progenitor and stem cells have been isolated and characterized in vitro from various regions of the adult CNS. Adapted with permission from Taupin and Gage 2002.

characterized in vitro and in situ, NSCs are still elusive cells in the adult CNS. They remain to be unequivocally identified and characterized (Kornblum, Geschwind 2001; Suslov, Kukekov, Ignatova et al. 2002; Fortunel, Out, Ng et al. 2003).

In all, neurogenesis occurs in the adult brain and NSCs reside in the adult CNS, in mammals. It is a functional neurogenesis and NSCs remain to be unequivocally identified and characterized in the adult CNS. The confirmation that neurogenesis occurs in the adult brain and NSCs reside in the adult CNS has tremendous implications for our understanding of the development and functioning of the nervous system, particularly for our understanding of the etiology and pathogenesis of neurological diseases and disorders, as well as for therapy.

ADULT NEUROGENESIS IN NEUROLOGICAL DISEASES AND DISORDERS

Adult neurogenesis is modulated in a broad range of neurological diseases and disorders, such as Alzheimer's disease, depression, epilepsy, and Huntington's and Parkinson's diseases, and in animal models of these conditions (Table 10.1).

Alzheimer's Disease

Alzheimer's disease (AD) is a progressive neurodegenerative disease that starts with mild memory problems and ends with severe brain damage. It is associated with the loss of nerve cells in areas of the brain that are vital to memory and other mental abilities, such as the hippocampus. AD is characterized by amyloid plaque deposits and neurofibrillary tangles in the brain (Caselli, Beach, Yaari et al. 2006). There are two forms of the disease: the early-onset, or familial, form, and the late-onset, or sporadic, form of AD. The early-onset form of AD is a rare form of the disease. Approximately 10% of patients with AD have the familial form. It is the genetic form of the disease and is inherited. It appears at a young age. Mutations in three genes, *presenilin 1*, *presenilin 2*, and *amyloid precursor protein* (*APP*), have been identified as causes of the early-onset form of AD (St George-Hyslop, Petit 2005). The late-onset form is not inherited. It appears generally at an older age (above age 65). The origin of the late-onset form of AD remains unknown; risk factors include expression of different forms of the gene *apolipoprotein* (Raber, Huang, Ashford et al. 2004) and reduced expression of neuronal sortilin-related receptor gene (Rogaeva, Meng, Lee et al. 2007). The late-onset form of AD is the most common type of dementia among older people. AD is the fourth

Table 10.1 Modulation of Adult Neurogenesis in Neurological Diseases and Disorders

Disease/Model	Regulation	References
Alzheimer's disease		
Autopsies	Increase	Jin (2004a)
Transgenic mice, Swedish and Indiana APP mutations	Increase	Jin (2004b)
Knockout/deficient mice for presenilin 1 (PS-1) and APP	Decrease	Feng (2001) Wen (2002)
Depression		
Autopsies	Not altered	Reif (2006)
Epilepsy		
Animal model— pilocarpine treatment	Increase	Parent (1997)
Huntington's disease		
Autopsies	Increase	Curtis (2003)
R6/1 transgenic mouse model of HD	Decrease	Lazic (2004)
Quinolinic acid striatal lesion	Increase	Tattersfield (2004)
Parkinson's disease		
MPTP lesion	Increase	Zhao (2003)
6-Hydroxydopamine lesion	Not altered	Frielingsdorf (2004)

Adult neurogenesis is modulated in a broad range of neurological diseases and disorders, and in animal models, such as Alzheimer's disease, depression, epilepsy, and Huntington's and Parkinson's diseases. The contribution and significance of this modulation is yet to be elucidated. Newborn neuronal cells may be involved in regenerative attempts and plasticity of the nervous system.

highest cause of death in the developed world. There is currently no cure for AD. Actual treatments consist of drug therapy, physical support, and assistance (Caselli, Beach, Yaari et al. 2006).

Neurogenesis is increased in the hippocampus of brains of patients with AD, as revealed after autopsies by an increase in the expression of markers for immature neuronal cells, such as doublecortin and polysialylated nerve cell adhesion molecule, in hippocampal regions (Jin, Peel, Mao et al. 2004). In animal models of AD, neurogenesis is increased in the DG of transgenic mice expressing the Swedish and Indiana APP mutations, mutant forms of human APP (Jin, Galvan, Xie et al. 2004), and decreased in the DG and SVZ of knockout mice for presenilin 1 and APP (Feng, Rampon, Tang et al. 2001; Wen, Shao, Shao et al. 2002).

Hence, there are discrepancies in the data observed on adult neurogenesis in brain autopsies of patients with AD and animal models of AD. These discrepancies may originate from the limitations of animal models, particularly transgenic mice, as representative models of complex diseases, particularly AD (Dodart, Mathis,

Bales et al. 2002), and for studying adult phenotypes, such as adult neurogenesis. Further, high levels (4% to 10%) of tetraploid nerve cells have been reported in regions in which degeneration occurs in AD, such as in the hippocampus (Yang, Geldmacher, Herrup et al. 2001). It is proposed that cell cycle reentry and DNA duplication, without cell proliferation, precede neuronal death in degenerating regions of the CNS (Herrup, Neve, Ackerman et al. 2004). Some of the data, observed by means of immunohistochemistry for cell cycle proteins and bromodeoxuridine (BrdU) labeling, may therefore represent not adult neurogenesis but rather labeled nerve cells that may have entered the cell cycle and undergone DNA replication without completing the cell cycle (Taupin 2007). In the end, though adult neurogenesis is increased in the adult brain with AD, these data remain to be further investigated and confirmed.

Depression

Depression is a major public health issue; 8% of adolescents and 25% of adults will have a major depressive episode sometime in their life (Kessler, McGonagle, Zhao et al. 1994). The hippocampus of patients with depression shows signs of atrophy and neuronal loss (Sheline, Wang, Gado et al. 1996; Colla, Kronenberg, Deuschle et al. 2007). Current treatments consist of drug therapy and psychological support (Wong, Licinio 2001). Among the drugs used to treat depression are selective serotonin reuptake inhibitors, such as fluoxetine.

Chronic administration of antidepressants such as fluoxetine increases neurogenesis in the DG but not in the SVZ in adult rats (Malberg, Eisch, Nestler et al. 2000; Malberg, Duman 2003). Stress is an important causal factor in precipitating episodes of depression, and it decreases hippocampal neurogenesis in adult monkeys (Gould, Tanapat, McEwen et al. 1998). It is proposed that the waning and waxing of hippocampal neurogenesis are important causal factors in the precipitation of and recovery from episodes of clinical depression (Jacobs, Praag, Gage 2000) (Fig. 10.2).

Further support for the role of adult neurogenesis in depression has come from pharmacological studies (Santarelli, Saxe, Gross et al. 2003). These show that adult neurogenesis may be important in the etiology of depression and for the mediation of the activity of drugs such as selective serotonin reuptake inhibitors to treat depression. However, the importance of the hippocampus and adult neurogenesis in depression has been challenged by others (Campbell, Macqueen 2004; Reif, Fritzen, Finger 2006). In particular, some studies report that hippocampal volume and neurogenesis remain unchanged in depressive patients.

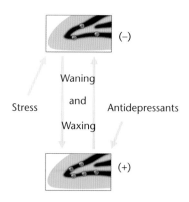

Figure 10.2 Adult neurogenesis, depression, and the effects of antidepressants. Stress is an important causal factor in precipitating episodes of depression and decreases hippocampal neurogenesis in adult monkeys. It is proposed that the waning and waxing of hippocampal neurogenesis are important causal factors in the precipitation and recovery from episodes of clinical depression. Chronic administration of antidepressants, such as fluoxetine, increases neurogenesis in the dentate gyrus. Hence, adult neurogenesis may be important in the etiology of depression and for the mediation of drug activity to treat of depression. However, the importance of the hippocampus and adult neurogenesis in the depression remain to be established.

Hence, the links among the hippocampus, adult neurogenesis, and depression remain to be further established.

Epilepsy

Epilepsy is a brain disorder in which populations of neurons signal abnormally. In the individual, this translates into a variety of seizures with symptoms that range from mild changes in behavior to more severe symptoms, such as convulsions, muscle spasms, and loss of consciousness. The hippocampal formation is a critical area in the pathology of epilepsy. Patients suffering from temporal lobe epilepsy show a hippocampal formation with a dispersed granular cell layer and ectopic granule-like cells in the hilus (Houser 1990). Dentate granule cells give rise to abnormal axonal projections, or mossy fiber (MF) sprouting, in the supragranular inner molecular layer of the DG and basal dendrites of CA3 pyramidal cells in the stratum oriens (Sutula, Cascino, Cavazos et al. 1989; Represa, Tremblay, Ben-Ari 1990). Epilepsy is one of the most prevalent neurological disorders, affecting approximately 1% of Americans.

Neurogenesis is increased in the DG of animal models of epilepsy, such as after pilocarpine treatment (Parent, Yu, Leibowitz et al. 1997). In this model, ectopic granule-like cells in the hilus of the DG and the CA3 cell layer are labeled for BrdU. The authors present data suggesting that MF remodeling derives from newborn granule-like cells rather than from preexisting mature dentate granule cells. These data indicate that neurogenesis is enhanced in the brain following limbic-induced seizures and that newborn cells in the DG contribute to hippocampal plasticity associated with seizures, such as the generation of ectopic granule-like cells and MF sprouting.

These data have been challenged by subsequent studies (Parent, Tada, Fike et al. 1999). Low-dose, whole-brain, X-ray irradiation in adult rats inhibits dentate granule cell neurogenesis (Tada, Parent, Lowenstein et al. 2000). Low-dose, whole-brain, X-ray irradiation in adult rats, after pilocarpine treatment, does not prevent the induction of recurrent seizures or the generation of seizure-induced ectopic granule-like cells and MF sprouting. These data show that seizure-induced ectopic granule-like cells and MF sprouting arise not only from newborn neuronal cells, as previously reported (Parent, Tada, Fike et al. 1999), but also from mature dentate granule cells. These data provide a strong argument against a critical role of adult neurogenesis in epileptogenesis. However, although increased hippocampal neurogenesis may not be critical to epileptogenesis, it could be a contributing factor to limbic seizures when present.

Huntington's Disease

Huntington's disease (HD) results from genetically programmed degeneration of neuronal cells in certain areas of the brain (Sawa, Tomoda, Bae et al. 2003). This degeneration causes uncontrolled movements, loss of intellectual faculties, and emotional disturbance. The caudate nucleus is the most severely and preferentially affected region of the brain in HD. HD is a familial disease, inherited through a mutation—a polyglutamine repeat/expansion that lengthens a glutamine segment in the huntingtin protein (Li, Li 2004).

Immunohistochemistry and confocal microscopy analysis at autopsies for markers of the cell cycle and neuronal differentiation, such as proliferating cell nuclear antigen and β-tubulin, show that cell proliferation and neurogenesis are increased in the SVZ of brains of patients with HD (Curtis, Penney, Pearson et al. 2003). In the adult R6/1 transgenic mouse model of HD, neurogenesis decreases in the DG (Lazic, Grote, Armstrong et al. 2004). Tattersfield et al. (2004) reported that after quinolinic acid striatal lesioning of adult brain, neurogenesis is increased in the SVZ, leading to the migration of neuroblasts and formation of new neurons in damaged areas of the striatum, as observed in brains of HD patients (Curtis, Penney, Pearson et al. 2003).

These data provide evidence that adult neurogenesis is increased in the SVZ of brains with HD. It also shows that neural progenitor cells from the SVZ migrate toward the site of degeneration in HD. Data from an R6/1 transgenic mouse model of HD are difficult to interpret in the context of adult neurogenesis in HD, as mutated forms of huntingtin affect brain development (White, Auerbach, Duyao et al. 1997). This could underlie the decrease of neurogenesis reported in adult R6/1 transgenic mice.

Parkinson's Disease

Parkinson's disease (PD) is a chronic and progressive neurodegenerative disease, primarily associated with the loss of a specific type of dopamine neuron in the SN (Fernandez-Espejo 2004). The four primary symptoms of PD are tremors, rigidity, bradykinesia, and postural instability. The disease is considerably more common in the above-50 age group. The cause of PD is mostly unknown. Certain mutations in genes such as *α-synuclein* and *Parkin* have been associated with a risk of developing PD, but PD is not usually inherited (Douglas, Lewthwaite, Nicholl 2007). A variety of medications provide relief from the symptoms. However, no drug yet can stop the progression of the disease, and in many cases medications lose their benefit over time. In such cases, surgery, such as deep brain stimulation, pallidotomy, or transplantation, may be considered (Volkmann 2007).

One study reports that the rate of neurogenesis, measured by BrdU labeling, is stimulated in the SN following lesion induced by a systemic dose of MPTP (1-methyl-4-phenyl-1,2,3,6-tetrahydropyridine) (Zhao, Momma, Delfani et al. 2003). Another study reports no evidence of new dopaminergic neurons in the SN of 6-hydroxydopamine-lesioned hemi-parkinsonian rodents (Frielingsdorf, Schwarz, Brundin et al. 2004).

Hence, neurogenesis in the SN is the source of debate and controversy. Therefore, reports that neurogenesis can be stimulated in the SN must be approached with caution, and need to be confirmed.

In all, neurogenesis is enhanced in many neurological diseases and disorders. However, these data remain to be further evaluated and confirmed. The role, contribution, and significance of enhanced neurogenesis in the etiology and pathogenesis of neurological diseases and disorders remain to be established.

THERAPEUTIC POTENTIAL OF ADULT NEURAL STEM CELLS

Cellular therapy is the replacement of unhealthy or damaged cells or tissues by new ones. Because of their potential to generate the different cell types of the nervous system, NSCs hold the promise to cure a broad range of CNS diseases and injuries. The recent confirmation that neurogenesis occurs in the adult brain and that NSCs reside in the adult mammalian CNS suggests that the CNS may be amenable to repair, and offers new opportunities for cellular therapy in the CNS (Taupin 2006a). Cell therapeutic intervention may involve the stimulation or transplantation of neural progenitor and stem cells of the adult CNS.

Stimulation of Neural Progenitor or Stem Cells of the Adult CNS

Self-renewing multipotent neural progenitor and stem cells have been isolated and characterized in vitro from various regions of the adult mammalian CNS, including the spinal cord (Reynolds, Weiss 1992; Gage, Coates, Palmer et al. 1995; Gritti, Parati, Cova et al. 1996; Palmer, Takahashi, Gage et al. 1997; Shihabuddin, Horner, Ray et al. 2000). This suggests that neural progenitor and stem cells reside throughout the adult CNS in mammals. The stimulation of endogenous neural progenitor or stem cells locally would represent a strategy to promote regeneration of the diseased and/or injured nervous system. The administration of platelet-derived growth factor (PDGF) and brain-derived neurotrophic factor (BDNF) induces neurogenesis in the striatum in adult rats with 6-hydroxydopamine lesions, with no indications of any newborn neuronal cells displaying a dopaminergic phenotype (Mohapel, Frielingsdorf, Haggblad et al. 2005). The administration of glial cell line–derived neurotrophic factor (GDNF) increases cell proliferation in the SN significantly, with new cells displaying glial features, and none of the newborn BrdU-positive cells co-label for the dopamine neuronal marker tyrosine hydroxylase (TH) (Chen, Ai, Slevin et al. 2005). The increase in TH activity observed after administration of GDNF results not from neurogenic activity but from a restorative activity of GDNF (Slevin, Gerhardt, Smith et al. 2005). Hence, stimulation of endogenous neural progenitor and stem cells locally remains to be validated as a strategy for repairing the nervous system.

New neuronal cells are generated at sites of degeneration in the diseased brain and after CNS injuries, such as in HD and experimental models of cerebral strokes (Arvidsson, Collin, Kirik et al. 2002; Curtis, Penney, Pearson et al. 2003; Jin, Sun, Xie et al. 2003). These cells originate from the SVZ and migrate partially through the RMS to the sites of degeneration. This suggests that strategies to promote regeneration and repair may focus on stimulating SVZ neurogenesis. The intracerebroventricular administration of

Table 10.2 Stimulation of Endogenous Neural Progenitor or Stem Cells in the Adult Brain

Trophic Factors	Neurogenic Activity	References
PDGF/BDNF	Neurogenesis in striatum, after 6-hydroxydopamine lesions	Mohapel (2005)
GDNF	Proliferation in substantia nigra	Chen (2005)
GDNF	Increased TH activity	Slevin (2005)
EGF	SVZ neurogenesis	Craig (1996), Kuhn (1997)

The stimulation of endogenous neural progenitor or stem cells represents a strategy to promote regeneration of the diseased and injured nervous system. Various trophic factors and cytokines have been studied for their activity in promoting endogenous neurogenesis in the adult brain and in animal models of neurological diseases.

BDNF, brain-derived neurotrophic factor; EGF, epidermal growth factor; GDNF, glial cell line–derived neurotrophic factor; PDGF, platelet-derived growth factor.

trophic factors provides a strategy to promote SVZ neurogenesis in the diseased or injured nervous system (Craig, Tropepe, Morshead et al. 1996; Kuhn, Winkler, Kempermann et al. 1997). Newborn neuronal cells in the adult brain undergo programmed cell death before achieving maturity (Morshead, van der Kooy 1992; Cameron, McKay 2001). Thus, administration of factors preventing cell death, such as caspases, would also be potentially beneficial for cellular therapy to promote SVZ neurogenesis, alone or in combination with the administration of trophic factors (Ekdahl, Mohapel, Elmer et al. 2001).

To summarize, various strategies can be considered to stimulate endogenous neurogenesis to promote brain repair in the diseased and/or injured brain (Table 10.2). These strategies have yet to be experimentally validated before their potential use for therapeutic applications can be proved. However, two trophic factors/cytokines, human chorionic gonadotropin and erythropoietin, are currently in clinical trial (phase IIa) in Canada for the treatment of cerebral strokes. The aim of this clinical trial is to promote the proliferation and differentiation of endogenous neural progenitor and stem cells into mature nerve cells, to promote functional recovery in patients suffering from cerebral stroke. This study carries a lot of hope for cellular therapy, particularly that aimed at stimulating endogenous neural progenitor and stem cells to promote functional recovery.

Transplantation of Neural Progenitor and Stem Cells of the Adult CNS

Neural progenitor and stem cells can be isolated from the adult brain and cultured in vitro from various regions of the CNS, including from human biopsies and postmortem tissues (Roy, Wang, Jiang et al. 2000; Palmer, Schwartz, Taupin et al. 2001), providing valuable sources of tissue for cellular therapy. Experimental studies reveal that adult-derived neural progenitor and stem cells engraft the host tissues and express mature neuronal and glial markers when transplanted in the brain (Gage, Coates, Palmer et al. 1995; Shihabuddin, Horner, Ray et al. 2000), providing proof of principle of the potential of adult-derived neural progenitor and stem cells for therapy.

Intracerebral transplantation aims at replacing unhealthy or damaged tissues at sites of degeneration (Fig. 10.3). Such a strategy may not be applicable for injuries or diseases where the degeneration is widespread, particularly for neurodegenerative diseases such as AD, HD, and multiple sclerosis. Neural progenitor and stem cells, administered intravenously, migrate to diseased and injured sites of the brain (Brown, Yang, Schmidt et al. 2003; Pluchino, Quattrini, Brambilla et al. 2003). Experimental studies reveal that systemic injection of neural progenitors and stem cells promote functional recovery in an animal model of multiple sclerosis (Pluchino, Quattrini, Brambilla et al. 2003). This shows that systemic injection provides a model of choice for delivering adult-derived neural progenitor and stem cells for the treatment of neurological diseases and injuries where the degeneration is widespread. Hence, adult-derived neural progenitor and stem cells provide a promising model for cellular therapy for a broad range of neurological

diseases and injuries. In addition, systemic injection provides a noninvasive strategy for delivering neural progenitor and stem cells in the adult CNS.

The potential of neural progenitor and stem cells to promote functional recovery has been studied in animal models, mostly with fetal-derived neural progenitor and stem cells. Studies from fetal tissues have revealed that grafted neural progenitor and stem cells induce functional recovery in animal models. In this process, the release of trophic factors by the grafted neural progenitor and stem cells is believed to play a major role in the recovery process (Ourednik, Ourednik, Lynch et al. 2002; Yan, Welsh, Bora et al. 2004; Bjugstad, Redmond, Teng et al. 2005). In a study where human fetal-derived neural progenitor and stem cells were injected after spinal cord injury in mice, the improvements in walking disappeared following treatment with diphtheria toxin, which kills only human cells and not mouse cells (Cummings, Uchida, Tamaki et al. 2005). This shows that neural progenitor and stem cells have a beneficial effect after transplantation and that the grafted cells themselves contribute to the recovery process, by both trophic activities and their integration to the network. However, ex vivo studies have revealed that grafted neural progenitor and stem cells derived from the spinal cord adopt the fate of the stem cells in the niches into which they are transplanted (Shihabuddin, Horner, Ray et al. 2000). Hence, the microenvironment is also a determining factor for the efficiency of transplantation (Taupin 2006b). The understanding of all these mechanisms will contribute to the optimization of therapeutic applications involving the transplantation of neural progenitor and stem cells.

Neural stem and progenitor cells derived from human fetal tissues are currently in clinical trial for the treatment of Batten's disease, a childhood neurodegenerative disorder (Taupin 2006c). Preclinical data reveal that grafted neural progenitor and stem cells survive in damaged brain tissues and migrate to specific sites of degeneration, where they differentiate into neural lineages. This study carries a lot of hope for cellular therapy. However, the use of human fetal tissue is associated with ethical and political constraints. Hence, adult-derived neural progenitor and stem cells offer an alternative to the use of fetal-derived neural progenitor and stem cells for therapy. Adult-derived neural progenitor and stem cells can be isolated from postmortem tissues, providing multiple sources or tissues for therapy (Palmer, Schwartz, Taupin et al. 2001).

In summary, adult-derived neural progenitor and stem cells provide a promising strategy for cellular therapy to treat a broad range of neurological diseases and injuries. However, the mechanisms underlying the integration of neural progenitor and stem cells in

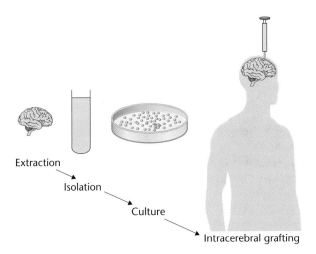

Figure 10.3 Adult neural stem cells and cellular therapy. Neural progenitor and stem cells can be isolated from the adult brain and cultured in vitro from various regions of the CNS, providing valuable sources of tissue for cellular therapy. Adult-derived neural progenitor and stem cells engraft the host tissues and express mature neuronal and glial markers when transplanted in the brain, providing proof of principle of the potential of adult-derived neural progenitor and stem cells for therapy.

the host and their potential for recovery remain to be established.

NEUROINFLAMMATION AND THE THERAPEUTIC POTENTIAL OF ADULT NSCs

Neuroinflammation in Neurological Diseases and Injuries

Inflammation is a process in which the body's white blood cells and chemicals protect the individual from infections, foreign substances, and injuries. In the CNS, neuroinflammation occurs following traumatic brain injuries, spinal cord injuries, and cerebral strokes (Ghirnikar, Lee, Eng 1998; Stoll, Jander, Schroeter 1998; Nencini, Sarti, Innocenti et al. 2003; Schmidt, Heyde, Ertel et al. 2005). There are two types of immune cells that are activated following injury to the CNS: microglial cells, a population of glial cells of the CNS (Stoll, Jander 1999; Streit, Walter, Pennell 1999), and cells from the hematopoietic system, such as lymphocytes, monocytes, and macrophages. Neuroinflammation disrupts the blood–brain barrier (BBB), allowing cells from the hematopoietic system to leave the blood stream and come in contact with the injury site (Lossinsky, Shivers 2004). The immune cells respond to injury by eliminating debris and releasing a host of powerful regulatory substances, such as the complements, glutamate, interleukins, nitric oxide, reactive oxygen species, and transforming growth factors (Ghirnikar, Lee, Eng 1998; Stoll, Jander 1999; Jander, Schroeter, Stoll 2002; Stoll, Schroeter, Jander et al. 2004; Hensley, Mhatre, Mou et al. 2006; Bonifati, Kishore 2007). These chemicals are both beneficial and harmful to the cellular environment, thereby creating further damage to the CNS (Stoll Jander, Schroeter 2002). Mature astrocytes are also activated following injury to the CNS (Latov, Nilaver, Zimmerman et al. 1979; Miyake, Hattori, Fukuda et al. 1988). Astrocytic activation is believed to be necessary for containing the immune response, repairing the BBB, and attenuating further neuronal death (Bush, Puvanachandra, Horner et al. 1999; Lossinsky, Shivers 2004).

It is now well documented that neuroinflammation is actively involved in neurological diseases and disorders such as AD, depression, HD, PD, amyotrophic lateral sclerosis, and multiple sclerosis (Minghetti 2005; Arnaud, Robakis, Figueiredo-Pereira 2006; Eikelenboom, Veerhuis, Scheper et al. 2006; Hensley, Mhatre, Mou et al. 2006; Sivaprakasam 2006; Klegeri, Schulzer, Harper et al. 2007). In AD, there is a correlation between local inflammation and amyloid plaques and neurofibrillary tangles (Zilka, Ferencik,

Hulin 2006). Chronic inflammation is considered as a causative factor in the pathogenesis of neurological diseases and disorders (Eikelenboom, Veerhuis, Scheper et al. 2006; Zilka, Ferencik, Hulin 2006; Whitton 2007). It is proposed that the immune cells and proinflammatory chemicals involved in neuroinflammation underlie the mechanisms of neurodegeneration. The activation or overactivation of immune cells involved in neuroinflammation and release of proinflammatory chemicals would result in reduced neuroprotection and neuronal repair, and increased neurodegeneration, leading to neurodegenerative diseases (Bonifati, Kishore 2007; Donnelly, Popovich 2008). Interestingly, depression is a common antecedent to many neurological diseases, particularly AD and PD (Karceski 2007; Potter, Steffens 2007). Hence, chronic inflammation during depressive episodes could predispose depressive patients to neurodegenerative diseases later in life (Leonard 2007).

Neuroinflammation in Adult Neurogenesis

Neuroinflammation inhibits neurogenesis in the adult hippocampus (Ekdahl, Mohapel, Elmer et al. 2003; Monje, Toda, Palmer 2003) (Table 10.3). The function, significance, and mechanisms of the modulation of neurogenesis during inflammatory processes remain to be elucidated. The function and significance of the modulation of neurogenesis during inflammatory processes remain to be particularly elucidated during neurological diseases and disorders, such as AD and depression. On the cellular level, neurological diseases and disorders are associated with microglia activation (Stoll, Jander 1999), a component of the inflammation reaction known to impair hippocampal neurogenesis in adult rats (Ekdahl, Mohapel, Elmer et al. 2003; Monje, Toda, Palmer 2003). On the molecular level, substances such as interleukin (Vallieres, Campbell, Gage et al. 2002) and nitric oxide (Packer, Stasiv, Benraiss et al. 2003), released by the immune cells, regulate adult neurogenesis negatively. Hence,

Table 10.3 Adult Neurogenesis and Neuroinflammation

Disease/Model	Regulation	References
Neuroinflammation	Decrease	Ekdahl (2003), Monje (2003)
Microglia activation	Decrease	Ekdahl (2003), Monje (2003)
Interleukins	Decrease	Vallieres (2002)
Nitric oxide	Decrease	Packer (2003)

Neuroinflammation inhibits neurogenesis in the adult hippocampus. Chronic inflammation is associated with neurological diseases and disorders, such as Alzheimer's and Parkinson's diseases, and is thought to be a causative factor for these diseases. The involvement and significance of the modulation of adult neurogenesis in neurological diseases and disorders remain to be established.

neuroinflammation may contribute to the effects of neurological diseases and disorders on adult neurogenesis. The contribution and involvement of neuroinflammation with regard to the effects of neurological diseases and disorders on adult neurogenesis remain to be determined.

X-ray irradiation has been used to study the function and involvement of adult neurogenesis in various neurological diseases and disorders, such as epilepsy and depression (Parent, Tada, Fike et al. 1999; Santarelli, Saxe, Gross et al. 2003). Brain irradiation induces inflammatory responses. The effect of brain irradiation on adult neurogenesis in animal models, particularly of neurological diseases and disorders, is therefore difficult to interpret in light of these data.

Neuroinflammation and Neural Progenitor and Stem Cell Transplantation

Neural progenitor and stem cells express receptors and respond to trophic factors and cytokines. Hence, the inflammatory process involved in the pathological processes to be treated by the transplantation of neural progenitor and stem cells may have adverse effects on the success of the graft. On the one hand, adult-derived neural progenitor and stem cells promote neuroprotection via an immunomodulatory mechanism (Pluchino, Zanotti, Rossi et al. 2005). This shows that grafted neural progenitor and stem cells interact with the host to promote functional recovery. This also suggests that neural progenitor and stem cells may provide clinical benefit for the treatment of autoimmune diseases. On the other hand, the timing of transplantation in the diseased brain or after injuries may be critical for successful transplantation of neural progenitor and stem cell therapy (Mueller, McKercher, Imitola et al. 2005). This suggests that preclinical studies involving immunosuppressed mice to study the engraftment of neural progenitor and stem cells for future therapy may not represent an appropriate model to characterize and validate sources of human-derived neural progenitor and stem cells for therapy (Taupin 2006c).

In summary, neuroinflammation is involved in the pathogenesis of neurological diseases and disorders, but its contribution and involvement with regard to these pathological processes remain to be elucidated. It may be involved in the modulation of neurogenesis in neurological diseases and disorders, but the contribution and significance of this modulation remain to be understood. Neuroinflammation may affect the success of therapeutic strategies involving the transplantation of neural progenitor and stem cells. Hence, therapeutic strategies for promoting neurogenesis after injuries or in neurological diseases and disorders and for promoting the engraftment of neural progenitor and stem cells may involve the use of anti-inflammatory treatments to reduce the adverse effects of neuroinflammation on adult neurogenesis and transplants, respectively (Craft, Watterson, Van Eldik 2005; Hernan, Logroscino, Garcia Rodriguez 2006; Ho, Qin, Stetka et al. 2006; Vardy, Hussain, Hooper 2006).

LIMITATIONS AND PITFALLS OF BrdU LABELING FOR STUDYING NEUROGENESIS

BrdU is a thymidine analogue that incorporates DNA of dividing cells during the S-phase of the cell cycle and is used for birthdating and monitoring cell proliferation (Miller, Nowakowski 1988). There are limitations and pitfalls regarding the use of BrdU for studying neurogenesis. BrdU is a toxic and mutagenic substance (Nowakowski, Hayes 2001; Taupin 2007). It triggers cell death and formation of teratomes. It alters DNA stability, lengthens the cell cycle. It also has mitogenic, transcriptional, and translational effects on cells that incorporate it. BrdU is not a marker for cell proliferation but a marker for DNA synthesis. In addition, many physiological and pathological processes affect the permeability of the BBB and cerebral flow, particularly exercise; neurological diseases and injuries such as AD, PD, and cerebral strokes; and neuroinflammation and drug treatments (Lossinsky, Shivers 2004; Deane, Zlokovic 2007; Desai, Monahan, Carvey et al. 2007; Pereira, Huddleston, Brickman et al. 2007), all of which can affect the bioavailability of BrdU in the brain. Hence, studies involving the use of BrdU for studying adult neurogenesis must be carefully assessed, and their conclusions carefully weighted (Taupin 2007).

CONCLUSION AND PERSPECTIVES

The confirmation that adult neurogenesis occurs in the adult brain and that NSCs reside in the adult CNS suggests that the adult brain may be amenable to repair and raises the question of the function of newborn neuronal cells in the physiology and pathology of the adult nervous system. The modulation of adult neurogenesis in neurological diseases and disorders suggests that it may be involved in the etiology and pathogenesis of the diseases. The contribution and significance of this modulation is yet to be elucidated. Newborn neuronal cells may be involved in regenerative attempts and plasticity of the nervous system. The stimulation of endogenous neural progenitor or stem cells or the transplantation of adult-derived neural progenitor and stem cells offers new opportunities for cellular therapy. Particularly, intrinsic properties of adult NSCs provide new strategies to treat a broad range of neurological diseases and injuries, as well as brain tumors. However, NSCs are still elusive cells, and will have to be fully and unequivocally characterized before adult NSCs are brought to therapy.

Chronic inflammation is associated with neurological diseases and disorders such as AD and PD, and is thought to be a causative factor for these diseases. Neuroinflammation modulates adult neurogenesis, particularly in the hippocampus. However, the significance of this modulation and its impact on adult neurogenesis in neurological diseases remain to be established. Chronic inflammation and proinflammatory substances have tremendous implications for cellular therapy involving adult NSCs, both in vivo and ex vivo. Neuroinflammation may affect the potential of NSC therapy and provide new perspectives for NSC therapy. Therapeutic strategies for promoting neurogenesis after injuries or in neurological diseases and disorders and for promoting the engraftment of neural progenitor and stem cells may involve the use of anti-inflammatory treatments to reduce the adverse effects of neuroinflammation on adult neurogenesis and NSC transplants. Future studies will aim at elucidating the contribution and involvement of chronic inflammation with regard to neurological diseases, disorders, and injuries; its underlying mechanism; and its potential for cellular therapy. These investigations will result in new therapeutic strategies to treat neurological diseases, disorders, and injuries.

REFERENCES

Arnaud L, Robakis NK, Figueiredo-Pereira ME. 2006. It may take inflammation, phosphorylation and ubiquitination to "tangle" in Alzheimer's disease. *Neurodegener Dis.* 3(6):313–319.

Arvidsson A, Collin T, Kirik D, Kokaia Z, Lindvall O. 2002. Neuronal replacement from endogenous precursors in the adult brain after stroke. *Nat Med.* 8(9):963–970.

Belluzzi O, Benedusi M, Ackman J, LoTurco JJ. 2003. Electrophysiological differentiation of new neurons in the olfactory bulb. *J Neurosci.* 23(32):10411–10418.

Bjugstad KB, Redmond DE Jr, Teng YD et al. 2005. Neural stem cells implanted into MPTP-treated monkeys increase the size of endogenous tyrosine hydroxylase-positive cells found in the striatum: A return to control measures. *Cell Transplant.* 14(4):183–192.

Bonifati DM, Kishore U. 2007. Role of complement in neurodegeneration and neuroinflammation. *Mol Immunol.* 44(5):999–1010.

Brown AB, Yang W, Schmidt NO et al. 2003. Intravascular delivery of neural stem cell lines to target intracranial and extracranial tumors of neural and non-neural origin. *Hum Gene Ther.* 14(18):1777–1785.

Bush TG, Puvanachandra N, Horner CH et al. 1999. Leukocyte infiltration, neuronal degeneration, and neurite outgrowth after ablation of scar-forming, reactive astrocytes in adult transgenic mice. *Neuron.* 23(2):297–308.

Cajal Santiago Ramon y. 1928. *Degeneration and Regeneration of the Nervous System.* New York: Hafner.

Cameron HA, Woolley CS, McEwen BS, Gould E. 1993. Differentiation of newly born neurons and glia in the dentate gyrus of the adult rat. *Neuroscience.* 56(2):337–344.

Cameron HA, McKay RD. 2001. Adult neurogenesis produces a large pool of new granule cells in the dentate gyrus. *J Comp Neurol.* 435(4):406–417.

Campbell S, Macqueen G. 2004. The role of the hippocampus in the pathophysiology of major depression. *J Psychiatry Neurosci.* 29(6):417–426.

Caselli RJ, Beach TG, Yaari R, Reiman EM. 2006. Alzheimer's disease a century later. *J Clin Psychiatry.* 67(11):1784–1800.

Chen Y, Ai Y, Slevin JR, Maley BE, Gash DM. 2005. Progenitor proliferation in the adult hippocampus and substantia nigra induced by glial cell line-derived neurotrophic factor. *Exp Neurol.* 196(1):87–95.

Chiasson BJ, Tropepe V, Morshead CM, van der Kooy D. 1999. Adult mammalian forebrain ependymal and subependymal cells demonstrate proliferative potential but only subependymal cells have neural stem cell characteristics. *J Neurosci.* 19(11):4462–4471.

Colla M, Kronenberg G, Deuschle M et al. 2007. Hippocampal volume reduction and HPA-system activity in major depression. *J Psychiatr Res.* 41(7):553–560.

Craft JM, Watterson DM, Van Eldik LJ. 2005. Neuroinflammation: a potential therapeutic target. *Expert Opin Ther Targets.* 9(5):887–900.

Craig CG, Tropepe V, Morshead CM, Reynolds BA, Weiss S, van der Kooy D. 1996. In vivo growth factor expansion of endogenous subependymal neural precursor cell populations in the adult mouse brain. *J Neurosci.* 16(8):2649–2658.

Cummings BJ, Uchida N, Tamaki SJ et al. 2005. Human neural stem cells differentiate and promote locomotor recovery in spinal cord-injured mice. *Proc Natl Acad Sci U S A.* 102(39):14069–14074.

Curtis MA, Penney EB, Pearson AG et al. 2003. Increased cell proliferation and neurogenesis in the adult human Huntington's disease brain. *Proc Natl Acad Sci U S A.* 100(15):9023–9027.

Curtis MA, Kam M, Nannmark U et al. 2007. Human neuroblasts migrate to the olfactory bulb via a lateral ventricular extension. *Science.* 315(5816):1243–1249.

Deane R, Zlokovic BV. 2007. Role of the blood-brain barrier in the pathogenesis of Alzheimer's disease. *Curr Alzheimer Res.* 4(2):191–197.

Desai BS, Monahan AJ, Carvey PM, Hendey B. 2007. Blood-brain barrier pathology in Alzheimer's and Parkinson's disease: implications for drug therapy. *Cell Transplant.* 16(3):285–99.

Garcia-Verdugo, JM, Alvarez-Buylla, A. Dodart JC, Mathis C, Bales KR, Paul SM 2002. Does my mouse have Alzheimer's disease? *Genes Brain Behav.* 1(3):142–155.

Doetsch F, Caille I, Lim DA, Garcia-Verdugo JM, Alvarez-Buylla A. 1999. Subventricular zone astrocytes are neural stem cells in the adult mammalian brain. *Cell.* 97(6):703–16.

Donnelly DJ, Popovich PG. 2008. Inflammation and its role in neuroprotection, axonal regeneration and functional recovery after spinal cord injury. *Exp Neurol.* 209(2):378–388.

Douglas MR, Lewthwaite AJ, Nicholl DJ. 2007. Genetics of Parkinson's disease and parkinsonism. *Expert Rev Neurother.* 7(6):657–666.

Eikelenboom P, Veerhuis R, Scheper W, Rozemuller AJ, van Gool WA, Hoozemans JJ. 2006. The significance of neuroinflammation in understanding Alzheimer's disease. *J Neural Transm.* 113(11):1685–1695.

Ekdahl CT, Mohapel P, Elmer E, Lindvall O. 2001. Caspase inhibitors increase short-term survival of progenitor-cell progeny in the adult rat dentate gyrus following status epilepticus. *Eur J Neurosci.* 14(6):937–945.

Ekdahl CT, Claasen JH, Bonde S, Kokaia Z, Lindvall O. 2003. Inflammation is detrimental for neurogenesis in adult brain. *Proc Natl Acad Sci U S A.* 100(23):13632–13637.

Eriksson PS, Perfilieva E, Bjork-Eriksson T et al. 1998. Neurogenesis in the adult human hippocampus. *Nat Med.* 4(11):1313–1317.

Feng R, Rampon C, Tang YP et al. 2001. Deficient neurogenesis in forebrain-specific presenilin-1 knockout mice is associated with reduced clearance of hippocampal memory traces. [published erratum appears in *Neuron.* 2002 33(2):313]. *Neuron.* 32(5):911–926.

Fernandez-Espejo E. 2004. Pathogenesis of Parkinson's disease: prospects of neuroprotective and restorative therapies. *Mol Neurobiol.* 29(1):15–30.

Fortunel NO, Out HH, Ng HH et al. 2003. Comment on "'Stemness': transcriptional profiling of embryonic and adult stem cells" and "a stem cell molecular signature". *Science.* 302(5644):393.

Karceski, S. 2007. Early Parkinson disease and depression. *Neurology.* 69(4):E2–E3.

Frielingsdorf H, Schwarz K, Brundin P, Mohapel P. 2004. No evidence for new dopaminergic neurons in the adult mammalian substantia nigra. *Proc Natl Acad Sci U S A.* 101(27):10177–10182.

Gage FH. 2000. Mammalian neural stem cells. *Science.* 287(5457):1433–1438.

Gage FH, Coates PW, Palmer TD et al. 1995. Survival and differentiation of adult neuronal progenitor cells transplanted to the adult brain. *Proc Natl Acad Sci U S A.* 92(25):11879–11883.

Ghirnikar RS, Lee YL, Eng LF. 1998. Inflammation in traumatic brain injury: role of cytokines and chemokines. *Neurochem Res.* 23(3):329–340.

Gould E, Tanapat P, McEwen BS, Flugge G, Fuchs E. 1998. Proliferation of granule cell precursors in the dentate gyrus of adult monkeys is diminished by stress. *Proc Natl Acad Sci U S A.* 95(6):3168–3171.

Gould E, Reeves AJ, Graziano MS, Gross CG. 1999. Neurogenesis in the neocortex of adult primates. *Science.* 286(5439):548–552.

Gritti A, Parati EA, Cova L et al. 1996. Multipotential stem cells from the adult mouse brain proliferate and self-renew in response to basic fibroblast growth factor. *J Neurosci.* 16(3):1091–1100.

Gross CG. 2000. Neurogenesis in the adult brain: death of a dogma. *Nat Rev Neurosci.* 1(1):67–73.

Hensley K, Mhatre M, Mou S et al. 2006. On the relation of oxidative stress to neuroinflammation: lessons learned from the G93A-SOD1 mouse model of amyotrophic lateral sclerosis. *Antioxid Redox Signal.* 8(11–12):2075–2087.

Hernan MA, Logroscino G, Garcia Rodriguez LA. 2006. Nonsteroidal anti-inflammatory drugs and the incidence of Parkinson disease. *Neurology.* 66(7):1097–1099.

Herrup K, Neve R, Ackerman SL, Copani A. 2004. Divide and die: cell cycle events as triggers of nerve cell death. *J Neurosci.* 24(42):9232–9239.

Ho L, Qin W, Stetka BS, Pasinetti GM. 2006. Is there a future for cyclo-oxygenase inhibitors in Alzheimer's disease? *CNS Drugs.* 20(2):85–98.

Houser CR. 1990. Granule cell dispersion in the dentate gyrus of humans with temporal lobe epilepsy. *Brain Res.* 535(2):195–204.

Jacobs BL, Praag H, Gage FH. 2000. Adult brain neurogenesis and psychiatry: a novel theory of depression. *Mol Psychiatry.* 5(3):262–269.

Jander S, Schroeter M, Stoll G. 2002. Interleukin-18 expression after focal ischemia of the rat brain: association with the late-stage inflammatory response. *J Cereb Blood Flow Metab.* 22(1):62–70.

Jin K, Sun Y, Xie L et al. 2003. Directed migration of neuronal precursors into the ischemic cerebral cortex and striatum. *Mol Cell Neurosci.* 24(1):171–189.

Jin K, Galvan V, Xie L et al. 2004. Enhanced neurogenesis in Alzheimer's disease transgenic (PDGF-APPSw, Ind) mice. *Proc Natl Acad Sci U S A.* 101(36):13363–13367.

Jin K, Peel AL, Mao XO et al. 2004. Increased hippocampal neurogenesis in Alzheimer's disease. *Proc Natl Acad Sci U S A.* 101(1):343–347.

Johansson CB, Momma S, Clarke DL, Risling M, Lendahl U, Frisen J. 1999. Identification of a neural stem cell in the adult mammalian central nervous system. *Cell.* 96(1):25–34.

Kaplan MS. 2001. Environment complexity stimulates visual cortex neurogenesis: death of a dogma and a research career. *Trends Neurosci.* 24(10):617–620.

Kato T, Yokouchi K, Fukushima N, Kawagishi K, Li Z, Moriizumi T. 2001. Continual replacement of newly-generated olfactory neurons in adult rats. *Neurosci Lett.* 307(1):17–20.

Kempermann G, Kuhn HG, Gage FH. 1997. More hippocampal neurons in adult mice living in an enriched environment. *Nature.* 386(6624):493–495.

Kessler RC, McGonagle KA, Zhao S et al. 1994. Lifetime and 12-month prevalence of DSM-III-R psychiatric disorders in the United States. Results from the National Comorbidity Survey. *Arch Gen Psychiatry.* 51(1):8–19.

Klegeris A, Schulzer M, Harper DG, McGeer PL. 2007. Increase in core body temperature of Alzheimer's disease patients as a possible indicator of chronic neuroinflammation: a meta-analysis. *Gerontology.* 53(1):7–11.

Kornack DR, Rakic P. 1999. Continuation of neurogenesis in the hippocampus of the adult macaque monkey. *Proc Natl Acad Sci U S A.* 96(10):5768–5773.

Kornack DR, Rakic P. 2001. Cell proliferation without neurogenesis in adult primate neocortex. *Science.* 294(5549):2127–2130.

Kornblum HI, Geschwind DH. 2001. Molecular markers in CNS stem cell research: hitting a moving target. *Nat Rev Neurosci.* 2(11):843–846.

Kuhn HG, Winkler J, Kempermann G, Thal, LJ, Gage FH. 1997. Epidermal growth factor and fibroblast growth factor-2 have different effects on neural progenitors in the adult rat brain. *J Neurosci.* 17(15):5820–5829.

Latov N, Nilaver G, Zimmerman EA et al. 1979. Fibrillary astrocytes proliferate in response to brain injury: a study combining immunoperoxidase technique for glial fibrillary acidic protein and radioautography of tritiated thymidine. *Dev Biol.* 72(2):381–384.

Lazic SE, Grote H, Armstrong RJ et al. 2004. Decreased hippocampal cell proliferation in R6/1 Huntington's mice. *Neuroreport.* 15(5):811–813.

Leonard BE. 2007. Inflammation depression and dementia: are they connected? *Neurochem Res.* 32(10):1749–1756.

Li SH, Li XJ. 2004. Huntingtin-protein interactions and the pathogenesis of Huntington's disease. *Trends Genet.* 20(3):146–154.

Lois C, Alvarez-Buylla A. 1994. Long-distance neuronal migration in the adult mammalian brain. *Science.* 264(5162):1145–1148.

Lossinsky AS, Shivers RR. 2004. Structural pathways for macromolecular and cellular transport across the blood-brain barrier during inflammatory conditions. *Histol Histopathol.* 19(2):535–564.

Luskin MB. 1993. Restricted proliferation and migration of postnatally generated neurons derived from the forebrain subventricular zone. *Neuron.* 11(1):173–189.

Malberg JE, Eisch AJ, Nestler EJ, Duman RS. 2000. Chronic antidepressant treatment increases neurogenesis in adult rat hippocampus. *J Neurosci.* 20(24):9104–9110.

Malberg JE, Duman RS. 2003. Cell proliferation in adult hippocampus is decreased by inescapable stress: reversal by fluoxetine treatment. *Neuropsychopharmacol.* 28(9):1562–1571.

Markakis EA, Gage FH. 1999. Adult-generated neurons in the dentate gyrus send axonal projections to field CA3 and are surrounded by synaptic vesicles. *J Comp Neurol.* 406(4):449–460.

Miller MW, Nowakowski RS. 1988. Use of bromodeoxyuridine-immunohistochemistry to examine the proliferation, migration and time of origin of cells in the central nervous system. *Brain Res.* 457(1):44–52.

Minghetti L. 2005. Role of inflammation in neurodegenerative diseases. *Curr Opin Neurol.* 18(3):315–321.

Miyake T, Hattori T, Fukuda M, Kitamura T, Fujita S. 1988. Quantitative studies on proliferative changes of reactive astrocytes in mouse cerebral cortex. *Brain Res.* 451(1–2):133–138.

Mohapel P, Frielingsdorf H, Haggblad J, Zachrisson O, Brundin P. 2005. Platelet-derived growth factor (PDGF-BB) and brain-derived neurotrophic factor (BDNF) induce striatal neurogenesis in adult rats with 6-hydroxydopamine lesions. *Neurosci.* 132(3):767–776.

Monje ML, Toda H, Palmer TD. 2003. Inflammatory blockade restores adult hippocampal neurogenesis. *Science.* 302(5651):1760–1765.

Morshead CM, van der Kooy D. 1992. Postmitotic death is the fate of constitutively proliferating cells in the subependymal layer of the adult mouse brain. *J Neurosci.* 12(1):249–256.

Mueller FJ, McKercher SR, Imitola J et al. 2005. At the interface of the immune system and the nervous system: how neuroinflammation modulates the fate of neural progenitors in vivo. *Ernst Schering Res Found Workshop.* (53):83–114.

Nencini P, Sarti C, Innocenti R, Pracucci G, Inzitari D. 2003. Acute inflammatory events and ischemic stroke subtypes. *Cerebrovasc Dis.* 15(3):215–221.

Nowakowski RS, Hayes NL. 2001. Stem cells: the promises and pitfalls *Neuropsychopharmacol.* 25(6):799–804.

Ourednik J, Ourednik V, Lynch WP, Schachner M, Snyder EY. 2002. Neural stem cells display an inherent mechanism for rescuing dysfunctional neurons. *Nat Biotechnol.* 20(11):1103–1110.

Packer MA, Stasiv Y, Benraiss A et al. 2003. Nitric oxide negatively regulates mammalian adult neurogenesis. *Proc Natl Acad Sci U S A.* 100(16):9566–9571.

Palmer TD, Takahashi J, Gage FH. 1997. The adult rat hippocampus contains primordial neural stem cells. *Mol Cell Neurosci.* 8(6):389–404.

Palmer TD, Schwartz PH, Taupin P, Kaspar B, Stein SA, Gage FH. 2001. Cell culture. Progenitor cells from human brain after death. *Nature.* 411(6833):42–43.

Parent JM, Yu TW, Leibowitz RT, Geschwind DH, Sloviter RS, Lowenstein DH. 1997. Dentate granule cell neurogenesis is increased by seizures and contributes to aberrant network reorganization in the adult rat hippocampus. *J Neurosci.* 17(10):3727–3738.

Parent JM, Tada E, Fike JR, Lowenstein DH. 1999. Inhibition of dentate granule cell neurogenesis with brain irradiation does not prevent seizure-induced mossy fiber synaptic reorganization in the rat. *J Neurosci.* 19(11):4508–4519.

Pereira AC, Huddleston DE, Brickman AM et al. 2007. An in vivo correlate of exercise-induced neurogenesis in the adult dentate gyrus. *Proc Natl Acad Sci U S A.* 104(13):5638–5643.

Pluchino S, Quattrini A, Brambilla E et al. 2003. Injection of adult neurospheres induces recovery in a chronic model of multiple sclerosis. *Nature.* 422(6933):688–694.

Pluchino S, Zanotti L, Rossi B et al. 2005. Neurosphere-derived multipotent precursors promote neuroprotection by an immunomodulatory mechanism. *Nature.* 436(7048):266–271.

Potter GG, Steffens DC. 2007. Contribution of depression to cognitive impairment and dementia in older adults. *Neurologist.* 13(3):105–117.

Raber J, Huang Y, Ashford JW. 2004. ApoE genotype accounts for the vast majority of AD risk and AD pathology. *Neurobiol Aging.* 25(5):641–650.

Rakic P. 1985. Limits of neurogenesis in primates. *Science.* 227(4690):1054–1056.

Reif A, Fritzen S, Finger M. 2006. Neural stem cell proliferation is decreased in schizophrenia, but not in depression. *Mol Psychiatry.* 11(5):514–522.

Represa A, Tremblay E, Ben-Ari Y. 1990. Sprouting of mossy fibers in the hippocampus of epileptic human and rat. *Adv Exp Med Biol.* 268:419–424.

Reynolds BA, Weiss S. 1992. Generation of neurons and astrocytes from isolated cells of the adult mammalian central nervous system. *Science.* 255(5052):1707–1710.

Rietze R, Poulin P, Weiss S. 2000. Mitotically active cells that generate neurons and astrocytes are present in multiple regions of the adult mouse hippocampus. *J Comp Neurol.* 424(3):397–408.

Rogaeva E, Meng Y, Lee JH et al. 2007. The neuronal sortilin-related receptor SORL1 is genetically associated with Alzheimer disease. *Nat Genet.* 39(2):168–177.

Roy NS, Wang S, Jiang L et al. 2000. In vitro neurogenesis by progenitor cells isolated from the adult human hippocampus. *Nat Med.* 6(3):271–277.

Santarelli L, Saxe M, Gross C et al. 2003. Requirement of hippocampal neurogenesis for the behavioral effects of antidepressants. *Science.* 301(5634):805–809.

Sawa A, Tomoda T, Bae BI. 2003. Mechanisms of neuronal cell death in Huntington's disease. *Cytogenet Genome Res.* 100(1–4):287–295.

Schmidt OI, Heyde CE, Ertel W, Stahel PF. 2005. Closed head injury—An inflammatory disease? *Brain Res Brain Res Rev.* 48(2):388–399.

Seri B, Garcia-Verdugo JM, McEwen BS, Alvarez-Buylla A. 2001. Astrocytes give rise to new neurons in the adult mammalian hippocampus. *J Neurosci.* 21(18):7153–7160.

Sheline YI, Wang PW, Gado MH, Csernansky JG, Vannier MW. 1996. Hippocampal atrophy in recurrent major depression. *Proc Natl Acad Sci U S A.* 93(9):3908–3913.

Shihabuddin LS, Horner PJ, Ray J, Gage FH. 2000. Adult spinal cord stem cells generate neurons after transplantation in the adult dentate gyrus. *J Neurosci.* 20(23):8727–8735.

Sivaprakasam K. 2006. Towards a unifying hypothesis of Alzheimer's disease: cholinergic system linked to plaques, tangles and neuroinflammation. *Curr Med Chem.* 13(18):2179–2188.

Slevin JT, Gerhardt GA, Smith CD, Gash DM, Kryscio R, Young B. 2005. Improvement of bilateral motor functions in patients with Parkinson disease through the unilateral intraputaminal infusion of glial cell line-derived neurotrophic factor. *J Neurosurg.* 102(2):216–222.

St George-Hyslop PH, Petit A. 2005. Molecular biology and genetics of Alzheimer's disease. *C R Biol.* 328(2):119–130.

Stanfield BB, Trice JE. 1988. Evidence that granule cells generated in the dentate gyrus of adult rats extend axonal projections. *Exp Brain Res.* 72(2):399–406.

Stoll G, Jander S, Schroeter M. 1998. Inflammation and glial responses in ischemic brain lesions. *Prog Neurobiol.* 56(2):149–171.

Stoll G, Jander S. 1999. The role of microglia and macrophages in the pathophysiology of the CNS. *Prog Neurobiol.* 58(3):233–247.

Stoll G, Jander S, Schroeter M. 2002. Detrimental and beneficial effects of injury-induced inflammation and cytokine expression in the nervous system. *Adv Exp Med Biol.* 513:87–113.

Stoll G, Schroeter M, Jander S et al. 2004. Lesion-associated expression of transforming growth factor-beta-2 in the rat nervous system: evidence for down-regulating the phagocytic activity of microglia and macrophages. *Brain Pathol.* 14(1):51–58.

Streit WJ, Walter SA, Pennell NA. 1999. Reactive microgliosis. *Prog Neurobiol.* 57(6):563–581.

Suslov ON, Kukekov VG, Ignatova TN, Steindler DA. 2002. Neural stem cell heterogeneity demonstrated by molecular phenotyping of clonal neurospheres. *Proc Natl Acad Sci U S A.* 99(22):14506–14511.

Sutula T, Cascino G, Cavazos J, Parada I, Ramirez L. 1989. Mossy fiber synaptic reorganization in the epileptic human temporal lobe. *Ann Neurol.* 26(3):321–330.

Tada E, Parent JM, Lowenstein DH, Fike JR. 2000. X-irradiation causes a prolonged reduction in cell proliferation in the dentate gyrus of adult rats. *Neuroscience.* 99(1):33–41.

Tattersfield AS, Croon RJ, Liu YW, Kells AP, Faull RL, Connor B. 2004. Neurogenesis in the striatum of the quinolinic acid lesion model of Huntington's disease. *Neuroscience.* 127(2):319–332.

Taupin P. 2006a. The therapeutic potential of adult neural stem cells. *Curr Opin Mol Ther.* 8(3):225–231.

Taupin. P. 2006b. Adult neural stem cells, neurogenic niches and cellular therapy. *Stem Cell Reviews.* 2(3):213–220.

Taupin P. 2006c. HuCNS-SC (StemCells). *Curr Opin Mol Ther.* 8(2):156–163.

Taupin P. 2007. BrdU immunohistochemistry for studying adult neurogenesis: paradigms, pitfalls, limitations, and validation. *Brain Res Rev.* 53(1):198–214.

Taupin P, Gage FH. 2002. Adult neurogenesis and neural stem cells of the central nervous system in mammals. *J Neurosci Res.* 69(6):745–749.

Toni N, Teng EM, Bushong EA et al. 2007. Synapse formation on neurons born in the adult hippocampus. *Nat Neurosci.* 10(6):727–734.

Vallieres L, Campbell IL, Gage FH, Sawchenko PE. 2002. Reduced hippocampal neurogenesis in adult transgenic mice with chronic astrocytic production of interleukin-6. *J Neurosci.* 22(2):486–492.

van Praag H, Schinder AF, Christie BR, Toni N, Palmer TD, Gage FH. 2002. Functional neurogenesis in the adult hippocampus. *Nature.* 415(6875):1030–1034.

Vardy ER, Hussain I, Hooper NM. 2006. Emerging therapeutics for Alzheimer's disease. *Expert Rev Neurother.* 6(5):695–704.

Volkmann J. 2007. Update on surgery for Parkinson's disease. *Curr Opin Neurol.* 20(4):465–469.

Wen PH, Shao X, Shao Z et al. 2002. Overexpression of wild type but not an FAD mutant presenilin-1 promotes neurogenesis in the hippocampus of adult mice. *Neurobiol Dis.* 10(1):8–19.

White JK, Auerbach W, Duyao MP et al. 1997. Huntingtin is required for neurogenesis and is not impaired by the Huntington's disease CAG expansion. *Nat Genet.* 17(4):404–410.

Whitton PS. 2007. Inflammation as a causative factor in the aetiology of Parkinson's disease. *Br J Pharmacol.* 150(8):963–976.

Wong ML, Licinio J. 2001. Research and treatment approaches to depression. *Nat Rev Neurosci.* 2(5):343–351.

Yan J, Welsh AM, Bora SH, Snyder EY, Koliatsos VE. 2004. Differentiation and tropic/trophic effects of exogenous neural precursors in the adult spinal cord. *J Comp Neurol.* 480(1):101–114.

Yang Y, Geldmacher DS, Herrup K. 2001. DNA replication precedes neuronal cell death in Alzheimer's disease. *J Neurosci.* 21(8):2661–2668.

Zhao M, Momma S, Delfani K et al. 2003. Evidence for neurogenesis in the adult mammalian substantia nigra. *Proc Natl Acad Sci U S A.* 100(13):7925–7930.

Zilka N, Ferencik M, Hulin I. 2006. Neuroinflammation in Alzheimer's disease: protector or promoter? *Bratisl Lek Listy.* 107(9–10):374–383.

Chapter **11**

GLUTAMATERGIC SIGNALING IN NEUROGENESIS

Noritaka Nakamichi and Yukio Yoneda

ABSTRACT

In this chapter, we have summarized recent studies on the functional expression of ionotropic (iGluR) and metabotropic (mGluR) glutamate receptors by neural progenitor cells isolated from embryonic rat and mouse brains. Cells are cultured in the presence of growth factors toward the formation of round spheres termed as *neurospheres* for different periods under floating conditions, whereas a reverse transcription polymerase chain reaction (RT-PCR) analysis reveals expression of mRNA for particular iGluR and mGluR subtypes in undifferentiated cells and neurospheres formed with clustered cells during the culture with growth factors. Moreover, sustained exposure to an agonist for the *N*-methyl-D-aspartate receptor (NMDAR) not only inhibits the formation of neurospheres but also promotes spontaneous and induced differentiation of neurospheres into cells immunoreactive to a neuronal marker protein on immunocytochemistry and Western blot analyses. On the other hand, sustained exposure to an agonist for the group III mGluR subtype similarly leads to suppression of proliferation activity in these neurospheres along with facilitation of the subsequent differentiation into astroglial cells, irrespective of the differentiation inducers used. Accordingly, glutamate could play a pivotal role in mechanisms underlying proliferation for self-renewal, together with determination of the subsequent differentiation fate toward particular progeny lineages through activation of NMDAR and group III mGluR subtypes expressed by neural progenitor cells in developing brains.

Keywords: neural progenitors, neurospheres, NMDAR, mGluR.

Neural stem cells are primitive cells with the self-renewal capacity as well as the multipotentiality to generate different neural lineages including neurons, astroglia, and oligodendroglia (Fig. 11.1). Cells with these characteristics are enriched in the subventricular zone (SVZ) during development of the brain (Doetsch, Caille, Lim et al. 1999; Johansson, Momma, Clarke et al. 1999; Haydar, Wang, Schwartz et al. 2000), while in the adult brain progenitor cells are also localized to the dentate gyrus (DG) of hippocampus as well as to the SVZ (Altman, Das 1967; Kaplan, Hinds 1977; Kaplan, Bell 1983, 1984; Gage, Kempermann, Palmer et al. 1998; Garcia-Verdugo, Doetsch, Wichterle et al. 1998) (Fig. 11.2). These neural progenitors indeed undergo cellular proliferation, commitment, and differentiation into neurons and glia in vitro (Gage, Coates, Palmer et al. 1995), suggesting that cells are indeed derived from multipotential neural stem cells (Temple, Alvarez-Buylla 1999). The fact that on transplantation of neural stem cells into the brain, cells develop into mature neurons or glia with morphological and biochemical features similar to those of neighboring cells gives rise to an idea that cellular commitment and/or differentiation is at least in part under control by microenvironments around the stem cells in vivo (Suhonen, Peterson, Ray et al. 1996).

Emerging evidence that endogenous factors regulate the self-renewal capacity and the multipotentiality

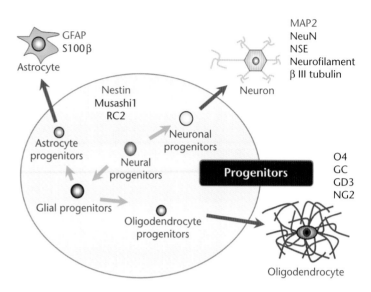

Figure 11.1 Cellular markers. Neural stem cells are primitive cells with the self-renewal capacity and multipotentiality to generate different neural lineages including neurons, astroglia and oligodendroglia. Neural progenitor cells are a group of cells with an ability to differentiate into neuronal progenitors toward neurons and glial progenitors toward both astroglia and oligodendroglia, along with the constitutive expression of nestin. Once they are destined to differentiate into one of the progeny lineages, nestin disappears with expression of the individual marker proteins.

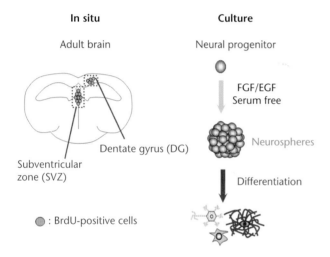

Figure 11.2 Experimental techniques. In adult brains, BrdU is heavily incorporated into neural progenitor cells predominantly enriched in the DG and SVZ in vivo. Neural progenitor cells could be isolated from developing and matured brains for subsequent culture in the presence of growth factors such as bFGF and EGF. Under floating culture conditions in vitro, round spheres are formed by clustered cells derived from neural progenitor cells under self-replication. These floating neurospheres are able to differentiate into a particular progeny lineage after the removal of growth factors under adherent culture conditions.

of neural progenitors expressed in the developing and matured brains is available in the literature. Several extracellular molecules, such as growth factors and neurotransmitters, have been implicated in the extrinsic regulation of cell proliferation in the developing telencephalon. For example, basic fibroblast growth factor (bFGF) prolongs the proliferation of progenitor cells with concomitant increases in the number of neurons in rat neocortex when either added to cultured cells in vitro (Cavanagh, Mione, Pappas et al. 1997) or microinjected into embryonic rat brains in vivo (Vaccarino, Schwartz, Raballo et al. 1999). The

neurotransmitters glutamate and γ-amino butyric acid (GABA) reduce the number of proliferating cells in dissociated or organotypic cultures of rat neocortex (LoTurco, Owens, Heath et al. 1995). Systemic administration of the glutamate analog N-methyl-D-aspartate (NMDA) not only increases DNA-binding activity of the transcription factor activator protein 1 (AP1) (Yoneda, Ogita, Azuma et al. 1999) but also decreases cellular proliferation activity determined by the incorporation of the thymidine analog 5-bromo-2'-deoxyuridine (BrdU) in a manner sensitive to the NMDA receptor antagonist dizocilpine (MK-801) (Kitayama, Yoneyama, Yoneda 2003) in the DG of the adult murine hippocampus. Systemic administration of NMDA also markedly reduces expression of the neural progenitor marker protein nestin and proliferating cell nuclear antigen in the DG, without significantly affecting that in the SVZ (Kitayama, Yoneyama, Yoneda 2003). Moreover, sustained activation of NMDA receptors not only decreases the size of neurospheres formed by clustered cells but also facilitates the neuronal commitment induced by all-*trans*-retinoic acid (ATRA) in cultured neural progenitor cells isolated from adult mouse hippocampus (Kitayama, Yoneyama, Tamaki et al. 2004).

Alternatively, glutamatergic signals are mediated by iGluR and mGluR glutamate receptors in the developing and matured brains. The iGluRs are categorized into three different cation channel subtypes according to the nucleotide sequential homology and intracellular signaling systems. These include NMDA receptor (NMDAR), DL-α-amino-3-hydroxy-5-methyl-4-isoxasolepropionate receptor (AMPAR), and kainate receptor (KAR) subtypes. By contrast, the mGluRs are a family of type III G protein–coupled receptors activated by glutamate, and divided into three major subtypes (group I, mGluR1 and 5 isoforms; group II,

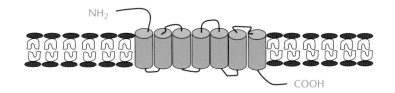

Subtype	Isoform	Effector	Agonist	Antagonist
Group I	mGluR1 mGluR5	Phospholipase C ▲	DHPG	AIDA
Group II	mGluR2 mGluR3	Adenylyl cyclase ▼	DCG-IV	APICA
Group III	mGluR4 mGluR6 mGluR7 mGluR8	Adenylyl cyclase ▼	L-AP4	CPPG

Figure 11.3 Classification of mGluRs. The mGluRs are a family of type III G protein–coupled receptors activated by glutamate, and divided into three major subtypes (group I, mGluR1 and 5 isoforms; group II, mGluR2 and 3 isoforms; group III, mGluR4, 6, 7, and 8 isoforms) based on sequence homology, signal transduction pathway, and pharmacology. The group I mGluR subtype is coupled to stimulatory Gq proteins to activate phospholipase C, which catalyzes the production of diacylglycerol and inositol (1,4,5)-triphosphate for subsequent activation of protein kinase C and release of Ca^{2+} from intracellular stores, respectively. Both group II and III mGluR subtypes are coupled to the inhibitory Gi/o protein to negatively regulate the activity of adenylyl cyclase, which induces a decrease in intracellular cAMP concentrations.

mGluR2 and 3 isoforms; group III, mGluR4, 6, 7, and 8 isoforms) on the basis of sequence homology, signal transduction pathway, and pharmacology (Conn, Pin 1997; Schoepp, Jane, Monn 1999; Zhai, George, Zhai et al. 2003). Group I mGluR subtype is coupled to stimulatory G_q proteins to activate phospholipase C, which catalyzes the production of diacylglycerol and inositol (1,4,5)-triphosphate for subsequent activation of protein kinase C and release of Ca^{2+} from intracellular stores, respectively. Both group II and III mGluR subtypes are coupled to the inhibitory $G_{i/o}$ protein to negatively regulate the activity of adenylyl cyclase, which decreases intracellular concentrations of cyclic adenosine monophosphate (cAMP) (Cartmell, Schoepp 2000; Schoepp 2001; Moldrich, Chapman, De Sarro et al. 2003; Kenny, Markou 2004) (Fig. 11.3).

In this chapter, therefore, we will outline recent findings on the importance of the signal inputs mediated by different glutamate receptor subtypes in mechanisms related to the self-replication and multipotentiality in neural progenitor cells isolated from fetal rodent brains.

ISOLATION OF NEURAL PROGENITOR CELLS FROM FETAL RODENT BRAINS

Neocortex is isolated from 18-day-old embryonic Wistar rats (Kitayama, Yoneyama, Yoneda 2003) and 15.5-day-old embryonic Std-ddY mice (Yoneyama, Fukui, Nakamichi et al. 2007), followed by treatment with an enzyme cocktail solution containing 2.5 U/mL papain, 250 U/mL DNAse, and 1 U/mL neutral protease in phosphate-buffered saline (PBS) at 37°C for 30 minutes (Fig. 11.4). Cells are washed three times with Dulbecco's modified Eagle's medium: Nutrient Mixture F-12 (DMEM/F-12) supplemented with 10% fetal bovine serum (FBS) and then mixed with an equal volume of the percoll solution made by mixing nine parts percoll with one part 10-fold condensed PBS. Cell suspensions are centrifuged at 20,000 g for 30 minutes at 18°C, followed by collection of cell fractions in the lower layer and subsequent washing three times with DMEM/F-12 containing 10% FBS (Kitayama, Yoneyama, Tamaki et al. 2004). Cell suspensions (15,000 cells) are seeded in 0.5 mL on each well in a culture plate (1.9 cm^2, 24 wells; Nalge Nunc International). Cells are usually cultured for a period of around 10 days in the absence of FBS in DMEM/F12 growth medium containing 0.6% glucose, 15 mM sodium bicarbonate, 250 mM N-acetyl-L-cysteine, 20 nM progesterone, 30 nM sodium selenite, 60 nM putrescine, 25 μg/mL insulin, and 100 μg/mL apo-transferrin, together with growth factors such as bFGF (20 ng/mL) for rat brains and epidermal growth factor (EGF) (10 ng/mL) for mouse brains, under floating conditions as described previously (Kitayama, Yoneyama, Tamaki et al. 2004). Cells are cultured at 37°C under 5% CO_2 in a humidified CO_2 incubator with a half medium change every 2 days.

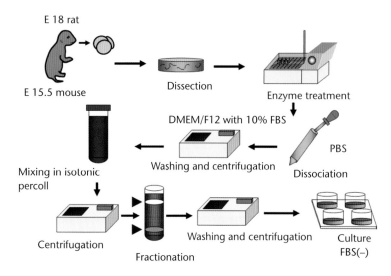

Figure 11.4 Isolation procedures of neural progenitor cell. Neocortex is isolated from 18-day-old embryonic rats or 15.5-day-old embryonic mice, followed by treatment with an enzyme cocktail solution containing papain, DNAse, and neutral protease. Cells are washed with DMEM/F-12 supplemented with 10% FBS and then mixed with the percoll solution for subsequent centrifugation. Neural progenitor cells are collected in the lower cell layer after centrifugation. Cells are cultured in the absence of FBS in DMEM/F12 medium with growth factors at 37°C in 5% CO_2 incubator under floating conditions.

In the upper cell layer prepared from fetal mouse neocortex, for example, particular cells are immunoreactive for either the neuronal marker microtubule associated protein 2 (MAP2) or the astroglial marker glial fibrillary acidic protein (GFAP) on double immunocytochemistry analysis but not for the neural progenitor marker nestin (Fig. 11.5A, upper panels). In the lower cell layer, by contrast, several cells are immunoreactive for nestin, but expression of either MAP2 or GFAP is not detected (Fig. 11.5A, lower panels). The lower cell layer is thus collected as a source of progenitors expressing nestin, followed by culture in either the presence or absence of EGF for 10 days and subsequent double immunocytochemical detection of MAP2 and GFAP. In the presence of EGF, round spheres are formed within 4 days with increasing sizes proportional to culture durations up to 10 days. In these neurospheres cultured for 10 days, cells are immunoreactive for nestin but not for either MAP2 or GFAP (Fig. 11.5B, upper panels).

Floating neurospheres are dispersed on day 10, followed by seeding on wells previously coated with poly-L-lysine and subsequent culture in the absence of EGF for an additional 4 days toward the spontaneous differentiation. Removal of EGF leads to a complete abolition of immunoreactive nestin together with a drastic increase in the number of cells immunoreactive for either MAP2 or GFAP on day 14 (Fig. 11.5B, lower panels). Dispersed cells are also cultured for an additional 4 days in the presence of either the neuronal inducer ATRA or the astroglial inducer ciliary neurotrophic factor (CNTF) to facilitate commitment toward a neuronal or astroglial lineage, respectively, after the removal of EGF on day 10. As shown in Figure 11.5C, sustained exposure to ATRA markedly increases the number of cells immunoreactive

for MAP2 compared to that found in the presence of CNTF. Neurospheres are dispersed on day 10, followed by the further culture in the presence of EGF for 10 days under floating conditions and subsequent dispersion toward culture in the absence of EGF for an additional 4 days. Round spheres are again formed with clustered cells immunoreactive for nestin, but not for either MAP2 or GFAP, within an additional 10 days (Fig. 11.5D, upper panel). Removal of EGF leads to a marked increase in the number of cells immunoreactive for either MAP2 or GFAP, but not for nestin, on day 24 (Fig. 11.5D, lower panels). Accordingly, the lower cell layer indeed contains neural progenitor cells endowed with the ability to proliferate for self-replication sensitive to a growth factor and to differentiate into neuronal and astroglial lineages in response to the respective differentiation inducers.

IONOTROPIC GLUTAMATE RECEPTORS IN PROGENITORS

Expression of Glutamate Receptor Isoforms

In the rat neocortical lower cell layer before culture, mRNA expression is seen for NR1, NR2A-2C, and NR2D subunits of the NMDAR subtype, GluR1–4 subunits of the AMPAR subtype, and GluR5, GluR6, GluR7, KA1, and KA2 subunits of the KAR subtype on RT-PCR analysis. In neocortical neurospheres cultured for 12 days, by contrast, mRNA expression is similarly seen for NR2A-2C subunits of NMDAR, GluR1–4 subunits of AMPAR, and GluR5, GluR6, KA1, and KA2 subunits of KAR, but not for NR1 and NR2D subunits of NMDAR and GluR7 subunit of KAR (Table 11.1).

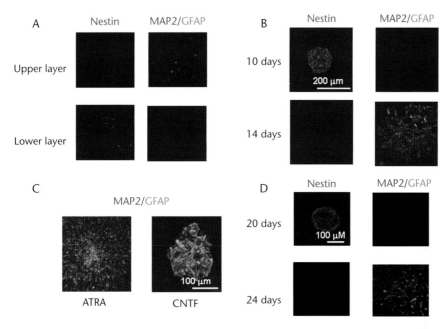

Figure 11.5 Neural progenitor cells isolated from fetal mouse brains. (A) Fetal mouse neocortex was triturated with a Pasteur pipette, followed by the percoll density gradient centrifugation and subsequent gentle aspiration of upper and lower cell layers for immunocytochemical detection of nestin, or double immunocytochemistry on MAP2 and GFAP. (B) The lower cell layer was prepared from fetal mouse neocortex, followed by culture in the presence of EGF under floating conditions for 10 consecutive days toward neurosphere formation and subsequent removal of EGF for culture under adherent conditions for an additional 4 days. (C) After removal of EGF, cells were cultured in the presence of either ATRA or CNTF under adherent conditions for an additional 4 days, followed by double immunocytochemistry on MAP2 and GFAP. (D) After removal of EGF, dispersed cells were again cultured in the presence of EGF for an additional 10 days under floating conditions, followed by immunohistochemical detection of nestin, MAP2, and GFAP. These cells were again dispersed and cultured in the absence of EGF for an additional 4 days for immunocytochemical detection of nestin, MAP2, and GFAP. Typical micrographic pictures are invariably shown with similar results in at least four independent sets of experiments.

Table 11.1 Expression Profile of mRNA for Ionotropic Glutamate Receptor Subtypes in Neural Progenitor Cells

Subtype	Subunit	Neurospheres	
		0 DIV	*12 DIV*
NMDAR	NR1	+	−
	NR2A-C	+	+
	NR2D	+	−
AMPAR	GluR1–4	+	+
KAR	GluR5	+	+
	GluR6	−	+
	GluR7	+	−
	KA 1	+	+
	KA 2	+	+

Total RNA was extracted from the lower cell layer after the percoll centrifugation and neurospheres cultured for 12 days, and then subjected to the synthesis of cDNA. The individual cDNA species were amplified in a reaction mixture containing a cDNA aliquot, PCR buffer, dNTPs, relevant sense and antisense primers, and rTaq DNA polymerase.

Cells are thus cultured in either the presence or absence of different glutamate receptor agonists at 100 μM for 12 consecutive days, followed by determination of mitochondrial activity with 3-(4,5-dimethyl-2-thiazolyl)-2,5-diphenyl-2H-tetrazolium bromide (MTT) reduction and accumulation of lactate dehydrogenase (LDH) released in culture medium. Sustained exposure to either the NMDAR agonist NMDA or the group III mGluR agonist l-2-amino-4-phosphonobutyrate (l-AP4) leads to a significant decrease in the MTT reduction activity (Fig. 11.6A), without significantly affecting LDH release during culture (Fig. 11.6B). However, other GluR agonists do not significantly affect either the MTT reduction activity or LDH release even when persistently exposed to neurospheres for 12 days. These include the AMPAR agonist AMPA, the KAR agonist KA, the group I mGluR agonist 3,5-dihydroxyphenylglycine (DHPG), and the group II mGluR agonist (2S,2'R,3'R)-2-(2,'3'-dicarboxycyclopropyl)glycine (DCG-IV). Therefore, subsequent experiments focus on temporal expression profiles of group III mGluR and NMDAR subtypes in neurospheres cultured in the presence of bFGF for 12 consecutive days.

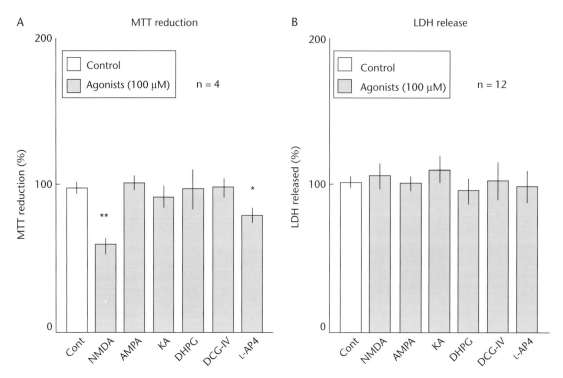

Figure 11.6 Proliferative activity of fetal rat brain progenitor cells. Neocortex was dissected from fetal rat brain, followed by preparation of the lower cell layer. (A) Cells were then cultured in the growth medium containing bFGF in either the presence or absence of an agonist for each glutamate subtype at 100 μM for 12 consecutive days, followed by the determination of activities of (A) MTT reduction and (B) LDH released into culture medium. Values are the mean ± S.E. in four or twelve independent sets of experiments. *$P < 0.05$, **$P < 0.01$, significantly different from each control value obtained in cells not exposed to any GluR agonists.

The expression of mGluR4 mRNA is almost constant in neurospheres cultured up to 12 days (Fig. 11.7), while a drastic increase is seen in mRNA expression of both mGluR6 and mGluR7 isoforms in proportion to increasing culture periods from 2 to 12 days. The expression of mGluR8 mRNA is doubled in neurospheres cultured for 2 days with a constant expression level up to 12 days. Expression levels are not significantly different with mRNA for all group III mGluR subtype isoforms examined in cells further cultured in the absence of bFGF for an additional 6 days from those seen in neurospheres cultured for 12 days. For further evaluation of mRNA expression of each NMDAR subunit, specific primers are designed and used for semiquantitative RT-PCR analysis. In contrast to the temporal expression profile of mRNA for group III mGluR isoforms, transient expression is seen with the NR1 subunit absolutely essential for the heteromeric assemblies toward the functional NMDAR channels in neurospheres cultured for 2 to 6 days, with subsequent disappearance during the culture with bFGF under floating conditions. In dispersed cells cultured for an additional 6 days after the removal of bFGF, however, marked expression is seen in NR1 subunit mRNA at the level similar to that found in pre-neurospheres before culture. By contrast, NR2A subunit mRNA is not

expressed in pre-neurospheres before culture with a gradual increase proportional to the culture duration from 2 to 12 days. Constitutive expression is seen for NR2B subunit mRNA in neurospheres cultured up to 12 days with a sudden 3-fold increase for 2 to 4 days. A gradual decrease is found in the expression of mRNA for both NR2C and NR2D subunits during the culture periods up to 12 days. Marked mRNA expression is seen for all NMDAR subunits examined in dispersed cells cultured after the removal of bFGF up to 18 days. Accordingly, functional NMDAR seems to be transiently expressed during a culture period of 2 to 6 days, but not for 8 to 12 days, in neurospheres cultured in the presence of bFGF under floating conditions.

Responses to NMDA

For further confirmation of the transient expression of functional NMDAR, neurospheres are exposed to 100 μM NMDA for 5 minutes every 2 days, followed by exposure to MK-801 at 10 μM for 10 minutes and subsequent addition of the calcium ionophore A23187 at 10 μM for Ca^{2+} imaging analysis. Cells are then fixed with 4% paraformaldehyde (PA) for the immunocytochemical detection of nestin. Brief exposure to

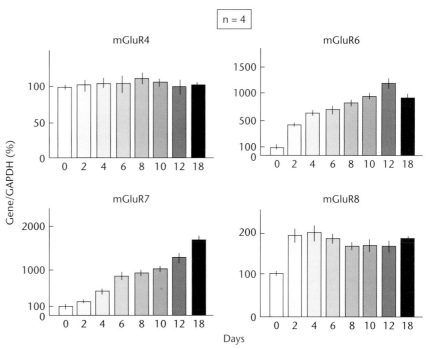

n = 4

mGluR4

mGluR6

mGluR7

mGluR8

Gene/GAPDH (%)

Days

Figure 11.7 Expression profiles of mGluR mRNA in fetal rat brain progenitor cells. The lower cell layer was cultured in the growth medium containing bFGF, followed by cell harvest on different days after plating up to 12 days and subsequent extraction of RNA for semiquantitative RT-PCR analysis. Cells were also dispersed on day 12 and further cultured in the absence of bFGF for an additional 6 days under adherent conditions. Cells were then harvested on day 18, followed by the extraction of RNA for the semiquantitative RT-PCR analysis. Values are the mean ± S.E. in four independent sets of experiments.

NMDA leads to a marked increase in the fluorescence intensity in neurospheres cultured for 2 to 6 days in an MK-801–sensitive manner, but not in those cultured for a period longer than 8 days. The calcium ionophore A23187 is invariably active in drastically increasing the Ca^{2+} fluorescence in neurospheres cultured for 2 to 12 days, however, while marked expression is also seen with nestin in neurospheres throughout the culture period. In cells cultured for 18 days with spontaneous differentiation after the removal of bFGF, NMDA markedly increases the fluorescence in an MK-801–sensitive manner. The addition of A23187 profoundly increases fluorescence in these differentiated cells, where immunoreactive nestin is not expressed at all. Repetition and quantification clearly reveal transient expression of functional NMDAR in neurospheres during culture in the presence of bFGF.

To evaluate the transient expression of functional NMDAR, neurospheres are similarly exposed to 50 mM potassium chloride for determination of intracellular free Ca^{2+} ions every 2 days. In contrast to the response to NMDA, exposure to potassium chloride at a high concentration invariably increases the fluorescence intensity in neurospheres irrespective of the culture duration up to 12 days. Quantification of these data clearly confirms the constant responsiveness to depolarization by potassium chloride with respect to the increased intracellular free Ca^{2+} level in both neurospheres cultured in the presence of bFGF and cells spontaneously differentiated after the removal of bFGF.

Proliferation Modulation by NMDAR

Exposure to NMDA alone markedly decreases the size of neurospheres throughout the culture period up to 12 days in a manner sensitive to prevention by MK-801. To confirm these observations on the size of neurospheres formed, mitochondrial activity is determined by MTT reduction as a measure of the proliferative activity. In proportion to increasing culture durations, mitochondrial activity is drastically increased in neurospheres cultured in the presence of bFGF for 2 to 12 days. However, the activity is significantly decreased in neurospheres cultured in the presence of NMDA alone as seen in phase contrast micrographs. Cells are next cultured in either the presence or absence of NMDAR ligands for different periods up to 12 days, followed by incubation with the thymidine analog BrdU for 24 hours and subsequent determination of the incorporation of BrdU by an enzyme-linked immunosorbent assay (ELISA) kit. The incorporation is drastically increased in proportion to increasing culture periods from 2 to 12 days in the absence of NMDAR ligands, while sustained exposure to NMDA at 100 μM significantly decreases the activity of BrdU incorporation in neurospheres cultured for 2 to 12 days. The aforementioned decreases by NMDA are not seen in neurospheres cultured in the presence of both NMDA and MK-801 irrespective of the culture period up to 12 days. An attempt is then made to determine whether NMDAR ligands affect the incidence of cell death in neurospheres during the culture of up to 12 days. However, no significant difference is seen in the release of LDH from neocortical neurospheres cultured for 2 to 12 days into the culture medium, irrespective of the sustained exposure to any NMDAR ligands examined. Therefore, tonic activation of NMDAR could lead to a significant decrease in the proliferation activity in neural progenitor cells before commitment and/or differentiation without affecting the cellular viability.

Differentiation Modulation by NMDAR

An attempt is next made to determine whether prior activation of NMDAR affects subsequent differentiation of neural progenitor cells after the suppression of cellular proliferation. For this purpose, neurospheres are cultured in either the presence or absence of NMDA at 100 μM for 2 to 12 days, followed by the removal of bFGF and the addition of ATRA or CNTF on 12 days, and subsequent dispersion toward the culture for an additional 6 days. Cells are finally harvested on day 18 for the determination of MAP2 and GFAP on Western blotting analysis. In cells cultured in the absence of differentiation inducers for an additional 6 days, marked expression is seen for the neuronal marker MAP2 and the astroglial marker GFAP. Addition of ATRA significantly increases the expression of MAP2 in cells not exposed to NMDA with a concomitant decrease in GFAP expression, while the exposure to CNTF significantly decreases MAP2 expression with a concurrent increase in GFAP expression vice versa. In cells previously exposed to NMDA for 2 to 12 days, by contrast, a significant increase is seen in MAP2 expression with a concomitant significant decrease in GFAP expression irrespective of the presence of any differentiation inducers.

For further evaluation of the property of cells differentiated after the removal of bFGF, neurospheres are cultured in either the presence or absence of 100 μM NMDA for 2 to 12 days, followed by the removal of bFGF for spontaneous differentiation and subsequent culture for an additional 6 days toward the determination of intracellular free Ca^{2+} levels by fluorescence imaging. Prior exposure to NMDA leads to a significant increase in the number of cells with high fluorescence in response to the second brief exposure to NMDA in an MK-801–sensitive manner on spontaneous differentiation compared to neurospheres not exposed to NMDA when determined on day 18. Therefore, activation of NMDAR would invariably lead to suppression of the proliferative activity toward self-renewal and subsequent promotion of the neuronal differentiation with a concomitant diminution of the astroglial differentiation in neural progenitors isolated from fetal rat neocortex.

Role of NMDAR in Neurogenesis

The essential importance is that sustained exposure to NMDA leads to marked inhibition of the formation of neurospheres and subsequent facilitation of the differentiation to cells immunoreactive for different neuronal marker proteins irrespective of the presence of the neuronal inducer ATRA in cultured neural progenitor cells (Goncalves, Boyle, Webber et al. 2005). The data obtained in both immunocytochemistry and RT-PCR analyses give rise to an idea that functional heteromeric NMDAR channels would be expressed in neural progenitor cells before commitment and/or differentiation to neurons. The fact that brief exposure to NMDA induces marked expression of c-Fos, Fos-B, Fra-2 and c-Jun proteins in a manner sensitive to MK-801 (Kitayama, Yoneyama, Tamaki et al. 2004) is also favorable for the high functionality of NMDAR subunits expressed in neurospheres composed of neural progenitor cells before differentiation. It is highly likely that heteromeric NMDAR channels are functionally expressed by undifferentiated neural progenitor cells. Neural progenitor cells are shown to express particular adhesion molecules including neural cell adhesion molecule (NCAM), cadherin, and integrin α5β1, α6aβ1, αvβ1, αvβ8, α5β1 and low level α6bβ1 (Jacques, Relvas, Nishimura et al. 1998). Moreover, an AP1-binding site exists on the promoter regions of NCAM (Feng, Li, Ng et al. 2002) and integrin α6 (Nishida, Kitazawa, Mizuno et al. 1997). The cell adhesion molecules NCAM and integrin are believed to play an important role in mechanisms underlying cellular proliferation (Jacques, Relvas, Nishimura et al. 1998), migration (Prestoz, Relvas, Hopkins et al. 2001), and differentiation (Amoureux, Cunningham, Edelman et al. 2000) in neural progenitor cells. The administration of an NMDA receptor antagonist leads to the upregulation of NCAM expression in granular cells of the adult rat DG (Nacher, Rosell, Alonso-Llosa et al. 2001). Notch is a signal of differentiation in cell adhesion (Coffman, Skoglund, Harris et al. 1993), while sustained activation of Notch inhibits both commitment and differentiation to either neurons or glia in neural progenitor cells (Yamamoto, Nagao, Sugimori et al. 2001).

Rapid responsiveness of AP1 member proteins (Yoneda, Ogita, Azuma et al. 1999; Kitayama, Yoneyama, Tamaki et al. 2004) argues in favor of a speculation that brief exposure to NMDA could induce transient expression of AP1 complex via functional NMDAR channels assembled by heteromeric subunits expressed by neural progenitor cells toward the modulation of de novo synthesis of inducible target proteins responsible for the regulation of cellular proliferation, commitment, differentiation, and/or maturation. Activation of NMDAR would play a key role in mechanisms associated with the commitment and differentiation of neural progenitor cells at an early developmental stage in neurogenesis. The exact mechanism as well as physiological significance of early and transient expression of functional heteromeric NMDAR channels in neural progenitor cells before differentiation, however, remains to be elucidated in future studies. The possibility that in vitro culture would alter original properties in neural progenitor cells in vivo, moreover, is not ruled out.

The present work also deals with the direct demonstration of facilitation of the subsequent commitment and differentiation to neurons of neural progenitor cells through prior activation of NMDAR. Under conditions that promote differentiation, cultures of dissociated neurospheres show a dose-dependent increase in the number of neurons in response to ATRA (Wohl, Weiss 1998). By contrast, CNTF is required for neural progenitor cells to differentiate into type II astrocytes, and the differentiation is specifically mediated via signal transducer and activator of transcription 3 (Aberg, Ryttsen, Hellgren et al. 2001). Accordingly, both inducers could regulate proliferation and differentiation of neural stem cells after commitment. The presence of ATRA would be favorable for the commitment to neuronal progenitor cells and that of CNTF for astroglial progenitor cells, respectively. Similarly, FBS induces an increase in the number of living cells as well as of astrocytes during differentiation. By contrast, bFGF is shown to facilitate proliferation with reduced differentiation to neurons in neural stem cells at a relatively high concentration as used in the present study (Qian, Davis, Goderie et al. 1998). These previous findings could account for marked expression of GFAP even in the presence of ATRA in cells previously exposed to NMDA. A great part of neural progenitor cells would have been already rendered to differentiate into astrocytes, rather than neurons, during culture under conditions favorable for cell proliferation. Culture conditions would be a determinant for the fate of commitment to neuronal or astroglial progenitor cells in neural progenitor cells. Neural stem cells commit differentiation to specific functional cells in subregions of brain at an early developmental stage in vitro (Retaux, Rogard, Bach et al. 1999; Xiao, Xu, Wang et al. 2000; Bachler, Neubuser 2001). The interaction between CNTF and CNTF receptor α leads to heightened expression of connexin 43 mRNA through the Janus tyrosine kinase/signal transducer and activator of transcription pathway in cultured murine cortical astrocytes (Ozog, Bernier, Bates et al. 2004).

The data cited are all suggestive of the proposal that NMDA signal input may suppress the proliferation toward self-renewal along with the promotion of subsequent commitment and differentiation to neurons in neural progenitor cells (Fig. 11.8). It thus

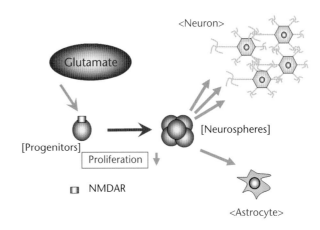

Figure 11.8 Modulation by NMDA signaling. Activation of NMDAR leads to suppressed proliferation activity toward self-replication together with promotion of commitment and differentiation into neurons in neural progenitor cells.

appears that functional heteromeric NMDA receptor channels are expressed by neural progenitor cells before commitment toward the regulation of subsequent differentiation to neurons through a mechanism associated with cellular adhesion. Modulation of the functionality of NMDAR channels would thus be of great benefit for the regeneration of central neurons without surgical implantations in patients with a variety of neurodegenerative disorders in a particular situation.

METABOTROPIC GLUTAMATE RECEPTORS IN PROGENITORS

Expression of mGluRs

In the mouse neocortical lower cell layer before culture, mRNA expression is seen for mGluR1 and mGluR5 isoforms of the group I subtype, mGluR2 and mGluR3 isoforms of the group II subtype, and mGluR4 and mGluR8 isoforms of the group III subtype, but not for mGluR6 and mGluR7 isoforms of the group III subtype, on RT-PCR analysis. In neocortical neurospheres cultured for 10 days, however, mRNA expression is seen for mGluR5, mGluR2, mGluR3, and mGluR8 isoforms, but not for mGluR1, mGluR4, mGluR6, and mGluR7 isoforms.

Cells are then cultured in either the presence or absence of an agonist for the three different mGluR subtypes for 10 consecutive days, followed by observation under a phase contrast microscope and subsequent determination of the total area of neurospheres in visual fields selected at random on computer imaging. The group III mGluR subtype agonist L-AP4 is effective in markedly decreasing the size of neurospheres at 100 μM, while sustained exposure to

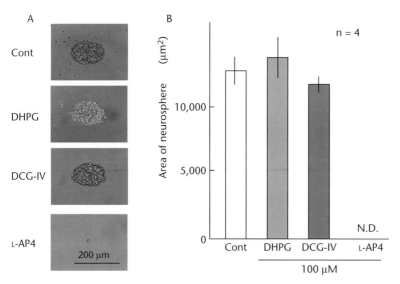

Figure 11.9 Effects of mGluR agonists. Cells were collected from the lower layer, followed by culture with EGF in either the presence or absence of different mGluR subtype agonists at 100 µM for 10 consecutive days. (A) Cell growth was observed under a phase contrast micrograph. (B) The sum of areas of neurospheres was calculated under a phase contrast micrograph on day 10. Each value represents the mean ± S.E.M. in four independent experiments. N.D, not detectable.

either the group I mGluR subtype agonist DHPG or the group II mGluR subtype agonist DCG-IV does not markedly affect the size of neurospheres formed during 10 days at 100 µM (Fig. 11.9A). The total area of neurospheres is almost completely abolished after sustained exposure to L-AP4 at 100 µM, but not to either DHPG or DCG-IV at the same concentration (Fig. 11.9B). Cells are further subjected to the determination of the mitochondrial activity by MTT reduction as a measure of the proliferative activity. In proportion to increasing durations, the mitochondrial activity is drastically increased in neurospheres cultured in the presence of EGF for 2 to 10 days. The activity is significantly decreased in neurospheres cultured in the presence of L-AP4, but not in the presence of either DHPG or DCG-IV, at 100 µM 10 days after plating, as seen by measurement of the total area.

The inhibition by L-AP4 is seen at concentrations above 1 µM when exposed to neurospheres for 10 consecutive days (Fig. 11.10A). Sustained exposure to L-AP4 significantly decreases the MTT reduction activity and the total area of neurospheres (Fig. 11.10B) in a concentration-dependent manner at a concentration range of 1 to 100 µM. No neurospheres are formed in the presence of L-AP4 at 50 µM on day 10, while no significant difference is seen in the cumulative release of LDH from neurospheres cultured for 10 days into culture medium irrespective of the sustained exposure to L-AP4 at concentrations effective in significantly inhibiting the MTT reduction activity. A negligibly little number of cells is reactive with the membrane-impermeable dye PI for DNA staining in neurospheres exposed to 5 µM L-AP4 for 10 days, but most cells are stained with the membrane-permeable dye Hoeschst33342. Cells are also exposed to 5 µM L-AP4 for different periods from 2 to 10 days, followed by the determination of total area of neurospheres on day 10. A significant decrease is seen in the total area

of neurospheres exposed to L-AP4 for a period of 4 to 10 days (Fig. 11.10C). Therefore, sustained exposure to L-AP4 would lead to a significant decrease in the proliferation activity toward self-replication in neural progenitor cells before commitment and/or differentiation, without affecting the cellular viability.

Involvement of Group III mGluR Subtype

Sustained exposure to 5 µM L-AP4 leads to a marked decrease in the size of neurospheres cultured for 10 days, which is blocked by the group III mGluR antagonist RS-α-cyclopropyl-4-phosphonophenyl glycine (CPPG) at 10 µM (Fig. 11.11A). In fact, L-AP4 significantly inhibits the MTT reduction activity and the total area of neurospheres (Fig. 11.11B) in a CPPG-sensitive manner. Moreover, CPPG alone significantly increases the MTT reducing activity and the total area of neurospheres at 10 µM. As the group III mGluR subtype is responsible for the negative regulation of adenylyl cyclase through inhibitory $G_{i/o}$ proteins, an attempt is made to determine whether the adenylyl cyclase activator forskolin affects the MTT reduction activity and the total area of neurospheres cultured for 10 days. Sustained exposure to 10 µM forskolin results in significant increases in the MTT reduction activity and the total area of neurospheres (Fig. 11.11C), which are both prevented by L-AP4. Accordingly, the inhibition by L-AP4 is indeed mediated by the group III mGluR subtype negatively linked to adenylyl cyclase in undifferentiated neural progenitor cells.

cAMP/Protein Kinase A (PKA) Pathway

In addition to forskolin, both dibutyryl cAMP and pituitary adenylyl cyclase–activating peptide (PACAP)

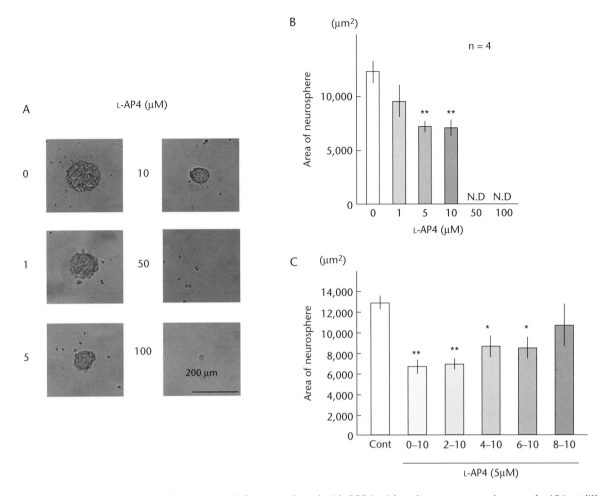

Figure 11.10 Effects of a group III mGluR agonist. Cells were cultured with EGF in either the presence or absence of L-AP4 at different concentrations for 10 consecutive days toward (A) the observation under a phase contrast micrograph and (B) the calculation of the total area of neurospheres. (C) L-AP4 at 5 μM was also added on different days after plating, followed by culture with EGF for 10 days. The total area of neurospheres was calculated in each culture well under a phase contrast micrograph. Each value represents the mean ± S.E.M. in four independent experiments. $*P < 0.05$, $**P < 0.01$, significantly different from each control value obtained in neurospheres grown in the absence of L-AP4. N.D, not detectable.

are effective in significantly increasing the MTT reduction activity and the total area (Fig. 11.12A) in neurospheres cultured for 10 days, with adrenaline being ineffective. The PKA inhibitor H89 significantly prevents the increases by forskolin in the MTT reduction activity and the total area (Fig. 11.12B) in neurospheres cultured for 10 days. H89 alone is also efficient in significantly inhibiting the MTT reduction activity and the total area of neurospheres.

L-AP4 markedly decreases the number of cells immunoreactive for BrdU in a manner sensitive to CPPG when exposed for 9 hours to neurospheres cultured for 6 days. Repetition of these experiments for quantitative analysis clearly confirms a significant decrease in the number of BrdU-positive cells in neurospheres exposed to L-AP4 alone and the significant prevention by CPPG. By contrast, forskolin significantly increases the number of cells immunoreactive for BrdU in neurospheres, which is significantly

blocked by L-AP4. The increase by forskolin is significantly inhibited by H89, while H89 alone significantly decreases the number of cells immunoreactive for BrdU. Thus, the cAMP/PKA pathway would be indeed involved in mechanisms underlying the regulation of proliferation activity toward self-replication in undifferentiated neural progenitor cells.

Cyclin D1 Gene Expression

To investigate the possible mechanism underlying the decreased proliferation by L-AP4, mRNA expression is altogether assessed with different adhesion molecules, in addition to cyclin D1 that is a key regulator of the cell cycle, by semiquantitative RT-PCR analysis. Marked expression is seen for cyclin D1 mRNA in neurospheres cultured for 10 days, while sustained exposure to L-AP4 at 5 μM leads to a

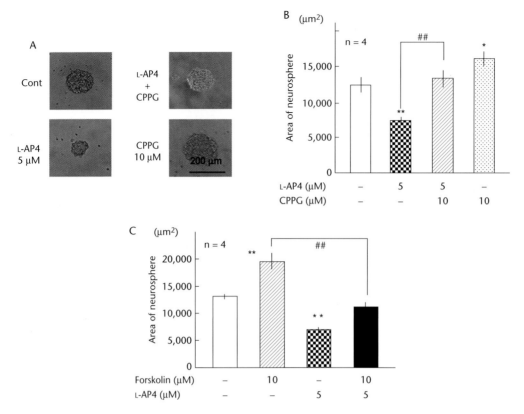

Figure 11.11 Possible involvement of group III mGluR subtype. Cells were cultured with EGF in either the presence or absence of 5 µM L-AP4 and 10 µM CPPG for 10 consecutive days toward (A) the observation under a phase contrast micrograph and (B) the calculation of the total area of neurospheres. (C) Cells were also cultured with EGF in either the presence or absence of 5 µM L-AP4 and 10 µM forskolin for 10 consecutive days for the calculation of the total area of neurospheres. Each value represents the mean ± S.E.M. in four independent experiments. *$P < 0.05$, **$P < 0.01$, significantly different from each control value obtained in neurospheres grown in the absence of added drugs. ## $P < 0.01$, significantly different from the value obtained in neurospheres grown in the presence of either L-AP4 or forskolin alone.

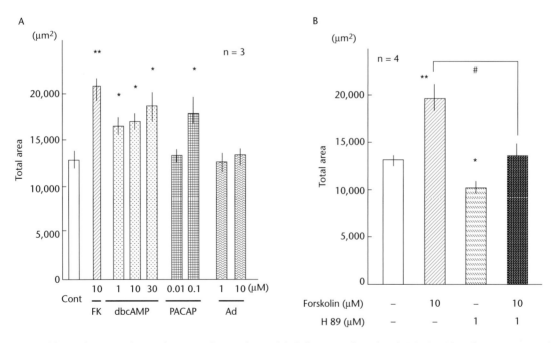

Figure 11.12 Possible involvement of cAMP/PKA signaling pathway. (A) Cells were cultured with EGF in either the presence or absence of forskolin (FK), dibutyryl cAMP (dbcAMP), PACAP, and adrenaline (Ad) at different concentrations for 10 consecutive days toward the calculation of the total area of neurospheres. (B) Cells were also cultured with EGF in either the presence or absence of 10 µM FK and 1 µM H89 for 10 consecutive days for the calculation of the total area of neurospheres. Each value represents the mean ± S.E.M. in three to four independent experiments. *$P < 0.05$, **$P < 0.01$, significantly different from each control value obtained in neurospheres grown in the absence of any added drugs. #$P < 0.05$, significantly different from the value obtained in neurospheres grown in the presence of FK alone.

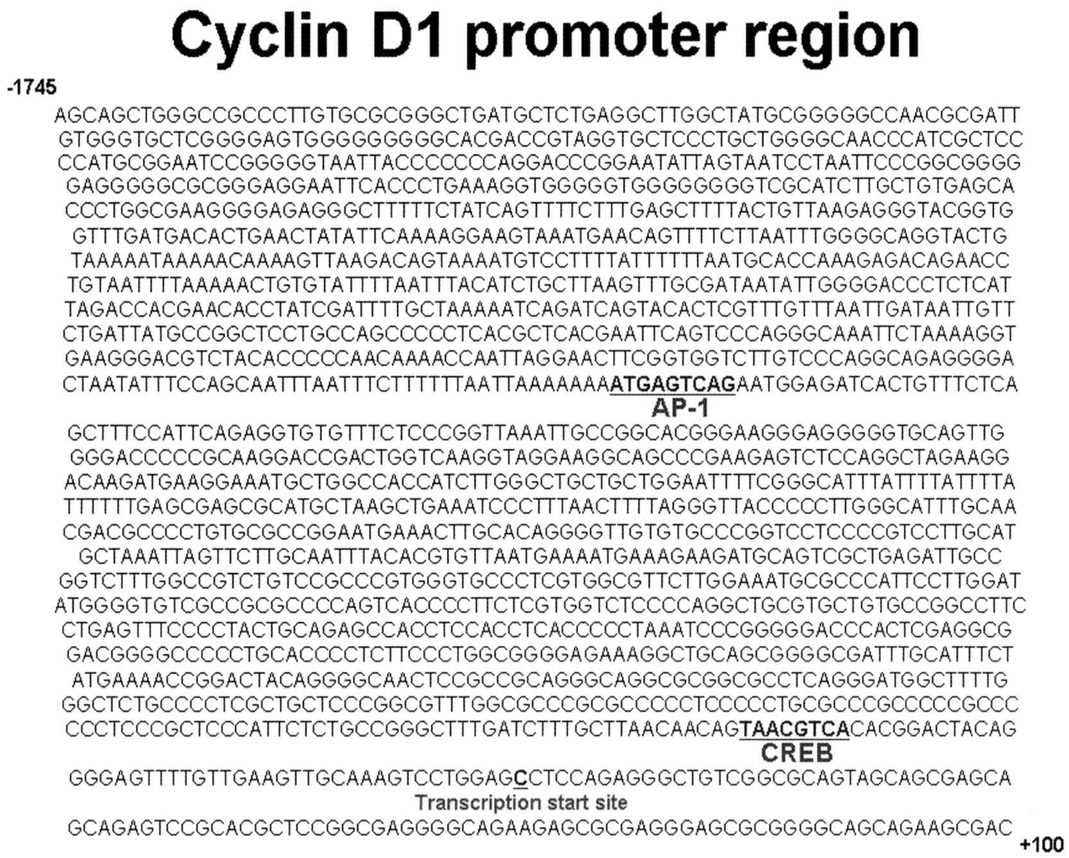

Cyclin D1 promoter region

-1745

```
AGCAGCTGGGCCGCCCTTGTGCGCGGGCTGATGCTCTGAGGCTTGGCTATGCGGGGGGCCAACGCGATT
GTGGGTGCTCGGGGAGTGGGGGGGGGGCACGACCGTAGGTGCTCCCTGCTGGGGCAACCCATCGCTCC
CCATGCGGAATCCGGGGGTAATTACCCCCCCAGGACCCGGAATATTAGTAATCCTAATTCCCGGCGGGG
GAGGGGGCGCGGGAGGAATTCACCCTGAAAGGTGGGGGTGGGGGGGGTCGCATCTTGCTGTGTGAGCA
CCCTGGCGAAGGGGAGAGGGCTTTTTCTATCAGTTTTCTTTGAGCTTTTACTGTTAAGAGGGTACGGTG
GTTTGATGACACTGAACTATATTCAAAAGGAAGTAAATGAACAGTTTTCTTAATTTGGGGCAGGTACTG
TAAAAATAAAAACAAAAGTTAAGACAGTAAAATGTCCTTTTATTTTTTAATGCACCAAAGAGACAGAACC
TGTAATTTTAAAAACTGTGTATTTTAATTTACATCTGCTTAAGTTTGCGATAATATTGGGGACCCTCTCAT
TAGACCACGAACACCTATCGATTTTGCTAAAAATCAGATCAGTACACTCGTTTGTTTAATTGATAATTGTT
CTGATTATGCCGGCTCCTGCCAGCCCCCTCACGCTCACGAATTCAGTCCCAGGGCAAATTCTAAAAGGT
GAAGGGACGTCTACACCCCCAACAAAACCAATTAGGAACTTCGGTGGTCTTGTCCCAGGCAGAGGGGA
CTAATATTTCCAGCAATTTAATTTCTTTTTTAATTAAAAAAAA{ATGAGTCAG}AATGGAGATCACTGTTTCTCA
```
AP-1
```
GCTTTCCATTCAGAGGTGTGTTTCTCCCGGTTAAATTGCCGGCACGGGAAGGGAGGGGGTGCAGTTG
GGGACCCCCGCAAGGACCGACTGGTCAAGGTAGGAAGGCAGCCCGAAGAGTCTCCAGGCTAGAAGG
ACAAGATGAAGGAAATGCTGGCCACCATCTTGGGCTGCTGCTGGAATTTTCGGGCATTTATTTTATTTTA
TTTTTTGAGCGAGCGCATGCTAAGCTGAAATCCCTTTAACTTTTAGGGTTACCCCCTTGGGCATTTGCAA
CGACGCCCCTGTGCGCCGGAATGAAACTTGCACAGGGGTTGTGTGCCCGGTCCTCCCCGTCCTTGCAT
GCTAAATTAGTTCTTGCAATTTACACGTGTTAATGAAAATGAAAGAAGATGCAGTCGCTGAGATTGCC
GGTCTTTGGCCGTCTGTCCGCCCGTGGGTGCCCTCGTGGCGTTCTTGGAAATGCGCCCATTCCTTGGAT
ATGGGGTGTCGCCGCGCCCCAGTCACCCCTTCTCGTGGTCTCCCCAGGCTGCGTGCTGTGCCGGCCTTC
CTGAGTTTCCCCTACTGCAGAGCCACCTCCACCTCACCCCCTAAATCCCGGGGGACCCACTCGAGGCG
GACGGGGCCCCCTGCACCCCTCTTCCCTGGCGGGGAGAAAGGCTGCAGCGGGGCGATTTGCATTTCT
ATGAAAACCGGACTACAGGGGCAACTCCGCCGCAGGGCAGGCGCGGCGCCTCAGGGATGGCTTTTG
GGCTCTGCCCCTCGCTGCTCCCGGCGTTTGGCGCCCGCGCCCCCTCCCCCTGCGCCCGCCCCCGCCC
CCCTCCCGCTCCCATTCTCTGCCGGGCTTTGATCTTTGCTTAACAACAG{TAACGTCA}CACGGACTACAG
```
CREB
```
GGGAGTTTTGTTGAAGTTGCAAAGTCCTGGAG{C}CTCCAGAGGGCTGTCGGCGCAGTAGCAGCGAGCA
```
Transcription start site
```
GCAGAGTCCGCACGCTCCGGCGAGGGGCAGAAGAGCGCGAGGGAGCGCGGGGCAGCAGAAGCGAC
```
+100

Figure 11.13 Full-length promoter region of cyclin D1. On in silico analysis, the cyclin D1 promoter region contains particular nucleotide sequences recognized by the nuclear transcription factors AP1 and CREB, respectively.

profound decrease in cyclin D1 mRNA expression. Semiquantification of these data clearly reveals that cyclin D1 mRNA expression is significantly inhibited by L-AP4 but promoted by forskolin at 10 μM. The decrease by L-AP4 is significantly prevented by CPPG at 10 μM. Similarly, marked expression is seen with mRNA for NCAM, N-cadherin, integrin-β1, and laminin-β1 in neurospheres cultured for 10 days. However, no significant alterations are found in mRNA expression of these adhesion molecules in neurospheres cultured for 10 days irrespective of the presence of those test drugs used.

Cyclin D1 Promoter Activity

In silico analysis clearly shows the presence of particular nucleotide sequences recognized by the nuclear transcription factors AP1 and cAMP response element binding protein (CREB) upstream of the cyclin D1 promoter region (Fig. 11.13). Therefore, we at first examined the similarity of the murine embryonic carcinoma stem cell line P19 cells to murine neural progenitor cells. The pluripotent P19 cells are cultured

in the presence of ATRA for 4 days under floating conditions toward neurosphere formation, followed by immunostaining for nestin, MAP2, and GFAP. The formation is seen with neurospheres immunoreactive for nestin, but neither for MAP2 nor for GFAP, in P19 cells cultured with ATRA within 4 days. In P19 cells before culture with ATRA, mRNA expression is seen for mGluR4 and mGluR8 isoforms of the group III subtype, but not for mGluR1 and mGluR5 isoforms of the group I subtype, mGluR2 and mGluR3 isoforms of the group II subtype, or mGluR6 and mGluR7 isoforms of the group III subtype on RT-PCR analysis. In P19 cells cultured for 4 days with ATRA, however, mRNA expression is seen for mGluR5, mGluR2, mGluR4, mGluR7, and mGluR8 isoforms, but not for mGluR1, mGluR3, or mGluR6 isoform. Therefore, mRNA expression is also seen with the group III mGluR subtype in undifferentiated P19 cells as seen in neural progenitor cells.

Accordingly, P19 cells are similarly exposed to the group III mGluR subtype agonist L-AP4 in the presence of ATRA for 4 days. Sustained exposure to 5 μM L-AP4 invariably leads to a decreased size of neurospheres, while a marked increase is seen in the size of neurospheres exposed to 10 μM forskolin. Determination of the area reveals that L-AP4 significantly decreases the total area of neurospheres in a CPPG-sensitive manner. Forskolin alone significantly increases the total area of neurospheres, while the increase by forskolin is significantly decreased by L-AP4 and H89. H89 alone significantly decreases the total area. These data clearly indicate the high similarity between neural progenitors and P19 cells in terms of the responsiveness to intracellular cAMP signals.

The pluripotent P19 cells are thus plated at a density of 2×10^5 cells/mL in alpha minimal essential medium (αMEM) supplemented with 10% FBS in a culture plate, followed by culture for 2 days and subsequent dispersion with trypsin-EDTA. Cells are then suspended in αMEM containing 10% FBS for centrifugation at 400 g for 5 minutes. Cells are collected for plating at 1×10^5 cells/mL in a plate previously coated with 0.2% agarose in DMEM/F12 supplemented with 10% FBS, followed by the addition of 0.5 μM ATRA and subsequent culture for 4 days under floating conditions in a humidified 5% CO_2 incubator with medium change every 2 days. Moreover, cells are transfected with a reporter plasmid containing the full-length promoter region of cyclin D1 (D'Amico, Wu, Fu et al. 2004) or four tandems of CRE along with the TK-Renilla luciferase construct, with an internal control vector phRL-SV40, by the calcium phosphate method. In brief, plasmid DNA was dissolved in 0.25 M $CaCl_2$, followed by the addition of 2×BES (11.76 g/L N,N-bis(2-hydroxyethyl)-2-aminoethanesulfonic acid sodium salt, 16.36 g/L NaCl, 0.21 g/L Na_2HPO_4, pH 6.95) and subsequent standing for 20 minutes before subsequent addition to cultured cells as a droplet. Cells are further cultured at 35°C under 3% CO_2 for an additional 24 hours, followed by dispersion with trypsin-EDTA and subsequent suspension in αMEM containing 10% FBS for centrifugation at 400 g for 5 minutes. Cells are collected for plating at 1×10^5 cells/mL in a plate previously coated with 0.2% agarose, followed by the culture in DMEM/F12 supplemented with 10% FBS and 0.5 μM ATRA in either the presence or absence of a test drug for 24 hours. Cells are lysed for the determination of luciferase activity using specific substrates in a luminometer. Transfection efficiency is normalized by determining the activity of Renilla luciferase. Approximately 30% of cells express green fluorescent protein in P19 cells transfected with the EGFP-C2 plasmid under the transfection condition employed.

The mouse embryonic carcinoma stem cell line P19 cells transfected with a reporter plasmid of the full-length promoter region of cyclin D1 or four tandems of CRE are thus exposed to a test drug for 24 hours in the presence of ATRA, followed by determination of the luciferase activity. Exposure to L-AP4 significantly decreases the cyclin D1 promoter activity in a CPPG-sensitive manner. Forskolin alone significantly increases the promoter activity, while the increase by forskolin is significantly decreased by L-AP4 and H89. Moreover, H89 alone is effective in significantly decreasing the promoter activity of cyclin D1. Similarly significant alterations are invariably seen with the promoter activity in P19 cells transfected with a reporter plasmid containing the CRE tandem construct. Therefore, activation of group III mGluR subtype would lead to suppression of the proliferation activity toward self-replication through downregulation of the cell cycle regulator cyclin D1 in neural progenitor cells.

Differentiation by Group III mGluR

Neural progenitor cells are cultured in the presence of EGF for 10 consecutive days and subsequent dispersion after the removal of EGF to initiate spontaneous differentiation. Cells are cultured with EGF in either the presence or absence of a test drug for 10 days, followed by further culture in the absence of those test drugs for an additional 4 days toward spontaneous differentiation and subsequent double immunocytochemical detection of both MAP2 and GFAP. Quantification is done by counting the number of cells immunoreactive for either MAP2 or GFAP on double immunocytochemistry analysis, followed by the calculation of percentages over the number of total cells. Irrespective of the exposure to a test drug, cells cultured for an additional 4 days are immunoreactive for either the neuronal marker MAP2 or the astroglial marker GFAP. Prior exposure to L-AP4 induces a marked increase in the number of cells immunoreactive for GFAP with a concomitant decrease in that for MAP2, however, whereas forskolin increases the number of cells immunoreactive for MAP2 together with a decrease in that for GFAP. For quantitative analysis, the number is counted with cells immunoreactive to either MAP2 or GFAP for the calculation of percentages over the total number of cells. Around 60% of cells are immunoreactive for GFAP and less than 40% for MAP2, respectively, on spontaneous differentiation. Prior exposure to L-AP4 alone significantly increases the number of cells immunoreactive for GFAP with a significant decrease in that for MAP2 in a CPPG-sensitive fashion. By contrast, forskolin significantly increases the number of cells immunoreactive for MAP2 along with a significant decrease in that for GFAP.

Neurospheres are cultured in the presence of EGF for 10 days, followed by the further culture in either the presence or absence of ATRA and CNTF for an additional 4 days and subsequent double immuno-cytochemical detection of both MAP2 and GFAP as mentioned. The addition of ATRA markedly increases the number of cells expressing MAP2 with a concomitant decrease in the number of GFAP-expressing cells, while CNTF decreases MAP2 expression with a concurrent increase in GFAP expression. As seen with spontaneous differentiation, prior sustained exposure to L-AP4 alone for 10 days significantly increases the number of cells immunoreactive for GFAP with a concomitant significant decrease in that for MAP2 in a CPPG-sensitive manner irrespective of the differentiation inducers added. Forskolin alone significantly increases the number of cells immunoreactive for MAP2 along with a significant decrease in that for GFAP in cells differentiated by either ATRA or CNTF. Accordingly, the group III mGluR subtype could be functionally expressed to play a pivotal role not only in the proliferation toward self-replication through the modulation relevant to a cAMP/PKA signaling pathway of *cyclin D1* gene expression but also in the subsequent differentiation toward particular cell lineages in undifferentiated neural progenitor cells.

Role of Group III mGluR Subtype in Neurogenesis

Tonic activation of the group III mGluR subtype leads to a significant decrease in the capability to form neurospheres in cultured neural progenitor cells. The data cited all give support to an idea that activation of the group III mGluR subtype leads to suppression of the proliferation activity in neural progenitors through the inhibition of cAMP/PKA signaling processes as shown in the literature (Cartmell, Schoepp 2000; Schoepp 2001; Moldrich, Chapman, De Sarro et al. 2003; Kenny, Markou 2004). As the group III mGluR subtype is negatively linked to adenylyl cyclase through the inhibitory $G_{i/o}$ protein, the formation of cAMP should be under the basic and/or tonic stimulation by some endogenous signals for a group III mGluR agonist to elicit its pharmacological actions in undifferentiated neural progenitor cells. From this point of view, it should be noted that PACAP significantly increases the MTT reduction and the total area of neurospheres in the present study. This polypeptide is shown to regulate the proliferation and differentiation in neural progenitor cells during embryonic development (Dicicco-Bloom, Lu, Pintar et al. 1998). In our hands, by contrast, mRNA expression is not detected for any isoforms of adrenergic β-receptors known to be positively coupled to adenylyl cyclase in undifferentiated neural progenitor cells. Accordingly, the group III mGluR subtype could play a pivotal role in mechanisms underlying the regulation of cellular

proliferation toward self-replication, in association with particular endogenous signals positively coupled to cAMP formation, in undifferentiated neural progenitor cells.

To our knowledge, this is the first direct demonstration of a significant decrease in mRNA expression of cyclin D1 after sustained activation of the group III mGluR subtype in neural progenitors. Cyclin D1 is a major cell cycle regulator responsible for promoted transition to a proliferative stage, while overexpression of cyclin D1 leads to shortening of the G1 phase and subsequent rapid entry into the S phase (Sherr 1994). *Cyclin D1* gene expression is mainly regulated at the transcriptional level with less involvement of the posttranscriptional processes (Yan, Nakagawa, Lee et al. 1997). In fact, CRE is shown to be required for the basal and inducible expression of *cyclin D1* gene in association with the cAMP/PKA signaling pathway in the pancreatic β-cell line INS-1 cells (Kim, Kang, Park et al. 2006). Our present findings from promoter analysis thus argue in favor of a proposal that activation of the group III mGluR subtype would suppress self-replication through the decreased *cyclin D1* gene expression due to reduction of promoter activity in response to the attenuation of the cAMP/PKA signaling pathway after decreased intracellular cAMP levels in undifferentiated neural progenitors.

Nevertheless, the reason why group II and group III mGluR subtypes differentially affect the self-replication activity in undifferentiated neural progenitor cells is not clear so far. The view that both mGluR subtypes are negatively coupled to adenylyl cyclase through the inhibitory $G_{i/o}$ protein in almost all cells is prevailing (Cartmell, Schoepp 2000; Schoepp 2001; Moldrich, Chapman, De Sarro et al. 2003; Kenny, Markou 2004), whereas several independent lines of evidence indicate differential properties between group II and group III mGluR subtypes (Neugebauer, Chen, Willis 2000; Capogna 2004). Similar differentiation between the group II and group III mGluR subtypes is also seen with the inducible expression of AP1 complex in cultured rat neocortical neurons (Sugiyama, Nakamichi, Ogura et al. 2007). The present data are suggestive of the proposal that signals mediated by the group III mGluR subtype may promote the subsequent differentiation of neural progenitor cells into an astroglial lineage. The group III mGluR subtype is not required for the expression of particular adhesion molecules responsible for the cellular proliferation, commitment, and/or differentiation toward a particular lineage in undifferentiated neural progenitor cells. Functional group III mGluR subtype could be constitutively expressed in undifferentiated neural progenitor cells before commitment for the regulation of cellular proliferation toward self-replication and subsequent differentiation into

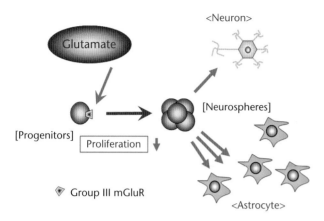

Figure 11.14 Metabotropic glutamatergic modulation. Activation of the group III mGluR subtype leads to the suppressed self-replication activity together with the promotion of commitment and differentiation into astroglia in neural progenitor cells.

particular lineages in fetal mouse brains. Sustained activation of the group III mGluR subtype would result in the suppression of proliferation activity toward self-renewal, together with the facilitation of subsequent differentiation into astroglia (Fig. 11.14).

BALANCING WITH GABAergic SIGNAL INPUTS

In the signal transduction mediated by the inhibitory neurotransmitter GABA, extracellular signals are transformed into intracellular signals through ionotropic (GABA$_A$R and GABA$_C$R) and metabotropic (GABA$_B$R) GABA receptor subtypes in the brain. The GABA$_A$R subtype is orchestrated by the heteromeric assembly of five different proteins, such as α, β, and γ subunits, toward anion channels permeable to chloride ions, whereas the GABA$_C$R subtype is formed from the homomeric assembly of five ρ subunits for chloride channels. In contrast to other metabotropic receptors, however, the metabotropic GABA$_B$R subtype is a heteromeric dimer from the assembly between GABA$_B$R1 and GABA$_B$R2 subunits with the functional linkage to the inhibitory G$_{i/o}$ protein to negatively regulate the activity of adenylyl cyclase, which in turn leads to a decrease in intracellular concentrations of cAMP, opening of potassium channels, and closing of calcium channels (Fig. 11.15).

Alternatively, GABA is shown to partially block the bFGF-induced increase in cell proliferation (Antonopoulos, Pappas, Parnavelas et al. 1997), but promotes cell proliferation in cultures of rat cerebellar progenitors (Fiszman, Borodinsky, Neale 1999). Signal inputs mediated by the ionotropic GABA$_A$R subtype promote the neuronal differentiation after depolarization in neural progenitors of adult mouse

hippocampal slices (Tozuka, Fukuda, Namba et al. 2005). In our previous study, by contrast, sustained activation of the GABA$_A$R subtype leads to increased proliferation along with subsequent facilitation of the commitment and/or differentiation toward an astroglial lineage in the presence of CNTF in neural progenitor cells isolated from fetal rat neocortex (Yoneyama, Fukui, Nakamichi et al. 2007). Moreover, we have attempted to evaluate the possible modulation of functionality by metabotropic GABA$_B$R subtype expressed in neural progenitor cells prepared from fetal mouse neocortex under similar conditions.

In the neocortical lower cell layer before culture, indeed, mRNA expression is seen for α1, α2, α3, α4, α5, β1, β2, β3, γ2, γ3, and δ subunits of GABA$_A$R, GABA$_B$R1a, 1b, and GABA$_B$R2 subunits of GABA$_B$R, and ρ1, ρ2, and ρ3 subunits of GABA$_C$R, but not for α6 or γ1 subunit of GABA$_A$R, on RT-PCR analysis. In neocortical neurospheres grown for 10 days, however, mRNA expression is seen for α2, α3, α4, α5, β1, β2, β3, γ1, γ2, and γ3 subunits of GABA$_A$R and GABA$_B$R1a, 1b, and GABA$_B$R2 subunits of GABA$_B$R, and ρ1, ρ2 subunit of GABA$_C$R, but not for α1, α6, and δ subunits of GABA$_A$R or ρ3 subunit of GABA$_C$R (Table 11.2). Moreover, mRNA expression is seen for Mgat1, Mgat3, and Mgat4, but not Mgat2, isoforms of GABA transporters, vesicular GABA transporter required for the condensation of GABA, and both GAD65 and GAD67 isoforms of glutamate decarboxylase responsible for the synthesis of GABA from glutamate, in the lower cell layer prepared from fetal mouse neocortex. Similar expression profiles are found with mRNA for these GABAergic signaling molecules, except Mgat2 isoform, in neurospheres cultured for 10 days. The GABA$_B$R subtype agonist baclofen significantly increases the mitochondrial activity and the total areas of neurospheres in a manner sensitive to a GABA$_B$R subtype antagonist when exposed for 10 consecutive days. By contrast, a significant decrease is seen in the total areas of neurospheres prepared from Balb/c mice defective of the GABA$_B$R1 subunit essential for the dimeric assembly to the functional GABA$_B$R subtype linked to the inhibitory G$_{i/o}$ protein toward negative regulation of the activity of adenylyl cyclase, which decreases intracellular concentrations of cAMP as seen with the group II and group III mGluR subtypes of glutamate receptors.

In neurospheres prepared from GABA$_B$R1-null mice, in fact, a significant increase is induced in the number of cells immunoreactive for GFAP, with a concomitant decrease in that of MAP2, after the removal of a growth factor. It is thus likely that the GABA$_B$R subtype may preferentially promote the commitment of neural progenitor cells toward a neuronal lineage after the activation of cellular proliferation in the developing mouse brain. In addition to glutamate,

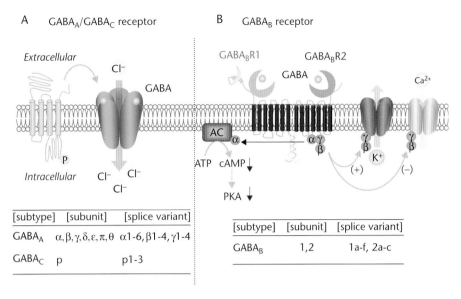

Figure 11.15 Classification of GABA receptors. GABAR is classified into three different subtypes according to the signal transduction system, nucleotide sequential homology, and pharmacology as seen with glutamate receptors. (A) The GABA$_A$R subtype is composed of the heteromeric assembly of five different proteins, such as α, β, and γ subunits, toward the orchestration of anion channels permeable to chloride ions, whereas the GABA$_C$R subtype is formed from the homomeric assembly of five ρ subunits for chloride channels. (B) The metabotropic GABA$_B$R subtype is a heteromeric dimer constructed from the assembly between GABA$_B$R1 and GABA$_B$R2 subunits with the functional linkage to the inhibitory Gi/o protein to negatively regulate the activity of adenylyl cyclase, which in turn leads to a decrease in intracellular concentrations of cAMP, opening of potassium channels, and closing of calcium channels. Expression of either GABA$_B$R1 or GABA$_B$R2 subunit alone is not functional as a GABA$_B$R subtype for the signal transformation at cell surfaces.

Table 11.2 Expression Profile of mRNA for GABA Receptor Subtypes in Neural Progenitor Cells

Subtype	Subunit	Neurospheres	
		0 DIV	*10 DIV*
GABA$_A$R	α1	+	−
	α2	+	+
	α3	+	+
	α4	+	+
	α5	+	+
	α6	−	−
	β1	+	+
	β2	+	+
	β3	+	+
	γ1	−	+
	γ2	+	+
	γ3	+	+
	δ	+	−
GABA$_B$R	1a, 1b	+	+
	2	+	+
GABA$_C$R	ρ1, ρ2	+	+
	ρ3	−	+

Total RNA was extracted from the lower cell layer after the percoll centrifugation and neurospheres cultured for 10 days, and then subjected to the synthesis of cDNA. The individual cDNA species were amplified in a reaction mixture containing a cDNA aliquot, PCR buffer, dNTPs, relevant sense and antisense primers, and rTaq DNA polymerase.

therefore, GABA could also play a pivotal role in the regulation of cellular proliferation through activation of ionotropic GABA$_A$R and metabotropic GABA$_B$R subtypes expressed by undifferentiated neural progenitor cells endowed with self-replication and multipotentiality. Taken together, one fascinating but hitherto unidentified speculation is that self-replication and multipotentiality would be under control by the delicate balancing between GABAergic and glutamatergic signals through the respective ionotropic and metabotropic receptors expressed by neural progenitor cells before differentiation as seen in matured neurons. In undifferentiated progenitors, GABA could positively regulate the proliferation through ionotropic GABA$_A$R and metabotropic GABA$_B$R subtypes, but glutamate would negatively modulate the proliferation through the group III mGluR subtype, in addition to the ionotropic NMDAR subtype (Kitayama, Yoneyama, Yoneda 2003; Kitayama, Yoneyama, Tamaki et al. 2004). The possibility that in vitro culture may artifactitiously alter original properties of neural progenitor cells in vivo, however, is not ruled out so far.

CONCLUDING REMARKS

Activation of the NMDAR subtype could lead to the suppressed self-replication activity in neural

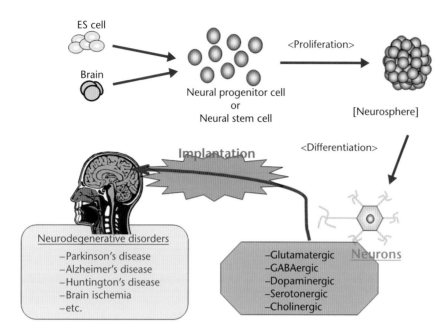

Figure 11.16 Possible clinical trials. Modulation of the functionality of either NMDAR or group III mGluR subtype would be of great benefit for regeneration and supplementation without surgical implantations of progenitor cells in patients suffering from a variety of brain diseases relevant to neuronal and/or astroglial dysfunctions. Alternatively, prior modulation of the activity of either glutamate receptor subtype could be a novel strategy for the subsequent regulation of the differentiation toward a neuronal lineage of neural progenitors implanted.

progenitor cells along with the promotion of subsequent differentiation into neurons, while activation of the group III mGluR subtype would result in the similarly efficient suppression of self-renewal activity together with the facilitation of subsequent differentiation into astroglia. Therefore, modulation of the functionality of particular glutamate receptor subtypes would be of a great benefit for the regeneration and supplementation of neuronal and/or astroglial lineages without surgical implantations of neural progenitor cells in patients suffering from a variety of brain diseases relevant to neuronal and/or astroglial dysfunctions. Alternatively, prior modulation of the activity of glutamate receptors could be a novel strategy for the subsequent regulation of the differentiation toward a particular progeny cell lineage of neural progenitor cells implanted (Fig. 11.16).

ACKNOWLEDGMENTS   This work was supported in part by Grants-in-Aid for Scientific Research to Y.Y. and N.N. from the Ministry of Education, Culture, Sports, Science and Technology, Japan.

REFERENCES

Aberg MA, Ryttsen F, Hellgren G et al. 2001. Selective introduction of antisense oligonucleotides into single adult CNS progenitor cells using electroporation demonstrates the requirement of STAT3 activation for CNTF-induced gliogenesis. *Mol Cell Neurosci.* 17:426–443.

Altman J, Das G. 1967. Postnatal neurogenesis in the guinea-pig. *Nature.* 214:1098–1101.

Amoureux MC, Cunningham BA, Edelman GM, Crossin KL. 2000. N-CAM binding inhibits the proliferation of hippocampal progenitor cells and promotes their differentiation to a neuronal phenotype. *J Neurosci.* 20:3631–3640.

Antonopoulos J, Pappas IS, Parnavelas JG. 1997. Activation of the GABAA receptor inhibits the proliferative effects of bFGF in cortical progenitor cells. *Eur J Neurosci.* 9:291–298.

Bachler M, Neubuser A. 2001. Expression of members of the Fgf family and their receptors during midfacial development. *Mech Dev.* 100:313–316.

Capogna M. 2004. Distinct properties of presynaptic group II and III metabotropic glutamate receptor-mediated inhibition of perforant pathway-CA1 EPSCs. *Eur J Neurosci.* 19:2847–2858.

Cartmell J, Schoepp DD. 2000. Regulation of neurotransmitter release by metabotropic glutamate receptors. *J Neurochem.* 75:889–907.

Cavanagh JF, Mione MC, Pappas IS, Parnavelas JG. 1997. Basic fibroblast growth factor prolongs the proliferation of rat cortical progenitor cells in vitro without altering their cell cycle parameters. *Cereb Cortex.* 7:293–302.

Coffman CR, Skoglund P, Harris WA, Kintner CR. 1993. Expression of an extracellular deletion of Notch diverts cell fate in Xenopus embryos. *Cell.* 73:659–671.

Conn PJ, Pin JP. 1997. Pharmacology and functions of metabotropic glutamate receptors. *Ann Rev Pharmacol Toxicol.* 37:205–237.

D'Amico M, Wu K, Fu M et al. 2004. The inhibitor of cyclin-dependent kinase 4a/alternative reading frame (INK4a/ARF) locus encoded proteins p16INK4a and p19ARF repress cyclin D1 transcription through distinct *cis* elements. *Cancer Res.* 64:4122–4130.

Dicicco-Bloom E, Lu N, Pintar JE, Zhang J. 1998. The PACAP ligand/receptor system regulates cerebral cortical neurogenesis. *Ann N Y Acad Sci.* 865:274–289.

Doetsch F, Caille I, Lim DA, Garcia-Verdugo JM, Alvarez-Buylla A. 1999. Subventricular zone astrocytes are neural stem cell in the adult mammalian brain. *Cell.* 97:703–716.

Feng ZF, Li L, Ng PY, Porter AG. 2002. Neuronal differentiation and protection from nitric oxide-induced apoptosis require c-Jun-dependent expression of NCAM 140. *Mol Cell Biol.* 22:5357–5366.

Fiszman ML, Borodinsky LN, Neale JH. 1999. GABA induces proliferation of immature cerebellar granule cells grown in vitro. *Brain Res Dev Brain Res.* 115:1–8.

Gage FH, Coates PW, Palmer TD et al. 1995. Survival and differentiation of adult neuronal progenitor cells transplanted to the adult brain. *Proc Natl Acad Sci U S A.* 92:11879–11883.

Gage FH, Kempermann G, Palmer TD, Peterson DA, Ray J. 1998. Multipotent progenitor cells in the adult dentate gyrus. *J Neurobiol.* 36:249–266.

Garcia-Verdugo JM, Doetsch F, Wichterle H, Lim DA, Alvarez-Buylla A. 1998. Architecture and cell types of the adult subventricular zone: in search of the stem cells. *J Neurobiol.* 36:234–248.

Goncalves MBCV, Boyle J, Webber DJ, Hall S, Minger SL, Corcoran JPT. 2005. Timing of the retinoid-signalling pathway determines the expression of neuronal markers in neural progenitor cells. *Dev Biol.* 278:60–70.

Haydar TF, Wang F, Schwartz ML, Rakic P. 2000. Differential modulation of proliferation in the neocortical ventricular and subventricular zones. *J Neurosci.* 20:5764–5774.

Jacques TS, Relvas JB, Nishimura S et al. 1998. Neural precursor cell chain migration and division are regulated through different β1 integrins. *Development.* 125:3167–3177.

Johansson CB, Momma S, Clarke DL, Risling M, Lendahl U, Frisen J. 1999. Identification of a neural stem cell in the adult mammalian central nervous system. *Cell.* 96:25–34.

Kaplan MS, Hinds JW. 1977. Neurogenesis in adult rat: electron microscopic analysis of light radioautographs. *Science.* 197:1092–1094.

Kaplan MS, Bell DH. 1983. Neuronal proliferation in the 9-month-old rodent: radioautographic study of granule cells in the hippocampus. *Exp Brain Res.* 52:1–5.

Kaplan MS, Bell DH. 1984. Mitotic neuroblasts in the 9-day-old and 11-month-old rodent hippocampus. *J Neurosci.* 4:1429–1441.

Kenny PJ, Markou A. 2004. The ups and downs of addiction: role of metabotropic glutamate receptors. *Trends Pharmacol Sci.* 25:265–272.

Kim M-J, Kang J-H, Park YG et al. 2006. Extendin-4 induction of cyclin D1 expression in INS-1 β-cells: involvement of cAMP-responsive element. *J Endocrinol.* 188:623–633.

Kitayama T, Yoneyama M, Yoneda Y. 2003. Possible regulation by N-methyl-D-aspartate receptors of proliferative progenitor cells expressed in adult mouse hippocampal dentate gyrus. *J Neurochem.* 84:767–780.

Kitayama T, Yoneyama M, Tamaki K, Yoneda Y. 2004. Regulation of neuronal differentiation by N-methyl-D-aspartate receptors expressed in neural progenitor cells isolated from adult mouse hippocampus. *J Neurosci Res.* 76:599–612.

LoTurco JJ, Owens DF, Heath MJS, Davis MBE, Kriegstein AR. 1995. GABA and glutamate depolarize cortical progenitor cells and inhibit DNA synthesis. *Neuron.* 15:1287–1298.

Moldrich RX, Chapman AG, De Sarro G, Meldrum BS. 2003. Glutamate metabotropic receptors as targets for drug therapy in epilepsy. *Eur J Pharmacol.* 476:3–16.

Nacher J, Rosell D, Alonso-Llosa G, McEwen B. 2001. NMDA receptor antagonist treatment induces a long-lasting increase in the number of proliferating cells, PSA-NCAM-immunoreactive granule neurons and radial glia in the adult rat dentate gyrus. *Eur J Neurosci.* 13:512–520.

Neugebauer V, Chen PS, Willis WD. 2000. Groups II and III metabotropic glutamate receptors differentially modulate brief and prolonged nociception in primate STT cells. *J Neurophysiol.* 84:2998–3009.

Nishida K, Kitazawa R, Mizuno K, Maeda S, Kitazawa S. 1997. Identification of regulatory elements of human alpha 6 integrin subunit gene. *Biochem Biophys Res Commun.* 241:258–263.

Ozog MA, Bernier SM, Bates DC, Chatterjee B, Lo CW, Naus CC. 2004. The complex of ciliary neurotrophic-ciliary neurotrophic receptor alpha up-regulates connexin 43 and intercellular coupling in astrocytes via the Janus tyrosine kinase/signal transducer and activator of transcription pathway. *Mol Biol Cell.* 15:4761–4774.

Prestoz L, Relvas JB, Hopkins K et al. 2001. Association between integrin-dependent migration capacity of neural stem cells in vitro and anatomical repair following transplantation. *Mol Cell Neurosci.* 18:473–484.

Qian X, Davis AA, Goderie SK, Temple S. 1998. FGF2 concentration regulates the generation of neurons and glia from multipotent cortical stem cells. *Neuron.* 18:81–93.

Retaux S, Rogard M, Bach I, Failli V, Besson MJ. 1999. Lhx9: a novel LIM-homeodomain gene expressed in the developing forebrain. *J Neurosci.* 19:783–793.

Schoepp DD. 2001. Unveiling the functions of presynaptic metabotropic glutamate receptors in the central nervous system. *J Pharmacol Exp Ther.* 299:12–20.

Schoepp DD, Jane DE, Monn JA. 1999. Pharmacological agents acting at subtypes of metabotropic glutamate receptors. *Neuropharmacol.* 38:1431–1476.

Sherr CJ. 1994. G1 phase progression: cycling on cue. *Cell.* 79:551–555.

Sugiyama C, Nakamichi N, Ogura M et al. 2007. Activator protein-1 responsive to the group II metabotropic glutamate receptor subtype in association with intracellular calcium in cultured rat cortical neurons. *Neurochem Int.* 51:467–475.

Suhonen JO, Peterson DA, Ray J, Gage FH. 1996. Differentiation of adult hippocampus-derived progenitors into olfactory neurons in vivo. *Nature.* 383:624–627.

Temple S, Alvarez-Buylla A. 1999. Stem cells in the adult mammalian central nervous system. *Curr Opin Neurobiol.* 9:135–141.

Tozuka Y, Fukuda S, Namba T, Seki T, Hisatsune T. 2005. GABAergic excitation promotes neuronal differentiation in adult hippocampal progenitor cells. *Neuron.* 47:803–815.

Vaccarino FM, Schwartz MI, Raballo R et al. 1999. Changes in cerebral cortex size are governed by fibroblast growth factor during embryogenesis. *Nature Neurosci.* 3:246–253.

Wohl CA, Weiss S. 1998. Retinoic acid enhances neuronal proliferation and astroglial differentiation in culture of CNS stem cell-derived precursors. *J Neurobiol.* 37:281–290.

Xiao Q, Xu HY, Wang SR, Lazar G. 2000. Developmental changes of NADPH-diaphorase positive structures in the isthmic nuclei of the chick. *Anat Embryol. (Berl).* 201:509–519.

Yamamoto S, Nagao M, Sugimori M et al. 2001. Transcription factor expression and Notch-dependent regulation of neural progenitors in the adult rat spinal cord. *J Neurosci.* 21:9814–9823.

Yan Y-X, Nakagawa H, Lee M-H, Rustgi AK. 1997. Transforming growth factor-α enhances cyclin D1 transcription through the binding of early response protein to a *cis*-regulatory element in the cyclin D1 promoter. *J Biol Chem.* 272:33181–33190.

Yoneda Y, Ogita K, Azuma Y, Kuramoto N, Manabe T, Kitayama T. 1999. Predominant expression of nuclear activator protein-1 complex with DNA binding activity following systemic administration of N-methyl-D-aspartate in dentate granule cells of murine hippocampus. *Neuroscience.* 93:19–31.

Yoneyama M, Fukui M, Nakamichi N, Kitayama T, Taniura H, Yoneda Y. 2007. Activation of GABA$_A$ receptors facilitates astroglial differentiation induced by ciliary neurotrophic factor in neural progenitors isolated from fetal rat brain. *J Neurochem.* 100:1667–1679.

Zhai Y, George CA, Zhai J, Nisenbaum ES, Johnson MP, Nisenbaum LK. 2003. Group II metabotropic glutamate receptor modulation of DOI-induced c-fos mRNA and excitatory responses in the cerebral cortex. *Neuropsychopharmacol.* 28:45–52.

PART III

Elucidating Inflammatory Mediators of Disease

Chapter **12**

NEUROIMMUNE INTERACTIONS THAT OPERATE IN THE DEVELOPMENT AND PROGRESSION OF INFLAMMATORY DEMYELINATING DISEASES: LESSONS FROM PATHOGENESIS OF MULTIPLE SCLEROSIS

Enrico Fainardi and Massimiliano Castellazzi

ABSTRACT

Multiple sclerosis (MS) is considered an autoimmune chronic inflammatory disease of the central nervous system (CNS) characterized by demyelination and axonal damage. It is widely accepted that MS immune response compartmentalized within the CNS is mediated by autoreactive major histocompatibility complex (MHC) class II–restricted $CD4^+$ T cells trafficking across the blood–brain barrier (BBB) after activation and secreting T helper 1 (Th1)-type pro-inflammatory cytokines. These cells seem to regulate a combined attack of both innate and acquired immune responses directed against myelin proteins, which includes macrophages, MHC class I–restricted $CD8^+$ T cells, B cells, natural killer (NK) cells, and $\gamma\delta$ T cells. This coordinated assault is also directed toward neurons and results in axonal loss. However, although the understanding of the mechanisms that orchestrate the development and the progression of the disease has recently received increasing attention, the sequence of events leading to myelin and axonal injury currently remains uncertain. Failure of peripheral immunologic tolerance is hypothesized to play a crucial role in the initiation of MS, but evidence for a single triggering factor is lacking. In addition, the different theories proposed to explain this crucial step, suggesting the involvement of an infectious agent, a dysfunction of regulatory pathways in the periphery and a primary neurodegeneration, are difficult to reconcile. On the other hand, the view of MS as a "two-stage disease," with a predominant inflammatory demyelination in the early phase (relapsing–remitting MS form) and a subsequent secondary neurodegeneration in the late phase (secondary or primary progressive MS) of the disease, is now challenged by the demonstration that axonal destruction may occur independently of inflammation and may also produce it. Therefore, as CNS inflammation and degeneration can coexist throughout the course of the disease, MS may be a "simultaneous two-component disease," in which the combination of neuroinflammation and neurodegeneration promotes irreversible disability.

Keywords: central nervous system, immune surveillance, inflammation, tissue damage, multiple sclerosis.

IMMUNE RESPONSES WITHIN THE CENTRAL NERVOUS SYSTEM

The central nervous system (CNS) has traditionally been considered as an immunologically privileged site in which the immune surveillance is lacking and where the development of an immune response is more limited compared to other non-CNS organs. This view was based on the results obtained in earlier transplantation studies demonstrating that a relative tolerance to grafts is present in the brain (Medawar 1948; Barker, Billingham 1977). In addition, the immunologically privileged status of the CNS was further supported by the following complementary observations (Ransohoff, Kivisäkk, Kidd 2003; Engelhardt, Ransohoff 2005; Bechmann 2005; Carson, Doose, Melchior et al. 2006): (a) the existence of a blood–brain barrier (BBB), a mechanical diffusion barrier for hydrophilic molecules, immune cells, and mediators, which is formed by specialized endothelial cells with tight junctions located at the level of brain capillaries and by the surrounding basement membrane and astroglial end-feet (glia limitans); (b) the absence of a lymphatic drainage of the brain parenchyma; (c) the lack of a constitutive expression of major histocompatibility complex (MHC) class I and class II antigens on neural cells; and (d) no occurrence of professional antigen-presenting cells (APCs) in the CNS. However, a growing body of evidence coming from experimental and human investigations now suggests that this paradigm should be modified.

CNS as an Immunologically Specialized Site

As indicated in Table 12.1, the immune privilege of the CNS has recently been challenged by several findings showing that (a) rejection of tissue grafts (Mason, Charlton, Jones et al. 1986) and delayed type hypersensitivity reactions (Matyszak, Perry

Table 12.1 Data Supporting the View of the Central Nervous System (CNS) as Immunospecialized Site

Evidence	References
Occurrence of tissue graft rejection and delayed type hypersensitivity responses in the CNS	Mason et al. 1986 Matyszac, Perry 1996a
Existence of a lymphocyte traffic into the brain across the blood–brain barrier (BBB) in the noninflamed normal CNS	Hickey et al. 1991
Drainage of brain antigens into cervical lymph nodes through the CSF	Cserr, Knopf 1992 Kida et al. 1993
Detection of CNS-associated cells acting as resident antigen-presenting cells (APC) in the Virchow-Robin perivascular spaces, the leptomeninges, and the choroid plexus	Matyszac, Perry 1996b McMenamin 1999
Expression of MHC class I and II molecules on all brain cell types after activation in the inflamed CNS	Hemmer et al. 2004

1996a) can be observed in the CNS; (b) activated lymphocytes are able to enter the brain trafficking across the BBB in the noninflamed CNS (Hickey, Hsu, Kimura 1991); (c) brain antigens are efficiently drained into cervical lymph nodes via the cribroid plate and perineural sheaths of cranial nerves (Cserr, Knopf 1992; Kida, Pantazis, Weller 1993); (d) CNS-associated cells acting as APCs are detectable in the Virchow-Robin perivascular spaces, the leptomeninges and the choroid plexus (Matyszak, Perry 1996b; McMenamin 1999); and (e) all brain cell types can express MHC class I and II molecules after activation in the inflamed CNS (Hemmer, Cepok, Zhou et al. 2004). In particular, it has been documented that foreign tissue grafts are rejected when injected into the ventricular system, whereas bystander demyelination and axonal loss are triggered by a delayed type hypersensitivity response after intraventricular bacterial injection (Galea, Bechmann, Perry 2007). In addition, migration of activated T cells from the intravascular compartment into the CNS can occur using different routes of entry (Ransohoff, Kivisäkk, Kidd 2003): (a) from blood to cerebrospinal fluid (CSF) across the choroid plexus; (b) from blood to subarachnoid space; and (c) from blood to parenchyma. In the first pathway, which is currently believed to be the main route by which T cells infiltrate the CNS under normal conditions, T cells penetrate fenestrated endothelial cells and specialized epithelial cells with tight junctions of the choroid plexus stroma and then move into the CSF. In the second pathway, T cells extravasate through the postcapillary venules at the pial surface of the brain and then arrive in the subarachnoid and perivascular spaces. In the third pathway, T cells traverse the postcapillary venules, pass into the subarachnoid and perivascular spaces, cross the BBB, and then gain direct access to brain tissue. In this setting, it is important to note that, in absence of ongoing CNS inflammation only activated T cells travel into the brain since resting T lymphocytes fail to transit across the BBB. On the other hand, the subarachnoid and perivascular spaces of the nasal olfactory artery are connected, via the cribriform plate, with nasal lymphatics and cervical lymph nodes, thus allowing CSF drainage into the cervical lymphatics (Harling-Berg, Park, Knopf 1999; Aloisi, Ria, Adorini 2000; Ransohoff, Kivisäkk, Kidd 2003; Engelhardt, Ransohoff 2005; Galea, Bechmann, Perry 2007). In this way, after their migration in CSF from white matter through the ependyma and from grey matter along perivascular spaces, brain-soluble proteins can be transported to local peripheral lymph nodes where they can trigger priming and activation of naïve T lymphocytes. Nevertheless, these interactions require local APCs capable of expressing specific antigens associated to MHC molecules on cell surface after engulfment. Resident APCs of the CNS include a variety of myeloid-lineage cells such as perivascular cells (macrophages), meningeal macrophages and dendritic cells, intraventricular macrophages (epiplexus or Kolmer cells), and choroid plexus macrophages and dendritic cells (Aloisi, Ria, Adorini 2000; Ransohoff, Kivisäkk, Kidd 2003; Engelhardt, Ransohoff 2005). Moreover, also microglial cells acquire APC properties in the course of CNS inflammation (Aloisi, Ria, Adorini 2000; Carson, Doose, Melchior et al. 2006). In this regard, the presence of meningeal and choroid plexus dendritic cells, which are the most effective APCs for initiating T-cell responses, is of relevance. In fact, these cells could capture CSF soluble proteins coming from brain parenchyma and transport them to draining cervical lymph nodes. Furthermore, dendritic cells may present such antigens to naïve T cells at the level of local lymph nodes (Galea, Bechmann, Perry 2007). In normal brain, a constitutive expression of MHC antigens is present on endothelial cells, perivascular, meningeal, and choroid plexus macrophages, and some microglial cells for MHC class I molecules (Hoftberger, Aboul-Enein, Brueck et al. 2004). Conversely, MHC class II molecules result constitutively expressed only on perivascular, meningeal, and choroid plexus cells since their expression on resting microglia still remains a controversial issue (Becher, Prat, Antel 2000; Aloisi, Ria, Adorini 2000; Aloisi 2001; Hemmer, Cepok, Zhou et al. 2004; Becher, Beckmann, Greter 2006). During intrathecal inflammatory responses, microglial cells and astrocytes become MHC-I and MHC-II positive, whereas oligodendrocytes and neurons upregulate MHC class I molecules (Dong, Benveniste 2001; Aloisi 2001; Neumann, Medana, Bauer 2002). Notably, while CD4$^+$ T cells recognize antigens bound to MHC class II molecules, CD8$^+$ T cells respond to peptides associated to MHC class I molecules. Therefore, in inflamed CNS, all brain cell types are theoretically susceptible to attack by CD8$^+$ T cells, whereas only microglial cells and astrocytes react with CD4$^+$ T cells (Hemmer, Cepok, Zhou et al. 2004). As given in Table 12.2, these data indicate that an immune reaction can take place in the CNS because both the afferent and the efferent arms of this response exist there (Harling-Berg, Park, Knopf

Table 12.2 Afferent and Efferent Arms of Immune Responses of the Central Nervous System (CNS)

Pathway	Features	References
Afferent arm	Migration of brain-soluble antigens from parenchyma to cerebrospinal fluid (CSF) through the ependyma for white matter and along perivascular spaces for grey matter	Harling-Berg et al. 1999 Ransohoff et al. 2003 Engelhardt, Ransohoff 2005 Galea et al. 2007
	Capture and transport of CSF brain-soluble antigens to draining cervical lymph nodes operated by meningeal and choroid plexus dendritic cells	
Efferent arm	Presentation of brain soluble antigens released from the CNS to naive T cells performed by dendritic cells at the level of cervical lymph nodes	Harling-Berg et al. 1999 Ransohoff et al. 2003 Engelhardt, Ransohoff 2005 Galea et al. 2007
	Priming and activation of naive T cells in cervical lymph nodes	
	Migration of activated T cells from blood to CSF across the choroid plexus	
	Presentation of cognate antigen to activated T cells carried out by perivascular macrophages	

1999; Ransohoff, Kivisäkk, Kidd 2003; Engelhardt, Ransohoff 2005; Galea, Bechmann, Perry 2007). The afferent limb is provided by the circulation of brain antigens from parenchyma to CSF where dendritic cells associated to meninges and choroid plexus provide for the transfer of these proteins to the cervical lymph nodes. Priming of immunocompetent cells in the peripheral lymphoid tissue due to the presentation of neural proteins released from the CNS by dendritic cells, the migration of activated immune cells into the CSF, and the presentation of cognate antigen operated by resident APCs constitute the efferent limb. Thus, it is reasonable to assume that the CNS could represent an immunospecialized site, rather than an organ with an immune privilege status, in which neural antigens are not segregated and the events related to immune surveillance can occur (Hickey 2001; Becher, Beckmann, Greter 2006). However, rejection of tissue grafts and delayed type hypersensitivity reactions do not arise when injection of the material is performed in the brain parenchyma (Mason, Charlton, Jones et al. 1986; Matyszak, Perry 1996a; Galea, Bechmann, Perry 2007). In addition, in normal CNS, activated T cells are retained in the CSF after entry because they do not traverse glia limitans (Becher, Beckmann, Greter 2006; Bechmann, Galea, Perry 2007) and the cellular route of the afferent arm of immune responses is lacking in the brain parenchyma since dendritic cells are confined within the CSF (Galea, Bechmann, Perry 2007). Therefore, in absence of pathologic conditions, the interactions between the immune system and the CNS occur within the CSF, whereas brain parenchyma maintains a relative immune privilege. For this reason, the immune specialization of the CNS should be assumed to be a dynamic process regulated by functional characteristics of the intrathecal compartment (Becher, Beckmann, Greter 2006; Galea, Bechmann, Perry 2007).

Immune Surveillance in the CNS

Under physiologic circumstances, it is widely accepted that immune surveillance is performed at the level of perivascular spaces (Becher, Prat, Antel 2000; Hickey 2001; Ransohoff, Kivisäkk, Kidd 2003; Engelhardt, Ransohoff 2005; Becher, Beckmann, Greter 2006; Bechmann, Galea, Perry 2007). In fact, the intrathecal compartment is constantly patrolled by T cells that have already been activated by the primary encounter with neural antigens in cervical lymph nodes. These cells penetrate the CSF across the choroid plexus and, to a lesser extent, the vessel wall of postcapillary venules located in Virchow-Robin spaces and then accumulate principally in the perivascular spaces

where they interact with the corresponding local APCs. At this point, if perivascular cells do not present the cognate antigen to T lymphocytes, these activated immunocompetent cells do not progress across the glia limitans and recirculate into the blood stream or undergo apoptotic death. On the contrary, if T cells recognize the related antigen presented by perivascular macrophages, they cross the glia limitans, invade the CNS parenchyma, and promote the activation of microglial cells that release several soluble factors, leading to the development of an inflammatory response. In both these cases, the mechanisms of lymphocyte recruitment are largely unknown, although it has been hypothesized that the egress of T cells into the CSF is regulated by chemokines and adhesion molecules such as selectins (Rebenko-Moll, Liu, Cardona et al. 2006), whereas the migration of T cells into the brain could be due to proteolytic enzymatic activity of matrix metalloproteinases (MMPs) (Bechmann, Galea, Perry 2007). The occurrence of a CNS immune surveillance in the CSF of the subarachnoid spaces seems to be confirmed by the demonstration that, in patients with noninflammatory neurological manifestations, central memory CD4$^+$ T lymphocytes trafficking into the CSF across choroid plexus and meninges (Kivisäkk, Mahad, Callahan et al. 2003) are present in identical amounts within ventricular and lumbar CSF (Provencio, Kivisäkk, Tucky et al. 2005). This concept is reinforced by the data coming from animal studies in which the induction of a monophasic brain inflammation in immunocompetent transgenic mice after transfer of CD8$^+$ T cells suggest the potential role of these lymphocytes in CNS immune surveillance (Cabarrocas, Bauer, Piaggio et al. 2003). The fact that not only T cells but also B cells can contribute to CNS immune surveillance since their entry into the CSF has been described (Uccelli, Aloisi, Pistoia 2005). The presence of immune mechanisms that provide a continuous monitoring of CNS microenvironment plays a fundamental role in protecting the brain. In fact, immune responses contribute to host defense against pathogens and preservation of tissue homeostasis since they aim to eliminate dangerous infectious agents invading the CNS, remove irreversible damaged cells and their products, and promote tissue repair (Becher, Prat, Antel 2000; Hickey 2001; Becher, Beckmann, Greter 2006). Moreover, immune reactions to foreign antigens are self-limited because, after the eradication of the antigens, the immune system returns to its basal resting state because of apoptotic deletion of activated T cells (Jiang, Chess 2006). However, when the antigen is difficult to clear from the CNS or a self–brain protein is recognized as non-self, there is a persistent antigenic stimulation of the immune system that favors the development of a chronic intrathecal inflammatory response leading

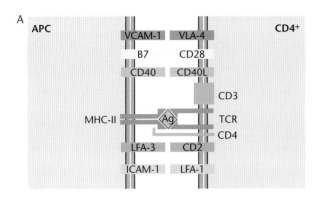

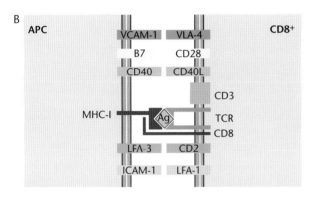

Figure 12.1 Signals implicated in antigen presentation: (A) recognition of the cognate antigen (Ag) by specific-T lymphocyte-associated T-cell receptor (TCR) after presentation in the context of major histocompatibility complex (MHC) molecules (class I for CD8+ T cells and class II for CD4+ T cells) expressed by perivascular antigen-presenting cells (APC) and in presence of associated molecules such as CD3; (B) co-stimulatory signals for T-cell activation provided by binding between accessory molecules expressed by T cells and APC. ICAM, intercellular adhesion molecule; LFA, leukocyte function–associated antigen; VCAM, vascular cell adhesion molecule.

to tissue destruction. Thus, immune surveillance can exert not only beneficial but also detrimental effects (Becher, Prat, Antel 2000; Hickey 2001; Becher, Beckmann, Greter 2006). In this scenario, it becomes clear that the recognition of the cognate antigens on APCs by activated T cells infiltrating the perivascular spaces is the fundamental prerequisite for CNS immune surveillance (Becher, Beckmann, Greter 2006; Bechmann, Galea, Perry 2007). More precisely, as depicted in Figure 12.1, in the process of antigen presentation two types of signal are needed (Hart, Fabry 1995; Becher, Prat, Antel 2000). Initially, the T lymphocyte–associated T-cell receptor (TCR) specific for a brain peptide can identify the related antigen only when it is presented in the context of MHC molecules expressed by perivascular APCs and in presence of associated molecules such as CD3 (signal 1). Subsequently, T cells and APCs express accessory molecules that provide co-stimulatory signals for T-cell activation and that are represented

by co-receptors that bind their matching ligands (signal 2). In absence of costimulation, T lymphocytes do not respond to antigen presentation and are either eliminated by apoptosis or enter a state of unresponsiveness called *anergy*. The co-stimulatory pathways include (a) CD4 and CD8 molecules expressed by T cells that bind MHC class I (CD8) and class II (CD4) molecules positioned on APCs; (b) CD40 ligand (CD40L) expressed by T cells that engages CD40 expressed by APCs; (c) CD28 molecule expressed by T cells that reacts with CD80 (B7–1) and CD86 (B7–2) on the surface of APCs; (d) leukocyte function–associated antigen 1 (LFA-1) expressed by T cells that interacts with intercellular adhesion molecule 1 (ICAM-1) expressed by APCs; (e) very late activation-4 (VLA-4) antigen expressed by T cells that binds vascular cell adhesion molecule 1 (VCAM-1) on APCs; and (f) CD2 molecule expressed by T cells that binds leukocyte function-associated antigen 3 (LFA-3) expressed by APCs. In particular, the engagement of T-cell co-receptor CD28 with its ligand CD80 (B7–1)/CD86 (B7–2) on APCs, stimulated by CD40L-CD40 interactions, induces the full activation of T lymphocytes that acquire effector functions. Therefore, in the course of CNS immune surveillance, two distinct phases can be identified (Bechmann, Galea, Perry 2007). The first step implies the migration of activated T cells from blood to perivascular spaces through choroid plexus and postcapillary vessels, which is not necessarily associated to pathological conditions involving the brain since it can occur when the appearance of a strong immune response in the body promotes the priming of T cells at the level of the secondary lymphoid organs (Hickey 2001). The second step is characterized by the penetration of activated T cells from perivascular spaces to brain parenchyma across the glia limitans, which is a restricted phenomenon because it depends on antigen presentation performed by perivascular cells. In fact, activated T cells are able to invade the CNS only when they re-encounter their cognate antigen in the context of appropriate MHC molecules associated to perivascular APCs. Conversely, activated T cells monitor the subarachnoid space and rapidly leave the CNS. Table 12.3 summarizes the mechanisms of CNS immune surveillance.

Immune Sentinels of the CNS

Given their ability to act as resident APCs for T cells in normal brain, perivascular cells can be viewed as sentinels at the gate of the CNS parenchyma (Becher, Beckmann, Greter 2006). Under inflammatory conditions, the same role can be imagined for the other CNS-associated cells, such as meningeal

Table 12.3 The Biphasic Nature of Immune Surveillance in the Central Nervous System (CNS)

Phases	Location	Mechanisms	References
Migration of activated T cells from blood to perivascular spaces (step 1)	Choroid plexus and postcapillary vessel wall	Activation of T cells in the secondary lymphoid organs due to a strong immune response in the body	Becher et al. 2000 Hickey 2001 Ransohoff et al. 2003 Engelhardt, Ransohoff 2005 Becher et al. 2006 Bechmann et al. 2007
Migration of activated T cells from perivascular spaces to brain parenchyma (step 2)	Glia limitans (astroglial end-feet)	Recognition of the cognate antigens by activated T cells after presentation in the context of appropriate MHC molecules expressed on perivascular cells	Becher et al. 2000 Hickey 2001 Becher et al. 2006 Bechmann et al. 2007

MHC, major histocompatability complex.

and choroid plexus macrophages and dendritic cells, which increase in number and exhibit APC properties in the inflamed brain (Hickey 2001; Becher, Beckmann, Greter 2006). Considering their importance in CNS immune surveillance, perivascular cells and other resident APCs are persistently repopulated by bone marrow–derived monocytes (Becher, Beckmann, Greter 2006). Although this peculiarity is absent in microglial cells and astrocytes, during intrathecal inflammation these cells may exert APC functions and can, therefore, be considered as sentinels within the CNS parenchyma (Aloisi, Ria, Adorini 2000; Dong, Benveniste 2001; Aloisi 2001; Becher, Beckmann, Greter 2006). Microglia is composed of cells of hematopoietic lineage that derive from mesodermal precursor cells and likely originate from monocytes entering the brain parenchyma from the blood compartment (Becher, Beckmann, Greter 2006). In the inflamed CNS, there is an activation of microglial cells that upregulate MHC class I and class II molecules and co-stimulatory molecules at their cell surface and then acquire the ability to present antigen to previously primed CD8+ and CD4+ T lymphocytes. Therefore, like meningeal and choroid plexus dendritic cells and perivascular cells, microglial cells also are resident APCs. However, while dendritic cells are professional APCs that are able to initiate a primary immune response by the presentation of brain antigens to naïve T cells in the secondary lymphoid organs, perivascular and microglial cells are nonprofessional APCs that trigger a secondary immune reaction by the presentation of neural antigens to already activated T cells in the Virchow-Robin space and within the brain, respectively (Aloisi, Ria, Aloisi 2001; Adorini 2000; Becher, Prat, Antel 2000; Becher, Beckmann, Greter 2006). Astrocytes are cells of neuroectodermal origin, which are fundamental for brain homeostasis and neuronal function since they contribute to the induction and maintenance of BBB by their foot processes, induce scar formation and tissue repair by astrogliosis, produce neurotrophic

factors, and regulate neuronal functions by providing metabolic support and uptake of neurotransmitters (Dong, Benveniste 2001). During inflammation, astroglia become MHC class I-positive and can express low levels of MHC class II and co-stim ulatory molecules (Becher, Prat, Antel 2000; Aloisi, Ria, Adorini 2000; Dong, Benveniste 2001; Hemmer, Cepok, Zhou et al. 2004; Becher, Beckmann, Greter 2006). Therefore, the effective involvement of these cells in intrathecal antigen presentation still remains uncertain and, at present, is believed to be restricted to CD4+ T helper with Th2 phenotype (Aloisi, Ria, Adorini 2000). On the other hand, the activation of microglia and astrocytes due to the presence of an inflammatory response within the brain is associated to increased cellular expression of pattern recognition receptors (PRPs) that can identify a broad spectrum of microbial proteins and pathogenic insults (Farina, Aloisi, Meinl 2007). Toll-like receptors (TLRs), dsRNA-dependent protein kinase (PKR), CD14, nucleotide-binding oligomerization domain (NOD) proteins, complement, mannose receptor (MR), and scavenger receptors (SRs) mediate an innate immune response that represents a trigger factor aimed at informing the immune system about brain tissue injury formation. Intriguingly, evidence for the constitutive expression of PRPs in meningeal, choroid plexus, and perivascular macrophages under normal circumstances indicate a potential role of these molecules as a first-line defense against danger signals (Aloisi 2001; Farina, Aloisi, Meinl 2007). In addition, microglial cells and astroglia share with neurons and endothelial cells the ability to eliminate T cells invading the CNS through Fas (CD95)/Fas ligand (FasL or CD95L)-dependent apoptosis under both physiologic and pathologic circumstances. In fact, while the expression of FasL on these cells is constitutive in the normal brain and is enhanced in the inflamed CNS, infiltrating T cells exhibit the receptor Fas on their surface (Bechmann, Mor, Nilsen et al 1999; Pender, Rist 2001; Choi, Benveniste 2004). The interaction between FasL expressed by resident brain cells and Fas expressed by immune cells trafficking across the BBB can induce apoptotic deletion of T cells migrating into the CNS. Apoptosis is an active suicide program leading to cell death in response to external stimuli (Krammer 2000). This process appears particularly efficient in astrocytes, neurons, and endothelial cells in which the low expression of co-stimulatory molecules activates the Fas/FasL pathway (Pender, Rist 2001; Dietrich, Walker, Saas 2003). Therefore, resident CNS cells, by using Fas/FasL-mediated mechanisms, are able to limit the penetration of immune cells into the brain at two different sites: at the BBB and within the brain parenchyma. Consequently, microglia, astroglia, neurons, and endothelial cells form an immunological brain barrier that preserves the brain against the infiltration of immunocompetent cells by the maintenance of a state of immune suppression within the CNS (Bechmann, Mor, Nilsen et al. 1999; Choi, Benveniste 2004). The characteristics of CNS immune sentinels are reported in Table 12.4.

Regulation of Immune Responses in the Inflamed CNS

In the course of brain inflammation, after the interactions with activated T cells entering the CNS parenchyma, microglial cells and astrocytes produce a series of pro-inflammatory and anti-inflammatory soluble mediators, such as cytokines and chemokines, which influence both innate and acquired (or adaptive) immune responses within the CNS (Becher, Prat, Antel 2000; Aloisi, Ria, Adorini 2000; Dong, Benveniste 2001; Aloisi 2001; Becher, Beckmann, Greter 2006). The innate immune system comprises

of epithelial barriers, monocytes, macrophages, NK cells, complement pathways, and cytokines and provides an early immune response directed against foreign antigens, which is characterized by low specificity and no memory. Conversely, the acquired immune system consists of humoral immunity mediated by B cells and cell-mediated immunity driven by MHC class I–restricted CD8$^+$ T cells and MHC class II–restricted CD4$^+$ T cells and triggers a late immune reaction targeting foreign antigens, which is able to respond more vigorously to repeated exposures to the same antigen because of its high specificity and memory (Medzhitov, Janeway 1997). Among the cellular players of adaptive immunity, CD4$^+$ T helper (Th) cells can be divided into two different populations with two distinct cytokine profiles and effector functions (Mosmann, Sad 1996). Th1 subset secreting interleukin (IL)-2, tumor necrosis factor (TNF)-α, and interferon (IFN)-γ (Th1-type cytokines) are implicated in macrophage activation, production of opsonizing and complement-fixing antibodies, and delayed hypersensitivity. Th2 cells producing IL-4, IL-5, IL-10, and IL-13 (Th2-type cytokines) antagonize Th1-mediated reaction and are involved in the production of neutralizing antibodies and allergic conditions. For these reasons, Th1 and Th2 polarized responses are believed to have opposite functions. Th1 response is judged as a pro-inflammatory reaction promoting cell-mediated immunity, whereas Th2 response is regarded as an anti-inflammatory reaction that mediates humoral immunity. Microglia and astroglia can release pro-inflammatory chemokines of the CXC or α-family chemokines, such as IL-8 (CXCL8) and IP-10 (CXCL10), and of the CC or β-family, including MIP-1α (CCL3), MIP-1β (CCL4), MCP-1 (CCL2), and RANTES (CCL5), which facilitate the intracerebral recruitment of additional

Table 12.4 Features of Central Nervous System (CNS) Cells acting as Immune Sentinels in the Normal and Inflamed Brain

Cell Type	Functions	Mechanisms	References
CNS-associated cells (meningeal and choroid plexus macrophages and dendritic cells, perivascular cells)	Immune sentinels at the gate of the CNS parenchyma	Expression of MHC class I and II antigens, co-stimulatory molecules and pattern recognition receptors	Becher et al. 2000 Aloisi 2001 Becher et al. 2006 Farina et al. 2007
Microglia	Immune sentinels within the CNS parenchyma	Expression of MHC class I and II antigens, co-stimulatory molecules, pattern recognition receptors and, along with neurons and endothelial cells, Fas ligand	Bechmann et al 1999 Aloisi 2000 Aloisi 2001 Choi, Benveniste 2004 Farina et al. 2007
Astroglia	Immune sentinels within the CNS parenchyma	Expression of MHC class I and II antigens, co-stimulatory molecules at low levels, pattern-recognition receptors and, along with neurons and endothelial cells, Fas ligand	Bechmann et al 1999 Aloisi 2000 Dong, Benveniste 2001 Choi, Benveniste 2004 Farina et al. 2007

immunocompetent cells (Aloisi, Ria, Adorini 2000; Dong, Benveniste 2001; Aloisi 2001). However, while microglia principally produce chemokines facilitating Th1-polarized responses, such as MIP-1α (CCL3), astrocytes generate chemokines stimulating an immune reaction with a Th2 phenotype, such as MCP-1 (CCL2) (Aloisi, Ria, Adorini 2000). Microglial cells and astroglia can liberate pro-inflammatory cytokines that regulate phenotype, recruitment, and activation of immune cells operating in both innate and acquired immunity (Becher, Prat, Antel 2000; Aloisi, Ria, Adorini 2000; Aloisi 2001; Becher, Beckmann, Greter 2006). IL-1 and TNF-α contribute to leukocyte extravasation into the CNS, IL-6 stimulates growth of B cells and their differentiation into antibody-secreting plasma cells, IL-15 activates NK and CD8$^+$ T cells, and IL-18 promotes the synthesis of IFN-γ by NK and T cells. Nevertheless, the key inducers of CNS inflammation are IL-12 and IL-23. IL-12 elicits the secretion of IFN-γ by NK cells and T lymphocytes, enhances the cytolytic activity of NK cells and CD8$^+$ cytotoxic T cells and, more important, generates an immune deviation toward Th1 direction because it drives the differentiation of CD4$^+$ Th cells into Th1 lymphocytes producing IFN-γ (Trinchieri 2003). IL-23 triggers the production of IL-17 in CD8$^+$ T cells, in NK cells, and in a novel T subset of CD4$^+$ Th cells distinct from Th1 and Th2 populations that are indicated as Th17 cells, and also releases IL-6 and TNF-α (McKenzie, Kastelein, Cua 2006). IL-17 represents a potent pro-inflammatory cytokine that induces a strong inflammatory response by favoring neutrophil recruitment and local macrophage activation. Therefore, IL-12 and IL-23 promote two different immunological pathways that play separate but complementary roles. However, IL-23 but not IL-12 is essential for the activation of CNS-associated macrophages in inflamed CNS (Cua, Sherlock, Chen et al. 2003). In addition, IFN-γ, the most important cytokine secreted by Th1 cells under the influence of IL-12, suppresses the differentiation of CD4$^+$ Th cells into Th17 cells induced by IL-23 (McKenzie, Kastelein, Cua 2006). Accordingly, it is currently presumed that the development of brain inflammation is critically dependent on the IL-23/IL-17 axis rather than on the IL-12/ IFN-γ circuit, which probably exerts immunoregulatory functions (Iwakura, Ishigame 2006). Microglial cells and astrocytes are also producers of anti-inflammatory cytokines such as IL-10 and transforming growth factor (TGF)-β (Aloisi, Ria, Adorini 2000; Aloisi 2001). IL-10 inhibits IL-12 synthesis and the expression of MHC class II and co-stimulatory molecules in activated macrophages and dendritic cells. TGF-β suppresses the proliferation and differentiation of T cells and the activation of macrophages. In general,

it is postulated that microglia exert pro-inflammatory functions because it mainly releases IL-12 and IL-23, which stimulate Th1 and Th17 immune responses. In contrast, astroglia seem to exhibit immunoregulatory properties because it mainly synthesizes anti-inflammatory cytokines, such as IL-10 and TGF-β, which downregulate Th1-polarized reactions suppressing IL-12 production by microglial cells. In addition, astrocytes interact with Th2 cells promoting the release of IL-4 that is crucial for the development of Th2-type responses (Becher, Prat, Antel 2000; Aloisi, Ria, Adorini 2000; Dong, Benveniste 2001; Aloisi 2001; Becher, Beckmann, Greter 2006). However, microglial cells can regulate Th2 responses by the secretion of IL-10 and TGF-β, whereas astroglia can trigger an intense inflammatory response by the shedding of IL-6 and the expression of PRPs (Aloisi, Ria, Adorini 2000; Dong, Benveniste 2001; Aloisi 2001; Farina, Aloisi, Meinl 2007). Interestingly, microglia and astroglia activation can be controlled by neurons, the electrical activity of which suppresses the expression of MHC class II molecules on microglial cells and astrocytes through cell-to-cell contact and the delivery of several substances including neurotrophins, neuropeptides, and neurotransmitters (Aloisi 2001). Thus, the final outcome of immune responses in the CNS depends on the activation state of microglia and astroglia, which regulates the balance between Th1 and Th17 pro-inflammatory and Th2 anti-inflammatory signals and is influenced by intrathecal microenvironment resulting from antigen presentation within the brain parenchyma (Becher, Prat, Antel 2000; Aloisi, Ria, Adorini 2000; Aloisi 2001; Schwartz, Butovsky, Brück et al. 2006). The immunoregulatory functions of microglia and astroglia are listed in Table 12.5.

Initiation of Th1-Mediated Immune Reactions in the Inflamed CNS

As discussed, the initiation of intrathecal immune responses is represented by the migration of T cells into the brain across the glia limitans (Becher, Beckmann, Greter 2006; Bechmann, Galea, Perry 2007). After entry into CNS parenchyma, T cells meet a decidedly inhospitable and hostile microenvironment that suppresses immune responses because the secretion of Th2 anti-inflammatory cytokines, such as IL-10 and TGF-β, by glial cells and, particularly, by astrocytes (Dong, Benveniste 2001; Hickey 2001; Becher, Beckmann, Greter 2006) and Fas/FasL-mediated apoptosis induced mainly by astroglia and also by microglia, neurons, and endothelial cells (Bechmann, Mor, Nilsen et al. 1999; Choi, Benveniste 2004) predominate. In this setting, the activation of microglia by T cells invading the brain parenchyma

Table 12.5 Main Regulatory Pathways of the Immune Response in the Inflamed Central Nervous System (CNS)

Cellular Players	Principal Functions	Soluble Mediators	References
Microglia	Recruitment of immunocompetent cells promoting Th1-mediated immune responses	Pro-inflammatory chemokines: MIP-1α (CCL3)	Aloisi 2000 Dong, Benveniste 2001 Aloisi 2001
	Immune deviation toward Th1-mediated immune responses	Pro-inflammatory cytokines: IL-12/ IFN-γ	Aloisi 2000 Becher et al. 2000 Aloisi 2001 Becher et al. 2006
	Immune deviation toward Th17-mediated immune responses	Pro-inflammatory cytokines: IL-23/IL-17	Becher et al. 2006
Astroglia	Recruitment of immunocompetent cells promoting Th2-mediated immune responses	Pro-inflammatory chemokines: MCP-1 (CCL2)	Aloisi 2000 Dong, Benveniste 2001 Aloisi 2001
	Immune deviation toward Th2-mediated immune responses	Anti-inflammatory cytokines: IL-10 TGF-β	Aloisi 2000 Becher et al. 2000 Dong, Benveniste 2001

IL, interleukin; IFN, interferon; TGF-β, tumor growth factor β.

represents the central event leading to the development of the intrathecal inflammation (Aloisi, Ria, Adorini 2000; Becher, Prat, Antel 2000; Aloisi 2001; Becher, Beckmann, Greter 2006; Schwartz, Butovsky, Brück et al. 2006; Galea, Bechmann, Perry 2007). In supposed Th1-mediated inflammatory diseases, such as MS, the recognition of the cognate antigen by CD4$^+$ Th1 cells, after presentation in the context of MHC class II molecules expressed by microglial cells, activates microglia that produces pro-inflammatory chemokines and pro-inflammatory cytokines such as IL-12 and IL-23, stimulating the massive recruitment of additional activated immune cells from blood to CNS and activating Th1- and Th17-mediated immune responses. In this stage, the homing of immune cells into the brain parenchyma occurs principally through the BBB of postcapillary venules and follows a multistep process that is tightly controlled by leukocyte–endothelial interactions based on the expression of adhesion molecules, chemokines, and their receptors on the surface of leukocytes and endothelial cells (Ransohoff, Kivisäkk, Kidd 2003; Engelhardt, Ransohoff 2005). The model of the extravasation of immune cells includes a series of different functional phases indicated as tethering/rolling to the vascular endothelium, leukocyte activation, adhesion to endothelial cells, and leukocyte diapedesis (Fig. 12.2). In the first step, an initial transient contact of circulating leukocytes with the vascular endothelium, called *tethering*, is followed by the rolling of blood leukocytes along the vascular wall that is regulated by adhesion molecules such as integrins and selectins and implies a reduction of leukocyte velocity. In particular, while CD8$^+$ T lymphocytes roll via the connection between leukocyte P-selectin glycoprotein ligand-1 (PSGL-1) and endothelial

P-selectin, the other immune cells roll through the binding between leukocyte α$_4$β$_1$ integrin VLA-4 and endothelial VCAM-1, an adhesion molecule of the immunoglobulin (Ig) superfamily. The interactions between L-selectin and E-selectin ligands expressed on leukocytes and L-selectin ligands and E-selectin expressed on cytokine-activated endothelial cells are also involved in this phase of leukocyte transendothelial migration. The second step is characterized by the binding of endothelial chemokines with their receptor expressed on rolling leukocytes, which leads to the delivery of a G protein–mediated signal into the leukocytes. The result is the functional activation of leukocytes that express integrins VLA-4 and LFA-1 on their surface. In the third step, there is the firm adhesion of leukocytes to the vascular endothelium because of the interactions between leukocyte VLA-4 and LFA-1 and their endothelial ligands VCAM-1 and ICAM-1, both belonging to the Ig-superfamily. The fourth and final step is represented by diapedesis that consists of the migration of leukocytes through interendothelial cell junctions, or directly across endothelial cells, mediated by junctional Ig-superfamily adhesion molecules such as platelet-endothelial cell adhesion molecule 1 (PECAM-1). However, the definitive penetration of immune cells into the brain parenchyma requires the trafficking of these cells across the basement membranes associated to endothelial cells and glia limitans that separate the vascular compartment from perivascular space and the perivascular space from CNS, respectively (Bechmann, Galea, Perry 2007). These membranes are the inner vascular basal lamina surrounding endothelial cells, the outer vascular basal lamina covering the media, and the basal lamina located on the top of astrocytic end-feet. For this reason, extravasating immune cells release

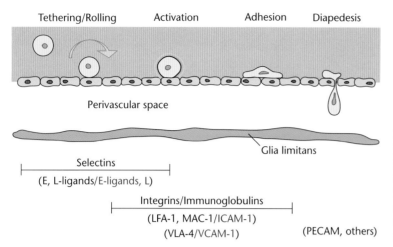

Figure 12.2 Schematic illustration showing the multistep paradigm of transendothelial migration of immune cells into the brain parenchyma in inflamed central nervous system (CNS). ICAM-1, intercellular adhesion molecule 1; LFA-1, leukocyte function–associated antigen 4; PECAM, platelet-endothelial cell adhesion molecule; VCAM-1, vascular cell adhesion molecule 1; VLA-4, very late activation-4 antigen.

MMPs, a family of zinc-containing and calcium-requiring endopeptidases, which are capable of remodeling and degrading the extracellular matrix (ECM) constituents contained in subendothelial basement membranes (Yong, Power, Forsyth et al. 2001; Rosenberg 2002). Among the various MMPs secreted by immune cells, MMP-9 (gelatinase B) is currently thought to be the most important enzyme implicated in the proteolytic breakdown of the basal lamina ECM components and then in the ultimate opening of the BBB occurring during ongoing intrathecal inflammation (Kieseier, Seifert, Giovannoni et al. 1999; Sellebjerg, Sørensen 2003), especially in MS (Opdenakker, Nelissen, Van Damme 2003; Yong, Zabad, Arawal et al. 2007). This hypothesis seems to be confirmed by recent data indicating that CSF mean levels and an intrathecal synthesis of active MMP-9, the only form of the enzyme that exerts catalytic activity, are more elevated in MS than in some noninflammatory conditions and in the course of MS inflammatory disease activity (Fainardi, Castellazzi, Bellini et al. 2006a). In fact, these findings suggest that a shift toward proteolytic activity of MMP-9 could be relevant in modulating immune responses operating in MS.

Immunocompetent Cells Infiltrating the Inflamed CNS during the Development of Th1-Mediated Immune Responses

After entry into the CNS, immigrating immune cells are involved in a cascade of inflammatory events, which remains compartmentalized at intrathecal level and depends on the specific properties of each cellular population (Hemmer, Cepok, Zhou et al. 2004). Activated macrophages infiltrating the brain act as effector cells of Th1-mediated responses since, under the influence of IFN-γ produced by CD4+ Th1

lymphocytes and IL-17 released by CD4+ Th17 cells, they direct phagocytic reactions and secrete inflammatory mediators such as TNF-α, IFN-γ, reactive oxygen intermediates, nitric oxide (NO), and MMPs. On the other hand, these cells exert an APC function expressing MHC class I antigens specific for CD8+ T cells and MHC class II molecules specific for CD4+ T cells (Hemmer, Archelos, Hartung 2002; Sospedra, Martin 2005). After recognition of the specific antigens presented by APCs in the context of MHC class II molecules, activated CD4+ Th1 cells invading the CNS produce pro-inflammatory cytokines such as IFN-γ, which promotes macrophage activation together with CD4+ Th17 cells and B cell synthesis of opsonizing and complement-binding antibodies (Hemmer, Archelos, Hartung 2002; Sospedra, Martin 2005). Conversely, activated CD4+ Th2 cells penetrating into the brain exert their effector functions by secreting anti-inflammatory cytokines such as IL-4, which stimulates the release of neutralizing antibodies by B cells, and IL-10, which inhibits macrophage activation induced by Th1-polarized responses (Sospedra, Martin 2005; Delgado, Sheremata 2006). Activated CD8+ T cells trafficking the BBB identify the specific antigen presented by MHC class I molecules expressed on APCs and differentiate into cytotoxic T lymphocytes (CTLs) with the help of pro-inflammatory cytokines produced by CD4+ T cells. CTLs act as effector cells by promoting apoptosis-dependent mechanisms—cytolysis via activation of Fas/FasL or perforin/granzymes pathways—and by shedding pro-inflammatory cytokines that trigger macrophage activity (Lassmann, Ransohoff 2004; Friese, Fugger 2005). Activated B cells entering the CNS differentiate into antibody-secreting plasma cells owing to the modulatory influence of CD4+ T cells. In fact, after the internalization of the antigen due to its binding with B-cell receptor (BCR) via CD80 (B7–1)/CD86

(B7–2) interactions, B cells present the specific anti-gen to TCR of CD4$^+$ T cells through CD40/CD40L pathway. These mechanisms favor the release of cytokines by CD4$^+$ T cells which, in turn, induces B-cell reactivation. CD4$^+$ Th1 cells secrete pro-inflammatory cytokines such as IFN-γ that stimu-lates the production of IgG1 and IgG3 subclasses that promote macrophage phagocytosis. IL-4 and IL-10 anti-inflammatory cytokines released by CD4$^+$ Th2 cells support the synthesis of the IgG4 isotype that exhibits neutralizing properties on target anti-gens (Abbas, Murphy, Sher 1996; Archelos, Storch, Hartung 2000; Archelos, Hartung 2000; Hemmer, Archelos, Hartung 2002; Hemmer, Cepok, Zhou et al. 2004; Meinl, Krumbholz, Hohlfeld 2006). Accordingly, CSF antibodies are predominantly composed of IgG1 subclass in a postulated Th1-mediated disease like MS (Greve, Magnusson, Melms et al. 2001). Activated $\gamma\delta$ T cells migrating into the brain are effector cells that induce cytotoxicity by using MHC independent-mechanisms and contribute to macrophage recruitment via pro-inflammatory cytokine and chemokine production (Sospedra, Martin 2005). In addition, $\gamma\delta$ T cells could have APC functions (Moser, Eberl 2007). Activated NK cells homing into the CNS differentiate into two dis-tinct functional subsets providing opposite effects. Type 1 NK (NK1) cells develop in response to a Th1-polarized milieu and, in particular, to IL-12 produced by macrophages. They represent an effector subset that activates Th1-mediated reactions by the secre-tion of pro-inflammatory cytokines, such as IFN-γ, and kills target cell by a MCH class I–restricted cytolytic apoptosis and antibody-dependent cell-mediated cytotoxicity (ADCC). In contrast, type 2 NK (NK2) cells constitute a regulatory subset since their formation, driven by a Th2-directed environment, is characterized by the release of anti-inflammatory cytokines, such as IL-10 and TGF-β, stimulating Th2-polarized responses and by the cytotoxic killing of APCs (Johansson, Berg, Hall et al. 2005; Shi, Van Kaer 2006). In this regard, immune cells infiltrat-ing the brain during an intrathecal inflammatory response also comprise other regulatory cells that suppress immune responses by blocking the activa-tion and function of effector T lymphocytes. These cells include CD4$^+$ T regulatory (Treg) cells, CD8$^+$ Treg cells, and NK T cells. CD4$^+$ Treg can be divided into three different subgroups that downregulate Th1-mediated responses by the production of anti-inflammatory cytokines. Among these, CD4$^+$CD25$^+$ Treg cells secrete IL-10 and TGF-β, type 1 regulatory T (Tr1) cells release IL-10, and type 3 regulatory T (Tr3) cells synthesize TGF-β. CD8$^+$ Treg cells sup-press CD8$^+$ cytotoxic T cells expressing human leuko-cyte antigen-E (HLA-E) molecules that interact with

TCR of effector cells, whereas NK T cells antagonize Th1-polarized response by producing IL-4, IL-10, and TGF-β (Friese, Fugger 2005; Jiang, Chess 2006; Baecher-Allan, Hafler 2006). Recently, a novel sub-population of CD4$^+$ and CD8$^+$ Treg cells expressing HLA-G has been identified in the CSF of MS patients (Feger, Tolosa, Huang et al. 2007). HLA-G molecules and their soluble isoforms are nonclassical class Ib HLA antigens structurally related to classical class Ia HLA products (HLA-I) that exert tolerogenic func-tions since they mediate apoptosis of cytotoxic CD8$^+$ T cells and NK cells by Fas/FasL interactions, inhibit proliferation of CD4$^+$ T cells and drive them into an immunosuppressive profile, promote a shift in Th1/Th2 balance toward Th2 polarization, control APC maturation, and are protective for pregnancy by maintaining tolerance at the feto–maternal interface (Carosella, Moreau, Aractingi et al. 2001; LeMaoult, Le Discorde, Rouas-Freiss et al. 2003; Hunt, Petroff, McIntire et al. 2005). Intriguingly, in MS, HLA-G expression is upregulated on CSF monocytes and on microglia, macrophages, and endothelial cells located in demyelinating areas (Wiendl, Feger, Mittelbronn et al. 2005), whereas CSF levels and an intrathecal synthesis of soluble HLA-G (sHLA-G) are higher in MS than in inflammatory and noninflammatory disorders (Fainardi, Rizzo, Melchiorri et al. 2003; Fainardi, Rizzo, Melchiorri et al. 2006b).

Amplification of Th1-Mediated Immune Responses in Inflamed CNS and Tissue Damage

Under the influence of IL-12 and IL-23 produced by activated microglial cells, immune cells infiltrating the inflamed brain activate immune responses with a Th1 and Th17 polarization, resulting in an accumu-lation of pro-inflammatory chemokines and cytok-ines and other soluble mediators such as MMPs that induce profound perturbation and derangement of the CNS microenvironment. In fact, there is the for-mation of a pro-inflammatory intrathecal milieu, which is not sufficiently counterbalanced by Th2 anti-inflammatory cytokines (Hemmer, Archelos, Hartung 2002; Hemmer, Cepok, Zhou et al. 2004; Delgado, Sheremata 2006) and is characterized by a massive recruitment of activated macrophages, CD4$^+$ Th1 cells, CD8$^+$ T cells, B cells, $\gamma\delta$ T cells, and NK1 cells from blood into the CNS (Sospedra, Martin 2005; Hauser, Oksenberg 2006; Dhib-Jalbut 2007). Therefore, the balance between pro-inflammatory Th1-type cytokines and anti-inflammatory Th2-type cytokines is currently believed to be relevant in immune deregulation occurring in inflamed brain (Özenci, Kouwenhoven, Link 2002; Imitola, Chitnis,

Khuory 2005). The transformation of the CNS microenvironment from being anti-inflammatory to pro-inflammatory results in an amplification of intrathecal immune response, triggering myelin and axon injury. The two principal events arising in this stage of intrathecal inflammation are the activation of CNS-resident and infiltrating APC functions and the priming of effector immune pathways (Sospedra, Martin 2005; Hauser, Oksenberg 2006; Dhib-Jalbut 2007). The elevated levels of pro-inflammatory cytokines produced by immune cells invading the brain restimulate APC properties of microglial cells, which further express MHC class II and co-stimulatory molecules by enhancing their ability to present the specific antigen to $CD4^+$ Th1 cells (Becher, Prat, Antel 2000; Aloisi 2001; Becher, Beckmann, Greter 2006; Frohman, Racke, Raine 2006; Schwartz, Butovsky, Brück et al. 2006). This reactivation also implies the release of cytokines implicated in IL-12/IFN-γ and IL-23/IL-17 axis, which provide a supplementary polarization of CNS immune reactions toward a pro-inflammatory direction (Becher, Prat, Antel 2000; Aloisi 2001; Becher, Beckmann, Greter 2006), as well as the secretion of several myelin and axonal toxic factors such as TNF-α, IFN-γ, reactive oxygen species, NO, and MMPs (Becher, Prat, Antel 2000; Hauser, Oksenberg 2006; Dhib-Jalbut 2007). In the same way, macrophages trafficking into the CNS exhibit the complete APC machinery for $CD4^+$ Th1 cells and synthesize pro-inflammatory cytokines and toxic mediators (Hemmer, Cepok, Zhou et al. 2004; Frohman, Racke, Raine 2006), perivascular cells, and the other CNS-associated cells, such as meningeal and choroid plexus macrophages and dendritic cells, and increase the expression of MHC class II and co-stimulatory molecules (Hickey 2001; Becher, Beckmann, Greter 2006), whereas astrocytes acquire a Th1 phenotype since they become MHC class II-positive (Becher, Prat, Antel 2000; Dong, Benveniste 2001; Becher, Beckmann, Greter 2006) and producers of pro-inflammatory cytokines such as IL-6 (Dong, Benveniste 2001; Farina, Aloisi, Meinl 2007), probably because of a loss of β_2-adrenergic receptor that mediates the suppression of MHC class II expression by norephinephrine (Keyser, Zeinstra, Frohman 2003). In this scenario, there is a diffuse activation of immune cells immigrating into the CNS, which leads to tissue damage through various effector mechanisms involving $CD4^+$ Th1 cells, B cells, cytotoxic $CD8^+$ T cells, $\gamma\delta$ T cells, and NK cells. $CD4^+$ Th1 cells determine IFN-γ-induced macrophage and microglia activation with the consequent liberation of TNF-α and IFN-γ, which have demonstrated myelinotoxic effects (Özenci, Kouwenhoven, Link 2002). Macrophages and microglial cells stimulated by

IFN-γ-secreting Th1 cells can also produce oxygen free radicals and NO, which direct the attack to myelin and neurons via calcium (Ca^{2+})-dependent glutamate excitotoxicity pathways and are responsible for an additional recruitment of circulating immune cells into the brain by promoting vasodilatation and increased permeability of the BBB (Smith, Lassmann 2002; Hauser, Oksenberg 2006). In addition, IFN-γ-activated macrophages and microglia generate MMPs that are able to disrupt the myelin sheath through proteolytic cleavage and the conversion of TNF-α precursor into their activated forms (Kieseier, Seifert, Giovannoni et al. 1999; Yong, Power, Forsyth et al. 2001). In MS, the effector functions of $CD4^+$ T cells are further supported by the demonstration that the activation of memory $CD4^+$ T cells in CSF and in peripheral blood is associated to disease activity and severity (Barrau, Montalban, Sáez-Torres et al. 2000; Okuda, Okuda, Apatoff et al. 2005; Krakauer, Sorensen, Sellebjerg 2006). On the other hand, $CD4^+$ Th1 cells help the differentiation of B cells into plasma cells that produce opsonizing and complement-binding IgG1 and IgG3 (Hemmer, Archelos, Hartung 2002; Hemmer, Cepok, Zhou et al. 2004). These antibodies cause demyelination via opsonization, consisting of the stimulation of macrophage-mediated phagocytosis by binding to Fc receptors expressed on the surface of phagocytes, and complement activation, in which they act as chemoattractants for lymphocytes and macrophages. In addition, antibodies are myelinotoxic also by means of NK-dependent ADCC, due to interactions between antibodies and Fc receptors expressed on NK cells, and by the production of proteolytic enzymes such as MMPs (Archelos, Storch, Hartung 2000; Archelos, Hartung 2000; Meinl, Krumbholz, Hohlfeld 2006). The intense release of antibodies restricted to the CNS by B cells confined within the brain is referred to as *intrathecal IgG synthesis,* which is a hallmark of MS since such antibodies can be identified in the CSF of MS patients as oligoclonal bands (Correale, Bassani Molinas 2002). In this phase of the CNS inflammatory response, activated astrocytes also contribute to intrathecal production of antibodies by the secretion of the B-cell activating factor of the TNF family (BAFF) that is an important survival factor during B-cell maturation (Hauser, Oksenberg 2006; Farina, Aloisi, Meinl 2007). The intrathecal release of antibodies is further facilitated by the development of ectopic lymphoid follicles in the inflamed meninges, a phenomenon indicated as lymphoid neogenesis or tertiary lymphoid organ formation (Uccelli, Aloisi, Pistoia 2005; Aloisi, Pujol-Borrell 2006). During CNS inflammation, persistent antigen stimulation leads to a continual activation of B cells infiltrating the

CNS, which increases their expression of cytokines, such as linfotoxin-$\alpha_1\beta_2$, and homeostatic chemokines migrate into and colonize the meningeal layers where these activated B cells organize themselves forming ectopic lymphoid tissue, undergo the same recapitulation occurring in the secondary lymphoid organ, and differentiate into memory B cells and plasma cells. The evidence of an accumulation of memory B cells and short-lived plasma cells in the CSF during neuroinflammation seems to corroborate the assumption that B cells play a significant role as effector cells of immune responses in inflamed brain (Cepok, Rosche, Grummel et al. 2005; Cepok, von Geldern, Grummel et al. 2006). Cytotoxic CD8$^+$ T cells can induce both myelin and axonal injury because they are able to promote apoptosis-dependent cytolysis of oligodendrocytes and neurons that express MHC class I molecules in the context of intrathecal inflammation. In fact, it has been reported that these cells outnumber CD4$^+$ T cells in MS lesions, cause demyelination in animal models of MS, and determine neurite transection in vitro (Neumann, Medana, Bauer 2002; Lassmann, Ransohoff 2004; Friese, Fugger 2005; McDole, Johnson, Pirko 2006). Moreover, a clonal expansion of CD8$^+$ T cells is present in demyelinating areas (Babbe, Roers, Waisman et al. 2000; Skulina, Schmidt, Dornmair et al. 2004), as well as in CSF and serum (Jacobsen, Cepok, Quak et al. 2002; Skulina, Schmidt, Dornmair et al. 2004) of MS patients, whereas blood levels of cytokines produced by CD8$^+$ T lymphocytes are strictly correlated to radiological signs of myelin and axonal damage (Killestein, Eikelenboom, Izeboud et al. 2003). Thus, cytotoxic CD8$^+$ T cells are currently considered the most important effector cells that mediate axonal loss (Friese, Fugger 2005; McDole, Johnson, Pirko 2006). On the other hand, CD8$^+$ T cells contribute to the recruitment of immune cells from blood to brain since they increase CNS vascular permeability by favoring the opening of the tight junctions of the BBB through the activation of astrocyte processes that form the glia limitans and, under inflammatory conditions, express MHC class I antigens (Suidan, Pirko, Johnson 2006). Among the effector cells involved in brain tissue injury, $\gamma\delta$ T cells and NK cells are suggested to be myelinotoxic. While $\gamma\delta$ T cells induce apoptosis through the release of perforin (Sospedra, Martin 2005; Dhib-Jalbut 2007), oligondrocyte killing is performed by NK1 cells via apoptosis and ADCC (Johansson, Berg, Hall et al. 2005; Shi, Van Kaer 2006). The effector functions of NK cells in intrathecal immune reactions seem to be proven in animal models of MS where the administration of IL-21 produced by activated CD4$^+$ T cells enhances the secretion of IFN-γ by NK cells and the severity of the disease. Conversely, the effect of IL-21 is abrogated by the depletion of NK cells (Vollmer, Liu, Price et al. 2005).

Termination of Th1-Mediated Immune Responses in Inflamed CNS

The resolution of immune events associated to the intrathecal inflammation is substantially driven by astrocytes that trigger the development of anti-inflammatory Th2-polarized responses through the release of IL-10 and TGF-β and the activation of infiltrating CD4$^+$ Th2 cells (Sospedra, Martin 2005; Delgado, Sheremata 2006; Dhib-Jalbut 2007). In fact, while IL-10 inhibits IL-12 production and MHC class II expression in resident microglial cells and in macrophages migrating into the brain, TGF-β suppresses the activation of migrating macrophages and CD4$^+$ Th1 cells. In addition, after antigen presentation occurs in the context of MHC class II molecules expressed by microglia, CD4$^+$ Th2 cells produce abundant amounts of IL-4 that counteracts Th1-mediated reactions. When the effects of ongoing Th2-type responses overcome those of Th1-dependent stimulation, microglial cells become producers of IL-10 and TGF-β, and there is a progressive immune deviation from Th1 to Th2 responses. At the end of this process, the original anti-inflammatory intrathecal microenvironment is re-established (Aloisi, Ria, Adorini 2000; Aloisi 2001; Schwartz, Butovsky, Brück et al. 2006). Therefore, initiation, amplification, and termination of CNS immune reactions ultimately depend on the interplay between microglia and astroglia that regulate the balance between Th1 pro-inflammatory and Th2 anti-inflammatory signals (Xiao, Link 1999). However, other mechanisms participate in the recovery from brain inflammation including apoptotic removal of immune cells invading the CNS and the activity of regulatory cells that are trafficking the BBB. The elimination of infiltrating immune cells occurs both at the gate of the CNS parenchyma and within the CNS parenchyma (Bechmann, Mor, Nilsen et al. 1999; Choi, Benveniste 2004). In the first case, the penetration of immune cells into the brain is prevented by the binding between FasL expressed by endothelial cells and astroglial end-feet and Fas expressed by immune cells that undergo apoptosis. In the second case, the CNS is protected by immune cells already entering the brain through microglial cells and neurons expressing FasL, which interact with immune cells presenting Fas on their surface. As a consequence, immune cells do not leave the intrathecal compartment where they perish by apoptotic pathway and are subsequently cleared by phagocytosis. Endothelial cells and astrocytes constitutively express Fas, but they are resistant to Fas/FasL-dependent apoptosis. In contrast, CNS inflammatory stimulation elicits the expression of Fas on microglia, oligodendrocytes, and neurons that are susceptible to apoptotic cell death via Fas/FasL system. In addition, the expression of FasL can be detected on infiltrating activated $CD8^+$ T and NK cells (Dietrich, Walker, Saas 2003; Choi, Benveniste 2004). Thus, $CD8^+$ T and NK cells contribute to the termination of intrathecal immune responses using Fas/FasL-mediated mechanisms to kill microglial cells, but are also implicated in myelin and neuronal injury by Fas/FasL-induced killing of oligodendrocytes and neurons (Sabelko-Downes, Russell, Cross 1999; Pender, Rist 2001; Choi, Benveniste 2004). In conclusion, the activation of Fas/FasL pathway plays a dual role in neuroinflammation since it could be both beneficial and detrimental by promoting the elimination of T cells invading the CNS as well as myelin and axonal damage (Sabelko-Downes, Russell, Cross 1999; Choi, Benveniste 2004). On the other hand, among the regulatory cells penetrating the CNS, $CD4^+CD25^+$ Treg cells inhibit infiltrating $CD4^+$ Th1 cells by cell contact or by secretion of IL-10 and TGF-β and exert their suppressor function mainly by the expression of the transcription factor FOXP3, whereas Tr1 and Tr3 cells have an immunosuppressive role on the same cells by the release of IL-10 and TGF-β, respectively (Jiang, Chess 2006; Baecher-Allan, Hafler 2006). The activity of invading $CD4^+$ Th1 cells is also downregulated by NK T cells through the liberation of IL-4, IL-10, and TGF-β (Jiang, Chess 2006) and by NK2 cells through the delivery of IL-10 and TGF-β and the cytolysis of APCs (Johansson, Berg, Hall et al. 2005; Shi, Van Kaer 2006). The protective functions of NK2 cells have recently been underlined in MS animal models in which the depletion of NK cells increases the severity of the disease (Xu, Fazekas, Hara et al. 2005; Huang, Shi, Jung et al. 2006), as well as in human studies that demonstrate that the overproduction of NK2 is related to disease remission (Takahashi, Aranami, Endoh et al. 2004; Aranami, Miyake, Yamamura et al. 2006). $CD8^+$ Treg cells block the activation of $CD8^+$ cytotoxic T cells by the recognition of the antigen presented by TCR of activated $CD8^+$ T cells in the context of nonclassical class Ib molecules HLA-E, but this inhibitory effect is also obtained by rendering APCs tolerogenic and by producing IL-10 (Friese, Fugger 2005). $HLA\text{-}G^+$ Treg cells and HLA-G–expressing microglia, endothelial cells, and immigrating macrophages may suppress CD4$^+$ Th1 cell pro-inflammatory signals and CD$^+$ T and NK cell cytotoxicity via release of sHLA-G and/or Fas/FasL interactions (Wiendl 2007). In fact, in MS, high CSF levels and an intrathecal synthesis of

sHLA-G seem to be associated to the resolution of inflammatory activity (Fainardi, Rizzo, Melchiorri et al. 2003; Fainardi, Rizzo, Melchiorri et al. 2006b). Overall, the course of immune responses within the inflamed CNS can be described as a biphasic phenomenon: (a) the development of neuroinflammation, initiated by the activation of microglia and amplified by the plentiful recruitment of immune cells from the systemic to the intrathecal compartments; (b) The termination of inflammatory storm promoted by resident and blood-derived regulatory mechanisms. These stages seem to be reciprocally controlled by microglia and astroglia acting on the balance Th1/Th2. The features of these two phases of Th1-mediated immune responses in inflamed CNS are shown in Table 12.6 and illustrated in Figure 12.3.

THE AUTOIMMUNE NATURE OF MS

MS is currently postulated to be an autoimmune chronic inflammatory disease of the CNS of unclear etiology in which both demyelination and axonal loss occur (Sospedra, Martin 2005; Frohman, Racke, Raine 2006; Hauser, Oksenberg 2006).

Clinical Characteristics of MS

MS commonly affects young adults and women more frequently than men and is clinically characterized by the dissemination in space and time of relapses, also called clinical attacks or exacerbations, which consist in the occurrence of neurological symptoms and signs. In fact, in MS, relapses typically affect different CNS functional systems (dissemination in space) in different periods of time separated by phases of recovery and remission (dissemination in time) (Compston, Coles 2002). Clinical expression of the disease is highly variable, but three main courses of MS are generally recognized (Noseworthy, Lucchinetti, Rodriguez et al. 2000; Compston, Coles 2002). About 80% of MS patients begin with an initial relapsing–remitting (RR) course characterized by self-limited acute exacerbations followed by periods of clinical stability which, in many patients, evolves into a secondary progressive (SP) phase characterized by a steady worsening in neurological function unrelated to acute attacks. Less often (20%), a primary progressive (PP) form with a slow and inexorable deterioration of clinical condition without acute attacks represents the onset of the disease. However, according to the recently proposed criteria (McDonald, Compston, Edan et al. 2001; Polman, Reingold, Edan et al. 2005; Swanton, Rovira, Tintore et al. 2007) the diagnosis of MS requires

Table 12.6 The Two Phases of Th1-Mediated Immune Responses in Inflamed Central Nervous System (CNS)

Phases	Mechanisms	References
Initiation and amplification	Presentation of cognate antigen to activated CD+ Th1 cells in the context of MHC class II molecules by microglial cells resulting in the activation of microglia that releases Th1 pro-inflammatory chemokines and cytokines	Aloisi 2000 Becher et al. 2000 Aloisi 2001 Becher et al. 2006 Schwartz et al. 2006
	Massive recruitment of immune cells secreting Th1-associated mediators from the blood to the CNS and formation of an intrathecal pro-inflammatory microenvironment	Hemmer et al. 2002 Sospedra, Martin 2005 Hauser, Oksenberg 2006 Dhib-Jalbut 2007
	Overstimulation of CNS-resident and infiltrating APC cells, activation of effector immune cells immigrating into the brain and development of meningeal lymphoid follicles containing B cells	Keyser et al. 2003 Sospedra, Martin 2005 Uccelli et al. 2005 Becher et al. 2006 Frohman et al. 2006
	Myelin damage and axonal loss mediated by toxic factors (TNF-α, IFN-γ, reactive oxygen species, NO and MMPs) for microglial cells and CD4+ Th1 cell-activated macrophages, antibodies for B cells, and cytolysis for CD8+ T cells, $\gamma\delta$ T cells and NK1 cells	Becher et al. 2000 Archelos, Hartung 2000 Hemmer et al. 2004 Friese, Fugger 2005 Hauser, Oksenberg 2006 Shi, Van Kaer 2006
Termination	Presentation of cognate antigen to activated CD4+ Th2 cells in the context of MHC class II molecules by astrocytes leading to the production of Th2 anti-inflammatory cytokines by activated astroglia and CD4+ Th2 cells	Sospedra, Martin 2005 Hauser, Oksenberg 2006 Dhib-Jalbut 2007
	Elimination of infiltrating immune cells by endothelial cells, astrocytes, microglia and neurons through Fas/FaL-dependent pathway	Bechmann et al 1999 Choi, Benveniste 2004
	Suppression of activity of invading immune cells by regulatory cells (CD4+CD25+ Treg, Tr1, Tr3, NK T, NK2, CD8+ Treg, and HLA-G+ Treg cells)	Friese, Fugger 2005 Johansson et al. 2005 Jiang, Chess 2006 Wiendl 2006
	Re-establishment of an intrathecal anti-inflammatory microenvironment	Aloisi 2000 Aloisi 2001

APC, antigen-presenting cells; IFN-γ, interferon γ; MHC-II, major histocompatibility complex II; MMP, matrix metalloproteinases; NK1 cells, natural killer 1 cells; NO, nitric oxide; TNF, tumor necrosis factor.

additional radiological and laboratory findings. In particular, more than 95% of MS patients show multifocal lesions in the periventricular white matter on T2-weighted magnetic resonance imaging (MRI) scans with or without gadolinium (Gd) enhancement on T1-weighted MRI scans (Fig. 12.4A and B), which are able to demonstrate dissemination in space and time. On the other hand, in more than 90% of cases isoelectric focusing (IEF) identifies oligoclonal IgG bands only in CSF and not in the corresponding serum reflecting an intrathecal synthesis of IgG sustained by few clones of antibody-secreting B cells sequestrated into the CNS (Fig. 12.4C). In the original diagnostic criteria for MS described by McDonald (2001), the diagnosis is reached through a combination of clinical, MRI, and CSF findings. Clinical dissemination in space is defined as the occurrence of neurological symptoms and signs (relapses) involving different CNS functional systems. Clinical dissemination in time is considered as the appearance

of neurological symptoms and signs (relapses) in different periods of time separated by phases of recovery and remission. MRI dissemination in space is designated as the presence of at least three of the following criteria: (1) one Gd-enhancing brain lesion or nine T2-weighted hyperintense brain lesions; (2) one infratentorial lesion; (3) one juxtacortical lesion; (4) three periventricular lesions. Notably, one spinal cord lesion can replace one brain lesion. MRI dissemination in time is regarded as the occurrence of at least one of the following criteria: (a) a Gd-enhancing lesion demonstrated in a scan done at least three months after the onset of a relapse at a site different from attack; (b) a Gd-enhancing lesion or a new T2 lesion identified in a follow-up scan done after additional 3 months. Recently, the recommended diagnostic MRI criteria have been modified by two different international panels. In the first revision (Polman, Reingold, Edan et al. 2005), a spinal cord lesion is equivalent to an infratentorial lesion and any spinal

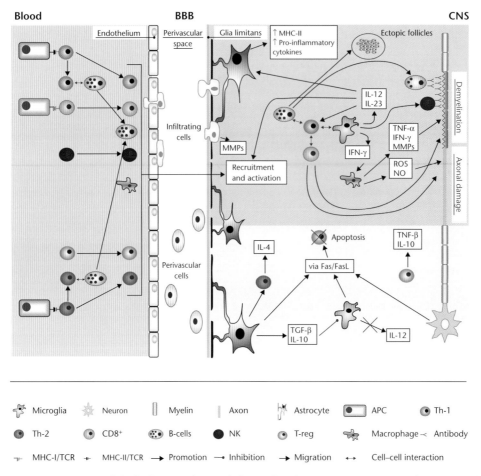

Figure 12.3 Schematic representation of the biphasic evolution of Th1-mediated immune responses in inflamed central nervous system (CNS). At intrathecal level, the grey area represents the mechanisms involved in the initiation and amplification whereas the white area corresponds to those mediating the termination of these reactions. APC, antigen-presenting cells; BBB, blood–brain barrier; IFN-γ, interferon γ; IL, interleukin; MHC-II, major histocompatibility complex II; MMP, matrix metalloproteinases; NO, nitric oxide; ROS, reactive oxygen species; TCR, T-cell receptor; TGF, transforming growth factor; TNF, tumor necrosis factor (see Table 12.6).

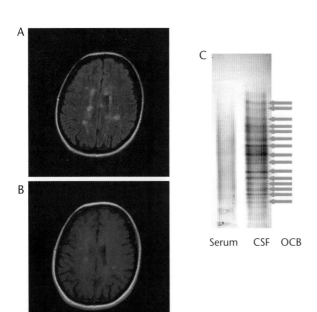

Figure 12.4 Magnetic resonance imaging (MRI) appearance of multiple sclerosis (MS) brain lesions disseminating the periventricular white matter (A) as hyperintense foci on T2-weighted fluid attenuated inversion recovery (FLAIR) scans and (B) as gadolinium (Gd)-enhanced small areas on post-contrast T1-weighted images. (C) shows oligoclonal IgG bands (OCB) only in CSF and not in the corresponding serum, reflecting an intrathecal synthesis of IgG as detected by isoelectric focusing (IEF).

cord lesions can be included in total lesion count in the demonstration of MRI dissemination in space, whereas the evidence of a new T2 lesion in a follow-up scan done after an additional 1 month is sufficient to confirm MRI dissemination in time. The second revision further simplifies MRI criteria (Swanton, Rovira, Tintore et al. 2007) since MRI dissemination in space is proven by the presence of at least one lesion in at least two characteristic locations (periventricular, juxtacortical, infratentorial, spinal cord) and by the occurrence of all lesions in the symptomatic region excluded in brainstem and spinal cord syndromes, whereas MRI dissemination in time is documented by the appearance of a new T2 lesion in a follow-up scan irrespective of timing of baseline scan. MRI criteria for dissemination in space and time are summarized in Table 12.7. In any case, the diagnosis of RR MS is obtained when there is the demonstration of at least one of these conditions: (a) two or more attacks and objective evidence of two or more lesions; (b) two or more attacks, objective evidence of one lesion, and, as additional data, MRI evidence of dissemination in space or detection of two or more MS-related MRI lesions, plus evidence of CSF-restricted oligoclonal IgG bands by IEF (positive CSF) or a second clinical exacerbation indicating a different site of tissue damage compared to the first one; (c) one attack, objective evidence of two lesion and, as additional data, dissemination in time or a second clinical attack; (d) one attack, objective evidence of one lesion and, as additional data, MRI evidence of dissemination

in space and/or time or detection of two or more MS-related MRI lesions, plus positive CSF or a second clinical relapse. Concerning PP MS, the diagnosis is differently achieved in McDonald and Polman criteria. In McDonald's criteria (McDonald, Compston, Edan et al. 2001), the occurrence of at least one of the following circumstances is needed: (a) positive CSF plus MRI evidence of dissemination in space or other additional findings detected by MRI and visual-evoked potential; (b) positive CSF plus MRI evidence of dissemination in time or 1 year of disease progression. Conversely, Polman criteria (Polman, Reingold, Edan et al. 2005) include 1 year of disease progression plus MRI evidence of lesions in brain or spine or positive CSF. In this setting, clinical evidence of disease activity is considered as the presence of relapse at neurological examination, whereas MRI appearance of disease activity is defined as the occurrence of lesions with Gd enhancement on T1-weighted MRI scans. Nevertheless, it is well known that MRI studies are more sensitive in measuring disease activity than clinical examination since several MRI active lesions are asymptomatic (Barkhof 2002).

Development of Autoimmunity in MS

The complex approach adopted for the diagnosis of MS reflects the uncertainty about disease pathogenesis. MS is currently hypothesized to be an autoimmune disease directed by autoreactive CD4+ Th1

Table 12.7 Diagnostic Magnetic Resonance Imaging (MRI) Criteria for Dissemination in Space and Time in Multiple Sclerosis (MS)

Dissemination in Space	Dissemination in Time	References
Presence of at least three of the following: (1) one Gd-enhancing brain lesion or nine T2-weighted hyperintense brain lesions (2) one infratentorial lesion (3) one juxtacortical lesion (4) three periventricular lesions One spinal cord lesion = one brain lesion	At least one of the following: (1) a Gd-enhancing lesion demonstrated in a scan done at least 3 months after the onset of a relapse at a different site from attack (2) a Gd-enhancing lesion or a new T2 lesion identified in a follow-up scan done after additional 3 months	McDonald et al. 2001
Presence of at least three of the following: (1) one Gd-enhancing brain lesion or nine T2-weighted hyperintense brain lesions (2) one infratentorial lesion (3) one juxtacortical lesion (4) three periventricular lesions One spinal cord lesion = one brain infratentorial lesion Any spinal cord lesion can be included in total lesion count	A new T2 lesion identified in a follow-up scan done after additional 1 month	Polman et al. 2005
(1) At least one lesion in at least two characteristic locations (periventricular, juxtacortical, infratentorial, spinal cord) (2) All lesions in symptomatic region excluded in brainstem and spinal cord syndromes	A new T2 lesion identified in a follow-up scan irrespective of timing of baseline scan	Swanton et al. 2007

cells that traffic across the BBB and migrate into the CNS after activation (Hemmer, Archelos, Hartung 2002; Hemmer, Cepok, Zhou et al. 2004; Sospedra, Martin 2005; Frohman, Racke, Raine 2006, Hauser, Oksenberg 2006; Dhib-Jalbut 2007). These cells seem to regulate a coordinated attack of both innate and acquired immune responses directed against myelin proteins that includes monocytes, macrophages, NK cells, B cells, and CD8+ T cells and results in CNS inflammation promoting myelin damage and axonal injury. In this context, it is generally believed that the initiation of MS autoimmunity takes place in the periphery because of failure of self-tolerance since T and B cells are primed in the peripheral lymphoid tissue after the presentation of neural antigens released from the CNS performed by meningeal and choroid plexus-associated dendritic cells that provide for transfer of these proteins from the brain to the cervical lymph nodes via the nasal lymphatics of the cribriform plate (Hemmer, Archelos, Hartung 2002; Hemmer, Cepok, Zhou et al. 2004; Sospedra, Martin 2005; Hauser, Oksenberg 2006). Under physiologic circumstances, myelin-specific autoreactive T cells are detectable in peripheral blood of healthy individuals since they are part of normal T-cell repertoire (Hemmer, Archelos, Hartung 2002; Sospedra, Martin 2005; Frohman, Racke, Raine 2006). These autoaggressive T cells are usually eliminated or inactivated through the mechanisms of peripheral immunologic tolerance by which autoreactive T cells that recognize self-antigens become incapable of responding to these proteins. This result is obtained through (Abbas, Lohr, Knoechel et al. 2004) (a) anergy that consists in the induction of a functional unresponsiveness of autoreactive T cells because of antigen recognition without adequate costimulation; (b) apoptotic deletion of autoreactive T cells; and (c) suppression of the activation of autoaggressive T cells promoted by regulatory cells. Therefore, brain antigens can be recognized as non-self by a dysfunction of regulatory immune cells ("autoimmune hypothesis") or by a reaction with proteins released from the CNS after primary degeneration ("degeneration hypothesis") or infection ("infection hypothesis") (Hemmer, Archelos, Hartung 2002; Hemmer, Cepok, Zhou et al. 2004; Sospedra, Martin 2005; Frohman, Racke, Raine 2006).

Infection Theory in MS

Epidemiological studies indicate that exposure to an environmental factor, such as an infectious agent, in combination with genetic predisposition could be implicated in MS pathogenesis (Casetta Granieri 2000; Marrie 2004; Sospedra, Martin 2005; Ascherio, Munger 2007). The risk of MS is enhanced by the presence of specific genes on chromosome 6 in the area of MHC, HLA in humans. In particular, *HLA-DR* and *HLA-DQ* genes, which are involved in antigen presentation, are strongly associated to the development of the disease. However, although the risk of the disease is higher in monozygotic than in dizygotic twins (about 30% and 5%, respectively), the low concordance rate obtained in identical twins suggests that nongenetic factors can contribute to the initiation of the disease. In this setting, the potential role for an infectious agent in MS pathogenesis is supported by descriptive epidemiological studies showing a nonhomogeneous geographical distribution, a variation in trend in some areas of the world, the evidence of possible clusters, and a change of risk in migrants. A primary encounter with this microbial agent could occur in young genetically susceptible adults, who subsequently develop the disease. This antecedent infection is believed to trigger autoimmune events operating in MS after reactivation. There is also substantial clinical and experimental evidence supporting the possible involvement of an infectious agent in the pathogenesis of MS (Scarisbrick, Rodriguez 2003; Gilden 2005; Lipton, Liang, Hertzler et al. 2007). First, nonspecific systemic infections, particularly those affecting the upper respiratory tract, represent a risk factor for relapse in MS patients (Buljevac, Flach, Ho et al. 2002; Correale, Fiol, Gilmore 2006) and are associated with increased MRI activity and T cells activation (Correale, Fiol, Gilmore 2006). Second, CSF oligoclonal bands are present not only in MS, but also in chronic bacterial, fungal, parasite, and viral CNS infections in which this intrathecal oligoclonal antibody response is directed against the causative agent (Contini, Fainardi, Cultrera et al. 1998; Fainardi, Contini, Benassi et al. 2001; Scarisbrick, Rodriguez 2003; Gilden 2005). Nevertheless, in CNS infections only 20% to 30% of intrathecally produced antibodies are directed against the causative agent, whereas the remaining 70% represent a polyspecific intrathecal immune response directed to many different pathogens not related to the cause of the disease (Conrad, Chiang, Andeen et al. 1994). Third, treatment with an antiviral agent, such as interferon-β, is beneficial in MS patients (Javed, Reder 2006). Fourth, CNS viral infections are able to induce inflammation and demyelination in humans and in MS animal models, as demonstrated by JC papovavirus-mediated multifocal leukoencephalopathy and measles-induced subacute sclerosing panencephalitis in man and by Theiler's murine encephalomyelitis virus in experimental studies (Scarisbrick, Rodriguez 2003; Sospedra, Martin 2005; Gilden 2005; Lipton, Liang, Hertzler et al. 2007). Finally, MHC class I–restricted

CD8$^+$ T-cell response, usually triggered by viruses, takes part in MS immune deregulation (Scarisbrick, Rodriguez 2003; Skulina, Schmidt, Dornmair et al. 2004). Infectious agents could generate an autoimmune response within the CNS by various mechanisms including antigen-specific and non–antigen-specific pathways such as (a) molecular mimicry; (b) epitope spreading; (c) bystander activation; (d) cryptic epitopes; and (e) superantigens (Vanderlugt, Miller 2002; Scarisbrick, Rodriguez 2003; Christen, von Herrat 2004; Sospedra, Martin 2005). Molecular mimicry is a cross-reactive T cell immune response between microbial and CNS self-antigens, due to their sequence homology, and is antigen specific. Epitope spreading describes a spreading of an antigen-specific T-cell immune response from infectious antigens to multiple CNS self-epitopes that are released as a consequence of microbe-mediated brain inflammation. Bystander activation consists of a non–antigen-specific T-cell immune reaction targeting CNS self-antigens promoted by infected T cells secreting pro-inflammatory cytokines and chemokines. Cryptic epitopes are antigens usually sequestered in the brain tissue that are unveiled and recognized as non-self by antigen-specific T cells after direct infection of target cells. Superantigens are microbial molecules originating primarily from bacteria or viruses that stimulate the activation of T cells cross-reacting with CNS self-antigens in an antigen-independent manner. In this way, infectious agents may initiate and maintain intrathecal inflammatory response of MS by reactivation of a chronic persistent latent infection occurring within the CNS or in the periphery (Scarisbrick, Rodriguez 2003). In the first circumstance, the microorganism infects the brain and promotes a local inflammation mediated by immune response involved in microbial clearance from CNS ("hit–hit hypothesis"). In the second condition, the pathogen infects the systemic compartment and produces an intrathecal inflammation by an immune reaction that develops after clearance of the infectious agent from the brain or as primary event because the microbial agent may never enter the CNS ("hit–run hypothesis"). In both cases, the prerequisite for the development and the perpetuation of MS autoimmunity is the presence of a latent infection in which the microorganism persists in a noninfectious, viable, but noncultivable form that can be periodically reactivated. This state differs from chronic infection characterized by permanent expression of infectious antigens (Lipton, Liang, Hertzler et al. 2007). In the past few decades, different infectious agents, mainly viruses, have been associated to MS because of their detection at protein and molecular levels in serum, peripheral blood, CSF, and brain tissue samples of patients with MS (Scarisbrick,

Rodriguez 2003; Gilden 2005; Sospedra, Martin 2005). These pathogens could operate by hit–hit mechanisms, such as human herpes virus-6 (HHV-6) (Swanborg, Whittum-Hudson, Hudson 2003; Stüve, Rache, Hemmer 2004), human T-lymphotropic virus type-I (HTLV-I) and MS-associated retrovirus (MSRV) (Scarisbrick, Rodriguez 2003; Gilden 2005), JC polyomavirus (Khalili, White, Lublin et al. 2007), and *Chlamydia pneumoniae* (Stratton, Sriram 2003; Fainardi, Castellazzi, Casetta et al. 2004; Contini, Cultrera, Seraceni et al. 2004; Stratton, Wheldon 2006) or by hit–run pathways, such as Epstein-Barr virus (EBV) (Giovannoni, Cutter, Lunemann et al. 2006; Ascherio, Munger 2007). However, although several efforts have been made to identify a possible link between various pathogens and the disease, direct evidence for an infectious etiology in MS is still lacking (Sospedra, Martin 2005). It follows that infection may not be the causative agent of the disease but can act as (a) a cofactor enhancing a preexisting autoimmune response; (b) an epiphenomenon due to overactive MS immune responses that reactivate an innocent bystander microbial reaction; and (c) a silent passenger trafficking into the CNS within activated immune cells (Stratton, Sriram 2003). Nevertheless, excluding a potential role of infection in MS pathogenesis may be an oversimplification since direct evidence of CNS infection is difficult to demonstrate. First, most healthy adults meet the infectious agent in their lifetime and show microbial-specific antibodies in body fluids, reflecting memory responses to this previous encounter, which can represent a possible confounding factor in serological studies (Swanborg, Whittum-Hudson, Hudson 2003). Second, the pathogen could be cleared from the CNS at the time of the diagnosis (hit–run hypothesis) (Christen, von Herrat 2004). Third, culture is considered the best method to isolate the microorganisms from CSF and brain tissue, but it is complicated to perform and rather insensitive because of technical issues (Lipton, Liang, Hertzler et al. 2007).

Autoimmune Theory in MS

The detection of myelin-specific autoreactive CD4$^+$ T cells, CD8$^+$ T cells, and autoantibodies directed against myelin basic protein (MPB), myelin oligodendrocyte glycoprotein (MOG), and proteolipid protein (PLP) in peripheral blood of MS patients argues for the possibility that the initiation of disease autoimmunity may be mediated by a disturbance of mechanisms that govern peripheral immunologic tolerance (Sospedra, Martin 2005). This view is in agreement with recent data suggesting that CD4$^+$ T cells with regulatory properties could be implicated in MS pathogenesis since a dysfunction of CD4$^+$CD25$^+$ Treg cells has been reported in peripheral blood samples of MS patients as compared to those of healthy donors (Viglietta, Baecher-Allan C, Weiner et al. 2004; Haas, Hug, Viehöver et al. 2005; Feger, Tolosa, Huang et al. 2007). More precisely, a decrease in suppressive effect of peripheral CD4$^+$CD25$^+$ Treg cells may cause the supposed loss of immune tolerance occurring in MS (Hafler et al. 2005). In the same way, a functional impairment of CD8$^+$ Treg cells (Friese, Fugger 2005), NK2 cells (Takahashi, Aranami, Endoh et al. 2004; Aranami, Miyake, Yamamura et al. 2006), and HLA-G$^+$CD4$^+$, and CD8$^+$ Treg cells (Feger, Tolosa, Huang et al. 2007) may contribute to the development of autoimmune response in MS. In fact, the presence of such immunoregulatory defects could allow the recognition of myelin antigens by autoaggressive T cells that become activated, undergo clonal expansion, and recirculate into the CNS, triggering an intrathecal immune response directed against the specific target represented by brain proteins (Hafler et al. 2005).

Degeneration Theory in MS

The potential significance of neurodegeneration as the primary mechanism that promotes the development of MS autoimmunity derives from the analysis of classical neurodegenerative disorders, such as Alzheimer's disease (AD) and Parkinson's disease (PD), which share some common molecular pathways of tissue damage with MS (Zipp, Aktas 2006; Aktas, Ullrich, Infante-Duarte et al. 2007). More precisely, while in MS neurodegeneration is presumed to be secondary to neuroinflammation, in AD and PD neurodegeneration induces neuroinflammation through microglial activation. The ability of neurodegenerative processes to promote a CNS inflammatory response is further supported by recent evidence showing that in nascent evolving MS plaques, a prephagocytic apoptotic death of oligodendrocytes can precede inflammation and demyelination and is associated with microglial activation (Barnett, Prineas 2004). These findings imply that oligodendrocyte apoptotic damage may be the primary event of the disease because it results in a release of myelin debris that could stimulate microglial phagocytic functions. As a consequence, the activation of microglia could determine the amplification of brain tissue damage by triggering the massive recruitment of immune cells from blood to CNS and then the intense intrathecal inflammatory response leading to myelin and axonal injury (Barnett, Sutton 2006; Barnett, Henderson, Prineas 2006). In this model, oligodendrocyte apoptosis may represent a primary degenerative phenomenon or, alternatively, it may be produced by a foreign antigen such as an infectious pathogen. In either case, the initial myelin insult could promote the exposition and release of cryptic epitopes that can be transported to local peripheral lymph nodes by dendritic cells associated to meninges and choroid plexus through the nasal lymphatics of the cribriform plate. Within the cervical lymph nodes, naive autoreactive T lymphocytes can recognize these neural proteins as non-self after presentation, operated by dendritic cells in the context of MHC molecules, and can recirculate into the brain where they participate and intensify the intrathecal immune response already generated by activated microglia (Barnett, Sutton 2006; Barnett, Henderson, Prineas 2006). The current hypotheses for MS pathogenesis are described in Table 12.8 and in Figure 12.5.

Progression of the Disability in MS

Whatever the mechanisms promoting the initiation of the disease, two different temporally distinct stages can classically be identified in MS (Steinman 2001): (1) an early inflammatory phase due to autoimmune-mediated demyelination leading to clinical recurrence of relapses and remissions (RR MS form); (2) a late degenerative phase due to axonal loss leading to clinical chronic progression (SP and PP MS forms). This model assumes that, in early RR MS clinical course, Th1-mediated inflammatory responses induce clinical relapses promoting demyelination mainly through the release of toxic mediators by activated macrophages and microglia and the production of antibodies by B cells. As axonal injury is present early in the disease, neurodegeneration begins in the same period because of Th1-related inflammatory mechanisms such as cytotoxic activity of CD8$^+$ T cells and Ca^{2+}-dependent glutamate excitotoxicity driven by activated macrophages and microglial cells. On the contrary, the resolution of neuroinflammation is followed by clinical remissions. Over time, the recurrence of several inflammatory events creates a persistent pro-inflammatory intrathecal microenvironment maintaining a permanent axonal loss in association with the reduced support for the axons and the destabilization of axon membrane potentials that follow myelin damage. When the compensatory immunoregulation fails, cumulative axonal injury leads to the irreversible progression of neurological disability (Bjartmar, Kidd, Ransohoff 2001; Hemmer, Archelos, Hartung 2002; Sospedra, Martin 2005; Brück, Stadelmann 2005; Frohman, Filippi, Stuve et al. 2005; Frohman, Racke, Raine 2006; Hauser, Oksenberg

Table 12.8 Immunopathogenetic Theories Currently Proposed for the Development of Autoimmunity in Multiple Sclerosis (MS)

Hypothesis	Mechanisms	References
Autoimmune	The initiation of MS autoimmunity takes place in the periphery since T and B cells are primed in the peripheral lymphoid tissue by neural antigens released from CNS. Brain antigens can be recognized as non-self by a dysfunction of regulatory immune cells. In this setting, neuroinflammation is the primary pathogenetic mechanism, whereas demyelination and neurodegeneration are secondary to neuroinflammation	Hemmer et al. 2002 Hemmer et al. 2004 Sospedra, Martin 2005 Hafler et al. 2005 Hauser, Oksenberg 2006
Infectious	The development of MS autoimmunity occurs in the periphery because brain antigens can be recognized as non-self by a reaction with proteins released from CNS after infection. Also in this case, neuroinflammation is the primary pathogenetic mechanism, whereas demyelination and neurodegeneration are secondary to neuroinflammation. Infectious agents could generate an autoimmune response within the CNS by various mechanisms such as molecular mimicry, epitope spreading, and/or bystander activation. In this way, infectious agents may initiate and maintain intrathecal inflammatory response of MS by reactivation of a chronic persistent latent infection occurring within the CNS ("hit–hit hypothesis") or in the periphery ("hit–run hypothesis")	Hemmer et al. 2002 Vanderlugt, Miller 2002 Scarisbrick, Rodriguez 2003 Hemmer et al. 2004 Christen, von Herrat 2004 Hafler et al. 2005 Sospedra, Martin 2005 Gilden 2005 Hauser, Oksenberg 2006 Lipton et al. 2007
Degenerative	MS autoimmunity is triggered in the periphery since brain antigens can be recognized as non-self by a reaction with proteins released from CNS after primary degeneration. In this view, neurodegeneration is the primary pathogenetic mechanism, whereas neuroinflammation and demyelination are secondary to neurodegeneration	Hemmer et al. 2002 Hemmer et al. 2004 Maggs, Palace 2004 Barnett, Prineas 2004 Sospedra, Martin 2005 Barnett, Sutton 2006 Barnett et al 2006

CNS, central nervous system.

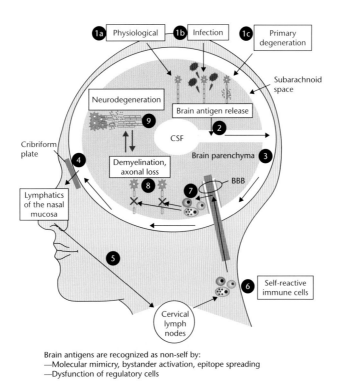

Figure 12.5 A schematic view of the current hypotheses on the mechanisms responsible for the initiation of multiple sclerosis (MS) autoimmunity. Under normal conditions, brain proteins are released in the cerebrospinal fluid (CSF) as the result of physiological processes of remodeling and tissue repair (1a). In MS, tissue injury due to infection (1b) or degeneration (1c) increases the shedding of central nervous system (CNS) antigens in the CSF including cryptic epitopes that are unknown for the immune system. These neural CSF proteins are captured by meningeal and choroid plexus dendritic cells (2) that transport them (3) to perivascular spaces of the nasal olfactory artery (4) and then, via nasal lymphatics of the cribriform plate, to peripheral cervical lymph nodes (5). Within the secondary lymphoid organs, brain protein coming from the CNS can be recognized as non-self by infection-mediated interactions (molecular mimicry, epitope spreading, bystander activation) or a dysfunction of regulatory immune cells. It follows the priming of naive autoreactive T and B cells that become activated and undergo clonal expansion (6). Subsequently, these cells recirculate into the CNS where the re-encounter and the recognition of the cognate antigen lead to the development of an intrathecal inflammatory response (7) that produces demyelination and axonal loss (8). Over time, inflammatory microenvironment promotes the progression of neurodegeneration, generating irreversible disability. Conversely, cumulative axonal destruction can occur independently of neuroinflammation and may cause irreversible disability (9). For details, see Table 12.8.

2006). Accordingly, axonal loss with clinical progression could be related to multiple waves of inflammation, involving various CNS locations at different times ("multiple hits hypothesis") (Pratt, Antel 2005; Imitola, Chitnis, Khuory 2006). Therefore, both demyelination and axonal damage are secondary to Th1-mediated neuroinflammation that plays a pivotal role in both the development and progression of MS (Zipp, Aktas 2006; Aktas, Ullrich, Infante-Duarte et al. 2007). In humans, this concept only seems to be partially supported by data coming from neuropathological studies, indicating that three types of MS lesions, all oriented on the long axis of periventricular postcapillary venules, can occur: (1) the acute active demyelinating plaques; (2) the chronic active demyelinating plaques; and (3) the chronic inactive demyelinating plaques (Hichey 1999; Hafler 2004; Frohman, Racke, Raine 2006). The acute active demyelinated lesions are characterized by an extensive myelin and oligodendrocyte loss involving the whole damaged area, reactive astrocytes, and a perivascular infiltration consisting of macrophages, CD4[+] T cells, CD8[+] T cells, and occasional B and plasma cells. In the chronic active demyelinated lesions, an ongoing myelin and oligodendrocyte loss and an astrocyte reactivity prevail at the edge of the plaques that surrounds the already demyelinated centre of the lesions. In addition, in comparison to acute active lesions, this type of plaque is associated to a less pronounced inflammatory cell infiltrate containing more abundant B and plasma cells. In the chronic inactive demyelinated lesions there is the predominance of glial scar tissue with the absence of an ongoing destruction of myelin sheaths. Oligodendroglial cells are not detectable, whereas only few macrophages, T and B cells, infiltrate the perivascular cuffs. In this setting, axonal injury is a constant feature of every demyelinated lesion type since, while a profound axonal damage is present in actively demyelinating lesions, a continuous axonal loss is also visible in inactive plaques (Lassmann 2004; Brück, Stadelmann 2005; Hauser, Oksenberg 2006; Brück 2007). Analysis of the chronological distribution of these type of lesions suggests that active lesions predominate in the early stage of MS (RR MS form), whereas chronic lesions are principally found in the late stage of the disease (SP and PP MS forms) (Brück 2007). Thus, the transition from acute to chronic stage is accompanied by a progressive decline of inflammatory responses producing demyelination and axonal loss in presence of a constant axonal degeneration (Frohman, Filippi, Stuve et al. 2005). The central role of neuroinflammation in MS demyelination and axonal injury has recently been strengthened by the demonstration that, while the early RR MS phase is associated to white matter focal inflammatory demyelinating lesions, the late SP and PP MS stages are marked by a diffuse axonal injury and cortical demyelination that develop in an inflammatory background involving the whole brain (Kutzelnigg, Lucchinetti, Stadelmann 2005; Lassmann 2007). However, there is increasing evidence indicating that, in MS, the interplay between neuroinflammation and neurodegeneration is more complex than previously presumed since the great extent of axonal damage in the late stage of the disease argues for the contribution of mechanisms other than inflammatory demyelination in the progression of neurodegeneration (Frohman, Filippi, Stuve et al. 2005; Brück 2007; Esiri 2007). In fact, in active MS lesions four distinct patterns of myelin destruction can be identified, suggesting that the pathology of the disease is heterogeneous (Lucchinetti, Brück, Prisi et al. 2000). In pattern I, demyelination is due to the cytotoxic activity of CD8[+] T cells together with the release of toxic mediators by CD4[+] T cell-activated macrophages and microglia. In pattern II, myelin dissolution is mainly mediated by antibody and complement deposition. In pattern III, myelin loss is driven by hypoxia-like mechanisms inducing oligondrocyte apoptosis. In pattern IV, typical of PP MS form, myelin impairment is the consequence of a periplaque nonapoptotic oligondrocyte degeneration.All these patterns of demyelination arise from a similar inflammatory background sustained by T-cell and macrophage-directed immune responses (Lassmann 2004). Hence, patterns I and II are linked to an immune-mediated attack, whereas patterns III and IV are related to a primary gliopathy (Brück 2007). Interestingly, it was initially believed that different patterns could only be detected in different patients at different stages of the disease (interindividual heterogeneity), but not in the same patient (intra-individual heterogeneity) (Lucchinetti, Brück, Prisi et al. 2000). Nevertheless, the presence of an intra-individual heterogeneity was later documented in MS patients with newly forming MS plaques (Barnett, Prineas 2004), favouring the idea that the heterogeneity found in MS lesions may reflect the temporal evolution of the lesions rather than the existence of distinct mechanisms of myelin damage (Barnett, Sutton 2006; Barnett, Henderson, Prineas 2006). More important, during the formation of acute MS lesions apoptotic depletion of oligodendrocytes can lead to the activation of microglial cells, resulting in inflammation and demyelination (Barnett, Prineas 2004). On the other hand, it has been reported that axonal loss is poorly correlated to demyelinating plaque load and can induce neuroinflammation (Maggs, Palace 2004; DeLuca, Williams, Evangelou 2006). These observations are consistent with the possibility that axonal damage may be independent of inflammation that, in turn, may be secondary to neurodegeneration

(Maggs, Palace 2004; Barnett, Henderson, Prineas 2006; Barnett, Sutton 2006; DeLuca, Williams, Evangelou 2006). These conclusions are partially in agreement with epidemiological studies proving that the accumulation of irreversible disability during the progression of MS is not related to frequency of inflammation-related relapses (Confavreux, Vukusic, Moreau et al. 2000; Kremenchutzky, Rice, Baskerville et al. 2006). Collectively taken (Fig. 12.6), these data underscore that the relationship between neuroinflammation and neurodegeneration still remains to be clarified since (a) CNS inflammation may promote demyelination that, in turn, leads to axonal loss; (b) axonal damage may induce CNS inflammation that, in turn, produces demyelination; and (c) axonal injury may occur independently of CNS inflammatory demyelination (Maggs, Palace 2004; Hauser, Oksenberg 2006; Brück 2007). The traditional view of MS as a "two-stage disease" is further challenged by radiological studies that confirm the heterogeneity of MS, because of the occurrence of different lesional patterns underlying distinct mechanisms of tissue injury, and show that inflammatory and degenerative phases can coexist (Lee, Smith, Palace 1999; Charil, Filippi 2007). For this reason, it has been proposed that MS may be a "simultaneous two-component disease" (Charil, Filippi 2007) in which neuroinflammation and neurodegeneration could represent two distinct events occurring separately.

CONCLUSIONS

Currently, little is known about the etiology and pathogenesis of MS, a chronic inflammatory demyelinating and neurodegenerative disease of the CNS that is commonly assumed to represent the prototypic autoimmune disorder of the brain. In particular, although a growing body of evidence suggests that MS inflammation could be mediated by autoreactive $CD4^+$ T cells secreting Th1 pro-inflammatory cytokines that infiltrate the CNS after activation and orchestrate a combined attack of both innate and acquired immune responses directed against myelin proteins, the mechanisms promoting the development and the progression of the disease are largely elusive. In fact, it has been hypothesized that the initiation of MS could occur in the periphery as a consequence of a failure of immunologic tolerance. However, the question whether this primary event is attributable to an infectious agent, a dysfunction of peripheral regulatory pathways, or neurodegeneration still remains poorly understood (Hemmer, Archelos, Hartung 2002; Hemmer, Cepok, Zhou et al. 2004; Sospedra, Martin 2005; Frohman, Racke, Raine 2006, Hauser, Oksenberg 2006). In addition, the conventional view of MS as a "two-stage disease," with a predominant inflammatory demyelination in the early phase and a subsequent secondary neurodegeneration in the late phase of the disease (Steinman 2001), is now under

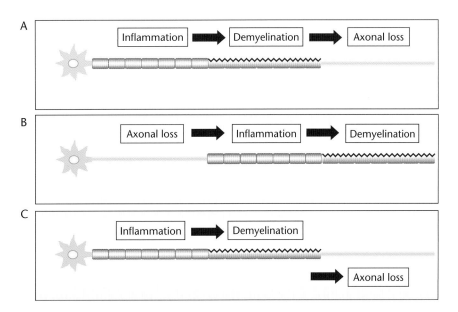

Figure 12.6 The interplay between neuroinflammation and neurodegeneration. In the conventional view of MS pathogenesis, CNS inflammation may promote demyelination that, in turn, leads to axonal loss (A). In this context, two different temporally distinct stages can be classically identified: (1) an early inflammatory phase due to autoimmune-mediated demyelination leading to clinical recurrence of relapses and remissions (RR MS form); (2) a late degenerative phase due to axonal loss leading to clinical chronic progression (SP and PP MS forms). (B and C) show the alternative hypotheses: axonal damage may induce CNS inflammation that, in turn, produces demyelination (A); axonal injury may occur independently of CNS inflammatory demyelination (C).

debate after the discovery that, in MS, neurodegeneration is not always produced by neuroinflammation but, conversely, it may be independent of CNS inflammation or may trigger intrathecal inflammatory responses. Therefore, the processes underlying the progression of neurological irreversible disability still require intensive investigation (Maggs, Palace 2004; Frohman, Filippi, Stuve et al. 2005; Imitola, Chitnis, Khuory 2006; Aktas, Ullrich, Infante-Duarte et al. 2007). In this setting, the evidence of coexistence between CNS inflammation and degeneration suggests that MS may be a "simultaneous two-component disease" in which both neuroinflammation and neurodegeneration contribute to clinical disability (Charil, Filippi 2007). For this reason, future studies are warranted to provide a better understanding of the exact mechanisms leading to the initiation and perpetuation of MS since the improvement of our knowledge on these crucial aspects of the disease may help us identify therapeutic strategies that are more efficient than the currently available treatments in ameliorating the disease.

REFERENCES

Abbas AK, Murphy KM, Sher A. 1996. Functional diversity of helper T lymphocytes. *Nature.* 383:787–793.

Abbas AK, Lohr J, Knoechel B, Nagabhushanam V. 2004. T cell tolerance and autoimmunity. *Autoimmun Rev.* 3:471–475.

Aktas O, Ullrich O, Infante-Duarte C, Nitsch R, Zipp F. 2007. Neuronal damage in brain inflammation. *Arch Neurol.* 64:185–189.

Aloisi F. 2001. Immune function of microglia. *Glia.* 36:165–179.

Aloisi F, Ria F, Adorini L. 2000. Regulation of T-cell responses by CNS antigen-presenting cells: different roles for microglia and astrocytes. *Immunol Today.* 21:141–147.

Aloisi F, Pujol-Borrell R. 2006. Lymphoid neogenesis in chronic inflammatory diseases. *Nat Rev Immunol.* 6:205–217.

Aranami T, Miyake S, Yamamura T. 2006. Differential expression of CD11c by peripheral blood NK cells reflects temporal activity of multiple sclerosis. *J Immunol.* 177:5659–5667.

Archelos JJ, Storch MK, Hartung HP. 2000. The role of B cells and autoantibodies in multiple sclerosis. *Ann Neurol.* 47:694–706.

Archelos JJ, Hartung HP. 2000. Pathogenetic role of autoantibodies in neurological diseases. *Trends Neurosci.* 23:317–327.

Ascherio A, Munger KL. 2007. Environmental risk factor for multiple sclerosis. Part I: role of infection. *Ann Neurol.* 61:288–299.

Babbe H, Roers A, Waisman A et al. 2000. Clonal expansion of CD8+ T cells dominate the cell infiltrate in active multiple sclerosis lesions as shown by micromanipulation and single cell polymerase chain reaction. *J Exp Med.* 192:393–404.

Baecher-Allan C, Hafler DA. 2006. Human regulatory T cells and their role in autoimmune disease. *Immunol Rev.* 212:203–216.

Barker CF, Billingham RE. 1977. Immunologically privileged sites. *Adv Immunol.* 25:1–54.

Barkhof F. 2002. The clinico-radiological paradox in multiple sclerosis revisited. *Curr Opin Neurol.* 15:239–245.

Barnett MH, Prineas JW. 2004. Relapsing an remitting multiple sclerosis: pathology of the newly forming lesions. *Ann Neurol.* 55:458–468.

Barnett MH, Henderson APD, Prineas JW. 2006. The macrophage in MS: just a scavenger after all? Pathology and pathogenesis of the acute MS lesion. *Mult Scler.* 12:121–132.

Barnett MH, Sutton I. 2006. The pathology of multiple sclerosis: a paradigm shift. *Curr Opin Neurol.* 19:242–247.

Barrau MA, Montalban X, Sáez-Torres I, Brieva L, Barberá N, Martinez-Cáceres EM. 2000. CD4+CD45RO+CD49d^high cells are involved in the pathogenesis of relapsing-remitting multiple sclerosis. *J Neuroimmunol.* 111:215–223.

Becher B, Prat A, Antel JP. 2000. Brain-immune connection: immuno-regulatory properties of CNS-resident cells. *Glia.* 29:293–304.

Becher B, Beckmann I, Greter M. 2006. Antigen presentation in autoimmunity and CNS inflammation: how T lymphocytes recognize the brain. *J Mol Med.* 84:532–543.

Bechmann I. 2005. Failed central nervous system regeneration: a downside of immune privilege? *Neuromolecular Med.* 7:217–228.

Bechmann I, Mor G, Nilsen I, Eliza M, Nitsch R, Naftolin F. 1999. FasL (CD95L, Ap01L) is expressed in the normal rat and human brain: evidence for the existence of an immunological brain barrier. *Glia.* 27:62–74.

Bechmann I, Galea I, Perry VH. 2007. What is the blood-brain barrier (not)? *Trends Immunol.* 28:5–11.

Bjartmar C, Kidd G, Ransohoff RM. 2001. A real-time insight into disease progression and the role of axonal injury in multiple sclerosis. *Arch Neurol.* 58:37–39.

Brück W. 2007. New insights into the pathology of multiple sclerosis: towards an unified concept? *J Neurol.* 254(Suppl 1):I/3–I/9.

Brück W, Stadelmann C. 2005. The spectrum of multiple sclerosis: new lessons from pathology. *Curr Opin Neurol.* 18:221–224.

Buljevac D, Flach HZ, Ho WC et al. 2002. Prospective study on the relationship between infections and multiple sclerosis exacerbations. *Brain.* 125:952–960.

Cabarrocas J, Bauer J, Piaggio E, Liblau R, Lassmann H. 2003. Effective and selective immune surveillance of the brain by MHC class I-restricted cytotoxic T lymphocytes. *Eur J Immunol.* 33:1174–1182.

Carosella ED, Moreau P, Aractingi S, Rouas-Freiss N. 2001. HLA-G: a shield against inflammatory aggression. *Trends Immunol.* 22:553–555.

Carson MJ, Doose JM, Melchior B, Schmid CD, Ploix CC. 2006. CNS immune privilege: hiding in plain sight. *Immunol Rev.* 213:48–65.

Casetta I, Granieri E. 2000. Clinical infections and multiple sclerosis: contribution from analytical epidemiology. *J Neurovirol.* 6(Suppl 2):S147–S151.

Cepok S, Rosche B, Grummel V et al. 2005. Short-lived plasma blasts are the main B cell effector subset during the course of multiple sclerosis. *Brain.* 128:1667–1676.

Cepok S, von Geldern G, Grummel V et al. 2006. Accumulation of class switched IgD-IgM-memory B cells in the cerebrospinal fluid during neuroinflammation. *J Neuroimmunol.* 180:33–39.

Charil A, Filippi M. 2007. Inflammatory demyelination and neurodegeneration in early multiple sclerosis. *J Neurol Sci.* 259:7–15.

Choi C, Benveniste EN. 2004. Fas ligand/Fas system in the brain: regulator of immune and apoptotic responses. *Brain Res Rev.* 44:65–81.

Christen U, von Herrat MG. 2004. Initiation of autoimmunity. *Curr Opin Immunol.* 16:759–767.

Compston A, Coles A. 2002. Multiple sclerosis. *Lancet.* 359:1221–1231.

Confavreux C, Vukusic S, Moreau T, Adeleine P. 2000. Relapses and progression of disability in multiple sclerosis. *N Engl J Med.* 343:1430–1438.

Conrad AJ, Chiang EY, Andeen LE et al. 1994. Quantitation of intrathecal measles virus IgG antibody synthesis rate: subacute sclerosing panencephalitis and multiple sclerosis. *J Neuroimmunol.* 54:99–108.

Contini C, Fainardi E, Cultrera R et al. 1998. Advanced laboratory techniques for diagnosing Toxoplasma Gondii encephalitis in AIDS patients: significance of intrathecal production and comparison with PCR and ECL-western blotting. *J Neuroimmunol.* 92:29–37.

Contini C, Cultrera R, Seraceni S, Castellazzi M, Granieri E, Fainardi E. 2004. Cerebrospinal fluid molecular demonstration of Chlamydia pneumoniae DNA is associated to clinical and brain magnetic resonance imaging activity in a subset of patients with relapsing-remitting multiple sclerosis. *Mult Scler.* 10:360–369.

Correale J, Bassani Molinas M. 2002. Oligoclonal bands and antibody responses in multiple sclerosis. *J Neurol.* 249:375–389.

Correale J, Fiol M, Gilmore W. 2006. The risk of relapses in multiple sclerosis during systemic infections. *Neurology.* 67:652–659.

Cserr HF, Knopf PM. 1992. Cervical lymphatics, the blood-brain barrier and the immunoreactivity of the brain: a new view. *Immunol Today.* 13:507–512.

Cua DJ, Sherlock J, Chen Y et al. 2003. Interleukin-23 rather than interleukin-12 is the critical cytokine for autoimmune inflammation of the brain. *Nature.* 421:744–748.

Delgado S, Sheremata WA. 2006. The role of CD4+ T-cells in the development of MS. *Neurol Res.* 28:245–249.

DeLuca GC, Williams K, Evangelou N, Ebers GC, Esiri MM. 2006. The contribution of demyelination to axonal loss in multiple sclerosis. *Brain.* 129:1507–1516.

Dhib-Jalbut S. 2007. Pathogenesis of myelin/oligodendrocyte damage in multiple sclerosis. *Neurology.* 68(Suppl 3): S13–S21.

Dietrich P-Y, Walker PR, Saas P. 2003. Death receptors on reactive astrocytes. A key role in the fine tuning of brain inflammation? *Neurology.* 60:548–554.

Dong Y, Benveniste EN. 2001. Immune function of astrocytes. *Glia.* 36:180–190.

Engelhardt B, Ransohoff RM. 2005. The ins and outs of T-lymphocytes trafficking to the CNS: anatomical sites and molecular mechanisms. *Trends Immunol.* 26:485–495.

Esiri MM. 2007. The interplay between inflammation and neurodegeneration in CNS disease. *J Neuroimmunol.* 184:4–16.

Fainardi E, Contini C, Benassi N et al. 2001. Assessment of HIV intrathecal humoral immune response in AIDS-related neurological disorders. *J Neuroimmunol.* 119:278–286.

Fainardi E, Rizzo R, Melchiorri L et al. 2003. Presence of detectable levels of soluble HLA-G molecules in CSF of relapsing-remitting multiple sclerosis: relationship with CSF soluble HLA-I and IL-10 concentrations and MRI findings. *J Neuroimmunol.* 142:149–158.

Fainardi E, Castellazzi M, Casetta I et al. 2004. Intrathecal production of Chlamydia pneumoniae-specific high-affinity antibodies is significantly associated to a subset of multiple sclerosis patients with progressive forms. *J Neurol Sci.* 217:181–188.

Fainardi E, Castellazzi M, Bellini T et al. 2006a. Cerebrospinal fluid and serum levels and intrathecal production of active matrix metalloproteinase-9 (MMP-9) as markers of disease activity in patients with multiple sclerosis. *Mult Scler.* 12:294–301.

Fainardi E, Rizzo R, Melchiorri L et al. 2006b. Intrathecal synthesis of soluble HLA-G and HLA-I molecules are reciprocally associated to clinical and MRI activity in patients with multiple sclerosis. *Mult Scler.* 12:2–12.

Farina C, Aloisi F, Meinl E. 2007. Astrocytes are active players in cerebral innate immunity. *Trends Immunol.* 28:138–145.

Feger U, Tolosa E, Huang YH et al. 2007. HLA-G expression defines a novel regulatory T cell subset present in human peripheral blood and sites of inflammation. *Blood.* 110:568–577.

Friese MA, Fugger L. 2005. Autoreactive CD8+ T cells in multiple sclerosis: a new target for therapy? *Brain.* 128:1747–1763.

Frohman EM, Filippi M, Stuve O et al. 2005. Characterizing the mechanisms of progression in multiple sclerosis. Evidence and new hypotheses for future directions. *Arch Neurol.* 62:1345–1356.

Frohman EM, Racke MK, Raine CS. 2006. Multiple sclerosis—the plaque and its pathogenesis. *N Engl J Med.* 354:942–955

Galea I, Bechmann I, Perry VH. 2007. What is immune privilege (not)? *Trends Immunol.* 28:12–18.

Gilden DH. 2005.Infectious causes of multiple sclerosis. *Lancet Neurol.* 4:195–202.

Giovannoni G, Cutter GR, Lunemann J et al. 2006. Infectious causes of multiple sclerosis. *Lancet Neurol.* 5:887–894.

Greve B, Magnusson CGM, Melms A, Wiessert R. 2001. Immunoglobulin isotypes reveal a predominant role of type 1 immunity in multiple sclerosis. *J Neuroimmunol.* 121:120–125.

Haas J, Hug A, Viehöver A et al. 2005. Reduced suppressive effect of CD4+CD25high regulatory T cells on the T cell immune response against myelin oligodendrocyte glycoprotein in patients with multiple sclerosis. *Eur J Immunol.* 35:3343–3352.

Hafler DA. 2004. Multiple sclerosis. *J Clin Invest.* 113:788–794.

Hafler, DA, Slavik JM, Anderson DE, O'Connor KC, De Jager P, Baecher-Allan C. 2005. Multiple sclerosis. *Immunol Rev.* 204: 208–231.

Harling-Berg CJ, Park JT, Knopf PM. 1999. Role of the cervical lymphatics in the Th2-type hierarchy of CNS immune regulation. *J Neuroimmunol.* 101:111–127.

Hart MN, Fabry Z. 1995. CNS antigen presentation. *Trends Neurosci.* 18:475–481.

Hauser SL, Oksenberg JR. 2006. The neurobiology of multiple sclerosis: genes, inflammation, and neurodegeneration. *Neuron.* 52:61–76.

Hemmer B, Archelos JJ, Hartung HP. 2002. New concepts in the immunopathogenesis of multiple sclerosis. *Nat Rev Neurosci.* 3:291–301.

Hemmer B, Cepok S, Zhou D, Sommer N. 2004. Multiple sclerosis—a coordinate immune attack across the blood brain barrier. *Curr Neurovasc Res.* 1:141–150.

Hickey WF. 1999. The pathology of multiple sclerosis: a historical perspective. *J Neuroimmunol.* 98:37–44.

Hickey WF. 2001. Basic principles of immunological surveillance of the normal central nervous system. *Glia.* 36:118–124.

Hickey WF, Hsu BL, Kimura H. 1991. T-lymphocyte entry into the central nervous system. *J Neurosci Res.* 28:254–260.

Hoftberger R, Aboul-Enein F, Brueck W et al. 2004. Expression of major histocompatibility complex class I molecules on the different cell types in multiple sclerosis lesions. *Brain Pathol.* 14:43–50.

Huang D, Shi FD, Jung S et al. 2006. The neuronal chemokine CX3CL1/fractalkine selectively recruits NK cells that modify experimental autoimmune encephalomyelitis within the central nervous system. *FASEB J.* 20:896–905.

Hunt JS, Petroff MG, McIntire RH, Ober C. 2005. HLA-G and immune tolerance in pregnancy. *FASEB J.* 19:681–693.

Imitola J, Chitnis T, Khuory AJ. 2006. Insights into molecular pathogenesis of progression in multiple sclerosis. *Arch Neurol.* 63:25–33.

Iwakura Y, Ishigame H. 2006. The IL-23/IL-17 axis in inflammation. *J Clin Invest.* 116:1218–1222.

Jacobsen M, Cepok S, Quak E et al. 2002. Oligoclonal expansion of memory CD8+ cells in cerebrospinal fluid from multiple sclerosis patients. *Brain.* 125:538–550.

Javed A, Reder AT. 2006. Therapeutic role of beta-interferons in multiple sclerosis. *Pharmacol Ther.* 110:35–56.

Jiang H, Chess L. 2006. Regulation of immune response by T cells. *N Engl J Med.* 354:1166–1176.

Johansson S, Berg L, Hall H, Höglund P. 2005. NK cells: elusive players in autoimmunity. *Trends Immunol.* 26:613–618.

Keyser J, Zeinstra E, Frohman E. 2003. Are astrocytes central players in the pathophysiology of multiple sclerosis? *Arch Neurol.* 60:132–136.

Khalili K, White MK, Lublin F, Ferrante P, Berger JR. 2007. Reactivation of JC virus and development of PML in patients with multiple sclerosis. *Neurology.* 68:985–990.

Kida S, Pantazis A, Weller RO. 1993. CSF drains directly from the subarachnoid space into nasal lymphatics in the rat. Anatomy, histology and immunological significance. *Neuropathol Appl Neurobiol.* 19:480–488.

Kieseier BC, Seifert T, Giovannoni G, Hartung HP. 1999. Matrix metalloproteinases in inflammatory demyelination. Targets for treatment. *Neurology.* 53:20–25.

Killestein J, Eikelenboom MJ, Izeboud T et al. 2003. Cytokine producing CD8+ T cells are correlated to MRI features of tissue destruction in MS. *J Neuroimmunol.* 142:141–148.

Kivisäkk P, Mahad DJ, Callahan MK et al. 2003. Human cerebrospinal fluid central memory CD4+ T cells: evidence for trafficking through choroid plexus and meninges via P-selectin. *Proc Natl Acad Sci U S A.* 100:8389–8394.

Krakauer Mm, Sorensen PS, Sellebjerg F. 2006. CD4+ memory T cells with high CD26 surface expression are enriched for Th1 markers and correlate with clinical severity of multiple sclerosis. *J Neuroimmunol.* 181:157–164.

Krammer PH. 2000. CD95's deadly mission in immune system. *Nature.* 407:789–795.

Kremenchutzky M, Rice GP, Baskerville J, Wingerchuk DM, Ebers GC. 2006. The natural history of multiple sclerosis: a geographically study 9: observations on the progressive phase of the disease. *Brain.* 129:584–594.

Kutzelnigg A, Lucchinetti CF, Stadelmann C et al. 2005. Cortical demyelination and diffuse white matter injury in multiple sclerosis. *Brain.* 128:2705–2712.

Lassmann H. 2004. Recent neuropathological findings in MS—implications for diagnosis and therapy. *J Neurol.* 251(Suppl 4):IV/2–IV/5.

Lassmann H. 2007. Multiple sclerosis: is there neurodegeneration independent from inflammation? *J Neurol Sci.* 259:3–6.

Lassmann H, Ransohoff RM. 2004. The CD4-Th1 model for multiple sclerosis: a critical re-appraisal. *Trends Immunol.* 25:132–137.

Lee MA, Smith S, Palace J et al. 1999. Spatial mapping of T_2 and gadolinium-enhancing T_1 lesion volumes in multiple sclerosis: evidence for distinct mechanisms of lesion genesis? *Brain.* 122:1261–1270.

LeMaoult J, Le Discorde M, Rouas-Freiss N et al. 2003. Biology and functions of human leukocyte antigen-G in health and sickness. *Tissue Antigens.* 62:273–284.

Lipton HL, Liang Z, Hertzler S, Son K-N. 2007. A specific viral cause of multiple sclerosis: one virus, one disease. *Ann Neurol.* 61:514–523.

Lucchinetti C, Brück W, Prisi J, Scheithauer B, Rodriguez M, Lassmann H. 2000. Heterogeneity of multiple sclerosis lesions: implications for pathogenesis of demyelination. *Ann Neurol.* 47:707–717.

Maggs FG, Palace J. 2004. The pathogenesis of multiple sclerosis: is it really a primary inflammatory process? *Mult Scler.* 10:326–329.

Marrie RA. 2004. Environmental risk factors in multiple sclerosis aetiology. *Lancet Neurol*. 3:709–718.

Mason DW, Charlton HM, Jones AJ, Lavy CB, Puklavec M, Simmonds SJ. 1986. The fate of allogeneic and xenogeneic neuronal tissue transplanted into the third ventricle of rodents. *Neuroscience*. 19:685–694.

Matyszak MK, Perry VH. 1996a. A comparison of leukocyte responses to heat-killed bacillus Calmette-Guérin in different CNS compartments. *Neuropathol Appl Neurobiol*. 22:44–53.

Matyszak MK, Perry VH. 1996b. The potential role of dendritic cells in immune-mediate inflammatory diseases in the central nervous system. *Neuroscience*. 74:599–608.

McDole J, Johnson AJ, Pirko I. 2006. The role of CD8$^+$ T cells in lesion formation and axonal dysfunction in multiple sclerosis. *Neurol Res*. 28:256–261.

McDonald WI, Compston A, Edan G et al. 2001. Recommended diagnostic criteria for multiple sclerosis: guidelines from the International Panel on the Diagnosis of Multiple Sclerosis. *Ann Neurol*. 50:121–127.

McKenzie BS, Kastelein RA, Cua DJ. 2006. Understanding the IL-23-IL-17 immune pathway. *Trends Immunol*. 27:17–23.

McMenamin PG. 1999. Distribution and phenotype of dendritic cells and resident tissue macrophages in the dura mater, leptomeninges, and choroid plexus of the rat brain as demonstrated in the wholemount preparation. *J Comp Neurol*. 405:553–562.

Medawar PB. 1948. Immunity to homologous grafted skin. III. The fate of skin homografts transplanted to the brain, to subcutaneous tissue, and to anterior chamber of the eye. *Br J Exp Pathol*. 29:58–69.

Medzhitov R, Janeway CAJ. 1997. Innate immunity: impact on the adaptive immune response. *Curr Opin Immunol*. 9:4–9.

Meinl E, Krumbholz M, Hohlfeld R. 2006. B lineage cells in the inflammatory central nervous system environment: migration, maintenance, local antibody production, and therapeutic modulation. *Ann Neurol*. 59:880–892.

Moser B, Eberl M. 2007. γδ T cells: a novel initiators of adaptive immunity. *Immunol Rev*. 215:89–102.

Mosmann TR, Sad S. 1996. The expanding universe of T-cell subsets: Th1, Th2 and more. *Immunol Today*. 17:138–146.

Neumann H, Medana IM, Bauer J, Lassmann H. 2002. Cytotoxic T lymphocytes in autoimmune and degenerative CNS diseases. *Trends Neurosci*. 25:313–319.

Noseworthy JH, Lucchinetti C, Rodriguez M, Weinshenker BG. 2000. Multiple sclerosis. *N Engl J Med*. 43:938–952.

Okuda Y, Okuda M, Apatoff BR, Posnett DN. 2005. The activation of memory CD4$^+$ T cells and CD8$^+$ T cells in patients with multiple sclerosis. *J Neurol Sci*. 235:11–17.

Opdenakker G, Nelissen I, Van Damme J. 2003. Functional roles and therapeutic targeting of gelatinase B and chemokines in multiple sclerosis. *Lancet Neurol*. 2:747–756.

Özenci V, Kouwenhoven M, Link H. 2002. Cytokines in multiple sclerosis: methodological aspects and pathogenetic implications. *Mult Scler*. 8:396–404.

Pender M, Rist MJ. 2001. Apoptosis of inflammatory cells in immune control of nervous system: role of glia. *Glia*. 36:137–144.

Polman CH, Reingold SC, Edan G et al. 2005. Diagnostic criteria for multiple sclerosis: 2005 revisions to the "McDonald criteria." *Ann Neurol*. 58:840–846.

Prat A, Antel J. 2005. Pathogenesis of multiple sclerosis. *Curr Opin Neurol*. 18:225–230.

Provencio JJ, Kivisäkk P, Tucky BH, Luciano MG, Ransohoff RM. 2005. Comparison of ventricular and lumbar cerebrospinal fluid T cells in non-inflammatory neurological disorder (NIND) patients. *J Neuroimmunol*. 163:179–184.

Ransohoff RM, Kivisäkk P, Kidd G. 2003. Three or more routes for leukocyte migration into the central nervous system. *Nat Rev Immunol*. 3:569–581.

Rebenko-Moll NM, Liu L, Cardona A, Ransohoff RM. 2006. Chemokines, mononuclear cells and the nervous system: heaven (or hell) is in the details. *Curr Opin Immunol*. 18:683–689.

Rosenberg GA. 2002. Matrix metalloproteinases in neuroinflammation. *Glia*. 39:279–291.

Sabelko-Downes KA, Russell JH, Cross AH. 1999. Role of Fas-FasL interactions in the pathogenesis and regulation of autoimmune demyelinating disease. *J Neuroimmunol*. 100:42–52.

Scarisbrick IA, Rodriguez M. 2003. Hit-hit and hit-run: viruses in the playing field of multiple sclerosis. *Curr Neurol Neurosci Rep*. 3:265–271.

Schwartz M, Butovsky O, Brück W, Hanisch UK. 2006. Microglial phenotype: is the commitment reversible? *Trends Neurosci*. 29:68–74.

Sellebjerg F, Sørensen TL. 2003. Chemokines and matrix metalloproteinase-9 in leukocyte recruitment to the central nervous system. *Brain Res Bull*. 61:347–355.

Shi F-D, Van Kaer L. 2006. Reciprocal regulation between natural killer cells and autoreactive T cells. *Nat Rev Immunol*. 6:751–760.

Skulina C, Schmidt S, Dornmair K et al. 2004. Multiple sclerosis: brain-infiltrating CD8$^+$ T cells persist as clonal expansion in the cerebrospinal fluid and blood. *Proc Natl Acad Sci U S A*. 101:2428–2243.

Smith KJ, Lassmann H. 2002. The role of nitric oxide in multiple sclerosis. *Lancet Neurol*. 1:232–241.

Sospedra M, Martin R. 2005. Immunology of multiple sclerosis. *Annu Rev Immunol*. 23:683–747.

Steinman L. 2001. Multiple sclerosis: a two-stage disease. *Nat Immunol*. 2:762–764.

Stratton CW, Sriram S. 2003. Association of Chlamydia pneumoniae with central nervous system disease. *Microbes Infect*. 5:1249–1253.

Stratton CW, Wheldon DB. 2006. Multiple sclerosis: an infectious syndrome involving Chlamydophila pneumoniae. *Trends Microbiol*. 14:474–479.

Stüve O, Rache M, Hemmer B. 2004. Viral pathogens in multiple sclerosis. An intriguing (hi)story. *Arch Neurol*. 61:1500–1502.

Suidan GL, Pirko I, Johnson AJ. 2006. A potential role for CD8$^+$ T-cells as regulators of CNS vascular permeability. *Neurol Res*. 28:250–255.

Swanborg RH, Whittum-Hudson JA, Hudson AP. 2003. Infectious agent and multiple sclerosis-are Chlamydia pneumoniae and human herpes virus 6 involved? *J Neuroimmunol.* 136:1–8.

Swanton JK, Rovira A, Tintore M et al. 2007. MRI criteria for multiple sclerosis in patients presenting with clinically isolated syndromes: a multicentre retrospective study. *Lancet Neurol.* 6:677–686.

Takahashi K, Aranami T, Endoh M, Miyake S, Yamamura T. 2004. The regulatory role of natural killer cells in multiple sclerosis. *Brain.* 127:1917–1927.

Trinchieri G. 2003. Interleukin-12 and the regulation of innate resistance and adaptive immunity. *Nat Rev Immunol.* 3:133–146.

Uccelli A, Aloisi F, Pistoia V. 2005. Unveiling the enigma of the CNS as a B-cell fostering environment. *Trends Immunol.* 26:254–259.

Vanderlugt CL, Miller SD. 2002. Epitope spreading in immune-mediated diseases: implications for immunotherapy. *Nat Rev Immunol.* 2:85–95.

Viglietta V, Baecher-Allan C, Weiner HI, Hafler DA. 2004. Loss of functional suppression by CD4$^+$CD25$^+$ regulatory T cells in patients with multiple sclerosis. *J Exp Med.* 199:971–979.

Vollmer TL, Liu R, Price M, Rhodes S, La Cava A, Shi F-D. 2005. Differential effects of IL-21 during initiation and progression of autoimmunity against neuroantigen. *J Immunol.* 174:2696–2701.

Wiendl H. 2007. HLA-G in the nervous system. *Hum Immunol.* 68:286–293.

Wiendl H, Feger U, Mittelbronn M et al. 2005. Expression of the immune-tolerogenic major histocompatibility molecule HLA-G in multiple sclerosis: implications for CNS immunity. *Brain.* 128:2689–2704.

Xiao B-G, Link H. 1999. Is there a balance between microglia and astrocytes in regulating Th1/Th2-cell responses and neuropathologies? *Immunol Today.* 20:477–479.

Xu W, Fazekas G, Hara H, Tabira T. 2005. Mechanism of natural killer (NK) cells regulatory role in experimental autoimmune encephalomylitis. *J Neuroimmunol.* 163:24–30.

Yong VW, Power C, Forsyth P, Edwards DR. 2001. Metalloproteinases in biology and pathogenesis of the nervous system. *Nat Rev Neurosci.* 2:502–511.

Yong VW, Zabad RK, Arawal S, Goncalves DaSilva A, Metz LM. 2007. Elevation of matrix metalloproteinases (MMPs) in multiple sclerosis and impact of immunomodulators. *J Neurol Sci.* 259:79–84.

Zipp F, Aktas O. 2006. The brain as a target of inflammation: common pathways link inflammatory and neurodegenerative diseases. *Trends Neurosci.* 29:518–527.

Chapter *13*

BRAIN INFLAMMATION AND THE NEURONAL FATE: FROM NEUROGENESIS TO NEURODEGENERATION

Maria Antonietta Ajmone-Cat, Emanuele Cacci, and Luisa Minghetti

ABSTRACT

Inflammation is a self-defensive reaction that may, under specific circumstances, develop into a chronic state and become a causative factor in the pathogenesis of a broad range of disabling diseases. For many of these pathologies, regardless of the nature of the primary pathogenic event, inflammation remains the best therapeutic target, and the development of novel strategies to treat inflammation is one of the major task of medical research and the pharmaceutical industry. Similar to peripheral inflammation, brain inflammation is increasingly being viewed as a target for treating neurological diseases, not only infectious and immune-mediated disorders such as meningitis or multiple sclerosis but also stroke, trauma and neurodegenerative diseases that were originally not considered to be inflammatory. Microglial cells, the resident macrophages of brain parenchyma, are generally viewed as major sources of proinflammatory and potentially neurotoxic molecules in the damaged brain. However, a direct link between activated microglia and tissue damage has not been univocally demonstrated in vivo, and recent studies have rather documented exacerbation of injury following selective microglial ablation or anti-inflammatory treatments. Intense research over the last two decades has shown that inflammation may in many ways affect neuronal activity and survival. Recent evidence indicates that inflammation is also implicated in controlling adult neurogenesis, thus broadening the therapeutic potential of strategies aimed at controlling neuroinflammation. In this chapter, an overview of the main evidence supporting both detrimental and protective roles of inflammation in acute and chronic brain diseases is presented, highlighting the need for innovative approaches to overcome the experimental constraints that still limit our knowledge of the molecular mechanisms underlying microglial activation and brain inflammation. Further understanding of brain inflammation will be instrumental for the development of effective treatments for highly disabling neurological disorders.

Keywords: brain macrophages, inflammation, microglia, neurogenesis, neurodegeneration, neuroprotection.

Inflammation is a self-defensive reaction that can arise in any tissue in response to traumatic, infectious, or toxic injury. This natural, although painful, process normally leads to healing and restored tissue integrity. In some instances, however, it might develop into a chronic state and cause more damage than the primary injurious event per se (Fig. 13.1). Chronic inflammation is associated with tissue damage in disabling conditions such as arthritis, multiple sclerosis, or cancer. Uncontrolled inflammation may ultimately lead to major organ failure and death. On the other hand, a deficient inflammatory response is equally undesirable as it increases the susceptibility to infections, exposing the organism to life-threatening conditions. The double-faceted nature of inflammation—beneficial and detrimental—explains the paramount effort of biomedical research in developing therapeutic strategies aimed at both preventing and inducing inflammation. In several and diverse disabling diseases, inflammation is one of the main therapeutic targets regardless of the nature of the primary pathogenic event. The development of novel strategies to treat inflammation is still the primary task for medical research and the pharmaceutical industry, for which anti-inflammatory drugs represent a multibillion dollar market (Rainsford 2007). Besides inhibition, generation of a robust inflammatory response has great therapeutic potential, for example, for efficacious prophylactic immunization against infectious diseases or for immune therapy for tumors (Nathan 2002).

Inflammation is being increasingly viewed as a target for treating neurological diseases, not only in classical infectious and immune-mediated disorders such as meningitis or multiple sclerosis but also in stroke, trauma, and neurodegenerative diseases that were not originally considered to be inflammatory (Minghetti, Ajmone-Cat, De Berardinis et al. 2005; Esiri 2007). The intense research over the last two decades has shown that inflammation may in many ways affect neuronal activity and survival. More recently, inflammation has been suggested to have a role in controlling neurogenesis in the adult brain. Further understanding of how to control brain inflammation will be instrumental for preventing and limiting neurodegeneration, as well as for promoting regeneration and functional recovery in highly disabling, and still untreatable, neurological diseases.

BRAIN INFLAMMATION

The central nervous system (CNS) is an enormously complex organ system, particularly sensitive to inflammatory and oxidant injury and having poor regenerative capacity. In comparison with other organ systems of the body, the CNS is endowed with unique anatomical and physiological features including the bony enclosure of the skull and spinal column, which not only contains and protects it but also limits the space for brain parenchymal expansion; a specialized system of autoregulation of the cerebral blood flow; the absence of a conventional lymphatic system; a special cerebrospinal fluid circulation; and a limited immunological surveillance. As a result of these peculiarities, the brain is vulnerable to unique pathological processes, and reactions to injury and healing in this organ differ considerably from elsewhere in the body. The uniqueness of brain reactions, which is indispensable for limiting damage during inflammation, is generally referred as to the *immune privilege* of the CNS.

The concept of the immune privilege of the CNS dates back to the beginning of 20th century, when,

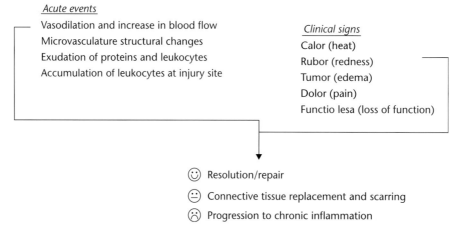

Figure 13.1 Major events and clinical signs of inflammation in vascularized tissues of peripheral organs. As indicated in the lower part of the figure, the outcome of these events could be the complete resolution of the inflammatory process and the regain of function; the replacement of the damaged tissue with connective tissue, scar formation, and partial functional recovery; or, in the worst case, progression to chronic inflammation.

on the basis of the observation that tumor cells survived well when transplanted into the mouse brain parenchyma but not when implanted in peripheral tissues, it was suggested that foreign antigens could evade the immune surveillance when present within the brain parenchyma (Shirai 1921). As reviewed by Galea et al. (2007), we now know that the brain's immune privilege is not an absolute or an immutable state. Rather, it is confined to the brain parenchyma proper (meninges, choroid plexus, circumventricular organs, and ventricles show an immune reactivity similar to that in the periphery). It is the result of the active interplay among specialized cellular elements and specific microenvironment characteristics, and it can be overcome in several instances.

One of the major factors contributing to the brain's immune privilege is the blood–brain barrier (BBB), a functional barrier between the brain parenchyma and the vascular system that regulates the movement of fluid, molecules, and cells in and out of the brain (Bechmann, Galea, Perry 2007). The functional unit of the BBB relies on three compartments: (1) the brain parenchyma or neuropil, which is delimited by glia limitans (consisting of astrocytic endfeet, few microglial endfeet, and a basement membrane); (2) the perivascular space (or Virchow-Robin space), containing fluid (from the lymphatic drainage of the neuropil) and cells (mainly macrophages, although many immune cells may invade the space under inflammatory conditions); and (3) the vessel walls, consisting of endothelial cells, smooth muscle cells, pericytes, and the outer basement membranes, facing the perivascular space. The presence of tight junctions in the endothelium of capillaries is crucial for the functional properties of the BBB, but specialized membrane channels and transport systems also contribute to the active control of exchanges between blood and brain. Solute diffusion is regulated at capillary levels, where the vessel walls and basement membranes of the glia limitans are in intimate contact, whereas immune cell infiltration occurs mainly at postcapillary venules, where the perivascular space separates the vessel wall and the glial limitans. The integrity of the BBB strongly impacts the immune-privilege status of the brain, but other elements play important roles in restraining the infiltration of immune cells and in the development of unrestricted inflammatory reactions.

Several features of brain parenchyma render it a hostile and repressive environment for the cells of innate and adaptive immune responses. All cells in the CNS express the death-inducing ligand (CD95L or fasL), which enables them to induce apoptosis of T cells expressing the cognate death receptor CD95. The constitutive expression of CD95L on the astrocytic endfeet may also limit the crossing of the glia limitans (Bechmann, Mor, Nilsen et al. 1999), contributing to the apoptosis of immune cells in the perivascular

space during inflammatory states of the brain when the recruitment of immune cells to this compartment is facilitated. Then, once T cells infiltrate the parenchyma, their activation requires the interaction of the cognate antigens in the context of the major histocompatibility complex (MHC) molecules, but the expression of MHC molecules is very low or absent in the healthy brain parenchyma. Activation of T cells can be further restrained by the regulatory activities of astrocytes, the most abundant glial cell population, and microglia, the resident macrophages of brain parenchyma, through the release of soluble factors that inhibit T-cell proliferation and cytokine production (Meinl, Aloisi, Ertl et al. 1994; Aloisi, Ria, Adorini 2000). In addition, microglial cells can control T cells through the expression of a homolog of the costimulatory molecule B7 (B7 homolog 1), which induces T-cell apoptosis (Magnus, Schreiner, Korn et al. 2005).

A further important aspect contributing to the peculiarity of brain inflammation is the effector cells of the innate system in this organ, namely the microglial cells. These cells belong to the myeloid lineage and their myeloid progenitors enter the nervous system primarily during embryonic and fetal periods of development. Recent evidence suggests that microglial progenitors may derive from a lineage of myeloid cells that is independent of the monocyte lineage and that is endowed with the unique property to home to the nervous system (Chan, Kohsaka, Rezaie 2007). Microglia comprise approximately 10% of cells in the human and rodent brain and their density varies by brain region, with the highest concentrations in the hippocampus, olfactory telencephalon, basal ganglia, and substantia nigra (Lawson, Perry, Dri et al. 1990). In the normal adult brain, microglia are characterized by a slow turnover and a downregulated phenotype when compared to other macrophage populations of peripheral tissues (Lawson, Perry, Gordon 1992; Kreutzberg 1996). Interaction with neurons and astrocytes, as well as BBB-dependent exclusion of activating molecules from the brain parenchyma, is the main factor contributing to the downregulated immunophenotype of microglia. Neuronal electric activity and neurotransmitters, such as noradrenaline and acetylcholine, have been shown to suppress MHC expression and prevent the release of proinflammatory products in microglia (Neumann, Misgeld, Matsumuro et al. 1998; De Simone, Ajmone-Cat, Carnevale et al. 2005; Carnevale, De Simone, Minghetti 2007). Several "ligand–receptor" type interactions between neurons and microglia, important for maintaining microglia in a nonactivated state, have been identified so far. Among these are the glycoprotein CD200 expressed on neurons and the cognate ligand CD200L expressed on microglia (Wright, Puklavec, Willis et al. 2000), and the neuronal chemokine fractalkine and its microglial receptor CXCR1 (Hughes, Botham, Frentzel et al.

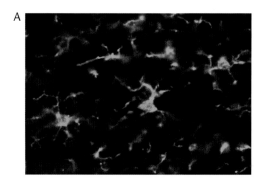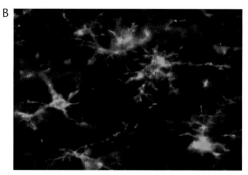

Figure 13.2 Typical morphology of resting (A) or activated (B) microglia in mouse hippocampus. Coronal sections were immunolabeled for the specific microglia/macrophage marker ionized calcium-binding adaptor molecule-1 (Iba-1).

2002; Cardona, Pioro, Sasse et al. 2006). The down-regulated (resting) phenotype that microglia acquire under physiological conditions should not be taken as a state of quiescence and inactivity. Using transgenic mice showing specific expression of enhanced green fluorescent protein in microglia and in vivo two-photon microscopy, it has been demonstrated that resting microglia constantly survey the surrounding microenvironment with extremely motile processes and protrusions, contacting other cellular elements and sensing alterations in the nearby parenchyma (Nimmerjahn, Kirchhoff, Helmchen 2005). In response to an injury or disease, microglia rapidly react by changing their morphology (Fig. 13.2), upregulating most of the molecular markers typical of macrophages, and acquiring the functions necessary to sustain the development of local innate immune responses.

In addition to microglia, astrocytes also play an important role in the innate immunity of the brain, as they express several, although fewer than microglial cells, pattern-recognition receptors (PRRs), such as Toll-like receptors, that recognize not only invading pathogens but also endogenous "danger signals" and release cytokines and chemokines, which can trigger or amplify the local inflammatory response (Farina, Aloisi, Meinl 2007).

From this brief overview, it is clear that inflammation in the brain follows distinctive rules, particularly in those diseases in which, in the absence of significant blood-borne cell infiltration, the resident cells are major players such as in chronic neurodegenerative diseases (Perry, Cunningham, Boche 2002). At molecular levels, however, most of the mediators and the signaling pathways are the same as those encountered in inflammatory processes of peripheral organs. The levels of most of the proinflammatory molecules such as cytokines, chemokines, and PGs found during inflammation in peripheral organs are increased in the inflamed brain, although there are important differences in their patterns of expression, cell sources, and targets.

INFLAMMATION AND NEURODEGENERATION

Microglial Activation and Inflammation

It is commonly accepted that activated microglia play a key pathogenic role in the tissue damage consequent to stroke or brain trauma, as well as in chronic neurodegenerative disorders. When activated, microglia may become a prominent source of oxidants, free radicals, inflammatory cytokines, chemokines, and lipid mediators, which in turn can promote neuronal dysfunction and tissue damage, and further activate microglia. This could result in a vicious cycle driving chronic inflammation and neurodegeneration. This view of activated microglia and inflammation as causative factors of neurodegeneration is however challenged by recent observations.

Morphologically activated microglia, characterized by cell body enlargement, loss of ramified processes, and upregulation of cell surface and/or cytoplasmic antigens, can be found in virtually all brain pathological states. However, the functional roles of these cells, fulfilling the morphological criteria of activation, may be diverse depending on the precise nature of the injurious stimulus, its intensity, the time for which it is present, and many other factors.

The functional properties of activated microglia have been extensively studied in in vitro models, which albeit very useful, present some intrinsic drawbacks that have to be taken into account when extending the in vitro observations to human pathologies. Among these is the partial activation of microglial cultures even in the absence of any additional stimulation, which can be most likely ascribed to the loss of cell-to-cell interactions and may account for higher reactivity of cultured microglia when compared to the in vivo counterpart. Other experimental constraints include the relatively short time of stimulation and the abrupt addition of activators (bacterial endotoxin, viral proteins, fibrillogenic peptides, or others) that only partially model the conditions of microglial activation occurring in vivo, particularly in chronic diseases such as neurodegenerative diseases.

In the recent years, thanks to the development of in vitro, ex vivo, and in vivo models more closely mimicking specific aspects of neurodegenerative diseases, the complexity of microglial activation has begun to unravel. As opposed to a linear model of activation, proceeding through a graded transformation of resting microglia into potentially cytotoxic cells, a plasticity model proposes that in different forms of injury or disease, activated microglia might synthesize a range of different molecules, including neurotrophic factors, whose typical profile will determine the outcome of microglial activation in terms of repair or injury. Importantly, the different states of activation can be switched between one state and another during the course of disease in the presence of a further stimulus or in response to signals from the periphery (Perry, Cunningham, Holmes 2007). According to this recent view, activated microglia are likely to play a complex and multifaceted role, which needs to be defined within each disease or each disease state. A deeper knowledge of microglial biology and the development of experimental models that replicate the relevant features of chronic degenerative diseases is crucial for finding new molecular targets and developing the long-awaited disease-modifying drugs necessary for effective treatment of these neurological disorders.

Besides adult neurological diseases, brain inflammation during gestation and the perinatal period is ever more recognized as the risk factor for developmental brain disorders, which involve damage or abnormalities of either the developing grey matter, as in epilepsy and autism, or white matter, as for example in cerebral palsy and periventricular leukomalacia (Chew, Takanohashi, Bell 2006; Leviton, Gressens 2007). Increased number of activated microglia have been found in children with autism, in the periventricular lesions of children with early signs of periventricular leukomalacia, and in several animal models of neonatal brain hypoxia-ischemia. Although the causal link between inflammation and brain damage is still missing, strong evidence suggests that activated microglia are profoundly involved in these processes and deciphering their roles in developmental brain injuries is presently considered essential for formulating therapeutic strategies for these diseases.

The increasing interest for the pathogenic role of inflammation/microglial activation in neurodegeneration is exemplified by the growing number of studies on this topic over the last few years (Klegeris, McGeer, McGeer 2007). Because of the impossibility to cover such a vast literature, we focus here on the role of inflammation in Alzheimer's disease (AD) and brain ischemia as representative examples of chronic and acute neurodegenerative diseases, respectively.

Alzheimer's Disease

Chronic degenerative diseases consist of high social impact disorders, including AD, Parkinson's Disease (PD), Huntington's disease, Creutzfeldt–Jakob disease, and amyotrophic lateral sclerosis, and are characterized by having diverse etiologies, clinical signs, and incidences but sharing some common features. The most striking feature is the aggregation of misfolded proteins, which regardless of the primary cause of misfolding, accumulate in the CNS in disease-specific and protein-specific ways, leading to progressive amyloidosis. The second common feature of neurodegenerative diseases is neuroinflammation, defined as the presence of activated microglia, reactive astrocytes, and inflammatory mediators in the absence of obvious blood-borne cell infiltration.

AD is one of the most studied neurodegenerative disorders, characterized by progressive loss of neurons of the basal forebrain cholinergic system, memory and cognitive performance decline, and ultimately, dementia. The two major hallmarks of disease, which mainly affects the hippocampus, the amygdala, and several cortical areas, are the extracellular deposits of β-amyloid (Aβ) in the brain parenchyma (senile plaques) and the neurofibrillary tangles consisting of intracellular aggregates of aberrantly phosphorylated tau protein. Deposits of Aβ are often also found around blood vessels. The presence of activated microglia surrounding the senile plaques and the increased levels of elements of the complement system—cytokines, chemokines, and free radicals (see Table 13.1)—in the affected areas (McGeer, McGeer 2001; Eikelenboom, Veerhuis, Scheper et al. 2006) led to the postulation of the neuroinflammatory hypothesis of AD, according to which neuronal injury and Aβ deposition are the primary events responsible for microglial activation and secretion of harmful substances that may drive a self-propagating toxic cycle, exacerbating neurodegeneration and Aβ deposition (Mrak, Griffin 2005). This "autotoxic" hypothesis (Fig. 13.3A) is supported by a large body of in vitro evidence showing that Aβ peptides are proinflammatory and that they activate microglia to release potentially neurotoxic factors, such as cytokines (interleukin 1β [IL-1β] and tumor necrosis factor α [TNF-α]), and free radicals, such as nitric oxide (NO) and superoxide (Akiyama, Barger, Barnum et al. 2000; Eikelenboom, Veerhuis, Scheper et al. 2006). Nonetheless, there is evidence that microglia persistently exposed to inflammatory agents such as bacterial endotoxin (lipopolysaccharide [LPS]) or cytokines undergo a process of adaptation

Table 13.1 Inflammatory Cells and Soluble Mediators Reported to Be Associated with Alzheimer's Disease or Experimental Models of the Disease

	Effects	*References*
Cell types		
Inflammatory cells		
Microglia	Detrimental (source of cytotoxic and/or inflammatory mediators)	Akiyama et al. 2000; Mrak, Griffin 2005
	Beneficial (amyloid clearance)	
Astrocytes	Glial scarring, source of inflammatory mediators	
Monocytes/macrophages	Beneficial (amyloid clearance)	Simard et al. 2006
Mediators		
Elements of complement system		
C1-C9	Proinflammatory Favoring amyloid clearance	Reviewed in Akiyama et al. 2000; McGeer, McGeer 2001; Eikelenboom et al. 2006; Wyss-Coray et al. 2002
Free radicals		
ROS, NO	Cytotoxic	Reviewed in Akiyama et al. 2000; McGeer, McGeer 2001; Eikelenboom et al. 2006
Cytokines and chemokines		
IL-1, TNF-α, IL-6 TGF-β	Proinflammatory, cytotoxic pleiotropic effects (anti-inflammatory, inducer of amyloid deposition)	
MCP-1, MIP-1α, MIP-1β	Recruiting inflammatory cells	
Adhesion molecules		
ICAM-1, ICAM-2, NCAM	Proinflammatory	
Growth factors		
NGF, FGF, BDNF, PDGF	Anti-inflammatory, neuroprotective	
Receptors and cognate ligands		
CD40/CD40L	Impeding amyloid clearance	Togo et al. 2000; Calingasan et al. 2002; Townsend et al. 2005
Acute phase proteins		
Serum amyloid P α_1-Antichymotrypsin	Promoting amyloid load	Nilsson et al. 2001; Veerhuis et al. 2003
Inducible enzymes		
COX-2	Controversial findings	Reviewed in Minghetti 2007

ROS, reactive oxygen species; NO, nitric oxide; IL, interleukin; TNF, tumor necrosis factor; TGF, transforming growth factor; MCP, monocyte chemotactic protein; MIP, macrophage inflammatory protein; ICAM, intracellular adhesion molecule; NCAM, neural cell adhesion molecule; NGF, neural growth factor; FGF, fibroblast growth factor; BDNF, brain-derived neurotrophic factor; PDGF, platelet-derived growth factor; COX, cyclooxygenase.

by which some functions are gained and other are lost (Fig. 13.3B), as previously demonstrated for peripheral macrophages (West, Heagy 2002). Persistent activation of cultured rat microglia with LPS induces significant alterations in the signaling network downstream from the LPS receptor, with the progressive downregulation of the release of potentially cytotoxic products, such as TNF-α and NO, but not of an immunoregulatory molecule such as prostaglandin (PG) E$_2$ (Ajmone-Cat, Nicolini, Minghetti et al. 2003). A similar anti-inflammatory phenotype has been described for microglia phagocytosing apoptotic but not necrotic neurons (De Simone, Ajmone-Cat, Minghetti et al. 2004; Minghetti, Ajmone-Cat, De Berardinis et al. 2005) and in few animal models of chronic neurodegenerative diseases including prion disease and PD (Perry, Cunningham, Boche et al. 2002; Depino, Earl, Kaczmarczyk et al. 2003). In addition, in vivo chronic expression of IL-1 in rat striatum has been reported to induce transient neutrophil infiltration, activation of astrocytes and microglia, BBB disruption, and demyelination. These effects were indeed largely resolved

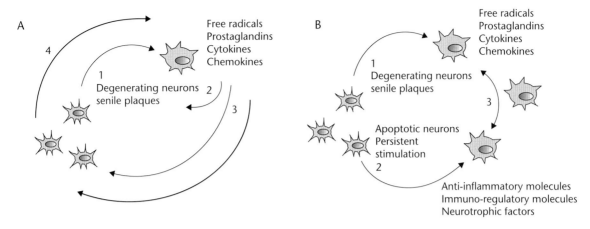

Figure 13.3 (A) Schematic representation of the "autotoxic hypothesis" of AD. Degenerating neurons and/or accumulation of Aβ and amyloid-associated proteins into senile plaques (1) will trigger microglial activation and the release of proinflammatory and potentially neurotoxic molecules, which will further induce neurodegeneration and plaque formation (2) as well as directly sustain microglial recruitment and activation (3), giving rise to a vicious autotoxic loop (4). (B) Alternative model of microglial activation in chronic neurodegenerative diseases. In addition to the proinflammatory activation of microglia by degenerating neurons and senile plaques (1), the presence of apoptotic neurons and the persistent stimulation of microglia in the vicinity of the plaque (2) will induce an alternative phenotype in microglial cells, characterized by the expression of anti-inflammatory and immunomodulatory molecules (IL-10, TGF-β, PGE$_2$) and neurotrophic factors (nerve growth factor). The different states of activation (pro- or anti-inflammatory) can be switched between one state and another during the course of disease, or in the presence of further stimuli or local factors, through multiple intermediate states of activation (3).

after a few weeks in spite of the still significantly elevated IL-1 levels, suggesting that, in vivo, astrocytes and microglia can become refractory to chronic exposure to IL-1 and adopt a nontoxic phenotype (Ferrari, Depino, Prada et al. 2004). On the other hand, the anti-inflammatory phenotype can be rapidly turned into aggressive proinflammatory phenotype by additional stimuli, as demonstrated in mice with prion disease that are challenged with an intraperitoneal dose of LPS to mimic a systemic infection (Combrinck, Perry, Cunningham et al. 2002). This suggests that systemic inflammation may trigger proinflammatory functions in atypical activated microglia that have been "primed" by the degenerative process. Such a phenomenon could be highly relevant in elderly people affected by AD, since the recurrent systemic infections in these patients could exacerbate the neurodegenerative processes (Perry 2004).

According to the dynamic model of microglial activation it can be predicted that in AD, as well as in other neurodegenerative disorders, activated microglia are present in distinct functional phenotypes, differently contributing to neuroprotection or neurodegeneration. In the brain in case of AD, microglia, displaying the typical morphology associated with activation, are often located between the core of the senile plaque and the corona of neuritic processes. Such a location and the ultrastructural appearances suggest their involvement in phagocytosis and in the removal of amyloid fibrils. Cultured microglia effectively phagocyte Aβ fibrils (Giulian, Haverkamp, Li et al. 1995), but the persistence of amyloid plaques in AD brain suggests that microglial phagocytic activity may be impaired in vivo (Rogers, Strohmeyer, Kovelowski et al. 2002). Using transgenic mouse models of AD, Simard et al. have demonstrated that many of the microglia within the core of amyloid plaques originate from the bone marrow and that these newly recruited cells, rather than the resident counterpart, effectively restrict the formation of amyloid deposits (Simard, Soulet, Gowing et al. 2006). The reasons for the reduced phagocytic activity of microglia in AD have not yet been clearly understood. The microglia could be overwhelmed by the increasing amount of amyloid or they could be in a state of activation characterized by a low phagocytic capacity, possibly related to local factors specifically associated with the plaque microenvironment. In line with this hypothesis, it has been suggested that the involvement of the microglial CD40 receptor, expressed together with its cognate ligand (CD40L) around the senile plaques (Togo, Akiyama, Kondo et al. 2000; Calingasan, Erdely, Altar 2002), is one of the mechanisms that render these cells ineffective for Aβ removal, shifting their state of activation toward antigen presentation and release of proinflammatory Th1-type cytokines, which further impede the phagocytosis of Aβ peptides (Townsend, Town, Mori et al. 2005). Alternatively, or additionally, the low efficiency in removing the amyloid deposits could be a characteristic of microglia of the aged brain, as suggested by the presence of abnormal or "dystrophic" microglial cells in healthy aged people and in AD patients (Streit 2004).

The reduced phagocytic activity and clearance capacity of microglia in several models of AD open the possibility that treatments that could stimulate or restore microglial phagocytic activity might be beneficial (Gelinas, DaSilva, Fenili et al. 2004; Sadowski, Wisniewski 2004; Town, Nikolic, Tan 2005). Both active vaccination and passive immunization in transgenic mouse models have been shown to result in reduction of Aβ deposits, and microglial activation appeared instrumental in enhancing Aβ clearance (Schenk, Barbour, Dunn et al. 1999; Wilcock, Munireddy, Rosenthal et al. 2004). Complement factors seem to play an active role in Aβ clearance. Double transgenic mice overexpressing the human amyloid precursor protein (hAPP) and the soluble complement inhibitor, Crry, show a two- to three-fold increase in Aβ burden and augmented inflammation (Wyss-Coray, Yan, Lin et al. 2002). On the contrary, acute-phase proteins, which are found in virtually all senile plaques in addition to Aβ, are crucial factors in amyloid plaque formation. Serum amyloid P component and complement factor C1q enhance fibril formation of Aβ peptides (Veerhuis, Van Breemen, Hoozemans et al. 2003), and overexpression of hAPP and $α_1$-antichymotrypsin, whose serum levels are associated with cognitive decline in older persons (Dik, Jonker, Hack et al. 2005), causes increased amyloid load and plaque density compared to mice carrying hAPP alone (Nilsson, Bales, DiCarlo et al. 2001). Interestingly, the tetracycline derivative minocycline, which has been shown to be neuroprotective in various neurodegenerative settings, attenuated the release of TNF-α by human microglia upon exposure to a mixture of Aβ, serum amyloid P component, and complement factor C1q without affecting Aβ fibril phagocytosis (Familian, Eikelenboom, Veerhuis 2007).

Further evidence fueling the neuroinflammatory hypothesis of AD comes from genetic and epidemiological studies. Genetic analyses have shown that specific polymorphisms of cytokines, including IL-1β and TNF-α, influence the risk of late-onset AD (Licastro, Veglia, Chiappelli et al. 2004; Lio, Annoni, Licastro et al. 2006), although conflicting results have been reported (Rainero, Bo, Ferrero et al. 2004; Ravaglia, Paola, Maioli et al. 2006). Retrospective epidemiological studies have shown an association between long-term nonsteroidal anti-inflammatory drug (NSAID) use and reduced risk of AD, although not every investigation has proved the same protective effect (Aisen 2002). The presumed mechanism of protection by NSAIDs is the inhibition of cyclooxygenase (COX), the limiting enzyme in PG synthesis. These lipid mediators are considered as being among the most potent proinflammatory substances, being involved in all the major events of inflammation. Nonetheless, PGs should be more correctly considered as immune modulators, since they affect important functions of virtually all the cells involved in innate and adaptive immunity and their activities are also crucial for the resolution of inflammation (Harris, Padilla, Koumas et al. 2002). In particular, the protective effect of NSAIDs has been attributed to the inhibition of the inducible isoform of COX (COX-2), which in the normal brain is expressed by specific neuronal populations in the cortex and hippocampus. The overexpression of COX-2 under pathological conditions has been associated with the cascade of events leading to excitotoxicity. Several studies have analyzed COX-2 expression at mRNA and protein levels in animal models and postmortem AD, but the involvement of COX-2 in AD remains controversial (Minghetti 2007). In a recent longitudinal study, the levels of prostaglandin E_2 (PGE_2) in the cerebral spinal fluid (CSF) of AD patients were found to decline with increasing dementia severity (Combrinck, Williams, De Berardinis et al. 2006). Interestingly, patients with higher initial PGE_2 levels survived longer, even when cognitive score, sex, and age were taken into account. These observations weigh against the idea that PGE_2 and/or COX activity are neurotoxic in AD and suggest that CSF PGE_2 may reflect the survival of COX-positive neurons. Alternatively, PGE_2 levels could reflect early inflammatory processes that may impede the later progression of AD.

Recent clinical trials have failed to demonstrate a beneficial effect of the selective COX-2 inhibitor rofecoxib on AD progression (Aisen, Schafer, Grundman et al. 2003; Reines, Block, Morris et al. 2004), and a number of experimental studies indicate that NSAIDs could exert their effects on alternative targets. A subset of NSAIDs—including indomethacin, ibuprofen, flurbiprofen, and sulindac—affects Aβ metabolism and reduces amyloid deposition (Gasparini, Ongini, Wenk 2004) independently from COX inhibition. Some NSAIDs also display free radical scavenging activity or bind to the nuclear receptor peroxisome proliferator–activated receptor-γ, whose activation has been demonstrated to suppress inflammation in animal models of brain disorders (Heneka, Landreth, Hull 2007).

Beneficial effects of chronic NSAID use have been reported for other neurodegenerative diseases such as PD. The high degree of variability in the effectiveness of various NSAIDs in reducing neurodegeneration in cellular and animal models of PD argues against the hypothesis that the protective effects are based on the shared COX-inhibiting property, although COX-2–dependent formation of dopamine-quinone may represent a disease-specific mechanism of neurotoxicity (Asanuma, Miyazaki 2006; Esposito, Di Matteo, Benigno et al. 2007).

Acute Brain Ischemia

Ischemic stroke, which is typically provoked by the sudden occlusion of a major cerebral artery (focal cerebral ischemia), is the most frequent cause of persistent neurological disabilities in industrialized countries and the third leading cause of death after ischemic heart disease and cancer. In the acute phase, the severity and duration of reduction in blood flow through the cerebral tissue determine the extent of cell death and white matter damage, as well as the magnitude of associated inflammatory processes. A large body of evidence suggests that stroke-induced brain damage progresses during subacute stages for up to several days after the insult, causing clinical worsening or impaired recovery. Local brain inflammation is a pathologic hallmark of ischemic stroke lesions (Table 13.2), which correlates with the occurrence of delayed apoptotic cell death. The modality of cell death after ischemia, which is in the first few

days most necrotic in the core of the lesion and is later apoptotic mainly in the outer boundaries of the lesion (penumbra), confers ischemia-induced inflammation with distinctive features of inflammation associated with chronic neurodegenerative diseases. Resident brain cell populations, including microglia, astrocytes, endothelium, and even neurons, become rapidly activated after the ischemic event and acquire inflammatory functions, while peripheral leukocytes home to the lesion, recruited by secreted inflammatory mediators and adhesion molecules whose expression is upregulated on the walls of the blood vessels (Wang, Tang, Yenari 2007). Microglia are activated within minutes of ischemia onset, whereas blood-derived macrophages are recruited with a delay of at least 24 to 48 hours (Schroeter, Jander, Huitinga et al. 1997; Schilling, Besselmann, Leonhard et al. 2003; Tanaka, Komine-Kobayashi, Mochizuki et al. 2003). Expression of inflammatory mediators peaks with the extensive activation of microglia. Within few hours or

Table 13.2 Inflammatory Pathways in Ischemic Stroke

	Effects/Modification	*References*
Cell types		
Microglia	Detrimental (source of cytotoxic and/or inflammatory mediators)	Wood 1995; Zhang et al. 1997; Schroeter et al. 1997; Yrjaneheikki et al. 1998, 1999; Zhang et al. 2005; Wang et al. 2007
Astrocytes	Beneficial	Lalancette-Hebert et al. 2007
Endothelial cells	Source of cytotoxic and/or inflammatory mediators	Reviewed in Wang et al. 2007
Neurons	Detrimental	Barone et al. 1992; Hallenbeck 1996; Zheng, Yenari 2004
Peripheral leukocytes		
Neutrophils	Detrimental	Arumugam et al. 2005; Gee et al. 2007
T lymphocytes	Beneficial	Offner et al. 2006; Dirnagl et al. 2007
Monocytes/macrophages	Detrimental	Giulian et al. 1993; Saleh et al. 2004, 2007; Nighoghossian et al. 2007
Mediators		
Adhesion molecules Selectins, integrins	Up-regulated	All reviewed in Wang et al. 2007
Cytokines IL-1, TNF-α, IL-6, IL-10, TGF-β		
Chemokines IL-8, IP-10, MCP-1, MIP-1α		
Transcriptional regulators NF-κB, AP-1; MAPK		
Immediate early genes COX-2, iNOS		
Free radicals ROS, NO		
Matrix metalloproteinases MPP-9	Up-regulated	Zhao et al. 2007

IL, interleukin; TNF, tumor necrosis factor; TGF, transforming growth factor; IP, interferon-inducible protein; MCP, monocyte chemotactic protein; MIP, macrophage inflammatory protein; AP, activator protein; MAPK, mitogen-activated protein kinases; COX, cyclooxygenase; iNOS, inducible nitric oxide synthase; ROS, reactive oxygen species; NO, nitric oxide; MPP, metalloproteinases.

earlier, immediate early genes, transcription factors (e.g., NF-κB, activator protein 1 [AP-1] and mitogen-activated protein kinases [MAPK] are activated and upregulated locally in brain tissue, leading to the enhancement of proinflammatory gene expression, including cytokines (e.g., IL-1, TNF-α, and IL-6) and chemokines (e.g., IL-8, interferon-inducible protein [IP-10], and monocyte chemotactic protein [MCP-1]). This pattern of expression appears to be progressively substituted by a much less inflammatory profile, and it is tempting to speculate that the exposure of microglia to the delayed wave of apoptotic cell death in the penumbra might be a contributing factor for such a functional reorientation. In addition, factors such as matrix metalloproteinases (MMP), which are thought to contribute to BBB disruption, cell death, and tissue damage early after stroke, have been recently reported to mediate tissue repair and remodeling in later stages, likely participating in proteolytic processing of growth factors such as the vascular endothelial growth factor (VEGF) (Zhao, Tejima, Lo 2007) to their mature active forms, and promoting their release from matrix-bound compartments or cell surface. The duality of MMP's action once again outlines the dynamism and complexity of the inflammatory process. In the secondary damage following ischemia, microglial and infiltrating macrophages are traditionally viewed as major causes of neuron loss, through the relase of inflammatory products (Wood 1995). The administration of agents such as edaravone, a novel free radical scavenger, or the tetracycline minocycline restrained microglial activation and provided significant neuroprotection and reduced the infarct volume in ischemic rodents (Yrjanheikki, Keinanen, Pellikka et al. 1998; Yrjanheikki, Tikka, Keinanen et al. 1999; Zhang, Komine-Kobayashi, Tanaka et al. 2005). In several ischemia models, tissue injury was exacerbated in the presence of microglia/macrophages (Giulian, Corpuz, Chapman et al. 1993; Zhang, Chopp, Powers et al. 1997; Lehnardt, Massillon, Follett et al. 2003). The observation that depletion of peripheral macrophages by liposome-encapsulated clodronate (Schroeter, Jander, Huitinga et al. 1997) did not affected infarct size suggests that resident microglia rather than infiltrating macrophages play a pathogenic role. However, a direct link between microglial activation and tissue damage has not been demonstrated in vivo, not even in stroke, and a recent study rather documented exacerbation of injury following selective microglial ablation (Lalancette-Hebert, Gowing, Simard et al. 2007).

Besides the role of resident and peripheral macrophages in tissue responses to ischemic stroke, most attention has been reserved to the possible role of neutrophils, whose infiltration is observed within few hours of damage. In animal models of focal ischemia induced by permanent middle cerebral artery occlusion (MCAO), neutrophil accumulation is moderate and localized within and adjacent to blood vessels bordering the ischemic cortex, whereas it is massive and distributed over the entire lesion after transient MCAO followed by reperfusion (Barone, Schmidt, Hillegass et al. 1992). Reactive oxygen species (ROS) generated during reperfusion and/or by resident and infiltrated cells contribute to amplify damage and cell recruitment. Neutrophil-derived inflammatory mediators could lead to secondary injury of potentially salvageable tissue in the penumbra (Hallenbeck 1996). Several studies demonstrated ameliorated neurological outcome following neutrophil depletion or inhibition of adhesion molecules, which facilitate their recruitment, in experimental stroke (Zheng, Yenari 2004). However, therapeutic strategies aimed at inhibition of neutrophil chemotaxis failed to show benefit in clinical trials.

T lymphocytes also accumulate in the postischemic brain and might further harm the infarcted tissue directly, by secreting cytotoxic molecules or proinflammatory cytokines, or indirectly, through activation of other circulating blood cells and/or extravascular cells (Arumugam, Granger, Mattson 2005). In addition, BBB and tissue disruption after stroke would expose CNS-specific antigens to recognition by T cells, thereby generating the possibility of autoimmune responses (Gee, Kalil, Shea et al. 2007). In line with this hypothesis, circulating antibodies to brain antigens, such as neurofilaments, have been detected within 48 hours of and up to 6 months following human stroke (Bornstein, Aronovich, Korczyn et al. 2001). Whether these responses induce autoregulatory, anti-inflammatory, and potentially protective T cells (Schwartz, Kipnis 2005) or rather result in a further threat to CNS, is unclear. Interestingly, after an early activation phase of the peripheral immune system, stroke brings about a drastic state of immunosuppression. This well-documented phenomenon, characterized by the depletion of T-cell populations, the shift from T helper (Th)1 to Th2 cytokine production within few hours of stroke, and an increased presence of CD4+FoxP3+ regulatory T cells (Treg), could represent a CNS-protective response against "nonprotective" autoimmunity, although at the expense of increased risk of infections (Offne, Subramanian, Parker et al. 2006; Dirnagl, Klehmet, Braun et al. 2007). The Th2 shift may also counterbalance excessive activation of resident microglia, as these cells exposed to Th2 cytokines are induced to acquire an anti-inflammatory phenotype. As is discussed later in this chapter, there is some evidence that such an anti-inflammatory microglial phenotype can favour neurogenesis and tissue remodelling (Butovsky, Landa, Kunis et al. 2006a; Butovsky, Ziv, Schwartz et al. 2006b).

The spatial–temporal pattern of cellular accumulation in the infarcted human brain has been addressed by means of postmortem histology and CSF examination or by advanced imaging techniques exploiting radioisotope tagging of specific cellular subpopulations, which allow longitudinal studies and dynamic description (Price, Warburton, Menon et al. 2003; Muir, Tyrrell, Sattar et al. 2007). Single photon emission computed tomography (SPECT) and [111]Indium-troponolate-labeling of neutrophils have been used to identify the recruitment of these cells to the infarct area, peaking within 19 hours of the ischemic event and attenuating over time (Price, Menon, Peters et al. 2004). Positron emission tomography (PET) scan and [11]C-(R)-PK11195 (a peripheral benzodiazepine receptor ligand) labeling of activated microglia provided evidence of increased binding as early as 3 days around the core region and of subsequent involvement of neighboring and distal areas up to 30 days (Gerhard, Schwarz, Myers et al. 2005; Price, Wang, Menon et al. 2006). Ultrasmall superparamagnetic particles of iron oxide (USPIO)-enhanced magnetic resonance imaging (MRI) studies identified macrophage infiltration into the lesion approximately 6 days after stroke, with a heterogeneous spatial–temporal pattern at earlier stages likely reflecting individual predisposition to initiate the inflammatory response (Saleh, Schroeter, Jonkmanns et al. 2004; Saleh, Schroeter, Ringelstein et al. 2007). Heterogeneity in USPIO-related MRI enhancement was recently found in a similar study, highlighting the need for further validation of this promising technique as a marker for neuroinflammation after stroke (Nighoghossian, Wiart, Cakmak et al. 2007).

Beyond individual susceptibility, studies in human stroke are complicated by the difficulty of discriminating between inflammation as a trigger for acute stroke and inflammation as a response to brain damage and by the multiplicity of pathological processes that can underlie this syndrome. In spite of these difficulties, inflammation remains a promising therapeutic target in subacute ischemic stages, although the beneficial effects of anti-inflammatory and/or immunomodulatory treatments observed in animal models have not yet given positive results in clinical applications. Therapeutic interventions such as hypothermia simultaneously affecting multiple aspects of ischemia-induced damage/inflammation, including gene expression associated with neuroprotection (Ohta, Terao, Shintani et al. 2007), could be preferable, as indicated by the positive outcome of a few small-sized clinical trials (van der Worp, Sena, Donnan et al. 2007). The therapeutic efficacy and safety of hypothermia is also currently under evaluation for the treatment of neonates who have experienced significant hypoxic–ischemic events (Blackmon, Stark 2006).

INFLAMMATION AND NEUROGENESIS

Generation of Neurons in the Adult Mammalian Brain

For a long time the adult mammalian brain has been considered entirely postmitotic. However, over the past few years many authors have contributed to establish the fundamental concept that neural stem cells (NSCs) exist in the adult mammalian brain and that new neurons are continuously added to the CNS during the entire life (Gage 2000).

Pioneer works from Altmann and Das (1965), based on proliferating cell ^{3}H-thymidine labeling, autoradiography, and light microscopy tissue analysis, showed the presence of new cells with neuronal morphology in some areas of the adult brain of rats . Subsequently, identification of newly formed neurons in the adult brain has been pursued by alternative experimental approaches, and neurogenesis in the adult mammalian brain, including the human brain (Altman, Das 1965), has been ascertained. Although some controversies remain on specific brain areas (Gould 2007), a general consensus has so far been reached about the existence of neurogenesis in two regions of the adult mammalian brain: the hippocampus and the olfactory bulb (OB).

The subventricular zone (SVZ), a layer of cells lining the lateral wall of the lateral ventricle (Doetsch, Caille, Lim et al. 1999), and the subgranular zone (SGZ) in the hippocampal dentate gyrus (Gage, Kempermann, Palmer et al. 1998) are considered privileged sites where NSCs/progenitor cells reside and give rise to new neurons destined to the OB and granular cell layer, respectively. The organization of the rodent SVZ has been extensively described. Type B cells, located in the SVZ and expressing the glial fibrillar acidic protein (GFAP), are considered to be the adult NSCs (Doetsch, Caille, Lim et al. 1999; Laywell, Rakic, Kukekov et al. 2000; Garcia, Doan, Imura et al. 2004) and have been shown to derive from the radial glia of the neonatal mouse brain (Merkle, Mirzadeh, Alvarez-Buylla 2007). Type B cells generate (via transit amplifying type C cells) type A cells or neuroblasts, which migrate from the SVZ to the OB through the rostral migratory stream (RMS). Neuroblasts, expressing the polysialylated-neural cell adhesion molecule (PSA-NCAM) (Altman, Das 1965; Doetsch, Garcia-Verdugo, Alvarez-Buylla 1997; Bedard, Levesque, Bernier et al. 2002), migrate to the OB where they terminally differentiate into periglomerular and granular interneurons. It has been proposed in a recent paper that adult NSCs located in discrete regions of the SVZ retain their capacity to generate astrocytes and oligodendrocytes but only specific types of OB neurons. Based on SVZ NSC labeling by adenovirus stereotactic injection, the authors suggest that NSCs from SVZ are spatially restricted in the types of neurons they generate and that they retain their positional information even if they are heterotopically grafted (Merkle, Mirzadeh, Alvarez-Buylla 2007). These data argue against the existence of homogeneous NSC populations in the CNS, and in contrast with previous findings (Suhonen, Peterson, Ray et al. 1996; Shihabuddin, Horner, Ray et al. 2000), they outline the reduced plasticity of adult NSCs. Importantly, neurogenesis persists in the adult human brain (Eriksson, Perfilieva, Bjork-Eriksson 1998) and NSCs can also be isolated from the adult human brain (Johansson, Svensson, Wallstedt et al. 1999; Kukekov, Aldskogius, Ulfhake 1999; Roy, Benraiss, Wang et al. 2000; Nunes, Roy, Keyoung et al. 2003). Moreover, the existence of a human SVZ germinal region (Sanai, Tramontin, Quinones-Hinojosa et al. 2004) and, more recently, the presence of a human rostral migratory stream have been demonstrated (Curtis, Kam, Nannmark et al. 2007b).

Physiological and Pathological Regulation of Adult Neurogenesis

The physiological and pathological regulation of neurogenesis involves a wide spectrum of converging and instructive signals from the microenvironment in which NSCs reside, the so called neurogenic niche. Besides astrocytes and endothelial cells (Song, Stevens, Gage 2002; Shen, Goderie, Jin et al. 2004), microglia and T cells (Aarum, Sandberg, Haeberlein et al. 2003; Walton, Sutter, Laywell et al. 2006; Ziv, Ron, Butovsky et al. 2006) are emerging as important components of the niche, although the exact nature of the signal they provide under different conditions is unclear.

Several physiological stimuli have been shown to regulate adult neurogenesis. Specific living conditions seem to trigger locally specific neurogenic signals in definite brain regions. Enriched environment, learning, and physical activity stimulate hippocampal but not OB neurogenesis (Kempermann, Kuhn, Gage 1998; Gould, Beylin, Tanapat et al. 1999; van Praag, Christie, Sejnowski et al. 1999a; van Praag, Kempermann, Gage 1999b; Brown, Cooper-Kuhn, Kempermann et al. 2003). T cells, through local interactions with microglia within the SGZ, seem to participate in the regulation of hippocampal progenitor proliferation induced by the enriched environment (Ziv, Ron, Butovsky et al. 2006). Circumstantial evidence suggests that hippocampal neurogenesis might be relevant to brain plasticity and cognitive function. Newborn neurons in the dentate gyrus have been shown to functionally integrate into the appropriate neuronal circuits (Carlen, Cassidy, Brismar et al. 2002; van Praag, Schinder, Christie et al. 2002; Brown, Cooper-Kuhn, Kempermann et al. 2003), raising the possibility that they might contribute to the better performance evoked by enriched environment or physical activity. In line with these results, it has been proposed that decreases in neurogenesis result in cognitive impairment (Shors, Miesegaes, Beylin et al. 2001). Similarly, "odor enrichment" of the environment enhances neurogenesis in the olfactory bulb by increasing the survival of progenitors and newly formed neurons (Rochefort, Gheusi, Vincent et al. 2002). The newly generated OB neurons display mature electrophysiological features and receive afferent synaptic inputs (Belluzzi, Benedusi, Ackman et al. 2003; Carleton, Petreanu, Lansford et al. 2003).

Neurogenesis is also modulated by pathological conditions (Curtis, Faull, Eriksson 2007a), most of which are associated with or caused by inflammatory processes. A number of studies have shown that epileptic seizures, focal and global ischemia, and brain trauma increase neurogenesis (Bengzon, Kokaia, Elmer et al. 1997; Parent, Yu, Leibowitz et al. 1997; Dash, Mach, Moore 2001; Arvidsson, Collin, Kirik et al. 2002; Braun, Schafer, Hollt 2002; Nakatomi, Kuriu, Okabe et al. 2002; Parent, Valentin, Lowenstein 2002; Thored, Arvidsson, Cacci et al. 2006). As a consequence of brain insults and neurogenesis enhancement, new neurons can be added into areas that are normally not neurogenic. It has been shown in an animal model of focal brain ischemia that SVZ-derived neuroblasts migrate into the poststroke adult striatum (Yamashita, Ninomiya, Hernandez et al. 2006) where they differentiate into striatal medium-sized spiny neurons (Arvidsson, Collin, Kirik et al. 2002). Newly formed cells with characteristics of striatal neurons can partially replace damaged or dead neurons in the ischemic striatum, and even if their role is not completely understood, they could contribute to the spontaneous recovery of sensorimotor functions following the ischemic event (Kokaia, Lindvall 2003). Cells expressing markers associated with newborn neurons have been detected near the ischemic damaged areas in human brain specimens (Jin, Wang, Xie et al. 2006).

These findings fuel the hope that the identification of tools able to enforce endogenous neurogenesis might be of therapeutic relevance in the treatment of acute or even chronic neurodegenerative diseases. Nonetheless, newly generated neurons might display altered properties when differentiating in a pathological environment and might aberrantly integrate in pre-existing circuits, further impairing brain function. Following status epilepticus (SE), new hippocampal granule neurons, migrating ectopically into the hilus or aberrantly extending their basal dendrites toward the hilar region, are likely to participate in recurrent seizure generation and cognitive disturbances (Parent, Yu, Leibowitz et al. 1997; Scharfman, Sollas, Goodman 2002; Scharfman 2004; Parent, Elliott, Pleasure et al. 2006; Jessberger, Zhao, Toni et al. 2007). However, recent evidence shows that new granule cells that integrate in the granule cell layer (GCL) circuitry under seizure conditions can acquire intrinsic membrane properties similar to physiologically produced neurons but exhibit modified synaptic connectivity that could be responsible for their reduced excitability in the epileptic brain (Jakubs, Nanobashvili, Bonde et al. 2006). As clearly demonstrated in this study, the development of functional properties by adult-born hippocampal neurons are then specifically influenced by the local physiological or pathological microenvironment they face. Cytokines and neurotrophic molecules released by activated microglia following SE might contribute to shape the characteristics of newly formed neurons. Whether increased neurogenesis constitutes a restorative response after the epileptic insult or whether it aggravates pathology remains to be demonstrated and is still a controversial issue (Kempermann 2006).

The effectiveness of endogenous neurogenesis as a self-repair mechanism in epilepsy and in other brain pathologies is minimized by the poor survival of the vast majority of newly formed neurons. Many new striatal neurons die between 2 and 5 weeks after stroke (Arvidsson, Collin, Kirik et al. 2002). Similarly, new SGZ cells are reduced in number by about 65% after 5 weeks following severe epileptic insult (Ekdahl, Mohapel, Elmer et al. 2001). This might be due to the disruption of tissue integrity following insult and/or due to the inflammatory events that accompany brain injury, which could generate an adverse environment for newly formed cells (see Table 13.3). One of the first studies addressing the role of inflammatory mediators in the regulation of neurogenesis was from Vallières et al. (Vallières, Campbell, Gage et al. 2002). They provided the first evidence that a proinflammatory cytokine, such as IL-6, compromises proliferation, survival, and differentiation of hippocampal progenitor cells when chronically overexpressed in the astrocytes of adult transgenic mice. Subsequently, a number of studies have indicated that the inflammatory process, sustained by activated microglia and infiltrating immune cells, primarily has a detrimental effect for neurogenesis, according to the hypothesis that the release of proinflammatory molecules (cytokines, free radicals) may be noxious to newborn cells (Monje, Mizumatsu, Fike et al. 2002; Ekdahl, Claasen, Bonde, Ekdahl, Lindvall 2003; Monje, Toda, Palmer et al. 2003; Liu, Fan, Won et al. 2007). An inverse correlation between microglial activation and hippocampal neurogenesis was shown in the rat hippocampus following prolonged intracortical infusion of the prototypical inflammogen LPS, which induced a major increase in the number of ED1 immunopositive cells (taken as an index of microglial activation) in the SGZ/GCL while abating the number of newly formed neurons (Ekdahl, Claasen, Bonde et al. 2003). The same study demonstrated that following electrically induced SE, the higher the seizures severity, the higher the number of activated microglia and the lower the survival of newly formed neurons within the first 5 weeks of insult. The idea that inflammation impairs both basal and insult-induced neurogenesis was consolidated by parallel studies from Palmer's group showing that systemic inflammation, achieved by intraperitoneal injection of LPS, also resulted in decreased hippocampal neurogenesis and finding a striking inverse correlation between the number of activated microglia and the number of newborn neurons in the dentate gyrus of rats exposed to cranial irradiation (Monje, Toda, Palmer et al. 2003). In both studies, neurogenesis was restored by systemic administration of anti-inflammatory drugs, such as minocycline and indomethacin, which increased newborn neuron survival and/or progenitors differentiation (Ekdahl, Claasen, Bonde et al. 2003; Monje, Toda, Palmer et al. 2003). These findings have been subsequently confirmed in different experimental paradigms, including rat models of focal cerebral ischemia (Hoehn, Palmer, Steinberg 2005; Liu, Fan, Won et al. 2007) and focal brain photothrombotic infarct (Kluska, Witte, Bolz et al. 2005). On the contrary, anti-inflammatory drugs such as acetylsalicylic acid, indomethacin, or the selective COX-2 inhibitor NS398 reduced ischemia-induced proliferation of neural progenitor cells in the SGZ in gerbil and mouse models (Kumihashi, Uchida, Miyazaki et al. 2001; Sasaki, Kitagawa, Sugiura et al. 2003). Furthermore, the NSAID flurbiprofen, administered 1 week after the induction of SE in adult rats to prevent interference with the progenitor cell proliferation, did not affect the survival of new neurons few weeks after the administration of the drug (Ajmone-Cat, Iosif, Ekdahl et al. 2006). The apparent discrepancy among the effects of anti-inflammatory agents can be reconciled by considering the differences in the experimental designs adopted (timing and duration of drug administration, injury model, etc.) and the variety of targets hit by these drugs. To mention a few examples, NSAIDs and minocycline can exert direct anti-apoptotic effects on newborn cells through the inhibition of the mitogen-activated protein kinase p38 or NF-κB–related pathways (Da Silva, Pierrat, Mary et al. 1997). The attenuation of the hypothalamic–pituitary adrenal (HPA) axis activation may represent a further pharmacological property by which NSAIDs could promote the restoration

Table 13.3 Inflammatory Pathways Affecting Neurogenesis

	Effects	References
Cell types		
Microglia	Detrimental	Monje et al. 2002; Monje et al. 2003; Ekhdal et al. 2003; Hoehn et al. 2005; Kluska et al. 2005; Liu et al. 2005; Cacci et al. 2005; Liu et al. 2007
	Beneficial and/or permissive	Aarum et al. 2003; Battista et al. 2006; Ziv et al. 2006; Walton et al. 2006; Butovsky et al. 2006a, 2006b; Cacci et al. 2008.
Astrocytes	Pro-neurogenic	Song et al. 2002
Endothelial cells		Shen et al. 2004; Palmer et al. 2000
T lymphocytes	Pro-neurogenic	Ziv et al. 2006
Monocytes/macrophages	Detrimental	Monje et al. 2003
Soluble mediators		
Cytokines		
TNF-α	Detrimental	Monje et al. 2003; Cacci et al. 2005; Liu et al. 2005
IL-18	Detrimental	Liu et al. 2005
IL-6	Detrimental	Vallières et al. 2002; Monje et al. 2003
TGF-β	Detrimental	Buckwalter 2006
	Beneficial	Battista et al. 2006
Complement-derived anaphylotoxins	Beneficial	Rahpeymai et al. 2006
Stress hormones	Detrimental	Reviewed by Tanapat et al. 1998; Cameron, McKay 1999; Mirescu, Gould 2006
Drugs		
Minocycline	Beneficial	Ekhdal et al. 2003; Liu et al. 2007
Indomethacin	Beneficial	Hoehn et al. 2005; Monje et al. 2003; Kluska et al. 2005
	Decreased NPC proliferation	Sasaki et al. 2003
Acetylsalicylic acid	Decreased NPC proliferation	Kumihashi et al. 2001
NS398	Decreased NPC proliferation	Sasaki et al. 2003
Flurbiprofen	No effects	Ajmone-Cat et al. 2006

TNF, tumor necrosis factor; IL, interleukin; TGF, transforming growth factor.

of neurogenesis (Gould, McEwen, Tanapat et al. 1997; Tanapat, Galea, Gould 1998). The stimulation of HPA is indeed a significant consequence of inflammation, leading to the elevation of serum glucocorticoid levels, whose antineurogenic effects have been described in several experimental models (Mirescu, Gould 2006).

Consistent with the assumption that activated microglia may exert a direct harmful effect on neurogenesis, a number of in vitro studies demonstrate that the survival and/or neuronal differentiation of hippocampal progenitors or NSCs is reduced when they are co-cultivated with activated microglia or when exposed to their conditioned medium (Monje, Toda, Palmer et al. 2003; Cacci, Claasen, Kokaia 2005; Liu, Lin, Tzeng et al. 2005). The microglia-derived cytokines IL-6, LIF, TNF-α, and IL-18 have been identified as key negative modulators of neural cell fate in these models. However, the pleiotropic functions potentially

exerted by these molecules, which depend on local concentrations, subtypes of expressed receptors, and cell targets, do not allow, till date, a conclusive view of their role in neurogenesis modulation in vivo. Although these studies strengthen the notion of a detrimental effect of inflammation on neurogenesis, the specific contribution of microglia and their products to these processes remains relatively unresolved, as it is the dichotomy between microglial neurotoxic and neuroprotective functions in brain pathology. What are the arrays of functions and mediators expressed by the ED1 immunopositive cells along the course of inflammation and how can they affect neurogenesis? Could microglia contribute to repair and regeneration through the release of mitogenic and/or neurotrophic factors, anti-inflammatory cytokines, or other soluble molecules, at different time points from the insult? Interestingly, the production of newborn neurons in the dentate gyrus following electrically induced SE, although initially compromised by the acute inflammatory response accompanying the damage (Ekdahl, Claasen, Bonde et al. 2003), is not further prevented by chronic inflammation after 6 months. This observation raises the possibility that chronically activated microglia may turn into a beneficial or at least non-detrimental phenotype for the survival and differentiation of newborn neurons (Bonde, Ekdahl, Lindvall et al. 2006). According to a recently proposed plasticity model, microglial activation is sensitive to the nature, intensity, and persistence of the stimuli around them and to other signals from the local environment that confer them the ability of synthesizing a range of different mediators in different pathological contexts (Schwartz, Butovsky, Bruck et al. 2006; Perry, Cunningham, Holmes et al. 2007). The relevance of the distinct microglial phenotypes for the outcome of neurogenesis is now beginning to be investigated, although a clear consistent picture is still lacking. It has been shown that microglia exposed to specific ranges of T helper–associated cytokines express the activation MHC-II antigens but do not release TNF-α, and promote neurogenesis and/or oligodendrogenesis from neural progenitor cells in vitro and in vivo (Butovsky, Landa, Kunis et al. 2006a; Butovsky, Ziv, Schwartz et al. 2006b). The dialogue between microglia and CNS-specific T lymphocytes has been proposed as an important positive factor for neurogenesis induced by physiological stimuli (Ziv, Ron, Butovsky et al. 2006), raising the possibility that similar interactions may also occur under certain pathological conditions and favor insult-induced neurogenesis.

Recently, Battista et al. proposed that the beneficial or detrimental nature of the neurogenic niche would depend on the degree of microglial activation and on the balance between the locally produced pro- and anti-inflammatory cytokines (Battista, Ferrari, Gage et al. 2006). By using a model of adrenalectomy that causes massive apoptotic neuronal death and increases NSC proliferation in the dentate gyrus, the authors observed a positive correlation between the number of activated microglia and the extent of neurogenesis and NSC proliferation. Interestingly, the activation profile of microglia was peculiar in that it did not proceeded to the fully phagocytic ED1+ state and was characterized by upregulation of the anti-inflammatory cytokine transforming growth factor β (TGF-β). Low levels of TNF-α, IL-1α, and IL-1β mRNAs were detected in the area. TGF-β contributed to the generation of a proneurogenic environment as its neutralization partially reduced neurogenesis, without affecting NSC proliferation. The microglial phenotype described in this model is reminiscent of the atypical phenotype that is acquired on interaction with apoptotic neurons in other in vivo and in vitro models (Perry, Cunningham,

Boche 2002; Depino, Earl, Kaczmarczyk et al. 2003; Minghetti, Ajmone-Cat, De Berardinis et al. 2005). More recently, such atypical activated microglia have been shown to support the neurogenic response in NSCs/progenitor cells isolated from embryonic mouse cortex or adult SVZ (Cacci, Ajmone-Cat, Anelli et al. 2008). The manifold facets of microglial activation and their repercussions on the neurogenic process need further investigations and underlie the importance of identifying specific tools that are able to direct or redirect microglial functions toward the potentially protective proneurogenic ones.

In addition to microglia, a variety of other cell-to-cell interactions and/or diffusible signals can determine the fate of adult-born cells. As an example, modified interactions of NSCs/progenitors with cells of the microvasculature could be of crucial importance (Monje, Mizumatsu, Fike et al. 2002). Endothelial cell expression of chemokines and adhesion molecules can indeed be altered during inflammation and can influence the neurogenic vascular microenvironment (Leventhal, Rafii, Rafii et al. 1999; Palmer, Willhoite, Gage 2000; Louissaint, Rao, Leventhal et al. 2002) and the recruitment of monocytes and other immune cells from periphery. The reported beneficial effects of anti-inflammatory compounds on neurogenesis, besides deactivation of microglia, could result from the normalization of the activation status of the endothelium and from the decreased extravasation of immune cells (Reichman, Farrell, Del Maestro et al. 1986). Other important components of the neurogenic niche are astrocytes and the extracellular matrix constituents (Song, Stevens, Gage 2002), as well as factors present in the surrounding parenchyma, which can be profoundly affected by brain injury and onset of inflammation. Among these is the complement system, leading either to neurodegeneration or to neuroprotection depending on the pathophysiological context (van Beek, Elward, Gasque 2003). Interestingly, several lines of evidence point to the involvement of complement-derived anaphylotoxins in regenerative processes in many organs, including the brain. It has recently been shown that basal and ischemia-induced neurogenesis are both impaired in mice with disrupted C3 signaling (Rahpeymai, Hietala, Wilhelmsson et al. 2006). In conclusion, a multiplicity of mechanisms taking place along with neuroinflammation contributes to defining the outcome of neurogenesis; their deep knowledge will help in successfully harnessing endogenous NSCs for brain repair.

Neurogenesis in Ageing Brain

Ageing is a physiological process characterized by decreased tissue homeostasis and repair capacity in response to damage. Brain does not make exceptions and it frequently undergoes a number of changes, possibly contributing to memory and learning deficits. The risk of developing neurodegenerative pathologies increases enormously with age, even if the rate of the ageing process and the incidence of specific brain disorders show strong variability, outlining the involvement of many additional genetic and/or epigenetic risk factors.

The aged brain displays gross anatomical modifications, such as shrinkage, decrease in weight, and histological and biochemical changes. Microarray analysis of the aged rodent brains has revealed altered expression of genes linked to inflammation, oxidative stress, and neurotrophic support (Table 13.4), which could have a role in cerebral function decline (Lee, Weindruch, Prolla 2000; Blalock, Chen, Sharrow et al. 2003). Many studies have shown increased proinflammatory cytokine expression in the healthy aged brain with respect to the adult brain (Bodles, Barger 2004) and enhanced mRNA expression of proinflammatory cytokines such as IL-6, IL-1β, and TNF-α after peripheral or central LPS injections (Godbout, Chen, Abraham et al. 2005; Huang, Henry, Dantzer et al. 2007), or following LPS stimulation of microglial cultures from aged brains (Xie, Morgan, Rozovsky et al. 2003; Ye, Johnson 1999). Furthermore, LPS-induced gene expression in the aged mice was protracted with respect to adult healthy mice and was associated with an exaggerated sickness behavior response, characterized by anorectic and reduced locomotor and social behaviors (Godbout, Chen, Abraham et al. 2005; Huang, Henry, Dantzer et al. 2007). Conversely, the levels of anti-inflammatory cytokines such as IL-10 and IL-4, which keep proinflammatory cytokine expression under control, have been found to be decreased in the elderly (Ye, Johnson 2001; Nolan, Maher, Martin et al. 2005).

Consistent with the reported biochemical alterations, histological analyses have demonstrated increased aged-related glial reactivity (Huang, Henry, Dantzer et al. 2007), and phenotypic and morphological changes of microglia in the healthy aged brain of different mammalian species, including humans. The phenotypical changes associated with microglial activation include increased immunoreactivity for the MHC-II antigens and elevated expression of the ED1 and CD14 surface antigens, and scavenger and complement receptors (Perry, Matyszak, Fearn 1993; Ogura, Ogawa, Yoshida 1994; Streit, Sparks 1997; Morgan et al. 1999; Kullberg, Aldskogius, Ulfhake 2001). Microglia with abnormal morphology, referred to as *dystrophic microglia*, have been described in the aged brain (Conde, Streit 2006). These observations, together with the already mentioned findings of exaggerated neuroinflammation and sickness behavior in aged mice in response to peripheral or central LPS (Godbout, Chen, Abraham et al. 2005; Huang, Henry, Dantzer et al. 2007), and evidence of hippocampal learning deficits induced by LPS in aged but not adult mice (Barrientos, Higgins, Biedenkapp 2006), reinforce the idea of a possible link between increased microglial reactivity (primed microglia) and alterations of cognitive functions during ageing. Nonetheless, the exact functional significance of morphologically activated glial cells and their consequences for the aging process, as well as for age-related pathologies, remain to be deciphered.

Neurogenesis is one of the functions that could be affected by the increased activation and reactivity of microglia in the elderly. Indeed, the decreased number of newly formed neurons observed in the aged brain (Kuhn, Dickinson-Anson, Gage et al. 1996; Cameron, McKay 1999; Jin, Sun, Xie et al. 2003; Heine, Maslam, Joels et al. 2004; Jin, Minami, Xie et al. 2004b) can be seen as a consequence of the

Table 13.4 Age-Related Modification of Inflammatory Pathways

	Modifications	*References*
Cell types		
Glial cells	Increased reactivity Morphological modification	Perry et al. 1993; Ogura et al. 1994; Streit, Sparks 1997; Morgan et al. 1999; Lee et al. 2000; Kullberg et al. 2001; Blalock et al. 2003; Godbout et al. 2005; Conde, Streit 2006; Huang et al. 2007
Soluble mediators		
IL-1β, IL-6, TNF-α	Upregulated	Ye, Johnson 1999; Xie et al. 2003; Bodles, Barger 2004; Godbout et al. 2005; Huang et al. 2007
IL-4, IL-10, bFGF, IGF-1, VEGF	Downregulated	Ye, Johnson 2001; Anderson et al. 2002; Shetty et al. 2005; Nolan et al. 2005

IL, interleukin; TNF, tumor necrosis factor; bFGF, basic fibroblast growth factor; IGF, insulin-like growth factor; VEGF, vascular endothelial growth factor.

altered brain milieu besides the intrinsic ageing of the NSC pool. A reduced supply of diffusible mitogenic and growth factors, such as basic fibroblast growth factor (bFGF), insulin-like growth factor (IGF-1), and vascular endothelial growth factor (VEGF), to the aged hippocampal neurogenic niche (Anderson, Aberg, Nilsson et al. 2002; Shetty, Hattiangady, Shetty 2005) could be responsible for decreased stem/progenitor cell proliferation (Kuhn, Dickinson-Anson, Gage 1996; Hattiangady, Shetty 2006). Notably, chronic exposure to TGF-β1, whose levels are increased in the aged brain, dramatically reduces the generation of newly formed neurons in the adult hippocampus (Buckwalter, Yamane, Coleman et al. 2006), as opposed to the beneficial effect of acute exposure (Battista, Ferrari, Gage et al. 2006). Several other extrinsic changes in the brain milieu, including increase of glucocorticoid levels, or the state of the vascular niche could be responsible for neurogenesis decline (Tanapat, Galea, Gould et al. 1998; Cameron, McKay 1999; Monje, Mizumatsu, Fike et al. 2002; Palmer 2002; Wurmser, Palmer, Gage 2004). Together with these factors, intrinsic NSC changes might lead to impairment of NSC properties, such as self-renewal, and hence, to senescence (Harley, Futcher, Greider 1990; Stewart, Ben-Porath, Carey et al. 2003; Villa, Navarro-Galve, Bueno et al. 2004).

Similar to basal neurogenesis, injury-induced neurogenesis is impaired or altered by aging. The results of recent studies, extensively reviewed by Popa-Wagner et al. (2007), have shown that several cellular and genetic responses to stroke, such as neuronal loss, cell proliferation, phagocytosis, scar formation, and production of neurotoxic or neuroprotective factors, are temporally dysregulated in aged animals, further compromising functional recovery . By using a model of global forebrain ischemia, Yagita et al. (2001) found that, despite the lower basal cell proliferation in the aged SGZ, the number of newborn neurons increased significantly in both young and old animals following damage, indicating that neural progenitor cells from old brains might retain the capacity to respond to environmental changes such as those produced by ischemia. However, newborn cells in the aged brain showed reduced survival with respect to the young rats, suggesting the presence of a hostile environment in the aged brain. In a different model of focal cerebral ischemia, Darsalia et al. (2005) found that newly formed neurons of the SGZ, but not SVZ-derived striatal neurons, were fewer in old rats than in young rats. The number of activated microglial cells was similar in young and old animals, either after stroke or sham surgery, suggesting an intrinsic age-related alteration of neurogenesis. However, the possibility that activated microglia in the aged brain impair SGZ neurogenesis more effectively than that in young animals

could not be excluded. These and other studies demonstrating increased cell proliferation and generation of neuroblasts in the SVZ of aged rats after stroke, as well as maturation of the newly formed striatal neurons (Sato, Hayashi, Sasaki et al. 2001; Jin, Minami, Xie et al. 2004b; Darsalia, Heldmann, Lindvall et al. 2005), indicate that the potentially beneficial mechanisms compensating cell loss after brain ischemia, although diminished, persist in the aged brain and foster the possibility of restorative therapeutic strategies in aged patients. As a matter of fact, evidence for stroke-induced neurogenesis in aged human brain has been reported (Macas, Nern, Plate et al. 2006).

It is important to note that human neurogenesis has been addressed by using different approaches, including labeling of proliferating cells with bromodeoxyuridine (BrdU) (Eriksson, Perfilieva, Bjork-Eriksson et al. 1998), or immunocytochemical detection of Ki67, considered as reliable markers for proliferating cells (Kee, Sivalingam, Boonstra et al. 2002). However, re-expression of cell-cycle regulators and evidence of a loss of cell-cycle control have been observed in mature neurons in the presence of acute or chronic neurodegenerative diseases such as stroke, AD, and PD. These findings have been interpreted as the initiation of a cell death program rather than a pathology-associated neurogenic response. Consequently, possible pathogenic alterations of mechanisms presiding to cell-cycle regulation in mature neurons have to be taken into account when adult neurogenesis is studied (Herrup, Yang 2007). An alternative approach is the immunochemical detection of the microtubule associated protein doublecortin (DCX), which is transiently expressed in migrating newly formed immature neurons (Couillard-Despres, Winner, Schaubeck et al. 2005).

Evidence for augmented neurogenesis in AD hippocampus comes from a recent study showing increased immunoreactivity for DCX and PSA-NCAM in postmortem AD brain specimens, with a tendency of positive correlation between neurogenesis and AD severity (Jin, Peel, Mao et al. 2004c). Similarly, the same group reported enhanced neurogenesis in a transgenic mouse model of AD (Jin, Galvan, Xie et al. 2004a). However, the increased neurogenesis has not been confirmed in studies on different AD animal models (Haughey, Nath, Chan et al. 2002b; Wang, Dineley, Sweatt et al. 2004; Donovan, Yazdani, Norris et al. 2006) or on human specimens (Boekhoorn, Joels, Lucassen 2006). Boekhoorn et al. reported an increased Ki67 immunoreactivity in AD, but they did not find differences in DCX staining between controls and AD cases. The authors suggested that augmented cell proliferation observed in the hippocampus was most likely due to astrocyte proliferation and vasculature-associated changes.

The discrepancies among studies on neurogenesis in AD could be partially reconduced to the intrinsic limitations of the experimental models adopted, each one recapitulating only few aspects of AD pathogenesis. The generation of single- or double-mutant mice knocked-in in *APP* (Swedish KM670/671 mutation) and/or *PS-1* (P264L mutation) genes it is worth mentioning. Different from other transgenic models (Haughey, Nath, Chan et al. 2002b; Jin, Galvan, Xie et al. 2004a; Wen, Hof, Chen et al. 2004; Chevallier, Soriano, Kang et al. 2005), the mutated *APP* is under the control of an endogenous promoter allowing its "physiological" temporal and spatial expression. Moreover, overexpression of mutated proteins is avoided. The double knock-in animals develop aging- and region-dependent amyloid deposition and microgliosis. By using this model, Zhang et al. (2007) found that the number of neuroblasts (DCX-positive cell) in the double knock-in mice dropped to 50% to 60% of wild type mice and at the same time the pool of the stem/progenitor cells reduced to 70%, accounting for the reduction of immature neurons. The impairment of neurogenesis was limited to the hippocampus, whereas no evidence for changes in OB neurogenesis was found. Interestingly, in these mice amyloid deposition was observed in the outer molecular layer of the dentate gyrus (DG) but not in the striatum and corpus callosum near the SVZ, raising the possibility that Aβ deposition could play a role in altering neurogenesis. Consistent with this view is the fact that injection of Aβ in the lateral ventricles has been reported to affect both proliferation and migration of neural progenitor cells (Haughey, Liu, Nath et al. 2002a), and the number of SVZ progenitors has been found diminished in AD patients (Ziabreva, Perry, Perry et al. 2006). A few reports highlighted a positive correlation between severity of dementia and degree of olfactory dysfunction (Murphy, Gilmore, Seery et al. 1990).

Further investigations are warranted to assess the mechanisms leading to neurogenesis alterations in AD and to develop strategies to manipulate resident adult NSC, which would allow the replacement of cells lost during brain disease.

CONCLUSIONS

The last decade has witnessed an increasing interest in inflammation as a determinant factor in many brain pathologies. Signs indicative of ongoing inflammatory processes and activation of microglia have been detected in pathological conditions traditionally not included in the category of "inflammatory diseases." This is the case not only of chronic neurodegenerative diseases, such as AD, but also of neurodevelopmental and psychiatric disorders such as autism and depression. Although the neurobiological basis for autism—a complex neurodevelopmental disorder characterized by cognitive and behavioral impairments—remains poorly understood, it has been proposed that immune dysfunctions contribute to the pathogenesis of this disorder (Pardo, Vargas, Zimmerman 2005). As previously mentioned, the number of activated microglia and astrocytes is increased in the cerebral cortex, white matter, and cerebellum of autistic patients (Vargas, Nascimbene, Krishnan et al. 2005). In addition, CSF from autistic subjects shows a unique proinflammatory profile of cytokines, including a marked increase in MCP-1. The lack of specific T-cell responses or antibody-mediated reactions suggests that the adaptive immune response does not play a significant role in this disease. Thus, microglial and astroglial reactions appear to be the main features of the innate immune responses in autism, suggesting that future therapies might involve modifying neuroglial responses. Inflammation have frequently been found to be associated with depression, although some studies did not find evidence for a direct correlation between the two events, pointing out that inflammation is not contributing to depression in all patients. Few reports have suggested that antidepressants can inhibit microglial proinflammatory cytokine production (Obuchowicz, Kowalski, Labuzek et al. 2006; Hashioka, Klegeris, Monji et al. 2007). Interestingly, data from animal models suggest that hippocampal neurogenesis is involved in depression and it is required for the behavioral effects of antidepressants (Santarelli, Saxe, Gross et al. 2003), raising the possibility that antidepressants affect neurogenesis through the modulation of microglial activation.

Although a substantial body of evidence supports the notion of detrimental effects of inflammation, the specific contributions of the many aspects of inflammatory processes remain relatively unresolved, as it is the dichotomy between microglial neurotoxic and neuroprotective functions in brain pathology. As a recent example of protective activities of microglia, it has been shown that intra-arterial injection of immortalized microglia protected CA1 neurons against global ischemia. The exogenous microglial cells homed to the brain and accumulated in the hippocampus after ischemia, significantly preventing neuronal degeneration, synaptic deficits, and decrease in brain-derived neurotrophic factor levels (Hayashi, Tomimatsu, Suzuki et al. 2006). Finally, the ability of hematopoietic cells to enter the CNS and differentiate into microglia after bone marrow transplantation suggests that microglia might serve as natural cellular vehicles for gene therapy for brain diseases (Priller, Flugel, Wehner et al. 2001; Neumann 2006).

The identification of molecular mechanisms governing the beneficial arm of microglial activation and neuroinflammation could help in designing novel therapeutic strategies aimed at fostering neuronal survival and neurogenesis and regaining function in disabling and high–social impact brain disorders.

REFERENCES

Aarum J, Sandberg K, Haeberlein SL, Persson MA. 2003. Migration and differentiation of neural precursor cells can be directed by microglia. *Proc Natl Acad Sci U S A.* 100(26):15983–15988.

Aisen PS. 2002. The potential of anti-inflammatory drugs for the treatment of Alzheimer's disease. *Lancet Neurol.* 1(5):279–284.

Aisen PS, Schafer KA, Grundman M et al. 2003. Effects of rofecoxib or naproxen vs placebo on Alzheimer disease progression: a randomized controlled trial. *JAMA.* 289(21):2819–2826.

Ajmone-Cat MA, Nicolini A, Minghetti L. 2003. Prolonged exposure of microglia to lipopolysaccharide modifies the intracellular signaling pathways and selectively promotes prostaglandin E2 synthesis. *J Neurochem.* 87(5):1193–1203.

Ajmone-Cat MA, Iosif RE, Ekdahl CT, Kokaia Z, Minghetti L, Lindvall O. 2006. Prostaglandin E2 and BDNF levels in rat hippocampus are negatively correlated with status epilepticus severity: no impact on survival of seizure-generated neurons. *Neurobiol Dis.* 23(1):23–35.

Akiyama H, Barger S, Barnum S et al. 2000. Inflammation and Alzheimer's disease. *Neurobiol Aging.* 21(3):383–421.

Aloisi F, Ria F, Adorini L. 2000. Regulation of T-cell responses by CNS antigen-presenting cells: different roles for microglia and astrocytes. *Immunol Today.* 21(3):141–147.

Altman J, Das GD. 1965. Autoradiographic and histological evidence of postnatal hippocampal neurogenesis in rats. *J Comp Neurol.* 124(3):319–335.

Anderson MF, Aberg MA, Nilsson M, Eriksson PS. 2002. Insulin-like growth factor-I and neurogenesis in the adult mammalian brain. *Brain Res Dev Brain Res.* 134(1–2):115–122.

Arumugam TV, Granger DN, Mattson MP. 2005. Stroke and T-cells. *Neuromolecular Med.* 7(3):229–242.

Arvidsson A, Collin T, Kirik D, Kokaia Z, Lindvall O. 2002. Neuronal replacement from endogenous precursors in the adult brain after stroke. *Nat Med.* 8(9):963–970.

Asanuma M, Miyazaki I. 2006. Nonsteroidal anti-inflammatory drugs in Parkinson's disease: possible involvement of quinone formation. *Expert Rev Neurother.* 6(9):1313–1325.

Barone FC, Schmidt DB, Hillegass LM et al. 1992. Reperfusion increases neutrophils and leukotriene B4 receptor binding in rat focal ischemia. *Stroke.* 23(9):1337–1347; discussion 1347–8.

Barrientos RM, Higgins EA, Biedenkapp JC et al. 2006. Peripheral infection and aging interact to impair hippocampal memory consolidation. *Neurobiol Aging.* 27(5):723–732.

Battista D, Ferrari CC, Gage FH, Pitossi FJ. 2006. Neurogenic niche modulation by activated microglia: transforming growth factor beta increases neurogenesis in the adult dentate gyrus. *Eur J Neurosci.* 23(1):83–93.

Bechmann I, Mor G, Nilsen J, Eliza M, Nitsch R, Naftolin F. 1999. FasL (CD95L, Ap01L) is expressed in the normal rat and human brain: evidence for the existence of an immunological brain barrier. *Glia.* 27(1):62–74.

Bechmann I, Galea I, Perry VH. 2007. What is the blood-brain barrier (not)? *Trends Immunol.* 28(1):5–11.

Bedard A, Levesque M, Bernier PJ, Parent A. 2002. The rostral migratory stream in adult squirrel monkeys: contribution of new neurons to the olfactory tubercle and involvement of the antiapoptotic protein Bcl-2. *Eur J Neurosci.* 16(10):1917–1924.

Belluzzi O, Benedusi M, Ackman J, LoTurco JJ. 2003. Electrophysiological differentiation of new neurons in the olfactory bulb. *J Neurosci.* 23(32):10411–10418.

Bengzon J, Kokaia Z, Elmer E, Nanobashvili A, Kokaia M, Lindvall O. 1997. Apoptosis and proliferation of dentate gyrus neurons after single and intermittent limbic seizures. *Proc Natl Acad Sci U S A.* 94(19):10432–10437.

Blackmon LR, Stark AR. 2006. Hypothermia: a neuroprotective therapy for neonatal hypoxic-ischemic encephalopathy. *Pediatrics.* 117(3):942–948.

Blalock EM, Chen KC, Sharrow K et al. 2003. Gene microarrays in hippocampal aging: statistical profiling identifies novel processes correlated with cognitive impairment. *J Neurosci.* 23(9):3807–3819.

Bodles AM, Barger SW. 2004. Cytokines and the aging brain - what we don't know might help us. *Trends Neurosci.* 27(10):621–626.

Boekhoorn K, Joels M, Lucassen PJ. 2006. Increased proliferation reflects glial and vascular-associated changes, but not neurogenesis in the presenile Alzheimer hippocampus. *Neurobiol Dis.* 24(1):1–14.

Bonde S, Ekdahl CT, Lindvall O. 2006. Long-term neuronal replacement in adult rat hippocampus after status epilepticus despite chronic inflammation. *Eur J Neurosci.* 23(4):965–974.

Bornstein NM, Aronovich B, Korczyn AD et al. 2001. Antibodies to brain antigens following stroke. *Neurology.* 56(4):529–30.

Braun H, Schafer K, Hollt V. 2002. BetaIII tubulin-expressing neurons reveal enhanced neurogenesis in hippocampal and cortical structures after a contusion trauma in rats. *J Neurotrauma.* 19(8):975–983.

Brown J, Cooper-Kuhn CM, Kempermann G et al. 2003. Enriched environment and physical activity stimulate hippocampal but not olfactory bulb neurogenesis. *Eur J Neurosci.* 17(10):2042–2046.

Buckwalter MS, Yamane M, Coleman BS et al. 2006. Chronically increased transforming growth factor-beta1 strongly inhibits hippocampal neurogenesis in aged mice. *Am J Pathol.* 169(1):154–164.

Butovsky O, Landa G, Kunis G et al. 2006a. Induction and blockage of oligodendrogenesis by differently activated microglia in an animal model of multiple sclerosis. *J Clin Invest.* 116(4):905–915.

Butovsky O, Ziv Y, Schwartz A et al. 2006b. Microglia activated by IL-4 or IFN-gamma differentially induce neurogenesis and oligodendrogenesis from adult stem/progenitor cells. *Mol Cell Neurosci.* 31(1):149–160.

Cacci E, Claasen JH, Kokaia Z. 2005. Microglia-derived tumor necrosis factor-alpha exaggerates death of newborn hippocampal progenitor cells in vitro. *J Neurosci Res.* 80(6):789–797.

Cacci E, Ajmone-Cat MA, Anelli T, Biagioni S, Minghetti L.. 2008. Neuronal and glial differentiation from embryonic or adult neural precursor cells are differently affected by chronic or acute activation of microglia. *Glia.* 56(4):412–425.

Calingasan NY, Erdely HA, Altar CA. 2002. Identification of CD40 ligand in Alzheimer's disease and in animal models of Alzheimer's disease and brain injury. *Neurobiol Aging.* 23(1):31–39.

Cameron HA, McKay RD. 1999. Restoring production of hippocampal neurons in old age. *Nat Neurosci.* 2(10):894–897.

Cardona AE, Pioro EP, Sasse ME et al. 2006. Control of microglial neurotoxicity by the fractalkine receptor. *Nat Neurosci.* 9(7):917–924.

Carlen M, Cassidy RM, Brismar H, Smith GA, Enquist LW, Frisen J. 2002. Functional integration of adult-born neurons. *Curr Biol.* 12(7):606–608.

Carleton A, Petreanu LT, Lansford R, Alvarez-Buylla A, Lledo PM. 2003. Becoming a new neuron in the adult olfactory bulb. *Nat Neurosci.* 6(5):507–518.

Carnevale D, De Simone R, Minghetti L. 2007. Microglia-neuron interaction in inflammatory and degenerative diseases: role of cholinergic and noradrenergic systems. *CNS Neurol Disord Drug Targets.* 6(6):388–397.

Chan WY, Kohsaka S, Rezaie P. 2007. The origin and cell lineage of microglia: new concepts. *Brain Res Rev.* 53(2):344–354.

Chevallier NL, Soriano S, Kang DE, Masliah E, Hu G, Koo EH. 2005. Perturbed neurogenesis in the adult hippocampus associated with presenilin-1 A246E mutation. *Am J Pathol.* 167(1):151–159.

Chew LJ, Takanohashi A, Bell M. 2006. Microglia and inflammation: impact on developmental brain injuries. *Ment Retard Dev Disabil Res Rev.* 12(2):105–112.

Combrinck MI, Perry VH, Cunningham C. 2002. Peripheral infection evokes exaggerated sickness behaviour in pre-clinical murine prion disease. *Neuroscience.* 112(1):7–11.

Combrinck M, Williams J, De Berardinis MA et al. 2006. Levels of CSF prostaglandin E2, cognitive decline, and survival in Alzheimer's disease. *J Neurol Neurosurg Psychiatry.* 77(1):85–88.

Conde JR, Streit WJ. 2006. Microglia in the aging brain. *J Neuropathol Exp Neurol.* 65(3):199–203.

Couillard-Despres S, Winner B, Schaubeck S et al. 2005. Doublecortin expression levels in adult brain reflect neurogenesis. *Eur J Neurosci.* 21(1):1–14.

Curtis MA, Faull RL, Eriksson PS. 2007a. The effect of neurodegenerative diseases on the subventricular zone. *Nat Rev Neurosci.* 8(9):712–723.

Curtis MA, Kam M, Nannmark U et al. 2007b. Human neuroblasts migrate to the olfactory bulb via a lateral ventricular extension. *Science.* 315(5816):1243–1249.

Da Silva J, Pierrat B, Mary JL, Lesslauer W. 1997. Blockade of p38 mitogen-activated protein kinase pathway inhibits inducible nitric-oxide synthase expression in mouse astrocytes. *J Biol Chem.* 272(45):28373–28380.

Darsalia V, Heldmann U, Lindvall O, Kokaia Z. 2005. Stroke-induced neurogenesis in aged brain. *Stroke.* 36(8):1790–1795.

Dash PK, Mach SA, Moore AN. 2001. Enhanced neurogenesis in the rodent hippocampus following traumatic brain injury. *J Neurosci Res.* 63(4):313–319.

De Simone R, Ajmone-Cat MA, Minghetti L. 2004. Atypical antiinflammatory activation of microglia induced by apoptotic neurons: possible role of phosphatidylserine-phosphatidylserine receptor interaction. *Mol Neurobiol.* 29(2):197–212.

De Simone R, Ajmone-Cat MA, Carnevale D, Minghetti L. 2005. Activation of alpha7 nicotinic acetylcholine receptor by nicotine selectively up-regulates cyclooxygenase-2 and prostaglandin E2 in rat microglial cultures. *J Neuroinflammation.* 2(1):4.

Depino AM, Earl C, Kaczmarczyk E et al. 2003. Microglial activation with atypical proinflammatory cytokine expression in a rat model of Parkinson's disease. *Eur J Neurosci.* 18(10):2731–2742.

Dik MG, Jonker C, Hack CE, Smit JH, Comijs HC, Eikelenboom P. 2005. Serum inflammatory proteins and cognitive decline in older persons. *Neurology.* 64(8):1371–1377.

Dirnagl U, Klehmet J, Braun JS et al. 2007. Stroke-induced immunodepression: experimental evidence and clinical relevance. *Stroke.* 38(Suppl 2) 770–773.

Doetsch F, Garcia-Verdugo JM, Alvarez-Buylla A. 1997. Cellular composition and three-dimensional organization of the subventricular germinal zone in the adult mammalian brain. *J Neurosci.* 17(13):5046–5061.

Doetsch F, Caille I, Lim DA, Garcia-Verdugo JM, Alvarez-Buylla A. 1999. Subventricular zone astrocytes are neural stem cells in the adult mammalian brain. *Cell.* 97(6):703–716.

Donovan MH, Yazdani U, Norris RD, Games D, German DC, Eisch AJ. 2006. Decreased adult hippocampal neurogenesis in the PDAPP mouse model of Alzheimer's disease. *J Comp Neurol.* 495(1):70–83.

Eikelenboom P, Veerhuis R, Scheper W, Rozemuller AJ, van Gool WA, Hoozemans JJ. 2006. The significance of neuroinflammation in understanding Alzheimer's disease. *J Neural Transm.* 113(11):1685–1695.

Ekdahl CT, Mohapel P, Elmer E, Lindvall O. 2001. Caspase inhibitors increase short-term survival of progenitor-cell progeny in the adult rat dentate gyrus following status epilepticus. *Eur J Neurosci.* 14(6):937–945.

Ekdahl CT, Claasen JH, Bonde S, Kokaia Z, Lindvall O. 2003. Inflammation is detrimental for neurogenesis in adult brain. *Proc Natl Acad Sci U S A.* 100(23):13632–13637.

Eriksson PS, Perfilieva E, Bjork-Eriksson T et al. 1998. Neurogenesis in the adult human hippocampus. *Nat Med.* 4(11):1313–1317.

Esiri MM. 2007. The interplay between inflammation and neurodegeneration in CNS disease. *J Neuroimmunol.* 184(1–2):4–16.

Esposito E, Di Matteo V, Benigno A, Pierucci M, Crescimanno G, Di Giovanni G. 2007. Non-steroidal anti-inflammatory drugs in Parkinson's disease. *Exp Neurol.* 205(2):295–312.

Familian A, Eikelenboom P, Veerhuis R. 2007. Minocycline does not affect amyloid beta phagocytosis by human microglial cells. *Neurosci Lett.* 416(1):87–91.

Farina C, Aloisi F, Meinl E. 2007. Astrocytes are active players in cerebral innate immunity. *Trends Immunol.* 28(3):138–145.

Ferrari CC, Depino AM, Prada F et al. 2004. Reversible demyelination, blood-brain barrier breakdown, and pronounced neutrophil recruitment induced by chronic IL-1 expression in the brain. *Am J Pathol.* 165(5):1827–1837.

Gage FH, Kempermann G, Palmer TD, Peterson DA, Ray J. 1998. Multipotent progenitor cells in the adult dentate gyrus. *J Neurobiol.* 36(2):249–266.

Gage FH. 2000. Mammalian neural stem cells. *Science.* 287(5457):1433–1438.

Galea I, Bechmann I, Perry VH. 2007. What is immune privilege (not)? *Trends Immunol.* 28(1):12–18.

Garcia AD, Doan NB, Imura T, Bush TG, Sofroniew MV. 2004. GFAP-expressing progenitors are the principal source of constitutive neurogenesis in adult mouse forebrain. *Nat Neurosci.* 7(11):1233–1241.

Gasparini L, Ongini E, Wenk G. 2004. Non-steroidal anti-inflammatory drugs (NSAIDs) in Alzheimer's disease: old and new mechanisms of action. *J Neurochem.* 91(3):521–536.

Gee JM, Kalil A, Shea C, Becker KJ. 2007. Lymphocytes: potential mediators of postischemic injury and neuroprotection. *Stroke.* 38(2 Suppl):783–788.

Gelinas DS, DaSilva K, Fenili D, St George-Hyslop P, McLaurin J. 2004. Immunotherapy for Alzheimer's disease. *Proc Natl Acad Sci U S A.* 101 (Suppl 2):14657–14662.

Gerhard A, Schwarz J, Myers R, Wise R, Banati RB. 2005. Evolution of microglial activation in patients after ischemic stroke: a [11C](R)-PK11195 PET study. *Neuroimage.* 24(2):591–595.

Giulian D, Corpuz M, Chapman S, Mansouri M, Robertson C. 1993. Reactive mononuclear phagocytes release neurotoxins after ischemic and traumatic injury to the central nervous system. *J Neurosci Res.* 36(6):681–693.

Giulian D, Haverkamp LJ, Li J et al. 1995. Senile plaques stimulate microglia to release a neurotoxin found in Alzheimer brain. *Neurochem Int.* 27(1):119–137.

Godbout JP, Chen J, Abraham J et al. 2005. Exaggerated neuroinflammation and sickness behavior in aged mice following activation of the peripheral innate immune system. *FASEB J.* 19(10):1329–1331.

Gould E, McEwen BS, Tanapat P, Galea LA, Fuchs E. 1997. Neurogenesis in the dentate gyrus of the adult tree shrew is regulated by psychosocial stress and NMDA receptor activation. *J Neurosci.* 17(7):2492–2498.

Gould E, Beylin A, Tanapat P, Reeves A, Shors TJ. 1999. Learning enhances adult neurogenesis in the hippocampal formation. *Nat Neurosci.* 2(3):260–265.

Gould E. 2007. How widespread is adult neurogenesis in mammals? *Nat Rev Neurosci.* 8(6):481–488.

Hallenbeck JM. 1996. Significance of the inflammatory response in brain ischemia. *Acta Neurochir Suppl.* 66:27–31.

Harley CB, Futcher AB, Greider CW. 1990. Telomeres shorten during ageing of human fibroblasts. *Nature.* 345(6274):458–460.

Harris SG, Padilla J, Koumas L, Ray D, Phipps RP. 2002. Prostaglandins as modulators of immunity. *Trends Immunol.* 23(3):144–150.

Hashioka S, Klegeris A, Monji A et al. 2007. Antidepressants inhibit interferon-gamma-induced microglial production of IL-6 and nitric oxide. *Exp Neurol.* 206(1):33–42.

Hattiangady B, Shetty AK. 2006. Aging does not alter the number or phenotype of putative stem/progenitor cells in the neurogenic region of the hippocampus. *Neurobiol Aging.* 29(1):129–147.

Haughey NJ, Liu D, Nath A, Borchard AC, Mattson MP. 2002a. Disruption of neurogenesis in the subventricular zone of adult mice, and in human cortical neuronal precursor cells in culture, by amyloid beta-peptide: implications for the pathogenesis of Alzheimer's disease. *Neuromolecular Med.* 1(2):125–135.

Haughey NJ, Nath A, Chan SL, Borchard AC, Rao MS, Mattson MP. 2002b. Disruption of neurogenesis by amyloid beta-peptide, and perturbed neural progenitor cell homeostasis, in models of Alzheimer's disease. *J Neurochem.* 83(6):1509–1524.

Hayashi Y, Tomimatsu Y, Suzuki H et al. 2006. The intra-arterial injection of microglia protects hippocampal CA1 neurons against global ischemia-induced functional deficits in rats. *Neuroscience.* 142(1):87–96.

Heine VM, Maslam S, Joels M, Lucassen PJ. 2004. Prominent decline of newborn cell proliferation, differentiation, and apoptosis in the aging dentate gyrus, in absence of an age-related hypothalamus-pituitary-adrenal axis activation. *Neurobiol Aging.* 25(3):361–375.

Heneka MT, Landreth GE, Hull M. 2007. Drug insight: effects mediated by peroxisome proliferator-activated receptor-gamma in CNS disorders. *Nat Clin Pract Neurol.* 3(9):496–504.

Herrup K, Yang Y. 2007. Cell cycle regulation in the postmitotic neuron: oxymoron or new biology? *Nat Rev Neurosci.* 8(5):368–378.

Hoehn BD, Palmer TD, Steinberg GK. 2005. Neurogenesis in rats after focal cerebral ischemia is enhanced by indomethacin. *Stroke.* 36(12):2718–2724.

Huang Y, Henry CJ, Dantzer R, Johnson RW, Godbout JP. 2007. Exaggerated sickness behavior and brain proinflammatory cytokine expression in aged mice in response to intracerebroventricular lipopolysaccharide. *Neurobiol Aging.* [Epub ahead of print.]

Hughes PM, Botham MS, Frentzel S, Mir A, Perry VH. 2002. Expression of fractalkine (CX3CL1) and its receptor, CX3CR1, during acute and chronic inflammation in the rodent CNS. *Glia.* 37(4):314–327.

Jakubs K, Nanobashvili A, Bonde S et al. 2006. Environment matters: synaptic properties of neurons born in the epileptic adult brain develop to reduce excitability. *Neuron.* 52(6):1047–1059.

Jessberger S, Zhao C, Toni N, Clemenson GD Jr., Li Y, Gage FH. 2007. Seizure-associated, aberrant neurogenesis in adult rats characterized with retrovirus-mediated cell labeling. *J Neurosci.* 27(35):9400–9407.

Jin K, Sun Y, Xie L et al. 2003. Neurogenesis and aging: FGF-2 and HB-EGF restore neurogenesis in hippocampus and subventricular zone of aged mice. *Aging Cell.* 2(3):175–183.

Jin K, Galvan V, Xie L et al. 2004a. Enhanced neurogenesis in Alzheimer's disease transgenic (PDGF-APPSw,Ind) mice. *Proc Natl Acad Sci U S A.* 101(36):13363–13367.

Jin K, Minami M, Xie L et al. 2004b. Ischemia-induced neurogenesis is preserved but reduced in the aged rodent brain. *Aging Cell.* 3(6):373–377.

Jin K, Peel AL, Mao XO et al. 2004c. Increased hippocampal neurogenesis in Alzheimer's disease. *Proc Natl Acad Sci U S A.* 101(1):343–347.

Jin K, Wang X, Xie L et al. 2006. Evidence for stroke-induced neurogenesis in the human brain. *Proc Natl Acad Sci U S A.* 103(35):13198–13202.

Johansson CB, Svensson M, Wallstedt L, Janson AM, Frisen J. 1999. Neural stem cells in the adult human brain. *Exp Cell Res.* 253(2):733–736.

Kee N, Sivalingam S, Boonstra R, Wojtowicz JM. 2002. The utility of Ki-67 and BrdU as proliferative markers of adult neurogenesis. *J Neurosci Methods.* 115(1):97–105.

Kempermann G, Kuhn HG, Gage FH. 1998. Experience-induced neurogenesis in the senescent dentate gyrus. *J Neurosci.* 18(9):3206–3212.

Kempermann G. 2006. They are not too excited: the possible role of adult-born neurons in epilepsy. *Neuron.* 52(6):935–937.

Klegeris A, McGeer EG, McGeer PL. 2007. Therapeutic approaches to inflammation in neurodegenerative disease. *Curr Opin Neurol.* 20(3):351–357.

Kluska MM, Witte OW, Bolz J, Redecker C. 2005. Neurogenesis in the adult dentate gyrus after cortical infarcts: effects of infarct location, N-methyl-D-aspartate receptor blockade and anti-inflammatory treatment. *Neuroscience.* 135(3):723–735.

Kokaia Z, Lindvall O. 2003. Neurogenesis after ischaemic brain insults. *Curr Opin Neurobiol.* 13(1):127–132.

Kreutzberg GW. 1996. Microglia: a sensor for pathological events in the CNS. *Trends Neurosci.* 19(8):312–318.

Kuhn HG, Dickinson-Anson H, Gage FH. 1996. Neurogenesis in the dentate gyrus of the adult rat: age-related decrease of neuronal progenitor proliferation. *J Neurosci.* 16(6):2027–2033.

Kukekov VG, Laywell ED, Suslov O et al. 1999. Multipotent stem/progenitor cells with similar properties arise from two neurogenic regions of adult human brain. *Exp Neurol.* 156(2):333–344.

Kullberg S, Aldskogius H, Ulfhake B. 2001. Microglial activation, emergence of ED1-expressing cells and clusterin upregulation in the aging rat CNS, with special reference to the spinal cord. *Brain Res.* 899(1–2):169–186.

Kumihashi K, Uchida K, Miyazaki H, Kobayashi J, Tsushima T, Machida T. 2001. Acetylsalicylic acid reduces ischemia-induced proliferation of dentate cells in gerbils. *Neuroreport.* 12(5):915–917.

Lalancette-Hebert M, Gowing G, Simard A, Weng YC, Kriz J. 2007. Selective ablation of proliferating microglial cells exacerbates ischemic injury in the brain. *J Neurosci.* 27(10):2596–2605.

Lawson LJ, Perry VH, Dri P, Gordon S. 1990. Heterogeneity in the distribution and morphology of microglia in the normal adult mouse brain. *Neuroscience.* 39(1):151–170.

Lawson LJ, Perry VH, Gordon S. 1992. Turnover of resident microglia in the normal adult mouse brain. *Neuroscience.* 48(2):405–415.

Laywell ED, Rakic P, Kukekov VG, Holland EC, Steindler DA. 2000. Identification of a multipotent astrocytic stem cell in the immature and adult mouse brain. *Proc Natl Acad Sci U S A.* 97(25):13883–13888.

Lee CK, Weindruch R, Prolla TA. 2000. Gene-expression profile of the ageing brain in mice. *Nat Genet.* 25(3):294–297.

Lehnardt S, Massillon L, Follett P et al. 2003. Activation of innate immunity in the CNS triggers neurodegeneration through a Toll-like receptor 4-dependent pathway. *Proc Natl Acad Sci U S A.* 100(14):8514–8519.

Leventhal C, Rafii S, Rafii D, Shahar A, Goldman SA. 1999. Endothelial trophic support of neuronal production and recruitment from the adult mammalian subependyma. *Mol Cell Neurosci.* 13(6):450–464.

Leviton A, Gressens P. 2007. Neuronal damage accompanies perinatal white-matter damage. *Trends Neurosci.* 30(9):473–478.

Licastro F, Veglia F, Chiappelli M, Grimaldi LM, Masliah E. 2004. A polymorphism of the interleukin-1 beta gene at position +3953 influences progression and neuro-pathological hallmarks of Alzheimer's disease. *Neurobiol Aging.* 25(8):1017–1022.

Lio D, Annoni G, Licastro F et al. 2006. Tumor necrosis factor-alpha -308A/G polymorphism is associated with age at onset of Alzheimer's disease. *Mech Ageing Dev.* 127(6):567–571.

Liu YP, Lin HI, Tzeng SF. 2005. Tumor necrosis factor-alpha and interleukin-18 modulate neuronal cell fate in embryonic neural progenitor culture. *Brain Res.* 1054(2):152–158.

Liu Z, Fan Y, Won SJ et al. 2007. Chronic treatment with minocycline preserves adult new neurons and reduces functional impairment after focal cerebral ischemia. *Stroke.* 38(1):146–152.

Louissaint A Jr, Rao S, Leventhal C, Goldman SA. 2002. Coordinated interaction of neurogenesis and angiogenesis in the adult songbird brain. *Neuron.* 34(6):945–960.

Macas J, Nern C, Plate KH, Momma S. 2006. Increased generation of neuronal progenitors after ischemic injury in the aged adult human forebrain. *J Neurosci.* 26(50):13114–13119.

Magnus T, Schreiner B, Korn T et al. 2005. Microglial expression of the B7 family member B7 homolog 1 confers strong immune inhibition: implications for immune responses and autoimmunity in the CNS. *J Neurosci.* 25(10):2537–2546.

McGeer PL, McGeer EG. 2001. Inflammation, autotoxicity and Alzheimer disease. *Neurobiol Aging.* 22(6):799–809.

Meinl E, Aloisi F, Ertl B et al. 1994. Multiple sclerosis. Immunomodulatory effects of human astrocytes on T cells. *Brain.* 117 (Pt 6):1323–1332.

Merkle FT, Mirzadeh Z, Alvarez-Buylla A. 2007. Mosaic organization of neural stem cells in the adult brain. *Science.* 317(5836):381–384.

Minghetti L, Ajmone-Cat MA, De Berardinis MA, De Simone R. 2005. Microglial activation in chronic neurodegenerative diseases: roles of apoptotic neurons and chronic stimulation. *Brain Res Brain Res Rev.* 48(2):251–256.

Minghetti L. 2007. Role of COX-2 in inflammatory and degenerative brain diseases. *Subcell Biochem.* 42:127–141.

Mirescu C, Gould E. 2006. Stress and adult neurogenesis. *Hippocampus.* 16(3):233–8.

Monje ML, Mizumatsu S, Fike JR, Palmer TD. 2002. Irradiation induces neural precursor-cell dysfunction. *Nat Med.* 8(9):955–962.

Monje ML, Toda H, Palmer TD. 2003. Inflammatory blockade restores adult hippocampal neurogenesis. *Science.* 302(5651):1760–1765.

Morgan TE, Xie Z, Goldsmith S et al. 1999. The mosaic of brain glial hyperactivity during normal ageing and its attenuation by food restriction. *Neuroscience.* 89(3):687–699.

Mrak RE, Griffin WS. 2005. Glia and their cytokines in progression of neurodegeneration. *Neurobiol Aging.* 26(3):349–354.

Muir KW, Tyrrell P, Sattar N, Warburton E. 2007. Inflammation and ischaemic stroke. *Curr Opin Neurol.* 20(3):334–342.

Murphy C, Gilmore MM, Seery CS, Salmon DP, Lasker BR. 1990. Olfactory thresholds are associated with degree of dementia in Alzheimer's disease. *Neurobiol Aging.* 11(4):465–469.

Nakatomi H, Kuriu T, Okabe S et al. 2002. Regeneration of hippocampal pyramidal neurons after ischemic brain injury by recruitment of endogenous neural progenitors. *Cell.* 110(4):429–441.

Nathan C. 2002. Points of control in inflammation. *Nature.* 420(6917):846–852.

Neumann H, Misgeld T, Matsumuro K, Wekerle H. 1998. Neurotrophins inhibit major histocompatibility class II inducibility of microglia: involvement of the p75 neurotrophin receptor. *Proc Natl Acad Sci U S A.* 95(10):5779–5784.

Neumann H. 2006. Microglia: a cellular vehicle for CNS gene therapy. *J Clin Invest.* 116(11):2857–2860.

Nighoghossian N, Wiart M, Cakmak S et al. 2007. Inflammatory response after ischemic stroke: a USPIO-enhanced MRI study in patients. *Stroke.* 38(2):303–307.

Nilsson LN, Bales KR, DiCarlo G et al. 2001. Alpha-1-antichymotrypsin promotes beta-sheet amyloid plaque deposition in a transgenic mouse model of Alzheimer's disease. *J Neurosci.* 21(5):1444–1451.

Nimmerjahn A, Kirchhoff F, Helmchen F. 2005. Resting microglial cells are highly dynamic surveillants of brain parenchyma in vivo. *Science.* 308(5726):1314–1318.

Nolan Y, Maher FO, Martin DS et al. 2005. Role of interleukin-4 in regulation of age-related inflammatory changes in the hippocampus. *J Biol Chem.* 280(10):9354–9362.

Nunes MC, Roy NS, Keyoung HM et al. 2003. Identification and isolation of multipotential neural progenitor cells from the subcortical white matter of the adult human brain. *Nat Med.* 9(4):439–447.

Obuchowicz E, Kowalski J, Labuzek K, Krysiak R, Pendzich J, Herman ZS. 2006. Amitriptyline and nortriptyline inhibit interleukin-1 release by rat mixed glial and microglial cell cultures. *Int J Neuropsychopharmacol.* 9(1):27–35.

Offner H, Subramanian S, Parker SM, Afentoulis ME, Vandenbark AA, Hurn PD. 2006. Experimental stroke induces massive, rapid activation of the peripheral immune system. *J Cereb Blood Flow Metab.* 26(5):654–665.

Ogura K, Ogawa M, Yoshida M. 1994. Effects of ageing on microglia in the normal rat brain: immunohistochemical observations. *Neuroreport.* 5(10):1224–1226.

Ohta H, Terao Y, Shintani Y, Kiyota Y. 2007. Therapeutic time window of post-ischemic mild hypothermia and the gene expression associated with the neuroprotection in rat focal cerebral ischemia. *Neurosci Res.* 57(3):424–433.

Palmer TD, Willhoite AR, Gage FH. 2000. Vascular niche for adult hippocampal neurogenesis. *J Comp Neurol.* 425(4):479–494.

Palmer TD. 2002. Adult neurogenesis and the vascular Nietzsche. *Neuron.* 34(6):856–858.

Pardo CA, Vargas DL, Zimmerman AW. 2005. Immunity, neuroglia and neuroinflammation in autism. *Int Rev Psychiatry.* 17(6):485–495.

Parent JM, Yu TW, Leibowitz RT, Geschwind DH, Sloviter RS, Lowenstein DH. 1997. Dentate granule cell neurogenesis is increased by seizures and contributes to aberrant network reorganization in the adult rat hippocampus. *J Neurosci.* 17(10):3727–3738.

Parent JM, Valentin VV, Lowenstein DH. 2002. Prolonged seizures increase proliferating neuroblasts in the adult rat subventricular zone-olfactory bulb pathway. *J Neurosci.* 22(8):3174–3188.

Parent JM, Elliott RC, Pleasure SJ, Barbaro NM, Lowenstein DH. 2006. Aberrant seizure-induced neurogenesis in experimental temporal lobe epilepsy. *Ann Neurol.* 59(1):81–91.

Perry VH, Matyszak MK, Fearn S. 1993. Altered antigen expression of microglia in the aged rodent CNS. *Glia.* 7(1):60–67.

Perry VH, Cunningham C, Boche D. 2002. Atypical inflammation in the central nervous system in prion disease. *Curr Opin Neurol.* 15(3):349–354.

Perry VH. 2004. The influence of systemic inflammation on inflammation in the brain: implications for chronic neurodegenerative disease. *Brain Behav Immun.* 18(5):407–413.

Perry VH, Cunningham C, Holmes C. 2007. Systemic infections and inflammation affect chronic neurodegeneration. *Nat Rev Immunol.* 7(2):161–167.

Popa-Wagner A, Carmichael ST, Kokaia Z, Kessler C, Walker LC. 2007. The response of the aged brain to stroke: too much, too soon? *Curr Neurovasc Res.* 4(3):216–227.

Price CJ, Warburton EA, Menon DK. 2003. Human cellular inflammation in the pathology of acute cerebral ischaemia. *J Neurol Neurosurg Psychiatry.* 74(11):1476–1484.

Price CJ, Menon DK, Peters AM et al. 2004. Cerebral neutrophil recruitment, histology, and outcome in acute ischemic stroke: an imaging-based study. *Stroke.* 35(7):1659–1664.

Price CJ, Wang D, Menon DK et al. 2006. Intrinsic activated microglia map to the peri-infarct zone in the subacute phase of ischemic stroke. *Stroke.* 37(7):1749–1753.

Priller J, Flugel A, Wehner T et al. 2001. Targeting gene-modified hematopoietic cells to the central nervous system: use of green fluorescent protein uncovers microglial engraftment. *Nat Med.* 7(12):1356–1361.

Rahpeymai Y, Hietala MA, Wilhelmsson U et al. 2006. Complement: a novel factor in basal and ischemia-induced neurogenesis. *EMBO J.* 25(6):1364–1374.

Rainero I, Bo M, Ferrero M, Valfre W, Vaula G, Pinessi L. 2004. Association between the interleukin-1alpha gene and Alzheimer's disease: a meta-analysis. *Neurobiol Aging.* 25(10):1293–1298.

Rainsford KD. 2007. Anti-inflammatory drugs in the 21st century. *Subcell Biochem.* 42:3–27.

Ravaglia G, Paola F, Maioli F et al. 2006. Interleukin-1beta and interleukin-6 gene polymorphisms as risk factors for AD: a prospective study. *Exp Gerontol.* 41(1):85–92.

Reichman HR, Farrell CL, Del Maestro RF. 1986. Effects of steroids and nonsteroid anti-inflammatory agents on vascular permeability in a rat glioma model. *J Neurosurg.* 65(2):233–237.

Reines SA, Block GA, Morris JC et al. 2004. Rofecoxib: no effect on Alzheimer's disease in a 1-year, randomized, blinded, controlled study. *Neurology.* 62(1):66–71.

Rochefort C, Gheusi G, Vincent JD, Lledo PM. 2002. Enriched odor exposure increases the number of newborn neurons in the adult olfactory bulb and improves odor memory. *J Neurosci.* 22(7):2679–2689.

Rogers J, Strohmeyer R, Kovelowski CJ, Li R. 2002. Microglia and inflammatory mechanisms in the clearance of amyloid beta peptide. *Glia.* 40(2):260–269.

Roy NS, Benraiss A, Wang S et al. 2000. Promoter-targeted selection and isolation of neural progenitor cells from the adult human ventricular zone. *J Neurosci Res.* 59(3):321–331.

Sadowski M, Wisniewski T. 2004. Vaccines for conformational disorders. *Expert Rev Vaccines.* 3(3):279–290.

Saleh A, Schroeter M, Jonkmanns C, Hartung HP, Modder U, Jander S. 2004. In vivo MRI of brain inflammation in human ischaemic stroke. *Brain.* 127(Pt 7):1670–1677.

Saleh A, Schroeter M, Ringelstein A et al. 2007. Iron oxide particle-enhanced MRI suggests variability of brain inflammation at early stages after ischemic stroke. *Stroke.* 38(10):2733–2737.

Sanai N, Tramontin AD, Quinones-Hinojosa A et al. 2004. Unique astrocyte ribbon in adult human brain contains neural stem cells but lacks chain migration. *Nature.* 427(6976):740–744.

Santarelli L, Saxe M, Gross C et al. 2003. Requirement of hippocampal neurogenesis for the behavioral effects of antidepressants. *Science.* 301(5634):805–809.

Sasaki T, Kitagawa K, Sugiura S et al. 2003. Implication of cyclooxygenase-2 on enhanced proliferation of neural progenitor cells in the adult mouse hippocampus after ischemia. *J Neurosci Res.* 72(4):461–471.

Sato K, Hayashi T, Sasaki C et al. 2001. Temporal and spatial differences of PSA-NCAM expression between young-adult and aged rats in normal and ischemic brains. *Brain Res.* 922(1):135–139.

Scharfman HE, Sollas AL, Goodman JH. 2002. Spontaneous recurrent seizures after pilocarpine-induced status epilepticus activate calbindin-immunoreactive hilar cells of the rat dentate gyrus. *Neuroscience.* 111(1):71–81.

Scharfman HE. 2004. Functional implications of seizure-induced neurogenesis. *Adv Exp Med Biol.* 548:192–212.

Schenk D, Barbour R, Dunn W et al. 1999. Immunization with amyloid-beta attenuates Alzheimer-disease-like pathology in the PDAPP mouse. *Nature.* 400(6740):173–177.

Schilling M, Besselmann M, Leonhard C, Mueller M, Ringelstein EB, Kiefer R. 2003. Microglial activation precedes and predominates over macrophage infiltration in transient focal cerebral ischemia: a study in green fluorescent protein transgenic bone marrow chimeric mice. *Exp Neurol.* 183(1):25–33.

Schroeter M, Jander S, Huitinga I, Witte OW, Stoll G. 1997. Phagocytic response in photochemically induced infarction of rat cerebral cortex. The role of resident microglia. *Stroke.* 28(2):382–386.

Schwartz M, Kipnis J. 2005. Protective autoimmunity and neuroprotection in inflammatory and noninflammatory neurodegenerative diseases. *J Neurol Sci.* 233(1–2):163–166.

Schwartz M, Butovsky O, Bruck W, Hanisch UK. 2006. Microglial phenotype: is the commitment reversible? *Trends Neurosci.* 29(2):68–74.

Shen Q, Goderie SK, Jin L et al. 2004. Endothelial cells stimulate self-renewal and expand neurogenesis of neural stem cells. *Science.* 304(5675):1338–1340.

Shetty AK, Hattiangady B, Shetty GA. 2005. Stem/progenitor cell proliferation factors FGF-2, IGF-1, and VEGF exhibit early decline during the course of aging in the hippocampus: role of astrocytes. *Glia.* 51(3):173–186.

Shihabuddin LS, Horner PJ, Ray J, Gage FH. 2000. Adult spinal cord stem cells generate neurons after transplantation in the adult dentate gyrus. *J Neurosci.* 20(23):8727–8735.

Shirai Y. 1921. On the transplantation of the rat sarcoma in adult heterogenous animals. *Jap Med World.* 1:14–15.

Shors TJ, Miesegaes G, Beylin A, Zhao M, Rydel T, Gould E. 2001. Neurogenesis in the adult is involved in the formation of trace memories. *Nature.* 410(6826):372–376.

Simard AR, Soulet D, Gowing G, Julien JP, Rivest S. 2006. Bone marrow-derived microglia play a critical role in restricting senile plaque formation in Alzheimer's disease. *Neuron.* 49(4):489–502.

Song H, Stevens CF, Gage FH. 2002. Astroglia induce neurogenesis from adult neural stem cells. *Nature.* 417(6884):39–44.

Stewart SA, Ben-Porath I, Carey VJ, O'Connor BF, Hahn WC, Weinberg RA. 2003. Erosion of the telomeric single-strand overhang at replicative senescence. *Nat Genet.* 33(4):492–496.

Streit WJ, Sparks DL. 1997. Activation of microglia in the brains of humans with heart disease and hypercholesterolemic rabbits. *J Mol Med.* 75(2):130–138.

Streit WJ. 2004. Microglia and Alzheimer's disease pathogenesis. *J Neurosci Res.* 77(1):1–8.

Suhonen JO, Peterson DA, Ray J, Gage FH. 1996. Differentiation of adult hippocampus-derived progenitors into olfactory neurons in vivo. *Nature.* 383(6601):624–627.

Tanaka R, Komine-Kobayashi M, Mochizuki H et al. 2003. Migration of enhanced green fluorescent protein expressing bone marrow-derived microglia/macrophage into the mouse brain following permanent focal ischemia. *Neuroscience.* 117(3):531–539.

Tanapat P, Galea LA, Gould E. 1998. Stress inhibits the proliferation of granule cell precursors in the developing dentate gyrus. *Int J Dev Neurosci.* 16(3–4):235–239.

Thored P, Arvidsson A, Cacci E et al. 2006. Persistent production of neurons from adult brain stem cells during recovery after stroke. *Stem Cells.* 24(3):739–747.

Togo T, Akiyama H, Kondo H et al. 2000. Expression of CD40 in the brain of Alzheimer's disease and other neurological diseases. *Brain Res.* 885(1):117–121.

Town T, Nikolic V, Tan J. 2005. The microglial "activation" continuum: from innate to adaptive responses. *J Neuroinflammation.* 2:24.

Townsend KP, Town T, Mori T et al. 2005. CD40 signaling regulates innate and adaptive activation of microglia in response to amyloid beta-peptide. *Eur J Immunol.* 35(3):901–910.

Vallières L, Campbell IL, Gage FH, Sawchenko PE. 2002. Reduced hippocampal neurogenesis in adult transgenic mice with chronic astrocytic production of interleukin-6. *J Neurosci.* 22(2):486–492.

van Beek J, Elward K, Gasque P. 2003. Activation of complement in the central nervous system: roles in neurodegeneration and neuroprotection. *Ann N Y Acad Sci.* 992:56–71.

van der Worp HB, Sena ES, Donnan GA, Howells DW, Macleod MR. 2007. Hypothermia in animal models of acute ischaemic stroke: a systematic review and meta-analysis. *Brain.* 130(12):3063–3074.

van Praag H, Christie BR, Sejnowski TJ, Gage FH. 1999a. Running enhances neurogenesis, learning, and long-term potentiation in mice. *Proc Natl Acad Sci U S A.* 96(23):13427–13431.

van Praag H, Kempermann G, Gage FH. 1999b. Running increases cell proliferation and neurogenesis in the adult mouse dentate gyrus. *Nat Neurosci.* 2(3):266–270.

van Praag H, Schinder AF, Christie BR, Toni N, Palmer TD, Gage FH. 2002. Functional neurogenesis in the adult hippocampus. *Nature.* 415(6875):1030–1034.

Vargas DL, Nascimbene C, Krishnan C, Zimmerman AW, Pardo CA. 2005. Neuroglial activation and neuroinflammation in the brain of patients with autism. *Ann Neurol.* 57(1):67–81.

Veerhuis R, Van Breemen MJ, Hoozemans JM et al. 2003. Amyloid beta plaque-associated proteins C1q and SAP enhance the Abeta1–42 peptide-induced cytokine secretion by adult human microglia in vitro. *Acta Neuropathol. (Berl).* 105(2):135–144.

Villa A, Navarro-Galve B, Bueno C, Franco S, Blasco MA, Martinez-Serrano A. 2004. Long-term molecular and cellular stability of human neural stem cell lines. *Exp Cell Res.* 294(2):559–570.

Walton NM, Sutter BM, Laywell ED et al. 2006. Microglia instruct subventricular zone neurogenesis. *Glia.* 54(8):815–825.

Wang Q, Tang XN, Yenari MA. 2007. The inflammatory response in stroke. *J Neuroimmunol.* 184(1–2):53–68.

Wang R, Dineley KT, Sweatt JD, Zheng H. 2004. Presenilin 1 familial Alzheimer's disease mutation leads to defective associative learning and impaired adult neurogenesis. *Neuroscience.* 126(2):305–312.

Wen PH, Hof PR, Chen X et al. 2004. The presenilin-1 familial Alzheimer disease mutant P117L impairs neurogenesis in the hippocampus of adult mice. *Exp Neurol.* 188(2):224–237.

West MA, Heagy W. 2002. Endotoxin tolerance: a review. *Crit Care Med.* 30(Suppl 1) S64–S73.

Wilcock DM, Munireddy SK, Rosenthal A, Ugen KE, Gordon MN, Morgan D. 2004. Microglial activation facilitates Abeta plaque removal following intracranial anti-Abeta antibody administration. *Neurobiol Dis.* 15(1):11–20.

Wood PL. 1995. Microglia as a unique cellular target in the treatment of stroke: potential neurotoxic mediators produced by activated microglia. *Neurol Res.* 17(4):242–248.

Wright GJ, Puklavec MJ, Willis AC et al. 2000. Lymphoid/neuronal cell surface OX2 glycoprotein recognizes a novel receptor on macrophages implicated in the control of their function. *Immunity.* 13(2):233–242.

Wurmser AE, Palmer TD, Gage FH. 2004. Neuroscience. Cellular interactions in the stem cell niche. *Science.* 304(5675):1253–1255.

Wyss-Coray T, Yan F, Lin AH et al. 2002. Prominent neurodegeneration and increased plaque formation in complement-inhibited Alzheimer's mice. *Proc Natl Acad Sci U S A.* 99(16):10837–10842.

Xie Z, Morgan TE, Rozovsky I, Finch CE. 2003. Aging and glial responses to lipopolysaccharide in vitro: greater induction of IL-1 and IL-6, but smaller induction of neurotoxicity. *Exp Neurol.* 182(1):135–141.

Yagita Y, Kitagawa K, Ohtsuki T et al. 2001. Neurogenesis by progenitor cells in the ischemic adult rat hippocampus. *Stroke.* 32(8):1890–1896.

Yamashita T, Ninomiya M, Hernandez Acosta P et al. 2006. Subventricular zone-derived neuroblasts migrate and differentiate into mature neurons in the post-stroke adult striatum. *J Neurosci.* 26(24):6627–6636.

Ye SM, Johnson RW. 1999. Increased interleukin-6 expression by microglia from brain of aged mice. *J Neuroimmunol.* 93(1–2):139–148.

Ye SM, Johnson RW. 2001. An age-related decline in interleukin-10 may contribute to the increased expression of interleukin-6 in brain of aged mice. *Neuroimmunomodulation.* 9(4):183–192.

Yrjanheikki J, Keinanen R, Pellikka M, Hokfelt T, Koistinaho J. 1998. Tetracyclines inhibit microglial activation and are neuroprotective in global brain ischemia. *Proc Natl Acad Sci U S A.* 95(26):15769–15774.

Yrjanheikki J, Tikka T, Keinanen R, Goldsteins G, Chan PH, Koistinaho J. 1999. A tetracycline derivative, minocycline, reduces inflammation and protects against focal cerebral ischemia with a wide therapeutic window. *Proc Natl Acad Sci U S A.* 96(23):13496–13500.

Zhang C, McNeil E, Dressler L, Siman R. 2007. Long-lasting impairment in hippocampal neurogenesis associated with amyloid deposition in a knock-in mouse model of familial Alzheimer's disease. *Exp Neurol.* 204(1):77–87.

Zhang N, Komine-Kobayashi M, Tanaka R, Liu M, Mizuno Y, Urabe T. 2005. Edaravone reduces early accumulation of oxidative products and sequential inflammatory responses after transient focal ischemia in mice brain. *Stroke*. 36(10):2220–2225.

Zhang Z, Chopp M, Powers C. 1997. Temporal profile of microglial response following transient (2 h) middle cerebral artery occlusion. *Brain Res*. 744(2):189–198.

Zhao BQ, Tejima E, Lo EH. 2007. Neurovascular proteases in brain injury, hemorrhage and remodeling after stroke. *Stroke*. 38(Suppl 2):748–752.

Zheng Z, Yenari MA. 2004. Post-ischemic inflammation: molecular mechanisms and therapeutic implications. *Neurol Res*. 26(8):884–892.

Ziabreva I, Perry E, Perry R et al. 2006. Altered neurogenesis in Alzheimer's disease. *J Psychosom Res*. 61(3):311–316.

Ziv Y, Ron N, Butovsky O et al. 2006. Immune cells contribute to the maintenance of neurogenesis and spatial learning abilities in adulthood. *Nat Neurosci*. 9(2):268–275.

Chapter *14*

IMMUNOMODULATION IN THE NERVOUS AND VASCULAR SYSTEMS DURING INFLAMMATION AND AUTOIMMUNITY: THE ROLE OF T REGULATORY CELLS

Kokona Chatzantoni and Athanasia Mouzaki

ABSTRACT

Because the human body is an ideal habitat for microbes, it confronts a large variety of invading organisms such as bacteria, viruses, fungi, and parasites. The immune system, a system that nears the complexity of the nervous system, has evolved to bar the entry of such microbes, or detect and destroy them in case of infection.

The immune system is characterized by a complex network of cells and organs specialized to extinguish foreign invaders or malfunctioning cells of the organism. Its ability to not only distinguish between self and nonself but also remember previous experiences and react accordingly provides for an enormous amount of diversity and specificity of function.

In order for this complicated function to be effective, a dynamic regulatory communication network is necessary. This necessity appears not only during ontogeny within the thymus but also later in the periphery. Without regulation, such a complex system could lead to problems such as inflammation, autoimmunity, oversensitivity, and general functional destabilization.

Although innate immunity, B-cell function via antibody responses, and cytotoxic T lymphocytes are very important for protection of the body, T cells play a central role in the immune system and are more important for its regulation.

In this chapter, T-cell regulation within the immune system is analytically discussed. Central and peripheral tolerance mechanisms of positive and negative selection, anergy and deletion, are described, together with a detailed analysis of regulatory T-cell types and function. Immunomodulation in the nervous and vascular systems during inflammation and autoimmunity is then discussed using the paradigms of two complex pathological conditions: multiple sclerosis and atherosclerosis. The role of T cells and T regulatory cells in breaking or maintaining tolerance is underlined, together with an appraisal of the proposed ways of their therapeutic manipulations to ameliorate disease progression.

Keywords: immune regulation, T regulatory cells, multiple sclerosis, atherosclerosis.

IMMUNOREGULATION OF THE IMMUNE SYSTEM

Among T cells, T helper cells (Th) play the most important role in immune regulation. In order to sustain the large diversity of T-cell receptors (TCRs) that characterizes these components of the immune system, as well as the system's effectiveness, T cells go through a maturation process during ontogeny in the thymus, as well as in the periphery, to control self-reactive T-cell formation and development. The control of self-reactive T cells that occurs within the thymus is known as *central tolerance*, while the regulatory mechanisms in the periphery that control self-reactive T cells that have escaped central tolerance are referred to as *peripheral tolerance*.

Central Tolerance

Hemopoietic precursors migrate from the bone marrow to the thymus through an ordered process regulated by chemokines. At the thymus, precursor cells are directed toward the random development of numerous types of TCRs that are able to recognize almost any peptide epitope presented by an antigen-presenting cell (APC) through the major histocompatibility complex (MHC) (Fig. 14.1) (Annunziato, Romagnani, Cosmi et al. 2001).

Positive Selection

The first step of T-cell regulation and selection occurs during T-cell maturation in the thymic cortex. MHC–peptide complexes are presented through APCs in the thymic cortex to double-positive CD4+CD8+ thymocytes. Less than 5% of these thymocytes has the necessary affinity for these complexes and is able to survive, be positively selected, and migrate to the medullary areas of the thymus, where they differentiate to single-positive CD4+ or CD8+ thymocytes. Those thymocytes that do not have the appropriate affinity for the peptide–MHC complex are not positively selected and die of neglect (Starr, Jameson, Hogquist 2003).

Negative Selection

The thymocytes that are positively selected go through a second level of selection called *negative selection*. These cells carry an enormous variety of TCRs that are able to recognize almost every exogenous peptide that will be encountered; they also carry receptors that are able to react with self-peptides. The elimination of

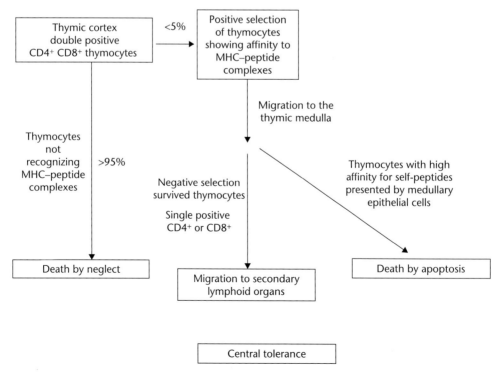

Figure 14.1 Central tolerance. MHC, major histocompatibility complex.

cells that have the capacity to recognize self-peptides occurs as a result of negative selection. MHC–self-peptide complexes are presented to these cells on the surface of medullary epithelial cells. The thymocytes that show a relatively high avidity for these complexes undergo apoptotic death. Only 3% of the T-cell precursors survive both positive and negative selection.

These cells then migrate to the secondary lymphoid organs in the periphery, where they bind to foreign peptides although they have the ability to bind to self-peptides with low avidity (Starr, Jameson, Hogquist 2003; Kyewski, Derbinski 2004).

Peripheral Tolerance

Not all self-reactive T cells can be deleted during thymic maturation; autoreactive mature T cells are present in secondary lymphoid organs and must therefore be regulated to avoid the development of an autoimmune response (Romagnani 2006). Three main pathways of peripheral self-tolerance are known thus far:

1. Anergy: Anergy occurs when the antigen-presentation process takes place through a nonprofessional APC—a cell that has the correct MHC formulation for the TCR to recognize the presented peptide but lacks the costimulatory molecules CD80 and CD86. Therefore, the correct activation signal that should be provided through the CD28 molecule is not available. A T cell that goes through such a process cannot be activated and loses the ability of being correctly activated when it encounters the same peptide through a proper presentation process. Cells that are anergized do not die but persist as functionally inactive effector cells (Powell 2006).

2. Deletion: When T cells encounter a very high dose of antigen and are strongly activated, they express Fas and FasL on their surface; this leads to the activation of the caspase enzyme cascade and, finally, to the deletion of the T cells through a process called *activation-induced cell death* (Worth, Thrasher, Gaspar 2006).

3. Immune suppression by T regulatory cells: Although the mechanisms mentioned in the preceding text are essential for the survival of an organism, they are imperfect, and autoreactive T cells can still be found in the periphery. To keep these potentially harmful T cells under control, the immune system develops a form of dominant tolerance that involves regulatory T cells (Tregs). Tregs refers to a specialized group of T cells that suppresses the activation of other cells of the immune system to maintain self-tolerance; they also control excessive responses to foreign antigens (Le, Chao 2007).

The molecular characterization of Tregs has led to the identification of many populations with immunosuppressive capabilities (Table 14.1). The main population of Tregs characterized so far is natural Tregs, which are $CD4^+$ T cells that arise in the thymus during thymic development and constitutively express the CD25 cell marker. Another major group of Tregs is the inducible Tregs, which can be induced in the periphery from naive T cells. Inducible Tregs are subdivided into two major populations: (1) Th3 cells, which have a main role in oral tolerance through the secretion of transforming growth factor β (TGF-β), and (2) Tr1 cells, which are similar to Th3 cells but secrete IL-10 and play a major role in controlling autoimmunity (Chen, Kuchroo, Inobe et al. 1994; Levings, Sangregorio, Galbiati et al. 2001; Barrat, Cua, Boonstra et al. 2002). Other T-cell populations have also been characterized as having an immunosuppressive role. These include $CD8^+$ Tregs and natural killer (NK) Tregs, which have been shown to possess a role in controlling autoimmunity and transplantation tolerance (Zhou, Carr, Liwski et al. 2001; Seino, Fukao, Muramoto et al. 2001; Gilliet, Liu 2002; Scalzo, Magdalena Plebanski, Apostolopoulos 2006).

Natural Tregs

Natural Tregs are thought to originate from a group of thymocytes that recognizes self-antigens with avidities between the lower end of the negative selection spectrum and the higher end of the positively selected cells (Schwartz 2005). $CD4^+$ Tregs constitutively express a number of cell markers that are associated with the activation or memory phase of these cells. These markers mainly include CD25, $CD45RB_{low}$, CD62L, and CTLA-4 or CD152, as well as GITR. The usefulness of these markers depends on the level of their expression, since they are not uniquely expressed on natural Tregs. The definition of the Treg population was based on the expression of CD4 and CD25 until Foxp3, the forkhead family transcription factor, was identified. The identification of this factor has proved to be critical in the development and function of Tregs (Fontenot, Rudensky 2005; Sakaguchi 2005; Ziegler 2006). Developing thymocytes with intermediate avidity for self-antigens express Foxp3 and commit to the Treg lineage (Hsieh, Liang, Tyznik et al. 2004). As previously shown, mutations in this factor result in autoimmune diseases in humans; this has also been demonstrated in animal models. Humans with such mutations and dysfunction of Foxp3 present with autoimmune diseases characterized by immune deregulation, polyendocrinopathy, and enteropathy X-linked syndrome (IPEX). Ectopic expression of this factor can convert T effector cells to Treg cells, both at the phenotypical and at the functional level (Ziegler 2006). Nevertheless, Foxp3 expression alone is not sufficient to substantiate the regulatory action of $CD4^+CD25^+$ cells, since abundant Foxp3 mRNA

Table 14.1 Regulatory T-cell Populations

Cell Type	Generation/Location	Markers	Properties and Function	References
Natural Tregs	Generated in the thymus, predominantly located in lymphoid organs, migrate toward sites of inflammation	CD4, CD25, Foxp3, CD45RB$_{low}$, CD62L, CTLA-4 or CD152, GITR, ±CD127, ±CD38	Antigen specific, secrete IL-10 and/or TGF-β, suppressive activity, inhibit effector T-cell functions, contact dependent, require CD80 and CD86 ligands on target T cells	Hsieh et al. 2004; Fontenot, Rudensky 2005; Ziegler 2006; Scalzo et al. 2006
Inducible or adaptive Tregs: (1) Tr1 (2) Th3	Generated in the periphery, migrate toward sites of inflammation	CD4, CD25, CD45RO	Target APC and T cells; prevent autoimmune colitis and inflammation of the digestive track mainly the gut, and are mainly involved in oral tolerance	Groux et al. 1997; Graca et al. 2002; Chen et al. 2003; Apostolou et al. 2004; Cottrez, Groux 2004
Tr1	From naive CD4 T cells in the presence of IL-10 and IFN-α		Secrete mainly IL-10, but also TGF-β, IL-5, and IFN-γ; do not secrete IL-2 or IL-4; inhibit Th1 and Th2 cell responses, regulate both naive and memory T cells, inhibit T-cell-mediated responses to pathogens and alloantigens and cancer; target APC	Groux et al. 1997; Foussat et al. 2003; Roncarolo et al. 2003; Scalzo et al. 2006
Th3	Through oral antigen administration		Produce mainly TGF-β but also IL-10; suppress APC and T-cells, mainly Th2	Weiner 1997; Scalzo et al. 2006
T helper 1 cells (Th1)	Generated in the periphery from Th0 or Th2 cells mainly in the presence of IL-12	CD4, CD25, STAT-4, T-bet	Produce IL-2, IFN-γ, lymphotoxin-α; target Th2 cells; activate phagocytosis, opsonization, and complement protection against intracellular antigens; responsible for autoimmunity and inflammation	Mosmann, Coffman 1989; Boom et al. 1990; Le Gros et al. 1990; Romagnani 1991, 1994, 1997; Hsieh et al. 1993
T helper 2 cells (Th2)	Generated in the periphery from Th0 cells or Th1 mainly in the presence of IL-4	CD4, CD25, STAT-6, GATA-3, c-maf	Secrete IL-4, IL-5, IL-9, IL-13; target Th1 cells; induce B-cell function and eosinophil activation; participate in allergic disorders	Abbas et al. 1996; Annunziato et al. 2001; Smits et al. 2001; Ghoreschi et al. 2003; Szabo et al. 2003; Skapenko et al. 2004; Scalzo et al. 2006
T helper 17 cells (Th17)	Generated in the periphery from naive T cells mainly in the absence of IFN-γ, IL-4, and IL-6 and in the presence of IL-β or TNF-α; IL-23 promotes their survival	CD4	Secrete IL-17A, F, IL-6, TNF-α, IL-22; protect against extracellular microbes, responsible for autoimmune disorders, inflammation, downregulate Treg function	Ye et al. 2001; Murphy et al. 2003; Nakae et al. 2003; Langrish et al. 2005; Bettelli et al. 2006; Harrington et al. 2006; Iwakura, Ishigame 2006; Liang et al. 2006; Reinhardt et al. 2006; Tato, O'Shea 2006; Annunziato et al. 2007
CD8 regulatory T cells	Generated in the thymus and also in the periphery (?), predominantly located in lymphoid organs, migrate toward sites of inflammation	CD8, Foxp3, CD28⁻, γδ subgroup	Induction of tolerance; inhibit T cells; antigen-specific (MHC class Ib APC-dependent) subgroup and IFN-γ-secreting, nonantigen-specific subgroup; CD8gdT cells secrete IFN-γ and IL-4 and inhibit APC and Th cells	Jiang et al. 1992; Hu et al. 2004; Scalzo et al. 2006
Natural Killer T cells (NKT)	Periphery	CD3, CD56	Secrete IFN-γ and IL-4; inhibit Th1/Th2 responses and DCs; tolerogenic but also proinflammatory in different pathological conditions	Boyson et al. 2002; Scalzo et al. 2006; Godfrey, Berzins 2007; Novak et al. 2007; Nowak, Stein-Streilein 2007

APC, antigen presenting cell; DC, dendritic cell; IL, interleukin; IFN, interferon; TGF, transforming growth factor; (?), not clear.

has also been detected in activated CD4$^+$CD25$^+$ cells with no regulatory action (Seidel, Ernst, Printz et al. 2006).

CD127 (IL-7 receptor α chain) has been shown to have a reverse relationship with the suppressive function of CD4$^+$ Foxp3 T cells and is downregulated in human T cells after activation. Cells separated on the basis of CD4 and CD127 expression were shown to be anergic and to possess suppressive action compared to CD4$^+$CD25$^+$ T cells (Huster, Busch, Schiemann et al. 2004; Fuller, Hildeman, Sabbaj et al. 2005; Boettler, Panther, Bengsch et al. 2006; Liu et al. 2006a; Seddiki, Santner-Nanan, Martinson et al. 2006). Natural Tregs develop in the thymus after positive selection on cortical medullary epithelial cells (Bensinger, Bandeira, Jordan et al. 2001). The selection of CD4$^+$CD25$^+$ thymocytes requires an intermediate affinity of TCRs for self-peptides, since thymocytes with low-affinity TCRs do not yet undergo selection (Jordan, Boesteanu, Reed et al. 2001). However, a defect in this selection process contributes to the enrichment of autoreactive Tregs, as these precursors seem to be resistant to clonal deletion (van Santen, Benoist, Mathis et al. 2004; Romagnoli, Hudrisier, van Meerwijk 2005). Nevertheless, this enrichment could be due to both positive selection by self-ligands and the absence of negative selection.

Antigen specificity is required for natural Treg activation. Studies with TCR-transgenic mice specific for ovalbumin (OVA) have shown that protection from graft-versus-host-disease (GVHD) is realized only when the host T cells used for immunization recognize the antigen (Albert, Liu, Anasetti et al. 2005). Tregs also recognize pathogen antigens. Tregs from mice infected with *Schistosoma* or *Leishmania* produce IL-10 in response to the same parasite antigens but not other pathogens (Belkaid, Piccirillo, Mendez et al. 2002; Hesse, Piccirillo, Belkaid et al. 2004). In human studies of asymptomatic human immunodeficiency virus–infected individuals, CD4$^+$CD25$^+$ peripheral blood Tregs showed immunosuppressive properties in an antigen-specific way (Kinter, Hennessey, Bell et al. 2004). The same phenomenon was observed in *Helicobacter pylori*–infected patients (Raghavan, Suri-Payer, Holmgren 2004).

The in vivo suppressive activity of Tregs requires close contact with T effectors with certain antigen specificity. Tregs seem to require strong localization to parts of the body where antigenic stimulation occurs, like draining lymph nodes. Furthermore, it has been shown that suppression of activated T cells occurs when the ratio of Tregs to T effectors is one third. Since the percentage of Tregs is only 2 to 3% of total T cells, selective homing, as well as expansion, is very important for a suppressive effect to be achieved. It has been shown in animal models that cells with

suppressive potential that are not able to accumulate and proliferate in the lymph nodes cannot suppress or prevent disease (Tang, Henriksen, Bi et al. 2004; Tarbell, Yamazaki, Olson et al. 2004; Jaeckel, von Boehmer, Manns 2005). Therefore, it seems that in vivo homing and proliferation of Tregs in the lymph nodes are important for these cells to exert their suppressive activity in the early phase of the immune response. The migration of Tregs toward sites of inflammation is essential for their suppression of T effector cells, and it has been shown that activated Tregs change their homing receptors to accomplish this task (Huehn, Siegmund, Lehmann et al. 2004). It has also been demonstrated that natural Tregs are predominantly located in lymphoid organs, whereas another group of Tregs, Tr1 cells, tends to migrate toward sites of inflammation (Graca, Cobbold, Waldmann 2002; Cottrez, Groux 2004).

Antigen exposure is very important for Tregs to initiate suppressive activity. Interestingly, in vitro studies have also shown that activated Tregs can inhibit the immune response, regardless of the antigen that causes it (Thornton, Shevach 2000). Furthermore, there is strong evidence that Foxp3-transduced CD4$^+$ T cells specific for the OVA antigen are able to protect OVA-specific TCR-transgenic mice from GVHD (Albert, Liu, Anasetti et al. 2005). There seems to be antigen specificity during the activation phase and a bystander suppression phenomenon in the effector suppressor phase.

Although the exact suppression mechanism remains largely unknown, in vitro and in vivo research has shown a relative contribution of both cell-to-cell contact and soluble cytokine mechanisms. Accessory molecules such as CTLA-4 and its ligands CD80, CD86, and GITR, which are expressed on the surface of Tregs, have been implicated (Takahashi, Kuniyasu, Toda et al. 1998; Takahashi, Tagami, Yamazaki et al. 2000; Suri-Payer, Cantor 2001; Piccirillo, Letterio, Thornton et al. 2002; Shimizu, Yamazaki, Takahashi et al. 2002). In the GVHD murine model, CD4$^+$CD25$^+$ or CD4$^+$CD25$^-$ T cells were unable to inhibit the development of disease caused by effector T cells deficient in CD80 or CD86 ligands, indicating that suppression of T-cell activation functions through CD80 and CD86 molecules on activated T cells and CTLA-4 on Tregs (Paust, Lu, McCarty et al. 2004). Furthermore, studies have implicated cell surface TGF-β1 in the immunosuppressive effect of Tregs (Nakamura, Kitani, Strober 2001).

Inducible or Adaptive Tregs

Another important group of regulatory T cells includes the T cells that can be induced by naive T cells in the periphery under low doses of antigenic stimulation or in the presence of immunosuppressive cytokines like TGF-β (Chen, Jin, Hardegen et al. 2003; Apostolou von Boehmer 2004; von Boehmer 2005). There are two subgroups of inducible Tregs, Tr1 and Th3, and they cannot be separated on the basis of their phenotype. In addition, they are better characterized on the basis of the cytokines they use as mediators. Tr1 and Th3 cells are similar—Tr1 cells are characterized by their large amount of IL-10 secretion and their role in preventing autoimmune colitis (Groux, O'Garra, Bigler et al. 1997) and Th3 cells play an important role in oral tolerance through the secretion of TGF-β (Chen, Kuchroo, Inobe et al. 1994). None of these subgroups expresses Foxp3, and the suppression effect on Th1 and Th2 cells mediated by TGF-β1 and IL-10 is MHC unrestricted and antigen nonspecific (Vieira, Christensen, Minaee et al. 2004).

TR1   Tr1 cells were first identified in a murine model in which CD4[+] transgenic T cells generated Tr1 cells after repetitive stimulation by their cognate peptide in the presence of IL-10 (Groux O'Garra, Bigler et al. 1997). Tr1 cells are characterized by the secretion of large amounts of IL-10 and moderate amounts of TGF-β, IL-5, and interferon γ (IFN-γ). These cells do not secrete IL-2 or IL-4 (Groux O'Garra, Bigler et al. 1997). Although they show poor proliferative ability after polyclonal or antigen-specific stimulation, they can inhibit T-cell responses in vitro and in vivo through mechanisms similar to bystander suppression, as has been shown in the case of colitis. Tr1 cells are capable of regulating the activation of naive and memory T cells and also inhibit T-cell–mediated responses to pathogens and alloantigens, as well as cancer (Foussat, Cottrez, Brun et al. 2003; Roncarolo, Gregori, Levings 2003). Neutralizing anti-IL-10 antibodies blocks most of the immunosuppressive effects of Tr1, demonstrating the importance of IL-10 in Tr1's immunosuppressive function (Roncarolo, Bacchetta, Bordignon et al. 2001). It has also been shown that complement can play a role in Tr1 induction. Resting CD4[+] T cells treated with anti-CD3 and anti-CD46 antibodies in the presence of IL-2 resulted in the induction of Tr1 cells. CD46 is an important complement regulator that induces Tr1 through an endogenous receptor–mediated event (Kemper, Chan, Green et al. 2003). Tr1 cells have been shown to be important in controlling autoimmunity. In the case of pemphigus vulgaris, desmoglein 3–specific Tr1 cells maintained and restored natural tolerance against the pemphigus vulgaris antigen (Veldman, Hohne, Dieckmann et al. 2004). Healthy individuals carrying the pemphigus-associated human leukocyte antigen (HLA) class II allele DRB1*0402 and DQB1*0503 were found to have desmoglein 3–responsive Tr1 cells that secreted IL-10 although these cells were rarely found in patients.

Furthermore, desmoglein 3–specific Tr1 cell induction requires the presence of IL-2; these cells function mainly through IL-10 and TGF-β secretion, indicating their critical involvement in tolerance homeostasis in response to the specific antigen (Beissert, Schwarz, Schwarz 2006).

TH3   It has been shown in an experimental allergic/autoimmune encephalomyelitis (EAE) model that the oral delivery of myelin basic protein (MBP) antigen generates a T-cell population that inhibits the inflammatory reaction. This population was identified as the Th3 cell subgroup of T regulatory cells and produces high amounts of TGF-β and moderate amounts of IL-10, and has the ability to inhibit the development of autoimmunity (Weiner 1997). Anti-TGF-β monoclonal antibodies inhibit the suppressive effects of Th3 cells, indicating the importance of TGF-β in immunosuppression through Th3 cells. Th3 cells have been shown to inhibit the proliferation and cytokine production of MBP-specific Th1 clones through TGF-β. This suppression is antigen nonspecific and is mediated through TGF-β, indicating a bystander suppression–based mechanism (Weiner 1997). Furthermore, suppression of Th2, as well as Th2 clones, by Th3 cells has also been demonstrated, suggesting a unique role for this orally induced Treg population.

Th1 and Th2 Regulation

For the last 20 years, the classical concept of the immune response included two main branches of the T-cell group, Th1 and Th2 cells, based mainly on the type of cytokines produced. Th1 cells were found to produce IL-2, IFN-γ, and lymphotoxin-α, and Th2 cells were found to produce IL-4, IL-5, IL-9, and IL-13 (Mosmann, Coffman 1989; Romagnani 1991). These two cell groups also differ in the transcription factors used for their regulation. Th1 cells are regulated by transcription factors that include STAT-4 and T-bet, whereas Th2 development is regulated by factors such as STAT-6, GATA-3, and c-maf, which are also antagonistic to the transcription factors belonging to the Th1 branch (Hsieh, Macatonia, Tripp et al. 1993; Szabo, Sullivan, Peng et al. 2003). Th1 transcription factors STAT-4 and T-bet are usually activated in the presence of IL-12 or IFN-γ. IL-12 is produced by dendritic cells and IFN-γ is produced by NK cells when activation by highly conserved microbial products occurs. Th2 transcription factors are activated when IL-4, instead of IL-12 or IFN-γ, is present (Le Gros, Ben-Sasson, Seder et al. 1990). Cytokines produced by Th1 cells activate phagocytosis, opsonization, and complement protection against intracellular parasites, whereas Th2 cytokines induce mainly B-cell function and eosinophil activation (Romagnani 1994; Abbas,

Murphy, Sher et al. 1996). Currently, the Th1 branch is considered to be mainly responsible for phenomena such as autoimmunity, whereas the Th2 branch participates in allergic disorders (Romagnani 1997). A process known as *immune deviation* reflects the mutual regulation between the Th1 and Th2 responses. The presence of IL-12, IL-18, IFN-γ, and IFN-α induces the development of Th1 cells while at the same time inhibiting the development of Th2 cells. Microbial products induce the secretion of IL-12 and IFNs, leading Th2 responses toward a Th0 or Th1 type of response (Maggi, Parronchi, Manetti et al. 1992; Parronchi, De Carli, Manetti et al. 1992; Manetti, Parronchi, Giudizi et al. 1993; Kips, Brusselle, Joos et al. 1996; Lack, Bradley, Hamelmann et al. 1996; Li, Chopra, Chou et al. 1996). The presence of IL-12 is important in the polarization of immune responses, since it can shift even established Th2 responses toward a Th1 response (Annunziato, Cosmi, Manetti et al. 2001; Smits, van Rietschoten, Hilkens et al. 2001). On the other hand, the presence of IL-4 inhibits Th1-cell type development and can in turn shift established Th1 responses toward a Th2 phenotype, although the opposite phenomenon can occur just as easily (Boom, Liebster, Abbas et al. 1990; Ghoreschi, Thomas, Breit et al. 2003; Skapenko, Niedobitek, Kalden et al. 2004). Furthermore, some chemokines can interact with Th1 or Th2 cells and shift their balance in either direction, thus inducing the production of certain cytokines (Karpus, Lujacs, Kennedy et al. 1997).

Th17: Treg Antagonists?

Beyond the initially polarized forms of Th effector T cells (Th1 and Th2, as well as Th0 CD4$^+$ cells), another subset has been identified. This subset, called *Th17*, is distinct from Th1, Th2, and Th0 cells. Th17 cells secrete IL-17A, IL-17F, IL-6, and tumor necrosis factor α (TNF-α) cytokines.

Th17 cells are protective against extracellular microbes but also seem to be responsible for autoimmune disorders in mice (Annunziato, Cosmi, Santarlasci et al. 2007). Recent studies show that these cells are probably a separate lineage of Th cells and that they do not represent just another Th1 population that has undergone further differentiation (Harrington, Mangan, Weaver 2006; Reinhardt, Kang, Liang et al. 2006). When naive CD4$^+$ T cells were cultured in the presence of anti-IFN-γ monoclonal antibody, induction of Th17 population was observed. This observation was stronger with IL-4 inhibition, which is an indication of Th17 inhibition in the presence of IFN-γ and IL-4 (Reinhardt, Kang, Liang et al. 2006). The T-bet transcription factor seems to play an important role in Th1 cell differentiation, but Th17 cell growth is not influenced

by lack of T-bet (Harrington, Mangan, Weaver 2006). Furthermore, TGF-β secreted from Tregs in the presence of IL-6 was responsible for the differentiation of Th17 cells, and IL-1β or TNF-α addition significantly increased the percentage of naïve T cells that differentiated into Th17. The presence of IL-23 seems to be important for the maintenance and survival of Th17 cells, although it was not necessary for their generation (Reinhardt, Kang, Liang et al. 2006).

Th17 cells are induced through the production of IL-23 from dendritic cells and are involved in the pathogenesis of inflammatory and autoimmune diseases such as rheumatoid arthritis, systemic lupus erythematosus, and EAE (Murphy, Langrish, Chen et al. 2003; Nakae, Nambu, Sudo et al. 2003; Langrish, Chen, Blumenschein et al. 2005). Th17 cells produce IL-17 and IL-22, which is a member of the IL-10 family (Ye, Rodriguez, Kanaly et al. 2001; Tato, O'Shea 2006; Liang, Tan, Luxenberg et al. 2006). These cytokines induce fibroblasts and endothelial and epithelial cells, as well as macrophages, to produce chemokines that result in the recruitment of polymorphonuclear leukocytes and the induction of inflammation (Ye, Rodriguez, Kanaly et al. 2001). Thus, IL-17 may play a protective role against extracellular bacteria, although, under certain circumstances, inflammation is induced by macrophages through the production of IL-1, IL-6, and metalloproteinases (Cua, Sherlock, Chen et al. 2003; Park, Li, Yang et al. 2005). Th17 cells do not express Th1 or Th2 transcription factors such as T-bet or GATA-3 (Dong 2006). Therefore, clarification of the pathogenetic role of Th17 cells may provide more information on the role of other Th cell groups in protecting against different pathogens. Murine model experiments have suggested that Th17 cells are involved in autoimmune phenomena like inflammatory bowel disease and EAE. Th17 originate through the production of IL-23 by dendritic cells, which has been shown to be due to the combined activity of IL-6 and TGF-β. TGF-β is also involved in the generation of Tregs. Furthermore, there is evidence for a functional antagonism between Th17 and Foxp3 Tregs (Bettelli, Carrier, Gao et al. 2006). Since the production of Th17 cells is inhibited by IL-6, IL-4, and IFN-γ, there must be a regulatory point that separates the generation of Th17 cells, which are pathogenic and induce autoimmunity, from Foxp3 Tregs, which inhibit autoimmunity (Iwakura, Ishigame 2006).

CD8$^+$ and NK T cells (or NKT cells)

CD8$^+$ T cells have also been shown to possess immunosuppressive activity; this also results in the inhibition of EAE (Jiang, Zhang, Pernis 1992) by inhibiting Th1 encephalitogenic cells. These CD8$^+$ T cells exert their suppressive activity only after being primed during the first episode of EAE. There are indications that these cells function through the nonclassical MHC class Ib pathway, since their suppressive function can be blocked by MHC class Ib Qa-1 antibodies. Qa-1 cells have the ability to present foreign and self-peptides to CD8$^+$ T cells (Hu, Ikizawa, Lu et al. 2004).

NK T cells are innate cells that can be induced to secrete both proinflammatory and anti-inflammatory cytokines immediately on exposure to activating signals and induced to regulate an ongoing immune response, usually in conjunction with other regulatory T-cell types. NK T cells recognize glycolipid antigens presented by a monomorphic glycoprotein CD1d. Numerous works have shown that NK T cells may serve as regulatory cells in autoimmune diseases and are tolerogenic in conditions of prolonged exposure to foreign antigen (e.g., in pregnancy) (Boyson, Rybalov, Koopman et al. 2002). However, recent studies have revealed that the presence of NK T cells accelerates some inflammatory conditions, implying that their protective role against autoimmunity is not predetermined (Godfrey, Berzins 2007; Novak, Griseri, Beaudoin et al. 2007; Nowak, Stein-Streilein 2007).

AUTOIMMUNITY AND T REGULATION

On the basis of what has been previously reported in this chapter, immune tolerance as a whole is the result of a very sensitive balance between naturally arising autoreactive cells and the regulatory mechanisms that regulate these autoreactive processes. In terms of immune regulation as discussed so far, autoimmunity can be considered to be manifested by a loss of balance among these functions. This lack of balance can result from either an increase in the number or function of autoreactive cells or a decrease in the function of regulatory mechanisms, leading to autoimmunity. However, a decrease in these regulatory mechanisms can lead to immunodeficiency.

Autoimmunity targeting the nervous system has been studied extensively in animal models and human subjects (Mouzaki, Tselios, Papathanassopoulos et al. 2004; Mouzaki, Deraos, Chatzantoni 2005; Owens, Babcock, Millward et al. 2005; Boscolo, Passoni, Baldas et al. 2006; Alaedini, Okamoto, Briani et al. 2007; Cabanlit, Wills, Goines et al. 2007; Cassan, Liblau 2007; Correa, Maccioni, Rivero et al. 2007; Krishnamoorthy, Holz, Wekerle 2007; Tschernatsch, Gross, Kneifel et al. 2007; Weber, Prod'homme, Youssef et al. 2007) and a plethora of experimental and clinical observations indicate that all major types of immune cells together with cells of the central nervous system (CNS) are involved in the resulting damage to the nervous system mediated through direct cell-to-cell cytotoxicity and/or soluble mediators that include cytokines, chemokines, and antibodies (Table 14.2).

In the following paragraph immunomodulation in the nervous system in relation to T-cell regulation will be analytically discussed with the use of multiple sclerosis (MS) as a prototype autoimmune disease of the nervous system (Toy 2006).

Immunomodulation in the Nervous System: The Paradigm of Multiple Sclerosis

MS is considered to be a chronic autoimmune demyelinating disease that results in axonal loss within the CNS.

MS is characterized by T cell and macrophage infiltrates that are triggered by CNS-specific CD4

Table 14.2 Immune Disorders that Affect the Nervous System

Immune Disorder	Implicated Cell Types	Mediators	References
Leukocyte recruitment to the CNS, axon terminal degeneration, hippocampal lesions, MS, EAE	CD4, CD8 T cells, NK cells, B cells, CD45CD11b MΦ, microglia	IFN-γ, TNF-α, IL-1β, Abs, chemokine MCP-1/CCL2 expression by blood–brain barrier–associated glial cells	Mouzaki et al. 2004; Owens et al. 2005; Toy 2006; Cassan, Liblau 2007
MS, EAE, reduced suppressive activity of Tregs	Th1 and Th17 cells recognizing MBP, PLP, MOG self-peptides	IFN-γ, TNF-α, IL-17	Mouzaki et al. 2004, 2005; Langrish et al. 2005; Haas et al. 2005; Huan et al. 2005; Bettelli et al. 2006; Cassan, Liblau 2007
Inflammation, Alzheimer's disease, MS, viral or bacterial infections, ischemia, stroke, encephalopathy	Brain/hypothalamus	*Agonists*: IL-1β, IFN-γ *Antagonists*: IL-4, TGF-β	Toy 2006; Correa et al. 2007
Myasthenia gravis, Lambert—Eaton myasthenic syndrome, Guillain—Barre syndrome, paraneoplastic cerebellar degeneration, generalized neuropathies	B cells	Antibrain Abs, antigliadin Abs, Abs to glial antigens	Boscolo et al. 2006; Alaedini et al. 2007; Cabanlit et al. 2007; Tschernatsch et al. 2007

CNS, central nervous system; MS, multiple sclerosis; EAE, experimentally induced autoimmune encephalomyelitis; MΦ, macrophage; Ab, antibody.

T cells. The prominent autoimmune etiology of MS is considered to be the aberrant activation of IFN-γ-producing Th1 cells that recognize self-peptides of the myelin sheath, such as MBP, proteolipid protein (PLP), and myelin oligodendrocyte glycoprotein (MOG) (Mouzaki, Tselios, Papathanassopoulos et al. 2004).

There is a heterogeneous pathophysiology of this disease that remains unclear and includes an inflammatory response characterized by CD4⁺ CD8⁺ T cells and macrophages. MBP, PLP, and MOG components of the myelin sheath are the main specific targets of T cells and B cells that are directed against these self-peptides (Olsson, Sun, Hillert et al. 1992; Genain, Cannella, Hauser et al. 1999; Bielekova, Goodwin, Richert et al. 2000; Berger, Rubner, Schautzer et al. 2003; Bielekova, Sung, Kadom et al. 2004; Sospedra, Martin 2005). The etiology for the immune system, triggering such an inflammatory response against self-antigens of the CNS, remains largely unknown, similar to most autoimmune diseases.

The proposed mechanism for the pathophysiology of this disease based on what we know so far is described in Figure 14.2 and Table 14.3.

Our knowledge of CNS dynamics and function so far gives the impression that the CNS is a privileged organ system for the induction of immune responses based on the following facts:

- The limited renewal and mitotic nature of neurons protect the CNS from immune pathology.
- The blood–brain barrier does not allow trafficking of resting lymphocytes, whereas it does allow the entrance of activated cells (Hickey, Hsu, Kimura 1991).
- The fact that only a few cells within the CNS constitutively express MHC molecules makes it difficult for immune responses to develop (Perry 1998).
- A functional silencing or elimination of T cells that manage to enter the CNS occurs through the expression of CNS Fas-ligand, TGF-β, and prostaglandin E_2 (Zhu, Anderson, Schubart et al. 2005; Liu, Teige, Birnir et al. 2006b).

Nevertheless, recent evidence has proved that there is access to the CNS, although limited, and naive T cells have been shown to traffic within the inflamed tissue (Krakowski, Owens 2000; Aloisi, Pujol-Borrell 2006). Studies in animal models have also shown that naive CD4⁺ and CD8⁺ T cells are able to patrol nonlymphoid tissues including the CNS (Brabb, von Dassow, Ordonez et al. 2000; Cose, Brammer, Khanna et al. 2006). Although these cells are allowed to circulate

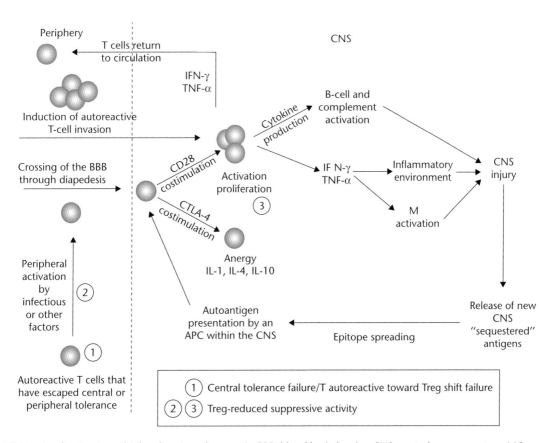

Figure 14.2 Treg implication in multiple sclerosis pathogenesis. BBB, blood brain barrier; CNS, central nervous system; MΦ, macrophage; APC, antigen presenting cell; IFN, interferon; TNF, tumor necrosis factor.

Table 14.3 Immune Cells and Soluble Mediators Involved in the Pathogenesis of Multiple Sclerosis

Cell Type	Mediator	Effect	References
Th1 cells, CD8 T cells, NK cells	IFN-γ	MΦ and MN activation, disease exacerbation	Mouzaki et al. 2004*; Chatzantoni et al. 2004; Scalzo et al. 2006; Cassan, Liblau 2007*; Krishamoorthy et al. 2007*
Th1 cells, MΦ	TNF-α	MΦ and T-cell activation, disease exacerbation	
Th2 cells	IL-4	Symptom alleviation, ±anaphylactic shock	
Th2 cells	IL-13	Symptom alleviation	
MN, MF	IL-1	EAE deterioration	
CD4CD25 ± Foxp3 T cells, Th3 cells	TGF-β	Th2 cell response, anti-inflammatory activity, differentiation of CD4 T-cells towards the Th17 lineage	Hafler 2004; Sakaguchi 2004; Langrish et al. 2005; Lim et al. 2005; Bettelli et al. 2006
CD4CD25 ± Foxp3 T cells, Tr1 cells, MΦ	IL-10	Th2 cell response, anti-inflammatory activity	Hafler 2004; Sakaguchi 2004; Lim et al. 2005
CD11b(+)CD11c(+)CD45(hi) myeloid dendritic cells (mDCs)	TGF-β1, IL-6, IL-23	Drive epitope spreading, enhance Th17 cell activity	Miller et al. 2007
DC	IL-23	Th17 cell production	Langrish et al. 2005; Bettelli et al. 2006
Th17 cells	IL-17	Disease exacerbation, anti-Foxp3 Treg activity	
In vivo and in vitro treatments	anti-CD25 Ab	Disease exacerbation in EAE, inactivation ±depletion of Tregs	Stephens et al. 2005; Cassan et al. 2006
	anti-CD3 Ab+anti-CD28 Ab+IL-2+IL-4, Ag-loaded DCs	Expansion of Tregs	Yamazaki et al. 2003; Thornton et al. 2004; Masteller et al. 2005; Fisson et al. 2006; Ochi et al. 2006; Tischner et al. 2006
	Glatiramer acetate, other copolymers	Expansion of Tregs	Stern et al. 2004; Hong et al. 2005
Immature DCs+Ag+CD4 T cells +TGF-β; murine neurons + encephalitogenic CD4 T-cells; human CD4 T-cells.		Conversion of CD4 T cells to Tregs	Chen et al. 2003; Kretschmer et al. 2005; Weber et al. 2006; Liu et al. 2006a,b

*Papers describing in detail the animal models used to study the pathogenesis of multiple sclerosis.

Ab, antibody; DC, dendritic cell; MΦ, macrophage.

within the CNS without causing an unwanted effect, their entry requires more than the activation of myelin-specific T cells, since additional signals are needed, such as those triggered by specific microbial components through the Toll-like receptors (TLRs) (Brabb, Goldrath, von Dassow et al. 1997; Waldner, Collins, Kuchroo 2004).

Although there are no professional APCs in the CNS, antigen presentation does occur in the CNS. There is evidence that MHC class I molecules are present on oligodendrocytes and neurons when they are exposed to an inflammatory environment that allows for antigen presentation to CD8[+] T cells. Presentation to both CD8[+] and CD4[+] T cells can be realized by astrocytes and microglial cells, which have been shown to express both MHC class I and class II molecules. As has been shown in an EAE model, dendritic-like cells are needed to reactivate CD4[+] T cells within the CNS (Greter, Heppner, Lemos et al. 2005).

Another dendritic cell phenomenon that has been shown to occur within the CNS is epitope spreading, which leads to the induction of immune reactivity against more self-epitopes during chronic inflammation (McMahon, Bailey, Castenada et al. 2005; Miller, McMahon, Schreiner et al. 2007). These data, along with the fact that vessel-associated dendritic cells have also been found in active MS lesions, indicate that reactivation of incoming T cells is possible within the CNS (Kivisakk, Mahad, Callahan et al. 2004; Greter, Heppner, Lemos et al. 2005). TGF-β is known to play an important regulatory role and is now being implicated in pathogenic processes. TGF-β has been shown to promote, in an inflammatory cytokine environment, the differentiation of CD4[+] T cells toward the pathogenic lineage Th17, which is characterized, as explained in the preceding text, by the secretion of IL-17 (Langrish, Chen, Blumenschein et al. 2005; Bettelli, Carrier, Gao et al. 2006).

The first step in CNS self-reactive regulation occurs in the thymus during thymic ontogeny where T cells expressing high-affinity receptors for self-antigens undergo apoptosis (Siggs, Makaroff, Liston 2006). Until recently, it has been thought that thymocytes specific for CNS-specific self-antigens were spared during negative thymic selection, whereas eliminated T cells recognized only ubiquitous or blood-born antigens. Current research data indicate that many of these self-antigens, which were once believed to be tissue restricted, are expressed in the thymus and are therefore eliminated by negative selection. These antigens are expressed by cortical and medullary thymic epithelial APCs (Derbinski, Schulte, Keywski et al. 2001). There are a variety of CNS self-antigens expressed in the thymus, several of which are related to MS pathogenesis. Several thymic cell types have been shown to synthesize MBP mRNA and proteins (Feng, Givogri, Bongarzone et al. 2000; Liu, MacKenzie-Graham, Kim et al. 2001). Experiments in animal models have clearly shown that MBP$^{+/+}$ mice demonstrate a strong negative selection of that particular self-antigen in the thymus, although it seems that bone marrow–derived cells play a more important role in this process (Huseby, Sather, Huseby et al. 2001; Perchellet, Stromnes, Pang et al. 2004). Expression of several MBP isoforms was shown to be associated with reduced development of EAE in animal models (Liu, MacKenzie-Graham, Kim et al. 2001). Nevertheless, MBP-specific T cells are present in the periphery of both mice and humans, which is an indication of the importance of not only the presence of thymic expression but also the extent of that expression (Kuchroo, Anderson, Waldner et al. 2002; Sospedra, Martin 2005).

DM20, a splice variant of PLP, was found to be constitutively expressed chiefly by cortical and medullary thymic cells (Anderson, Nicholson, Legge et al. 2000; Klein, Klugmann, Nave et al. 2000; Derbinski, Schulte, Kyewski et al. 2001). In SLJ mice, an animal model with susceptibility to PLP-induced EAE, CD4$^+$ encephalitogenic T cells are specific for the PLP139–151 peptide, which is not transcribed in the thymus (Anderson, Nicholson, Legge et al. 2000). Nevertheless, it has been shown that thymic stromal cells expressing PLP can induce the tolerance of PLP-specific T cells (Klein, Klugmann, Nave et al. 2000). Other experiments showing that the introduction of PLP peptides in the thymus can induce tolerance to these specific peptides indicate that there can be tolerance to PLP peptides as long as they are expressed in the thymus (Anderson, Nicholson, Legge et al. 2000). Although MOG does not represent an important percentage of the myelin proteins, it seems to be a very important target in cases of EAE in experimental models and MS in humans (Adelman, Wood, Benzel et al. 1995). There was limited detection of MOG expression in the thymus of both mice and humans (Derbinski, Schulte, Kyewski et al. 2001). Recent results in mice indicate that there is very limited expression in the thymus, and this expression does not seem to be sufficient to induce tolerance (Delarasse, Daubas, Mars et al. 2003; Linares, Mana, Goodyear et al. 2003; Fazilleau, Delarasse, Sweenie et al. 2006).

In addition to myelin oligodendrocyte antigens other CNS antigens are expressed in the thymus. For example, S100β, which is synthesized by astrocytes in the CNS, has been detected in the thymus of animal models (Kojima, Reindl, Lassmann et al. 1997). Thymic expression of αB-crystallin, a heat-shock protein expressed by astrocytes and oligodendrocytes, has been associated with the inability of peripheral lymphocytes to respond to autologous αB-crystallin (van Stipdonk, Willems, Plomp et al. 2000).

Although there seems to be a negative selection process for CNS antigens in the thymus, there are circulating CNS autoreactive T cells in the periphery, both in healthy individuals and MS patients, that are related to MS pathogenesis. Therefore, there must be another level of regulation in the secondary lymphoid organs that limit the action of these autoreactive cells in healthy individuals.

Experimental findings in the last few years have demonstrated the important role of Tregs in CNS autoimmunity (Hafler 2004; Sakaguchi 2004; Lim, Hillsamer, Banham et al. 2005). Recovery of EAE is accompanied by Treg accumulation within the CNS and, when isolated, these cells showed significant suppressive ability in vitro. Furthermore, transfer of these cells in low numbers reduced EAE (Kohm, Carpentier, Anger et al. 2002; McGeachy, Stephens, Anderton et al. 2005). Disease activity in Rag$^{-/-}$ MBP TCR-transgenic mice was reduced after the transfer of CD4$^+$ or CD4$^+$CD25$^+$ T cells from wild type animals (Hori, Haury, Coutinho et al. 2002). On the other hand, injection of anti-CD25 monoclonal antibody before EAE induction, which leads to the inactivation or depletion of Tregs, resulted in higher activation of autoaggressive T cells (Stephens, Gray, Anderton et al. 2005; Cassan, Piaggio, Zappulla et al. 2006). Typically resistant C57BL/6 mice become susceptible to reinduction of disease when depletion of Tregs is performed after the acute phase of EAE (McGeachy, Stephens, Anderton et al. 2005). The influence of Tregs on disease progression is also indicated by the fact that depletion of Tregs in remitting-relapsing EAE models increases acute phase severity and prevents secondary remissions (Zhang, Reddy, Ochi et al. 2006).

Research investigating the presence of a quantitative defect in the Treg population of MS patients has shown that there is no difference whatsoever, on the basis of CD4 CD25 expression, between the blood of MS patients and healthy individuals (Huan, Culbertson, Spencer et al. 2005; Venken, Hellings, Hensen et al. 2006). No difference has been shown for the proportion of Tregs in the peripheral blood and cerebrospinal fluid of MS patients (Haas, Hug, Viehover et al. 2005).

Tregs from remitting-relapsing MS patients showed reduced suppressive activity in vitro (Haas, Hug, Viehover et al. 2005; Huan, Culbertson, Spencer et al. 2005). This reduction in Treg activity is associated with reduced Foxp3 mRNA and protein expression in MS CD4$^+$CD25$^+$ peripheral blood T cells compared to those of healthy individuals (Huan, Culbertson, Spencer et al. 2005). It is not yet clear whether this defect is due to decreased expression at the cellular level or due to the lower incidence of Tregs among CD4$^+$CD25$^+$ T cells. This phase of the disease seems to be of great importance in Treg function, since patients with secondary progressive MS show normal levels of Foxp3 expression among CD4$^+$CD25^{high} T cells, and normal suppressive activity in vitro (Venken, Hellings, Hensen et al. 2006). In contrast, there is no correlation between relapses and the defective suppressive activity of Tregs from remitting-relapsing MS patients (Haas, Hug, Viehover et al. 2005).

As has been previously described and reported from experiments in animal models, the presence of self-antigen in the thymus is very important for the development and maintenance of Tregs for this antigen, as well as for the reduction of the ratio between T cells and Tregs (Kyewski, Klein 2006; Grajewski, Silver, Agarwal et al. 2006). It has been reported specifically for CNS antigens that SJL mice, which have a greater susceptibility to EAE than the B10.S strain, have stronger thymic expression of the PLP antigen and a lower frequency of Tregs specific for this antigen (Reddy, Illes, Zhang et al. 2004). This is an indication of the relationship between high thymic expression of an antigen and the generation of Tregs specific for this antigen. It can be concluded that thymus plays an important role in immune tolerance against CNS-restricted self-antigens, not only through negative selection but also through the induction of Tregs.

Although manipulation of the Treg population has proved to be quite difficult, such an attempt could be useful for the manipulation of CNS autoimmune diseases based on what is known so far about the function of this T-cell population.

Beyond the natural hyporesponsiveness of Tregs, their clonal expansion occurs upon stimulation with anti-CD3 and anti-CD28 monoclonal antibodies in the presence of IL-2 and IL-4 (Thornton, Piccirillo, Shevach 2004). Nevertheless, since antigen-specific Tregs have been shown to be better able to control autoimmunity, their expansion with antigen-loaded dendritic cells would be more useful and has already been achieved (Yamazaki, Iyoda, Tarbell et al. 2003; Masteller, Warner, Tang et al. 2005; Fisson, Djelti, Trenado et al. 2006). Another approach is aimed at the in vitro conversion of CD4$^+$ T cells to Tregs, which requires cultures of immature dendritic cells in the presence of low doses of antigen. The presence of TGF-β in this culture system seems to be of great importance for the switching of one cell type to another (Chen, Jin, Hardegen et al. 2003; Kretschmer, Apostolou, Hawiger et al. 2005; Weber, Harbertson, Godebu et al. 2006). It has also been reported that co-culturing murine neurons with encephalitogenic CD4$^+$ T cells can lead to their conversion to Tregs, which have been shown to be effective in controlling autoimmunity. The expression of TGF-β and CD80 CD86 costimulatory factors seems to be very important for this conversion, but the fact that neurons are able to produce factors that lead to such a conversion and thus induce a protective response is of great importance (Liu, Teige, Birnir et al. 2006b). There have also been attempts to induce the expression of Foxp3 on CD4$^+$ T cells to convert them to Tregs. Such an attempt in mice using a retroviral vector encoding Foxp3 resulted in cells with regulatory properties and protective function against autoimmunity (Bettelli, Dastrange, Oukka 2005). In the last few years, many similar attempts have focused on the human system and expansion of natural Tregs has been achieved (Liu, Putnam, Xu-Yu et al. 2006a). Polyclonal, as well as antigen-specific, conversion of CD4$^+$ T cells to Tregs has also been achieved in the human system, but the extent of the suppressive activity of these Foxp3-expressing cells requires further investigation (Grossman, Verbsky, Barchet et al. 2004; Allan, Passerini, Bacchetta et al. 2005; Walker, Carson, Nepom et al. 2005).

Despite the promising results of these attempts, the best way to use Treg properties as a possible therapeutic approach for autoimmunity is the direct expansion of Tregs in vivo. It has been observed that Tregs proliferate strongly when they encounter their specific antigen in vivo (Fisson, Djelti, Trenado et al. 2003). Glatiramer acetate , a drug approved and largely used for MS, seems to have the ability to induce Tregs. The expansion of Tregs after injection of copolymers has been shown to occur in both mice and humans (Stern, Illes, Reddy et al. 2004; Hong, Zhang, Zheng et al. 2005).

In animal models, oral administration of anti-CD3 monoclonal antibodies or treatment with anti-CD28 monoclonal antibodies led to prevention of EAE and induction of the Treg population, along with an increase in their regulatory properties (Ochi, Abraham, Ishikawa et al. 2006; Tischner, Weishaupt, van den Brandt et al. 2006).

Although selective induction and expansion of CNS-specific human Tregs has a strong potential for controlling the manifestations of CNS autoimmunity based on our knowledge so far, a few obstacles must be considered. The fine specificity of Tregs has an impact on their efficacy, especially when this population is very limited and hardly identified on the basis of the markers known so far. Autoantigens vary among patients and in the same patient during different phases of the disease. As Tregs have been shown to be nonfunctional in an inflammatory environment, they cannot be used to block an already ongoing disease (Cassan, Liblau 2007).

Immunomodulation in the Vascular System

Diseases of the vascular system such as atherosclerosis have been proved by experimental evidence to implicate aspects of the immune system that are important for innate immunity and inflammatory mechanisms (see Table 14.4).

These mechanisms are not only implicated in situations such as atherosclerosis, but can also initiate vascular ischemic damage to prevent and treat vascular disease and even induce ischemic tolerance. There is also evidence of autoimmune involvement in atherosclerotic individuals, since these patients have higher titers of autoantibodies against HSP60/65, which are related to ischemia. Such autoimmune situations are also involved in shaping the size and composition of the atherosclerotic lesions (Xu, Dietrich, Steiner et al. 1992; Xu, Willeit, Marosi et al. 1993; George, Afek, Gilburd et al. 1998; George, Shoenfeld, Afek et al. 1999; Frangogiannis, Smith, Entman 2002; Kariko, Weissman, Welsh 2004; Hahn, Grossmana, Chena et al. 2007). Further evidence showed a considerable number of Th1 cells present in human and murine plaques, some of which were reactive with oxidized low-density lipoprotein (LDL) (Jonasson, Holm, Skalli et al. 1986; Zhou, Stemme, Hansson 1996).

Attenuation of the induction of atherosclerosis has been shown to be possible through induction of Tregs; the extent of the disease can be reduced by induction of oral tolerance with proatherogenic antigens (Maron, Sukhova, Faria et al. 2002; Harats, Yacov, Gilburd et al. 2002; George, Yacov, Breitbart et al. 2004). Furthermore, cytokines secreted by Tregs are antiatherogenic (Hansson 2005).

Ischemic stroke and cardiovascular disease are mainly caused by atherosclerosis, which involves plaques and lesions of the arteries. These plaques and lesions are composed of cell debris and lipids, mainly cholesterol, as well as inflammatory cells such as macrophages and T cells, collagen and smooth muscle cells, and sites of old hemorrhage, angiogenesis, and calcium deposits (Stary 2005). Acute ischemia is created when a thrombus is formed, a phenomenon precipitated by activation of these plaques (Falk, Shah, Fuster 1995). Together with risk factors such as

Table 14.4 Immune System Involvement in Vascular Disorders

Immune Cells and Molecules	Function	References
Th1 cells	Reactive with oxidized LDL, Hsp, β2 glycoprotein 1; activation by specific antigens, secretion of IFN-γ leading to further activation of MΦ, EC	Jonasson et al. 1986; Zhou et al. 1996; Mach et al. 1998; Nicoletti et al. 1998; Stary 2005; Hahn et al. 2007
Tregs	Induction of oral tolerance with proatherogenic antigens leading to disease inhibition Antiatherogenic cytokine secretion, atherosclerosis inhibition through IL-10 and TGF-β secretion	Harats et al. 2002; Maron et al. 2002; Robertson et al. 2003; George et al. 2004; Hansson 2005
CD8 T cells, NK T cells	Disease acceleration, CTL activity	Shresta et al. 1998; Robertson et al. 2003
MΦ	Transformation to foam cells in atherosclerotic lesions; promotion of inflammation in the arteries	Schmitz, Drobnik 2002; Miller et al. 2003; Edfeldt et al. 2004; Stary 2005
MN	Recruited by secreted chemokines, transformation to MΦ	Schmitz, Drobnik 2002; Dai et al. 2004; Sheikine, Hansson 2004
EC	Activation by phospholipids, leading to MN and lymphocyte activation	Cybulsky, Gimbrone 1991; Witztum, Berliner 1998
B cells, systemic immunity	Abs to Hsp65, OxLDL, cardiolipin, β2-glycoprotein 1, DNA, HDL, Apolipoprotein A1, lipoprotein lipase, Abs to CNS antigens, myocardial Abs, complement activation, induction of acute phase proteins, release of proinflammatory cytokines IL-1, IL-6, IL-8, activation of neutrophils, microglia	Melguizo et al. 1997; Streit 2000; Hansson 2005; Hahn et al. 2007

MΦ, macrophage; MN, monocyte; EC, endothelial cell; Ab, antibody; Hsp, heat-shock protein.

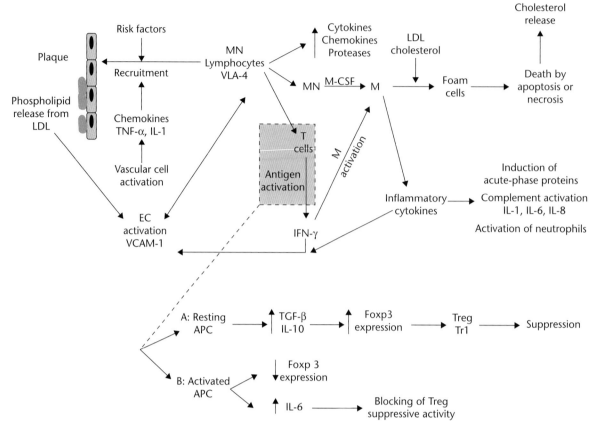

Figure 14.3 Cerebrovascular disease and implicated immune system mechanisms. MN, monocyte; MΦ, macrophage, EC, endothelial cell; APC, antigen presenting cell; TNF, tumor necrosis factor; IL, interleukin; VCAM, vascular cell adhesion molecule; M-CSF, monocyte colony stimulating factor; LDL, low-density lipoprotein; IFN, interferon, APC, antigen-presenting cell; TGF, transforming growth factor.

hypercholesterolemia, hypertension, and cigarette smoking, immunity also seems to play an important role in the pathogenesis of atherosclerosis (Hansson 2005) (Fig. 14.3).

During hypercholesterolemia and hypertension, levels of LDL, a major transport particle for cholesterol, are increased and vascular endothelium inflammation is initiated (Skalen, Gustafsson, Rydberg et al. 2002). Oxygen radicals and enzymes chemically modify LDL protein and lipids in the intima, and the resultant phospholipids that are released activate endothelial cells that express the vascular cell adhesion molecule-1 (VCAM-1) (Cybulsky, Gimbrone 1991; Witztum, Berliner 1998). Monocytes and lymphocytes that display the very late antigen (VLA-4) are recruited in this way to the endothelium. VCAM-1 expression is further induced by oscillating flow (Dai, Kaazempur-Mofrad, Natarajan et al. 2004). Activation of vascular cells induces the signals provided by secreted chemokines to recruit monocytes and T cells to the lesion. These include monocyte chemoattractant protein-1 (MCP-1), fractalkine, and others. Blocking of leukocyte adhesion molecules or chemokines by antibodies leads to reduction of atherosclerosis in animal

models (Sheikine, Hansson 2004). Under the influence of monocyte colony stimulating factor (M-CSF), monocytes migrating into vascular tissues transform to macrophages, which in turn take up the cholesterol contained in LDL particles. These particles accumulate in macrophages and induce their transformation to foam cells, the prototypic cells of atherosclerotic lesions (Schmitz, Drobnik 2002). In addition to these macrophages that transform into foam cells and die either from apoptosis or from necrosis and thus release cholesterol, other macrophages promote inflammation in the arteries. Toll-1-like receptors expressed in lesions bind to endotoxins and endogenous molecules. TNF and IL-1 produced by vascular and immune cells trigger signal transduction pathways that lead to the secretion of cytokines, chemokines, and proteases. The risk of atherothrombotic diseases and polymorphisms of TNF and IL-1 genes has been epidemiologically identified (Miller, Chang, Binder et al. 2003; Edfeldt, Bennet, Eriksson et al. 2004). Although T cells migrate similarly to macrophages, there is need for specific antigens for T cells to be activated. Th1 cells are the most common circulating T cells in the lesion and they are activated by antigens such as oxidized LDL and microbial antigens, leading to secretion of cytokines such as IFN-γ and further activation of macrophages and endothelial cells. Animal models that lack CD4$^+$ T cells and IFN-γ receptors or in which these are blocked in immune activation showed a reduction in atherosclerosis (Nicoletti, Kaveri, Caligiuri et al. 1998; Mach, Schonbeck, Sukhova et al. 1998). The disease process also includes NK T cells; CD8$^+$ T cells, which seem to accelerate the disease; and Tregs, which have been shown to inhibit atherosclerosis through secretion of IL-10 and TFG-β (Robertson, Rudling, Zhou et al. 2003). Tregs are altered numerically as well as functionally in patients with acute coronary syndromes (Hallenbeck, Hansson, Becker et al. 2005). Oral tolerance induction in animal models is associated with the attenuation of atherosclerotic lesions (Harats, Yacov, Gilburd et al. 2002; Maron, Sukhova, Faria et al. 2002; George, Yacov, Breitbart et al. 2004). Furthermore, cytokines classically secreted by Tregs are reduced in humans with unstable angina (Heeschen, Dimmeler, Hamm et al. 2003). Recent evidence from animal models is indicative of a possible protective role of Tregs in atherosclerosis (Ait-Oufella, Salomon, Potteaux et al. 2006). Purified Tregs from acute coronary syndrome patients showed reduced expression of Foxp3 along with downregulation of CTLA-4 mRNA expression (Hallenbeck, Hansson, Becker et al. 2005).

Systemic immune responses also occur. Antibodies reactive to oxidized LDL have been detected along with acute-phase reactants such as C-reactive protein (CRP), pentraxin, and others. (Hansson 2005). There are indications that proinflammatory cytokines produced in the plaques induce the acute phase proteins (Liuzzo, Biasucci, Gallimore et al. 1994; Peri, Introna, Corradi et al. 2000).

The progression of cellular injury during acute ischemia also includes the participation of immune mechanisms (Iadecola, Alexander 2001; Frangogiannis, Smith, Entman 2002). Activation of complement; release of proinflammatory cytokines such as IL-1, IL-6, and IL-8; as well as activation of neutrophils occurs. Microglial activation just after the episode induces neutrophil trafficking to the ischemic area. Inhibition of this response has been shown to decrease the infract volume and improve neurological outcome (Streit 2000). Although macrophages, monocytes, and lymphocytes were not thought to be involved in the immune response during such episodes until 2 to 3 days later, recent evidence has shown that there is a much earlier contribution of these mononuclear cells to the immune response, and when it occurs early enough it can improve neurological outcome (Becker, Kindrick, Relton et al. 2001).

The ability of immune system components to invade the CNS and encounter novel CNS antigens

in the CNS and periphery increases after stroke (Herrmann, Vos, Wunderlich et al. 2000). There is evidence of humoral immune responses to CNS antigens after a stroke and the possibility of autoimmunity occurrence is very strong. Furthermore, although myocardial antigens have unrestricted access to peripheral lymphoid organs, myocardial antibodies have been detected in patients after myocardial ischemia (Melguizo, Prados, Velez et al. 1997).

The microenvironment of the tissue at the time of immune response generation is very important. Under normal conditions, costimulatory signals necessary for lymphocyte priming are not expressed at adequate levels in the brain (Dangond, Windhagen, Groves et al. 1997). Immune responses in other areas, such as those after a microbial infection, might occur. This could lead to an induced expression of costimulatory molecules and a cytokine ratio shift phenomenon that increases the potential for autoimmunity (Becker, Kindrick, Relton et al. 2005). Treg suppression of the activation of antigen-specific T cells is inhibited by the induction of TLRs and IL-6 expression (Oyama, Blais, Liu et al. 2004). It has been shown in animal models that animals with the capacity for brain antigen recognition have the worst outcomes after brain injury as opposed to animals that do not have autoreactive T cells. Also, T lymphocytes from animals after spinal cord injury possess encephalitogenic properties when injected into naive animals (Jones, Basso, Sodhi et al. 2002). Immune damage in the brain or heart can also occur via direct cell killing by lysis or apoptosis through CTL action, or by the secretion of neurotoxic cytokines by activated lymphocytes (Shresta, Pham, Thomas et al. 1998).

CONCLUSIONS AND FUTURE DIRECTIONS

Owing to recent discoveries of the nature and function of Tregs and other regulatory T-cell populations, the scientific community has within grasp major natural controllers of various physiological and pathological immune responses. Regulatory T cells have been shown to have a central role in determining the balance between tolerance, inflammation, and autoimmunity. The reestablishment of tolerance to self-antigens by regulating Treg cell number and function can result in effective treatment strategies of autoimmune and inflammatory disorders, and recent attempts to harness the immunoregulatory activities of the different regulatory cell populations for therapeutic purposes have met with relative success.

Nevertheless, there are still many unknowns in the development and function of regulatory T cells. For example, population studies are needed to determine the influence of environmental and genetic factors on Treg types, numbers, and function. Although it seems so, it is not yet clear whether ageing provokes alterations that lead to loss of function of regulatory T cells, thus contributing to susceptibility to autoimmune or vascular system diseases.

The possibilities to modulate immune responses by manipulating immunoregulatory cells are hindered by many obstacles such as the antigenic specificity of Tregs, which influences their efficacy; the need for autologous Treg therapy; and their limited function in an inflammatory environment.

Beyond those difficulties, an optimal scenario for Treg usage in the treatment of autoimmune or inflammatory conditions exists. Thymus-derived or peripherally induced Tregs have the potential of being activated and expanded in the lymphoid tissue and migrate to the inflamed tissues to control the pathogenic immune responses.

The central role of Tregs in controlling the activation of effector T cells, and therefore, the worsening of inflammation and immune activation in vascular ischemic diseases, directs to a potential therapeutic role of these cells.

As underlined in this chapter, to reach a level of controlling regulatory T-cell numbers and activity, the mechanisms of their function need to be understood, more stable and exclusive markers need to be established, and Treg cellular frequency and function in the context of a given disease needs to be determined.

REFERENCES

Abbas AK, Murphy K, Sher A. 1996. Functional diversity of helper T lymphocytes. *Nature.* 383:787–793.

Adelmann M, Wood J, Benzel I et al. 1995. The N-terminal domain of the myelin oligodendrocyte glycoprotein (MOG) induces acute demyelinating experimental autoimmune encephalomyelitis in the Lewis rat. *J Neuroimmunol.* 63:17–27.

Ait-Oufella H, Salomon BL, Potteaux S et al. 2006. Natural regulatory T-cells control the development of atherosclerosis in mice. *Nat Med.* 12(2):178–180.

Alaedini A, Okamoto H, Briani C et al. 2007. Immune cross-reactivity in celiac disease: anti-gliadin antibodies bind to neuronal synapsin I. *J Immunol.* 178:6590–6595.

Albert MH, Liu Y, Anasetti C, Yu XZ. 2005. Antigen-dependent suppression of alloresponses by Foxp3-induced regulatory T-cells in transplantation. *Eur J Immunol.* 35:2598–2607.

Allan SE, Passerini L, Bacchetta R et al. 2005. The role of two FOXP3 isoforms in the generation of human CD4+ Tregs. *J Clin Invest.* 115:3276–3284.

Aloisi F, Pujol-Borrell R. 2006. Lymphoid neogenesis in chronic inflammatory diseases. *Nat Rev Immunol.* 6:205–217.

Anderson AC, Nicholson LB, Legge KL, Turchin V, Zaghouani H, Kuchroo VK. 2000. High frequency of autoreactive myelin proteolipid protein-specific T-cells in the periphery of naive mice: mechanisms of selection of the self-reactive repertoire. *J Exp Med.* 191:761–770.

Annunziato F, Cosmi L, Manetti R et al. 2001. Reversal of human allergen-specific CRTH2Th2 cells by IL-12 or the PS-DSP30 oligodeoxynucleotide. *J Allergy Clin Immunol.* 108:815–821.

Annunziato F, Romagnani P, Cosmi L et al. 2001. Chemokines and lymphopoiesis in human thymus. *Trends Immunol.* 22:277–281.

Annunziato F, Cosmi L, Santarlasci V et al. 2007. Phenotypic and functional features of human Th17 cells. *J Exp Med.* 204:1849–1861.

Apostolou I, von Boehmer H. 2004. In vivo instruction of suppressor commitment in naïve T-cells. *J Exp Med.* 199:1401–1408.

Barrat FJ, Cua DJ, Boonstra A et al. 2002. In vitro generation of interleukin 10- producing regulatory CD4(+) T-cells is induced by immunosuppressive drugs and inhibited by T helper type 1 (Th1)- and Th2-inducing cytokines. *J Exp Med.* 195:603–616.

Becker K, Kindrick D, Relton J, Harlan J, Winn R. 2001. Antibody to the a4 integrin decreases infarct size in transient focal cerebral ischemia in rats. *Stroke.* 32:206–211.

Becker KJ, Kindrick DL, Lester MP, Shea C, Ye ZC. 2005. Sensitization to brain antigens after stroke is augmented by lipopolysaccharide. *J Cereb Blood Flow Metab.* 25(12):1634–1644.

Beissert S, Schwarz A, Schwarz T. 2006. Regulatory T-cells. *Journal of Investigative Dermatology.* 126:15–24.

Belkaid Y, Piccirillo CA, Mendez S, Shevach EM, Sacks DL. 2002. CD4+CD25+ regulatory T-cells control Leishmania major persistence and immunity. *Nature.* 420:502–507.

Bensinger SJ, Bandeira A, Jordan MS, Caton AJ, Laufer TM. 2001. Major histocompatibility complex class II-positive cortical epithelium mediates the selection of CD4(+)25(+) immunoregulatory T-cells. *J Exp Med.* 194:427–438.

Berger T, Rubner P, Schautzer F et al. 2003. Anti-myelin antibodies as a predictor of clinically definite multiple sclerosis after a first demyelinating event. *N Engl J Med.* 349:139–145.

Bettelli E, Dastrange M, Oukka M. 2005. Foxp3 interacts with nuclear factor of activated T-cells and NF-κB to repress cytokine gene expression and effector functions of T helper cells. *Proc Natl Acad Sci U S A.* 102:5138–5143.

Bettelli E, Carrier Y, Gao W et al. 2006. Reciprocal developmental pathways for the generation of pathogenic effector TH17 and regulatory T-cells. *Nature.* 441:235–238.

Bielekova B, Goodwin B, Richert N et al. 2000. Encephalitogenic potential of the myelin basic protein peptide (amino acids 83–99) in multiple sclerosis: results of a phase II clinical trial with an altered peptide ligand. *Nat Med.* 6:1167–1175.

Bielekova B, Sung MH, Kadom N, Simon R, McFarland H, Martin R. 2004. Expansion and functional relevance of high avidity myelin-specific CD4+ T-cells in multiple sclerosis. *J Immunol.* 172:3893–3904.

Boettler T, Panther E, Bengsch B et al. 2006. Expression of the interleukin-7 receptor alpha chain (CD127) on virus-specific CD8+ T-cells identifies functionally and phenotypically defined memory T-cells during acute resolving hepatitis B virus infection. *J Virol.* 80:3532–3540.

Boom WH, Liebster L, Abbas AK, Titus RG. 1990. Patterns of cytokine secretion in murine leishmaniasis: correlation with disease progression or resolution. *Infect Immun.* 58:3863–3870.

Boscolo S, Passoni M, Baldas V et al. 2006. Detection of anti-brain serum antibodies using a semi-quantitative immunohistological method. *J Immunol Methods.* 309:139–349.

Boyson JE, Rybalov B, Koopman LA et al. 2002. CD1d and invariant NKT cells at the human maternal-fetal interface. *Proc Natl Acad Sci U S A.* 99:13741–13746.

Brabb T, Goldrath AW, von Dassow P, Paez A, Liggitt HD, Goverman J. 1997. Triggers of autoimmune disease in a murine TCR-transgenic model for multiple sclerosis. *J Immunol.* 159:497–507.

Brabb T, von Dassow P, Ordonez N, Schnabel B, Duke B, Goverman J. 2000. In situ tolerance within the central nervous system as a mechanism for preventing autoimmunity. *J Exp Med.* 192:871–880.

Cabanlit M, Wills S, Goines P, Ashwood P, Van de Water J. 2007. Brain-specific autoantibodies in the plasma of subjects with autistic spectrum disorder. *Ann N Y Acad Sci.* 1107:92–103.

Cassan C, Piaggio E, Zappulla JP et al. 2006. Pertussis toxin reduces the number of splenic Foxp3+ regulatory T-cells. *J Immunol.* 177:1552–1560.

Cassan C, Liblau RS. 2007. Immune tolerance and control of CNS autoimmunity: from animal models to MS patients *J Neurochem.* 100:883–892.

Chen W, Jin W, Hardegen N et al. 2003. Conversion of peripheral CD4+CD25- naive T-cells to CD4+CD25+ regulatory T-cells by TGF-β induction of transcription factor Foxp3. *J Exp Med.* 198:1875–1886.

Chen Y, Kuchroo VK, Inobe J, Hafler DA, Weiner HL. 1994. Regulatory T-cell clones induced by oral tolerance: suppression of autoimmune encephalomyelitis. *Science.* 265:1237–1240.

Correa SG, Maccioni M, Rivero VE, Iribarren P, Sotomayor CE, Riera CM. 2007. Cytokines and the immune-neuroendocrine network: what did we learn from infection and autoimmunity? *Cytokine Growth Factor Rev.* 18:125–134.

Cose S, Brammer C, Khanna KM, Masopust D, Lefrancois L. 2006. Evidence that a significant number of naive T-cells enter non-lymphoid organs as part of a normal migratory pathway. *Eur J Immunol.* 36:1423–1433.

Cottrez F, Groux H. 2004. Specialization in tolerance: innate CD(4+)CD(25+) versus acquired TR1 and TH3 regulatory T-cells. *Transplantation.* (Suppl 77):S12–S15.

Cua DJ, Sherlock J, Chen Y et al. 2003. Interleukin-23 rather than interleukin-12 is the critical cytokine for autoimmune inflammation of the brain. *Nature.* 421:744–748.

Cybulsky MI, Gimbrone MA. 1991. Endothelial expression of a mononuclear leukocyte adhesion molecule during atherosclerosis. *Science.* 251:788–791

Dai G, Kaazempur-Mofrad MR, Natarajan S et al. 2004. Distinct endothelial phenotypes evoked by arterial waveforms derived from atherosclerosis-susceptible and–resistant regions of human vasculature. *Proc Natl Acad Sci U S A.* 101:14871–14876.

Dangond F, Windhagen A, Groves CJ, Hafler DA. 1997. Constitutive expression of costimulatory molecules by human microglia and its relevance to CNS autoimmunity. *J Neuroimmunol.* 76:132–138.

Delarasse C, Daubas P, Mars LT et al. 2003. Myelin/oligodendrocyte glycoprotein-deficient (MOG-deficient) mice reveal lack of immune tolerance to MOG in wild-type mice. *J Clin Invest.* 112:544–553.

Derbinski J, Schulte A, Kyewski B, Klein L. 2001. Promiscuous gene expression in medullary thymic epithelial cells mirrors the peripheral self. *Nat Immunol.* 2:1032–1039.

Dong C. 2006. Diverisification of T-helper-cell lineages: finding of the family root of IL-17-producing cells. *Nat Rev Immunol.* 6:329–333.

Edfeldt K, Bennet AM, Eriksson P et al. 2004. Association of hypo-responsive Toll-like receptor 4 variants with risk of myocardial infarction. *Eur Heart J.* 25:1447–1453.

Falk E, Shah PK, Fuster V. 1995. Coronary plaque disruption. *Circulation.* 92:657–671.

Fazilleau N, Delarasse C, Sweenie CH et al. 2006. Persistence of autoreactive myelin oligodendrocyte glycoprotein (MOG)-specific T-cell repertoires in MOG-expressing mice. *Eur J Immunol.* 36:533–543.

Feng JM, Givogri IM, Bongarzone ER et al. 2000. Thymocytes express the golli products of the myelin basic protein gene and levels of expression are stage dependent. *J Immunol.* 165:5443–5450.

Fisson S, Darrasse-Jeze G, Litvinova E et al. 2003. Continuous activation of autoreactive CD4+ CD25+ regulatory T-cells in the steady state. *J Exp Med.* 198:737–746.

Fisson S, Djelti F, Trenado A et al. 2006. Therapeutic potential of self-antigen-specific CD4+ CD25+ regulatory T-cells selected in vitro from a polyclonal repertoire. *Eur J Immunol.* 36:817–827.

Fontenot JD, Rudensky AY. 2005. A well adapted regulatory contrivance: regulatory T cell development and the forkhead family transcription factor Foxp3. *Nat Immunol.* 6:331–337.

Foussat A, Cottrez F, Brun V, Fournier N, Breittmayer JP, Groux H. 2003. A comparative study between T regulatory type 1 and CD4+CD25+ T-cells in the control of inflammation. *J Immunol.* 171:5018–5026.

Frangogiannis NG, Smith CW, Entman ML. 2002. The inflammatory response in myocardial infarction. *Cardiovasc Res.* 53:31–47.

Fuller MJ, Hildeman DA, Sabbaj S et al. 2005. Cutting edge: emergence of CD127high functionally competent memory T-cells is compromised by high viral loads and inadequate T-cell help. *J Immunol.* 174:5926–5930.

Genain CP, Cannella B, Hauser SL, Raine CS. 1999. Identification of autoantibodies associated with myelin damage in multiple sclerosis. *Nat Med.* 5:170–175.

George J, Afek A, Gilburd B et al. 1998. Induction of early atherosclerosis in LDL-receptor-deficient mice immunized with beta2-glycoprotein I. *Circulation.* 98(11):1108–1115.

George J, Shoenfeld Y, Afek A et al. 1999. Enhanced fatty streak formation in C57BL/6J mice by immunization with heat shock protein-65. *Arterioscler Thromb Vasc Biol.* 19(3):505–510.

George J, Yacov N, Breitbart E et al. 2004. Suppression of early atherosclerosis in LDL-receptor deficient mice by oral tolerance with beta 2-glycoprotein I. *Cardiovasc Res.* 62(3):603–609.

Ghoreschi K, Thomas P, Breit S et al. 2003. Interleukin-4 therapy of psoriasis induces Th2 responses and improves human autoimmune disease. *Nat Med.* 9:40–46.

Gilliet M, Liu YJ. 2002. Generation of human CD8T regulatory cells by CD40 ligand-activated plasmacytoid dendritic cells. *J Exp Med.* 195:695–704.

Godfrey DI, Berzins SP. 2007. Control points in NKT-cell development. *Nat Rev Immunol.* 7:505–518.

Graca L, Cobbold SP, Waldmann H. 2002. Identification of regulatory T-cells in tolerated allografts. *J Exp Med.* 195:1641–1646.

Grajewski RS, Silver PB, Agarwal RK et al. 2006. Endogenous IRBP can be dispensable for generation of natural CD4+CD25+ regulatory T-cells that protect from IRBP-induced retinal autoimmunity. *J Exp Med.* 203:851–856.

Greter M, Heppner FL, Lemos MP et al. 2005. Dendritic cells permit immune invasion of the CNS in an animal model of multiple sclerosis. *Nat Med.* 11:328–334.

Grossman WJ, Verbsky JW, Barchet W, Colonna M, Atkinson JP, Ley TJ. 2004. Human T regulatory cells can use the perforin pathway to cause autologous target T-cell death. *Immunity.* 21:589–601.

Groux H, O'Garra A, Bigler M et al. 1997. A CD4+ T-cell subset inhibits antigen-specific T-cell responses and prevents colitis. *Nature.* 389:737–742.

Haas J, Hug A, Viehover A et al. 2005. Reduced suppressive effect of CD4+CD25high regulatory T-cells on the T-cell immune response against myelin oligodendrocyte glycoprotein in patients with multiple sclerosis. *Eur J Immunol.* 35:3343–3352.

Hafler DA. 2004. Multiple sclerosis. *J Clin Invest.* 113:788–794.

Hahn BH, Grossmana J, Chena W, McMahona M. 2007. The pathogenesis of atherosclerosis in autoimmune rheumatic diseases: roles of inflammation and dyslipidemia. *J Autoimmun.* 28:69–75.

Hallenbeck JM, Hansson GK, Becker KJ. 2005. Immunology of ischemic vascular disease: plaque to attack. *Trends Immunol.* 26:550–556.

Hansson GK. 2005. Inflammation, atherosclerosis, and coronary artery disease. *N Engl J Med.* 352:1685–1695.

Harats D, Yacov N, Gilburd B, Shoenfeld Y, George J. 2002. Oral tolerance with heat shock protein 65 attenuates Mycobacterium tuberculosis-induced and high-fat-diet-driven atherosclerotic lesions. *J Am Coll Cardiol.* 40:1333–1338.

Harrington LE, Mangan PR, Weaver CT. 2006. Expanding the effector CD4 T-cell repertoire: the Th17 lineage. *Curr Opin Immunol.* 18:349–356.

Heeschen C, Dimmeler S, Hamm CW et al. 2003. Serum level of the antiinflammatory cytokine interleukin-10 is an important prognostic determinant in patients with acute coronary syndromes. *Circulation.* 107:2109–2114.

Herrmann M, Vos P, Wunderlich MT, de Bruijn CH, Lamers KJ. 2000. Release of glial tissue-specific proteins after acute stroke: a comparative analysis of serum concentrations of protein S-100B and glial fibrillary acidic protein. *Stroke.* 31:2670–2677.

Hesse M, Piccirillo CA, Belkaid Y et al. 2004. The pathogenesis of schistosomiasis is controlled by cooperating IL-10-producing innate effector and regulatory T-cells. *J Immunol.* 172:3157–3166.

Hickey WF, Hsu BL, Kimura H. 1991. T-lymphocyte entry into the central nervous system. *J Neurosci Res.* 28:254–260.

Hong J, Li N, Zhang X, Zheng B, Zhang JZ. 2005. Induction of CD4+CD25+ regulatory T-cells by co-polymer-I through activation of transcription factor Foxp3. *Proc Natl Acad Sci U S A.* 102:6449–6454.

Hori S, Haury M, Coutinho A, Demengeot J. 2002. Specificity requirements for selection and effector functions of CD25+4+ regulatory T-cells in anti-myelin basic protein T-cell receptor transgenic mice. *Proc Natl Acad Sci U S A.* 99:8213–8218.

Hsieh CS, Macatonia SE, Tripp CS, Wolf SF, O'Garra A, Murphy KM. 1993. Development of TH1 CD41 T-cells through IL-12 produced by Listeria-induced macrophages. *Science.* 260:547–549.

Hsieh CS, Liang Y, Tyznik AJ, Self SG, Liggitt D, Rudensky AY. 2004. Recognition of the peripheral self by naturally arising CD25+ CD4+ T-cell receptors. *Immunity.* 21:267–277.

Hu D, Ikizawa K, Lu L, Sanchirico ME, Shinohara ML, Cantor H. 2004. Analysis of regulatory CD8 T-cells in Qa-1-deficient mice. *Nat Immunol.* 5:516–523.

Huan J, Culbertson N, Spencer L et al. 2005. Decreased FOXP3 levels in multiple sclerosis patients. *J Neurosci Res.* 81:45–52.

Huehn J, Siegmund K, Lehmann JC et al. 2004. Developmental stage, phenotype, and migration distinguish naive- and effector/memory-like CD4+ regulatory T-cells. *J Exp Med.* 199:303–313.

Huseby ES, Sather B, Huseby PG, Goverman J. 2001. Agedependent T-cell tolerance and autoimmunity to myelin basic protein. *Immunity.* 14:471–481.

Huster KM, Busch V, Schiemann M et al. 2004. Selective expression of IL-7 receptor on memory T-cells identifies early CD40L-dependent generation of distinct CD8+ memory T-cell subsets. *Proc Natl Acad Sci U S A.* 101:5610–5615.

Iadecola C, Alexander M. 2001. Cerebral ischemia and inflammation. *Curr Opin Neurol.* 14:89–94.

Iwakura Y, Ishigame H. 2006. The IL-23/Il-17 axis in inflammation. *J Clin Invest.* 116:1218–22.

Jaeckel E, von Boehmer H, Manns MP. 2005. Antigen-specific FoxP3-transduced T-cells can control established type 1 diabetes. *Diabetes.* 54:306–310.

Jiang H, Zhang SI, Pernis B. 1992. Role of CD8+ T-cells in murine experimental allergic encephalomyelitis. *Science.* 256:1213–1215.

Jonasson L, Holm J, Skalli O, Bondjers G, Hansson GK. 1986. Regional accumulations of T-cells, macrophages, and smooth muscle cells in the human atherosclerotic plaque. *Arteriosclerosis.* 6:131–138.

Jones TB, Basso DM, Sodhi A et al. 2002. Pathological CNS autoimmune disease triggered by traumatic spinal cord injury: implications for autoimmune vaccine therapy. *J Neurosci.* 22:2690–2700.

Jordan MS, Boesteanu A, Reed AJ et al. 2001. Thymic selection of CD4+CD25+ regulatory T-cells induced by an agonist self-peptide. *Nat Immunol.* 2:301–306.

Kariko K, Weissman D, Welsh FA. 2004. Inhibition of Toll-like receptor and cytokine signaling a unifying theme in ischemic tolerance. *J Cereb Blood Flow Metab.* 24:1288–1304.

Karpus WJ, Lujacs NW, Kennedy KJ, Smith WS, Hurst SD, Barrett TA. 1997. Differential CC chemokine-induced enhancement of T helper cell cytokine production. *J Immunol.* 158:4129–4136.

Kemper C, Chan AC, Green JM, Brett KA, Murphy KM, Atkinson JP. 2003. Activation of human CD4+ cells with CD3 and CD46 induces a T-regulatory cell 1 phenotype. *Nature.* 421:388–392.

Kinter AL, Hennessey M, Bell A et al. 2004. CD25(+)CD4(+) regulatory T-cells from the peripheral blood of asymptomatic HIV-infected individuals regulate CD4(+) and CD8(+) HIV-specific T-cell immune responses in vitro and are associated with favorable clinical markers of disease status. *J Exp Med.* 200:331–343.

Kips JC, Brusselle GJ, Joos GF et al. 1996. Interleukin-12 inhibits antigen-induced airway hyperresponsiveness in mice. *Am J Respir Crit Care Med.* 153:535–539.

Kivisakk P, Mahad DJ, Callahan MK et al. 2004. Expression of CCR7 in multiple sclerosis: implications for CNS immunity. *Ann Neurol.* 55:627–638.

Klein L, Klugmann M, Nave KA, Tuohy VK, Kyewski B. 2000. Shaping of the autoreactive T-cell repertoire by a splice variant of self protein expressed in thymic epithelial cells. *Nat Med.* 6:56–61.

Kohm AP, Carpentier PA, Anger HA, Miller SD. 2002. Cutting edge: CD4+CD25+ regulatory T-cells suppress antigenspecific autoreactive immune responses and central nervous system inflammation during active experimental autoimmune encephalomyelitis. *J Immunol.* 169:4712–4716.

Kojima K, Reindl M, Lassmann H, Wekerle H, Linington C. 1997. The thymus and self-tolerance: co-existence of encephalitogenic S100 b-specific T-cells and their nominal autoantigen in the normal adult rat thymus. *Int Immunol.* 9:897–904.

Krakowski ML, Owens T. 2000. Naive T lymphocytes traffic to inflamed central nervous system, but require antigen recognition for activation. *Eur J Immunol.* 30:1002–1009.

Kretschmer K, Apostolou I, Hawiger D, Khazaie K, Nussenzweig MC, von Boehmer H. 2005. Inducing and expanding regulatory T-cell populations by foreign antigen. *Nat Immunol.* 6:1219–1227.

Krishnamoorthy G, Holz A, Wekerle H. 2007. Experimental models of spontaneous autoimmune disease in the central nervous system. *J Molec Med.* 85:1161–1173.

Kuchroo VK, Anderson AC, Waldner H, Munder M, Bettelli E, Nicholson LB. 2002. T-cell response in experimental autoimmune encephalomyelitis (EAE): role of self and cross-reactive antigens in shaping, tuning, and regulating the autopathogenic T-cell repertoire. *Annu Rev Immunol.* 20:101–123.

Kyewski B, Derbinski J. 2004. Self representation in the thymus: an extended view. *Nat Rev Immunol.* 4:688–698.

Kyewski B, Klein L. 2006. A central role for central tolerance. *Annu Rev Immunol.* 24:571–606.

Lack G, Bradley KL, Hamelmann E et al. 1996. Nebulized IFN-gamma inhibits the development of secondary allergen responses in mice. *J Immunol.* 157:1432–1439.

Langrish CL, Chen Y, Blumenschein WM et al. 2005. IL-23 drives a pathogenic T-cell population that induces autoimmune inflammation. *J Exp Med.* 201:233–240.

Le Gros G, Ben-Sasson SZ, Seder R, Finkelman FD, Paul WE. 1990. Generation of interleukin 4 (IL-4)-producing cells in vivo and in vitro: IL-2 and IL-4 are required for in vitro generation of IL-4- producing cells. *J Exp Med.* 172:921–29.

Le NT, Chao N. 2007. Regulating regulatory T-cells. *Bone Marrow Transplant.* 39:1–9.

Levings MK, Sangregorio R, Galbiati F et al. 2001. IFN-alpha and IL-10 induce the differentiation of human type 1 T regulatory cells. *J Immunol.* 166:5530–5539.

Li XM, Chopra RK, Chou TY, Schofield BH, Wills-Karp M, Huang SK. 1996. Mucosal IFN-gamma gene transfer inhibits pulmonary allergic responses in mice. *J Immunol.* 157:3216–3219.

Liang SC, Tan XY, Luxenberg DP et al. 2006. Interleukin (IL)-22 and IL-17 are co-expressed by Th17 cells and cooperatively enhance expression of antimicrobial peptides. *J Exp Med.* 203:2271–2279.

Lim HW, Hillsamer P, Banham AH, Kim CH. 2005. Cutting edge: direct suppression of B-cells by CD4+ CD25+ regulatory T-cells. *J Immunol.* 175:4180–4183.

Linares D, Mana P, Goodyear M et al. 2003. The magnitude and encephalogenic potential of autoimmune response to MOG is enhanced in MOG deficient mice. *J Autoimmun.* 21:339–351.

Liu H, MacKenzie-Graham AJ, Kim S, Voskuhl RR. 2001. Mice resistant to experimental autoimmune encephalomyelitis have increased thymic expression of myelin basic protein and increased MBP-specific T-cell tolerance. *J Neuroimmunol.* 115:118–126.

Liu W, Putnam AL, Xu-Yu Z et al. 2006a. CD127 expression inversely correlates with FoxP3 and suppressive function of human CD4+ T reg cells. *J Exp Med.* 203:1701–1711.

Liu Y, Teige I, Birnir B, Issazadeh-Navikas S. 2006b. Neuronmediated generation of regulatory T-cells from encephalitogenic T-cells suppresses EAE. *Nat Med.* 12:518–525.

Liuzzo G, Biasucci LM, Gallimore JR et al. 1994. The prognostic value of C-reactive protein and serum amyloid a protein in severe unstable angina. *N Engl J Med.* 331:417–424.

Mach F, Schonbeck U, Sukhova GK, Atkinson E, Libby P. 1998. Reduction of atherosclerosis in mice by inhibition of CD40 signalling. *Nature.* 394:200–203.

Maggi E, Parronchi P, Manetti R et al. 1992. Reciprocal regulatory role of IFN-gamma and IL-4 on the in vitro development of human Th1 and Th2 cells. *J Immunol.* 148:2142–2147.

Manetti R, Parronchi P, Giudizi MG et al. 1993. Natural killer cell stimulatory factor (interleukin-12) induces T helper type 1 (Th1)- specific immune responses and inhibits the development of IL-4- producing Th cells. *J Exp Med.* 177:1199–204.

Maron R, Sukhova G, Faria AM et al. 2002. Mucosal administration of heat shock protein-65 decreases atherosclerosis and inflammation in aortic arch of low-density lipoprotein receptor-deficient mice. *Circulation.* 106:1708–1715.

Masteller EL, Warner MR, Tang Q, Tarbell KV, McDevitt H, Bluestone JA. 2005. Expansion of functional endogenous antigen- specific CD4+CD25+ regulatory T-cells from non-obese diabetic mice. *J Immunol.* 175:3053–3059.

McGeachy MJ, Stephens LA, Anderton SM. 2005. Natural recovery and protection from autoimmune encephalomyelitis: contribution of CD4+CD25+ regulatory cells within the central nervous system. *J Immunol.* 175:3025–3032.

McMahon EJ, Bailey SL, Castenada CV, Waldner H, Miller SD. 2005. Epitope spreading initiates in the CNS in two mouse models of multiple sclerosis. *Nat Med.* 11:335–339.

Melguizo C, Prados J, Velez C, Aránega AE, Marchal JA, Aránega A. 1997. Clinical significance of antiheart antibodies after myocardial infarction. *Jpn Heart J.* 38:779–786.

Miller YI, Chang MK, Binder CJ, Shaw PX, Witztum JL. 2003. Oxidized low density lipoprotein and innate immune receptors. *Curr Opin Lipidol.* 14:437–445.

Miller SD, McMahon EJ, Schreiner B, Bailey SL. 2007. Antigen presentation in the CNS by myeloid dendritic cells drives progression of relapsing experimental autoimmune encephalomyelitis. *Ann N Y Acad Sci.* 1103:179–191.

Mosmann TR, Coffman RL. 1989. TH1 and TH2 cells: different patterns of lymphokine secretion lead to different functional properties. *Adv Immunol.* 46:111–147.

Mouzaki A, Tselios T, Papathanassopoulos P, Matsoukas I, Chatzantoni K. 2004. Immunotherapy for multiple sclerosis: basic insights for new clinical strategies. *Curr Neurovasc Res.* 1:325–340.

Mouzaki A, Deraos S, Chatzantoni K. 2005. Advances in the treatment of autoimmune diseases; cellular activity, Type-1/Type-2 cytokine secretion patterns and their modulation by therapeutic peptides. *Curr Med Chem.* 12:1537–1550.

Murphy CA, Langrish CL, Chen Y et al. 2003. Divergent pro- and antiinflammatory roles for IL-23 and IL-12 in joint autoimmune inflammation. *J Exp Med.* 198:1951–1957.

Nakae S, Nambu A, Sudo K, Iwakura Y. 2003. Suppression of immune induction of collagen-induced arthritis in IL-17-deficient mice. *J Immunol.* 171:6173–6177.

Nakamura K, Kitani A, Strober W. 2001. Cell contact-dependent immunosuppression by CD4+CD25+ regulatory T-cells is mediated by cell surface-bound transforming growth factor b. *J Exp Med.* 194:629–644.

Nicoletti A, Kaveri S, Caligiuri G, Bariety J, Hansson GK. 1998. Immunoglobulin treatment reduces atherosclerosis in Apo E knockout mice. *J Clin Invest.* 102:910–918.

Novak J, Griseri T, Beaudoin L, Lehuen A. 2007. Regulation of type 1 diabetes by NKT cells. *Int Rev Immunol.* 26:49–72.

Nowak M, Stein-Streilein J. 2007. Invariant NKT cells and tolerance. *Int Rev Immunol.* 26:95–119.

Ochi H, Abraham M, Ishikawa H et al. 2006. Oral CD3-specific antibody suppresses autoimmune encephalomyelitis by inducing CD4+ CD25–LAP+ T-cells. *Nat Med.* 12:627–635.

Olsson T, Sun J, Hillert J et al. 1992. Increased numbers of T-cells recognizing multiple myelin basic protein epitopes in multiple sclerosis. *Eur J Immunol.* 22:1083–1087.

Owens T, Babcock AA, Millward JM, Toft-Hansen H. 2005. Cytokine and chemokine inter-regulation in the inflamed or injured CNS. *Brain Res Rev.* 48:178–184.

Oyama J, Blais C Jr, Liu X et al. 2004. Reduced myocardial ischemia-reperfusion injury in Toll-like receptor 4-deficient mice. *Circulation.* 109:784–789.

Park H, Li Z, Yang XO et al. 2005. A distinct lineage of CD4 T-cells regulates tissue inflammation by producing IL-17. *Nat Immunol.* 6:1133–1141.

Parronchi P, De Carli M, Manetti R et al. 1992. IL-4 and IFN(s) (alpha and gamma) exhibit opposite regulatory effects on the development of cytolytic potential by TH1 or TH2 human T-cell clones. *J Immunol.* 149:2977–2982.

Paust S, Lu L, McCarty N, Cantor H. 2004. Engagement of B7 on effector T-cells by regulatory T-cells prevents autoimmune disease. *Proc Natl Acad Sci U S A.* 101:10398–10403.

Perchellet A, Stromnes I, Pang JM, Goverman J. 2004. CD8+ T-cells maintain tolerance to myelin basic protein by 'epitope theft.' *Nat Immunol.* 5:606–614.

Peri G, Introna M, Corradi D et al. 2000. PTX3, A prototypical long pentraxin, is an early indicator of acute myocardial infarction in humans. *Circulation.* 102:636–641.

Perry VH. 1998. A revised view of the central nervous system microenvironment and major histocompatibility complex class II antigen presentation. *J Neuroimmunol.* 90:113–121.

Piccirillo CA, Letterio JJ, Thornton AM et al. 2002. CD4(+) CD25(+) regulatory T-cells can mediate suppressor function in the absence of transforming growth factor beta1 production and responsiveness. *J Exp Med.* 196:237–246.

Powell JD. 2006. The induction and maintenance of T-cell anergy. *Clin Immunol.* 120:239–246.

Raghavan S, Suri-Payer E, Holmgren J. 2004. Antigen-specific in vitro suppression of murine Helicobacter pylori-reactive immunopathological T-cells by CD4CD25 regulatory T-cells. *Scand J Immunol.* 60:82–88.

Reddy J, Illes Z, Zhang X et al. 2004. Myelin proteolipid protein-specific CD4+CD25+ regulatory cells mediate genetic resistance to experimental autoimmune encephalomyelitis. *Proc Natl Acad Sci U S A.* 101:15434–15439.

Reinhardt RL, Kang SJ, Liang HE, Locksley RM. 2006. T helper cell effector fates-who, how and where? *Curr Opin Immunol.* 18:271–277.

Robertson AK, Rudling M, Zhou X, Gorelik L, Flavell RA, Hansson GK. 2003. Disruption of TGF-β signaling in T-cells accelerates atherosclerosis. *J Clin Invest.* 112:1342–1350.

Romagnani S. 1991. Human TH1 and TH2 subsets: doubt no more. *Immunol Today.* 12:256–257.

Romagnani S. 1994. Lymphokine production by human T-cells in disease states. *Annu Rev Immunol.* 12:227–257.

Romagnani S. 1997. The Th1/Th2 paradigm. *Immunol Today.* 18:263–266.

Romagnani S. 2006. Regulation of the T-cell response. *Clin Exp Allergy.* 36:1357–1366.

Romagnoli P, Hudrisier D, van Meerwijk JP. 2005. Molecular signature of recent thymic selection events on effector and regulatory CD4+ T lymphocytes. *J Immunol.* 175:5751–5758.

Roncarolo MG, Bacchetta R, Bordignon C, Narula S, Levings MK. 2001. Type 1 T regulatory cells. *Immunol Rev.* 182:68–79.

Roncarolo MG, Gregori S, Levings M. 2003. Type 1 T regulatory cells and their relationship with CD4+CD25+ T regulatory cells. *Novartis Found Symp.* 252:115–127.

Sakaguchi S. 2004. Naturally arising CD4+ regulatory T-cells for immunologic self-tolerance and negative control of immune responses. *Annu Rev Immunol.* 22:531–562.

Sakaguchi S. 2005. Naturally arising Foxp3-expressing CD25+CD4+ regulatory T cells in immunological tolerance to self and non-self. *Nat Immunol.* 6:345–352.

Sakaguchi S, Ono M, Setoguchi R et al. 2006. Foxp3+ CD25+ CD4+ natural regulatory T cells in dominant self-tolerance and autoimmune disease. *Immunol Rev.* 212:8–27.

Scalzo K, Magdalena Plebanski M, Apostolopoulos V. 2006. Regulatory T-cells: immunomodulators in health and disease. *Curr Top Med Chem.* 6:1759–1768.

Schmitz G, Drobnik W. 2002. ATP-binding cassette transporters in macrophages: promising drug targets for treatment of cardiovascular disease. *Curr Opin Invest Drugs.* 3:853–858.

Schwartz RH. 2005. Natural regulatory T cells and self-tolerance. *Nat Immunol.* 6:327–330.

Seddiki N, Santner-Nanan B, Martinson J et al. 2006. Expression of interleukin (IL)-2 and IL-7 receptors discriminates between human regulatory and activated T-cells. *J Exp Med.* 203:1693–1700.

Seidel MG, Ernst U, Printz D et al. 2006. Expression of the putatively regulatory T-cell marker FOXP3 by CD4+CD25+ T-cells after pediatric hematopoietic stem cell transplantation. *Haematologica.* 91:566–569.

Seino KI, Fukao K, Muramoto K et al. 2001. Requirement for natural killer T (NKT) cells in the induction of allograft tolerance. *Proc Natl Acad Sci U S A.* 98:2577–2581.

Sheikine Y, Hansson GK. 2004. Chemokines and atherosclerosis. *Ann Med.* 36:98–118.

Shimizu J, Yamazaki S, Takahashi T, Ishida Y, Sakaguchi S. 2002. Stimulation of CD25(+)CD4(+) regulatory T-cells through GITR breaks immunological self-tolerance. *Nat Immunol.* 3:135–142.

Shresta S, Pham CT, Thomas DA, Graubert TA, Ley TJ. 1998. How do cytotoxic lymphocytes kill their targets? *Curr Opin Immunol.* 10:581–587.

Siggs OM, Makaroff LE, Liston A. 2006. The why and how of thymocyte negative selection. *Curr Opin Immunol.* 18:175–183.

Skalen K, Gustafsson M, Rydberg EK et al. 2002. Subendothelial retention of atherogenic lipoproteins in early atherosclerosis. *Nature.* 417:750–754.

Skapenko A, Niedobitek GU, Kalden JR, Lipsky PE, Schulze-Koops H. 2004. IL-4 exerts a much more profound suppression of Th1 immunity in humans than in mice. *J Immunol.* 172:6427–6434.

Smits HH, van Rietschoten JG, Hilkens CM et al. 2001. IL-12-induced reversal of human Th2 cells is accompanied by full restoration of IL-12 responsiveness and loss of GATA-3 expression. *Eur J Immunol.* 31:1055–1065.

Sospedra M, Martin R. 2005. Immunology of multiple sclerosis. *Annu Rev Immunol.* 23:683–747.

Starr TK, Jameson SC, Hogquist KA. 2003. Positive and negative selection of T-cells. *Annu Rev Immunol.* 21:139–176.

Stary HC. 2005. Histologic classification of human atherosclerotic lesions. In V Fuster,Topol EJ, Nabel EG, eds. *Atherothrombosis and Coronary Artery Disease.* USA: Lippincott Williams & Wilkins, 439–449.

Stephens LA, Gray D, Anderton SM. 2005. CD4+CD25+ regulatory T-cells limit the risk of autoimmune disease arising from T-cell receptor crossreactivity. *Proc Natl Acad Sci U S A.* 102:17418–17423.

Stern JN, Illes Z, Reddy J et al. 2004. Amelioration of proteolipid protein 139–151-induced encephalomyelitis in SJL mice by modified amino acid copolymers and their mechanisms. *Proc Natl Acad Sci. U S A.* 101:11743–11748.

Streit WJ. 2000. Microglial response to brain injury: a brief synopsis. *Toxicol Pathol.* 28:28–30.

Suri-Payer E, Cantor H. 2001. Differential cytokine requirements for regulation of autoimmune gastritis and colitis by CD4(+)CD25(+) T-cells. *J Autoimmun.* 16:115–123.

Szabo SJ, Sullivan BM, Peng SL, Glimcher LH. 2003. Molecular mechanisms regulating Th1 immune responses. *Annu Rev Immunol.* 21:713–758.

Takahashi T, Kuniyasu Y, Toda M et al. 1998. Immunologic self-tolerance maintained by CD25+CD4+ naturally anergic and suppressive T-cells: induction of autoimmune disease by breaking their anergic/ suppressive state. *Int Immunol.* 10:1969–1980.

Takahashi T, Tagami T, Yamazaki S et al. 2000. Immunologic self-tolerance maintained by CD25(+)CD4(+) regulatory T-cells constitutively expressing cytotoxic T lymphocyte-associated antigen 4. *J Exp Med.* 192:303–310.

Tang Q, Henriksen KJ, Bi M et al. 2004. In vitro-expanded antigen-specific regulatory T-cells suppress autoimmune diabetes. *J Exp Med.* 199:1455–1465.

Tarbell KV, Yamazaki S, Olson K, Toy P, Steinman RM. 2004. CD25+ CD4+ T-cells, expanded with dendritic cells presenting a single autoantigenic peptide, suppress autoimmune diabetes. *J Exp Med.* 199:1467–1477.

Tato CM, O'Shea JJ. 2006. What does it mean to be just 17? *Nature.* 441:166–168.

Thornton AM, Shevach EM. 2000. Suppressor effector function of CD4+CD25+ immunoregulatory T-cells is antigen nonspecific. *J Immunol.* 164:183–190.

Thornton AM, Piccirillo CA, Shevach EM. 2004. Activation requirements for the induction of CD4+CD25+ T-cell suppressor function. *Eur J Immunol.* 34:366–376.

Tischner D, Weishaupt A, van den Brandt J et al. 2006. Polyclonal expansion of regulatory T-cells interferes with effector cell migration in a model of multiple sclerosis. *Brain.* 129:2635–2647.

Toy R. 2006. Torgenson Regulatory T-cells in human auto-immune diseases. *Springer Semin Immun.* 28:63–76.

Tschernatsch M, Gross O, Kneifel N et al. 2007. Autoantibodies against glial antigens in paraneoplastic neurological diseases. *Ann N Y Acad Sci.* 1107:104–110.

van Santen HM, Benoist C, Mathis D. 2004. Number of T reg cells that differentiate does not increase upon encounter of agonist ligand on thymic epithelial cells. *J Exp Med.* 200:1221–1230.

van Stipdonk MJ, Willems AA, Plomp AC, van Noort JM, Boog CJ. 2000. Tolerance controls encephalitogenicity of αB-crystallin in the Lewis rat. *J Neuroimmunol.* 103:103–111.

Veldman C, Hohne A, Dieckmann D, Schuler G, Hertl M. 2004. Type I regulatory T-cells specific for desmoglein 3 are more frequently detected in healthy individuals than in patients with Pemphigus vulgaris. *J Immunol.* 172:6468–6475.

Venken K, Hellings N, Hensen K et al. 2006. Secondary progressive in contrast to relapsing-remitting multiple sclerosis patients show a normal CD4+CD25+ regulatory T-cell function and FOXP3 expression. *J Neurosci Res.* 83:1432–1446.

Vieira PL, Christensen JR, Minaee S et al. 2004. IL-10-secreting regulatory T-cells do not express Foxp3 but have comparable regulatory function to naturally occurring CD4+CD25+ regulatory T-cells. *J Immunol.* 172:5986–5993.

von Boehmer H. 2005. Mechanisms of suppression by suppressor T cells. *Nat Immunol.* 6:338–344.

Waldner H, Collins M, Kuchroo VK. 2004. Activation of antigen presenting cells by microbial products breaks self tolerance and induces autoimmune disease. *J Clin Invest.* 113:990–997.

Walker MR, Carson BD, Nepom GT, Ziegler SF, Buckner JH. 2005. De novo generation of antigen-specific CD4+CD25+regulatoryT-cellsfromhumanCD4+CD25-cells. *Proc Natl Acad Sci U S A.* 102:4103–4108.

Weber SE, Harbertson J, Godebu E et al. 2006. Adaptive islet-specific regulatory CD4 T-cells control autoimmune diabetes and mediate the disappearance of pathogenic Th1 cells in vivo. *J Immunol.* 176:4730–4739.

Weber MS, Prod'homme T, Youssef S et al. 2007. Type II monocytes modulate T cell-mediated central nervous system autoimmune disease. *Nat Med.* 13:935–943.

Weiner HL. 1997. Oral tolerance: immune mechanisms and treatment of autoimmune diseases. *Immunol Today.* 18:335–343.

Witztum JL, Berliner JA. 1998. Oxidized phospholipids and isoprostanes in atherosclerosis. *Curr Opin Lipidol.* 9:441–448.

Worth A, Thrasher AJ, Gaspar B. 2006. Autoimmune lymphoproliferative syndrome: molecular basis of disease and clinical phenotype. *Br J Haematol.* 133:124–140.

Xu Q, Dietrich H, Steiner HJ et al. 1992. Induction of arteriosclerosis in normocholesterolemic rabbits by immunization with heat shock protein 65. *Arterioscler Thromb.* 12:789–799.

Xu Q, Willeit J, Marosi M et al. 1993. Association of serum antibodies to heat-shock protein 65 with carotid atherosclerosis. *Lancet.* 341:255–259.

Yamazaki S, Iyoda T, Tarbell K et al. 2003. Direct expansion of functional CD25+ CD4+ regulatory T-cells by antigen-processing dendritic cells. *J Exp Med.* 198:235–247.

Ye P, Rodriguez FH, Kanaly S et al. 2001. Requirement of IL-17 receptor signalling for lung CXC chemokine and granulocyte colony stimulating factor expression, neutrophil recruitment, and host defense. *J Exp Med.* 194:519–527.

Zhang X, Reddy J, Ochi H, Frenkel D, Kuchroo VK, Weiner HL. 2006. Recovery from experimental allergic encephalomyelitis is TGF-β dependent and associated with increases in CD4+LAP+ and CD4+CD25+ T-cells. *Int Immunol.* 18:495–503.

Zhou J, Carr RI, Liwski RS, Stadnyk AW, Lee TD. 2001. Oral exposure to alloantigen generates intragraft CD8+ regulatory cells. *J Immunol.* 167:107–113.

Zhou X, Stemme S, Hansson GK. 1996. Evidence for a local immune response in atherosclerosis. CD4+ T-cells infiltrate lesions of apolipoprotein-E-deficient mice. *Am J Pathol.* 149:359–366.

Zhu C, Anderson AC, Schubart A et al. 2005. The Tim-3 ligand galectin-9 negatively regulates T helper type 1 immunity. *Nat Immunol.* 6:1245–1252.

Ziegler SF. 2006. FOXP3: of mice and men. *Annu Rev Immunol.* 24:209–226.

PART IV
Translating Novel Cellular Pathways into Viable Therapeutic Strategies

Chapter *15*

ALZHEIMER'S DISEASE—IS IT CAUSED BY CEREBROVASCULAR DYSFUNCTION?

Christian Humpel

ABSTRACT

Alzheimer's disease (AD) is a progressive chronic disorder and is characterized by β-amyloid plaques, tau pathology, cell death of cholinergic neurons, and inflammatory responses. The reasons for this disease are not known, but one hypothesis suggests that cerebrovascular dysfunctions play an important role. This chapter summarizes the most important hypotheses: the role of the β-amyloid cascade, tau pathology, the role of cerebrovascular damage, the influence of glutamate-induced cell death, silent stroke and acidosis, the cell death of cholinergic neurons, the neurovascular unit, growth factor effects, and inflammation. Vascular risk factors are discussed by focusing on the idea that the cerebrovascular dysfunction triggers the development of the disease. Finally, a common hypothesis tries to link the different pathologies of the disease. Different forms of dementia, such as mild cognitive impairment, vascular dementia, and finally AD may overlap at certain stages.

Keywords: vascular system, Alzheimer, vascular dementia, hypothesis, cascade.

ALZHEIMER'S DISEASE, VASCULAR DEMENTIA, AND OTHER FORMS OF DEMENTIA

Sporadic Alzheimer's disease (AD) is a progressive chronic neurodegenerative disorder (at least 95% of all cases are nongenetic), and is characterized by severe β-amyloid deposition (senile plaques), tau pathology, cell death of cholinergic neurons, microglial activation, and inflammation. The causes for AD are yet unknown, but several risk factors may trigger this disease. AD is the most aggressive form of dementia and is distinguished from vascular dementia (vaD). This differentiation of vaD from AD has been based on evidence of a cerebrovascular disorder. However, pure cases of vaD without neurodegenerative changes are very rare and autopsy of some cases clinically diagnosed as vaD showed that they had pathological signs for AD (Sadowski, Pankiewicz, Scholtzova et al. 2004). In addition, mild cognitive impairment (MCI) has been defined as the earliest form of dementia, which partly converts into AD (approximately 15% to 30% per year). Two additional forms of degenerative nonreversible forms of

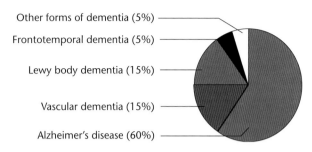

Figure 15.1 Etiology of degenerative forms of dementia. From Heinemann, Zerr 2007.

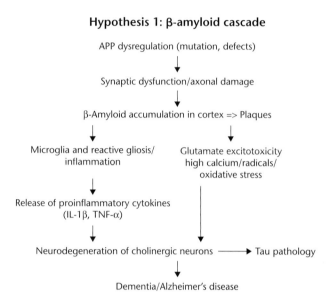

Figure 15.2 The β-amyloid cascade hypothesis suggests that a dysfunction of amyloid-precursor protein (APP), caused by mutation or other defects, results in axonal damage and synaptic dysfunction. This causes β-amyloid accumulation in cortex. Resulting from plaque deposition, inflammatory and excitatory processes occur, which result in neuronal cell death. The inflammatory processes include the release of interleukin-1β (IL-1β) and tumor necrosis factor α (TNF-α), microglial activation, and tau pathology, which are all symptoms of AD.

dementia have been described, Lewy body dementia and frontotemporal dementia, which can be distinguished from AD and vaD. In addition, other nonspecific forms of dementia are seen during, for example, HIV, Parkinson's disease, or alcohol-related diseases. Among all forms of dementia, AD is the most frequent pathological finding (approximately 60%), followed by vascular dementia (approximately 15%), Lewy body dementia (approximately 15%), frontotemporal dementia (approximately 5%), and other degenerative forms of dementia (Gearing, Mirra, Hedree et al. 1995; Barker, Luis, Kashuba et al. 2002; Heinemann, Zerr 2007) (Fig. 15.1).

This chapter discusses the most prominent hypotheses and tries to find a link, especially putting forward the role of the cerebrovascular system for vaD and AD.

β-AMYLOID CASCADE

So far, the β-amyloid cascade (Fig. 15.2) is the most prominent hypothesis (Selkoe 1998; Atwood, Obrenovich, Liu et al. 2003; Tanzi, Moir, Wagner 2004; Wirths, Multhaup, Bayer 2004; Marchesi 2005; Schroeder, Koo 2005) and is thought to be the primary event that triggers the pathological cascade in AD (Selkoe 1998). The amyloid-precursor protein (APP) is cleaved by secretases into β-amyloid peptides (40, 42, or 43 amino acids), and these peptides aggregate under certain conditions and are deposited as β-amyloid plaques (Figs. 15.3A, B). It is hypothesized that the accumulation of β-amyloid in the brain causes the AD pathology and a dysbalance between β-amyloid production and clearance results in other hallmarks of the disease. The β-amyloid cascade hypothesis (Hardy, Selkoe 2002; Tanzi, Bertram 2005) favors the model that insoluble fibrillar β-amyloid triggers the neuronal degeneration. Evidence is now accumulating that soluble activated monomers, soluble oligomers (dimer, trimer, tetramer), and protofibrils could be responsible for triggering the pathology in AD (Walsh, Klyubin, Fadeeva et al. 2002; Canevari, Abramov, Duchen 2004). The exact mechanism by which β-amyloid induces

cell death is not known, but "channel hypothesis" suggests that certain fibrillar forms of the peptide cause neurodegeneration by forming ion channels that are generally large, voltage independent, and relatively poor selective (Wirths, Multhaup, Bayer 2004; Marchesi 2005). Soluble β-amyloid levels in the cortex correlate with the degree of synaptic loss in dementia, and it becomes more and more clear that AD is primarily caused by dysfunction of nerve axons and synapses (Selkoe 2002). In AD, axonal degeneration may depend on β-amyloid levels, but not on plaque deposition, which means that nerve damage occurs before deposition of plaques.

TAUOPATHIES

Tau protein is a microtubule-associated protein that is highly expressed in neurons in the brain. Tau is enriched in axons, where it directly binds to microtubuli. In AD tau is hyperphosphorylated at a variety of serine and threonine residues and loses its ability to bind to microtubuli. Such abnormal hyperphosphorylated tau is a major event involved in the formation of neurofibrillary tangles (Figs. 15.3C, D) in the AD brain (Mandelkow, Mandelkow 1998; Spillantini, Goedert 1998; Smith, Drew, Nunomura et al. 2002; Iqbal, Alonso Adel, Chen et al. 2005). An imbalance between protein kinases and phosphatases may play a role in hyperphosphorylation (Fig. 15.4). Interestingly, enhanced tau is a diagnostic marker in cerebrospinal

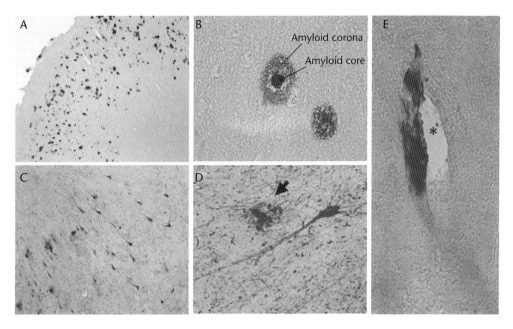

Figure 15.3 β-Amyloid depositions (plaques) are seen in an Alzheimer brain (A, B). Plaques consist of a dense amyloid core and an outer amyloid corona (B). Phospho-tau positive neurofibrillary tangles are intensively found in an Alzheimer brain (C, D). A typical tangle is shown close to dystrophic neurites (D, arrow). β-Amyloid is also concentrated along a brain vessel (E, star). Figures were kindly provided by Prof. Josef Marksteiner (Department of Psychiatry, Innsbruck).

Hypothesis 2: Tau pathology

Protein kinase activity enhanced or phosphatase activity reduced

↓

Hyperphosphorylated Tau

↓

Dsyfunctional binding to microtubuli

↓

Reduced neuronal transport

↓

Synaptic damage—cell death of cholinergic neurons

↓

β-Amyloid accumulation in cortex => plaques

↓

Microglia and reactive gliosis/inflammation/excitotoxicity

↓

Dementia/Alzheimer's disease

Figure 15.4 The tau hypothesis suggests that initially tau is hyperphosphorylated, caused by enhanced protein kinase or decreased phosphatase activity. Reduced axonal transport causes axonal damage and subsequent neuronal cell death. This results in β-amyloid accumulation and plaque deposition, accompanied by inflammatory and excitatory processes and finally AD.

fluid for different forms of neurodegeneration (e.g., Creutzfeldt-Jakob disease) and may strongly correlate to any other form of neurodegeneration and not just AD. Different forms of tau dysregulation (tauopathies) have been described in the literature and are thought to play a role not just in AD.

CEREBROVASCULAR DAMAGE AND BLOOD–BRAIN BARRIER BREAKDOWN

There is increasing evidence that vascular risk factors (Fig. 15.5) contribute to the pathogenesis of AD (de la Torre 1999, 2002; Kudo, Imaizumu, Tanimukai et al. 2000; Iadecola 2004; Zlokovic 2005) and a cerebrovascular hypoperfusion (decreased cerebral blood flow, lower metabolic rates of glucose and oxygen) could be the initial event in AD (Farkas, Luiten 2001; Iadecola 2004). Thus, cerebrovascular diseases and AD may share common risk factors (Fig. 15.5), which indicate that their pathogenic mechanism could be related (de la Torre 2002). Evidence comes from epidemiological studies that these risk factors are hypertension, diabetes, hypercholesterolemia, hyperhomocysteinemia, and the apolipoproteinE4 (ApoE4) genotype (de la Torre 2002). In fact it is hypothesized that neurodegeneration in AD may arise from a chronic mild cerebrovascular dysregulation (Fig. 15.6) caused by continuous exposure to the risk factors over years (Humpel, Marksteiner 2005), which precedes hypoperfusion (de la Torre, Stefano 2000; Iadecola 2004).

A very high percentage (70%–90%) of AD patients show amyloid pathology in their vessels (Fig. 15.3E), which narrow the vessels and produce hypoperfusion (Farkas, Luiten 2001; Cullen, Kocsi, Stone 2006; Hardy, Cullen 2006). This cerebral amyloid angiopathy can result in hemorrhagic and (possibly) ischemic forms of stroke (Armstrong 2006; Haglund, Kalaria, Slade et al. 2006; Soffer 2006; Boscolo, Folin, Nico et al. 2007). The cerebral amyloid angiopathy is common in AD and is also associated with cerebral atherosclerosis (Farkas, Luiten 2001; de la Torre 2002; Attems, Lintner, Jellinger 2004) and with the development of cognitive deficits (Thal, Ghebremedhin, Orantes et al. 2003; Solfrizzi, Panza, Colacicco et al. 2004). As a consequence of cerebrovascular dysfunction the breakdown of the blood–brain barrier (BBB) may occur. This breakdown may have several effects on neurons, such as cell death after influx of excitotoxic amino acids (e.g., glutamate) or enhanced APP

expression after cholesterol influx (see below). In addition, an enhanced influx of blood-derived serum albumin into the brain is seen after BBB disrupture and may induce neurodegeneration (see Moser, Humpel 2007).

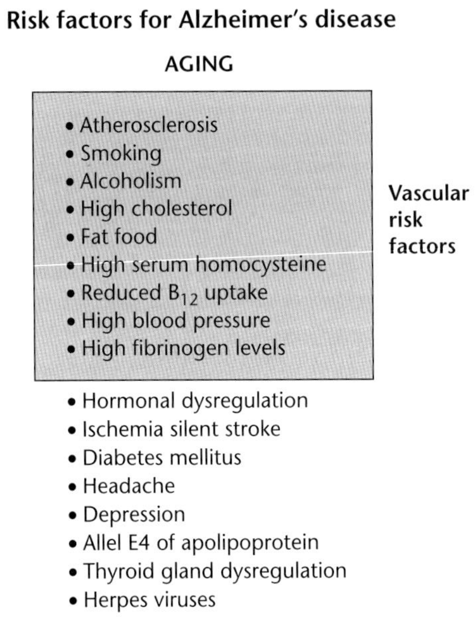

EXCITOTOXICITY

Glutamate is the most important excitatory neurotransmitter in the brain and plays an important role in learning and memory (Figs. 15.2, 15.5, 15.6). Enhanced activity of glutamatergic function, accompanied by massive intracellular calcium influx, is often related with cell death of neurons (Coyle, Puttfarcken 1993). In addition, a rapidly growing body of evidence indicates that increased oxidative stress from reactive oxygen radicals is associated with increased glutamate activity (Olanow 1993; Beal 1996). Oxidative damage induced by free radicals target intracellular structures such as DNA, lipids, or proteins and these free radicals, generated through mitochondrial metabolism, can act as causative factors of abnormal function and cell death. These oxidative changes can arise from the normal aging process, head trauma, increased levels of heavy metals (iron, aluminum, and mercury), and possibly the aggregation of β-amyloid. Thus, glutamate-excitotoxicity and oxidative stress play an important role during the aging process and in different age-related degenerative disorders (Aliev, Smith, Obrenovich et al. 2003; Hynd, Scott, Dodd et al. 2004) including AD.

In AD oxidation of DNA, proteins and fatty acids occur in different brain areas. Some of the oxidation

Risk factors for Alzheimer's disease

AGING

- Atherosclerosis
- Smoking
- Alcoholism
- High cholesterol
- Fat food
- High serum homocysteine
- Reduced B$_{12}$ uptake
- High blood pressure
- High fibrinogen levels

Vascular risk factors

- Hormonal dysregulation
- Ischemia silent stroke
- Diabetes mellitus
- Headache
- Depression
- Allel E4 of apolipoprotein
- Thyroid gland dysregulation
- Herpes viruses

Figure 15.5 Age (>65 years) is the most important risk factor for sporadic AD. Many risk factors have been identified and many of them are also vascular risk factors.

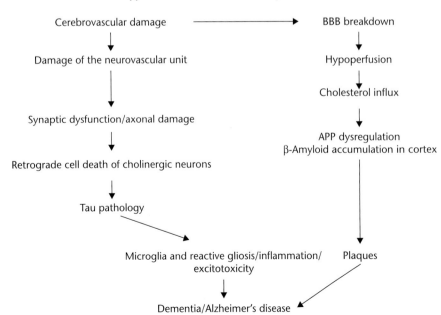

Hypothesis 3: Cerebrovascular dysfunction

Cerebrovascular damage → BBB breakdown

Damage of the neurovascular unit

Synaptic dysfunction/axonal damage

Retrograde cell death of cholinergic neurons

Tau pathology

Hypoperfusion

Cholesterol influx

APP dysregulation
β-Amyloid accumulation in cortex

Microglia and reactive gliosis/inflammation/excitotoxicity   Plaques

Dementia/Alzheimer's disease

Figure 15.6 The hypothesis of cerebrovascular dysfunction suggests that chronic cerebrovascular damage and/or BBB breakdown causes two events: damage of the NVU with subsequent axonal degeneration and cell death of cholinergic neurons and hypoperfusion of mainly cortical areas, resulting in cholesterol influx and subsequent dysregulation of the APP and subsequent β-amyloid dysfunction. Tau pathology and inflammatory and excitatory processes are caused by neuronal cell death ending finally in AD.

products have been found in the neurofibrillary tangles and senile plaques (Markesbery, Carney 1999) and these oxidative modifications are closely associated with an inflammatory process in the AD brain (Butterfield, Griffin, Munch et al. 2002). Markers of oxidative damage are increased in patients with AD (Engelberg 2004) and correlate with decreased levels of plasma antioxidants (Mecocci, Polidori, Cherubini et al. 2002). In fact, oxidative stress and vascular lesions may show an intimate relationship (Aliev, Smith, Obrenovich et al. 2003). It seems quite clear that vascular hypoperfusion induces dysfunction of mitochondria in AD with subsequent RNA oxidation, lipid peroxidation, or mitochondrial DNA deletion (Marcus, Thomas, Rodriguez et al. 1998; Nunomura, Perry, Pappolla et al. 1999; Engelberg 2004; Zhu, Smith, Perry et al. 2004). In fact, patients with AD and vaD showed similar plasma levels of antioxidants and levels of biomarkers of lipid peroxidation (Polidori, Mattioli, Aldred et al. 2004). It was suggested that β-amyloid induces oxidative stress (Behl 1997) and can exert a deleterious effect on endothelial nitric oxide by inhibiting nitric oxide synthetase activity (Venturini, Colasanti, Persichini et al. 2002), which can lead to an alteration of intracellular calcium homeostasis (Gentile, Vecchione, Maffei et al. 2004).

SILENT STROKE

Cerebrovascular disease and ischemic brain injury secondary to cardiovascular diseases are common causes of dementia and cognitive decline in the elderly (Erkinjuntti, Roman, Gauthier et al. 2004). Territorial infarct, old age, and low educational level were identified as predictors of cognitive disorders after stroke (Rasquin Verhey, van Oostenbrugge et al. 2004). Stroke may account for as many as 50% AD cases in old age (Kalaria 2000), and it is known that ischemic events induce APP, β-amyloid, and tau pathology (Kalaria 2000). Approximately 35% of AD patients show autopsy-proven vascular infarcts and 60% show white matter lesions. There exists an association between stroke and AD that may be due to an underlying systemic vascular disease process or, alternatively, due to the additive effects of stroke and AD pathologic features, leading to an earlier age at onset of disease (Honig, Tang, Albert et al. 2003). Several longitudinal studies report an association between stroke and cognitive decline (Langa, Foster, Larson 2004; Linden, Skoog, Fagerberg et al. 2004; Roman 2004; Zhou, Wang, Li et al. 2004). Such small ischemic lesions ("silent stroke," cortical microinfarcts; Kovari, Gold, Herrmann et al. 2007), which in isolation would not alter cognition, substantially aggravate dementia, indicating that cerebral ischemia may interact with AD pathology.

ACIDOSIS

It is now widely accepted that acidosis is an important component of the pathological event that leads to ischemic brain damage (Siesjo 1988, 1992). Acidosis is a result of either an increase in tissue CO_2 or an accumulation of acids produced by dysfunctional metabolism (Rehncrona 1985). Severe hypercapnia (arterial CO_2 around 300 mmHg) may cause a fall in tissue pH to around 6.6 without any morphological evidence of irreversible cell damage (Rehncrona 1985). In severe ischemia and tissue hypoxia, anaerobic glycolysis leads to accumulation of acids, for example, lactate, causing a decrease in pH to around 6.0 (Rehncrona 1985) with strong signs of irreversible damage. This cellular damage seems to be mediated by free radicals but not by a perturbation of cell calcium metabolism (Li, Siesjo 1997). It is well known that acidosis enhances iron-catalyzed production of reactive oxygen species, probably by releasing iron from its binding to transferrin, ferritin, or other proteins (Li, Siesjo 1997). At the cellular level, hypercapnic stimulation activates different transcription factors, which may play a role in counteracting acidosis. Hypercapnic stimulation activates c-jun terminal kinase cascade via influx of extracellular calcium through voltage-gated calcium channels (Shimokawa, Dikic, Sugama et al. 2005). Some transmembrane proteins have been implicated in regulation of H^+ sensitivity and brain acidosis-mediated metabolism (Shimokawa, Dikic, Sugama et al. 2005).

The role of lactate in the brain is divergent, it is a metabolic product and reduces pH, but it is also involved in neuronal metabolism and energy balance. In the brain, lactate is increased after various forms of mild stress (accumulation, handling, cold exposure) after 6 to 7 minutes, which slowly returns to baseline levels over a period of 40 minutes (Fillenz 2005). However, evidence from in vivo experiments does not support the postulate that lactate produced by astrocytes is oxidized by neurons (Fillenz 2005). There is no evidence that under physiological conditions, lactate serves as a significant source of energy for activated neurons (Fillenz 2005). Cerebral intracellular acidosis is endogenous and arises when lactate accumulates, which occurs after epileptic seizures, hypoxia, and ischemia, resulting in a moderate or pronounced decrease in pH (Siesjo 1982). In seizure states, accumulation of lactate is usually moderate (about 10 μmol/g), but in severe ischemia and hypoxia, the accumulation of lactate is markedly enhanced (30 to 60 μmol/g) accompanied by irreversible damage.

Acidosis occurs in the brain during ischemia and plays a role in damaging neuronal environments. We have shown that acidosis causes massive cell death of cholinergic neurons in vitro in brain slices (Pirchl, Marksteiner, Humpel 2006), pointing to a potent role of low pH in the AD brain. However, Cronberg et al. (2005) have shown that acidosis selectively protected CA3 pyramidal neurons during in vitro ischemia. Furthermore, it is highly interesting to note that β-amyloid processing is markedly affected by low pH, which could link acidosis to AD. Brewer (1997) reported that lactate caused a dose-dependent increase in cellular β-amyloid immunoreactivity in hippocampal neurons but acidosis did not affect secretion of β-APP. Atwood et al. (1998) showed that a marked Cu^{2+}-induced aggregation of β-amyloid emerged when the pH was lowered to 6.8, indicating that H^+ induced conformational changes unmask a metal-binding site on β-amyloid that mediates reversible assembly of the peptide that could have relevance for plaque deposition in AD. Matsunaga et al. (1994) showed that β-amyloid (15–22) may control both aggregation of β-amyloid (1–42) at acidic pH and its proteolytic activity at neutral pH. Prolonged acidosis may in fact contribute to the dysregulation of β-amyloid and subsequent plaque deposition and cell death of cholinergic neurons. We have recently shown that under acidic conditions (pH 6.0 + ApoE4) cholinergic neurons degenerate in brain slices that is accompanied by aggregated β-amyloid peptides (Marksteiner, Humpel 2007).

THE NEUROVASCULAR UNIT: THE MOST SENSITIVE NETWORK?

The neurovascular unit (NVU) (Fig. 15.7) defines the cellular interaction between brain capillary endothelial cells (forming the BBB), the astrocytic end feet, and neuronal axons (Iadecola 2004). Astrocytes are

involved in neuronal energy metabolism and synapse function (Iadecola 2004) and neuronal processes are closely associated with cerebral blood vessels (Iadecola 2004). Interestingly, nerve terminals from the cholinergic neurons of the basal nucleus of Meynert interact with astrocytic end feet of the BBB via muscarinic acetylcholine receptors (Vaucher, Hamel 1995; Farkas, Luiten 2001). Thus the NVU provides a direct link between the cerebrovascular system and cholinergic neurons in the brain (Fig. 15.7). Since the NVU provides the first line of defense against deleterious effects of cerebral ischemia and other forms of injury (Iadecola 2004), the NVU may display a very sensitive (pH dependent) link to the brain. In fact, conditioned medium collected from microvessels of AD patients has been shown to kill neurons in vitro, pointing to selective neurotoxic factors derived from brain capillary endothelial cells (Grammas, Moore, Weigel 1999). This is in agreement with our own previous study, where we found that rat primary capillary endothelial cells secreted factors into the medium, which killed cholinergic neurons (Moser, Reindl, Blasig et al. 2004).

It seems likely that the NVU is very sensitive for changes in pH, which may influence cholinergic neurons. In fact, cholinergic neurons interact with cortical microvessels in the rat (Vaucher, Hamel 1995; Farkas, Luiten 2001), and the interaction between vascular structures and cholinergic nerve fibers should be considered as a critical element in neurodegeneration, especially in the view of long-standing suggestions that vessels are lost in the aging brain and that low pH may mediate this cell death. In addition, brain capillary endothelial cells react very sensitively to pH changes, and it is known that acidosis regulates vascular endothelial growth factor (VEGF) expression and angiogenesis in human cancer cells (Fukumura,

The neurovascular unit

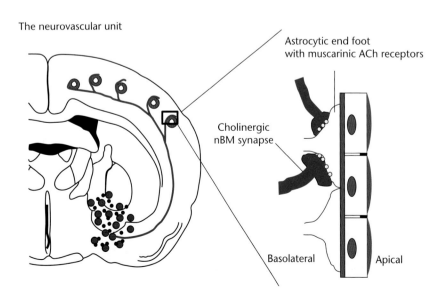

Figure 15.7 The NVU defines a network of the BBB with astrocytes and axonal processes. Cholinergic neurons in the basal nucleus of Meynert send their axons into the cortex, where they connect to the brain capillaries. Cholinergic nerve fibers interact with astrocytes on the endothelial cells via muscarinic cholinergic receptors.

Xu, Chen et al. 2001). It has been shown that in AD angiogenesis occurs accompanied by an upregulation of the transcription factor HIF 1α and subsequently VEGF (Vagnucci, Li 2003), which may be of importance for rearranging the NVU at the BBB. Thus it seems possible that lowering pH may play a role to maintain brain capillary endothelial cells in degenerative diseases, such as in AD and dementia. This is in agreement with a finding that acidosis blocks apoptosis of endothelial cells (D'Arcangelo, Facchiano, Barlucchi et al. 2000).

CELL DEATH OF CHOLINERGIC NEURONS

In AD a marked reduction of cholinergic neurons in the basal forebrain (septum and nucleus basalis of Meynert) is found in advanced stages (Whitehouse et al. 1983; Wilcock, Esiri, Bowen et al. 1982), which leads to cholinergic hypothesis in AD (Francis, Palmer, Snape et al. 1999; Humpel, Weis 2002). Cholinergic activity directly correlates with cognitive activity and a lack of acetylcholine is a hallmark in dementia and AD. It is not known, why these cholinergic neurons die, but it seems possible that the direct interaction with the cerebrovascular system may contribute to cholinergic decline. In fact, damage of the NVU possibly via oxidative stress or inflammation may result in degeneration of nerve terminals and subsequent retrograde cell death of cholinergic neurons. However, neurodegeneration in AD also results in dysregulation of other neurotransmitter systems in the brain, such as serotonin, noradrenaline, or glutamate.

GROWTH FACTORS

Among all growth factors, nerve growth factor (NGF) is the most potent growth factor to counteract cell death of cholinergic neurons in vitro and in vivo (Thoenen, Barde 1980; Levi-Montalcini 1987). In fact NGF was thought to play a role in development of AD, but transgenic NGF knockout mice did not show cognitive deficits. However, NGF was considered to be a candidate for treating AD and purified mouse NGF was infused in some AD patients (Seiger, Nordberg, Von Holst et al. 1993). Interestingly, NGF is upregulated in brains of AD patients (Fahnestock, Michalski, Xu et al. 2001) and in cerebrospinal fluid (Hock, Heese, Müller-Spahn et al. 2000), while the high-affinity NGF receptor trkA is downregulated (Mufson, Ma, Dills et al. 2002; Counts, Nadeem, Wuu et al. 2004). It can be explained that enhanced cortical (target-derived) NGF is enhanced but cannot be transported to neuronal somata, because the axonal transport is destructed and the receptors are not functional

(Mufson, Kroin, Sendera et al. 1999). Furthermore, angiogenic growth factors, such as VEGF (Fukumura, Xu, Chen et al. 2001; Tarkowski, Issa, Sjögren et al. 2002), are increased, resulting in enhanced microvascular density in developing AD. It has been shown that in AD angiogenesis occurs accompanied by an upregulation of the transcription factor HIF1-α and VEGF (Vagnucci, Li 2003), which may be of importance in rearranging the capillary network.

However, besides NGF and VEGF, other growth factors contribute to the AD pathology or are dysregulated. Platelet-derived growth factor (PDGF) has been found to upregulate APP in the hippocampus by inducing secretases (Gianni, Zambrano, Bimonte et al. 2003; Zambrano, Gianni, Bruni et al. 2004; Lim, Cho, Hong et al. 2007). Insulin-like growth factor-I (IGF-I) regulates β-amyloid levels and displays protective effects against β-amyloid toxicity (Carro, Trejo, Gomez-Isla et al. 2002; Aguado-Llera, Arilla-Ferreiro, Campos-Barros et al. 2005). Fibroblast growth factor-2 (FGF-2) has common binding sites with β-amyloid fibrils in heparan sulfate from cerebral cortex (Lindahl, Westling, Gimenez-Gallego et al. 1999) and plays a role in β-amyloid toxicity (Cantara, Ziche, Donnini 2005). Finally, members of the transforming growth factor-β (TGF-β) family interact with β-amyloid mediating its toxicity (TGF-β2; Hashimoto, Chiba, Yamada et al. 2005; Hashimoto, Nawa, Chiba et al. 2006) or are a risk for cerebral β-amyloid angiopathy due to polymorphism of the *TGF-β1* gene with cerebral amyloid (Greenberg, Cho, O'Donnell et al. 2000; Lesne, Docagne, Gabriel et al. 2003; Hamaguchi, Okino, Sodeyama et al. 2005).

INFLAMMATION AND MICROGLIA

Inflammation is an important trigger of neurodegeneration during aging ("Inflammaging") (Franceschi, Valensin, Bonafe et al. 2001) and is considered as a major factor of neurodegeneration in AD (Figs. 15.2, 15.4, 15.6). Inflammation is a potential target for AD therapy and anti-inflammatory drugs may delay AD (Perry, Bell, Brown et al. 1995; Moore, O'Banion 2002). Indeed, cholinergic neurons of the basal nucleus of Meynert are very sensitive for inflammatory insults (Wenk, McGann, Mencarelli et al. 2000; Wenk, McGann, Hauss-Wegrzyniak et al. 2003). Chronic release of pro-inflammatory cytokines, such as interleukin-1β, tumor necrosis factor α, or TGF-β1, indicate a powerful role in inflammation, pathology, and neuronal dysfunction associated with AD (Perry, Bell, Brown et al. 1995; Grammas, Ovase 2002; Wenk, McGann, Hauss-Wegrzyniak et al. 2003). These inflammatory processes include activation of microglia and subsequent neuroinflammatory processes (Gonzalez-Scarano, Baltuch 1999). However, it is not clear if inflammation is a result of β-amyloid dysregulation (Moore, O'Banion 2002) or if inflammation itself is the primary cause in initiation of AD. Inflammation of brain capillary endothelial cells may play a potent role, and it is well known that endothelial cells strongly respond to inflammatory stimuli (Moser, Reindl, Blasig et al. 2004), especially involving production of reactive oxygen species (Iadecola 2004).

WHAT IS THE TRIGGER FOR CEREBROVASCULAR DAMAGE?

The risk factors and the pathology in AD are well known; however, it is not clear which factors trigger the development of the different forms of dementia that finally may end in AD. On the basis of cerebrovascular hypothesis, different initial vascular triggers can be identified.

Hyperhomocysteinemia

Cerebrovascular diseases and AD share common risk factors, such as hyperhomocysteinemia, which indicate that their pathogenic mechanism could be connected. It is well established that elevated plasma levels of the amino acid homocysteine increase the risk for atherosclerosis, stroke, myocardial infarction, and AD (Shea, Lyons-Weiler, Rogers 2002; Faraci 2003; Flicker, Martins, Thomas et al. 2004; Gallucci, Zanardo, De Valentin et al. 2004; Skurk, Walsh 2004; Ravaglia, Forti, Maioli et al. 2005; rev. Troen 2005). It has been reported that plasma homocysteine levels >15 μM increase the risk for vaD and AD (Clarke, Smith, Jobst et al. 1998; McCaddon, Davies, Hudson et al. 1998; Hogervorst, Ribeiro, Molyneux et al. 2002; McIlroy, Dynan, Lawson et al. 2002; Seshadri, Beiser, Selhub et al. 2002; Luchsinger, Tang, Shea et al. 2004). In humans the effective concentration results from total levels of homocysteine and its oxidation product disulfide homocysteine (Lipton, Kim, Choi et al. 1997). In an in vivo rat model, hyperhomocysteinemia provokes a memory deficit in the Morris water maze task, clearly indicating that hyperhomocysteinemia causes cognitive dysfunction (Streck, Bavaresco, Netto et al. 2004). In rat models of hyperhomocysteinemia plasma levels vary between 19 and 26 μM, which highly correlates with plasma levels found in vaD and AD (Kim, Lee, Chang 2002; Lee, Borchelt, Wong et al. 2004).

Metabolism of Homocysteine

Homocysteine is a nonprotein forming sulfur amino acid involved in two important pathways: (1) methylation

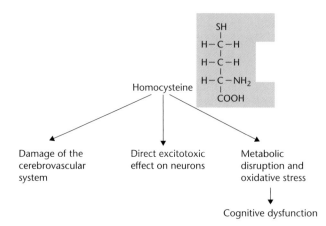

Figure 15.8 Effects of hyperhomocysteinemia in the brain.

and (2) trans-sulfuration (rev. Troen 2005). In the methylation pathway, homocysteine and 5-methyltetrahydrofolate generate methionine (vitamin B_{12} dependent), which is converted to S-adenosylmethionine and acts as a methyl donor. S-adenosylhomocysteine is then formed and hydrolyzed to homocysteine and adenosine. In the trans-sulfuration pathway, homocysteine and serine generate cystathionine, which is involved in generation of cysteine, taurine, and inorganic sulfates. The rapid removal of homocysteine is of importance to the maintenance of a normal methylation process.

Three hypothetical mechanisms of hyperhomocysteinemia have been reported (Fig. 15.8):

1. Damage of the cerebrovascular system: Hyperhomocysteinemia induces endothelial damage, mitochondrial swelling and disintegration, swelling of pericytes, basement membrane thickening, and perivascular detachment (Weir, Molloy 2000; Kim, Lee, Chang 2002; rev. Troen 2005); all pathologies are also seen in vaD and AD. The intracellular effects of homocysteine are very divergent: it induces, for example, caspase-8 and subsequent apoptosis, it stimulates monocyte chemoattractant protein-1/interleukin-8 and subsequent inflammation, and it enhances oxidative stress (via activation of different oxidases), inhibits endothelial nitric oxide synthetase, and generates peroxynitrite with subsequent cell death (Faraci 2003; Lee, Borchelt, Wong et al. 2004; Skurk, Walsh 2004). Furthermore, homocysteine decreases capillary endothelial nitric oxide synthetase (Faraci 2003) and glucose transporter and transiently changes different cell adhesion molecules (Lee, Borchelt, Wong et al. 2004).

2. Direct excitotoxic effect on neurons: Homocysteine and its derivative homocysteic acid are excitatory amino acids. Lipton et al. (1997) have shown that 10 μM homocysteine directly induces cell death of cerebrocortical-isolated neurons after 6 days. This cell death was blocked by 10 μM MK-801 and 12 μM memantine, indicating involvement of *N*-methyl-D-aspartate receptors in vitro. However, it is unclear if brain levels of homocysteine may reach µM concentrations and exert direct toxic effects. In fact, homocysteine levels in cerebrospinal fluid in the brain are in the nM range (rev. Troen 2005).

3. Metabolic disruption and oxidative stress: Accumulation of homocysteine increases intracellular *S*-adenosylhomocysteine, which is a potent inhibitor of many methylation reactions (rev. Troen 2005), including methylation of biogenic amines and inhibition of catechol-*O*-methyltransferase (Zhu 2002). Chronic hyperhomocysteinemia induced by methionine administration enhanced lipid peroxidation and decreased glutathione, suggesting the involvement of oxidative stress (Baydas, Ozer M, Yasar et al. 2005). These dysfunctions were accompanied by cognitive impairment and could be counteracted by the antioxidant melatonin (Baydas, Ozer, Yasar et al. 2005).

Hypercholesterolemia

Cholesterol is increasingly recognized to play a major role in the pathogenesis of AD (Raffai, Weisgraber 2003; Wellington 2004; Wolozin 2004). This is based on four lines of investigation: (1) the lipoprotein ApoE4 coordinates the mobilization and redistribution of cholesterol in the brain and

affects the age of onset, (2) intracellular cholesterol stimulates γ-secretase and APP/β-amyloid processing, (3) cholesterol-lowering drugs (statins) reduce the prevalence of AD, and (4) elevated plasma cholesterol in midlife is associated with an increased risk for AD. Interestingly, rabbits fed with a 2% cholesterol diet display an accumulation of intracellular immunolabeled β-amyloid after 4 to 8 weeks (Sparks, Scheff, Hunsaker et al. 1994) and hypercholesterolemia accelerates the amyloid pathology in a transgenic mouse model (Refolo, Pappolla, Malester et al. 2000; Shie, Jin, Cook et al. 2002).

Cholesterol does not pass the BBB and is synthesized locally in the brain and degraded to 24-hydroxy-cholesterol, which is transported outside the brain into the bloodstream (Fig. 15.9). Cholesterol regulates γ-secretase with enhanced processing of β-amyloid (1–42). It is hypothesized that a breakdown of the BBB causes influx of cholesterol, with subsequent activation of γ-secretase and enhanced β-amyloid (1–42) production (Fig. 15.9). Under specific conditions (high ApoE4, low pH, metals, and dysfunctional clearance) the β-amyloid (1–42) peptides may aggregate in the brain. β-amyloid is present in the brain and in the blood and is transported through the BBB via two important receptor transport systems (Fig. 15.9): the receptor for advanced glycosylation end products (RAGE) and low-density lipoprotein-related protein (LRP) (Tanzi, Moir,

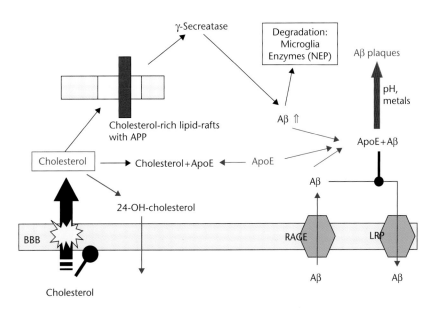

Figure 15.9 Role of cholesterol on metabolism of β-amyloid. Cholesterol does not pass the blood–brain barrier (BBB) and is synthesized locally in the brain and degraded to 24-OH-cholesterol, which is transported into the bloodstream. Cholesterol regulates γ-secretase with enhanced processing of the amyloid-precursor protein (APP) to β-amyloid (Aβ). This peptide is degraded by different enzymes (e.g., neutral endopeptidase [NEP]) or transported to the blood via low-density lipoprotein-related proteins (LRP). The concentration of β-amyloid in the brain is regulated by steady-state clearance of influx via receptor for advanced glycosylation end products (RAGE) and efflux via LRP. It is hypothesized that a breakdown of the BBB causes influx of cholesterol, with subsequent activation of γ-secretase and enhanced β-amyloid (1–42) production. Under specific conditions (high apolipoprotein E [ApoE], low pH, metals, and/or dysfunctional clearance) the β-amyloid (1–42) peptides may aggregate in the brain.

Wagner 2004). The influx of β-amyloid from blood into brain is mediated via RAGE, while the efflux from brain into blood is mediated via LRP (Tanzi, Moir, Wagner et al. 2004). This clearance from brain to blood is of pivotal importance for the regulation of β-amyloid levels in the brain (Tanzi, Moir, Wagner 2004) and a dysregulation of the BBB contributes to enhanced β-amyloid levels in the brain.

Hypo- and Hyperglycemia

Hypo- and hyperglycemia both have disruptive effects on the brain and markedly affect cognition and memory (for a review see Brands, Kessels, deHaan et al. 2004). Several reports showed a relation between recurrent episodes of severe hypoglycemia and cognitive deficits and patients who experienced multiple severe hypoglycemic episodes showed cortical atrophy. Severe and prolonged hypoglycemia provokes brain damage through uncontrolled release of excitatory amino acids such as glutamate and aspartate, which triggers calcium influx. Hyperglycemia leads to increased levels of glucose in the brain, by which excess glucose is converted into sorbitol and fructose, which influences several intracellular cascades. Elevated glucose is also associated with formation of toxic advanced glycation end products, reactive oxygen species, or hyperhomocysteinemia. Diabetes causes hyperglycemia due to defects in secretion of, or resistance to, insulin, or both; it is associated with both structural and functional alterations in the cerebral vascular system, which increases stroke. Cerebral blood flow has been reported to be decreased in diabetes increasing risk of "silent stroke." There was a strong interaction of diabetes and hypertension, such that the association between diabetes and cortical atrophy existed only in hypertensive but not in normotensive participants (Schmidt, Launer, Nilsson et al. 2004). In a prospective population-based cohort study among elderly subjects, it was found that diabetes significantly increased the risk for dementia (Ott, Stolk, van Harskamp et al. 1999).

RODENT MODELS FOR AD, vaD, AND OTHER FORMS OF DEMENTIA

Rodent models for AD allow the study of this progressive neurodegenerative chronic disease. Most models have been established in mice, by overexpression of β-amyloid (transgenic APP mice) and plaque deposition, which displays the severest endstage of pathology in AD (Lee, Borchelt, Wong et al. 1996). Transgenic mice that express large amounts of β-amyloid in the central nervous system is likely to

elucidate mechanisms by which the protein is selectively deposited in the brain in a parenchymal or microvascular form, and how it contributes to the pathogenesis of neurodegeneration (Vinters, Wang, Secor et al. 1996). Transgenic mice have been developed, which displayed a pathology very close to AD, and these mice were generated by overexpression of anti-NGF antibodies (Capsoni, Giannotta, Cattaneo 2002). Novak and colleagues (Axon Neuroscience, Vienna) developed the first rat with enhanced expression of tau ("Axon Alzheimer rat"). Several other models have been established to observe learning and aging in mice and rats, and especially cerebrovascular hypoperfusion (e.g., by common carotid occlusion) has been shown to result in dementia-like pathology (de la Torre, Mussivand 1993). The stroke-prone spontaneous hypertensive rats display pathology of vaD pointing to the importance of "silent stroke" or "multi-infarct dementia" in the development of AD (Kimura, Saito, Minami et al. 2000). Riederer and colleagues demonstrated gene expression profiled in a streptozotocin rat model for sporadic AD (Grünblatt, Hoyer, Riederer 2004). However, all these models do either show the endstage of the disease (including plaque deposition) or use severe invasive surgery (carotid occlusion or stereotaxic surgery), models which do not reflect the physiological chronic noninvasive neurodegenerative disease for AD or vaD.

CURRENT CLINICAL TRIALS

On the basis of experimental in vitro and in vivo approaches, different therapeutic clinical strategies have been developed that enter the clinical routine. Four important strategies are outlined in this chapter:

- **Acetylcholine esterase inhibitors:** To date the acetylcholine esterase inhibitors (Giacobini 2004), donepezil, galantamine, and rivastigmine, are the best medication to counteract the symptoms of AD.
- **Glutamate antagonist:** Alternatively to acetylcholine esterase inhibitors, the glutamate antagonist memantine is used to counteract glutamate-mediated toxicity in AD (Molinuevo, Llado, Rami 2005).
- **NGF therapy:** NGF was infused into AD patients directly into the brain at high dose to protect cholinergic neurons; however, this study failed due to severe side effects (Seiger, Nordberg, Von Holst et al. 1993). Alternatively, NGF secreting human skin cells were transplanted directly into the brain displaying some improvements in cognition (Tuszynski, Thal, Pay et al. 2005). The problem of such treatments is the severe invasive surgical procedure, which will only be possible for some

selected patients. As an alternative, noninvasive delivery methods need to be explored, such as the development of BBB permeable NGF agonists, or the use of delivery vehicles, such as NGF secreting blood cells, an approach that is also currently explored in our laboratory.

- β-**Amyloid immunization:** Finally, experiments in animals with β-amyloid immunization (Morgan 2006) were successful; however, the first clinical trials failed due to severe side effects. Recently a new clinical study in Vienna was again started for β-amyloid immunization. The number of international clinical trials is enormous and cannot be fully described in this chapter, however, two links to prominent databases may help to find specific clinical AD trials:

www.nia.nih.gov/Alzheimer
www.clinicaltrials.gov

A COMMON HYPOTHESIS–WHAT IS THE LINK?

How do all these puzzle stones fit into one model? It is not clear, how AD is caused and it is not clear how the different forms of dementia fit into one model. Is vaD another disease or is it an early stage of AD? Is MCI the earliest form of AD and of vaD? Many researchers favor the β-amyloid cascade hypothesis, and think that a dysregulation of β-amyloid metabolism is the primary cause for AD. Other researchers believe that only tau may account for the disease without affecting the β-amyloid processing. Putting several evidence together, it seems likely that the aging of the cerebrovascular system may trigger the development of dementia: age is the most important risk factor and different vascular risk factors correlate with the development of dementia and with cognitive deficits.

In this chapter it is hypothesized that the damage of the cerebrovascular system is the initial event in the development of dementia. This damage is a chronic long-lasting and mild event over years, which may dramatically affect the small brain capillaries (Fig. 15.10). Different vascular risk factors, such as hyperhomocysteinemia, hypercholesterolemia, hypertension, hypo- or hyperglycemia, may play an important role in such a chronic damage (Fig. 15.10). This chronic damage of the brain capillaries will result in hypoperfusion of the cortex (Fig. 15.10) and also in selective damage of the NVU (Fig. 15.10). As a result of the damage of the NVU cholinergic synapses lose contact with the NVU. It seems likely that such an event may cause retrograde-induced axonal damage and subsequent cell death of cholinergic neurons (Fig. 15.10). Such a loss of cholinergic neurons correlates with

lack of acetylcholine in cortex and hippocampus. On the other hand, hypoperfusion causes "silent stroke," which as a single small event does not cause massive cell death, but will cause small local lesions, which may correlate to short cognitive deficits (Fig. 15.10). Silent stroke results in release of glutamate, influx of calcium and reduction of pH (acidosis), which further contributes to the damage of the NVU (Fig. 15.10). Depending on the extent of lesion and cell death, these cognitive deficits might be regarded as MCI or in larger extent as vaD. However, if the extent of damage exceeds after BBB breakdown, cholesterol influx may dysregulate APP expression and enhance γ-secretase and subsequent β-amyloid (1–42) production (Fig. 15.10). Enhanced brain β-amyloid (1–42) cannot be effectively cleared by efflux through the BBB (Tanzi, Moir, Wagner 2004; Zlokovic 2004), resulting in enhanced β-amyloid (1–42) levels in the brain tissue (Fig. 15.10). Combined with reduced pH (6.0–6.6) β-amyloid may aggregate under specific conditions (e.g., in the presence of ApoE4 or metals) and form aggregates, which is the major hallmark seen in AD.

It seems likely that cell death of neurons and axonal damage correlates with tau pathology (Fig. 15.10). This cell death also mediates activation of microglia and subsequent inflammatory processes (Fig. 15.10). A dysregulated β-amyloid also affects brain capillaries and causes β-amyloid angiopathy. Last but not the least, several compensatory mechanisms are seen in the AD brains. The most potent protective growth factor NGF is enhanced, but since axonal transport systems are damaged, this protein cannot be transported to somata (Fig. 15.10). On the other hand, the reduced stimulation produces a downregulation of the high-affinity NGF receptor trkA (Fig. 15.10). Furthermore, other growth factors are enhanced, such as VEGF, which can be induced by the transcription factor HIF1-α after stroke and may play a role in repairing brain capillaries.

It seems possible that the different stages in dementia are defined as the extent of damage of the cerebrovascular system and all subsequent events in the brain. However, it cannot be excluded that the "final link" is still missing, which may favor another, or a modified, hypothesis.

CONCLUSION

It is not known if AD has a common origin with all other forms of dementia; however, if the damage of the cerebrovascular system is the major factor for cognitive decline, then it may be likely that the different forms of dementia may overlap and finally end in AD. Thus, it seems possible that mainly the extent of vascular lesion, silent stroke, cholinergic cell death, APP

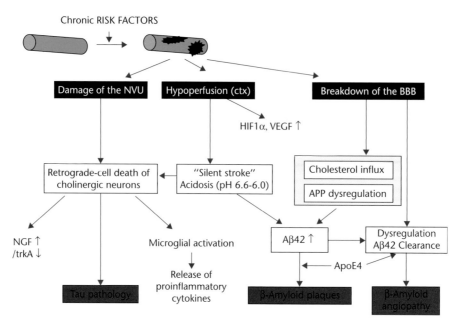

Figure 15.10 A common hypothesis for AD. It is hypothesized that small brain capillaries are the major target for initiation of dementia. Different risk factors (such as hyperhomocysteinemia, hypercholesterol, hypertension, hypoperfusion) chronically trigger damage of brain capillaries. This leads to (1) damage of the neurovascular unit (NVU), (2) hypoperfusion of the brain, especially the cortex (ctx), and (3) breakdown of the BBB. The damage of the NVU results in degeneration of synaptic nerve terminals at the NVU. The subsequent retrograde-induced cell death of cholinergic neurons correlates with lack of cortical acetylcholine as found in dementia. An upregulation of NGF in the cortex and downregulation of its high-affinity NGF receptor trkA contributes to axonal damage. The breakdown of the BBB of the cortex contributes to the damage of the NVU. Reduced glucose and cerebral blood flow causes silent stroke that may induce upregulation of the transcription factor HIF1α and subsequently vascular endothelial growth factor (VEGF) and subsequent angiogenic responses. Hypoperfusion may trigger APP dsyfunction possibly via cholesterol influx and β/γ-secretase stimulation, which results in enhanced generation of β-amyloid (1–42) (Aβ42). A combined dysregulation of (1) enhanced β-amyloid production, (2) reduced β-amyloid clearance through the blood–brain barrier (BBB), (3) reduced pH (acidosis), and (4) apolipoprotein E4 (ApoE4) binding to β-amyloid, favors the aggregation of β-amyloid and plaque deposition. The severe axonal damage and cell death of neurons lead to dysfunction of tau and hyperphosphorylation and subsequent tau pathology. Last but not the least microglia become massively activated and migrate to lesion sites and release proinflammatory cytokines. It seems reasonable that mild chronic changes in cerebrovascular dysfunction correlate to mild cognitive impairment; moderate damage is found in vascular dementia, while an extensive chronic damage results in β-amyloid and tau pathology as seen in AD.

dysfunction and β-amyloid deposition, tau pathology, and common neurodegeneration may define the different stages of aging, predementia stages, early stages of dementia, vaD, and AD.

ACKNOWLEDGMENT   C.H. was supported by the Austrian Science Funds (P19122-B05).

REFERENCES

Aguado-Llera D, Arilla-Ferreiro E, Campos-Barros A, Puebla-Jimenez L, Barrios V. 2005. Protective effects of insulin-like growth factor-I on the somatostatinergic system in the temporal cortex of beta-amyloid-treated rats. *J Neurochem.* 92:607–615.

Aliev G, Smith MA, Obrenovich ME, de la Torre JC, Perry G. 2003. Role of vascular hypoperfusion-induce oxidative stress and mitochondria failure in the pathogenesis of Alzheimer's disease. *Neurotox Res.* 5:491–504.

Armstrong RA. 2006. Classic beta-amyloid deposits cluster around large diameter blood vessels rather than capillaries in sporadic Alzheimer's disease. *Curr Neurovasc.* 3:89–94.

Attems J, Lintner F, Jellinger K. 2004. Amyloid beta peptide 1–42 highly correlates with capillary cerebral amyloid angiopathy and Alzheimer disease pathology. *Acta Neuropathol.* 107:283–291.

Atwood CS, Moir RD, Huang X et al. 1998. Dramatic aggregation of Alzheimer Abeta by Cu(II) is induced by conditions representing physiological acidosis. *J Biol Chem.* 273:12817–12826.

Atwood CS, Obrenovich ME, Liu T et al. 2003. Amyloid-beta: a chameleon walking in two worlds: a review of the trophic and toxic properties of amyloid-beta. *Brain Res Rev.* 43:1–16.

Barker WW, Luis CA, Kashuba A et al. 2002. Relative frequencies of Alzheimer disease, Lewy body, vascular and frontotemporal dementia, and hippocampal sclerosis in the State of Florida Brain Bank. *Alzheimer Dis Assoc Disord.* 16:203–212.

Baydas G, Ozer M, Yasar A, Tuzcu M, Koz ST. 2005. Melatonin improves learning and memory performances impaired by hyperhomo-cysteinemia in rats. *Brain Res.* 1046:187–194.

Beal MF. 1996. Mitochondria, free radicals, and neurodegeneration. *Curr Opinion Neurobiol.* 6:661–666.

Behl C. 1997. Amyloid beta-protein toxicity and oxidative stress in Alzheimer's disease. *Cell Tissue Res.* 290:471–480.

Boscolo E, Folin M, Nico B et al. 2007. Beta amyloid angiogenic activity in vitro and in vivo. *Int J Mol Med.* 19:581–587.

Brands AMA, Kessels RPC, deHaan EHF, Kappelle LJ, Biessels GJ. 2004. Cerebral dysfunction in type 1 diabetes; effects of insulin, vascular risk factors and blood-glucose levels. *Eur J Clin Pharmacol.* 490:159–168.

Brewer GJ. 1997. Effects of acidosis on the distribution of processing of the beta-amyloid precursor protein in cultured hippocampal neurons. *Mol Chem Neuropathol.* 31:171–186.

Butterfield DA, Griffin S, Munch G, Pasinetti GM. 2002. Amyloid beta-peptide and amyloid pathology are central to the oxidative stress and inflammatory cascades under which Alzheimer's disease brain exists. *J Alzheimers Dis.* 4:193–201.

Canevari L, Abramov AY, Duchen MR. 2004. Toxicity of amyloid beta peptides: tales of calcium, mitochondria, and oxidative stress. *Neurochem Res.* 29:637–650.

Cantara S, Ziche M, Donnini S. 2005. Opposite effects of beta amyloid on endothelial cell survival: role of fibroblast growth factor2 (FGF-2). *Pharmacol Rep.* 57:138–143.

Capsoni S, Giannotta S, Cattaneo A. 2002. Early events of Alzheimer-like neurodegeneration in anti-nerve growth factor transgenic mice. *Brain Aging.* 2:24–43.

Carro E, Trejo JL, Gomez-Isla T, LeRoith D, Torres-Aleman I. 2002. Serum insulin-like growth factor I regulates brain amyloid-beta levels. *Nat Med.* 8:1390–1397.

Clarke R, Smith AD, Jobst KA, Refsum H, Sutton L, Ueland PM 1998. Folate, vitamin B12, and serum total homocysteine levels in confirmed Alzheimer disease. *Arch Neurol.* 55:1449–1455.

Counts SE, Nadeem M, Wuu J, SD G, Saragovi HU, Mufson EJ. 2004. Reduction of cortical trkA but not p75NTR protein in early-stage Alzheimer's Disease. *Ann Neurol.* 56:520–531.

Coyle JT, Puttfarcken P. 1993. Oxidative stress, glutamate, and neurodegenerative disorders. *Science.* 262:689–695.

Cronberg T, Jensen K, Rytter A, Wieloch T. 2005. Selective sparing of hippocampal CA3 cells following in vitro ischemia is due to selective inhibition by acidosis. *Europ J Neurosci.* 22:310–316.

Cullen KM, Kocsi Z, Stone J. 2006. Microvascular pathology in the aging human brain: evidence that senile plaques are sites of microhaemorrhages. *Neurobiol Aging.* 27:1786–1796.

D'Arcangelo D, Facchiano F, Barlucchi LM et al. 2000. Acidosis inhibits endothelial cell apoptosis and function and induce basic fibroblast growth factor and vascular endothelial growth factor. *Circ Res.* 86:312–318.

de la Torre JC. 1999. Critical threshold cerebral hypoperfusion causes Alzheimer's disease. *Acta Neuropathol.* 98:1–8.

de la Torre JC. 2002. Alzheimer's disease as a vascular disorder. *Stroke.* 33:1152–1162.

de la Torre JC, Mussivand T. 1993. Can disturbed brain microcirculation cause Alzheimer's Disease? *Neurol Res.* 15:146–153.

de la Torre JC, Stefano GB. 2000. Evidence that Alzheimer's disease is a microvascular disorder, the role of constitutive nitric oxide. *Brain Res Brain Res Rev.* 34:119–136.

Engelberg H. 2004. Pathogenic factors in vascular dementia and Alzheimer's Disease, multiple actions of heparin that probably are beneficial. *Dement Geriatr Cogn Disord.* 18:278–298.

Erkinjuntti T, Roman G, Gauthier S, Feldman H, Rockwood K. 2004. Emerging therapies for vascular dementia and vascular cognitive impairment. *Stroke.* 35:1010–1017.

Fahnestock M, Michalski B, Xu B, Coughlin MD. 2001. The precursor pro-nerve growth factor is the predominant form of nerve growth factor in brain and is increased in Alzheimer's disease. *Mol Cell Neurosci.* 18:210–220.

Faraci FM. 2003. Hyperhomocysteinemia, A million ways to lose control. *Arterioscler Thromb Vasc Biol.* 23:371–373.

Farkas E, Luiten PGM. 2001. Cerebral microvascular pathology in aging and Alzheimer's disease. *Progr Neurobiol.* 64:575–611.

Fillenz M. 2005. The role of lactate in brain metabolism. *Neurochem Int.* 47:413–417.

Flicker L, Martins RN, Thomas J et al. 2004. Homocysteine, Alzheimer genes and proteins, and measures of cognition and depression in older men. *J Alzheimers Dis.* 6:329–336.

Franceschi C, Valensin S, Bonafe M et al. 2000. The network and the remodeling theories of aging, historical background and new perspectives. *Exp Gerontol.* 35:879–896.

Francis PT, Palmer AM, Snape M, Wilcock GK. 1999. The cholinergic hypothesis of Alzheimer's disease, a review of progress. *J Neurol Neurosurg Psychiatr.* 66:137–147.

Fukumura D, Xu L, Chen Y, Gohongi T, Seed B, Jain RK. 2001. Hypoxia and acidosis independently up-regulate vascular endothelial growth factor transcription in brain tumor in vivo. *Cancer Res.* 61:6020–6024.

Gallucci M, Zanardo A, De Valentin L, Vianello A. 2004. Homocysteine in Alzheimer disease and vascular dementia. *Arch Gerontol Geriatr.* Suppl 9:195–200.

Gearing M, Mirra SS, Hedree JC, Sumi SM, Hansen LA, Heyman A. 1995. The Consortium to Establish a Registry for Alzheimer's Disease (CERAD). Part X. Neuropathology confirmation of the clinical diagnosis of Alzheimer's disease. *Neurology.* 45:461–466.

Gentile MT, Vecchione C, Maffei A et al. 2004. Mechanisms of soluble beta-amyloid impairment of endothelial function. *J Biol Chem.* 279:48135–48142.

Giacobini E. 2004. Cholinesterase inhibitors: new roles and therapeutic alternatives. *Pharmacol Res.* 50:433–40.

Gianni D, Zambrano N, Bimonte M et al. 2003. Platelet-derived growth factor induces the beta-gamma-secretase-mediated cleavage of Alzheimer's amyloid precursor protein through a Src-Rac-dependent pathway. *J Biol Chem.* 278:9290–9297.

Gonzalez-Scarano F, Baltuch G. 1999. Microglia as mediators of inflammatory and degenerative diseases. *Annu Rev Neurosci.* 22:219–240.

Grammas P, Moore P, Weigel PH. 1999. Microvessels from Alzheimer's disease brains kill neurons in vitro. *Am J Pathol.* 154:337–342.

Grammas P, Ovase R. 2002. Cerebrovascular transforming growth factor-beta contributes to inflammation in the Alzheimer's disease brain. *Am J Pathol.* 160:1583–1587.

Greenberg SM, Cho HS, O'Donnell HC et al. 2000. Plasma beta-amyloid peptide, transforming growth factor-beta 1, and risk for cerebral amyloid angiopathy. *Ann N Y Acad Sci.* 903:144–149.

Grünblatt E, Hoyer S, Riederer P. 2004. Gene expression profile in streptozotocin rar model for sporadic Alzheimer's disease. *J Neural Transm.* 111:367–386.

Haglund M, Kalaria R, Slade JY, Englund E. 2006. Differential deposition of amyloid beta peptides in cerebral amyloid angiopathy associated with Alzheimer's disease and vascular dementia. *Acta Neuropathol.* 111:430–435.

Hamaguchi T, Okino S, Sodeyama N et al. 2005. Association of a polymorphism of the transforming growth factor-beta1 gene with cerebral amyloid angiopathy. *J Neurol Neurosurg Psychiatr.* 76:696–699.

Hardy J, Selkoe D. 2002. The amyloid hypothesis of Alzheimer's disease: progress and problems on the road to therapeutics. *Science.* 298:353–356.

Hardy J, Cullen K. 2006. Amyloid at the blood vessel wall. *Nat Med.* 12:756–757.

Hashimoto Y, Chiba T, Yamada M et al. 2005. Transforming growth factor beta2 is a neuronal death-inducing ligand for amyloid-beta precursor protein. *Mol Cell Biol.* 25:9304–9317.

Hashimoto Y, Nawa M, Chiba T, Aiso S, Nishimoto I, Matsuoka M. 2006. Transforming growth factor beta2 autocrinally mediates neuronal cell death induced by amyloid-beta. *J Neurosci Res.* 83:1039–1047.

Heinemann U, Zerr J. 2007. Demenzen: pathogenese, neurobiochemische diagose sowie reversible Demenz symptome. *NeuroForum.* 2:47–54.

Hock C, Heese K, Müller-Spahn F et al. 2000. Increased CSF levels of nerve growth factor in patients with Alzheimer's disease. *Neurology.* 54:2009–2011.

Hogervorst E, Ribeiro HM, Molyneux A, Budge M, Smith AD. 2002. Plasma homocysteine levels, cerebrovascular risk factors, and cerebral white matter changes (leukoaraiosis) in patients with Alzheimer disease. *Arch Neurol.* 59:787–793.

Honig LS, Tang MX, Albert S et al. 2003. Stroke and the risk of Alzheimer disease. *Arch Neurol.* 60:1707–1712.

Humpel C, Weis C. 2002. Nerve growth factor and cholinergic CNS neurons studied in organotypic brain slices, Implications in Alzheimer's disease. *J Neural Transm Suppl.* 62:253–263.

Humpel C, Marksteiner J. 2005. Cerebrovascular damage as a cause for Alzheimer's disease? *Curr Neurovas Res.* 2:341–347.

Hynd MR, Scott HL, Dodd PR. 2004. Glutamate-mediated excitotoxicity and neurodegeneration in Alzheimer's disease. *Neurochem Int.* 45:583–595.

Iadecola C. 2004. Neurovascular regulation in the normal brain and in Alzheimer's disease. *Nat Rev Neurosci.* 5:347–360.

Iqbal K, Alonso Adel C, Chen S et al. 2005. Tau pathology in Alzheimer disease and other tauopathies. *Biochim Biophys Acta.* 1739:198–210.

Kalaria RN. 2000. The role of cerebral ischemia in Alzheimer's disease. *Neurobiol Aging.* 21:321–330.

Kim J-M, Lee HJ, Chang N. 2002. Hyperhomocysteinemia due to short-term folate deprivation is related to electron microscopic changes in the rat brain. *J Nutr.* 132:3418–3421.

Kimura S, Saito H, Minami M et al. 2000. Pathogenesis of vascular dementia in stroke-prone spontaneously hypertensive rats. *Toxicology.* 153:167–178.

Kovari E, Gold G, Herrmann FR et al. 2007. Cortical microinfarcts and demyelination affect cognition in cases at high risk for dementia. *Neurology.* 68:927–931.

Kudo T, Imaizumu K, Tanimukai H et al. 2000. Are cerebrovascular factors involved in Alzheimer's disease? *Neurobiol Aging.* 21:215–224.

Langa KM, Foster NL, Larson EB. 2004. Mixed dementia, emerging concepts and therapeutic implications. *JAMA.* 292:2901–2908.

Lee H, Kim H-J, Kim J-M, Chang N. 2004. Effects of dietary folic acid supplementation on cerebrovascular endothelial dysfunction in rats with induced hyperhomocysteinemia. *Brain Res.* 996:139–147.

Lee MK, Borchelt DR, Wong PC, Sisodia SS, Price DL. 1996. Transgenic models of neurodegenerative diseases. *Curr Opin Neurobiol.* 6:651–660.

Lesne S, Docagne F, Gabriel C et al. 2003. Transforming growth factor-beta 1 potentiates amyloid-beta generation in astrocytes and in transgenic mice. *J Biol Chem.* 278:18408–18418.

Levi-Montalcini R. 1987. The nerve growth factor, thirty-five years later. *Biosci Rep.* 7:681–699.

Li PA, Siesjo BK. 1997. Role of hyperglycaemia-related acidosis in ischemic brain damage. *Acta Physiol Scand.* 161:567–580.

Lim JS, Cho H, Hong HS, Kwon H, Mook-Jung I, Kwon YK. 2007. Upregulation of amyloid precursor protein by platelet-derived growth factor in hippocampal precursor cells. *Neuroreport.* 6:1225–1229.

Lindahl B, Westling C, Gimenez-Gallego G, Lindahl U, Salmivirta M. 1999. Common binding sites for beta-amyloid fibrils and fibroblast growth factor-2 in heparan sulfate from human cerebral cortex. *J Biol Chem.* 274:30631–30635.

Linden T, Skoog I, Fagerberg B, Steen B, Blomstrand C. 2004. Cognitive impairment and dementia 20 months after stroke. *Neuroepidemiology.* 23:45–52.

Lipton SA, Kim W-K, Choi Y-B et al. 1997. Neurotoxicity associated with dual actions of homocysteine at the N-methyl-D-aspartate receptor. *Proc Natl Acad Sci U S A.* 94:5923–5928.

Luchsinger JA, Tang MX, Shea S, Miller J, Green R, Mayeux R. 2004. Plasma homocysteine levels and risk of Alzheimer disease. *Neurology.* 62:1972–1976.

Mandelkow EM, Mandelkow E. 1998. Tau in Alzheimer's disease. *Trends Cell Biol.* 8:425–427.

Marchesi VT. 2005. An alternative interpretation of the amyloid Abeta hypothesis with regard to the pathogenesis of Alzheimer's disease. *Proc Natl Acad Sci U S A.* 102:9093–9098.

Marcus DL, Thomas C, Rodriguez C et al. 1998. Increased peroxidation and reduced antioxidant enzyme activity in Alzheimer's disease. *Exp Neurol.* 150:40–44.

Markesbery WR, Carney JM. 1999. Oxidative alterations in Alzheimer's disease. *Brain Pathol.* 9:133–146.

Marksteiner J, Kaufmann WA, Gurka P, Humpel C. 2002. Synaptic proteins in Alzheimer's disease. *J Mol Neurosci.* 18:53–63.

Marksteiner J, Humpel C. 2007. Beta-amyloid expression, release and extracellular deposition in aged rat brain slices. *Mol Psychiatry.* [Epub ahead of print.]

Matsunaga Y, Fujii A, Awasthi A, Yokotani J, Takakura T, Yamada T. 1994. Eight residue amyloid beta peptides inhibit the aggregation and enzymatic activity of amyloid-beta42. *Regul Pept.* 120:227–236.

McCaddon A, Davies G, Hudson P, Tandy S, Cattell H. 1998. Total serum homocysteine in senile dementia of Alzheimer type. *Int J Geriatr Psychiatry.* 13:235–239.

McIlroy SP, Dynan KB, Lawson JT, Patterson CC, Passmore AP. 2002. Moderately elevated plasma homocysteine, methylenetetra-hydrofolate reductase genotype, and risk for stroke, vascular dementia, and Alzheimer disease in Northern Ireland. *Stroke.* 33:2351–2356.

Mecocci P, Polidori MC, Cherubini A et al. 2002. Lymphocyte oxidative DNA damage and plasma antioxidants in Alzheimer disease. *Arch Neurol.* 59:794–798.

Molinuevo JL, Llado A, Rami L. 2005. Memantine: targeting glutamate excitotoxicity in Alzheimer's disease and other dementias. *Am J Alzheimers Dis Other Demen.* 20:77–85.

Moore AH, O'Banion MK. 2002. Neuroinflammation and anti-inflammatory therapy for Alzheimer's disease. *Adv Drug Deliv Rev.* 54:1627–1656.

Morgan D. 2006. Immunotherapy for Alzheimer's disease. *J Alzheimers Dis.* 9:425–432.

Moser K, Reindl M, Blasig I, Humpel C. 2004. Brain capillary endothelial cells proliferate in response to NGF, express NGF receptors and secrete NGF after inflammation. *Brain Res.* 1017:53–60.

Moser KV, Humpel C. 2007. Blood-derived serum albumin contributes to neurodegeneration via astroglial stress fiber formation. *Pharmacology.* 80(4):286–292.

Mufson EJ, Kroin JS, Sendera TJ, Sobreviela T. 1999. Distribution and retrograde transport of trophic factors in the central nervous system, functional implications for the treatment of neurodegenerative diseases. *Prog Neurobiol.* 57:451–484.

Mufson EJ, Ma SY, Dills J et al. 2002. Loss of basal forebrain p75NTR immunoreactivity in subjects with mild cognitive impairment and Alzheimer's disease. *J Comp Neurol.* 443:136–153.

Nunomura A, Perry G, Pappolla MA et al. 1999. RNA oxidation is a prominent feature of vulnerable neurons in Alzheimer's disease. *J Neurosci.* 19:1959–1964.

Olanow CW. 1993. A radical hypothesis for neurodegeneration. *Trends Neurosci.* 16:439–444.

Ott A, Stolk RP, van Harskamp F, Pols HA, Hofman A, Breteler MM. 1999. Diabetes mellitus and the risk of dementia, the rotterdam Study. *Neurology.* 53:1937–1942.

Perry VH, Bell MD, Brown HC, Matyszak MK. 1995. Inflammation in the nervous system. *Curr Opin Neurobiol.* 5:636–641.

Pirchl M, Marksteiner J, Humpel C. 2006. Effects of acidosis on brain capillary endothelial cells and cholinergic neurons, relevance for vascular dementia and Alzheimer's disease. *Neurol Res.* 28:657–664.

Polidori MC, Mattioli P, Aldred S et al. 2004. Plasma antioxidant status, immunoglobulin g oxidation and lipid peroxidation in demented patients, relevance to Alzheimer disease and vascular dementia. *Dement Geriatr Cogn Disord.* 18:265–270.

Raffai RL, Weisgraber KH. 2003. Cholesterol, from heart attacks to Alzheimer's disease. *J Lipid Res.* 44:1423–1430.

Rasquin SM, Verhey FR, van Oostenbrugge RJ, Lousberg R, Lodder J. 2004. Demographic and CT scan features related to cognitive impairment in the first year after stroke. *J Neurol Neurosurg Psychiatr.* 75:1562–1567.

Ravaglia G, Forti P, Maioli F et al. 2005. Homocysteine and folate as risk factors for dementia and Alzheimer disease. *Am J Clin Nutr.* 82:636–643.

Refolo LM, Pappolla MA, Malester B et al. 2000. Hypercholesterolemia accelerates the Alzheimer's amyloid pathology in a transgenic mouse model. *Neurobiol Dis.* 7:321–331.

Rehncrona S. 1985. Brain acidosis. *Ann Emerg Med.* 14:770–776.

Rocca WA, Kokmen E. 1999. Frequency and distribution of vascular dementia. *Alzheimer Dis Assoc Disord.* 13:S9–S14.

Roman GC. 2004. Facts, myths, and controversies in vascular dementia. *J Neurol Sci.* 226:49–52.

Sadowski M, Pankiewicz J, Scholtzova H et al. 2004. Links between the pathology of Alzheimer's disease and vascular dementia. *Neurochem Res.* 29:1257–1266.

Schmidt R, Launer LJ, Nilsson LG et al. 2004. Magnetic resonance imaging of the brain in diabetes, the cardiovascular determinants of dementia (CASCADE) study. *Diabetes.* 53:687–692.

Schroeder BE, Koo EH. 2005. To think or not to think, synaptic activity and Abeta release. *Neuron.* 48:873–879.

Seiger A, Nordberg A, Von Holst H et al. 1993. Intracranial infusion of purified nerve growth factor to an Alzheimer patient, the first attempt of a possible future treatment strategy. *Beh Brain Res.* 57:255–261.

Selkoe DJ. 1998. The cell biology of beta-amyloid precursor protein and presenilin in Alzheimer's disease. *Trends Cell Biol.* 8:447–453.

Selkoe DJ. 2002. Alzheimer's disease is a synaptic failure. *Science.* 298:789–791.

Seshadri S, Beiser A, Selhub J et al. 2002. Plasma homocysteine as a risk factor for dementia and Alzheimer's disease. *N Engl J Med.* 346:476–483.

Shea TB, Lyons-Weiler J, Rogers E. 2002. Homocysteine, folate deprivation and Alzheimer neuropathology. *J Alzheimers Dis.* 4:261–267 Review.

Shie F-S, Jin L-W, Cook DG, Leverenz JB, LeBouef RC. 2002. Diet-induced hypercholesterolemia enhances brain Abeta accumulation in transgenic mice. *NeuroReport.* 13:455–459.

Shimokawa N, Dikic I, Sugama S, Koibuchi N. 2005. Molecular responses to acidosis of central chemosensitive neurons in brain. *Cell Signal.* 17:799–808.

Siesjo BK. 1982. Lactic acidosis in the brain, occurrence, triggering mechanisms and pathophysiological importance. *Ciba Found Symp.* 87:77–100.

Siesjo BK. 1988. Acidosis and ischemic brain damage. *Neurochem Pathol.* 9:31–88.

Siesjo BK. 1992. Pathophysiology and treatment of focal cerebral ischemia. Part I, Pathophysiology. *J Neurosurg.* 77:169–184.

Skurk C, Walsh K. 2004. Death receptor induced apoptosis, a new mechanism of homocysteine-mediated endothelial cell cytotoxicity. *Hypertension.* 43:1168–1170.

Smith MA, Drew KL, Nunomura A et al. 2002. Amyloid-beta, tau alterations and mitochondrial dysfunction in Alzheimer disease, the chickens or the eggs? *Neurochem Int.* 40:527–531.

Soffer D. 2006. Cerebral amyloid angiopathy—a disease or age-related condition. *Isr Med Assoc J.* 8:803–806.

Solfrizzi V, Panza F, Colacicco AM et al. 2004. Vascular risk factors, incidence of MCI, and rates of progression to dementia. *Neurology.* 63:1882–1891.

Sparks DL, Scheff SW, Hunsaker JC 3rd, Liu H, landers T, Gross DR. 1994. Induction of Alzheimer-like beta-amyloid immunoreactivity in the brains of rabbits with dietary cholesterol. *Exp Neurol.* 126:88–94.

Spillantini MG, Goedert M. 1998. Tau protein pathology in neurodegenerative diseases. *Trends Neurosci.* 21:428–433.

Streck EL, Bavaresco CS, Netto CA, de Souza Wyse AT. 2004. Chronic hyperhomocysteinema provokes a memory deficit in rats in the morris water maze task. *Beh Brain Res.* 153:377–381.

Tanzi RE, Moir RD, Wagner SL. 2004. Clearance of Alzheimer's Abeta peptide, The many roads to perdition. *Neuron.* 43:505–608.

Tanzi RE, Bertram L. 2005. Twenty years of the Alzheimer's disease amyloid hypothesis, a genetic perspective. *Cell.* 120:545–555.

Tarkowski E, Issa R, Sjögren M, et al. 2002. Increased intrathecal levels of the angiogenic factors VEGF and TGF-beta in Alzheimer's disease and vascular dementia. *Neurobiol Aging.* 23:237–243.

Thal DR, Ghebremedhin E, Orantes M, Wiestler OD. 2003. Vascular pathology in Alzheimer disease, correlation of cerebral amyloid angiopathy and arteriosclerosis/lipohyalinosis with cognitive decline. *J Neuropathol Exp Neurol.* 62:1287–1301.

Thoenen H, Barde Y-A. 1980. Physiology of nerve growth factor. *Physiol Rev.* 60:1284–1335.

Troen AM. 2005. The central nervous system in animal models of hyperhomocysteinemia. *Progr Neuro-Psychopharmacol. & Biological Psychiatry.* 29:1140–1151.

Tuszynski MH, Thal L, Pay M et al. 2005. A phase I clinical trial of nerve growth factor gene therapy for Alzheimer disease. *Nat Med.* 11:551–555.

Vagnucci AH, Li WW. 2003. Alzheimer's disease and angiogenesis. *Lancet.* 361:605–608.

Vaucher W, Hamel EC. 1995. Holinergic basal forebrain neurons project to cortical microvessels in the rat, electron microscopic study with anterograde transported *Phaesolus vulgaris* leucoagglutinin and choline acetyltransferase immunocytochemistry. *J Neurosci.* 15:7427–7441.

Venturini G, Colasanti M, Persichini T et al. 2002. Beta-amyloid inhibits NOS activity by subtracting NADPH availability. *FASEB J.* 16:1970–1972.

Vinters HV, Wang ZZ, Secor DL. 1996. Brain parenchymal and microvascular amyloid in Alzheimer's disease. *Brain Pathol.* 6:179–195.

Walsh DM, Klyubin I, Fadeeva JV, Rowan MJ, Selkoe DJ. 2002. Amyloid-beta oligomers: their production, toxicity and therapeutic inhibition. *Biochem Soc Trans.* 30:552–557.

Weir DG, Molloy AM. 2000. Microvascular disease and dementia in the elderly, are they related to hyperhomocysteinemia? *Am J Clin Nutr.* 71:859–860.

Wellington CL. 2004. Cholesterol at the crossroads, Alzheimer's disease and lipid metabolism. *Clin Genet.* 66:1–16.

Wenk GL, McGann K, Mencarelli A, Hauss-Wegrzyniak B, Soldato PD, Fiorucci S. 2000. Mechanisms to prevent the toxicity of chronic neuroinflammation on forebrain cholinergic neurons. *Eur J Pharmacol.* 402:77–85.

Wenk GL, McGann K, Hauss-Wegrzyniak B, Rosi S. 2003. The toxicity of tumor necrosis factor-alpha upon cholinergic neurons within the nucleus basalis and the role of norepinephrine in the regulation of inflammation, implications for Alzheimer's disease. *Neurosci.* 121:719–729.

Whitehouse PJ, Hedreen JC, White CL III, Price DL. 1983. Basal forebrain neurons in the dementia of Parkinson's disease. *Ann Neurol.* 13:243–248.

Wilcock GK, Esiri MM, Bowen DM, Smith CC. 1982. Alzheimer's disease Correlation of cortical choline acetyltransferase activity with the severity of dementia and histological abnormalities. *J Neurol Sci.* 57:407–417.

Wirths O, Multhaup G, Bayer TA. 2004. A modified beta-amyloid hypothesis, intraneuronal accumulation of beta-amyloid peptide—the first step of a fatal cascade. *J Neurochem.* 91:513–520.

Wolozin B. 2004. Cholesterol and the biology of Alzheimer's disease. *Neuron.* 41:7–10.

Zambrano N, Gianni D, Bruni P, Passaro F, Telese F, Russo T. 2004. Fe65 is not involved in the platelet-derived growth factor-induced processing of Alzheimer's amyloid precursor protein, which activates its caspase-directed cleavage. *J Biol Chem.* 279:16161–16169.

Zhou DH, Wang JY, Li J, Deng J, Gao C, Chen M. 2004. Study on frequency and predictors of dementia after ischemic stroke, the chongqing stroke study. *J Neurol.* 251:421–427.

Zhu BT. 2002. On the mechanism of homocysteine pathophysiology and pathogenesis, a unifying hypothesis. *Histol Histopathol.* 17:1283–1291.

Zhu X, Smith MA, Perry G, Aliev G. 2004. Mitochondrial failure in Alzheimer's disease. *Am J Alzheimers Dis Other Demen.* 19:345–352.

Zlokovic BV. 2004. Clearing amyloid through the blood-brain barrier. *J Neurochem.* 89:807–811.

Zlokovic BV. 2005. Neurovascular mechanisms of Alzheimer's neurodegeneration. *Trends Neurosci.* 28:202–208.

Chapter *16*

PROTEASES IN β-AMYLOID METABOLISM: POTENTIAL THERAPEUTIC TARGETS AGAINST ALZHEIMER'S DISEASE

Noureddine Brakch and Mohamed Rholam

ABSTRACT

Proteases are extremely important signaling molecules that are involved in numerous vital processes. By cleaving the proteins or peptides, proteases participate in the control of a large number of key physiological processes such as cell proliferation and cell death, DNA replication, tissue remodeling and haemostasis. Protease signaling pathways are strictly regulated, and therefore the dysregulation of their activity can lead to pathologies such as cardiovascular and inflammatory diseases, cancer, and neurological disorders. An illustration of the functional role of proteases in physiological processes is demonstrated in the metabolism of β-amyloid.

Under normal physiological conditions, the steady-state level of β-amyloid peptide in the brain is determined by the rate of production from amyloid precursor protein via β- and γ-secretases and rate of degradation by the activity of several known metallopeptidases. In conditions that affect the activity of these proteases (e.g., genetic mutations, environmental factors, or age), overactive secretases or underactive β-amyloid–degrading enzymes could shift the balance of amyloid metabolism toward abnormal β-amyloid deposition in the brain, an early and invariant feature of all forms of Alzheimer's disease (AD).

In view of this, these proteases represent potential therapeutic targets against AD, and consequently, regulation of their activity by drugs is now considered as an important strategy in the neuroprotection.

Keywords: β-amyloid, proteases, proteolytic processing, Alzheimer's disease.

A large number of debilitating human diseases such as Alzheimer's, Creutzfeld–Jacob, Huntington's, and Parkinson's diseases, type 2 diabetes mellitus, and various forms of systematic amyloidosis have in common the presence of characteristic lesions in affected tissues, consisting of intra- or extracellular aggregates of misfolded proteins. In these pathological conditions, the aggregation of misfolded proteins may arise from abnormalities in the ubiquitin–proteasome system for removing damaged proteins, problems with the chaperone systems, or increased levels of protein misfolding, or a combination of all three (Ohnishi, Takano 2004; Stefani 2004; Uversky, Fink 2004; Chiti, Dobson 2006; Glabe 2006). Generally, the misfolding process can occur sporadically or result from mutations to the gene that encodes the deposited protein or the related processing proteins. In Alzheimer's disease

(AD), sporadic disease is more common than inherited disease, suggesting that a spontaneous misfolding event, engendered by conformational changes in the deposited protein and/or by a deficiency in the cellular clearance mechanisms, can initiate aggregation (Selkoe 2004; Masters, Beyreuther 2006). It is noteworthy that the fate of proteins and peptides is generally affected by different events (e.g., posttranslational modifications, sorting to subcellular localization sites, and processing or degradation processes) that are noticeably controlled by partial amino acid sequences and cellular microenvironments (Nakai 2001; Brakch, El Abida, Rholam 2006).

AD, the most frequent form of amyloidosis that affects humans during aging, is a multifactorial and heterogeneous mental illness characterized by an age-dependent loss of memory and an impairment of cognitive functions (Ferri, Prince, Brayne et al. 2005; Dubois, Feldman, Jacova et al. 2007). The neuropathological features of AD are the extracellular neuritic plaques, composed of a dense amyloid core of β-amyloid peptides (Aβ), and the intracellular neurofibrillary tangles, composed of an abnormally phosphorylated form of the protein tau, in the brain (Selkoe 2004; Dubois, Feldman, Jacova et al. 2007). All the data provided by biochemical, cell biological, and genetic studies argue in favor of the upstream initiator of Aβ in the progression of AD (Dubois, Feldman, Jacova et al. 2007). Support for the importance of Aβ in AD etiology has been provided by genetic analysis of Down syndrome (DS) and the dominant forms of early-onset familial Alzheimer's disease (FAD). In DS, triplication of *APP* gene–containing chromosome 21 leads to increased APP expression (Mori, Spooner, Wisniewsk et al. 2002) while in FAD, mutations in the gene encoding the amyloid precursor protein (APP) or the γ-secretase enhance Aβ production (Selkoe 2004). In sporadic forms of AD, which account for more than 90% of all AD cases, or in certain forms of FAD, linked to hereditary cerebral hemorrhage with amyloidosis, a reduction in the catabolic activity toward Aβ has been the major cause for Aβ accumulation than an elevation of anabolic activity (Selkoe 2004; Dubois, Feldman, Jacova et al. 2007). Several risk factors such as age (Dubois, Feldman, Jacova et al. 2007), apolipoprotein E genotype (Raber, Huang, Ashford 2004), insulin-dependent diabetes (de la Monte, Wands 2005), and environmental conditions (Onyango, Khan 2006) are known for contributing to the development of late-onset AD.

FAD is caused by genetic mutations that directly lead to an overproduction of Aβ while sporadic AD is triggered by genetic and/or environmental factors that predispose the brain to an increased production or a reduced rate of clearance of Aβ. This review discusses the events involved in the proteolytic processing of APP, the modulation of Aβ production, and the clearance of Aβ. Altered protease activity and/or peptide conformation may have a strong association with the pathophysiology of AD.

AMYLOID PRECURSOR PROTEIN AND Aβ PRODUCTION

Aβ, the main component of senile plaques and cerebral amyloid angiopathy, is generated by sequential proteolytic cleavage of APP (Fig. 16.1). This precursor, expressed in brain and most other tissues, has features of an integral type I transmembrane glycoprotein containing a large extracytoplasmic domain, a membrane-spanning domain containing the Aβ peptide, and a short intracytoplasmic tail (De Strooper, Annaert 2000).

APP Functions

APP is a member of a multigene family that includes amyloid precursor-like proteins 1 and 2 (APLP1 and APLP2) having little homology to APP in the region corresponding to Aβ (Wasco, Bupp, Magendantz et al. 1992). APP occurs in numerous isoforms that arise from alternative splicing of a single gene located on chromosome 21. Of the two most commonly expressed isoforms (APP695 and APP751), APP695 lacks the Kunitz-type serine protease inhibitor domain (De Strooper, Annaert 2000).

The ubiquitous expression of APP in many tissues as well as the presence of homologues in a variety of species argues for an important physiological function of APP (De Strooper, Annaert 2000). Deletion of the APP protein gene in mice results in only minor deficits whereas combined knockouts (KOs) of *APP* gene family members in mice result in perinatal lethality and neurological deficits (Herms, Anliker, Heber et al. 2004; Wang, Yang, Mosier et al. 2005). Besides its importance in brain development, APP exhibits numerous subdomains that confer a variety of potential biological functions including axonal transport of vesicles (Gunawardena, Goldstein 2001) and metal ion homeostasis (Barnham, McKinstry, Multhaup et al. 2003).

Processing of APP

APP is proteolytically processed by α-, β- and γ-secretases via two distinct processing pathways (Panchal, Rholam, Brakch 2004). APP is cleaved by α-secretase (Fig. 16.1A) or at a separate site by β-secretase (Fig. 16.1B) to generate the soluble APP ectodomains

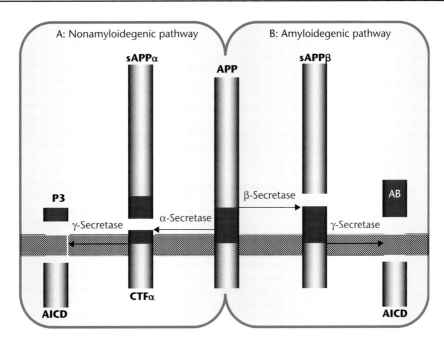

Figure 16.1 Proteolytic processing pathways of APP. APP can be processed through two main pathways. In the nonamyloidogenic pathway (A), α-secretase cleaves APP within the Aβ domain, releasing the large soluble APP fragment (sAPPα). The remaining C-terminal fragment (CTFα) is cleaved by the γ-secretase complex to generate the short p3 peptide. The remaining APP intracellular domain (AICD) is metabolized in the cytoplasm. In the amyloidogenic pathway (B), β-secretase cleaves APP at the N-terminus of the Aβ domain, releasing soluble sAPPβ. The remaining CTFβ is cleaved by the γ-secretase complex to generate the free Aβ40 and Aβ42 peptides. The remaining AICD is metabolized in the cytoplasm.

(sAPPα or sAPPβ) and the membrane-associated C-terminal fragments (CTFα or CTFβ). The CTFs then become substrates for the γ-secretase, which cleaves their transmembrane domain to release the p3 peptide from CTFα and the peptide Aβ from CTFβ. In both cases, an APP intracellular domain (AICD) is generated at the cytoplasmic side.

α-Secretase

The major physiological route of APP processing involves the protease α-secretase, which cleaves APP within its Aβ domain to generate the fragments sAPPα and CTFα (Fig. 16.1A). The α-secretase cleavage of APP is nonamyloidogenic because it not only precludes the production of Aβ but also generates the soluble and large fragment sAPPα, which has neuroprotective and memory-enhancing effects (Caillé, Allinquant, Dupont et al. 2004). Several members of the A disintegrin-like and metalloprotease (ADAM) family of proteases such as ADAM9, ADAM10, and ADAM17 have been reported to have α-secretase activity (Hotoda, Koike, Sasagawa et al. 2002; Allinson, Parkin, Turner et al. 2003). The emerging consensus is that ADAM10 is largely responsible for the constitutive basal α-secretase activity (Buxbaum, Liu, Luo et al. 1998) whereas the protein kinase C–stimulated α-secretase activity is essentially assigned to ADAM17

(Lammich, Kojro, Postina et al. 1999). Overexpression of ADAM10 in an animal model of AD prevented senile plaques accompanied by an increase in the secretion of sAPPα and a reduction in the production of Aβ (Postina, Schroeder, Dewachter et al. 2004). In contrast, overexpression of the inactive mutant of ADAM10 in the brain enhanced the formation of senile plaques (Postina, Schroeder, Dewachter et al. 2004).

β-Secretase

This protease is involved in the alternative processing pathway (amyloidogenic pathway) that generates the fragments sAPPβ and CTFβ (Fig. 16.1B). The β-secretase activity was identified as the transmembrane aspartic protease β-site APP-cleaving enzyme 1 (BACE1) (Vassar, Bennett, Babu-Khan et al. 1999) which, together with its homologue BACE2 (Hussain, Powell, Howlett et al. 1999), cleaves APP at the β-secretase site. BACE1 is expressed in the brain and more specifically in neuronal cells whereas BACE2 is mostly expressed in the heart and kidney. In vivo studies showed that BACE1-knockout mice are deficient in Aβ production and that there is no compensatory mechanism for β-secretase cleavage in the brain (Harrison, Harper, Hawkins et al. 2003; Luo, Bolon, Damore et al. 2003). Moreover, BACE1 deficiency prevents the learning and memory impairments and cholinergic dysfunction observed in a transgenic mouse model for AD (Ohno, Sametsky, Younkin et al. 2004). Besides BACEs, it was reported that the cysteine protease cathepsin B constitutes the major β-secretase for Aβ production in the regulatory secretory pathway whereas BACE1 is essentially involved in the constitutive secretory pathway (Hook, Toneff, Bogyo et al. 2005). In a recent report, it was, however, found that cathepsin B ablation had no effect on APP processing whereas cathepsin B inhibition increased Aβ levels and plaque deposition (Mueller-Steiner, Zhou, Arai et al. 2006).

γ-Secretase

As described in prior sections, the fragments CTFα and CTFβ, resulting from the α- and β-secretase cleavages respectively (Fig. 16.1), undergo proteolysis within their membrane domain by the γ-secretase to release p3 and Aβ, respectively, and the intracellular domain AICD that moves to the nucleus. γ-Secretase is a multiprotein complex consisting of at least the proteins presenilin 1 (PS1), presenilin 2 (PS2), nicastrin (NCT), anterior pharynx defective 1 homologue (APH1), and presenilin enhancer 2 (PEN2) (Kaether, Haass, Steiner 2006). All four proteins are both necessary and sufficient to reconstitute γ-secretase activity in yeast, which lacks this enzyme (Edbauer, Winkler, Regula et al. 2003). Either the mutation of two aspartates in PS1 (D^{257} and D^{385}) (Wolfe, Xia, Ostaszewski et al. 1999) or the knockout of both PSs (Herreman, Serneels, Annaert et al. 2000) resulted in complete loss of γ-secretase activity and Aβ production, indicating that the PSs are the catalytic components of γ-secretase. γ-Secretase belongs to the family of intramembrane-cleaving proteases, which all perform peptide bond cleavage within the interior of the lipid bilayer, suggesting that membrane instability may influence the proteolytic activity of γ-secretase (Weihofen, Martoglio 2003). Indeed, changes in the distribution of cellular cholesterol and sphingomyelin in transfected cells resulted in overproduction of total Aβ peptides (Kaether, Haass, Steiner 2006). This explains that γ-secretase is directly involved in Aβ biogenesis and determines the pathogenic potential of Aβ by its heterogeneous catalytic action, generating peptides of various lengths, particularly the amyloidogenic peptide Aβ42 (Grziwa, Grimm, Masters et al. 2003).

CLEARANCE OF β-AMYLOID PEPTIDE

Efficient clearance of Aβ is essential to prevent Aβ accumulation in the brain. Under normal physiological circumstances, Aβ is removed by multiple clearance pathways including transfer of Aβ from the brain tissue to the cerebrospinal fluid and plasma and direct proteolysis of Aβ by degradative enzymes (Selkoe 2004; Masters, Beyreuther 2006). Many proteases or peptidases have been reported with the capability of cleaving Aβ either in vitro or in vivo (Carson, Turner 2002).

Neprilysin

Neprilysin (NEP, enkephalinase) is a plasma membrane glycoprotein belonging to the neutral zinc metalloproteinases family. Widely expressed in many tissues including the brain areas vulnerable to amyloid plaque deposition (Akiyama, Kondo, Ikeda et al. 2001; Fukami, Watanabe, Iwata et al. 2002), NEP cleaves and inactivates a large number of peptide substrates such as enkephalins, bradykinin, and neuropeptide Y in addition to Aβ. In vitro, NEP cleaves Aβ between the residues Glu³↓Phe⁴, Gly⁹↓Tyr¹⁰, Phe¹⁹↓Phe²⁰, Ala³⁰↓Ile³¹, and Gly³³↓Leu³⁴. Evidence for NEP contribution to Aβ catabolism was provided by several studies. Indeed, rat brains infused with thiorphan, the more selective NEP inhibitor, show elevated levels of endogenous Aβ (Zou, Mouri, Iwata et al. 2006). Similarly, genetic knockout of NEP raises endogenous Aβ levels in murine brain (Eckman, Adams, Troendle et al. 2006; Madani, Poirier, Wolfer et al. 2006). In contrast, overexpression of human NEP in the brains of APP transgenic mice has been shown to lower Aβ levels, decrease amyloid plaque, and prevent premature lethality (Marr, Rockenstein, Mukherjee et al. 2003; Carter, Pedrini, Ghiso et al. 2006).

Insulin-Degrading Enzyme

Insulin-degrading enzyme (IDE, insulysin) is a thiol-dependent, Zn^{2+}-metalloprotease that not only occurs in soluble form in the cytoplasm (Selkoe 2001), but has also been observed as secreted and membrane-associated isoforms in neurons and microglia (Lynch, George, Eisenhauer et al. 2006). IDE has a broad substrate specificity, which allows it to hydrolyze multiple peptides including insulin and amylin in addition to the AICD and Aβ (Selkoe 2001; Farris, Mansourian, Chang et al. 2003). In vitro, IDE degrades Aβ40 between residues Val¹²↓His¹³, His¹³↓His¹⁴, His¹⁴↓Gln¹⁵, Gln¹⁵↓Lys¹⁶, Val¹⁸↓Phe¹⁹, Phe¹⁹↓Phe²⁰, Phe²⁰↓Ala²¹, and Lys²⁸↓Gly². Several studies provide evidence indicating that IDE is an Aβ degrading enzyme. Indeed, deficiency of IDE resulted in defects in the metabolic suppression of the endogenous Aβ peptide levels in the brain of IDE-knockout mice and in the degradation of the exogenous Aβ peptide by primary cultured neurons derived from these IDE-deficient mice (Farris, Mansourian, Chang et al. 2003). Moreover, overexpression of IDE in transgenic mice resulted in reduction of brain Aβ levels and prevented amyloid plaque formation while IDE-knockout mice showed a clear elevation of brain Aβ and AICD (Leissring, Farris, Chang et al. 2003).

Endothelin-Converting Enzyme

Endothelin-converting enzyme 1 (ECE-1) and endothelin-converting enzyme 2 (ECE-2), abundantly expressed in vascular and nonvascular cells of many tissues, are homologous enzymes belonging to the M13 family of zinc metalloproteases that includes NEP. The ECEs, known for their ability to catalyze the conversion of proendothelin into vasoactive endothelin, hydrolyze also a number of other biologically active peptides such as bradykinin, neurotensin, and angiotensin I. Recombinant soluble ECE-1 was shown to hydrolyze synthetic Aβ40 and Aβ42 in vitro between the residues $Lys^{16}\downarrow Leu^{17}$, $Leu^{17}\downarrow Val^{18}$, and $Phe^{19}\downarrow Phe^{20}$ (Eckman, Reed, Eckman 2001). Overexpression of ECE-1 in cultured cells lacking endogenous ECE activity was found to reduce extracellular Aβ concentration and this effect was completely abolished by treatment with phosphoramidon (Eckman, Reed, Eckman 2001). Both ECE-1 and ECE-2 are expressed in the brain regions that are relevant to AD pathology, suggesting that these proteases may contribute to the regulation of the steady-state levels of Aβ (Funalot, Ouimet, Claperon et al. 2004). Indeed, the brain of mice deficient for ECE-1 and ECE-2 or treated with ECE inhibitors shows a significant increase in the levels of both Aβ40 and Aβ42 (Eckman, Watson, Marlow et al. 2003; Eckman, Adams, Troendle 2006).

Angiotensin-Converting Enzyme

Angiotensin-converting enzyme 1 (ACE-1) and angiotensin-converting enzyme 2 (ACE-2) (dipeptidyl carboxypeptidases) are membrane-bound zinc metalloproteases, which play a role in the regulation of blood pressure (Coates 2003). For example, ACE hydrolyzes peptides by removing a dipeptide from the C-terminus as in the conversion of angiotensin I to angiotensin II or the inactivation of bradykinin. Previous studies using purified human plasma ACE and cultured cells showed that ACE degrades the peptide Aβ40 between the residues $Asp^{7}\downarrow Ser^{8}$ (Hu, Igarashi, Kamata et al. 2001; Oba et al. 2005). These studies also established that inhibition of ACE by captopril increases Aβ levels in APP- and ACE-transfected cells (Hu, Igarashi, Kamata et al. 2001; Hemming, Selkoe 2005). However, ACE-deficient mice or mice treated with ACE inhibitors did not show Aβ brain accumulation, suggesting that ACE does not have a physiological role in clearing Aβ (Eckman, Adams, Troendle et al. 2006). Interestingly, it was recently reported that purified ACE from mouse and human brain homogenates generates Aβ40 by carboxydipeptidyl cleavage of Aβ42 and that captopril treatment of Tg2576 mice enhances predominant Aβ42 deposition in the brain (Zou, Yamaguchi, Akatsu et al. 2007). These findings underline a novel catabolic pathway for modulating the levels of highly amyloidogenic Aβ42.

Other Candidate Aβ Degrading Enzymes

Besides NEP, IDE, ECEs, and ACEs, other peptidases have been proposed to act as Aβ metabolizing enzymes such as plasmin (Exley, Korchazhkina 2001), matrix metalloproteinases MMP-2 and MMP-9 (Yan, Hu, Song et al. 2006), cathepsin B (Mueller-Steiner, Zhou, Arai et al. 2006), and acyl peptide hydrolase (Yamin, Bagchi, Hildebrant et al. 2007).

Clearance of Aβ by Neuronal and Non-Neuronal Cells

As shown in prior sections, several nonrelated proteases originating from a variety of cell types degrade Aβ and this proteolytic process occurs in different cellular locations. In this context, we have analyzed the clearance of Aβ40 by several cell types in a systematic way to find out the relative importance of each of these proteases in the catabolic pathway of Aβ. For this purpose, the mammalian cell lines used were selected to originate from brain (SH-SY5Y, SK-N-BE, CHP-100, and U-373), bone marrow (K-562), skin (HFF), ovary (CHO), and kidney (COS-7). The ability of these cell types to deplete Aβ40 from their media was evaluated using enzyme-linked immunosorbent assay (ELISA), high-performance liquid chromatography (HPLC), and a combination of HPLC separation/online ESI-Q-TOF mass spectroscopy methods (Panchal, Lazar, Munoz et al. 2007).

As shown in Figure 16.2, the amount of radioactive Aβ40 (IAβ40), incubated with the cultured cells for 8 hours, decreases in all cell media accompanied by a concomitant appearance of two radioactive peaks PI and PII. Moreover, data in Figure 16.2 also indicate that all conditioned cell media exhibited almost no proteolytic activity on the IAβ40 substrate and that γ-counting of all the media fractions shows a complete conservation of counts. Together, these observations argue in favor of a proteolytic process

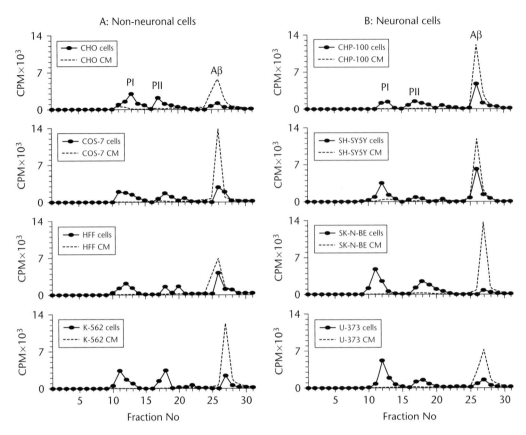

Figure 16.2 Degradation of IAβ40 by cultivated non-neuronal (A) and neuronal (B) cells. IAβ40 (20 pM) was incubated with each cell line (—●—) or with each cell 8 hour-conditioned medium (CM) (⋯⋯⋯⋯) for 8 hours. Aliquot of each supernatant was subjected to HPLC separation and the radioactivity of collected fractions was measured in a γ-counter.

in which Aβ40 clearance from these culture media is principally mediated by cell surface protease(s), ruling out the possibility of mechanisms involving an intracellular degradation of Aβ40 after its cellular uptake or an extracellular degradation of Aβ40 by the proteases secreted in cell media. To define the mechanisms involved in PI and PII formation, IAβ40 was incubated with each cell line for 8 hours and the withdrawn supernatants were subsequently incubated for 16 hours at 37°C. The results of these experiments (Panchal, Lazar, Munoz et al. 2007) have shown that the amount of peak PI components decreases, with a concomitant increase of peak PII area without any significant change in the residual IAβ40 amount. Since no extracellular degradation has been observed for IAβ40 (Fig. 16.2), this finding indicates that the membrane-associated proteases hydrolyze IAβ40 to release the peak PI, which in turn undergoes a cleavage by secreted proteases to generate the peak PII.

To characterize the proteases involved in the degradation of Aβ40 and peak PI, we have examined the influence of various protease-specific inhibitors and more specifically those known to inhibit Aβ-degrading metalloproteases like NEP, IDE, ECE, ACE, or MMPs. The results of these experiments (Panchal, Lazar, Munoz

et al. 2007) have shown that the cell surface proteases, implicated in Aβ40 degradation, are thiol-dependent metalloproteases (inhibition by 1,10-phenanthroline and N-ethylmaleimide) whereas the soluble proteases involved in the cleavage of PI components are serine proteases (inhibition by the compound AEBSF). To identify the cleavage sites of both proteolytic activities, the sequences of Aβ40 proteolytic products were precisely determined (without any off-line purification of Aβ fragments) by introducing a combination of HPLC separation/online ESI-Q-TOF-MS analysis. Figure 16.3 displays the LC-MS total ion current (TIC) chromatograms obtained from the cultured cell media in the absence or the presence of inhibitors. From the calculated mass spectra of fragments contained in each peak of these TIC chromatograms, we have deduced the sequences of proteolytic products enclosed in the peaks PI and PII and subsequently the cleavages sites of Aβ40 and PI peptides (Fig. 16.4).

The observations from our study provide data indicating that the proteolytic degradation of Aβ is primarily dictated by its conformational state, whatever the normal mechanisms for the removal of Aβ peptides and the contribution of each potent Aβ-degradation enzyme to this proteolytic process. It

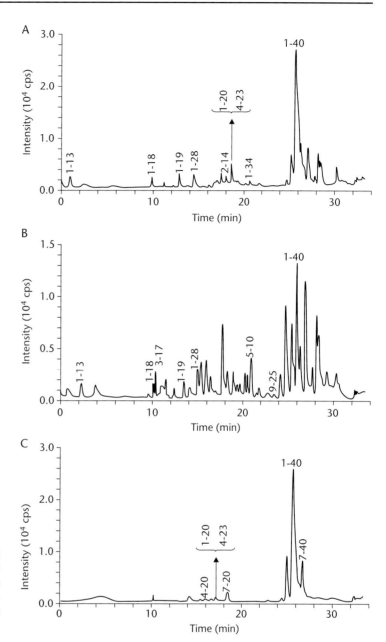

Figure 16.3 Total ion current chromatograms obtained from the cultured CHO media by LC-MS. Synthetic Aβ40 (5 μg/mL) was incubated with CHO cell line for 8 hours in the absence (A) or the presence of Pefabloc (B) or 1,10-phenanthroline (or NEM) (C). The column effluent was monitored by MS with positive ESI.

is noteworthy that multiple factors such as the peptide concentration, protein modifications, or physical properties of the extracellular medium influence the conformation of Aβ, which subsequently modulates the clearance and degradation of the peptide Aβ (Zhu, Lee, Casadesus et al. 2005; Onyango, Khan 2006; Walsh, Selkoe 2007).

THERAPEUTIC APPROACHES TO ALZHEIMER'S DISEASE

Inhibition of the accumulation of Aβ is the most active area of investigation for the development of AD therapies. Currently, three logical antiamyloidogenic strategies have been adopted (Fig. 16.5): (1) reduction of Aβ production, (2) promotion of the Aβ degrading catabolic pathway, and (3) inhibition of Aβ aggregation.

Reduction of Aβ Production

Aβ is generated from APP by two proteases, β- and γ-secretases (Fig. 16.1B), whereas a third protease, α-secretase, interferes with the production of Aβ by competing with β-secretase for the APP substrate (Fig. 16.1A). Therefore, two strategies to reduce Aβ production have been proposed: stimulation of α-secretase or inhibition of β- and/or γ-secretase.

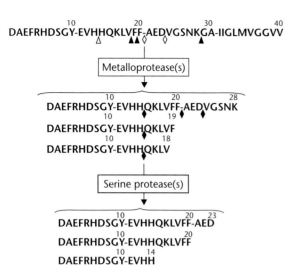

Figure 16.4 Schematic representation of cleavage sites observed for the degradation of Aβ40 by neuronal and non-neuronal cell types. Diamonds and triangles indicate the peptide bonds hydrolyzed by the secreted and cell surface proteases, respectively (black symbols: major cleavage, white symbols: minor cleavage).

α-Secretase Stimulation

As shown in Figure 16.1A, α-secretase prevents Aβ production by its participation in the nonamyloidogenic pathway of APP processing. Therefore, enhancing the activity of this secretase can be considered as a therapeutic target for AD modification. Several molecule drugs such as muscarinic agonists, specific protein kinase C (PKC) activators, and statins have been characterized to upregulate the activity of α-secretase (Kojro, Fahrenholz 2005).

Presently, the medications available with few side effects are donepezil and galantamine, which are selective inhibitors of acetylcholinesterase (AChEI) (Black, Doody, Li et al. 2007). These drugs act by promoting feedback effect that increases acetylcholinesterase transcripts that intracellularly interact with other proteins such as RACK1 and PKCβII (Birikh, Sklan, Shoham et al. 2003). Besides their activity as AChEI, donepezil and galantamine appear to enhance the α-secretase cleavage of APP by modulating the intracellular trafficking of ADAM10 and ADAM17 (Black, Doody, Li et al. 2007).

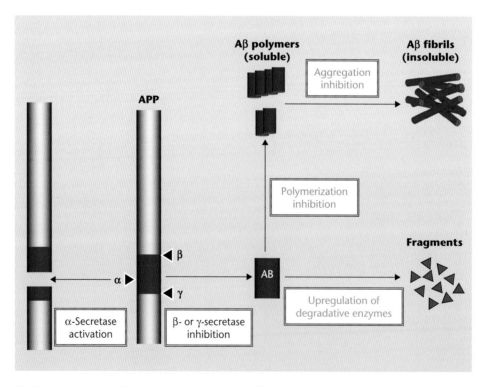

Figure 16.5 Potential therapeutic targets for Alzheimer's disease modification. Steady-state levels of Aβ monomer are controlled by its rates of production and degradation. Above a certain critical concentration or under some pathological conditions (aging, dementia, or stroke), Aβ monomers can self-associate to form different soluble oligomeric assemblies. Consequently, inhibition of Aβ production (enhancement of α-secretase or inhibition of β- and/or γ-secretase) or stimulation of Aβ degradation should decrease or prevent formation of oligomers and then amyloid fibrils. Small molecules that bind to and stabilize Aβ monomers should prevent oligomerization and allow for the natural removal of monomers by the brain's degradative machinery. Similarly, agents capable of disrupting preformed oligomers should reduce the concentration of toxic oligomers.

Moreover, previous studies have shown that PKC hypofunction has an important role in AD pathophysiology (Ercheberrigaray, Tan, Dewachter et al. 2004). Recently, it was shown that an amide bearing the benzolactam-based PKC activator (TPPB) directs APP processing toward the nonamyloidogenic pathway by increasing α-secretase activity (Yang, Pan, Ba et al. 2007). Specifically, TPPB promoted the secretion of sAPPα without affecting APP, NEP, and IDE expression and, interestingly, decreased expression and activity of BACE1. These findings suggest that TPPB can be a potential α-secretase-targeted drug for AD modification. All three candidate α-secretase proteins are usually synthesized in the form of preproproteins that must be cleaved to become active (Lopez-Perez, Seidah N, Checler 1999; Lopez-Perez, Zhang, Frank et al. 2001). This activation of ADAMs is mediated by proprotein convertases, enzymes known to participate in the processing of peptide hormone precursors and in the activation of zymogens (Nakai 2001; Brakch, El Abida, Rholam 2006). Recently, *N*-arginine dibasic convertase (NRDc), a further convertase (Chesneau, Pierotti, Barré et al. 1994), was shown to decrease the production of Aβ by enhancing the α-secretase cleavage of APP through activation of ADAM proteases (Hiraoka, Ohno, Yoshida et al. 2007). Since NRDc is expressed in cortical neurons of human brain, this convertase may be a novel target for the treatment of AD.

β-Secretase Inhibition

As shown in Figure 16.1B, β-secretase is the rate-limiting enzyme in the production of Aβ. Indeed, the membrane-bound fragment CTFβ, generated from APP cleavage by β-secretase, serves as substrate for γ-secretase to generate the peptides Aβ40/42. Consequently, inhibition of this secretase is an attractive therapeutic approach for AD treatment.

Several peptide-derived inhibitors, developed by using the sequence of the APP β-cleavage site P4-P'4 site or specific regions of the catalytic domain of BACE1 as templates, were able to decrease Aβ production in wild-type and transgenic mice (Asai, Hattori, Iwata et al. 2006; Yeon, Jeon, Hwang et al. 2007). Moreover, a selective nonpeptidic BACE1 inhibitor (GSK188909) was shown to reduce levels of secreted and intracellular Aβ in cells expressing APP, and its oral administration to transgenic mice results in a significant reduction in the level of Aβ40 and Aβ42 in the brain (Hussain, Hawkins, Harrison et al. 2007). Besides the direct inhibition of BACE itself by various synthetic molecules, the other reported strategy is based on the design of inhibitors that prevent production of Aβ by specific binding to the β-secretase cleavage site of APP. The advantage of this strategy is that the inhibitors do not interfere with the processing of other BACE1 substrates such as sialyltransferase, P-selectin glycoprotein ligand-1, low-density lipoprotein receptor–related protein, and β-subunit of voltage-gated sodium channels (Paris, Quadros, Patel et al. 2005). By using the hydropathic complementarity approach (Heal, Roberts, Raynes et al. 2002), several short peptides, mimicking the β-secretase cleavage site of APP, were synthesized (Na, Jeon, Zhang et al. 2007). Some of these peptides were able to inhibit cleavage of the APP substrate by the β-secretase without significantly affecting other BACE1 protein substrates (Na, Jeon, Zhang et al. 2007). Nevertheless, only a few reports about clinically useful BACE1 inhibitors have appeared.

A similar approach was demonstrated with antibodies that bind to the β-secretase cleavage site of APP (Arbel, Yacoby, Solomon 2005; Tampellini, Magrané, Takahashi et al. 2007). The concept adopted for inhibiting β-secretase activity principally affects Aβ generated through the endocytic pathway, which is responsible for the internalization and processing of cell surface APP. One can note that all the studies indicate that Aβ derives through processing of APP endocytosed from the cell surface in addition to the secretory pathway (Nixon, Mathews, Cataldo 2001). Indeed, these studies show that the blockage of the β-secretase cleavage site either by binding of antibodies to human APP overexpressed by cellular models or by active immunization of transgenic mice led to a considerable reduction in intracellular Aβ (Arbel, Yacoby, Solomon 2005; Tampellini, Magrané, Takahashi et al. 2007). It is noteworthy that antibody internalization into the cell after APP binding, together with the fact that it does not bind Aβ, avoids microglia and complement activation, as was reported for anti-Aβ antibodies that bind the senile plaques (Solomon 2004).

Moreover, some proteins such as prostate apoptosis response-4 and reticuon-3 have been described to act as BACE1 regulators. Their overexpression reduces Aβ production whereas their downregulation results in Aβ production increase (He, Lu, Qahwash et al. 2004). Drugs that may upregulate these regulators represent an additional viable strategy for the treatment of AD.

γ-Secretase Inhibition

Similar to BACE1, γ-secretase contributes to the pathology of AD (Fig. 16.1B) and therefore likely represents the other attractive therapeutic target to cure AD. However, γ-secretase also cleaves many other substrates such as Notch, and E-cadherins ErbB-4 and CD44 (De Strooper, Annaert, Cupers et al. 1999; Ni, Murphy, Golde et al. 2001; Lammich, Okochi, Takeda et al. 2002; Marambaud, Shioi, Serban et al. 2002), all of which are type I transmembrane proteins involved in a variety of vital cellular functions. In this context, inhibition of the γ-secretase processing of APP without any effect on the action of these precursors is required (Paris, Quadros, Patel et al. 2005). Several nonpeptidic compounds have been designed to inhibit γ-secretase (Beher, Clarke, Wrigley et al. 2004).

For example, treatment of APP transgenic animals with a benzodiazepine-containing analogue of the inhibitor DAPT (LY411575) lowered Aβ production in brain and plasma (Wong, Manfra, Poulet et al. 2004). However, the used doses affected lymphocyte development and induced drastic morphological changes in gastrointestinal tract tissue, resulting from impaired proteolytic processing of Notch by LY411575. Other drugs such as the benzodiazepine or sulphonamide derivatives (BMS-299897 and SCH 697466) were shown to reduce Aβ production in transgenic mice by a partial inhibition of γ-secretase without these side effects (Siemers, Quinn, Kaye et al. 2006). Owing to the complexity of the multisubunit γ-secretase and the lack of structural information, the mechanism explaining the selectivity of these molecules is presently lacking. Further studies are required to establish a more detailed mechanism of action for these compounds.

Other nonpeptidic potential inhibitors, named *JLK isocoumarin*, have been designed to selectively target the γ-secretase pathway (Petit, Pasini, Alves et al. 2003). Among these isocoumarin compounds, some impair γ-secretase–mediated Aβ production without triggering unwanted cleavages of other proteins. Indeed, these JLK inhibitors were unable not only to alter Notch pathway and E-cadherin processing but also to affect α- and β-secretase activities, the proteasome, and GSK3β kinase.

Several epidemiological studies indicate that the use of nonsteroidal anti-inflammatory drugs (NSAIDs) correlates with a lower risk of developing AD (Aisen 2002). Overexpression of cyclooxygenase (COX) correlates with the increased production of Aβ40 and Aβ42, indicating that cyclooxygenase inhibitors act as AD drug treatments (Weggen, Eriksen, Sagi et al. 2003). Among these COX inhibitors, various NSAIDs reduce the production of Aβ42 in transgenic mice by direct action on γ-secretase (Weggen, Eriksen, Sagi et al. 2003). The basis of NSAID modulation of APP processing derives probably from allosteric binding of inhibitors, which changes the conformation of the γ-secretase complex (Lleó, Greenberg, Growdon et al. 2006). In addition, it was reported that NSAIDs have the ability to lower Aβ42 through inhibition of Rho kinases, which constitute a target for drug development in multiple neurodegenerative diseases (Leuchtenberger, Kummer, Kukar et al. 2006). Finally, Aβ-lowering properties have been reported

for compounds isolated from ginseng, which is used in traditional Asian medicine for a wide variety of disorders, including neuroprotection and a broad range of antiaging effects (Chen, Eckman, Eckman 2006).

Numerous pharmacological products are currently developed but only a few are presently studied in clinical trials (Lundkvist, Naslund 2007).

Promotion of Aβ Degrading Catabolic Pathway

In sporadic AD, which accounts for more than 90% of all AD cases, an overproduction of Aβ is generally not observed. Therefore, the onset of sporadic AD may be attributed to an impaired clearance of Aβ. Under normal physiological circumstances, Aβ is removed by multiple clearance pathways including direct proteolysis by several proteases among which NEP and IDE are the prototypes. Therefore, activation of Aβ-degrading proteases for enhancing the clearance of Aβ in the brain represents an emerging therapeutic approach in the sporadic AD.

Activation of NEP

As shown in prior sections, NEP participates in a variety of physiological processes by cleaving a variety of substrates including Aβ. Cerebral NEP levels have been reported to decrease with age and in AD, particularly in amyloid-vulnerable regions of the brain (Fukami, Watanabe, Iwata et al. 2002; Caccamo, Oddo, Sugarman et al. 2005; Russo, Borghi, Markesbery et al. 2005). Therefore, the approaches that could upregulate NEP levels can be used as therapeutic tools to reduce Aβ levels in AD.

Supporting a therapeutic function for NEP in Aβ degradation, both transgenic overexpression and direct viral vector injection of NEP have been shown to noticeably lower Aβ levels (Leissring, Farris, Chang et al. 2003; Marr, Rockenstein, Mukherjee et al. 2003; Iwata, Mizukami, Shirotani et al. 2004). In a recent report, it was shown that a lentiviral vector carrying the human NEP gene was able to induce the expression of NEP in neuronal cells and that the expressed human NEP was able to degrade monomeric Aβ peptide (El-Amouri et al. 2007). Therefore, overexpression of NEP by a gene therapy approach in areas vulnerable to Aβ aggregation in AD brain may protect the neurons from the toxic effects of Aβ peptide.

In another report, the ex vivo gene delivery approach, which has already produced therapeutic improvements in experimental models of human diseases (Frim, Uhler, Galpern et al. 1994; Emerich, Winn, Hantraye et al. 1997; Tuszynski, Smith, Roberts et al. 1998), was used to elevate NEP levels into the brain of APP transgenic mice having advanced amyloid plaques (Hemming et al. 2007). In this study, it was shown that, after syngenic fibroblasts (modified to produce soluble NEP) were engrafted into the brain of APP transgenic mice, the amyloid plaques surrounding the graft were proteolytically cleared (Hemming et al. 2007). Because several of these potential treatments have advanced to human trials (Tuszynski, Thal Pay et al. 2005; Sieving, Caruso, Tao et al. 2006), these results indicate that the ex gene delivery of Aβ-degrading proteases such as NEP represents a very promising therapeutic tool to lower Aβ levels in AD.

In a previous report, it was demonstrated that NEP was regulated by a PS-dependent γ-secretase pathway via the amyloid precursor protein intracellular domain AICD, which acts as a transcriptional activator of NEP (Pardossi-Piquard, Petit, Kawarai et al. 2005). Indeed, this report shows that the expression and activity of NEP are lowered in PS-deficient cells or by γ-secretase inhibitors and by PS1/PS2 deficiency in mouse brain. Interestingly, the NEP gene promoters are not transactivated by Aβ or by the γ-secrctase cleavage products of Notch or N- or E-cadherins. Because AICD is cogenerated with Aβ during γ-secretase cleavage of APP (Fig. 16.1), the γ PS-dependent regulation of NEP, mediated by AICD, provides a physiological mechanism to modulate Aβ levels by varying levels of γ-secretase activity. Moreover, it was reported that NCT, a member of the γ-secretase complex, is also able to control the activity and expression of NEP (Pardossi-Piquard et al. 2006). Actually, NCT deficiency drastically lowers NEP expression, but, on the contrary, does not modulate the expression of the two other Aβ-cleaving enzymes, ECE and IDE. Interestingly, NCT was shown to restore NEP activity and expression in NCT-deficient fibroblasts, but not in PS-deficient fibroblasts, indicating that control of NEP requires the complete integrity of the γ-secretase complex.

Gleevec, a tyrosine kinase inhibitor, has been described to lower Aβ in cells expressing human APP, in neurons, or in animal brain without inhibiting Notch cleavage (Netzer, Dou, Cai et al. 2003). It has been proposed that Gleevec may act as a selective γ-secretase inhibitor (Netzer, Dou, Cai et al. 2003), whereas others found no direct inhibition of γ-secretase activity (Fraering et al. 2005). Recently, it was shown that Aβ-lowering effect of Gleevec is accompanied by an increase in the levels of both AICD and NEP, even in the presence of a potent γ-secretase inhibitor (Eisele et al. 2007). Given that AICD is cogenerated with Aβ during γ-secretase cleavage of APP (Fig. 16.1), the increase in AICD levels is due to Gleevec treatment that slows down the rate of AICD turnover. Because NEP is a target gene of AICD-regulated transcription (Pardossi-Piquard, Petit, Kawarai et al. 2005, 2006),

the increase of NEP expression is due to enhanced AICD signaling. Together, these observations underline a new possibility for controlling Aβ levels without directly affecting γ-secretase by using AICD or small molecules that mimic AICD as activators of NEP activity.

Activation of IDE

As indicated in a precedent section, IDE participates in a variety of physiological processes by cleaving a variety of bioactive peptides. Albeit IDE has a broad range of peptides, it was shown that IDE uses size and charge distribution of its substrate-binding cavity to cleave the substrates selectively (Shen, Joachimiak, Rosner et al. 2006). The solved structures of human IDE in complex with certain substrates reveal that its catalytic site is buried and is controlled by a closed–open conformational equilibrium (Shen, Joachimiak, Rosner et al. 2006; Im, Manolopoulou, Malito et al. 2007). Moreover, oligomerization of IDE regulates its activity by shifting this conformational equilibrium toward the closed state, corresponding to the low activity of IDE (Song, Juliano, Juliano et al. 2003). Therefore, compounds that could regulate the activity of IDE by favoring the open state or by reducing IDE oligomerization might facilitate the clearance of Aβ and other pathologically relevant IDE substrates.

Clinical and epidemiological studies have found that type 2 diabetes, and hyperinsulinemia in particular, increased the risk for developing AD in the elderly (Dubois, Feldman, Jacova et al. 2007). The link between hyperinsulinemia and AD may be IDE since both insulin and amylin, peptides related to the pathology of type 2 diabetes (Farris, Mansourian, Chang et al. 2003), are also degraded by this protease. Indeed, partial loss-of-function mutations in IDE lead to elevated circulating insulin and cerebral Aβ levels in rodents (Farris, Mansourian, Leissring et al. 2004) whereas enhancement of IDE activity reduces Aβ accumulation in AD mouse models (Leissring, Farris, Chang et al. 2003). Moreover, genetic studies have shown that genetic variations in the IDE region on chromosome 10 are associated with the clinical symptoms of late-onset AD (Leissring, Farris, Chang et al. 2003; Kim, Hersh, Leissring et al. 2007) as well as the risk of type 2 diabetes (Karamohamed, Demissie, Volcjak et al. 2003). Consistent with these observations, the dysfunctional IDE, which leads to Aβ increases, can be caused by either competition between insulin and Aβ for IDE or IDE genetic variations (Qiu, Folstein 2006).

Like NEP, IDE presents other avenues for prevention and/or treatment of AD. This may be performed through gene and/or enzyme replacement therapy as shown for NEP, or through drugs that induce enzyme expression and activity. It is noteworthy that ATP (Im, Manolopoulou, Malito et al. 2007), long-chain fatty acids (Song, Juliano, Juliano et al. 2003), oxidative stress (Shinall, Song, Hersh 2005), and endogenous peptide inhibitors (Saric, Muller, Seitz et al. 2003) have been reported to regulate the catalytic activity of IDE.

Inhibition of Aβ Aggregation

Aβ is released from its precursor protein as soluble monomeric species, but under certain conditions (aging, stress, stroke, or dementia) it self-aggregates to form soluble oligomers or insoluble fibrils that may be toxic to neurons and vascular cells. However, there is increasing evidence indicating that soluble oligomers of secreted Aβ cause substantial neuronal dysfunction before the appearance of amyloid deposits (Lansbury, Lashuel 2006; Ferreira, Vieira, De Felice et al. 2007; Haass, Selkoe 2007; Walsh, Selkoe 2007). Thus, amyloid fibril formation and deposition may be end stages of a process in which the key pathogenetic events, mediated by these oligomeric assemblies, occur early.

Accordingly, the role of soluble forms of aggregated Aβ has gained increasing attention as the most important mediator of neuronal toxicity in AD. Indeed, several studies on the aggregation, fibrillization, and toxicity of Aβ peptides indicate that oligomeric Aβ42 is more toxic than fibrillar Aβ42 (Dahlgren, Manelli, Stine et al. 2002), consistent with the observation that high expression of Aβ42 in transgenic mice produces synaptotoxicity without significant amyloid plaque formation (Mucke, Masliah, Yu et al. 2000). Moreover, some pathogenic mutations in Aβ such as Arctic APP mutation promote the formation of amyloid intermediates rather than fibrils (Nilsberth, Westlind-Danielsson, Eckman et al. 2001; Lashuel, Hartley, Petre et al. 2003). Demonstration of the important role that Aβ oligomers may play in neuronal dysfunction has been achieved by different studies. It has been reported that dysfunction of neurons does not correlate well with the distribution and density of fibrils in affected humans and mouse models of AD; rather, the amount of soluble Aβ, which includes diffusible Aβ aggregates, correlates with neural dysfunction (Lansbury, Lashuel 2006; Ferreira, Vieira, De Felice et al. 2007; Haass, Selkoe 2007; Walsh, Selkoe 2007). Moreover, diffusible Aβ aggregates also inhibit long-term potentiation (Walsh, Klyubin, Fadeeva et al. 2002) and disrupt memory (Kokubo, Kayed, Glabe et al. 2005;Lesné, Koh, Kotilinek et al. 2006) in mouse models. Because Aβ oligomerization acts as an upstream phenomenon leading to neuronal dysfunction and, ultimately, to dementia in AD, structures of amyloid intermediates (e.g., protofibrils, annular structures, Aβ-derived diffusible ligands (ADDLs) and globulomers) have attracted wide attention as potential therapeutic targets, particularly at early stages of amyloid diseases. Interestingly, it was shown that the neurotoxicity of amyloid aggregates is influenced not only by conformations of Aβ but also by morphology or supramolecular structures of Aβ aggregates (Hoshi, Sato, Matsumoto et al. 2003; Chromy, Nowak, Lambert et al. 2003; Kawarabayashi, Shoji, Younkin et al. 2004). It is noteworthy that larger deposits, such as compacted Aβ plaques, seem to be relatively inert but might serve as reservoirs of diffusible oligomers (Martins, Kuperstein, Wilkinson et al. 2008).

Since soluble oligomeric assemblies of Aβ initiate disease-specific cytopathology and subsequent symptoms, these oligomeric species are potential targets for therapeutic intervention. Aβ immunotherapy, Aβ-aggregation inhibitors, allosteric modulators of γ-secretase, and Aβ-degrading proteases (Fig. 16.5) can all reduce oligomeric Aβ, with consequent neuronal degeneration and behavioral deficits in mouse models of AD. Indeed, small peptides that interfere with oligomers of Aβ can prevent the conformational change of Aβ to β-sheet structure and subsequent fibrillization. These designed potential peptide-based aggregation inhibitors contain Aβ amino acid sequences (KLVFF) from part of the binding region responsible for Aβ self-association. Such peptides have been shown to reduce Aβ fibrillization in vitro and brain Aβ load in AD transgenic mice, without inducing an immune response (Permanne, Adessi, Saborio et al. 2002; Sadowski, Pankiewicz, Scholtzova et al. 2004; Walsh, Townsend, Podlisny et al. 2005; Austen, Paleologou, Ali et al. 2008). Moreover, it was shown that glycosaminoglycans bind Aβ and can promote its aggregation (van Horssen, Wesseling, van den Heuvel et al. 2003). The drug candidate NC-531 (Alzhemed) is a glycosaminoglycan mimetic designed to interfere with the association between glycosaminoglycans and Aβ (Geerts 2004), but more experiments are needed. A phase III clinical trial is ongoing. In addition, it was demonstrated that metals, and in particular copper and zinc ions, promote Aβ aggregation and toxic effects (Ha, Ryu, Park 2007). The metal chelator clioquinol (PBT-1) reduces brain Aβ deposition in AD transgenic mice (Cherny, Atwood, Xilinas et al. 2001). A small phase II trial showed marginal cognitive improvements with clioquinol (Ritchie, Bush, Mackinnon et al. 2003) but a new drug, PBT-2, without side effects, is currently undergoing clinical trials. Furthermore, several studies reported that antioxidants have a potential effect on the inhibition of Aβ deposition. There are several molecules developed for this purpose and have been showed to inhibit Aβ aggregate formation and its destabilization

(Hamaguchi, Ono, Yamada 2006). Curcumin, resveratrol, rosmarinic acid, nordihydroguaretic acid, ferulic acid, and tannic acid and other polyphenols represent some examples that are effective in destabilization of Aβ aggregates (Yang et al. 2005; Liu, Barkhordarian, Emadi et al. 2005; McLaurin, Kierstead, Brown et al. 2006). The isolation and development of their derivative molecules in addition to their clinical trial represents an important application that is presumed easily feasible, that may, if not cure it, delay AD (Durairajan, Yuan, Xie et al. 2007).

CONCLUSION

The metabolism of β-amyloid is an excellent example that illustrates the functional role of proteases in several physiological processes. Indeed, a dysregulation in the activity of proteases involved in the metabolism of β-amyloid leads to abnormal Aβ deposition in the brain, an invariant feature of all forms of AD. Although the clinical development of several drugs targeting the Aβ pathway is in progress, it is unlikely that a single class of compound or targeting a single mechanism of action will be sufficient to treat this illness. Given the multifactorial nature of AD, it seems likely that effective treatments will be based on the combined use of several therapeutic strategies to propose a rational therapy.

REFERENCES

Aisen PS. 2002. The potential of anti-inflammatory drugs for the treatment of Alzheimer's disease. *Lancet Neurol.* 1:279–284.

Akiyama H, Kondo H, Ikeda K, Kato M, McGeer PL. 2001. Immunohistochemical localization of neprilysin in the human cerebral cortex: inverse association with vulnerability to amyloid beta-protein (Abeta) deposition. *Brain Res.* 902:277–281.

Allinson TM, Parkin ET, Turner AJ, Hooper NM. 2003. ADAMs family members as amyloid precursor protein alpha-secretases. *J Neurosci Res.* 74:342–352.

Arbel M, Yacoby I, Solomon B. 2005. Inhibition of amyloid precursor protein processing by beta-secretase through site-directed antibodies. *Proc Natl Acad Sci U S A.* 102:7718–7723.

Asai M, Hattori C, Iwata N et al. 2006. The novel beta-secretase inhibitor KMI-429 reduces amyloid beta peptide production in amyloid precursor protein transgenic and wild-type mice. *J Neurochem.* 96:533–540.

Austen BM, Paleologou KE, Ali SAE, Qureshi MM, Allsop D, El-Agnaf OM. 2008. Designing Peptide Inhibitors for Oligomerization and Toxicity of Alzheimer's β-Amyloid Peptide. *Biochemistry.* 47(7):1984–1992.

Barnham KJ, McKinstry WJ, Multhaup G et al. 2003. Structure of the Alzheimer's disease amyloid precursor protein copper binding domain. A regulator of neuronal copper homeostasis. *J Biol Chem.* 278:17401–17407.

Beher D, Clarke EE, Wrigley JD et al. 2004. Selected nonsteroidal anti-inflammatory drugs and their derivatives target gamma-secretase at a novel site. Evidence for an allosteric mechanism. *J Biol Chem.* 279:43419–43426.

Birikh KR, Sklan EH, Shoham S, Soreq H. 2003. Interaction of "readthrough" acetylcholinesterase with RACK1 and PKCbeta II correlates with intensified fear-induced conflict behavior. *Proc Natl Acad Sci U S A.* 100:283–288.

Black SE, Doody R, Li H et al. 2007. Donepezil preserves cognition and global function in patients with severe Alzheimer disease. *Neurology.* 69:459–469.

Brakch N, El Abida B, Rholam M. 2006. Functional role of β-turn in polypeptide structure and its use as template to design therapeutic agents. *Current Medicinal Chemistry-Central Nervous System Agents.* 6:163–173.

Buxbaum JD, Liu KN, Luo Y et al. 1998. Evidence that tumor necrosis factor alpha converting enzyme is involved in regulated alpha-secretase cleavage of the Alzheimer amyloid protein precursor. *J Biol Chem.* 273:27765–27767.

Caccamo A, Oddo S, Sugarman MC, Akbari Y, LaFerla FM. 2005. Age- and region-dependent alterations in Aβ-degrading enzymes: implications for Aβ-induced disorders. *Neurobiol Aging.* 26:645–654.

Caillé I, Allinquant B, Dupont E et al. 2004. Soluble form of amyloid precursor protein regulates proliferation of progenitors in the adult subventricular zone. *Development.* 131:2173–2181.

Carson JA, Turner AJ. 2002. Beta-amyloid catabolism: roles for neprilysin (NEP) and other metallopeptidases? *J Neurochem.* 81:1–8.

Carter TL, Pedrini S, Ghiso J, Ehrlich ME, Gandy S. 2006. Brain neprilysin activity and susceptibility to transgene-induced Alzheimer amyloidosis. *Neurosci Lett.* 392:235–239.

Chen F, Eckman EA, Eckman CB. 2006. Reductions in levels of the Alzheimer's amyloid beta peptide after oral administration of ginsenosides. *FASEB J.* 20:1269–1271.

Cherny RA, Atwood CS, Xilinas ME et al. 2001. Treatment with a copper zinc chelator markedly and rapidly inhibits beta-amyloid accumulation in Alzheimer's disease transgenic mice. *Neuron.* 30:665–676.

Chesneau V, Pierotti AR, Barré N, Créminon C, Tougard C, Cohen P. 1994. Isolation and characterization of a dibasic selective metalloendopeptidase from rat testes that cleaves at the amino terminus of arginine residues. *J Biol Chem.* 269:2056–2061.

Chiti F, Dobson CM. 2006. Protein misfolding, functional amyloid, and human disease. *Annu Rev Biochem.* 75:333–366.

Chromy BA, Nowak RJ, Lambert MP et al. 2003. Self-assembly of Aβ(1–42) into globular neurotoxins. *Biochemistry.* 42:12749–12760.

Coates D. 2003. The angiotensin converting enzyme (ACE) *Int J Biochem Cell Biol.* 35:769–773.

Dahlgren KN, Manelli AM, Stine WB, Baker LK, Krafft GA, LaDu MJ. 2002. Oligomeric and fibrillar species of amyloid-beta peptides differentially affect neuronal viability. *J Biol Chem.* 277:32046–32053.

de la Monte SM, Wands JR. 2005. Review of insulin and insulin-like growth factor expression, signaling, and malfunction in the central nervous system: relevance to Alzheimer's disease. *J Alzheimers Dis.* 7:45–61.

De Strooper B, Annaert W, Cupers P et al. 1999. A presenilin-1-dependent gamma-secretase-like protease mediates release of notch intracellular domain. *Nature.* 398:518–522.

De Strooper B, Annaert W. 2000. Proteolytic processing and cell biological functions of the amyloid precursor protein. *J Cell Sci.* 113:1857–1870.

Dubois B, Feldman HH, Jacova C et al. 2007. Research criteria for the diagnosis of Alzheimer's disease: revising the NINCDS–ADRDA criteria. *Lancet Neurol.* 6:734–746.

Durairajan SS, Yuan Q, Xie L et al. 2007. Salvianolic acid B inhibits Abeta fibril formation and disaggregates preformed fibrils and protects against Abeta-induced cytotoxicity. *Neurochem Int.* 52(4–5):741–750.

Eckman EA, Reed DK, Eckman CB. 2001. Degradation of the Alzheimer's amyloid beta peptide by endothelin-converting enzyme. *J Biol Chem.* 276:24540–24548.

Eckman EA, Watson M, Marlow L, Sambamurti Z, Eckman CB. 2003. Alzheimer's disease beta-amyloid peptide is increased in mice deficient in endothelin-converting enzyme. *J Biol Chem.* 278:2081–2084.

Eckman EA, Adams SK, Troendle FJ et al. 2006. Regulation of steady-state β-amyloid levels in the brain by neprilysin and endothelin-converting enzyme but not angiotensin-converting enzyme. *J Biol Chem.* 281:30471–30478.

Edbauer D, Winkler E, Regula JT, Pesold B, Steiner H, Haass C. 2003. Reconstitution of γ-secretase activity. *Nat Cell Biol.* 5:486–488.

Eisele YS, Baumann M, Klebl B, Nordhammer C, Jucker M, Kilger E. 2007. Gleevec increases levels of the amyloid precursor protein intracellular domain and of the amyloid-beta degrading enzyme neprilysin. *Mol Biol Cell.* 18(9):3591–3600.

El-Amouri SS, Zhu H, Yu J, Gage FH, Verma IM, Kindy MS. 2007. Neprilysin protects neurons against Abeta peptide toxicity. *Brain Res.* 1152:191–200.

Elkins JS, Douglas VC, Johnston SC. 2004. Alzheimer disease risk and genetic variation in ACE: a meta-analysis. *Neurology.* 62:363–368.

Emerich DF, Winn SR, Hantraye PM et al. 1997. Protective effect of encapsulated cells producing neurotrophic factor CNTF in a monkey model of Huntington's disease. *Nature.* 386:395–399.

Ercheberrigaray R, Tan M, Dewachter I et al. 2004. Therapeutic effects of PKC activators in Alzheimer's disease transgenic mice. *Proc Natl Acad Sci U S A.* 101:11141–11146.

Exley C, Korchazhkina OV. 2001. Plasmin cleaves Abeta42 in vitro and prevents its aggregation into beta-pleated sheet structures. *Neuroreport.* 12:2967–2970.

Farris W, Mansourian S, Chang Y et al. 2003. Insulin-degrading enzyme regulates the levels of insulin, amyloid β-protein, and the β-amyloid precursor protein intracellular domain in vivo. *Proc Natl Acad Sci U S A.* 100:4162–4167.

Farris W, Mansourian S, Leissring MA et al. 2004. Partial loss-of-function mutations in insulin-degrading enzyme that induce diabetes also impair degradation of amyloid beta-protein. *Am J Pathol.* 164:1425–1434

Ferreira ST, Vieira MN, De Felice FG. 2007. Soluble protein oligomers as emerging toxins in Alzheimer's and other amyloid diseases. *IUBMB Life.* 59:332–345.

Ferri CP, Prince M, Brayne C et al. 2005. Alzheimer's Disease international global prevalence of dementia: a Delphi consensus study. *Lancet.* 366:2112–2117.

Fraering PC, Ye W, LaVoie MJ, Ostaszewski BL, Selkoe DJ, Wolfe MS. 2005. gamma-Secretase substrate selectivity can be modulated directly via interaction with a nucleotide-binding site. *J Biol Chem.* 280(51):41987–41996.

Frim DM, Uhler TA, Galpern WR, Beal MF, Breakefield XO, Isacson O. 1994. Implanted fibroblasts genetically engineered to produce brain-derived neurotrophic factor prevent 1-methyl-4-phenylpyridinium toxicity to dopaminergic neurons in the rat. *Proc Natl Acad Sci U S A.* 91:5104–5108.

Fukami S, Watanabe K, Iwata N et al. 2002. Abeta-degrading endopeptidase, neprilysin, in mouse brain: synaptic and axonal localization inversely correlating with Abeta pathology. *Neurosci Res.* 43:39–56.

Funalot B, Ouimet T, Claperon A et al. 2004. Endothelin-converting enzyme-1 is expressed in human cerebral cortex and protects against Alzheimer's disease. *Mol Psychiatry.* 9:1122–1128.

Geerts H. 2004. NC-531 (Neurochem). *Curr Opin Investig Drugs.* 5:95–100.

Glabe CG. 2006. Common mechanisms of amyloid oligomer pathogenesis in degenerative disease. *Neurobiol Aging.* 27:570–575.

Grziwa B, Grimm MO, Masters CL, Beyreuther K, Hartmann T, Lichtenthaler SF. 2003. The transmembrane domain of the amyloid precursor protein in microsomal membranes is on both sides shorter than predicted. *J Biol Chem.* 278:6803–6808.

Gunawardena S, Goldstein LS. 2001. Disruption of axonal transport and neuronal viability by amyloid precursor protein mutations in Drosophila. *Neuron.* 32:389–401.

Ha C, Ryu J, Park CB. 2007. Metal ions differentially influence the aggregation and deposition of Alzheimer's β-amyloid on a solid template. *Biochemistry.* 46:6118–6125.

Haass C, Selkoe DJ. 2007. Soluble protein oligomers in neurodegeneration: lessons from the Alzheimer's amyloid β-peptide *Nat Rev.* 8:101–112.

Hamaguchi T, Ono K, Yamada M. 2006. Anti-amyloidogenic therapies: strategies for prevention and treatment of Alzheimer's disease. *Cell Mol Life Sci.* 63:1538–1552.

Harrison SM, Harper AJ, Hawkins J et al. 2003. BACE1 (β-secretase) transgenic and knockout mice: identification of neurochemical deficits and behavioral changes. *Mol Cell Neurosci.* 24:646–655.

He W, Lu Y, Qahwash I, Hu XY, Chang A, Yan R. 2004. Reticulon family members modulate BACE1 activity and amyloid-beta peptide generation. *Nat Med.* 10:959–965.

Heal JR, Roberts GW, Raynes JG, Bhakoo A, Miller AD. 2002. Specific interactions between sense and complementary peptides: the basis for the proteomic code. *Chembiochem.* 3:136–151.

Hemming ML, Selkoe DJ. 2005. Amyloid β-protein is degraded by cellular angiotensin-converting enzyme (ACE) and elevated by an ACE inhibitor. *J Biol Chem.* 280:37644–37650.

Hemming ML, Patterson M, Reske-Nielsen C, Lin L, Isacson O, Selkoe DJ 2007. Reducing Amyloid Plaque Burden via Ex Vivo Gene Delivery of an Aβ-Degrading Protease: A Novel Therapeutic Approach to Alzheimer Disease. *PLoS Med.* 4(8):e262.

Herms J, Anliker B, Heber S et al. 2004. Cortical dysplasia resembling human type 2 lissencephaly in mice lacking all three APP family members. *EMBO J.* 23:4106–4115.

Herreman A, Serneels L, Annaert W, Collen D, Schoonjans L, De Strooper B. 2000. Total inactivation of γ-secretase activity in presenilin-deficient embryonic stem cells. *Nat Cell Biol.* 2:461–462.

Hiraoka Y, Ohno M, Yoshida K et al. 2007. Enhancement of alpha-secretase cleavage of amyloid precursor protein by a metalloendopeptidase nardilysin. *J Neurochem.* 102:1595–1605.

Hook V, Toneff T, Bogyo M et al. 2005. Inhibition of cathepsin B reduces beta-amyloid production in regulated secretory vesicles of neuronal chromaffin cells: evidence for cathepsin B as a candidate beta-secretase of Alzheimer's disease. *Biol Chem.* 386:931–940.

Hoshi M, Sato M, Matsumoto S et al. 2003. Spherical aggregates of (β-amyloid (amylospheroid) show high neurotoxicity and activate tau protein kinase I/glycogen synthase kinase-3β. *Proc Natl Acad Sci U S A.* 100:6370–6375.

Hotoda N, Koike H, Sasagawa N, Ishiura S. 2002. A secreted form of human ADAM9 has an α-secretase activity for APP. *Biochem Biophys Res Commun.* 293:800–805.

Hu J, Igarashi A, Kamata M, Nakagawa H. 2001. Angiotensin-converting enzyme degrades Alzheimer amyloid β-peptide (Aβ); retards Aβ aggregation, deposition, fibril formation, and inhibits cytotoxicity. *J Biol Chem.* 276:47863–47868.

Hussain I, Powell D, Howlett DR et al. 1999. Identification of a novel aspartic protease (Asp 2) as beta-secretase. *Mol Cell Neurosci.* 14:419–427.

Hussain I, Hawkins J, Harrison D et al. 2007. Oral administration of a potent and selective non-peptidic BACE-1 inhibitor decreases β-cleavage of amyloid precursor protein and amyloid-β production in vivo. *J Neurochem.* 100;802–809.

Im H, Manolopoulou M, Malito E et al. 2007. Structure of substrate-free human insulin-degrading enzyme (IDE) and biophysical analysis of ATP-induced conformational switch of IDE. *J Biol Chem.* 282:25453–25463.

Iwata N, Mizukami H, Shirotani K et al. 2004. Presynaptic localization of neprilysin contributes to efficient clearance of amyloid-beta peptide in mouse brain. *J Neurosci.* 24:991–998.

Kaether C, Haass C, Steiner H. 2006. Assembly, trafficking and function of gamma-secretase. *Neurodegener Dis.* 3:275–283.

Karamohamed S, Demissie S, Volcjak J et al. 2003. Polymorphisms in the insulin-degrading enzyme gene are associated with type 2 diabetes in men from the NHLBI Framingham Heart Study. *Diabetes.* 52:1562–1567.

Kawarabayashi T, Shoji M, Younkin LH et al. 2004. Dimeric amyloid beta protein rapidly accumulates in lipid rafts followed by apolipoprotein E and phosphorylated tau accumulation in the Tg2576 mouse model of Alzheimer's disease. *J Neurosci.* 24:3801–3809.

Khachaturian AS, Zandi PP, Lyketsos CG et al. 2006. Antihypertensive medication use and incident Alzheimer disease: the Cache County Study. *Arch Neurol.* 63:686–692.

Kim M, Hersh LB, Leissring MA et al. 2007. Decreased catalytic activity of the insulin-degrading enzyme in chromosome 10-linked Alzheimer disease families. *J Biol Chem.* 282:7825–7832.

Kojro E, Fahrenholz F. 2005. The non-amyloidogenic pathway: structure and function of alpha-secretases. *Subcell Biochem.* 38:105–127.

Kokubo H, Kayed R, Glabe CG, Yamaguchi H 2005. Soluble Abeta oligomers ultrastructurally localize to cell processes and might be related to synaptic dysfunction in Alzheimer's disease brain. *Brain Res* 1031:222–228.

Lammich S, Kojro E, Postina R et al. 1999. Constitutive and regulated alpha-secretase cleavage of Alzheimer's amyloid precursor protein by a disintegrin metalloprotease. *Proc Natl Acad Sci U S A.* 96:3922–3927.

Lammich S, Okochi M, Takeda M et al. 2002. Presenilin-dependent intramembrane proteolysis of CD44 leads to the liberation of its intracellular domain and the secretion of an Abeta-like peptide. *J Biol Chem.* 277:44754–44759.

Lansbury PT, Lashuel HA. 2006. A century-old debate on protein aggregation and neurodegeneration enters the clinic. *Nature.* 443:774–779.

Lashuel HA, Hartley DM, Petre BM et al. 2003. Mixtures of wild-type and a pathogenic (E22G) form of Aβ40 in vitro accumulate protofibrils, including amyloid pores. *J Mol Biol.* 332:795–808.

Lehmann DJ, Cortina-Borja M, Warden DR et al. 2005. Large meta-analysis establishes the ACE insertion-deletion polymorphism as a marker of Alzheimer's disease. *Am J Epidemiol.* 162:305–317.

Leissring MA, Farris W, Chang AY et al. 2003. Enhanced proteolysis of beta-amyloid in APP transgenic mice prevents plaque formation, secondary pathology, and premature death. *Neuron.* 40:1087–1093.

Lesné S, Koh MT, Kotilinek L et al. 2006. A specific amyloid-beta protein assembly in the brain impairs memory. *Nature.* 440:352–357.

Leuchtenberger S, Kummer MP, Kukar T et al. 2006. Inhibitors of Rho-kinase modulate amyloid-beta (Abeta) secretion but lack selectivity for Abeta42. *J Neurochem.* 96:355–365.

Liu R, Barkhordarian H, Emadi S, Park CB, Sierks MR. 2005. Trehalose differentially inhibits aggregation and neurotoxicity of beta-amyloid 40 and 42. *Neurobiol Dis.* 20:74–81.

Lleó A, Greenberg SM, Growdon JH. 2006. Current pharmacotherapy for Alzheimer's disease. *Annu Rev Med.* 57:513–533.

Lopez-Perez E, Seidah N, Checler F. 1999. Proprotein convertase activity contributes to the processing of the Alzheimer's beta-amyloid precursor protein in human cells: evidence for a role of the prohormone PC7 in the constitutive alpha-secretase pathway. *J Neurochem.* 73:2056–2062.

Lopez-Perez E, Zhang Y, Frank S, Creemers J, Seidah N, Checler F. 2001. Constitutive α-secretase cleavage of the β-amyloid precursor protein in the furin-deficient LoVo cell line: involvement of the prohormone convertase 7 and the disintegrin metalloprotease ADAM-10. *J Neurochem.* 76:1532–1539.

Lundkvist J, Näslund J. 2007. Gamma-secretase: a complex target for Alzheimer's disease. *Curr Opin Pharmacol.* 7:112–118.

Luo Y, Bolon B, Damore MA et al. 2003. BACE1 (β-secretase) knockout mice do not acquire compensatory gene expression changes or develop neural lesions over time. *Neurobiol Dis.* 14:81–88.

Lynch JA, George AM, Eisenhauer PB et al. 2006. Insulin degrading enzyme is localized predominantly at the cell surface of polarized and unpolarized human cerebrovascular endothelial cell cultures. *J Neurosci Res.* 83:1262–1270.

Madani R, Poirier R, Wolfer DP et al. 2006. Lack of neprilysin suffices to generate murine amyloid-like deposits in the brain and behavioral deficit in vivo. *J Neurosci Res.* 84:1871–1878.

Marambaud P, Shioi J, Serban G et al. 2002. A presenilin-1/gamma-secretase cleavage releases the E-cadherin intracellular domain and regulates disassembly of adherens junctions. *EMBO J.* 21:1948–1956.

Marr RA, Rockenstein E, Mukherjee A et al. 2003. Neprilysin gene transfer reduces human amyloid pathology in transgenic mice. *J Neurosci.* 23:1992–1996.

Martins IC, Kuperstein I, Wilkinson H et al. 2008. Lipids revert inert Aβ amyloid fibrils to neurotoxic protofibrils that affect learning in mice. *EMBO J.* 27:224–233.

Masters CL, Beyreuther K. 2006. Alzheimer's centennial legacy: prospects for rational therapeutic intervention targeting the Aβ amyloid pathway. *Brain.* 129:2823–2839.

McLaurin J, Kierstead ME, Brown ME et al. 2006. Cyclohexanehexol inhibitors of Aβ aggregation prevent and reverse Alzheimer phenotype in a mouse model. *Nat Med.* 12:801–809.

Mori C, Spooner ET, Wisniewsk KE et al. 2002. Intraneuronal Abeta42 accumulation in Down syndrome brain. *Amyloid.* 9:88–102.

Mucke L, Masliah E, Yu GQ et al. 2000. High-level neuronal expression of abeta 1–42 in wild-type human amyloid protein precursor transgenic mice: synaptotoxicity without plaque formation. *J Neurosci.* 20:4050–4058.

Mueller-Steiner S, Zhou Y, Arai H et al. 2006. Antiamyloidogenic and neuroprotective functions of cathepsin B: implications for Alzheimer's disease. *Neuron.* 51:703–714.

Na CH, Jeon SH, Zhang G, Olson GL, Chae C-B. 2007. Inhibition of amyloid β-peptide production by blockage of β-secretase cleavage site of amyloid precursor protein. *J Neurochem.* 101:1583–1595.

Nakai K. 2001. Prediction of in vivo fates of proteins in the era of genomics and proteomics. *J Struct Biol.* 134:103–116.

Netzer WJ, Dou F, Cai D et al. 2003. Gleevec inhibits beta-amyloid production but not Notch cleavage. *Proc Natl Acad Sci U S A.* 100:12444–12449.

Ni CY, Murphy MP, Golde TE, Carpenter G. 2001. Gamma-secretase cleavage and nuclear localization of ErbB-4 receptor tyrosine kinase. *Science.* 294:2179–2218.

Nilsberth C, Westlind-Danielsson A, Eckman CB et al. 2001. The 'Arctic' APP mutation (E693G) causes Alzheimer's disease by enhanced Aβ protofibril formation. *Nat Neurosci.* 4:887–893.

Nishi E, Hiraoka Y, Yoshida K, Okawa K, Kita T. 2006. Nardilysin enhances ectodomain shedding of heparin-binding epidermal growth factor-like growth factor through activation of tumor necrosis factor-alpha-converting enzyme. *J Biol Chem.* 281:31164–31172.

Nixon RA, Mathews PM, Cataldo AM. 2001. The neuronal endosomal-lysosomal system in Alzheimer's disease. *J Alzheimer's Dis.* 3:97–107.

Oba R, Igarashi A, Kamata M, Nagata K, Takano S, Nakagawa, H. 2005. The N-terminal active centre of human angiotensin-converting enzyme degrades Alzheimer amyloid β-peptide. *Eur J Neurosci.* 21:733–740.

Ohnishi S, Takano K. 2004. Amyloid fibrils from the viewpoint of protein folding. *Cell Mol Life Sci.* 61:511–524.

Ohno M, Sametsky EA, Younkin LH et al. 2004. BACE1 deficiency rescues memory deficits and cholinergic dysfunction in a mouse model of Alzheimer's disease. *Neuron.* 41:27–33.

Ohrui T, Tomita N, Sato-Nakagawa T et al. 2004. Effects of brain-penetrating ACE inhibitors on Alzheimer disease progression. *Neurology.* 63:1324–1325.

Onyango IG, Khan SM. 2006. Oxidative stress, mitochondrial dysfunction, and stress signaling in Alzheimer's disease. *Curr Alzheimer Res.* 3:339–349.

Panchal M, Rholam M, Brakch N. 2004. Abnormalities of Peptide Metabolism in Alzheimer Disease. *Curr Neurovas Res.* 1:269–281.

Panchal M, Lazar N, Munoz N et al. 2007. Clearance of amyloid-β peptide by neuronal and non-neuronal cells: proteolytic degradation by secreted and membrane associated proteases. *Curr Neurovas Res.* 4:240–251.

Pardossi-Piquard R, Petit A, Kawarai T et al. 2005. Presenilin-dependent transcriptional control of the Aβ-degrading enzyme neprilysin by intracellular domains of βAPP and APLP. *Neuron.* 46:541–554.

Pardossi-Piquard R, Dunys J, Yu G, St George-Hyslop P, Alves da Costa C, Checler F. 2006. Neprilysin activity and expression are controlled by nicastrin. *J Neurochem.* 97(4):1052–1056.

Paris D, Quadros A, Patel N, DelleDonne A, Humphrey J, Mullan M. 2005. Inhibition of angiogenesis and tumor growth by β and γ-secretase inhibitors. *Eur J Pharmacol.* 514:1–15.

Permanne B, Adessi C, Saborio GP et al. 2002. Reduction of amyloid load and cerebral damage in a transgenic mouse model of Alzheimer's disease by treatment with a beta-sheet breaker peptide. *FASEB J.* 16:860–862.

Petit A, Pasini A, Alves Da Costa C et al. 2003. JLK isocoumarin inhibitors: selective gamma-secretase inhibitors that do not interfere with notch pathway in vitro or in vivo. *J Neurosci Res.* 74:370–377.

Postina R, Schroeder A, Dewachter I et al. 2004. A disintegrin-metalloproteinase prevents amyloid plaque formation and hippocampal defects in an Alzheimer disease mouse model. *J Clin Invest.* 113:1456–1464.

Qiu WQ, Folstein MF. 2006. Insulin, insulin-degrading enzyme and amyloid-β peptide in Alzheimer's disease: review and hypothesis. *Neurobiol Aging.* 27:190–198.

Raber J, Huang Y, Ashford JW. 2004. ApoE genotype accounts for the vast majority of AD risk and AD pathology. *Neurobiol Aging.* 25:641–650.

Ritchie CW, Bush AI, Mackinnon A et al. 2003. Metalprotein attenuation with iodochlorhydroxyquin (clioquinol) targeting Abeta amyloid deposition and toxicity in Alzheimer disease: a pilot phase 2 clinical trial. *Arch Neurol.* 60:1685–1691.

Russo R, Borghi R, Markesbery W, Tabaton M, Piccini A. 2005. Neprylisin decreases uniformly in Alzheimer's disease and in normal aging. *FEBS Lett.* 579:6027–6030.

Sadowski M, Pankiewicz J, Scholtzova H et al. 2004. A synthetic peptide blocking the apolipoprotein E/beta-amyloid binding mitigates beta amyloid toxicity and fibril formation in vitro and reduces beta amyloid plaques in transgenic mice. *Am J Pathol.* 165:937–948.

Saric T, Muller D, Seitz HJ, Pavelic K. 2003. Non-covalent interaction of ubiquitin with insulin-degrading enzyme. *Mol Cell Endocrinol.* 204:11–20.

Selkoe DJ. 2001. Clearing the brain's amyloid cobwebs. *Neuron.* 32:177–180.

Selkoe DJ. 2004. Cell biology of protein misfolding: the examples of Alzheimer's and Parkinson's diseases. *Nat Cell Biol.* 6:1054–1061.

Shen Y, Joachimiak A, Rosner MR, Tang WJ. 2006. Structures of human insulin-degrading enzyme reveal a new substrate recognition mechanism. *Nature.* 443:870–874.

Shinall H, Song ES, Hersh LB. 2005. Susceptibility of amyloid beta peptide degrading enzymes to oxidative damage: a potential Alzheimer's disease spiral. *Biochemistry.* 44:15345–15350.

Siemers ER, Quinn JF, Kaye J et al. 2006. Effects of a gamma-secretase inhibitor in a randomized study of patients with Alzheimer disease. *Neurology.* 66:602–624.

Sieving PA, Caruso RC, Tao W et al. 2006. Ciliary neurotrophic factor (CNTF) for human retinal degeneration: phase I trial of CNTF delivered by encapsulated cell intraocular implants. *Proc Natl Acad Sci U S A.* 103:3896–3901.

Solomon B. 2004. Alzheimer's disease and immunotherapy. *Curr Alzheimer Res.* 1:149–163.

Song ES, Juliano MA, Juliano L, Hersh LB. 2003. Substrate activation of insulin-degrading enzyme (insulysin). A potential target for drug development. *J. Biol. Chem.* 278:49789–49794.

Stefani M. 2004. Protein misfolding and aggregation: new examples in medicine and biology of the dark side of the protein world. *Biochimica et Biophysica Acta.* 1739:5–25.

Tampellini D, Magrané J, Takahashi RH et al. 2007. Internalized antibodies to the Abeta domain of APP reduce neuronal Abeta and protect against synaptic alterations. *J Biol Chem.* 282:18895–18906.

Tuszynski MH, Smith DE, Roberts J, McKay H, Mufson E. 1998. Targeted intraparenchymal delivery of human NGF by gene transfer to the primate basal forebrain for 3 months does not accelerate beta-amyloid plaque deposition. *Exp Neurol.* 154:573–582.

Tuszynski MH, Thal L, Pay M et al. 2005. A phase 1 clinical trial of nerve growth factor gene therapy for Alzheimer disease. *Nat Med.* 11:551–555.

Uversky VN, Fink AL. 2004. Conformational constraints for amyloid fibrillation: the importance of being unfolded. *Biochimica et Biophysica Acta.* 1698:131–153.

van Horssen J, Wesseling P, van den Heuvel LP, de Waal RM, Verbeek MM. 2003. Heparan sulphate proteoglycans in Alzheimer's disease and amyloid-related disorders. *Lancet Neurol.* 2:482–492.

Vassar R, Bennett BD, Babu-Khan S et al. 1999. β-secretase cleavage of Alzheimer's amyloid precursor protein by the transmembrane aspartic protease BACE. *Science.* 286:735–741.

Walsh DM, Klyubin I, Fadeeva JV et al. 2002. Naturally secreted oligomers of amyloid beta protein potently inhibit hippocampal long-term potentiation in vivo. *Nature.* 416:535–539.

Walsh DM, Townsend M, Podlisny MB et al. 2005. Certain inhibitors of synthetic amyloid beta peptide (Abeta) fibrillogenesis block oligomerization of natural Abeta and thereby rescue long-term potentiation. *J Neurosci.* 25:2455–2462.

Walsh DM, Selkoe DJ. 2007. Aβ Oligomers–a decade of discovery. *J Neurochem.* 101:1172–1184.

Wang P, Yang G, Mosier DR et al. 2005. Defective neuromuscular synapses in mice lacking amyloid precursor protein (APP) and APP-Like protein 2. *J Neurosci.* 25:1219–1225

Wasco W, Bupp K, Magendantz M, Gusella JF, Tanzi RE, Solomon F. 1992. Identification of a mouse brain cDNA that encodes a protein related to the Alzheimer disease-associated amyloid beta protein precursor. *Proc Natl Acad Sci U S A.* 89:10758–10762.

Weggen S, Eriksen JL, Sagi SA, Pietrzik CU, Golde TE, Koo EH. 2003. Abeta42-lowering nonsteroidal anti-inflammatory drugs preserve intramembrane cleavage of the amyloid precursor protein (APP) and ErbB-4 receptor and signaling through the APP intracellular domain. *J Biol Chem.* 278:30748–30754.

Weihofen A, Martoglio B. 2003. Intramembrane-cleaving proteases: controlled liberation of proteins and bioactive peptides. *Trends Cell Biol.* 13:71–78.

Wolfe MS, Xia W, Ostaszewski BL, Diehl TS, Kimberly WT, Selkoe DJ. 1999. Two transmembrane aspartates in presenilin-1 required for presenilin endoproteolysis and γ-secretase activity. *Nature.* 398:513–517.

Wong GT, Manfra D, Poulet FM et al. 2004. Chronic treatment with the gamma-secretase inhibitor LY411575 inhibits beta-amyloid peptide production and alters lymphopoiesis and intestinal cell differentiation. *J Biol Chem.* 279:12876–12882.

Yamin R, Bagchi S, Hildebrant R, Scaloni A, Widom RL, Abraham CR. 2007. Acyl peptide hydrolase, a serine proteinase isolated from conditioned medium of neuroblastoma cells, degrades the amyloid-β peptide. *J Neurochem.* 100:458–467.

Yan P, Hu X, Song H et al. 2006. Matrix metalloproteinase-9 degrades amyloid-β fibrils in vitro and compact plaques in situ. *J Biol Chem.* 281:24566–24574.

Yang F, Lim GP, Begum AN, et al. 2005. Curcumin inhibits formation of amyloid beta oligomers and fibrils, binds plaques, and reduces amyloid in vivo. *J Biol Chem.* 280:5892–901.

Yang HQ, Pan J, Ba MW et al. 2007. New protein kinase C activator regulates amyloid precursor protein processing in vitro by increasing α-secretase activity. *Eur J Neurosci.* 26:381–391.

Yeon SW, Jeon YJ, Hwang EM, Kim TY. 2007. Effects of peptides derived from BACE1 catalytic domain on APP processing. *Peptides.* 28:838–844.

Zhu X, Lee HG, Casadesus G et al. 2005. Oxidative imbalance in Alzheimer's disease. *Mol Neurobiol.* 31:205–217.

Zou LB, Mouri A, Iwata N et al. 2006. Inhibition of neprilysin by infusion of thiorphan into the hippocampus causes an accumulation of amyloid β and impairment of learning and memory. *J Pharmacol Exp Ther.* 317:334–340.

Zou K, Yamaguchi H, Akatsu H et al. 2007. Angiotensin-converting enzyme converts amyloid β-protein 1–42 (Aβ$_{1-42}$) to Aβ$_{1-40}$, and its inhibition enhances brain Aβ deposition. *J Neurosci.* 27:8628–8635.

Chapter *17*

NEUROBIOLOGY OF POSTISCHEMIC RECUPERATION IN THE AGED MAMMALIAN BRAIN

Aurel Popa-Wagner, Adrian Balseanu, Leon Zagrean, Imtiaz M. Shah,Mario Di Napoli, Henrik Ahlenius, and Zaal Kokaia

ABSTRACT

Old age is associated with an enhanced susceptibility to stroke and poor recovery from brain injury, but the cellular processes underlying these phenomena are uncertain. Therefore studying the basic mechanism underlying functional recovery after brain ischemia in aged subjects is of considerable clinical interest.

Potential mechanisms include neuroinflammation, changes in brain plasticity–promoting factors, unregulated expression of neurotoxic factors, or differences in the generation of scar tissue that impedes the formation of new axons and blood vessels in the infarcted region. Available data indicate that behaviorally, aged rats were more severely impaired by ischemia than were young rats, and they also showed diminished functional recovery. Further, as compared to young rats, aged rats develop a larger infarct area, as well as a necrotic zone characterized by a higher rate of cellular degeneration, and a larger number of apoptotic cells. Both in old and young rats, the early intense proliferative activity following stroke leads to a precipitous formation of growth-inhibiting scar tissue, a phenomenon amplified by the persistent expression of neurotoxic factors. Finally, the regenerative potential of the rat brain is largely preserved up to 20 months of age but gene expression is temporally displaced, has lower amplitude, and is sometimes of relatively short duration. Most interestingly it has recently been shown that the human brain can respond to stroke with increased progenitor proliferation in aged patients, opening the possibilities of utilizing this intrinsic attempt for neuroregeneration of the human brain as a potential therapy for stroke.

Given the heterogeneity of stroke, a universal anti-inflammatory solution may be a distant prospect, but probably neuroprotective drug cocktails targeting inflammatory pathways in combination with thrombolysis may be a possibility for acute stroke treatment in the future.

Keywords: stroke, aging, gene expression, neurogenesis, regeneration, recuperation, neuroinflammation, neuroprotection.

With the rapid increase in the world's aging population, the societal burden of age-associated disorders of the nervous system will also grow. Stroke (cerebrovascular disease) is the third leading cause of death in the major industrialized countries and the second most common cause of death worldwide. Furthermore, stroke is responsible for more prolonged and expensive hospitalization compared to other neurological disorders in adults. The use of thrombolytic agents in acute ischemic stroke, which has a limited therapeutic time window, is currently the only effective therapeutic intervention (Xiong, Chu, Simon 2007). For these reasons one can assume that stroke is already, and will continue to be, one of the most challenging diseases (Durukan, Tatlisumak 2007).

FEATURES OF BRAIN METABOLISM AND CIRCULATION

The brain exhibits higher vulnerability to the demand for oxygen and glucose than any other tissue or organ of human body. To understand the vulnerability of the central nervous system (CNS) to the lack of continuous and adequate supply of oxygen and blood-borne glucose, we have to keep in mind that normal energy metabolism in the brain has several unusual features including a high metabolic rate, very limited intrinsic energy store, and a great dependence on aerobic metabolism of glucose (Dugan, Kim 2006).

The rate of oxygen consumption by the entire brain (average weight ≈1400 g) of normal conscious young subject amounts to 49 mL of O_2/min (Clarke, Sokoloff 1999). In the basal state, the brain, which represents almost 2% of total body weight, accounts for approximately 20% of the resting total body oxygen consumption (250 mL O_2/min). Cerebral oxygen consumption is almost entirely responsible for the oxidation of carbohydrates, which provides about 95% of the energy consumed by the normal adult human brain in resting metabolic rate conditions (Erecinska, Silver 1989). The fundamental role of oxygen for normal brain activity is sustained by the high extraction rate. Indeed, the average extraction rate of oxygen for the entire body is 25%, whereas that for the brain is 50% to 70% (Paulson 2002).

Glucose is the most important energy-yielding substrate and is essential for developing and, particularly, for adult brain activity. Under normal conditions, glucose utilization rate in resting brain (absence of excitation) is approximately 31 mmol/100 g/min (Aichner, Bauer 2005); 95% glucose that enters the brain is metabolized ultimately by mitochondria, where more than 95% adenosine triphosphate (ATP) is generated by oxidative phosphorylation. The average extraction rate of glucose in the normal brain is 10% and it can increase at higher metabolic rates.

Glucose and oxygen, the two main substances that provide the impressive, high brain metabolic rate, are continuously delivered by cerebral circulation. Since the amount of glucose and oxygen stored in the brain is very small compared with its high metabolic rate, the normal cerebral activity is strongly dependent on their supply via the cerebral blood flow (CBF). For the adult human brain, under normal resting conditions, the average of CBF is about 800 mL/min or 57 mL/100 g tissue/min, corresponding to approximately 15% of total basal cardiac output (Aichner, Bauer 2005). Any "supply and demand" imbalance of energy-yielding substrates has a very prompt effect on brain electric activity and consequently on cerebral function.

THE MEMBRANE ION TRANSPORT SYSTEM

Another important role of cerebral circulation, consistently connected with the brain activity, is to maintain local homeostasis such as pH, ionic concentration, and temperature. When deprived of oxygen the brain perishes first (Somjen 2004). Two particular functional features can justify the great vulnerability of the brain to the lack of oxygen. One feature is that the brain ensues environmental integration of the being and for this function, reaction time to stimulus is often the most important parameter. Another particular feature of the brain is that the energy required to support normal function is provided by glycolysis and mostly by oxidative phosphorylation. However, in sharp contrast to other cells, nerve cells generate and consume more energy in the resting state. This "paradoxical" energy metabolism is due to the preparation, during the resting state (absence of excitation), that conditions the nerve cells to promptly respond to stimuli. In other words, the resting brain spends a lot of energy to gain the speed of stimulus-induced response.

BASAL TRANSCRIPTIONAL ACTIVITIES IN THE CORTEX OF YOUNG AND AGED ANIMALS

Since baseline differences between gene expression in young and old control rats might affect levels found after infarction, we summarize age-related changes in gene expression in the normal aged brain (Buga, Sasacau, Herndon et al. 2008).

We studied a total of 442 genes representing stem cells (258 genes), hypoxia signaling pathway (96 genes), and apoptosis arrays (96 genes). In control animals, the levels of the apoptotic gene *Casp7* are increased in the sensorimotor cortex of aged rats (Table 17.1). Since Casp7 is implicated in the terminal stages of apoptosis, this result suggests that apoptosis is increased in the brains of aged rats. A similar observation has been made in the cortices of aged Fischer

Table 17.1 Ratio (+SD) of Baseline Gene Expression Levels in Old Versus Young Sham Control Rats

Gene	Category	Ratio (Old Versus Young)
Casp 7	Terminal phase of apoptosis	2.08 ± 0.13
Cat	Antioxidant; ROS scavenging	0.42 ± 0.01
Sod2	Antioxidant; ROS scavenging	0.51 ± 0.02
Fabp7	Fatty acid–binding protein 7; lipid metabolism	2.09 ± 0.28
Inhibin-β	Growth factor, also known as activin β	0.43 ± 0.05
Igf1r	Insulin-like growth factor receptor	0.27 ± 0.01
Cdh5	Vascular endothelial cadherin	1.93 ± 0.08
Icam5	Intercellular adhesion molecule 5	1.82 ± 0.07
Gjb1	Gap junction membrane channel protein β1	0.36 ± 0.04
Nkx2.2	Transcription factor; oligodendrocytes	0.39 ± 0.04

344 rats (Dorszewska, Adamczewska-Goncerzewicz, Szczech et al. 2004; Hiona, Leeuwenburgh 2004).

Changes in the mRNAs levels for two major enzymes responsible for reactive oxygen species (ROS) scavenging, catalase (CAT) and superoxide dismutase (SOD), were significantly decreased in the brains of aged rats (Table 17.1), which is indicative of a reduced capacity to remove radicals from the aging brain.

Fatty acid-binding protein 7 mRNA, which is produced by radial glia during development and which is involved in fatty acid (FA) uptake, transport, and targeting, was, on the contrary, increased in the aged rat brain (Table 17.1), suggesting, among other things, an intensification of lipid metabolism after injuries in the aged brain (Murphy, Owada, Kitanaka et al. 2005).

ANIMAL STROKE MODELS ENSUE THE PATHOPHYSIOLOGY OF CEREBRAL VASCULATURE

The meaning of term *stroke* can only be extracted from a puzzling mosaic of definitions of the term itself, mechanisms, signs, and diagnosis. Moreover, most times stroke is the endpoint of a longtime evolution of some complex biological processes bordering the frontier between normal and abnormal, such as aging and atherosclerosis (Hossmann 2006; Popa-Wagner, Carmichael, Kokaia et al. 2007).

The cerebral blood supply is provided by two pairs of arteries: the right and left internal carotid arteries, which supply the anterior two-thirds of the corresponding cerebral hemisphere, and the right and left vertebral arteries, which join together at the

pontomedullary junction to form the basilar artery that supplies the brain stem and posterior portion of the hemispheres (Zazulia 2002).

The two internal carotid arteries and the basilar artery unite via anastomotic channels at the base of the brain to form the circle of Willis. Each of the four arteries, before and after the circle of Willis, gives off branches that supply a territory with imprecise border. The cerebral tissue along the borders of the major arterial territories, between middle, posterior, and anterior cerebral arteries forms the border or "watershed" zone. The blood supply for the "watershed" zone is more reduced than for the neighboring major arterial territories, and it can have more than one arterial source. For this reason the "watershed" zone is more resistant to the decrease in the rate of blood flow.

The cerebral vasculature contains three collateral pathways that can supply blood to a vascular territory in the event of compromise of one of the major vessels. The first one of these is the circle of Willis, which allows for communication between all four major arteries supplying the brain. Others collateral pathways including communication between the extracranial and intracranial circulations or end-to-end arterial anastomoses of the superficial cortical branches of the anterior, middle, and posterior cerebral arteries have minor significance, being considered mostly in different models of experimental ischemia. This short description of cerebral vasculature is applicable to the human brain and for the majority of animals used for the "in vivo" study models of cerebral ischemia, excluding the gerbil (see subsequent text).

Global Ischemia Animal Models

According to brief data about the pathophysiology of cerebral circulation and metabolism provided in the previous section, different animal models can be used in the field of stroke research.

Although global cerebral ischemia has a more reduced correspondence in neurology than focal ischemia, there are numerous experiments and models carried out for their study. The four-vessel occlusion model (4-VO) in rats, most widely used for global cerebral ischemia, involves permanent electrocoagulation of vertebral arteries and temporary ligation of the two common arteries (Pulsinelli, Buchan 1988). The electroencephalogram (EEG) or the electrocorticogram (ECoG) becomes isoelectric for 30 to 40 seconds (Raffin, Harrison, Sick et al. 1991) or 15 to 20 seconds, respectively (Moldovan, Munteanu, Nita et al. 2000). The 4-VO model is easy to manipulate and induces a decrease of blood flow to <3% of control values in neocortex, hippocampus, and striatum (Pulsinelli,

Levy, Duffy 1982), and it can be used for the study of ischemic preconditioning in rats (Zagrean, Moldovan, Munteanu et al. 2000).

The two-vessel occlusion (2-VO) in rat consists in ligation of the common carotid arteries associated with blood pressure (BP) reduction to 50 mmHg (Smith, Bendek, Dalhgren et al. 1984). In this model, fall of blood flow to 1% of control values and EEG suppression are recorded within 15 to 25 seconds after onset of ischemia.

The two-vessel occlusion in gerbil models is performed by only temporary ligation of the common carotid arteries without reduction of blood pressure because there are no posterior communicating arteries in brain circulation. The induced changes by this model are similar to those in the rat models (Kirino, Tsujita, Tamura 1991).

Considering the collateral pathways by communication between the extracranial and intracranial circulations, experimental complete global brain ischemia, corresponding to clinical cardiorespiratory arrest, can be performed by neck-cuff, cardiac arrest, or clamping of the initial segment of aorta (for a review see Lipton 1999).

Focal Ischemia Animal Models

Animal ischemic stroke models contribute to our understanding of the complex pathogenic mechanisms induced by ischemia and reperfusion of the brain.

Experimental models for focal ischemia and reperfusion in different species have a common element, with the occlusion of a major cerebral artery or its branches. The middle cerebral artery (MCA) occlusion (MCAO) model in rats and in mice is the most frequently used because it most accurately mimics human stroke; the ischemic stroke accounts for approximately 80% of all strokes of human pathology (Durukan, Tatlisumak 2007).

The main outcome of experimental focal ischemia and reperfusion models, after the identification of underlying pathophysiological mechanisms, is to identify the mechanisms of neurological recovery involved in stroke evolution and to target these for clinical treatments. To accomplish this target it is necessary to select the most appropriate experimental stroke model.

According to arterial occlusion procedure there are two relevant animal models analogous to human stroke: embolic stroke models and intraluminal suture MCAO model (Durukan, Tatlisumak 2007). Thromboembolic models or nonclot embolic models can reproduce embolic stroke. The thromboembolic ischemia can be performed by injection of either human blood clot, or, most commonly, autologous thrombi into extracranial arteries.

Microsphere-induced stroke is most extensively studied for the testing of drug effects—nonclot embolus models (Zivin, DeGirolami, Kochhar 1987).

Photothrombosis model consists of systemic injection of a photoactive dye (most often Rose Bengal), which in combination with irradiation by a light beam at a specific wavelength, induces the singlet oxygen generation. Free radical formation leads to peroxidative focal endothelial damage and consecutively to platelet activation and aggregation and the coagulation cascade, leading to thrombotic occlusion of small vessels (Rosenblum, El-Sabban 1977; Watson, Dietrich, Busto 1985). Recently, a new photothrombosis model was published for study of ischemic stroke in infant piglets (Kuluz, Prado, Zhao et al. 2007).

Endothelin-1 middle cerebral artery occlusion (EMCAO) model causes a significant decrease of CBF when endothelin-1, a peptide produced by hypoxic endothelial cells with a potent and long-lasting vasoconstriction effect, is applied directly or nearly onto the MCA, inducing an ischemic lesion pattern similar to that induced by surgical MCAO (Sharkey, Butcher, Kelly 1993; Sharkey, Butcher, Kelly 1994). EMCAO is a more reliable model of thromboembolic stroke and is technically advantageous with respect to surgical or endovascular models of transient focal ischemia (Moyanova, Kortenska, Rumiana et al. 2007)

Intraluminal suture MCAO model in rats and in mice is considered the most frequently used model to perform both permanent and transient ischemia. The model involves inserting a monofilament into the internal carotid artery and advancing until it blocks blood flow to the MCA.

Others focal cerebral ischemia models requiring craniectomy such as ligation of the distal MCA, posterior cerebral circulation stroke models have been performed, but they are seldom used (for review see, Durukan, Tatlisumak 2007).

Electrophysiological Investigation in Animal Stroke Models

The earlier quantifiable changes induced by brain ischemia/hypoxia are the changes of membrane electric potentials. These changes are investigated by electrophysiological tools—many technical variants of electroencephalography (EEG) and somatosensory or motor evoked potentials.

EEG has a long history in clinical and experimental model evaluations of cerebrovascular disease. The great advantages of EEG consist in the real-time identification and easy storage of recordings. The long-term video EEG recordings (Kelly, Jukkola,

Kharamov et al. 2006) and quantitative EEG spectral analysis and topographic mapping have improved EEG use in experimental stroke (Tolonen, Sulg 1981; Lu, Williams, Tortella 2001).

The mechanisms involved in EEG suppression induced by brain ischemia/hypoxia represent a provocative target of modern neuroscience research because of interplay between energy metabolism and ion membrane transport alterations, on one side, and the EEG supporting electric activity and investigative function of EEG, on the other side. EEG suppression is regarded either as a mechanism induced by adenosine excess due to lack of oxygen (Fowler 1990; Fowler, Gervitz, Hamilton 2003; Ilie, Ciocan, Zagrean et al. 2006), or as a protective mechanism, considering that EEG suppression spares oxygen (Raffin, Harrison, Sick et al. 1991; Moldovan, Munteanu, Nita et al. 2000).

The evoked potentials (EPs) are used to establish functional alterations of the brain regions involved in processing specific stimulus such as repeated light flashes and acoustic stimulus (Nunez 2002). Other electrophysiological methods use deep electrodes to record electric activity of different nucleus or nervous centers.

Stroke Models Using Aged Animals Are Clinically More Relevant Than Stroke Models in Young Animals

Age and high BP are the most important risk factors for stroke. The risk for each BP value, moreover, multiplies in each decade of life (Lewington, Clarke, Qizilbash et al. 2002; Redon, Cea-Calvo 2007). Aging is associated with a decline in locomotor, sensory, and cognitive performance in humans (Grady, Craik 2000; Clayton, Mesches, Alvarez et al. 2002; Mesches, Gemma, Veng et al. 2004; Navarro, Carmen Gomez, Maria-Jesus Sanchez-Pino et al. 2005). Many of these changes are due to age-related functional decline of the brain.

Studies of stroke in experimental animals have demonstrated the neuroprotective efficacy of a variety of interventions, but most of the strategies that have been clinically tested failed to show benefit in aged humans. One possible explanation for this discrepancy between experimental and clinical studies may be the role that age plays in the recovery of the brain from insult. Indeed, age-dependent increase in conversion of ischemic tissue into infarction suggests that age is a biological marker for the variability in tissue outcome in acute human stroke (Ay, Koroshetz, Vangel et al. 2005).

Although it is well known that aging is a risk factor for stroke (Barnett 2002; Broderick 2004; American

Heart Association 2006; Seshadri, Beiser, Kelly-Hayes et al. 2006), the majority of experimental studies of stroke have been performed on young animals, and therefore may not fully replicate the effects of ischemia on neural tissue in aged subjects (Wang, Futrell, Wang et al. 1995; Popa-Wagner, Schroder, Walker et al. 1998; Markus, Tsai, Bollnow et al. 2005; Brown, Marlowe, Bjelke 2003). In the light of this, the aged postacute animal model is clinically most relevant to stroke rehabilitation and cellular studies, a recommendation put forward by the STAIR (The Stroke Therapy Academic Industry Roundtable) committee (Subramanyam, Pond, Eyles et al. 1999) and more recently by the Stroke Progress Review Group (Lindner, Gribkoff, Donlan et al. 2003).

RECUPERATION OF TISSUE FROM STROKE IS GOVERNED BY A COMPLEX CYTOLOGICAL RESPONSE

Poor recovery reflects the balance of factors leading to infarct progression (neuronal degeneration, apoptosis, phagocytosis), factors impeding tissue repair (astroglial scar, neurite inhibitory proteins), and factors promoting brain plasticity and repair.

Infarct Development Is Greatly Accelerated after Stroke in Aged Rats

Functional imaging studies after stroke have shown that the reorganization in the peri-infarcted cortex or connected cortical regions correlates closely with functional recovery (Price, Menon, Peters et al. 2004; Alarcón, Zijlmans, Dueñas et al. 2004; Ward, 2007). Therefore these regions are mostly studied at cellular and molecular levels.

There are a number of studies on the evolution of infarct volume in aged rats. Similar findings have been reported recently for senescence-prone mice (SAMP8). On the first day after hemorrhagic insult, there was no significant difference in the size of hemorrhagic injury in the SAMP8 and SAMR1 mice. Three days after hemorrhagic insult, however, a larger hemorrhagic injury was obtained in old SAMP8 mice. Seven days after intracerebral hemorrhage (ICH) induction, hemorrhagic injury was still present in old SAMP8 mice, but to a much lesser degree in young SAMP8 mice and young or old SAMR1 mice (Lee, Cho, Choi et al. 2006).

Recently it was found that aged rats usually develop an infarct within the first few days after ischemia. (Popa-Wagner, Badan, Walker et al. 2007a). In contrast to young animals, where the infarct area represented 7% of the ipsilateral hemisphere, on day 3, the necrotic zone of aged rats lacked NeuN immu-nopositivity in 28% of the ipsilateral cortical volume. The infarcted area continued to expand, and by day 7, reached 35% to 41% of the ipsilateral cortical volume in both young and aged rats. This suggests that the timing of neuronal loss in aged rats is accelerated, but the ultimate extent of brain cell loss is not signif-icantly different from that in young rats. It should be noted, however, that the greater number of degener-ating neurons in aged rats is seen only if the infarct area is relatively large; for small infarcts there is no age difference in the number of surviving neurons in the ischemic border zones (Sutherland, Dix, Auer 1996; Lindner, Gribkoff, Donlan et al. 2003).

Neuronal Degeneration and Loss through Postischemic Apoptosis Are Accelerated in Aged Rats

Fluoro JadeB-staining showed that aged rats had an unusually high number of degenerating neurons in the infarct core as early as day 3 while young rats had a lower number (3.5-fold vs. young rats; $P < 0.001$). Interestingly, the number of degenerating neurons did not rise further in aged animals, even though the infarcted area continued to expand, so that by day 7 the numbers of degenerating neurons were almost the same in both age-groups (Popa-Wagner, Schröder, Schmoll et al. 1999; Zhao, Puurunen, Schallert et al. 2005a.)

Aging increases the susceptibility of the CNS to apoptotic events (Hiona, Leeuwenburgh 2004). One possible mechanism of increased expression of pro-apoptotic proteins in aged animals is via increased NO production by constitutive NO synthase isoforms in a model of transient global ischemia (Martinez-Lara, Canuelo, Siles et al. 2005). The particular vul-nerability of the aged brain to apoptosis (Gozal, Row, Kheirandish et al. 2003) is confirmed by our find-ing that aged rats had considerably more apoptotic cells 3 days after ischemia than did young rats (2-fold increase over young rats, $P < 0.02$) (Popa-Wagner et al. 2007). At day 7, the ratio was unexpectedly reversed such that aged rats now had *fewer* apoptotic cells than young rats (1.7-fold difference; $P < 0.05$). However, if the damage to the cerebral cortex is extensive, there is no difference in infarct size or the number of cells undergoing apoptosis between aged and young adults (Sutherland, Dix, Auer 1996).

Genes related to apoptosis were not upregulated at day 3 after stroke. By day 14, however, the number of genes involved in apoptosis had increased in young rats. In contrast to young rats, at day 3, DNA dam-age–, cell cycle arrest–, and apoptosis-related genes were upregulated in the aged rats (Tables 17.2–17.4). In particular, aged rats rapidly upregulated genes such as *growth arrest and DNA-damaged inducible 45 α* (*Gadd45α*), a DNA damage-related gene, telangiecta-sis-mutated homolog (human) (*Atm_mapped*), *Hus1* homolog (*S. pombe*) (*Hus1_predicted*), and transformed mouse 3T3 cell double minute 2 (*Mdm2*) and tumor necrosis factor (TNF) receptor superfamily member 7 (*Tnfrsf7*, also called *CD27*) (Table 17.4).

It has been proposed that Mdm2 could be an indicator of DNA damage in the brain early after an ischemic insult in a way similar to Gadd45 α (Tu, Hou, Huang et al. 1998). The role of Hus1 and ATM in the post-stroke rat brain are not known. The pro-tein encoded by *Hus1* gene forms a heterotrimeric complex with checkpoint proteins RAD9 and RAD1. In response to DNA damage the trimeric complex interacts with another protein complex consisting of checkpoint protein RAD17 and four small sub-units of the replication factor C (RFC), which loads the combined complex onto the chromatin. The DNA damage–induced chromatin binding has been shown to depend on the activation of the checkpoint kinase ATM and is thought to be an early checkpoint signaling event (Roos-Mattjus, Vroman, Burtelow et al. 2002).

Tnfrsf7 plays an important role mediating CD27-binding protein–induced apoptosis (Prasad, Ao, Yoon et al. 1997). Interestingly, we found a strong upregula-tion of caspase 7 (*Casp7*) gene expression at 14 days post-stroke in aged rats. In young rats, however, *Casp7* was downregulated at this time point. However, in control aged rat brains, *Casp7* is already increased, suggesting that ischemia will exacerbate a death mech-anism that is already operational in aged brains.

ARE BRAIN CAPILLARIES IN THE AGED BRAIN MORE SUSCEPTIBLE TO BREAKDOWN?

Recent data show that not only do cells die earlier in the infarct zone of aged rats but there are also more newly generated cells at this time. Pulse-labeling with bromodeoxyuridine (BrdU) shortly before sacrifice revealed a dramatic increase in proliferating cells in the infarcted area. Significantly, at day 3, the number of BrdU-positive cells in the infarcted hemisphere of aged rats greatly exceeded that of young rats (Popa-Wagner et al. 2007). Similarly, BrdU-positive cell counts were significantly higher with severe global ischemia achieved by eight-vessel occlusion than with intermediate ischemia (four-vessel occlusion) or in sham-operated animals, respectively (He, Crook, Meschia et al. 2005). With double-labeling techniques,

Table 17.2 List of Expressed *Stem Cell Array* Genes in the Postischemic Rat Brain

Gene Name	Genbank Accession no.	Description	Fold Change							
			3-Months-Old Rat				18-Months-Old Rat			
			Day 3		Day 14		Day 3		Day 14	
			pi/ctrl	cl/ctrl	pi/ctrl	cl/ctrl	pi/ctrl	cl/ctrl	pi/ctrl	cl/ctrl
Stem cell–related genes										
Fabp7*	NM_021272	Fatty acid–binding protein 7, brain	3.40		4.17		7.48		8.07	
Fgf22	NM_023304	Fibroblast growth factor 22	2.28	2.15						
Fzd8	NM_008058	Frizzled homolog 8 (Drosophila)	4.61	2.37						0.61↓
Gata2	NM_008090	Gata binding protein 2	2.17			0.36↓			0.44↓	0.40↓
Igf1r*	NM_010513	Insulin-like growth factor 1 receptor	2.70		0.56↓		0.62↓			
Ngfb	NM_013609	Nerve growth factor, β	2.09	2.03	2.00					
Nkx2-2*	NM_010919	NK2 transcription factor related– locus 2 (Drosophila)	1.59	2.98	2.82					
Oligo1	NM_016968	Oligodendrocyte transcription factor 1	2.38	1.65	1.81		1.86		1.51	
Gjb1*	NM_008124	Gap junction membrane channel protein β1		2.35	3.12				0.38↓	
Ptch1	NM_008957	Patched homolog 1		1.81	0.36↓					
Cst3	NM_009976	Cystatin C			3.11				5.27	1.67
Gcm2	NM_008104	Glial cells missing homolog 2 (Drosophila)			2.04	2.21				
Igf2	NM_010514	Insulin-like growth factor 2			7.38				14.61	
Cdh5*	NM_009868	Cadherin 5					1.59		2.30	
Ptprc	NM_011210	Protein tyrosine phosphatase, receptor type, C					3.67		5.73	
Ptges3	NM_019766	Prostaglandin E synthase 3 (cytosolic)					2.60	1.56	2.09	0.66↓
Tgfbr1	NM_009370	Transforming growth factor, β receptor I					7.41		6.78	
Cdkn1b	NM_009875	Cyclin-dependent kinase inhibitor 1B						3.97		
Bmpr2*	NM_007561	Bone morphogenetic protein receptor, type 2	0.51↓						0.60↓	
Ctnna2	NM_009819	Catenin, α 2	0.41↓	0.41↓	0.17↓				0.35↓	
Ctnnd2	NM_008729	Catenin, δ2	0.50↓	0.33↓	0.27↓		0.26↓	0.57↓	0.17↓	
Fgfr1*	NM_010206	Fibroblast growth factor receptor 1			0.34↓		0.57↓		1.77	
Icam5*	NM_008319	Intercellular adhesion molecule 5, telecephalin	0.43↓	0.66↓					1.55	
Inhbb*	NM_008381	Inhibin β-B	0.58↓		2.30		0.65↓		0.60↓	0.53↓
Itgb5*	NM_010580	Integrin β 5	0.40↓							
Myh6	NM_010856	Myosin, heavy polypeptide 6, cardiac muscle, α	0.66↓	0.29↓	0.30↓					
Nefl	NM_010910	Neurofilament, light polypeptide	0.30↓	0.54↓			0.66↓		0.41↓	
Shh	NM_009170	Sonic hedgehog	0.22↓	0.22↓	0.22↓	0.22↓				0.51↓
Foxg1	NM_008241	Forkhead box G1							0.49↓	0.62↓

The "*" mark denotes that those genes changes have been confirmed by real time PCR.

Table 17.3 List of Expressed *Hypoxia Signalling Pathway Array* Genes in the Postischemic Rat Brain

Gene Name	Genbank Accession No.	Description	3-Months-Old Rat Day 3 pi/ctrl	3-Months-Old Rat Day 3 cl/ctrl	3-Months-Old Rat Day 14 pi/ctrl	3-Months-Old Rat Day 14 cl/ctrl	18-Months-Old Rat Day 3 pi/ctrl	18-Months-Old Rat Day 3 cl/ctrl	18-Months-Old Rat Day 14 pi/ctrl	18-Months-Old Rat Day 14 cl/ctrl
Hypoxia -related gene										
Col1a1	NM_007742	Procollagen, type I, α1	3.69		7.02		4.44		17.18	
cstb	NM_007793	Cystatin B	1.52	1.52			1.56			
Gpx1*	NM_008160	Glutathione peroxidase 1	5.38		5.18		3.07		3.01	
Mmp14	NM_008608	Matrix metallopeptidase 14 (membrane-inserted)	1.55							
Ucp2*	NM_011671	Uncoupling protein 2 (mitochondrial, proton carrier)	2.20	2.20	3.86		3.86		4.39	
Rps2	NM_008503	Ribosomal protein S2		2.43		0.65↓	2.47		1.93	
Sod2*	NM_013671	superoxide dismutase 2, mitochondrial		1.63			0.66↓		0.38↓	0.63↓
Cat*	NM_009804	Catalase			2.39					
Ssscal	NM_020491	Sjogren's syndrome/scleroderma autoantigen 1 homolog (human)			2.12					
Tgfb1	NM_011577	Transforming growth factor, β 1			2.33	2.33				
Pea15	NM_011063	Phosphoprotein enriched in astrocytes 15				1.57				
IL6	NM_031168	Interleukin 6					2.13			
Prpf40a	NM_018785	PRP40 pre-mRNA processing factor 40 homolog A (yeast)							2.25	2.65
Chga*	NM_007693	Chromogranin A	0.44↓				0.39↓		0.33↓	
Gap43*	NM_008083	Growth-associated protein 43	0.65↓						0.61↓	
Vegfa*	NM_009505	Vascular endothelial growth factor A	0.64↓	1.50			0.56↓			
Bhlhb2	NM_011498	Basic helix-loop-helix domain containing, class B2			0.23↓					
Gpi1	NM_008155	Glucose phosphate isomerase 1			0.57↓	0.61↓	0.54↓		0.42↓	
Npy	NM_023456	Neuropeptide Y			0.30↓		0.50↓		0.39↓	
Camk2g	NM_178597	Calcium/calmodulin-dependent protein kinase II gamma				0.41↓				
Plod3	NM_011962	Procollagen-lysine, 2-oxoglutarate 5-dioxygenase 3							0.41↓	
Tuba1*	NM_011653	Tubulin, α 1							0.59↓	

The "*" mark denotes that those genes changes have been confirmed by real time PCR.

the proliferating cells in the aged rat brain after stroke were identified as reactive microglia (45%), oligodendrocyte progenitors (17%), astrocytes (23%), CD8+ lymphocytes (4%), or apoptotic cells of indeterminate type (<1%)(Popa-Wagner, Badan, Walker et al. 2007a).

The reasons for the premature accumulation of BrdU-positive cells in the lesioned hemisphere of aged rats remain uncertain. We hypothesize that two age-associated factors could be important: (1) decreased plasticity of the cerebrovascular wall (reviewed in Riddle et al. 2003) and (2) an early, precipitous inflammatory reaction to injury.

The increased fragility of aged blood vessels due to decreases in the distensible components of the microvessels such as elastin (Hajdu, Heistad, Siems et al. 1990) may lead, upon ischemic stress, to a fragmentation of capillaries that would promote the leakage of hematogenous cells into the infarct area (Stoll, Jander, Schroeter et al. 1998; Justicia, Martin, Rojas et al. 2005). Similarly, the extravasation of the extent of Evans blue, a marker of the sealability of brain capillaries, was markedly increased 3 days after intracortical administration of autologous blood in aged SAMP8 mice (Lee, Cho, Choi et al. 2006). In another study conducted on postmortem human brain tissue, it was found that heme-like deposits that were rich in von Willebrand factor (vWF), fibrinogen, collagen IV, and red blood cells were found in the vicinity of brain capillaries, suggesting that microhemorrhages are a common feature of the aging cerebral cortex (Cullen, Kócsi, Stone et al. 2005).

Table 17.4 List of Expressed *Apoptosis Array* Genes in the Postischemic Rat Brain

Gene Name	Genbank Accession No.	Description	Fold Change							
			3-Months-Old Rat				18-Months-Old Rat			
			Day 3		Day 14		Day 3		Day 14	
			pi/ctrl	cl/ctrl	pi/ctrl	cl/ctrl	pi/ctrl	cl/ctrl	pi/ctrl	cl/ctrl
Apoptosis-related gene										
Atm	NM_007499	Ataxia telangiectasia mutated homolog (human)			2.64				1.97	
Gadd45a*	NM_007836	Growth arrest and DNA-damage-inducible 45 α			1.81		3.56		3.84	
Hus1	NM_008316	Hus1 homolog (S. pombe)			1.52		2.78		1.64	
Mdm2	NM_010786	Transformed mouse 3T3 cell double minute 2					2.67			
Tnfrsf7	NM_001033126	Tumor necrosis factor receptor superfamily, member 7					4.60			
Casp7*	NM_007611	Caspase 7			0.49↓	0.22↓			3.34	
Traf1	NM_009421	TNF receptor-associated factor 1					0.29↓	0.39↓	0.49↓	0.43↓
Traf4	NM_009423	TNF receptor-associated factor 4							0.50↓	
Trp53	NM_011640	Transformation-related protein 53					0.62↓			

The "*" mark denotes that those genes changes have been confirmed by real time PCR.

RAPID DELIMITATION OF THE INFARCT AREA BY SCAR-FORMING NESTIN- AND GFAP-POSITIVE CELLS

In aged animals the infarcted area was already visible at day 3 and was circumscribed by a rim of activated astrocytes. At this time point there was no accumulation of activated astrocytes in the peri-infarcted area of young rats.

The proliferating astrocytes lead to premature formation of scar in aged rats, a phenomenon that limits the recovery of function in aged animals. It should be noted that there are at least three cell types contributing to the formation of the astroglial scar: nestin-positive cells that are the first (day 3) to delineate the scar in the brains of aged rats, followed by GFAP-positive astrocytes (day 7) and finally by cells expressing the N-terminal fragment of β amyloid precursor protein (APP) (day 14) (Oster-Granite, McPhie, Greenan et al. 1996; Badan, Dinca, Buchhold et al. 2004; Zhao, Puurunen, Schallert et al. 2005a).

Capillaries of the Corpus Callosum Are a Major Source of Nestin-Positive Cells That Delimit the Infarct Site

Shortly after stroke, nestin-positive cells delimited the infarct core significantly earlier in aged rats than in young rats (Popa-Wagner, Dinca, Suofu et al. 2006). In light of the active cellular proliferation in nearby callosal capillaries and the apparent inability of lateral ventricle-derived nestin-positive cells to traverse the corpus callosum to reach the cortical infarct, we conclude that most of the nestin-positive cells are derived from capillaries in the corpus callosum. Some nestin-positive cells also could be supplied by disintegrating capillaries in the brain parenchyma. In aged rats in particular, nestin-positive cells migrate along corridor-like pathways from the corpus callosum to the infarct area and become primarily incorporated into the glial scar.

Aged rats had fewer nestin-BrdU double-labeled cells in the corpus callosum and periinfarcted area than did young animals, indicating that the proliferative potential of nestin cells in aged rats is reduced relative to that of young rats. Paradoxically, then, despite a lower number of proliferating nestin cells in aged rats, these cells envelope the infarct site in greater numbers soon after the ischemic event. A likely explanation for this phenomenon is that the steep upregulation of nestin mRNA shortly after stroke in aged rats leads to increased nestin that compensates for the lower proliferation rate of nestin-positive cells. In addition, the infarct core is delimited both by capillary-derived nestin cells originating in the corpus callosum, and nestin-expressing astrocytes from layers I and II of the neocortex that are chronically activated in aged rats (so-called reactive astrocytes) (Vaughan, Peters 1974; Jucker, Walker, Schwab et al. 1994; Peters 2002; Yu, Go, Guinn et al. 2002; Rozovsky, Wei, Morgan et al. 2005). This latter interpretation is supported by data showing that nestin is expressed in astrocytes forming the glial scar in the plaques of multiple sclerosis (Holley, Gveric, Newcombe et al. 2003).

Traditionally, neuroepithelial cells express nestin during development and reactive astrocytes do so after injury (Schwab, Beschorner, Meyermann et al. 2002). However, after stroke, nestin-positive cells arise from the capillary wall. According to the current model of vascular wall structure (Jain 2003), it is likely that nestin occupies the pericyte cell layer. This view has been shared by Yamashima, Tonchev, Vachkov et al. (2004) who showed that transient brain ischemia in monkeys induces an increase of the neuronal progenitor cells in the subgranular zone (SGZ). Ultrastructural analysis indicated that most of the neuronal progenitor cells and microglia originated from the pericytes of capillaries and/or adventitial cells of arterioles (called *vascular adventitia*). The detaching adventitial cells showed mitotic figures in the perivascular space, and the resultant neuronal progenitor cells made contact with dendritic spines associated with synaptic vesicles or boutons. These data implicate the vascular adventitia as a novel potential source of neuronal progenitor cells in the postischemic primate SGZ.

Although the finding that the vascular wall plays a dynamic role in post-infarct cytogenesis is novel and intriguing, in the stroke model it does not come as a surprise. In recent years, it has become increasingly apparent that the cerebral vascular wall is not just a mechanical highway for blood and nutrients but rather plays an active role in cellular proliferation. The vascular origin of nestin-positive scar cells is supported by previous data showing that nestin immunoreactivity is increased after stroke (Li, Chopp 1999), and that the upregulation of the protein persists for up to 13 months after damage to the spinal cord (Frisen, Johansson, Torok et al. 1995). Additionally, among the early vascular changes following stroke is the upregulation of the proliferative cell nuclear antigen (Gerzanich, Ivanova, Simard et al. 2003), a general marker of cell division, whereas adult blood vessels, upon transplantation (i.e., under initially hypoxic conditions), give rise to hematopoietic cells that incorporate BrdU (Montfort, Olivares, Mulcahy et al. 2002). The presence of BrdU-positive nuclei in nestin-immunoreactive cells following stroke, as we now have shown, suggests that these cells do not simply detach and differentiate from the vascular wall but rather arise via the active production of new cells.

THE ANTIOXIDANT DEFENSE SYSTEM IS COMPROMISED IN THE AGED POST-STROKE RAT BRAIN

One of the potential major causes of age-related destruction of neuronal tissue is toxic free radicals that result from aerobic metabolism after reperfusion. The main antioxidant enzyme of the brain is glutathione peroxidase (Gpx1). Gpx1 is usually considered to be primarily localized in glial cytoplasm. Counteracting oxidative stress through upregulation of mitochondrial antioxidants is one of the cell survival mechanisms operating shortly after cerebral ischemia. Failure to increase the expression of antioxidant systems may increase the sensitivity to oxidative stress (Kim, Piao, Lee et al. 2004; Van Remmen, Qi, Sabia et al. 2004) and contribute to poor recovery after cerebral ischemia. While Gpx1 was increased both in the young and aged animals, superoxide dismutase 2, mitochondrial (Sod2), another component of the antioxidant system, was downregulated in the peri-infarcted area of aged rats. In addition, CAT, which has been intensively studied as an antioxidant, was increased only in young but not in aged rats. Taken together, these data suggest that despite fulminant activation of the glial cells in the aged rat brain, the antioxidative system is not fully operational in aged rats.

Capacity to regulate energy production is crucial in the initial hours following stroke. We found that the mitochondrial uncoupling protein 2, (Ucp2) is strongly induced in aged rats as compared with young rats. This indicates that aged rats have less available energy to counteract the damaging effects of the oxidative stress. This hypothesis is in accordance with a recent study showing that at 3 days post-stroke, there was a massive induction of Ucp2 mRNA in the peri-infarct area of the wild-type mice (de Bilbao, Arsenijevic, Vallet et al. 2004). Ucp2 knockout mice, however, were less sensitive to ischemia as assessed by reduced brain infarct size, decreased densities of apoptotic cells in the peri-infarct area, and lower levels of lipid peroxidation as compared with wild-type mice (de Bilbao, Arsenijevic, Vallet et al. 2004).

NEUROINFLAMMATION IN ISCHEMIC STROKE

Stroke Triggers an Inflammatory Cascade

The pathophysiological consequences of acute ischemic stroke are still not fully understood. The extent of brain damage caused by the insult is ultimately determined by a combination of ischemic cell necrosis and detrimental host response. There is much evidence,

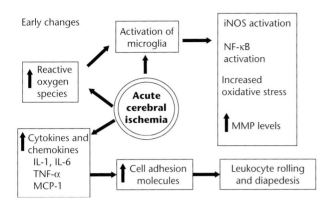

Early changes

Figure 17.1 Acute cerebral ischemia and neuroinflammation. Acute cerebral ischemia triggers an inflammatory cascade via the activation of a number of molecular pathways. The initial phase is associated with generation of reactive oxygen species (ROS) within the ischemic cerebral tissue, which is followed by release of inflammatory cytokines and chemokines. This subsequently results in activation of resident microglia and upregulation of cell adhesion molecules (CAMs). Chemokines are involved in the mobilization of leukocytes, and these inflammatory cells then interact with the CAMs. This leads to leukocyte infiltration of the ischemic tissue (diapedesis), which further exacerbates the inflammatory process. Activation of nuclear factor kappa B (NF-κB) and inducible nitric oxide synthase (iNOS) results in increased oxidative stress and further cytokine production. The release of matrix metalloproteinases (MMPs) from astrocytes and microglia leads to blood–brain barrier dysfunction, cerebral edema, and neuronal cell death.

largely derived from animal models, to suggest that inflammation plays a crucial role in the pathophysiology of acute cerebrovascular disease. Many aspects of this centrally derived inflammatory response to some extent parallel the nature of the reaction in the periphery, but the existence of the blood–brain barrier (BBB) and specific resident cells of the brain parenchyma offer characteristics unique to the CNS, and the evidence they provide has been persuasive.

Acute stroke triggers an inflammatory cascade that causes injury to the cerebral tissue, and this can continue for several days (Fig. 17.1). Research studies have also demonstrated that the secondary inflammatory response following a stroke plays an important role in exacerbating cerebral tissue damage (Montaner, Rovira, Molina et al, 2003b). This is associated with increased infarct size and worsens clinical outcome (Montaner, Rovira, Molina et al. 2003b; Smith, Emsley, Gavin et al, 2004; Rallidis, Vikelis, Panagiotakos et al. 2006). After occlusion of a cerebral blood vessel, the resulting brain ischemia leads to the generation of free radicals, which induce the expression of inflammatory cytokines and chemokines (Fig. 17.1). Cytokines upregulate the expression of adhesion molecules, which mediate the interaction

between endothelial cells and leukocytes leading to infiltration of leukocytes into the brain parenchyma, and also activate resident microglia, which leads to increased oxidative stress and release of matrix metalloproteinases (MMPs). Cytokines also cause systemic actions such as activation of the hypothalamic–pituitary–adrenal axis, hepatic synthesis of the acute-phase reactants, and marrow stimulation. Cytokine production is normally tightly regulated within cerebral tissue, but an ischemic insult can produce a massive and self-destroying inflammatory reaction. The chemokines mediate both leukocyte migration and microglial activation. These postischemic neuroinflammatory changes lead to BBB dysfunction, cerebral edema, and cell death (Danton, Dietrich 2003; Simard, Kent, Chen et al. 2007). Therefore, therapeutic targeting of the neuroinflammatory pathways in acute stroke is an important area of translational medicine research (Han, Yenari 2003).

Unfortunately, many anti-inflammatory agents that have shown successful results in treating animal models of stroke have failed to translate into clinical treatments (Savitz, Fisher 2007), and clinical trials of treatment aimed at reducing neuroinflammation have been unsuccessful, despite the recruitment of large numbers of patients (Durukan, Tatlisumak 2007). Only tissue-plasminogen activator (t-PA) is currently licensed for use in the treatment of acute ischemic stroke (Khaja, Grotta 2007; Adams, del Zoppo, Alberts et al. 2007). These failures of anti-inflammatory therapy form part of a larger picture, where experimental success with neuroprotection has not been translated into clinical practice (Ginsberg 2007; Durukan, Tatlisumak 2007).

Studies of cerebral ischemia in experimental animal models have demonstrated the neuroprotective efficacy of a variety of interventions, but most of the strategies that have been clinically tested failed to show benefit in aged humans. Several confounding variables may have contributed to the differences between animal and clinical studies (Table 17.5). It is also relevant that animal models of stroke are extremely heterogeneous, that the data on the spatial localization of inflammatory activation are sparse inflammation in the core infarct area may be of limited relevance as a therapeutic target and that age could play an important in the recovery of the brain from insult. Most experimental studies of stroke have been performed on young animals, and therefore may not fully replicate the effect of ischemia on neural tissue in aged subjects (Popa-Wagner, Carmichael, Kokaia et al. 2007b). There remains a need to describe the clinical pathophysiology of stroke more appropriately, and to identify how such information can be translated into clinical trials.

Table 17.5 Possible Causes of Failure Trials of Clinical Neuroprotection

Causes of Failure
Experimental demonstration of neuroprotection incomplete (functional end points?)
Inappropriate agent: mechanism of action not relevant in humans*
Inappropriate dose of agent (plasma concentrations suboptimal either globally or in subgroups)
Target process not active in critical areas of pathophysiology (penumbra)
Efficacy limited by side effects that worsen outcome (e.g., fever)
Inappropriate timing: mechanism of action not active at time of administration
Inappropriate or inadequate duration of treatment
Study population too sick to benefit
Study population too heterogeneous: efficacy only in an unidentifiable subgroup*
Study cohort too small to remove effect of confounding factors*
Failure of randomization to distribute confounding factors evenly*
Insensitive, inadequate, or poorly implemented outcome measures

*May benefit from small mechanistic studies in homogeneous well-characterized clinical subgroups.

Inflammation after Cerebral Ischemia

The entire spectrum of inflammatory processes is likely to act in concert in stroke. The inflammatory cascade comprises both cellular and molecular components and both local and systemic response. When cerebral ischemia occurs, an inflammatory response that involves enzyme activation, mediator release, inflammatory cell migration, glial activation, brain tissue breakdown, and repair follows (Iadecola, Alexander 2001). Recent animal and clinical studies have provided an understanding of the inflammatory process that occurs after cerebral ischemia.

Clinical studies of inflammation in ischemic stroke are usually limited to blood or cerebrospinal fluid (CSF) sampling after stroke. Relatively little histopathological data exist concerning ischemic stroke in human postmortem specimens.

Cellular Components of Inflammation

The major inflammatory cells that are activated and that accumulate within the brain after cerebral ischemia are blood-derived leukocytes, macrophages, and resident microglia. Leukocytes clearly perform important roles in normal host defense. Mounting evidence suggests that neutrophils in particular might

be mediators of secondary brain damage after cerebral ischemia. Microglia, which constitute as many as 12% of the cells in the CNS (Gonzalez-Scarano, Baltuch 1999), are the first non-neuronal cells to respond to CNS injury. When fully activated by either neuronal cell death or other processes, they become phagocytic. Infiltrating leukocytes, macrophages, and activated glial cells are the major CNS sources of cytokines, chemokines, and other immunomolecules (Arumugam, Granger, Mattson et al. 2005; Huang, Upadhyay, Tamargo et al. 2006).

Leukocytes

Research studies have demonstrated that peripheral inflammatory cells play an important role in the pathogenesis of cerebral ischemia. This has been demonstrated in numerous animal models of stroke, leading to several observations: (a) leukocytes are present within cerebral tissue after an ischemic insult (Bednar, Dooley, Zamani et al. 1995; Lehrmann, Christensen, Zimmer et al. 1997); (b) neutrophil inhibition is associated with reduced ischemic damage (Hartl, Schurer, Schmid-Schonbein et al. 1996; Shimakura, Kamanaka, Ikeda et al. 2000); (c) treatments that prevent leukocyte vascular adhesion and extravasation into the brain parenchyma, for example, anti-intercellular cell adhesion molecule 1 (ICAM-1) (Zhang, Chopp, Li et al. 1994b; Williams, Dave, Tortella et al. 2006) and anti-CD11/CD18 antibodies, can be neuroprotective in animal models of stroke (Vedder, Winn, Rice et al. 1990; Zhang, Chopp, Tang et al. 1995c; Yenari, Kunis, Sun et al. 1998); (d) studies using ICAM-1 knockout animals have demonstrated significant reduction in ischemic infarct size, relative to that of wild-type animals (Connolly, Winfree, Springer et al. 1996; Soriano, Lipton, Wang et al. 1996; Kitagawa, Matsumoto, Mabuchi et al. 1998).

Both models of permanent and transient focal ischemia are characterized by a massive infiltration of inflammatory cells. After permanent MCAO, neutrophils start to accumulate in cerebral vessels within a few hours and infiltrate into the infarct zone after 12 hours. This process peaks at 24 hours and then the number of neutrophils significantly decreases (Kochanek, Hallenbeck 1992; Garcia, Liu, Yoshida et al. 1994). Monocytes/macrophages start to infiltrate the parenchyma at 12 hours and further increase in numbers up to day 14 (Clark, Lee, Fish et al. 1993; Schroeter, Jander, Witte et al. 1994). The entire infarct area is covered by macrophages at 3 days after MCAO (Schroeter, Jander, Witte et al. 1994). In transient MCAO these processes seem to evolve more rapidly than after permanent MCAO. Despite the same temporal profile of neutrophil accumulation in the vessels, significant infiltration in parenchyma appears within 6 hours (Clark, Lee, White et al. 1994; Zhang, Chopp, Chen et al. 1994a). This would, therefore, be an important therapeutic target for reducing reperfusion injury following thrombolytic therapy in acute ischemic stroke (Pan, Konstas, Bateman et al. 2007). Accumulation of monocytes is observed during the first 7 days and then their numbers decrease by day 14 (Kato, Kogure, Liu et al. 1996). The accumulation of neutrophils can lead to obstruction of microvessels (*no-reflow* phenomenon) and exacerbate the area of ischemia (del Zoppo, Schmid-Schonbein, Mori et al. 1991). This was proven by observations that blocking neutrophil accumulation after transient MCAO significantly reduced infarct size, (del Zoppo, Schmid-Schonbein, Mori et al. 1991; Matsuo, Onodera, Shiga et al. 1994) but was ineffective after permanent MCAO (Zhang, Chopp, Jiang et al. 1995a; Morikawa, Zhang, Seko et al. 1996). The lymphocytes are generally intended to play a negative role in ischemic brain pathogenesis even though there are conflicting data. While neutrophils were significantly increased by 48 hours and remained elevated at 96 hours post occlusion, lymphocytes were increased relatively late (72 and 96 hours) post occlusion (Stevens, Bao, Hollis et al. 2002; Li, Zhong, Yang et al. 2005). Preventing lymphocyte trafficking into ischemic brain ameliorated injury, suggesting that like neutrophils, lymphocytes also play a deleterious role (Becker, Kindrick, Relton et al. 2001). Clinical studies also show that lymphocytes have strong proinflammatory and tissue-damaging properties, and the upregulation of circulating lymphocytes is correlated to an increased risk of stroke recurrence and death (Nadareishvili, Li, Wright et al. 2004).

Clinical studies have also provided evidence that supports the role of leukocytes in cerebral ischemia. Early studies showed that leukocyte counts in CSF, especially the polymorphonuclear neutrophilic leukocyte and monocytes/macrophages, were frequently elevated (Sornas, Ostlund, Muller 1972). Furthermore, necropsy studies showed significant increases in the density of granulocytes in cerebral microvessels of the most acute patients (Lindsberg, Carpen, Paetau et al. 1996a). Enhanced peripheral leukocyte activation (Endoh, Maiese, Wagner 1994; Elneihoum, Falke, Axelsson et al. 1996; Santos-Silva, Rebelo, Castro et al. 2002), increased leukocyte/platelet adhesiveness (Meiner, Arber, Liberman et al. 1997; Caimi, Ferrara, Montana et al. 2000), and prothrombotic mechanisms mediated by leukocytes (Prentice, Szatrowski, Kato et al. 1982; Noto, Barbagallo, Cavera et al. 2001) have also been documented in ischemic stroke. While these reports support leukocyte involvement in the disease process, they cannot provide information on the temporal profile of leukocyte recruitment, and in particular, they supply no information on the role of

these cells in early stroke. Such predictions and presumptions offer at best circumstantial evidence for a role in etiology, and few insights into mechanisms. Whether leukocytes are activated primarily in the periphery or in the CNS before sequestration is a question that remains to be established. In vivo imaging suggests white cell accumulation in human cerebral infarction using radiolabeled [111]Indium (^{111}In) leukocyte single photon emission computed tomography (SPECT) studies (Pozzilli, Lenzi, Argentino et al. 1985). Neutrophil accumulation was first detected at 6 hours after onset, peaking at 24 hours and remaining at high levels for up to 9 days before declining (Akopov, Simonian, Grigorian 1996), with a significant leukocyte recruitment occurring up to 5 weeks after onset, which was spatially correlated with areas of perfusion defect and associated with crudely defined poor neurological outcomes (Wang, Kao, Mui et al. 1993). The poor localization provided by SPECT dictates that the specific localization of inflammation to penumbral regions is likely to require new markers and other techniques to delineate the biology of cellular inflammatory responses following stroke (Price, Menon, Peters et al. 2004; Price, Wang, Menon et al. 2006; Jander, Schroeter, Saleh 2007; Muir, Tyrrell, Sattar et al. 2007). The use of small magnetic iron oxide and ultrasmall particles of iron oxide (USPIOs) with magnetic resonance imaging (MRI) showed that USPIOs are taken up by macrophages into infarcted brain parenchyma, the iron being colocalized to lysosomes within macrophages and visualized as a signal dropout with MRI (Jander, Schroeter, Saleh 2007; Muir, Tyrrell, Sattar et al. 2007). Whether this will provide an index of an important tool to address the role of macrophages for ischemic lesion is the subject of further studies.

Accumulation and infiltration of hematogenous cells in the brain is a complex process that requires the interaction between several cell adhesion molecules (CAMs) and chemokines. A number of animal studies have shown that after transient or permanent focal ischemia, the upregulation of adhesion molecules, especially ICAM-1 and P- and E-selectins preceded the invasion of neutrophils into the cerebral tissue (Okada, Copeland, Mori et al. 1994; Zhang, Chopp, Zaloga et al. 1995b; Haring, Berg, Tsurushita et al. 1996). It has been shown that treatment with anti-ICAM antibodies significantly reduced infarct size after transient MCAO (Zhang, Chopp, Li et al. 1994b). This process is also accompanied by expression of chemokines at the site of damage. After MCAO the levels of cytokine-induced neutrophil chemoattractant (CINC) mRNA becomes elevated after 6 hours, peaks at 12 hours and then rapidly decreases at 24 hours (Liu, Young, McDonnell et al. 1993b). It is known that CINC acts mainly as a neutrophil chemoattractant. The temporal expression of monocyte chemoattractant protein-1 (MCP-1) follows that of CINC (Yamagami, Tamura, Hayashi et al. 1999). High levels of MCP-1 mRNA have been found at 6 hours. The maximal expression of this chemokine is observed between 12 hours and 2 days (Kim, Gautam, Chopp et al. 1995; Wang, Yue, Barone et al. 1995a).

Antileukocyte strategies have been protective in various experimental ischemia models (Matsuo, Onodera, Shiga et al. 1994; Bowes, Rothlein, Fagan et al. 1995a; Jiang, Moyle, Soule et al. 1995b; Hartl, Schurer, Schmid-Schonbein et al. 1996). Inhibition of leukocyte activation and infiltration into the ischemic cerebral tissue has, therefore, been an important area of neuroprotection research (Wood 1995; Hartl, Schurer, Schmid-Schonbein et al. 1996; Sughrue, Mehra, Connolly et al. 2004). The neutrophil

inhibitory factor, UK-279276, a recombinant protein inhibitor of the CD11/CD18 receptor, demonstrated reduced infarct size in animal models of stroke. However, the Acute Stroke Therapy by Inhibition of Neutrophil (ASTIN) study did not show any patient benefit and was terminated for futility (Krams, Lees, Hacke et al. 2003) (Table 17.6).

Microglia/Macrophages

Most of the data pertaining to microglia in cerebral ischemia derive from animal, rather than human, studies. Microglia constitute 5% to 20% of the total CNS glial population, playing a critical role as resident immunocompetent and phagocytic cells in the CNS and serving as scavenger cells in the event of infection, inflammation, trauma, ischemia, and

Table 17.6 Selected Neuroprotective Agents Targeting the Inflammatory Pathways in Acute Cerebral Ischemia and their Results in Clinical Trials

Mechanism of Action	Neuroprotective Agent	Summary of Clinical Trials
Neutrophil inhibitory factor (Krams et al. 2003)	UK-279276	The phase II clinical trial, Acute Stroke Therapy by Inhibition of Neutrophils (ASTIN), was terminated for futility. This was an adaptive design, dose-ranging study. Patients were randomized to receive an infusion of either UK-279 276 or placebo within 6 hours of acute stroke symptom onset. No efficacy was reported on administration of study medication. Further drug development has been abandoned
Anti-ICAM -1 monoclonal antibody (Enlimomab 2001)	Enlimomab	The phase III clinical trial of enlimomab proved negative. Patients were randomized to receive either enlimomab or placebo within 6 hours of acute stroke symptom onset. At day 90 the modified Rankin scale was worse in patients treated with enlimomab ($P = 0.004$) and treatment was associated with higher mortality. Patients also experienced significantly more adverse drug reactions (infections and fever). This was possibly related to an antibody and inflammatory response to enlimomab. Further drug development has been abandoned
Lipid Peroxidation Inhibitor (The RANTTAS Investigators, 1996; Tirilazad International Steering Committee, 2000)	Tirilazad	The phase III clinical trial, Randomized Trial of Tirilazad Mesylate in Acute Stroke (RANTTAS) was negative. Patients were randomized to receive either tirilazad or placebo within 6 hours of acute stroke symptom onset. Tirilazad was associated with increased disability and mortality. Drug development for ischemic stroke has been terminated
Nitrone-based free radical trapping–agent (Shuaib et al. 2007; Lyden et al. 2007)	Cerovive (NXY-059)	The phase III clinical trial, Stroke—Acute Ischemic—NXY-059 Treatment II (SAINT II) proved negative. Patients were randomized to either an infusion of NXY-059 or placebo within 6 hours of acute stroke symptom onset. There was no significant reduction in stroke-related disability, as assessed by the modified Rankin scale ($P = 0.33$). The cerebral hemorrhage and NXY-059 Treatment (CHANT) trial also showed no treatment effect on functional outcome
Antipyretic effect (van Breda et al. 2005)	Acetaminophen (Paracetamol)	The phase III clinical trial, Paracetamol (Acetaminophen) in Stroke (PAIS) is ongoing. The aim of the study is to determine if early antipyretic therapy reduces the risk of death or dependency in patients with acute stroke. Patients presenting within 12 hours of acute stroke symptom onset are randomized to either acetaminophen 1 gm 6 times daily or matching placebo for three days. The primary outcome is functional assessment at 3 months via the modified Rankin scale.
Interleukin-1 receptor antagonist (Emsley et al. 2005)	Recombinant human IL-1 ra (rhIL-1ra)	The phase II clinical trial of rhIL-1ra has been completed. Patients within 6 hours of acute stroke symptom onset were randomized to either rhIL-1ra or matching placebo. Treatment was administered intravenously with 100 mg loading dose over 60 seconds, followed by a 2 mg/kg/h infusion over 72 hours. Treatment with rhIL-1ra was well tolerated with no adverse drug events. Inflammatory markers (WCC, IL-6 and CRP) were lower in the treatment group. In the rhIL-1ra–treated group, patients with cortical infarcts had a better clinical outcome. Further evaluation of the drug is ongoing.

neurodegeneration (del Zoppo, Milner, Mabuchi et al. 2007). After brain injury, the microglia become activated, a state that can be identified by changes in morphology. Such changes include enlarged size with stout processes, upregulation of specific genes or proteins such as major histocompatibility complex (MHC) class I and II and complement receptor 3 (CR3), a migratory and proliferative response, and phagocytic behavior (Lai, Todd 2006b; del Zoppo, Milner, Mabuchi et al. 2007). Although the primary role for microglial activation after cerebral ischemia is to clear necrotic cells (Wood 1995), these activated microglia also express and release a variety of cytokines, ROS, nitric oxide, proteinases, and other potentially toxic factors able to contribute to the postischemic brain damage, as well as several important messenger molecules that play a part in how these factors respond to extracellular signals during ischemic injuries (Lai, Todd 2006b; del Zoppo, Milner, Mabuchi et al. 2007).

Via CD4, microglial activation has also been associated with stimulation of the toll-like receptor 4 (TLR4). How microglia are activated following ischemia is not completely clear, but CD14 receptors have been documented in monocytes and have activated microglia in brains of stroke patients (Beschorner, Schluesener, Gozalan et al. 2002). Permanent MCAO models of TLR4-deficient mice were shown to have reduced infarct size (Caso, Pradillo, Hurtado et al. 2007b). TLR4 plays an important role in the initiation of the inflammatory response during cerebral ischemia and an important target for neuroprotective therapy (Kariko, Weissman, Welsh 2004). In addition, a greater degree of microglial activation has been found in aged rats after cerebral ischemia than in young rats, suggesting that activated microglia might be a contributing component to enhanced brain injury in aged rats (Popa-Wagner, Badan, Walker et al. 2007a). Also recently, it was shown that complement activation may affect inflammatory responses, including microglial activation and neutrophil infiltration, thereby contributing to postischemic induced brain injury (Pekny, Wilhelmsson, Bogestal et al. 2007).

Whether microglia/macrophages are necessarily damaging following brain ischemia is unclear, but several lines of evidence suggest that activated microglia may contribute to injury. In transient MCAO, phagocytic microglial were documented in the cerebral cortex of the ischemic hemisphere (Kim, Yu, Kim et al. 2005). It has been shown that systemic administration of edaravone, a novel free radical scavenger, significantly reduced infarct volume and improved neurological deficit scores for ischemic mice by reducing microglial activation (Banno, Mizuno, Kato et al. 2005; Zhang et al. 2005). Downregulation of the expression of TNF-α (a proinflammatory mediator)

produced by microglia appears to reduce infarct volume and improve neurological deficits of the animals after MCAO (Zawadzka, Kaminska 2005). Investigations have been undertaken to determine the time course of necrotic core clearance after cerebral ischemia. In a mouse model of transient focal cerebral ischemia, microglial cells rapidly became activated at day 1 and started to phagocytose neuronal material. Quantitative analysis showed maximum numbers of phagocytes of local origin within 2 days and of blood-borne macrophages on day 4. The majority of phagocytes in the infarct area were derived from local microglia (Schilling, Besselmann, Muller et al. 2005; Popa-Wagner, Badan, Walker et al. 2007a), preceding and predominating over phagocytes of hematogenous origin that are expressed only after a permanent MCAO, as suggested in the presence of an increased macrophage receptor with collagenous structure (MARCO) mRNA expression (Milne, McGregor, McCulloch et al. 2005). Considering these findings, we suggest that the role of microglial activation after cerebral ischemia might be time dependent. These combined findings indicate that microglial activation occurs very early after the onset of ischemia. Therefore, the time cutoff for microglial activation between harm and protection should be clarified in cerebral ischemia. Furthermore, the number of proliferating microglial cells and astrocytes is usually lower in aged rats than in young rats. Despite a robust reactive phenotype of microglia and astrocytes, the aged brain has the capability to mount a cytoproliferative response to injury, but the timing of the cellular and genetic response to cerebral insult is deregulated (Popa-Wagner, Badan, Walker et al. 2007a). Therefore, the age cutoff for microglial activation between harm and protection should be also clarified in cerebral ischemia and ischemic stroke patients.

In humans, using positron emission tomography (PET) and PK11195, a ligand that binds peripheral benzodiazepine binding sites, activation of microglia is not seen before 72 hours after ischemic stroke. Beyond this, binding potential rises in core infarction, peri-infarct zone, and contralateral hemisphere to 30 days (Price, Wang, Menon et al. 2006). However, while PK11195 allows access to the exquisite sensitivity provided by PET, one problem is its lack of specificity in imaging of the various cell types involved in neuroinflammation following stroke. Thus increases in PK11195 binding in the brain following stroke have been often interpreted as microglial activation (Stephenson, Schober, Smalstig et al. 1995; Banati, Myers, Kreutzberg 1997), but there is the theoretical possibility that this upregulation may represent granulocytes.

Given the proposed detrimental effect of microglial activation in postischemia–induced early brain injury, it is important to clarify the therapeutic potential of treatments based on the inhibition of microglial activation shortly after the onset of cerebral ischemia. Several experimental works have shown that the inhibition of microglial activation obtained with different substances and methods is able to reduce edema and injury size, decreased neuronal degeneration, and improved neurological functions (Table 17.7). Owing to its safety record and ability to penetrate the BBB, minocycline might be considered for human clinical trials to protect the brain against postischemia–induced early brain injury. Minocycline and doxycycline were shown to provide significant protection against brain ischemia (Yrjanheikki, Keinanen, Pellikka et al. 1998; Yrjanheikki, Tikka, Keinanen et al. 1999; Weng, Kriz 2007). These beneficial effects coincided with amelioration of microglial activation and downregulation of MMP-2 and MMP-9 expression, although other mechanisms, such as inhibition of cytochrome c, nitric oxide (NO), and interleukin (IL)-1β release could also underlie the benefits (del Zoppo, Milner, Mabuchi et al. 2007). However,

Table 17.7 Inhibitors of Microglial Activation in Cerebral Ischemia

Inhibitors	Production or Responses: Enhancing (↑) or Inhibiting (↓)	Effects in Cerebral Ischemia	References
cAMP related molecules			
cAMP (cell permeable)	↓ LPS-induced TNF-α, IL-1β, PMA-induced $O_2^{\bullet}$, proliferation	NA	
	↓ LPS-induced IL-12p40		
	*↑Aβ-induced NO		
PDE inhibitors	↓ LPS-induced TNF-α		
Propentofylline (PDE inhibitor)	↓ LPS-induced TNF-α, IL-1β, PMA-induced $O_2^{\bullet}$, proliferation	+	Haag et al. 2000; Ng, Ling 2001; Plaschke et al. 2001; Bath, Bath-Hextall 2004
Cilostazol (PDE inhibitor)	↑ p-CREB and Bcl-2, COX-2 ↓ LPS-induced TNF-α, proliferation	+	Lee et al. 2006; Watanabe et al. 2006
Vasoactive intestinal peptide (VIP)	↓ LPS-induced TNF-α mRNA	–	Tamas et al. 2002
Pituitary adenylyl cyclase-activating polypeptide (PACAP)	↓ LPS-induced TNF-α mRNA	+	Somogyvari-Vigh, Reglodi 2004; Suk et al. 2004; Chen et al. 2006
Prostaglandin E2 (PGE₂)	↓ LPS-induced NO, TNF-α, IL-1β cAMP accumulation	+/−	Gendron et al. 2005; Ahmad et al. 2006; Ahmad et al. 2007
15-Deoxy-Δ (12,14)-PGJ₂	↓ LPS-induced NO, TNF-α, IL-1β	+	Pereira et al. 2006; Lin et al. 2006b
Steroids			
Hydrocortisone	↓ LPS-induced iNOS	NA	
Dexamethasone (Lipocortin-1)	↓ LPS-induced NO, PGE₂	+/−	Bertorelli et al. 1998; Zausinger et al. 2003; Mulholland et al. 2005
Dehydroepiandrosterone (DHEA)	↓ Microglial apoptosis	NA	
17β-Estradiol	↓ LPS-induced iNOS, PGE₂, MMP-9 ↑ Aβ uptake	+/−	Theodorsson, Theodorsson 2005; Liu et al. 2007; Chiappetta et al. 2007
Opioids			
Endomorphines (m-opioids)	↓ Phagocytosis, chemotaxis *↑ PMA-induced $O_2^{\bullet}$	NA	
Naloxone (μ-antagonist)	↓ PMA-induced $O_2^{\bullet}$	+	Chang et al. 2000
Naloxone (μ-antagonist) in mixed culture	↓ LPS-induced NO, TNF-α	+	Chang et al. 2000
Dynorphin (κ-opioids) in mixed culture	↓ LPS-induced neurotoxicity	+	Chang et al. 2000

(Continued)

Table 17.7 Continued

Inhibitors	Production or Responses: Enhancing ($\uparrow$) or Inhibiting ($\downarrow$)	Effects in Cerebral Ischemia	References
Other endogenous molecules			
Adenosine (2Cl-adenosine)	Microglial apoptosis	NA	
Melatonin	$\downarrow$ Aβ-induced IL-1β, IL-6 (in brain slice)	+	Lee, Kuan, Chen 2007; Welin et al. 2007
α-Melanocyte stimulating hormone (MSH)	$\downarrow$ Ab/INF-induced NO/TNF-α	+	Catania, Lipton 1998
Apolipoprotein E	$\downarrow$ LPS-induced TNF-α and NO	+	Koistinaho et al. 2002
IL-10	$\downarrow$ LPS-induced IL-1β, TNF-α, IL-2R, IL-6R	NA	
Neurotrophins (NGF, BDNF, NT-3, NT-4)	$\downarrow$ LPS-induced NO	+	Lin et al. 2006a; Lai, Todd 2006b
	$\downarrow$ Urokinase type-plasminogen activator (uPA)		
Ceramide	$\downarrow$ Urokinase-type plasminogen activator (uPA)	NA	
Other exogenous molecules			
Cannabinoids	$\downarrow$ LPS-induced mRNAs for IL-1α, IL-1β, IL-6, TNF-α	–	Franklin et al. 2003
N-acetyl-*O*-methyldopamine (NAMDA)	$\downarrow$ LPS-induced mRNAs for IL-1β, TNF-α, iNOS	NA	
K252a (pyridazine-based CaMK inhibitor)	$\downarrow$ LPS-induced NO	NA	
Atratoglaucosides	$\downarrow$ LPS-induced TNF-α	NA	
Thalidomide	$\downarrow$ LPS-induced chemokine (IL-8)	+	Persson et al. 2005
Minocycline (Tetracycline derivative)	$\downarrow$ NMDA-induced proliferation, NO, IL-1β	+	Yrjanheikki, et al. 1998; Yrjanheikki et al. 1999; Lai, Todd 2006a; Weng, Kriz 2007; Chu et al. 2007
Doxycycline (Tetracycline derivative)	$\downarrow$ NMDA-induced proliferation, NO, IL-1β	+	Yrjanheikki et al. 1998; Yrjanheikki et al. 1999; Lai, Todd 2006a; Weng, Kriz 2007; Chu et al. 2007
Nicergoline	$\downarrow$ PMA or zymosan-induced $O_2^{\bullet}$	NA	
Diazepam (benzodiazepine)	$\downarrow$ Tat-induced Ca^{2+} elevation	NA	
Thapsigargin	$\downarrow$ Transformation (keeping ramified shape)	+	Matsuda et al. 2001
Agmatine (endogenous amine)	$\downarrow$ NOS activity	NA	

*Not simple inhibition; + indicates protective effects, +/− variable and not univocal effects, − negative and/or dangerous effects, NA not available.

long-term inhibition of microglial activation and macrophage infiltration may be unwarranted because of the potential to eliminate neuroprotective benefits of microglia/macrophages as phagocytes and suppliers of neuroprotective molecules.

Microglia–Astrocyte Interactions

Astrocytes are known to carry out critical functions (maintenance of ionic homeostasis, metabolism of toxins, regulation of scar tissue, prevention of neovascularization, and support of synaptogenesis and neurogenesis) that are vital for normal brain function and the outcome of stroke injury (Panickar, Norenberg 2005). Following ischemia brain astrocytes are activated, resulting in increased expression and a so called reactive gliosis, characterized by specific structural and functional changes (Pekny, Nilsson 2005). It has been shown that astrocytes have stronger antioxidative potential than neurons (Lucius, Sievers 1996). During brain injury, astrocytes can directly modulate neuronal survival by producing angiogenic and neurotrophic factors (Dhandapani, Mahesh, Brann 2003; Swanson, Ying, Kauppinen 2004), expression of the *N*-methyl-D-aspartate (NMDA) receptor subunit (Daniels, Brown 2001), and the glutamate transporter excitatory amino acid carrier (Canolle, Masmejean, Melon et al. 2004), which influences neuronal sensitivity to glutamate toxicity.

Astrocytes also participate in inflammation after postischemic brain injury by secreting inflammatory factors such as cytokines, chemokines, and inducible nitric oxide synthase (iNOS) (Endoh, Maiese, Wagner 1994). Astrocytes, together with neurons and endothelial cells, also produce TNF-like weak inducer of apoptosis (TWEAK) and can stimulate pro-inflammatory molecule production by interaction with its Fn14 receptor found on astrocytes (Saas, Boucraut, Walker et al. 2000). While astrocytes normally play important roles in neuron function and maintenance, activated astrocytes have the potential to create damage to ischemic brain. Thus, astrocytes likely influence neuronal survival in the postischemic period because neurons become resistant to oxidative stress in the presence of astrocytes (Swanson, Ying, Kauppinen 2004). In addition, astrocytes can indirectly affect neuronal injury by modulating brain inflammation, reducing the expression of microglial inflammatory mediators (Pyo, Yang, Jou et al. 2003). Finally, astrocytes could cooperate with microglia to prevent inflammatory responses in the brain by regulating microglial ROS production (Min, Yang, Kim et al. 2006). Therefore, modulating microglial activation through astrocytes could be a novel method to minimize the brain injury caused by postischemia induced inflammation.

Molecular Components of Inflammation and Inflammatory Mediators

Cytokines

Cytokines are upregulated in cerebral tissue during the acute stages of stroke. As well as being expressed by cells of the immune system, cytokines are also endogenously produced by resident brain cells, including microglia and neurons. Cytokines possess pro- and anti-inflammatory properties, both of which play a key role in the progression of stroke (Vila, Castillo, Davalos et al. 2000; Perini, Morra, Alecci et al. 2001; Offner, Subramanian, Parker et al. 2006). Cytokines are responsible for the initiation and regulation of the inflammatory response and play an important role in leukocyte and monocyte/macrophage infiltration into the ischemic regions of the brain (Kouwenhoven, Carlstrom, Ozenci et al. 2001). The main cytokines involved in neuroinflammation are the interleukins, IL-1, IL-6, and IL-10, transforming growth factor-α (TGF-α), and TNF-α. Among those cytokines, IL-1 and TNF-α appear to exacerbate cerebral injury; however, IL-6, IL-10, and TGF-α may be neuroprotective (Allan, Rothwell 2001). MCP-1 and CINC also play an important role and belong to a superfamily of structurally related small, inducible, pro-inflammatory cytokines, called *chemokines* (Chen, Hallenbeck, Ruetzler et al. 2003). These are potent chemoattractant factors that function as inflammatory mediators and have been implicated in many inflammatory and autoimmune diseases.

IL-1 The IL-1 family comprises the agonistic isoforms IL-1α and IL-1β, and their endogenous inhibitor, the IL-1 receptor antagonist (IL-1ra) (Boutin, LeFeuvre, Horai et al. 2001; Allan, Tyrrell, Rothwell 2005). The expression of IL-1β mRNA is rapidly observed, within 15 minutes after permanent MCAO and remains persistent for up to 4 days (Liu, McDonnell, Young et al. 1993a; Haqqani, Nesic, Preston, et al. 2005; Caso, Moro, Lorenzo et al. 2007a). A similar temporal profile of expression is observed for its corresponding receptor, IL-1r (Sairanen, Lindsberg, Brenner et al. 1997). The important role of IL-1β in the pathophysiology of brain injury after stroke has been demonstrated by the observation that treatment with IL-1ra decreases neuronal cell death in the peri-infarct zone and reduces infarct size after permanent focal cerebral ischemia (Garcia, Liu, Relton 1995; Mulcahy, Ross, Rothwell et al. 2003). Furthermore, transgenic mice overexpressing IL-1ra showed reduced infarct size after focal ischemia (Yang, Zhao, Davidson et al. 1997), while IL-1ra deficient mice showed a significant increase in infarct size (Pinteaux, Rothwell, Boutin 2006). Further research into recombinant human IL-1ra as a neuroprotective agent in acute stroke is ongoing (Emsley, Smith, Georgiou et al. 2005).

IL-6 IL-6 is a pro-inflammatory cytokine, which is secreted by monocytes in response to cerebral injury. It belongs to a family of factors that includes ciliary neurotrophic factor and IL-11, which act via the gp130 signal transducer. Elevated levels of IL-6 in acute stroke patients correlate with a larger infarct volume and poorer clinical outcome (Fassbender, Rossol, Kammer et al. 1994; Dziedzic, Bartus, Klimkowicz et al. 2002; Smith, Emsley, Gavin et al. 2004; Rallidis, Vikelis, Panagiotakos et al. 2006). IL-6 mRNA is rapidly activated during experimental focal cerebral ischemia. The expression of IL-6 mRNA is observed at 3 hours after permanent focal ischemia and peaks at 12 hours (Wang, Yue, Young et al. 1995b). The role of IL-6 in stroke, however, is far from clear because multiple regulatory levels are apparent (Acalovschi, Wiest, Hartmann et al. 2003). On one hand, IL-6 regulates synthesis and expression of several acute-phase reactants (e.g., CRP, fibrinogen) (Mackiewicz, Schooltink, Heinrich et al. 1992) and it also possesses anti-inflammatory effects and is shown to be protective in both in vitro and in vivo studies (Biber, Lubrich, Fiebich et al. 2001; Herrmann, Tarabin, Suzuki et al. 2003; Sotgiu, Zanda, Marchetti et al. 2006).

TNF-α   The increased expression of TNF-α has been demonstrated in experimentally induced stroke models (Barone, Arvin, White et al. 1997). The initial source of TNF-α within the brain appears to be the microglia and macrophages, although it has also been found in ischemic neurons (Barone, Arvin, White et al. 1997; Feuerstein, Wang, Barone 1998). TNF-α mRNA is upregulated within 20 minutes after permanent MCAO and is persistent for up to 5 days (Liu, Clark, McDonnell et al. 1994). The overexpression of TNF-α receptors p55 and p75 is observed after 6 and 12 hours, respectively (Liu, Clark, McDonnell et al. 1994; Wang, Yue, Barone et al. 1994). Transient MCAO animal models and clinical studies have also shown increased peripheral TNF-α levels (Offner, Subramanian, Parker et al. 2006; Emsley, Smith, Gavin et al. 2007). Intracerebral administration of TNF-α 24 hours before MCAO significantly enlarges lesion size and there is evidence that infarct size can be reduced by treatment with anti-TNF-α antibodies (Barone, Arvin, White et al. 1997; Lavine, Hofman, Zlokovic 1998).

Therapeutic targeting of the TNF-α converting enzyme (TACE) is also being explored as a potential method of reducing TNF-α expression in acute stroke (Lovering, Zhang 2005). Some studies, however, have shown some neuroprotective effects of TNF-α in brain injury and this needs to be further explored (Mattson, Cheng, Baldwin et al. 1995; Hallenbeck 2002). Finally, TNF-α appears to be involved in the phenomenon of ischemic tolerance (Ginis, Jaiswal, Klimanis et al. 2002), and mice deficient in TNF receptors have larger infarcts (Bruce, Boling, Kindy et al. 1996).

Both interleukins and TNF-α are also responsible for activation of iNOS, an enzyme involved in the formation of NO and cyclooxygenase 2 (COX-2), a free radical–producing enzyme (Bonmann, Suschek, Spranger et al. 1997; Iadecola, Alexander 2001). This increased oxidative stress further worsens neuronal injury. Another important pathway, which exacerbates cerebral damage induced by IL-6 and TNF-α, is apoptosis of neuronal and glial cells. It is known that TNF-α is an activator of apoptosis at various cell targets via its p55 receptor, which is shown to be overexpressed in ischemic lesions (Fehsel, Kolb-Bachofen, Kolb 1991; Zheng, Fisher, Miller et al. 1995). Another member of the TNF superfamily, TWEAK is thought to be produced by neuronal stress (Polavarapu, Gongora, Winkles et al. 2005), and an increase in the cytokine TWEAK at the mRNA level in a mouse model of focal cerebral ischemia was detected (Potrovita, Zhang, Burkly et al. 2004). This can activate astrocytes via the Fn14 receptor, leading to a proinflammatory response (Polavarapu, Gongora, Winkles et al. 2005; Yepes, Brown, Moore et al. 2005). Interestingly, a neutralizing anti-TWEAK antibody reduced the infarct size,

demonstrating an in vivo role of TWEAK in ischemic brain damage (Potrovita, Zhang, Burkly et al. 2004). This finding was confirmed using a soluble form of Fn14 (Yepes, Brown, Moore et al. 2005). In addition to the effect on infarct size, TWEAK increases the permeability of the BBB in cerebral ischemia (Polavarapu, Gongora, Winkles et al. 2005). Indeed, TWEAK stimulates the transcription factor nuclear factor kappa B (NF-κB) in primary cortical neurons through the inhibitory kappa B (IκB) kinase (IKK) complex (Potrovita, Zhang, Burkly et al. 2004).

IL-10   IL-10 is an anti-inflammatory cytokine that inhibits both IL-1β and TNF-α (Strle, Zhou, Shen et al. 2001). It reduces injury in experimentally induced stroke, cerebral hemorrhage, and ischemic stroke (Pelidou, Kostulas, Matusevicius et al. 1999; van Exel, Gussekloo, de Craen et al. 2002). IL-10 regulates a variety of signaling pathways and promotes neuronal and glial cell survival by blocking the effects of pro-apoptotic cytokines, as well as promoting expression of cell-survival signals (Strle, Zhou, Shen et al. 2001). IL-10 also limits inflammation in the brain by suppressing cytokine receptor expression and inhibiting receptor activation (Pelidou, Kostulas, Matusevicius et al. 1999; Strle, Zhou, Shen et al. 2001).

Patients with acute ischemic stroke have an elevated numbers of peripheral blood mononuclear cells secreting IL-10 (Pelidou, Kostulas, Matusevicius et al. 1999) and elevated concentrations in CSF (Tarkowski, Rosengren, Blomstrand et al. 1997). Furthermore, subjects with low IL-10 levels have an increased risk of stroke (van Exel, Gussekloo, de Craen et al. 2002).

TGF-β   TGF-β is present within microglia and seems to have a neuroprotective effect. Both in vitro and animal studies have demonstrated neuroprotective effects of TGF-β in cerebral ischemia (Pang, Ye, Che et al. 2001; Lu, Lin, Cheng et al. 2005). It is mainly expressed during the recovery phase of stroke and may contribute to cerebral remodeling (Lehrmann, Kiefer, Christensen et al. 1998).

Chemokines

Chemokines are a family of over 40 cytokines that are involved in chemotaxis and include both ligands and receptors (Fernandez, Lolis 2002) (Table 17.8). CC and CXC are the two main classes involved in neuroinflammation. The chemokines are chemotactic cytokines, which mediate both leukocyte migration and microglial activation, and are extensively expressed after cerebral ischemia (Pantoni, Sarti, Inzitari 1998; Yamagami, Tamura, Hayashi et al. 1999; McColl, Rothwell N J, Allan 2007). IL-6 and TNF-α regulate

Table 17.8 Chemokine Groups Relevant to Inflammation After Cerebral Ischemia

Group	Molecule
CXC group	IL-8, IP-10, CINC
CC group	MIP-1, 5, MCP-1, 2, 3, RANTES, SLC

CINC, cytokine-induced neutrophil chemoattractant; IL, interleukin; IP, interferon-inducible protein; MCP, monocyte chemoattractant protein; MIP, macrophage inflammatory protein; RANTES, regulated on activation, normal T cell expressed and secreted; SLC, secondary lymphoid tissue chemokine.

the expression of MCP-1 and CINC in the brain (Pantoni, Sarti, Inzitari 1998; Campbell, Perry, Pitossi et al. 2005; McColl, Rothwell, Allan 2007). Increased expression of MCP-1 and CINC was observed in experimental stroke models where infiltrated leukocytes were thought to induce tissue injury. Animal and cell culture studies have shown that MCP-1 and CINC may play an important role in ischemia-induced inflammatory response and in ischemic brain damage (Yamasaki, Matsuo, Matsuura et al. 1995; Yamagami, Tamura, Hayashi et al. 1999; Campbell, Perry, Pitossi et al. 2005; McColl, Rothwell, Allan 2007). These studies indicated that MCP-1 in cerebral ischemia actually plays a significant role in the migration of macrophages into the lesion, and CINC precedes neutrophil accumulation. Raised levels of MCP-1 have been reported in CSF 24 hours after ischemic stroke, while CSF levels (which may represent autochthonous CNS production) are not matched by corresponding levels in plasma (Losy, Zaremba 2001).

In MCAO the level of CINC-1 mRNA increased after 6 hours, peaked at 12 hours, and rapidly decreased at 24 hours (Liu, Young, McDonnell et al. 1993b). It is known that CINC acts mainly as a neutrophil chemoattractant and is associated with an acute-phase response (Liu, Young, McDonnell et al. 1993b; Campbell, Perry, Pitossi et al. 2005). The temporal expression of MCP-1 follows that of CINC. High levels of MCP-1 mRNA have been found at 6 hours. The maximal expression of this chemokine was observed between 12 hours and 2 days (Chen, Hallenbeck, Ruetzler et al. 2003; Arakelyan, Petrkova, Hermanova et al. 2005). The different temporal production of MCP-1 and CINC contributes to the regulation of infiltrated white blood cell subtypes and the inhibition of MCP-1 and CINC signaling (Yamagami, Tamura, Hayashi et al. 1999). These chemokines are also implicated in BBB dysfunction (Stamatovic, Shakui, Keep et al. 2005; Dimitrijevic, Stamatovic, Keep et al. 2006). IL-8 is also classed as a chemokine (CXCL8) and is thought to contribute to tissue damage by activating neutrophil infiltration (Garcia, Liu, Relton 1995; Kostulas, Kivisakk, Huang et al. 1998). Anti–IL-8 antibody significantly reduced brain edema and infarct size (Matsumoto, Ikeda, Mukaida et al. 1997). Levels of IL-8 mRNA in neutrophil and peripheral monocyte populations in ischemic stroke were significantly higher than in controls up to 7 days postictus. Plasma and CSF concentrations of IL-8 and peripheral monocyte levels of IL-8 mRNA expression increase 1 to 3 days after ischemic stroke, and peripheral numbers of monocytes expressing IL-8 mRNA appeared to correlate with functional outcome (Kostulas, Pelidou, Kivisakk et al. 1999). At the same time, CSF levels of IL-8 were significantly greater than controls in early stroke, and peaked on day 2 postictus; CSF levels were particularly high in patients in whom disease was confined to white matter (Tarkowski, Rosengren, Blomstrand et al. 1997).This contrasts with other molecules such as macrophage inflammatory protein (MIP)-1α, thought to be an important mediator of monocyte/macrophage accumulation, over the same time period (Kostulas, Kivisakk, Huang et al. 1998; Kostulas, Pelidou, Kivisakk et al. 1999).

The chemokines could, therefore, be an attractive target for potential neuroprotective treatments in acute ischemic stroke (Matsumoto, Ikeda, Mukaida et al. 1997; Pantoni, Sarti, Inzitari 1998; Dawson, Miltz, Mir et al. 2003). However, there are no data addressing these molecules in the context of clinical stroke, and the data are limited even in the setting of experimental models. It is important to recognize that any of these molecules may play a role in leukocyte recruitment, and further studies are needed. Furthermore, chemokines may also play an important role in the area of cell-based therapy for stroke in induced migration of stem cells to regions of injury (Newman, Willing, Manresa et al. 2005). MCP-1 and/or its receptor have been observed at the interface of ischemic tissue and cell transplants (Kelly, Bliss, Shah et al. 2004). MCP-1 and other chemokines seem to be involved in marrow-derived stromal cell migration into ischemic brain (Wang, Chen, Gautam et al. 2002a; Wang, Li, Chen et al. 2002b). Manipulation of these signals may be important in the successful application of such therapies.

Cell Adhesion Molecules

Adhesion molecules, which are important in the context of cellular inflammation in acute ischemic stroke, may be categorized in terms of the cells that express the molecule, the cells targeted for adhesion, or in the chronological order in which they are expressed. They are classified according to their molecular structure or in relation to their functional domain. A classification of adhesion molecules is given in Table 17.9. Three families of leukocyte endothelial adhesion molecules have been identified: the selectins, the immunoglobulin gene superfamily, and the integrins.

Table 17.9 Adhesion Molecule Grouped by Site of Expression and Ligand

Group	Molecule	Location and Type of Expression	Ligand
Mucin-like	PSGL-1	Neutrophil	E, P-selectin
Selectins	L-selectin	All leucocytes, constitutive	Gly-CAM
	E, P-selectin	Endothelium, inducible	
Ig superfamily	ICAM-1, 2,3	Endothelium, constitutive and inducible	CD18/11α(LFA-1, αLβ2)
	VCAM-1	Endothelium, constitutive and inducible	CD18/11β(Mac-1, αMβ2) VLA-4 (α4β1)
Integrins	CD18/11α(LFA-1, αLβ2)	Neutrophils/macrophages, constitutive	ICAM-1, 2
	CD18/11β(Mac-1, αMβ2)	Neutrophils/macrophages, constitutive	VCAM-1
	VLA-4 (α4β1)	Lymphocytes, neutrophils and monocytes	VCAM-1

ICAM, intercellular adhesion molecule; Ig, immunoglobulin; PSGL, P-selectin glycoproteins ligand; VCAM, vascular cell adhesion molecule.

The white blood cells or leukocytes adhere to the endothelium before tissue infiltration via a series of carefully orchestrated steps (Okada, Copeland, Mori et al. 1994; Zhang, Chopp, Zaloga et al. 1995b; Haring, Berg, Tsurushita et al. 1996). Accumulation and infiltration of the brain by leukocytes is a complex process that requires the interaction between several CAMs and chemokines. Leukocytes roll on the endothelial surface and then adhere to the endothelial cells, which is followed by diapedesis (Fig. 17.2). The rolling of leukocytes is mediated by interaction of E- and P-selectin (found on the surface of endothelial cells), and L-selectin (normally found on the surface of leukocytes) with their respective ligands (Okada, Copeland, Mori et al. 1994; Haring, Berg, Tsurushita et al. 1996). Firm adhesion and activation of leukocytes is mediated by binding of the CD11/CD18 complex to receptors of the immunoglobulin gene superfamily, such as ICAM-1, vascular cell adhesion molecule 1 (VCAM-1), platelet-endothelial cell adhesion molecule 1 (PECAM-1), and the mucosal addressin (Zhang, Chopp, Tang et al. 1995c; Yenari, Kunis, Sun et al. 1998; Frijns, Kappelle 2002; Kalinowska, Losy 2006). Leukocyte integrins (including CD11 [α-chain], CD18 [β2 chain] and CD29 [β1 chain]) are activated by chemokines and cytokines. Once leukocyte rolling has stopped, an interaction between CD11/CD18 and ICAM-1 causes the leukocytes to shed L-selectin and transmigrate across the vessels to the luminal side of the target tissue. IL-6 and TNF-α also regulate the expression of CAMs on the endothelial cells and induce infiltration of the cerebral tissue by leukocytes at the site of inflammation (Frijns, Kappelle 2002). Inflammatory CAM may also play a role in the pathogenesis of delayed cerebral ischemia after SAH. In animal models, increased expression

of CAMs has been observed in vasospastic arteries (Rothoerl, Schebesch, Kubitza et al. 2006).

A number of animal studies have documented that after transient or permanent focal ischemia the upregulation of CAMs, especially ICAM-1 and P- and E-selectins, preceded the invasion of neutrophils into brain (Okada, Copeland, Mori et al. 1994; Zhang, Chopp, Zaloga et al. 1995b; Haring, Berg, Tsurushita et al. 1996). There is ample evidence from animal models of MCAO that expression of CAMs is associated with cerebral infarct size. Thus, absence of CAMs in knockout animal models resulted in reduced infarct size (Kitagawa, Matsumoto, Mabuchi et al. 1998). When MCAO in experimental stroke was followed by reperfusion, administration of anti-CAM antibodies decreased infarct size (Zhang, Chopp, Li et al. 1994b; Zhang, Chopp, Jiang et al. 1995a). Clinical data on adhesion molecule responses in cerebral ischemia are limited when compared with experimental studies. The precise relation between such circulating molecules and their bioactive bound counterparts remains to be established in ischemic stroke. Postmortem brain tissue examinations have shown an early (15 hours) ICAM-1 expression within the infarct after clinical onset (Lindsberg, Carpen, Paetau et al. 1996a). Increased ICAM-1 and VCAM-1 have been documented in the plasma and CSF of subjects with recent cerebral ischemic patients, and correlated to stroke severity (Simundic, Basic, Topic et al. 2004; Ehrensperger, Minuk, Durcan et al. 2005).

However, anti-CAM treatment has not been successful in patients with acute ischemic stroke. The enlimomab study used a monoclonal antibody against ICAM-1, which was administered within 6 hours of ischemic stroke onset. The 3-month outcome mortality data and adverse events were worse in the enlimomab

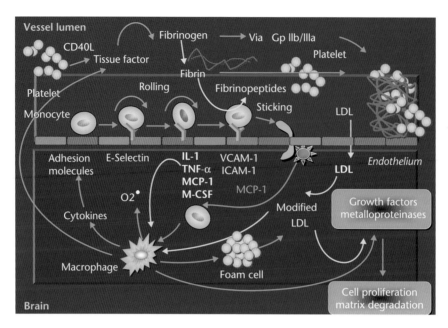

Figure 17.2 Accumulation and infiltration of the brain by leukocytes in acute cerebral ischemia. Leukocytes roll on the endothelial surface and then adhere to the endothelial cells, which is followed by diapedesis. The rolling of leukocytes is mediated by interaction of E- and P-selectins (found on the surface of endothelial cells), and L-selectin (normally found on the surface of leukocytes) with their respective ligands. Firm adhesion and activation of leukocytes is mediated by binding of the CD11/CD18 complex to receptors of the immunoglobulin gene superfamily, such as intercellular cell adhesion molecule 1 (ICAM-1), vascular cell adhesion molecule 1 (VCAM-1), platelet-endothelial cell adhesion molecule 1 (PECAM-1), and the mucosal addressin. Leukocyte integrins [including CD11 (α-chain), CD18 (β2 chain) and CD29 (β1 chain)] are activated by chemokines and cytokines. Once leukocyte rolling has stopped, an interaction between CD11/CD18 and ICAM-1 causes the leukocytes to shed L-selectin and transmigrate across the vessels to the luminal side of the target tissue. IL-6 and TNF-α also regulate the expression of CAMs on the endothelial cells and induce infiltration of the cerebral tissue by leukocytes at the site of inflammation.

group and it appears that there may have been a pro-inflammatory response (Enlimomab 2001). The interpretation of this study may have been confounded by the use of a murine antibody in humans, with subsequent neutrophil and complement activation (Vuorte, Lindsberg, Kaste et al. 1999). At the same time, few clinical studies examined the potential of anti-integrin therapies in acute stroke patients with a lack of efficacy (Becker 2002), despite positive results of blocking CD11β (Chen, Chopp, Zhang et al. 1994) as well as CD18 (Bowes, Rothlein, Fagan et al. 1995b) or both (Jiang, Moyle, Soule et al. 1995a; Yenari, Kunis, Sun et al. 1998) in models of cerebral ischemia. The lack of an obvious effect in humans could be due to study design not in line with laboratory data or inherent heterogeneity of clinical stroke. Another possibility is that neutrophil integrins are different in acute ischemic stroke patients compared to rodents. Therefore, some anti-adhesion approaches may not be appropriate in humans.

The Complement System

The complement system is one of major systems of innate immunity: it consists of more than 20 circulating proteins and a similar number of cell surface receptor and regulator proteins. The activation of complement by the classical, alternative, or lectin pathways generates opsonins, inflammatory mediators, and cytolytic protein complexes (Rus, Cudrici, David et al. 2006). It provides a first line of defense against infection, and so is a major component of innate immunity. However, undesirable complement activation contributes to the pathogenesis of many human diseases by damaging tissue and promoting inflammation. Complement plays a critical role in several stages of the processing of immune complexes. Incorporation of complement proteins into immune complexes modifies the lattice structure. Covalently incorporated cleavage products of the complement proteins, C3 and C4, then influence the fate of immune complexes by acting as ligands, first, for receptors on cells that transport immune complexes through the body and, second, for receptors on cells that take up and process circulating immune complexes (Rus, Cudrici, David et al. 2006).

The overlap of the complement cascade with other biochemical events occurring in stroke is quite complex and is only beginning to be elucidated (Lynch, Willis, Nolan et al. 2004; Ten, Sosunov, Mazer et al.

2005). In animal and cell culture models of stroke it has been shown that complement plays a key role in stroke outcome, and complement depletion improves neurological function after acute cerebral ischemia (Vasthare, Barone, Sarau et al. 1998; Huang, Kim, Mealey et al. 1999; De Simoni, Storini, Barba et al. 2003; Akita, Nakase, Kaido et al. 2003). As part of the classical complement pathway, the C1q component plays an important role in cerebral ischemia and C1 inhibitor treatment showed reduced infarct volumes (Schafer, Schwaeble, Post et al. 2000; De Simoni, Storini, Barba et al. 2003). As part of the alternative complement pathway, the factors C3a, C5a, and C4 are associated with increased CAM expression. C3a and C5a are also chemoattractant factors. The C3 complement component rises during the acute phase of stroke, and C3-deficient mice were shown to have reduced cerebral injury (Atkinson, Zhu, Qiao et al. 2006; Mocco, Mack, Ducruet et al. 2006a). The C5 component has also been shown to increase in cerebral ischemia/reperfusion models and inhibition with monoclonal antibody reduces cerebral tissue damage (Costa, Zhao, Shen et al. 2006). However, little research has been published in the pathogenesis of the complement system in stroke patients, particularly in acute ischemic injury (Pedersen, Waje-Andreassen, Vedeler et al. 2004; Mocco, Wilson, Komotar et al. 2006c). The complement component C3a has been shown to be elevated during the acute phase of ischemic stroke, with C5a rising during the recovery phase (Mocco, Wilson, Komotar et al. 2006c). A postmortem study of brain specimens taken from acute ischemic stroke patients showed deposition of complement membrane attack complex C5b–C9 in infarcted zones (Lindsberg, Ohman, Lehto et al. 1996b; Rus, Cudrici, David et al. 2006). Recent studies have suggested that systemic complement activation is dependent on stroke subtype (Di Napoli 2001b). Activation has been seen to be more prominent in cardioembolic stroke, compared to atherothrombotic or lacunar strokes. These results suggest that complement activation by both the classical and the alternative pathways could play an important role in the pathogenesis of ischemic stroke. Some potential therapeutic targets of the complement system have been identified, but more studies investigating its role in acute ischemic stroke and interaction with other inflammatory pathways is required (Mocco, Sughrue, Ducruet et al. 2006b).

Nitric Oxide Synthase and Oxidative Stress

NO possesses both neuroprotective and neurotoxic properties in cerebral ischemia. This is related to the activation of the three different isoforms of nitric oxide synthase (NOS) at different stages of the ischemic process. The three isoforms of NOS are termed *endothelial* (eNOS), *neuronal* (nNOS), and *inducible* (iNOS) isoforms (Andrew, Mayer 1999; Bredt 1999). NOS catalyzes the chemical conversion of L-arginine to NO and citrulline. Increased levels of intracellular calcium are able to activate the constitutive isoforms (eNOS and nNOS) during the acute phase of cerebral ischemia. Neuronal NOS has a much higher capacity for NO generation than eNOS, and this is responsible for neuronal damage during the early stages of ischemic stroke. Inducible NOS activation comes later on, usually 12 to 48 hrs after the initial ischemic insult (Iadecola, Zhang, Xu et al. 1995). This is associated with a much higher production of NO, and for a longer period, compared to its two isoforms. Studies using knockout and transgenic mice models have made an invaluable contribution to the pathophysiology of NOS in cerebral ischemia.

The role of eNOS is well-known for its vasodilatory properties, via the action of cyclic GMP. Studies using eNOS knockout mice have shown increased infarct size, following transient MCAO (Huang, Huang, Ma et al. 1996). Nonhemodynamic mechanisms have also been postulated for eNOS-related neuroprotection: inhibition of NF-κB activation, reduced leukocyte adhesion and infiltration, and diminished lipid peroxidation (Blais, Rivest 2001). Owing to the low generation of NO by eNOS, an antioxidant role has also been suggested, via the production of S-nitrosoglutathione (Chiueh 1999; Khan, Sekhon, Giri et al. 2005). The role of NO donors in early cerebral ischemia is an area of current research interest, both in improving cerebral perfusion and in potential neuroprotection (Willmot, Bath 2003; Khan, Jatana, Elango et al. 2006). The effect of NO-Aspirin (NCX-4016) in replenishing vascular NO is also under investigation (Burgaud, Riffaud, Del Soldato 2002; Di Napoli, Papa 2003a). The effect of statins in eNOS upregulation has provided an additional neuroprotective property to this class of lipid-lowering drugs (Vaughan, Delanty 1999; Endres, Laufs, Liao, et al. 2004). Adenovirus-mediated gene transfer is also currently being investigated in an attempt to augment the vasodilator effect of eNOS (Ooboshi, Ibayashi, Heistad et al. 2000). However, the practical aspects of virus exposure to cerebral vasculature will prove challenging. Recent advances in endovascular interventions may overcome this problem (Schumacher, Khaw, Meyers et al. 2004). On the contrary, nNOS knockout mice have been shown to develop smaller infarct volumes in MCAO (Hara, Huang, Panahian et al. 1996). There is a strong association between the activation of NMDA receptors and calcium-dependent increase in nNOS activity. Peroxynitrite (ONOO⁻) production from NO reactions has been associated with neuronal cell death, via lipid peroxidation and DNA damage (Eliasson, Huang, Ferrante et al. 1999).

A vasodilator component to peri-ischemic nNOS activation has also been investigated, but this has a minor effect compared to its neurotoxicity. The majority of nNOS-selective inhibitor studies have reported neuroprotective effects in animal models of stroke (O'Neill, Murray, McCarty et al. 2000).

Inducible NOS upregulation and further NO generation occur during the later stages of cerebral ischemia (Iadecola, Zhang, Xu et al. 1995). Leukocytes and endothelial and glial cells are the main sources of iNOS expression. Selective inhibitors of iNOS have been shown to display neuroprotection for up to 5 days postischemic insult (Zhang, Iadecola 1998). Smaller infarct volumes have also been observed in iNOS knockout mice (Zhao, Haensel, Araki et al. 2000). Again, peroxynitrite is the main ROS involved in neuronal cell death, and studies have shown prolonged activity in postmortem human cerebral tissue (Forster, Clark, Ross et al. 1999). Recent studies have investigated the role of peroxisome proliferator–activated receptor gamma (PPAR-) agonists in limiting the upregulation of iNOS (Tureyen, Kapadia, Bowen et al. 2007). The thiazolidinediones, a class of oral hypoglycemic agents, have been shown to activate these receptors and show potential neuroprotective properties (Luo, Yin, Signore et al. 2006). The cholesterol-lowering fibrates have also been shown to reduce iNOS activity via activation of the PPAR-α receptors (Deplanque, Gele, Petrault et al. 2003). These findings may provide these different drug classes with an additional role in acute stroke treatment. Interactions between iNOS and COX-2 have also been linked to penumbral cell death in late cerebral ischemia (Nishimura I, Uetsuki T, Dani 1998). Owing to this late and prolonged activation of iNOS, it remains an important therapeutic target for anti-inflammatory therapy. This would also be an attractive therapeutic target for reducing reperfusion injury following thrombolytic therapy in acute ischemic stroke (Pan, Konstas, Bateman et al. 2007).

Another important source of ROS is NADPH oxidase (Lambeth 2004). This enzyme predominantly produces the superoxide anion (O_2^-), which can further react with NO to generate peroxynitrite (Chan 2001). Owing to the destructive nature of ROS in cerebral ischemia, therapeutic interventions have been an important area of stroke research. The SAINT II (Stroke–Acute Ischemic–NXY-059 [Cerovive] Treatment) study was investigating the effect of the nitrone spin-trap agent, NXY-059, in patients presenting within 6 hours of symptom onset (Green, Ashwood, Odergren et al. 2003). This nitrone-derived free radical trapping agent was shown to be an effective neuroprotective agent in animal models of stroke and has a large therapeutic window of opportunity (Sydserff, Borelli, Green et al. 2002). In the phase III study, patients received a 1-hour loading dose of NXY-059 followed by 71 hours of hourly infusions. The primary outcome measure was recovery of motor function, as measured by the modified Rankin scale. Unfortunately, results from the phase III study were negative and among patients treated with alteplase, there was no difference between the NXY-059 group and the placebo group in the frequency of symptomatic or asymptomatic hemorrhage (Shuaib, Lees, Lyden et al. 2007). Any further development of the drug was abandoned (Ginsberg 2007).

Arachidonic Acid (AA) Metabolites

After cerebral ischemia another critical metabolic event is the activation of phospholipase A2 (PLA2), resulting in hydrolysis of membrane phospholipids and release of free fatty acids including arachidonic acid (AA), a metabolic precursor for important cell-signaling eicosanoids. PLA2 enzymes have been classified as calcium-dependent cytosolic (cPLA2) and secretory (sPLA2) and calcium-independent (iPLA2) forms. Consistent with a damaging role of this pathway, PLA2-deficient mice had smaller infarcts and developed less brain edema with fewer neurological deficits (Bonventre, Huang, Taheri et al. 1997). Other studies have separately demonstrated increased lipid peroxidation: AA metabolites contribute to postischemic brain inflammation and circulatory disorders (Sanchez-Moreno, Dashe, Scott et al. 2004).

COX enzymes convert AA released from brain phospholipids during ischemia/reperfusion to prostaglandin H2 (PGH2). There are two isoforms of COX; COX-1 is constitutively expressed in many cells types, including microglia and leukocytes during brain injury (Schwab, Beschorner, Meyermann et al. 2002). COX-1 deficient mice have increased vulnerability to brain ischemia, and would support a protective role possibly because of an effect on maintaining CBF (Iadecola, Sugimoto, Niwa et al. 2001b). COX-2 is upregulated and is present at the border of the ischemic territory following ischemia (Nogawa, Zhang, Ross et al. 1997a).

In ischemic stroke patients, COX-2 is upregulated not only in regions of ischemic injury (Iadecola, Forster, Nogawa et al. 1999) but also in regions remote from the infarct area (Sairanen, Carpen, Karjalainen-Lindsberg et al. 2001). The roles of various COX metabolites are variable, but accumulated data suggest that those downstream of COX-2 are likely harmful. Recent work has shown that prostaglandin E2 (PGE2) EP1 receptors may be the downstream effectors responsible for neurotoxicity in ischemic stroke (Kawano, Anrather, Zhou et al. 2006). COX-2 mediates its toxic effect through PGE2 rather than ROS, even though COX-2 can generate both toxics (Manabe, Anrather,

Kawano et al. 2004). Treatment with COX-2 inhibitors improve neurological outcome after stroke (Nogawa, Zhang, Ross et al. 1997b; Sugimoto, Iadecola 2003). Furthermore, COX-2–deficient mice have reduced injury after NMDA exposure (Iadecola, Niwa, Nogawa et al. 2001a), whereas COX-2 overexpression exacerbates brain injury (Dore, Otsuka, Mito et al. 2003).

Few data are available about the role of the lipoxygenase (LOX) pathway in brain ischemia. AA can be converted to 5-hydroperoxyeicosatetraenoic acid (5-HPETE) by 5-lipoxygenase (5-LOX), which is metabolized to leukotriene A4 (LTA4), a precursor of cysteinyl leukotrienes (cysLTs). Leukotriene C4 (LTC4) is a potent chemoattractant that has been implicated in the BBB dysfunction, edema, and neuronal death after ischemia/reperfusion. During brain ischemia/reperfusion, biphasic AA and LTC4 elevations have been documented and appear to correspond to biphasic patterns of BBB disruption (Rao, Hatcher, Kindy et al. 1999). 5-LOX has also been documented in autopsied ischemic human brains, with 5-LOX localizing to perivascular monocytes (Tomimoto, Shibata, Ihara et al. 2002).

Matrix Metalloproteinases

Cerebral ischemia is also associated with the release of MMPs as part of the neuroinflammatory response. These proteases are involved in the breakdown of the microvascular basal lamina, which results in the disruption of the BBB (Heo, Lucero, Abumiya et al. 1999). These changes are most prominent in the core infarct, where neuronal damage is maximal. The gelatinases (MMP-2 and MMP-9) are the main MMPs involved in destruction of the basal lamina. MMP-2 is expressed constitutively in the CNS, and is normally present within brain tissue. MMP-9 is normally absent and this is the major MMP associated with cerebral inflammation (Montaner, Alvarez-Sabin, Molina et al. 2001). These enzymes are released from endothelium, glia, and infiltrating leukocytes (Gottschall, Yu, Bing 1995). They target laminin, collagen IV, and fibronectin proteins, which are the major components of the basal lamina. This is associated with BBB dysfunction, leading to cerebral edema (Simard, Kent, Chen et al. 2007). Reduced infarct size has been shown in rat models of stroke treated with MMP inhibitors, and also in MMP-9 knockout mice studies (Romanic, White, Arleth et al. 1998; Asahi, Asahi, Jung et al. 2000; Svedin, Hagberg, Savman et al. 2007).

MMP-9 levels have been shown to be elevated in patients with spontaneous ICH (Abilleira, Montaner, Molina et al. 2003). It plays an important role in the development of cerebral edema and hemorrhagic transformation of infarcted brain tissue. Recent studies have shown a strong correlation between elevated plasma MMP-9 levels and risk of hemorrhagic transformation in the acute phase of ischemic stroke (Castellanos, Leira, Serena et al. 2003). Elevated MMP-9 concentrations have also been shown to be a predictor of thrombolysis-related ICH in patients treated with t-PA for acute ischemic stroke (Montaner, Molina, Monasterio et al. 2003a). The role of MMP inhibitors in combination with t-PA may be a future option in reducing this complication of thrombolytic therapy (Lapchak, Araujo 2001). MMP inhibitor research has been most active in the areas of rheumatology and oncology. Unfortunately, most of the clinical trials have been abandoned because of poor drug efficacy and side effects (Peterson 2004). Further clinical trials of new MMP inhibitors are in progress (Hu, Van den Steen, Sang et al. 2007).

Transcriptional Regulation of Inflammation

It is now well recognized that cerebral ischemia upregulates gene expression. Activation of several transcription factors has been documented in experimental stroke models (Lu, Williams, Yao et al. 2004) and in humans (Tang, Xu, Du et al. 2006). Some of these transcription factors are particularly involved in the inflammatory response. Previous DNA microarray analysis indicated that after cerebral ischemia, numerous pro-inflammatory genes are upregulated, including transcription factors, heat shock proteins, cytokines, chemokines, extracellular proteases, and adhesion molecules (Lu, Williams, Yao et al. 2004; Tang, Xu, Du et al. 2006). Many such genes, including TNF-α, IL-1β, NOS, and ICAM-1, are regulated in vitro by NF-κB (Emsley, Tyrrell 2002).

Nuclear Factor kappa B

Early gene expression, induced by increased oxidative stress and hypoxia, further exacerbates the inflammatory response (Irving, Bamford 2002; Schwaninger, Inta, Herrmann 2006). The transcription factor, NF-κB is a major mediator of the brain's response to ischemia and reperfusion, in the pathogenesis of acute stroke (Schwaninger, Inta, Herrmann 2006). NF-κB is a key regulator of the inflammatory cascade and many inflammatory mediators such as inflammatory cytokines, adhesion molecules, and iNOS have NF-κB–binding sequences in their promoters (Stephenson, Yin, Smalstig et al. 2000; Di Napoli, Papa 2003b; Williams, Dave, Tortella et al. 2006). NF-κB is activated by a number of factors that are present during cerebral ischemia, including activated glutamate receptors, ROS, TNF-α, and IL-1β (Schmedtje, Ji, Liu et al. 1997; Clemens 2000; Perkins 2000; Schwaninger, Inta, Herrmann 2006) (Fig. 17.3). NF-κB regulates

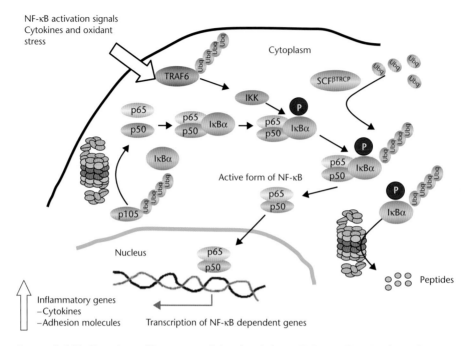

Figure 17.3 Nuclear factor κB (NF-κB) pathway. Upon extracellular signals (e.g., TNF-α, IL-2) or insults such as reactive oxygen species (ROS), a signaling cascade leads to the formation of Lys-63–linked chains on TRAF6, which mediates activation of IKK kinase. IKK phosphorylates IκBα bound to the p65/p50 NF-κB dimer in the cytoplasm. Phosphorylated NF-κB is ubiquitinated by the SCFβ^TRCP E3 complex and degraded by the 26S proteasome, releasing the p65/p50 dimer. The latter immediately translocates to the nucleus where it binds to specific promoter sequences initiating transcription of NF-κB-dependent genes, many of them mediators of the inflammatory response. The p50 itself is generated from a cytoplasmic p105 precursor by a unique mechanism involving partial proteolysis mediated by the 26S proteasome.

the expression of many genes that encode proteins involved in immunity, inflammation, oxidative damage, and apoptosis (Perkins 2000) and has several different targets and effects in various cell types and tissues, which can appear paradoxical (Schmedtje, Ji, Liu et al. 1997; Clemens 2000; Perkins 2000; Karin, Yamamoto, Wang 2004). In some studies, preventing NF-κB activation was shown to be protective, whereas in other studies, activation of NF-κB enhanced neuronal survival (Di Napoli, Papa 2003b; Luo, Kamata, Karin 2005). These conflicting results may be due to the fact that NF-κB can upregulate both pro-inflammatory and pro-survival factors and acts in different ways depending on cell subtype (Luo, Kamata, Karin 2005).

NF-κB inactivation is an attractive therapeutic option as a central target of the neuroinflammatory pathway, and proteasome inhibitors have shown promising results in animal models of acute stroke (Wojcik, Di Napoli 2004; Williams, Dave, Tortella et al. 2006; Zhang, Zhang, Liu et al. 2006). However, NF-κB activity may also be beneficial during the recovery phase of stroke and may be involved in cerebral remodeling (Mattson, Camandola 2001). Therefore, careful evaluation of the drugs targeting NF-κB is required.

The Systemic Inflammatory Response

In addition to the development of the local inflammatory processes in the brain, stroke evokes an immune response at the systemic level. The systemic inflammatory response is a well-known phenomenon caused by various toxic insults to the body, both infectious and noninfectious (Muckart, Bhagwanjee 1997). The clinical manifestation is called the *systemic inflammatory response syndrome* (SIRS). When an infective cause is associated with SIRS then this is referred to as *sepsis*. SIRS includes at least two of the following parameters (Table 17.10): (1) body temperature of >38°C or <36°C; (2) heart rate of >90 beats/min; (3) tachypnea, as manifested by a respiratory rate of >20 breaths/min or hyperventilation, as indicated by $PaCo_2$ of <4.3 kPa; (4) white blood cells count >12,000/mm³ or <4,000/mm³, or the presence of >10% immature neutrophils.

SIRS is evident in both ischemic (Coimbra, Drake, Boris-Moller et al. 1996; Di Napoli 2001a; Slowik, Turaj, Pankiewicz et al. 2002; Emsley, Smith, Gavin et al. 2003; Marchiori, Lino, Hirata et al. 2006) and hemorrhagic stroke (Yoshimoto, Tanaka, Hoya 2001; Godoy, Boccio, Hugo 2002; Castillo, Davalos, Alvarez-Sabin et al. 2002). The SIRS score is made up of each

Table 17.10 The Systemic Inflammatory Response Syndrome (SIRS)

Precipitating causes

Trauma, e.g., stroke

Burns

Pancreatitis

Prolonged shock

Diagnostic criteria—two or more of the following:

Temperature $>38°C$ or $<36°C$

Respiratory rate $>20/min$

Heart rate $>90/min$

White cell count $>12,000$ mm^3 or $<4,000$ mm^3 or $>10\%$ immature neutrophils

SIRS + infection = Sepsis.

diagnostic criterion (1 point for each with a maximum score of 4). A score of 2 or greater, which is diagnostic of SIRS, has been associated with poor outcome in trauma patients (Napolitano, Ferrer, McCarter et al. 2000). Similar results have been shown in acute stroke patients (Reith, Jorgensen, Pedersen et al. 1996; Yoshimoto, Tanaka, Hoya 2001). SIRS is characterized by the release of pro-inflammatory mediators into the systemic circulation, which has been demonstrated in numerous acute stroke studies (Di Napoli, Papa, Bocola 2001; Smith, Emsley, Gavin et al. 2004; Rallidis, Vikelis, Panagiotakos et al. 2006). The degree of the inflammatory response has been shown to be related to the size of infarct volume (Montaner, Rovira, Molina et al. 2003b). Recent SPECT studies have also shown neutrophil infiltration of the ischemic brain tissue (Price, Menon, Peters et al. 2004). The enlimomab neuroprotection study, using monoclonal antibodies against ICAM-1, attempted to attenuate this inflammatory response but was unsuccessful (Enlimomab 2001). The inflammatory response is also associated with the development of hyperthermia during the acute phase of stroke (Ginsberg, Busto 1998). This is related to stroke severity and is associated with poor patient outcome (Reith, Jorgensen, Pedersen et al. 1996; Boysen, Christensen 2001; Leira, Rodriguez-Yanez, Castellanos et al. 2006). Animal stroke models have also shown increased infarct size in hyperthermic conditions (Noor, Wang, Shuaib 2003). Current research studies have been investigating the neuroprotective effects of hypothermia (Han, Karabiyikoglu, Kelly et al. 2003; De Georgia, Krieger, Abou-Chebl et al. 2004). The effects of antipyretic treatment in hyperthermic acute stroke patients, as part of the Paracetamol (Acetaminophen) in Stroke (PAIS) trial, is also being investigated (van Breda, van der Worp, van Gemert et al. 2005) (Table 17.6). The role of prophylactic antibiotic use in acute stroke patients, in an attempt to reduce inflammatory

complications and treat infection, is another area of ongoing research (Vargas, Horcajada, Obach et al. 2006; Elewa, Hilali, Hess, Hill, Carroll et al. 2006).

Acute-Phase Reactants

Serum Amyloid A

Serum amyloid A (SAA) is an acute-phase protein complexed to high-density lipoproteins (HDL) as an apolipoprotein (apo SAA) (Shainkin-Kestenbaum, Zimlichman, Lis et al. 1996). It is mainly found in HDL$_3$ fraction, but small amounts can be found in other HDL fractions as well as in other lipoproteins. SAA occurs in different isoforms and the protein contains between 104 to 112 amino acids, with molecular weight 11.4 to 12.5 kDa (Uhlar, Whitehead 1999). There is a major rise in SAA levels within 24 hours of acute cerebral ischemia (Rallidis, Vikelis, Panagiotakos et al. 2006). SAA can influence lymphocytic responses to antigens and plays a role in cholesterol metabolism during the course of acute inflammation. It also induces the synthesis of collagenase and can inhibit fever induced by IL-1 or TNF-α (Rygg, Uhlar, Thorn et al. 2001). SAA can suppress thromboxane synthesis and platelet release of serotonin, and inhibit platelet aggregation and endothelial cell proliferation (Shainkin-Kestenbaum, Zimlichman, Lis et al. 1996). SAA levels are a sensitive indicator of clinical severity of ischemic stroke and an early indicator of possible infectious complications (Whicher, Biasucci, Rifai 1999; Rallidis, Vikelis, Panagiotakos et al. 2006).

C-Reactive Protein

C-reactive protein (CRP) is an indicator of underlying systemic inflammation. CRP, together with serum amyloid P protein (SAP), is a member of the family of proteins known as *pentraxins* (Pepys, Hirschfield 2003). It is one of the plasma proteins that are called *acute-phase reactants* because of a pronounced rise in concentration after tissue injury or inflammation; in the case of CRP the rise may be 1000-fold or more. CRP is composed of five identical, 21,500-molecular weight subunits. The liver produces CRP but small amounts are produced by lymphocytes. It is detectable on the surface of about 4% of normal peripheral blood lymphocytes (Kuta, Baum 1986).

On the basis of in vitro and in vivo studies, it has been postulated that the function of CRP is related to its ability to recognize specific foreign pathogens and damaged cells within the host. It initiates their elimination by interacting with humoral and cellular effector systems in the blood. Thus, the CRP molecule has both a recognition and an effector function (Pepys, Hirschfield 2003). It has been suggested that one of its major physiological functions is to act as a scavenger of chromatin released by dead cells during the acute inflammatory process (Du Clos 1996). CRP has a long plasma half-life and is now understood to be a mediator as well as a marker of cerebrovascular disease (Di Napoli, Schwaninger, Cappelli et al. 2005).

Recent research has focused on the involvement of CRP in the pathogenesis of cerebrovascular disease. The association of increased levels of CRP with ischemic stroke has been reported in several studies (Rallidis, Vikelis, Panagiotakos et al. 2006). It has been shown that increased levels of CRP are associated with a worse outcome in patients with ischemic stroke (Di Napoli, Papa, Bocola 2001; Winbeck, Poppert, Etgen et al. 2002; Smith, Emsley, Gavin et al. 2004). Increased levels of CRP are also associated with increased risk of future stroke in the elderly (Rost, Wolf, Kase et al. 2001; van Exel, Gussekloo, de Craen et al. 2002). The role of CRP in the pathogenesis of ischemic stroke is not completely understood. It is unclear whether CRP is just a marker of systemic inflammatory processes or is directly involved in pathogenesis of cerebral tissue damage (Di Napoli, Schwaninger, Cappelli et al. 2005). Further research is required to investigate any potential therapeutic effects of inhibiting CRP (Jialal, Devaraj, Venugopal 2004; Pepys, Hirschfield, Tennent et al. 2006).

AGED ANIMALS RECOVER MORE SLOWLY AND LESS COMPLETELY THAN DO YOUNG ANIMALS

Aging is associated with a decline in locomotor, sensory, and cognitive performance in humans (Grady, Craik 2000) and animals (Clayton, Mesches, Alvarez et al. 2002; Mesches, Gemma, Veng et al. 2004; Navarro, Carmen Gomez, Maria-Jesus Sanchez-Pino et al. 2005). While some of these changes may be owing to deficits in peripheral tissues, such as muscles and joints, age-related functional deterioration of the brain also plays a key role (Bachevalier, Landis, Walker et al. 1991).

Rehabilitation aims to improve the physical and cognitive impairments and disabilities of patients with stroke, but elderly individuals recover less effectively than do younger persons (Nakayama, Jørgensen, Raaschou et al. 1994). Therefore, studies on behavioral recuperation after stroke in aged animals are necessary and welcome. Various experimental settings have been used to assess the recovery of sensorimotor functions, spontaneous activity, and memory after stroke in aged rats (Lindner, Gribkoff, Donlan et al. 2003; Badan, Buchhold, Hamm et al. 2003; Markus, Tsai, Bollnow et al. 2005; Zhao, Puurunen, Schallert

et al. 2005a). Overall, the results indicate that aged rats have the capacity to recover behaviorally after cortical infarcts, albeit to a lesser extent than their young counterparts (Lindner, Gribkoff, Donlan et al. 2003; Badan, Buchhold, Hamm et al. 2003; Brown, Marlowe, Bjelke 2003; Markus, Tsai, Bollnow et al. 2005; Rosen, Dinapoli, Nagamine et al. 2005; Zhao, Puurunen, Schallert et al. 2005a).

It should be kept in mind that aged rats are impaired in certain domains, such as spontaneous activity (Badan, Buchhold, Hamm et al. 2003) and spatial memory (Zhao, Puurunen, Schallert et al. 2005a), even before stroke. In addition to their lower baseline level of performance, the ability of older rats to recover from stroke is significantly diminished relative to young animals. On the first postsurgical day, all rats have diminished performance, part of which is attributable to the surgery itself (Fig. 17.4). However, unlike young rats, which commence recovery by the first day after stroke, aged rats start recovery only after 3 to 4 days. Similar findings have been reported recently for post-stroke recovery of senescence-acceleration prone mice (Lee, Cho, Choi et al. 2006).

The extent of recovery in senescent rats was dependent on the complexity and difficulty of the test. For example, aged rats had difficulty mastering complex tasks such as neurological status (which measures a complex of motor, sensory, reflex, and balance functions), rotarod or the adhesive removal test (measures of somatosensory dysfunction), and the Morris water maze (a measure of spatial memory) (Badan, Buchhold, Hamm et al. 2003; Zhang, Komine-Kobayashi, Tanaka et al. 2005; Zhao, Puurunen, Schallert et al. 2005a). In contrast, old animals recovered well on simpler tasks such as the foot-fault test and corner test, which measure motor asymmetries. Finally, the performance level in aged rats is a function of the infarct size; that is, functional impairments in the group with the largest infarcts (20% tissue loss) were more severe than the functional impairments in rats with 4% tissue loss (Lindner, Gribkoff, Donlan et al. 2003). A schematic time course of functional recovery in aged and young rats is shown in Figure 17.4.

REGENERATIVE POTENTIAL OF BRAIN APPEARS TO BE COMPETENT UP TO 20 MONTHS OF AGE

After the infarct area is stabilized, repair mechanisms involving stem cells may become active. Our data on upregulated genes related to stem cell showed that in the first week post-stroke, there were 50% fewer transcriptionally active stem cell genes in the ipsilateral sensorimotor cortex of aged rats than in the same area of young rats, as expected. We also found that other

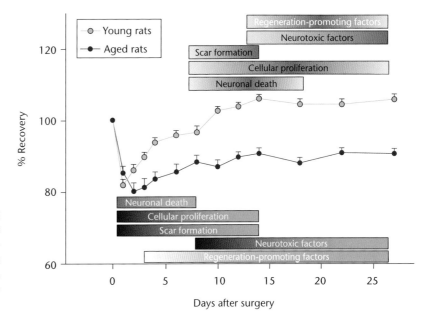

Figure 17.4 General time course of functional recovery after stroke in young and aged rats along with duration and intensity of underlying major cellular and molecular events such as neuronal death, phagocytosis, scar formation, neurotoxic factors, and regeneration-promoting factors.

factors implicated in cellular growth, survival, and neuroprotection, such as type 1 insulin-like growth factor receptor (IGF1R) and inhibin (activinβ), are already downregulated in the control (i.e., noninfarcted) aged rat brain (Florio, Gazzolo, Luisi et al 2007; Rochester et al. 2005).

Although the effect of age on cerebral ischemia has been the focus of several recent reports (Jin, Minami, Xie et al. 2004; He, Crook, Meschia et al. 2005; Badan, Dinca, Buchhold et al. 2004), the contribution of the contralateral hemisphere to neurorestoration has not been addressed at the gene expression level. Our study shows that the contralateral, healthy hemisphere in young rats is much more active at transcriptional level than that in the aged rats at day 3 postischemia, especially at the level of stem cell- and hypoxia-signaling coding genes. However, at this time point, tissue in the hypoperfusion region still struggles with survival, so it is unlikely that brain plasticity in the infracted area could support tissue regeneration and recovery of function. Instead, we hypothesize that activation of transcription in the contralateral sensorimotor cortex may contribute to functional recovery by taking over some function of the damaged hemisphere. It is tempting to speculate that genes involved in stem cell and hypoxia signaling are necessary in the contralateral hemisphere to take over some function of the damaged hemisphere. If so, it seems that oligodendrocyte activity is required in the contralateral hemisphere for the takeover action.

A number of genes implicated in remyelinization such as the NK2 transcription factor related, locus 2 (Nkx2–2) and oligodendrocyte transcription factor 1 (Olig1) were found that were upregulated in the contralateral hemisphere of young rats at 3 days postischemia, but not in the aged rats. Both Nkx2–2 and Olig1 are transcription factors, which play an important role in the differentiation of oligodendrocyte progenitor cell (OPC) into remyelinating oligodendrocytes, myelinogenesis, and axonal recognition (Floyd, Hensley 2000; Hoane, Lasley, Akstulewicz 2004). In this light, the aged rats are at a disadvantage in myelin repair because, as we found, *kx2–2* gene activity was substantially decreased even in intact aged rats as compared to their younger counterparts (Aliev, Smith, Seyidov et al. 2002).

Similarly, there was a downregulation of Gap junction membrane channel protein β1 (Gjb1) in the brains of control, aged rats. Consequently, Gjb1, a component of gap junctions, was strongly upregulated 3 days postischemia, but not in aged rats. Previous work showed that Gjb1, also known as Cx22, is expressed in oligodendrocytes and facilitates cell–cell communication (Oster-Granite, McPhie, Greenan et al. 1996).

Major transcriptional events after stroke included (a) upregulation of genes coding for growth factors such as fibroblast growth factor 22 (Fgf22), nerve growth factor β (Ngfb), frizzled homolog 8 (Fzd8) (Table 17.2); (b) reduction of energy availability by upregulating the uncoupling protein 2 (Ucp2) and upregulation of genes coding for proteins implicated in transport such as fatty acid-binding protein 7 or genes involved in neovasculogenesis like procollagen type Iα I that persisted through day 14 (Table 17.3).

Downregulated genes were mostly stem cell–associated genes and included genes implicated in cell adhesion such as catenin, intercellular adhesion molecule 5, and integrin β5.

The total number of genes that were regulated in response to ischemia was lower in aged rats as compared to that in young rats, but the overall difference between age-groups was not significant. However, if the data was analyzed by array type there were significant differences between young and aged animals in stem cell–related genes. The number of regulated stem cell–related genes increased gradually from day 3 to day 14 in the aged rats.

To explore the potential of older animals to initiate regenerative processes following cerebral ischemia, the expression of the juvenile-specific cytoskeletal protein, microtubule-associated protein 1B (MAP1B), the adult-specific protein, microtubule-associated protein 2 (MAP2), and the axonal growth marker, βIII-tubulin was studied in male Sprague-Dawley rats at 3 months and 20 months of age.

Focal cerebral ischemia, produced by reversible occlusion of the right middle cerebral artery, resulted in vigorous expression of both MAP1B penumbra of 3-month-old and, to a lesser extent, 20-month-old rats at 14d following the stroke (Popa-Wagner, Schröder, Schmoll et al. 1999; Badan, Dinca, Buchhold et al. 2004). Similarly, MAP2 protein and mRNAs were upregulated in the peri-infarcted area at almost the same levels both in young and aged rats. Somewhat lower levels of expression were noted for the axonal growth marker, βIII-tubulin, in the peri-infarcted area of aged rats as compared to young rats. Collectively, these results suggest that the regenerative potential of the brain at the structural level is competent up to 20 months of age.

Recent studies confirm that mechanisms for self-repair in the young brain also operate in the aged brain. For example, stroke causes increased numbers of new striatal neurons despite lower basal cell proliferation in the subventricular zone in the aged brain (Jin, Minami, Xie et al. 2001; Darsalia, Heldmann, Lindvall et al. 2005). However, despite conserved proliferative activity in the subventricular zone, the number of neurons that reach the injury site is quite modest, as was shown recently for doublecortin-positive neurons in the infarcted area of aged rats (Popa-Wagner, Carmichael, Kokaia et al. 2007b). One possible explanation is that lateral ventricle–derived nestin-positive cells do not pass the corpus callosum barrier, and therefore cannot contribute to generation of neurons in the neocortex. Indeed, current evidence indicates that the great majority of newly formed cells in the adult brain are non-neuronal (Priller, Persons, Klett et al. 2001; Vallieres, Sawchenko 2003; Hess, Hill, Carroll et al. 2004).

Recent studies also indicate that the molecular profile of growth-promoting genes is very different between aged and young adults during the sprouting response to lesions of the CNS. Aged individuals activate most growth-promoting genes at a later time

Table 17.11 Brief Description of Behavioural Tests Used to Evaluate Changes in Neurological Function Associated with Ischemia

Behavioral Test	Description
Neurological status	Rat is pulled gently by the tail and the presence or absence of circling is observed
Limb placement symmetry	Rat is held gently by the tail at the edge of a table. Symmetry or asymmetry of forelimb placement is observed
Body proprioception	Rat is touched lightly on each side of the body with a blunt probe. Tests sensorimotor responsiveness
Response to vibrissae touch	A blunt stick is brushed against the vibrissae on each side, and presence or absence of response is noted. Tests sensorimotor responsiveness
Beam walking test (Rotarod)	Rat is tested for its ability to maintain balance while walking on a rotating rod. Assesses fine vestibulomotor function
Inclined plane	The ability of each animal to maintain its position at a given angle on an inclined plane is determined
Spontaneous activity	Rat is placed in a large cage and the number of crossings of a bisecting line is determined. Assesses interest in exploration of a novel environment
T-mazes	Rat is placed in a T-maze in which one of the arms of the maze is baited with a reward. Tests working and reference memory
Radial arm maze	Rat is placed in an 8-arm radial maze, elevated 60 cm above the floor. Tests spatial working memory

point following stroke than do young adults. This includes a delayed induction of GAP43, CAP23, and the growth-promoting transcription factor c-jun. The growth-promoting cell guidance molecule L1 and the CDK5 inhibitor p21 are actually downregulated during the axonal sprouting process in aged individuals compared with a robust and early upregulation of these two molecules in young adults (Li, Penderis, Zhao et al. 2006; Carmichael, Archibeque, Luke et al. 2005). These results are summarized in Table 17.11.

FEW NEUROPROTECTANTS ARE EFFECTIVE IN AGED RODENTS

A major goal of clinical research is to limit the infarct size, and a principal line of investigation has involved the theory of excitotoxicity, which is based on the observation that large concentrations of glutamate can destroy neurons.

On the basis of this mechanism, several antiexcitotoxic candidates have emerged, including antagonists to the NMDA receptor (such as MK801), and to the AMPA receptor (NBQX). However, both MK-801 and NBQX were found to be less effective as neuro-protectants in aged rats than in young rats (Suzuki, Takagi, Nakamura et al. 2003). The failure to demonstrate the neuroprotective efficacy of such receptor antagonists in clinical trials has led investigators to search for other potential causative mechanisms. For example, a recent study showed that treatment of aged rats with sildenafil, a phosphodiesterase type 5 inhibitor that is used to enhance cGMP-mediated relaxation of the pulmonary vasculature, improves functional recovery in young and aged rats, possibly by promoting brain plasticity via enhancement of angiogenesis and synaptogenesis (Zhang, Komine-Kobayashi, Tanaka et al. 2005).

A more general method of neuroprotection that is efficacious in young rats is ischemic preconditioning. However, protection was diminished in aged rats as compared to young rats (He, Crook, Meschia et al. 2005), possibly because the brains of aged animals show a reduced stress response that is likely to act neuroprotectively to stroke (Li, Zhong, Yang et al. 2005).

Steroids recently have been shown to be effective as neuroprotective agents for ischemic stroke. Treatment with physiological concentrations of estradiol decreases ischemic injury by almost 50% in both young and aged rats, possibly by suppressing apoptosis (Wise 2006; Dubal, Rau, Shughrue et al. 2006). Thus, physiological concentrations of estradiol might be used to enhance neuronal survival in the penumbral region of the infarct (Wise, 2006; Dubal, Rau, Shughrue et al. 2006). In addition, progesterone can improve the outcome following traumatic brain injury (Cutler, Vanlandingham, Stein et al. 2006).

Finally, since calpain inhibitors appear to not only protect brain tissue from ischemia but also prevent neurotoxicity caused by such neurotoxins as Aβ or 3-nitropropionic acid, the currently available data suggest that calpain could be a useful therapeutic target (reviewed in Camins, Verdaguer, Folch et al. 2006).

Although environmental enrichment has been shown to improve the behavioral outcome of stroke in young animals, the effect of an enriched environment on behavioral and neuropathological recovery in *aged* animals is not known. Recently we have shown that the enriched environment significantly improved the rate and extent of recovery in aged animals. Correlation analysis revealed that the beneficial effect of the enriched environment on recovery, both in young and aged rats, correlated highly with a reduction in infarct size, in the number of proliferating astrocytes, and in the volume of the glial scar (Buchhold, Mogoanta, Suofu et al. 2007). These results suggest that temporally modulating astrocytic proliferation and the ensuing scar formation might be a fruitful approach to improving functional recovery after stroke in aged rats.

Acute cerebral ischemia results in a complex inflammatory cascade, resulting in the activation of a variety of inflammatory cells and chemical mediators. This is accompanied by a systemic inflammatory response and production of acute-phase reactants. The demonstration that inflammatory processes have a pathogenic role is dependent on showing improvement in outcome by treatment that antagonizes these processes. Different parts of the inflammatory cascade have been targeted in the setting of experimental cerebral ischemia, with variable results.

Animal models of stroke have demonstrated reduced infarct size on modification of the inflammatory response. Clinical studies have also suggested that infarct size and patient outcome may be affected by the inflammatory response. The evidence relates to leukocytes, and the molecular mechanisms involved in their recruitment in humans remains methodologically limited and broadly circumstantial, and a causal relation has yet to be established. This has prompted the suggestion that such models cannot be formally extrapolated to patients, and that our understanding of human pathophysiology remains incomplete. At present we do not have enough evidence to suggest that human inflammatory processes mimic animal models, and this should prompt a greater drive toward patient-based research. Clinical drug trials targeting the inflammatory pathways in acute ischemic stroke have thus far been disappointing (Table 17.6). However, with increasing knowledge of the inflammatory mechanisms involved during cerebral ischemia, new anti-inflammatory targets are continuing to be identified. With the success of thrombolysis in acute ischemic stroke and ongoing clinical trials of reperfusion therapies, for example, embolectomy, adjuvant neuroprotective therapy is an attractive option for minimizing reperfusion injury (Zhang, Zhang, Liu et al. 2006; Pan, Konstas, Bateman et al. 2007). However, such studies should place emphasis on the early stages of stroke pathogenesis when interventions are more likely to result in neuronal salvage. This should also account for interindividual and temporal and spatial heterogeneity in stroke, should quantify inflammatory responses, and should ideally examine critical relations between several different variables—for example, white cell invasion, chemokine response, adhesion molecules, penumbra, and outcome.

ADULT NEUROGENESIS

Neural stem cells (NSCs) are unspecialized cells, which have self-renewal capacity and can also, through differentiation, generate the specialized cells of the CNS (neurons, astrocytes and oligodendrocytes). Neural stem cells exist in the early embryo as neuroepitelial cells in the neural tube. These cells will transform into radial glial cells during embryogenesis. Radial glia persist in the early neonatal period and most likely transform into neural stem cells of the adult subventricular zone (SVZ) (Merkle, Alvarez-Buylla 2006).

Adult neurogenesis persists throughout adult life in all mammals investigated so far. Neural stem cells reside in at least two regions of the adult brain, namely, the SVZ and the dentate gyrus (DG) of the hippocampus. Stem cells in these regions ensure neurogenesis throughout adult life in the olfactory bulb and the subgranular layer respectively.

Relatively quiescent neural stem cells (NSCs) located in the SVZ (B-cells) proliferate and give rise to rapidly dividing transit-amplifying cells (C-cells). C-cells in turn divide and generate neuroblasts (A-cells), which then migrate using chain migration through the rostral migratory stream (RMS) to the olfactory bulb (OB). In a few days after birth, new neurons reach the OB and migrate radially to their final positions where they differentiate into inhibitory GABAergic or tyrosine hydroxylase (TH) interneurons in the glomerular and periglomerular layers and functionally integrate in the existing circuitry (Deacon, Pakzaban, Isacson 1994; Carleton, Rochefort, Morante-Oria J et al. 2002). The significance of OB neurogenesis is not totally clear. However, some studies suggest that OB neurogenesis could be associated with improved olfactory memory (Rochefort, Gheusi,Vincent et al. 2002).

Another neurogenic area in the adult brain is the hippocampal formation. Here, NSCs located in the SGZ proliferate and give rise to immature intermediate precursors (D cells) (Seri, Garcia-Verdugo, Collado-Morente et al. 2004), many of which die shortly after they are born. The surviving neurons then migrate into the dentate granule cell layer and differentiate into granule cells (Kempermann, Gast, Kronenberg et al. 2003; Seri, Garcia-Verdugo, Collado-Morente et al. 2004). Within few weeks, they send axons to the CA3 region and project dendrites to the outer molecular layer (Markakis, Gage 1999; Seri, Garcia-Verdugo, McEwen et al. 2001; van Praag, Schinder, Christie et al. 2002). At the same time, new neurons mature and start to generate action potentials and receive synaptic inputs from the cortex, thus becoming functionally integrated in the neuronal network (van Praag, Schinder, Christie et al. 2002). Although, to date there are no studies providing evidence for a direct link between behavioral performance and level of hippocampal neurogenesis, circumstantial data from several reports indicate that such link might exist (Shors, Miesegaes, Beylin et al. 2001; Kempermann, Gast Gage 2002; Drapeau, Mayo, Aurousseau et al. 2003; Raber, Fan, Matsumori et al. 2004).

Importantly, neurogenesis also occurs in adult humans. Gage and his colleagues investigated several years ago the postmortem brain of cancer patients who received BrdU, a marker of cell proliferation (Eriksson, Perfilieva Bjork-Eriksson et al. 1998). Many BrdU-positive neurons that were born after BrdU administration and before patients died (16 to 781 days) were detected in the hippocampal formation and SVZ, indicating that human brain also has the capacity to produce new neurons. Recently, it has been shown that NSCs exist in the SVZ of the human brain although the RMS toward the OB might be somewhat different as compared to that in rodents (Sanai, Tramontin, Quinones-Hinojosa et al. 2004).

Production of new hippocampal and SVZ cells is modulated by different physiological stimulations such as enriched environment (Kempermann, Kuhn, Gage 1997; Rochefort, Gheusi, Vincent et al. 2002), running (van Praag, Kempermann, Gage et al. 1999), training in hippocampus-dependent learning test (Gould, Beylin, Tanapat 1999), and several growth factors (Kuhn, Winkler, Kempermann 1997; Jin, Sun, Xie et al. 2003). Epileptic seizures (Bengzon, Kokaia, Nanobashvili et al. 1997; Parent, Yu, Leibowitz et al. 1997), brain trauma (Dash, Mach, Moore 2001; Braun, Schafer, Hollt 2002), chronic alcohol administration (Herrera, Yague, Johnsen-Soriano et al. 2003), and focal (Jin, Minami, Xie 2001; Zhang, Zhang, Zhang et al. 2001; Komitova, Perfilieva, Mattsson et al. 2002; Parent, Vexler, Gong et al. 2002; Takasawa, Kitagawa, Yagita et al. 2002) and global (Liu, Solway, Messing et al. 1998; Takagi, Nozaki, Takahashi et al. 1999; Kee, Preston, Woittowicz 2001; Yagita, Kitagawa, Ohtsuki et al. 2001) forebrain ischemia could also significantly alter neurogenesis in the adult brain. Another powerful regulator of adult neurogenesis is aging.

Neurogenesis and Aging

Neurogenesis declines with advanced age in both the SVZ and in the DG. Using BrdU incorporation and PSA-NCAM labeling Seki and Arai (1995) showed a decreased formation of newly formed neurons in the DG in rats with increased age. Further Kuhn et al. (1996) showed a reduced proliferation of progenitors in the DG, resulting in decreased neurogenesis and lower number of differentiating neuroblasts as assessed with BrdU and PSA-NCAM labeling. These findings were also reproduced later in the mouse (Kempermann, Kuhn, Gage 1998). These early studies did not show any age-dependent decline in neurogenesis within the SVZ. However, in 1997 Tropepe et al. showed decreased proliferation and lengthening of cell cycle time within the forebrain subependyma using sequential BrdU and tritiated tymidine labeling.

In the same study, the formation of neurospheres in vitro, reflecting number and/or proliferation of stem cells, from dissected subependyma was unchanged in aged animals compared to young animals. In recent years decline in SVZ progenitor proliferation and neurogenesis have been reported both in vivo and in vitro (Enwere, Shingo Gregg et al. 2004; Maslov, Barone, Plunkett et al. 2004; Luo, Daniels, Lennington et al. 2006).

Several studies support the hypothesis that an aging environment is the cause of age-dependent decline in neurogenesis. These environmental changes are most likely due to decreased growth factor signaling (Tropepe, Craig, Morshead et al. 1997; Enwere, Shingo Gregg et al. 2004; Shetty, Hattiangady, Shetty 2005) or increased corticosterone levels in aged animals (Cameron, Woolley, McEwen et al. 1993; Montaron, Petry, Rodriguez et al. 1999; Montaron, Drapeau, Dupret et al. 2006). Other possible explanations might be actual loss of stem cells in the SVZ and hippocampus (Maslov, Barone, Plunkett et al. 2004; Olariu, Cleaver, Cameron 2007). However, there are some conflicting reports (Hattiangady, Shetty 2008). Senescence of progenitors within the SVZ has also been put forward as an alternative explanation (Molofsky, Slutsky, Joseph et al. 2006). Clearly, there is a need for further studies within this field, especially regarding any intrinsic and functional changes in stem and progenitor cells in the SVZ and hippocampus with age.

Neural Stem Cells, Aging, and Disease

Since the discovery that neural stem cells exist in the adult brain and that neurogenesis persists throughout life intense research has been focused on exploring the possibility of using this discovery for treating neurodegenerative disease. Examples of neurodegenerative diseases where aging plays a crucial role are Alzheimer's disease and Parkinson's disease. Interestingly both amyloid β and α synuclein, proteins known to misfold and accumulate in Alzheimer's and Parkinson's disease, have been shown to have detrimental effects on neural stem/progenitor cells and neurogenesis (Uchida, Nakano, Gomi et al. 2007; Verret, Jankowsky, Xu et al. 2007; Winner, Rockenstein, Lie et al. 2008).

Another neurodegenerative disease that is highly increased in aged patients and where a potential stem cell–based therapy could be envisioned is stroke. Indeed it has been shown that after ischemic injury by MCAO in rats, progenitors within the SVZ proliferate and migrate toward the injured site and differentiate into neurons similar to the ones lost in the insult (Arvidsson, Collin, Kirik et al. 2002). Similarly, it has

been shown that after ischemia progenitors in the SGZ proliferate and replace neurons in the hippocampus (Nakatomi, Kuriu, Okabe et al. 2002). Interestingly, it has also been shown that ischemia-induced neural stem/progenitor proliferation is preserved although at reduced levels in aged animals. It has been shown using the MCAO model and BrdU labeling in young and aged rats that ischemia triggers proliferation in the aged SVZ. However, the increase in proliferation was 20% less than in young animals; further there was no increase in DG proliferation (Jin, Minami, Xie 2004). Darsalia et al showed in 2005 that MCAO in aged animals induces progenitor proliferation within both SVZ and in the DG although at lower levels than in young animals. Interestingly, the same study showed that cells, newly formed after stroke, develop into mature neurons both in striatum and in the hippocampus in aged animals. Further the number of newly formed striatal neurons after stroke was similar in young and aged animals.

There are no clear explanations to the decreased proliferation within SVZ or DG in aged animals either in steady state or after ischemic injury. Recently it was proposed that decrease in striatal neurogenesis after stroke in aged animals is attributed to increased death of progenitors and newborn neurons (Chen, Sun 2007). In this study the authors show increased colocalization of the apoptosis marker–active caspase-3 with markers of progenitors and immature neurons in aged animals compared to that in young animals after ischemia. However, another group published a report at the same time where they claim the opposite that there is more apoptosis in young SVZ and DG compared to the aged both under normal condition and after focal ischemia (Tang, Wang et al. 2007). This decrease in death of progenitors and newborn neurons was instead correlated to the age-dependent decline in proliferation. The discrepancy between these reports might be due to differences in the experimental setups.

Most interestingly, it has recently been shown that the human brain can respond to stroke with increased progenitor proliferation in aged patients (Jin, Wang, Xie 2006; Macas, Nern, Plate 2006), opening the possibilities to utilize this intrinsic attempt for neuroregeneration of the human brain as a potential therapy for stroke.

Neurogenesis is a complex process consisting of several steps such as cell proliferation, migration, differentiation, survival, and functional integration. Many environmental and cellular as well as genetic factors could influence each of these components, and in addition, physiological condition of the organism (age, physical condition, severity of the disease) could substantially alter the parameters and thus the outcome of this process. Especially, under such pathological conditions as stroke, where the degree of the disease and pathological consequences are extremely variable (e.g., depending on the extent and location of the damage in case of stroke), it requires individual approach to assess the possible extent of neurogenic response and possibilities to alter this response.

CONCLUSIONS

These results show that (a) compared to young rats, aged rats develop a larger infarct area, as well as a necrotic zone characterized by a higher rate of cellular degeneration and a larger number of apoptotic cells; (b) in both old and young rats, the early intense proliferative activity following stroke leads to a precipitous formation of growth-inhibiting scar tissue, a phenomemon amplified by the persistent expression of neurotoxic factors; and (c) the regenerative potential of the rat brain is largely preserved up to 20 months of age but gene expression is temporally displaced, has a lower amplitude, and is sometimes of relatively short duration.

Given the heterogeneity of stroke, a universal anti-inflammatory solution may be a distant prospect, but probably neuroprotective drug cocktails targeting inflammatory pathways in combination with thrombolysis may be a possibility for acute stroke treatment in the future (Sacco, Chong, Prabhakaran et al. 2007).

Most interestingly, it has recently been shown that the human brain can respond to stroke with increased progenitor proliferation in aged patients (Jin, Wang, Xie 2006; Macas, Nern, Plate 2006), opening up the possibilities to utilize this intrinsic attempt for neuroregeneration of the human brain as a potential therapy for stroke.

ACKNOWLEDGMENT   This work was supported by a grant from Prof. Dr. D.Platt Stiftung to APW and EU FP6 grant StemStroke to ZK.

REFERENCES

Abilleira S, Montaner J, Molina CA, Monasterio J, Castillo J, Alvarez-Sabin J. 2003. Matrix metalloproteinase-9 concentration after spontaneous intracerebral hemorrhage. *J Neurosurg.* 99:65–70.

Acalovschi D, Wiest T, Hartmann M et al. 2003. Multiple levels of regulation of the interleukin-6 system in stroke. *Stroke.* 34:1864–1869.

Adams HP, Jr, del Zoppo G, Alberts MJ et al. 2007. Guidelines for the early management of adults with Iichemic stroke: a guideline from The American Heart Association/American Stroke Association Stroke Council, Clinical Cardiology Council, Cardiovascular Radiology And Intervention Council, and the atherosclerotic peripheral vascular disease and quality of care outcomes In Research Interdisciplinary Working Groups: The American Academy of Neurology Affirms The Value of this Guideline as an Educational Tool for Neurologists. *Stroke.* 38:1655–1711.

Ahmad M, Saleem S, Zhuang H et al. 2006. 1-HydroxyPGE reduces infarction volume in mouse transient cerebral ischemia. *Eur J Neurosci.* 23:35–42.

Ahmad M, Ahmad AS, Zhuang H, Maruyama T, Narumiya S, Dore S. 2007. Stimulation of prostaglandin E2-EP3 receptors exacerbates stroke and excitotoxic injury. *J Neuroimmunol.* 184:172–179.

Aichner F, Bauer G. 2005. Cerebral anoxia. In E Niedermeyer, F Lopez da Silva, ed. *Electroencephalography: Basic Principles, Clinical Applications and Related Fields.* MD, Baltimore: Williams & Wilkins. 455–470.

Akita N, Nakase H, Kaido T, Kanemoto Y, Sakaki T. 2003. Protective effect of C1 esterase inhibitor on reperfusion injury in the rat middle cerebral artery occlusion model. *Neurosurgery.* 52:395–400.

Akopov SE, Simonian NA, Grigorian GS 1996. Dynamics of polymorphonuclear leukocyte accumulation in acute cerebral infarction and their correlation with brain tissue damage. *Stroke.* 27:1739–1743.

Alarcón F, Zijlmans JC, Dueñas G, Cevallos N. 2004. Poststroke movement disorders: report of 56 patients. *J Neurol Neurosurg Psychiatry.* 75:1568–1574.

Aliev G, Smith MA, Seyidov D et al. 2002. The role of oxidative stress in the pathophysiology of cerebrovascular lesions in Alzheimer's disease. *Brain Pathol.* 12:21–35.

Allan SM, Rothwell NJ. 2001. Cytokines and acute neurodegeneration. *Nat Rev Neurosci.* 2:734–744.

Allan SM, Tyrrell PJ, Rothwell NJ. 2005. Interleukin-1 and neuronal injury. *Nat Rev Immunol.* 5:629–640.

American Heart Association. 2006. *Heart Disease and Stroke Statistics—2006 Update.* Dallas, TX: American Heart Association.

Ando S, Tanaka Y, Toyoda Y, Kon K. 2003. Turnover of myelin lipids in aging brain. *Neurochem Res.* 28:5–13.

Andrew PJ, Mayer B. 1999. Enzymatic function of nitric oxide synthases. *Cardiovasc Res.* 43:521–531.

Arakelyan A, Petrkova J, Hermanova Z, Boyajyan A, Lukl J, Petrek M. 2005. Serum levels of the MCP-1 chemokine in patients with ischemic stroke and myocardial infarction. *Mediators Inflamm.* 3:175–179.

Arumugam TV, Granger DN, Mattson MP. 2005. Stroke and T-Cells. *Neuromolecular Med.* 7:229–242.

Arvidsson A, T Collin, Kirik D, Kokaia Z, Lindvall O. 2002. Neuronal replacement from endogenous precursors in the adult brain after stroke. *Nat Med.* 8:963–970.

Asahi M, Asahi K, Jung JC, del Zoppo GJ, Fini ME, Lo EH. 2000. Role for matrix metalloproteinase 9 after focal cerebral ischemia: effects of gene knockout and enzyme inhibition with BB-94. *J Cereb Blood Flow Metab.* 20:1681–1689.

Atkinson C, Zhu H, Qiao F et al. 2006. Complement-dependent P-selectin expression and injury following ischemic stroke *J Immunol.* 177:7266–7274.

Ay H, Koroshetz WJ, Vangel M et al. 2005. Conversion of ischemic brain tissue into infarction increases with age. *Stroke.* 36:2632–2636.

Bachevalier J, Landis LS, Walker LC et al. 1991. Aged monkeys exhibit behavioral deficits indicative of widespread cerebral dysfunction. *Neurobiol Aging.* 12:99–111.

Badan I, Buchhold B, Hamm A et al. 2003. Accelerated glial reactivity to stroke in aged rats correlates with reduced functional recovery. *J Cereb Blood Flow Metab.* 23:845–854.

Badan I, Dinca I, Buchhold B et al. 2004. Accelerated accumulation of N- and C-terminal betaAPP fragments and delayed recovery of microtubule-associated protein 1B expression following stroke in aged rats. *Eur J Neurosci.* 19:2270–2280.

Banati RB, Myers R, Kreutzberg GW. 1997. PK ('Peripheral Benzodiazepine')--binding sites in the CNS indicate early and discrete brain lesions: microautoradiographic detection of [3H]PK11195 binding to activated microglia. *J Neurocytol.* 26:77–82.

Banno M, Mizuno T, Kato H et al. 2005. The radical scavenger edaravone prevents oxidative neurotoxicity induced by peroxynitrite and activated microglia. *Neuropharmacology.* 48:283–290.

Barnett HJ. 2002. Stroke prevention in the elderly. *Clin Exp Hypertens.* 24:563–571.

Barone FC, Arvin B, White RF et al. 1997. Tumor necrosis factor-alpha. A mediator of focal ischemic brain injury. *Stroke.* 28:1233–1244.

Bath PM, Bath-Hextall FJ. 2004. Pentoxifylline, propentofylline and pentifylline for acute ischaemic stroke. *Cochrane Database Syst Rev.* CD000162.

Becker K, Kindrick D, Relton J, Harlan J, Winn R. 2001. Antibody to the alpha4 integrin decreases infarct size in transient focal cerebral ischemia in rats. *Stroke.* 32:206–211.

Becker KJ. 2002. Anti-leukocyte antibodies: leukArrest (Hu23F2G) and enlimomab (R6.5) in acute stroke. *Curr Med Res Opin.* 18 (Suppl 2) s18–s22.

Bednar MM, Dooley RH, Zamani M, Howard DB, Gross CE. 1995. Neutrophil and platelet activity and quantification following delayed TPA therapy in a rabbit model of thromboembolic stroke. *J Thromb Thrombolysis.* 1:179–185.

Bengzon J, Z Kokaia, Nanobashvili M, Kokaia Z, Lindvall O. 1997. Apoptosis and proliferation of dentate gyrus neurons after single and intermittent limbic seizures. *Proc Natl Acad Sci U S A.* 94:10432–10437.

Bertorelli R, Adami M, Di Santo E, Ghezzi P. 1998. MK 801 and dexamethasone reduce both tumor necrosis factor levels and infarct volume after focal cerebral ischemia in the rat brain. *Neurosci Lett.* 246:41–44.

Beschorner R, Schluesener HJ, Gozalan F, Meyermann R, Schwab JM. 2002. Infiltrating CD14+ monocytes and expression of CD14 by activated parenchymal microglia/macrophages contribute to the pool of CD14+ cells in ischemic brain lesions. *J Neuroimmunol.* 126:107–115.

Biber K, Lubrich B, Fiebich BL, Boddeke HW, van Calker D. 2001. Interleukin-6 enhances expression of adenosine A(1) receptor MRNA and signaling in cultured rat cortical astrocytes and brain slices. *Neuropsychopharmacology.* 24:86–96.

Blais V, Rivest S. 2001. Inhibitory action of nitric oxide on circulating tumor necrosis factor-induced NF-kappaB

activity and COX-2 transcription in the endothelium of the brain capillaries. *J Neuropathol Exp Neurol.* 60:893–905.

Bonmann E, Suschek C, Spranger M, Kolb-Bachofen V. 1997. The dominant role of exogenous or endogenous Interleukin-1 beta on expression and activity of inducible nitric oxide synthase in rat microvascular brain endothelial cells. *Neurosci Lett.* 230:109–112.

Bonventre JV, Huang Z, Taheri MR et al. 1997. Reduced fertility and postischaemic brain injury in mice deficient in cytosolic phospholipase A2. *Nature.* 390:622–625.

Boutin H, LeFeuvre RA, Horai R, Asano M, Iwakura Y, Rothwell NJ. 2001. Role of IL-1alpha and IL-1beta in ischemic brain damage. *J Neurosci.* 21:5528–5534.

Bowes MP, Rothlein R, Fagan SC, Zivin JA. 1995a. Monoclonal antibodies preventing leukocyte activation reduce experimental neurologic injury and enhance efficacy of thrombolytic therapy. *Neurology.* 45:815–819.

Boysen G, Christensen H. 2001. Stroke severity determines body temperature in acute stroke. *Stroke.* 32:413–417.

Braun H, K Schafer, Hollt V. 2002. Beta III tubulin-expressing neurons reveal enhanced neurogenesis in hippocampal and cortical structures after a contusion trauma in rats. *J Neurotrauma.* 19:975–983.

Bredt DS. 1999. Endogenous nitric oxide synthesis: biological functions and pathophysiology. *Free Radic Res.* 31:577–596.

Broderick JP. 2004. William M. Feinberg lecture: stroke therapy in the year 2025: burden, breakthroughs, and barriers to progress. *Stroke.* 35:205–211.

Brown AW, Marlowe KJ, Bjelke B. 2003. Age effect on motor recovery in a post-acute animal stroke model. *Neurobiol Aging.* 24:607–614

Bruce AJ, Boling W, Kindy MS et al. 1996. Altered neuronal and microglial responses to excitotoxic and ischemic brain injury in mice lacking TNF receptors. *Nat Med.* 2:788–794.

Buchhold B, Mogoanta L, Suofu Y et al. 2008. Environmental enrichment improves functional and neuropathological indices following stroke in young and aged rats. *Restorative Neurol Neurosci.* 25:1–18.

Buga AM, Sascau M, Herndon GJ, Kessler Ch, Popa-Wagner A. 2008. The genomic response of the contralateral cortex to stroke is diminished in the aged rats. *J Cel Mol Med.* (in press).

Burgaud JL, Riffaud JP, Del Soldato P. 2002. Nitric-oxide releasing molecules: a new class of drugs with several major indications. *Curr Pharm Des.* 8:201–213.

Caimi G, Ferrara F, Montana M et al. 2000. Acute ischemic stroke: polymorphonuclear leukocyte membrane fluidity and cytosolic Ca(2+) concentration at baseline and after chemotactic activation. *Stroke* 31: pp 1578–1582.

Cameron HA, CS Woolley, McEwen BS, Gould E. 1993. Differentiation of newly born neurons and glia in the dentate gyrus of the adult rat. *Neuroscience.* 56:337–344.

Camins A, Verdaguer E, Folch J, Pallas M. 2006. Involvement of calpain activation in neurodegenerative processes. *CNS Drug Rev.* 12:135–148.

Campbell SJ, Perry VH, Pitossi FJ et al. 2005. Central nervous system injury triggers hepatic CC and CXC chemokine expression that is associated with leukocyte mobilization and recruitment to both the central nervous system and the liver. *Am J Pathol.* 166:1487–1497.

Canolle B, Masmejean F, Melon C, Nieoullon A, Pisano P, Lortet S. 2004. Glial soluble factors regulate the activity and expression of the neuronal glutamate transporter EAAC1: implication of cholesterol. *J Neurochem.* 88:1521–1532.

Carleton A, C Rochefort, Morante-Oria J et al. 2002. Making scents of olfactory neurogenesis. *J Physiol (Paris).* 96:115–122.

Carmichael ST, Archibeque I, Luke L, Nolan T, Momiy J, Li S. 2005. Growth-associated gene expression after stroke: evidence for a growth-promoting region in periinfarct cortex. *Exp Neurol.* 193:291–311.

Caso JR, Moro MA, Lorenzo P, Lizasoain I, Leza JC. 2007a. Involvement of IL-1beta in acute stress-induced worsening of cerebral ischaemia in rats. *Eur Neuropsychopharmacol.* 17:600–607.

Caso JR, Pradillo JM, Hurtado O, Lorenzo P, Moro MA, Lizasoain I. 2007b. Toll-like receptor 4 is involved in brain damage and inflammation after experimental stroke. *Circulation.* 115:1599–1608.

Castellanos M, Leira R, Serena J et al. 2003. Plasma metalloproteinase-9 concentration predicts hemorrhagic transformation in acute ischemic stroke. *Stroke.* 34:40–46.

Castillo J, Davalos A, Alvarez-Sabin J et al. 2002. Molecular signatures of brain injury after intracerebral hemorrhage. *Neurology.* 58:624–629.

Catania A, Lipton JM. 1998. Peptide modulation of fever and inflammation within the brain. *Ann NY Acad Sci.* 856:62–68.

Chan PH. 2001. Reactive oxygen radicals in signaling and damage in the ischemic brain. *J Cereb Blood Flow Metab.* 21:2–14.

Chang RC, Rota C, Glover RE, Mason RP, Hong JS. 2000. A novel effect of an opioid receptor antagonist, naloxone, on the production of reactive oxygen species by microglia: a study by Electron paramagnetic resonance spectroscopy. *Brain Res.* 854:224–229.

Chen H, Chopp M, Zhang RL et al. 1994. Anti-CD11b monoclonal antibody reduces ischemic cell damage after transient focal cerebral ischemia in rat. *Ann Neurol.* 35:458–463.

Chen Y, Hallenbeck JM, Ruetzler C et al. 2003. Overexpression of monocyte chemoattractant protein 1 in the brain exacerbates ischemic brain injury and is associated with recruitment of inflammatory cells. *J Cereb Blood Flow Metab.* 23:748–755.

Chen Y, Samal B, Hamelink CR et al. 2006 Neuroprotection by endogenous and exogenous PACAP following stroke. *Regul Pept.* 137:4–19.

Chen Y, Sun FY. 2007. Age-related decrease of striatal neurogenesis is associated with apoptosis of neural precursors and newborn neurons in rat brain after ischemia. *Brain Res.* 29(1166):9–19.

Chiappetta O, Gliozzi M, Siviglia E et al. 2007. Evidence to implicate early modulation of Interleukin-1beta expression in the neuroprotection afforded by 17beta-estradiol in male rats undergone transient middle cerebral artery occlusion. *Int Rev Neurobiol.* 82:357–372.

Chiueh CC. 1999. Neuroprotective properties of nitric oxide. *Ann N Y Acad Sci.* 890:301–311.

Chu LS, Fang SH, Zhou Y et al. 2007. Minocycline inhibits 5-lipoxygenase activation and brain inflammation after focal cerebral ischemia in rats. *Acta Pharmacol Sin.* 28:763–772.

Clark RK, Lee EV, Fish CJ et al. 1993. Development of tissue damage, inflammation and resolution following stroke: an immunohistochemical and quantitative planimetric study. *Brain Res Bull.* 31:565–572.

Clark RK, Lee EV, White RF, Jonak ZL, Feuerstein GZ, Barone FC. 1994. Reperfusion following focal stroke hastens inflammation and resolution of ischemic injured tissue. *Brain Res Bull.* 35:387–392.

Clarke DD, Sokoloff L. 1999. Circulation and energy metabolism of the brain. In Siegel GJ, Albers RW, Fisher SK, Uhler MD, ed. *Basic Neurochemistry: Molecular, Cellular and Medical Aspects.* New York: Raven Press. 638–669.

Clayton DA, Mesches MH, Alvarez E, Bickford PC, Browning MD. 2002. A hippocampal NR2B deficit can mimic age-related changes in long-termpotentiation and spatial learning in the Fischer 344 rat. *J Neurosci.* 22:3628–3637.

Clemens JA. 2000. Cerebral ischemia: gene activation, neuronal injury, and the protective role of antioxidants. *Free Radic Biol Med.* 28:1526–1531.

Coimbra C, Drake M, Boris-Moller F, Wieloch T. 1996. Long-lasting neuroprotective effect of postischemic hypothermia and treatment with an anti-inflammatory/antipyretic Drug. evidence for chronic encephalopathic processes following ischemia. *Stroke.* 27:1578–1585.

Connolly ES, Jr, Winfree CJ, Springer TA et al. 1996. Cerebral protection in homozygous null ICAM-1 Mice after middle cerebral artery occlusion. Role of neutrophil adhesion in the pathogenesis of stroke. *J Clin Invest.* 97:209–216.

Costa C, Zhao L, Shen Y et al. 2006. Role of complement component C5 in cerebral ischemia/reperfusion injury. *Brain Res.* 1100:142–151.

Cullen KM, Kócsi Z, Stone J. 2005. Pericapillary haemrich deposits: evidence for microhaemorrhages in aging human cerebral cortex. *J Cereb Blood Flow Metab.* 25:1656–1667.

Cutler SM, Vanlandingham JW, Stein DG. 2006. Tapered progesterone withdrawal promotes long-term recovery following brain trauma. *Exp Neurol.* 200:378–385.

Daniels M, Brown DR. 2001. Astrocytes regulate N-Methyl-D-Aspartate receptor subunit composition increasing neuronal sensitivity to excitotoxicity. *J Biol Chem.* 276:22446–22452.

Danton GH, Dietrich WD. 2003. Inflammatory mechanisms after ischemia and stroke. *J Neuropathol Exp Neurol.* 62:127–136.

Darsalia V, Heldmann U, Lindvall O, Kokaia Z. 2005. Stroke-induced neurogenesis in aged brain. *Stroke.* 36:1790–1795.

Dash PK, SA Mach, Moore AN. 2001. Enhanced neurogenesis in the rodent hippocampus following traumatic brain injury. *J Neurosci Res.* 63:313–319.

Dawson J, Miltz W, Mir AK, Wiessner C. 2003. Targeting monocyte chemoattractant protein-1 signalling in disease. *Expert Opin Ther Targets.* 7:35–48.

de Bilbao F, Arsenijevic D, Vallet P et al. 2004. Resistance to cerebral ischemic injury in UCP2 knockout mice: evidence for a role of UCP2 as a regulator of mitochondrial glutathione levels. *J Neurochem.* 89:1283–1292.

De Georgia MA, Krieger DW, Abou-Chebl A et al. 2004. cooling for acute ischemic brain damage (COOL AID): a feasibility trial of endovascular cooling. *Neurology.* 63:312–317.

De Simoni MG, Storini C, Barba M et al. 2003. Neuroprotection by complement (C1) inhibitor in mouse transient brain ischemia. *J Cereb Blood Flow Metab.* 23:232–239.

Deacon TW, P Pakzaban, Isacson O. 1994. The lateral ganglionic eminence is the origin of cells committed to striatal phenotypes: neural transplantation and developmental evidence. *Brain Res.* 668:211–219.

del Zoppo GJ, Schmid-Schonbein GW, Mori E, Copeland BR, Chang CM. 1991. Polymorphonuclear leukocytes occlude capillaries following middle cerebral artery occlusion and reperfusion in baboons. *Stroke.* 22:1276–1283.

del Zoppo GJ, Schmid-Schonbein GW, Mori E, Copeland BR, Chang CM. 1991. Polymorphonuclear leukocytes occlude capillaries following middle cerebral artery occlusion and reperfusion in baboons. *Stroke.* 22:1276–1283.

del Zoppo GJ, Milner R, Mabuchi T et al. 2007. Microglial activation and matrix protease generation during focal cerebral ischemia. *Stroke.* 38:646–651.

Deplanque D, Gele P, Petrault O et al. 2003. Peroxisome proliferator-activated receptor-alpha activation as a mechanism of preventive neuroprotection induced by chronic fenofibrate treatment. *J Neurosci.* 23:6264–6271.

Dhandapani KM, Mahesh VB, Brann DW. 2003. Astrocytes and brain function: implications for reproduction. *Exp Biol Med (Maywood).* 228:253–260.

Di Napoli M. 2001a. Early inflammatory response in ischemic stroke. *Thromb Res.* 103:261–264.

Di Napoli M. 2001b. Systemic complement activation in ischemic stroke. *Stroke.* 32:1443–1448.

Di Napoli M, Papa F, Bocola V. 2001. C-reactive protein in ischemic stroke: an independent prognostic factor. *Stroke.* 32:917–924.

Di Napoli M, Papa F. 2003a. NCX-4016 NicOx. *Curr Opin Investig Drugs.* 4:1126–1139.

Di Napoli M, Papa F. 2003b. The proteasome system and proteasome inhibitors in stroke: controlling the inflammatory response. *Curr Opin Investig Drugs.* 4:1333–1342.

Di Napoli M, Schwaninger M, Cappelli R et al. 2005. Evaluation of C-reactive protein measurement for assessing the risk and prognosis in ischemic stroke: a statement for health care professionals from the CRP pooling project members. *Stroke.* 36:1316–1329.

Dimitrijevic OB, Stamatovic SM, Keep RF, Andjelkovic AV. 2006. Effects of the chemokine CCL2 on blood-brain barrier permeability during ischemia-reperfusion injury. *J Cereb Blood Flow Metab.* 26:797–810.

Dore S, Otsuka T, Mito T et al. 2003. Neuronal overexpression of cyclooxygenase-2 increases cerebral infarction. *Ann Neurol.* 54:155–162.

Dorszewska J, Adamczewska-Goncerzewicz Z, Szczech J. 2004. Apoptotic proteins in the course of aging of central nervous system in the rat. *Respir Physiol Neurobiol.* 139:145–155.

Drapeau E, W Mayo, Aurousseau C, Le Moal M, Piazza P-V, Nora Abrous D. 2003. Spatial memory performances of aged rats in the water maze predict levels of hippocampal neurogenesis. *Proc Natl Acad Sci U S A.* 100:14385–14390.

Du Clos TW. 1996. The interaction of C-reactive protein and serum amyloid P component with nuclear antigens. *Mol Biol Rep.* 23:253–260.

Dubal DB, Rau SW, Shughrue PJ et al. 2006. Differential modulation of estrogen receptors (ERs) in ischemic brain injury: arole for ERalpha in estradiol-mediated protection against delayed cell death. *Endocrinology.* 147:3076–3084.

Dugan LL, Kim-Han JS. 2006. Hypoxic-ischemic brain injury and oxidative stress. In Siegel GJ, Albers RW, Brady ST, Price DL, ed. *Basic Neurochemistry: Molecular, Cellular and Medical Aspects.* AP: Elsevier. 559–573.

Durukan A, Tatlisumak T. 2007. Acute ischemic stroke: overview of major experimental rodent models, pathophysiology, and therapy of focal cerebral ischemia. *Pharmacol Biochem Behav.* 87:179–197.

Dziedzic T, Bartus S, Klimkowicz A, Motyl M, Slowik A, Szczudlik A. 2002. Intracerebral hemorrhage triggers interleukin-6 and interleukin-10 release in blood. *Stroke.* 33:2334–2335.

Ehrensperger E, Minuk J, Durcan L, Mackey A, Wolfson C, Fontaine AM, Cote R. 2005. Predictive value of soluble intercellular adhesion molecule-1 for risk of ischemic events in individuals with cerebrovascular disease. *Cerebrovasc Dis.* 20:456–462.

Elewa HF, Hilali H, Hess DC, Machado LS, Fagan SC. 2006. Minocycline for short-term neuroprotection. *Pharmacotherapy.* 26:515–521.

Eliasson MJ, Huang Z, Ferrante RJ et al. 1999. Neuronal nitric oxide synthase activation and peroxynitrite formation in ischemic stroke linked to neural damage. *J Neurosci.* 19:5910–5918.

Elneihoum AM, Falke P, Axelsson L, Lundberg E, Lindgarde F, Ohlsson K. 1996. Leukocyte activation detected by increased plasma levels of inflammatory mediators in patients with ischemic cerebrovascular diseases. *Stroke.* 27:1734–1738.

Emsley HC, Tyrrell PJ. 2002. Inflammation and infection in clinical stroke. *J Cereb Blood Flow Metab.* 22:1399–1419.

Emsley HC, Smith CJ, Gavin CM et al. 2003. An early and sustained peripheral inflammatory response in acute ischaemic stroke: relationships with infection and atherosclerosis. *J Neuroimmunol.* 139:93–101.

Emsley HC, Smith CJ, Georgiou RF et al. 2005. A randomised phase ii study of interleukin-1 receptor antagonist in acute stroke patients. *J Neurol Neurosurg Psychiatry.* 76:1366–1372.

Emsley HC, Smith CJ, Gavin CM et al. 2007. Clinical outcome following acute ischaemic stroke relates to both activation and autoregulatory inhibition of cytokine production. *BMC Neurol.* 7:5.

Endoh M, Maiese K, Wagner J. 1994. Expression of the inducible form of nitric oxide synthase by reactive astrocytes after transient global ischemia. *Brain Res.* 651:92–100.

Endres M, Laufs U, Liao JK, Moskowitz MA. 2004. Targeting ENOS for stroke protection. *Trends Neurosci.* 27:283–289.

Enlimomab AST. 2001. Use of anti-ICAM-1 therapy in ischemic stroke: results of the Enlimomab acute stroke trial. *Neurology.* 57:1428–1434.

Enwere E, T Shingo, Gregg C, Fujikawa H, Ohta S, Weiss S. 2004. Aging results in reduced epidermal growth factor receptor signaling, diminished olfactory neurogenesis, and deficits in fine olfactory discrimination. *J Neurosci.* 24:8354–8365.

Erecinska M, Silver IA. 1989. ATP and brain function. *J Cereb Blood Flow Metab.* 9:2–19.

Eriksson PS, E Perfilieva, Bjork-Eriksson T et al. 1998. Neurogenesis in the adult human hippocampus. *Nat Med.* 4:1313–1317.

Fassbender K, Rossol S, Kammer T et al. 1994. Proinflammatory cytokines in serum of patients with acute cerebral ischemia: kinetics of secretion and relation to the extent of brain damage and outcome of disease. *J Neurol Sci.* 122:135–139.

Fehsel K, Kolb-Bachofen V, Kolb H. 1991. Analysis of TNF alpha-induced DNA strand breaks at the single cell level. *Am J Pathol.* 139:251–254.

Fernandez EJ, Lolis E. 2002. Structure, function, and inhibition of chemokines. *Annu Rev Pharmacol Toxicol.* 42:469–499.

Feuerstein G, Wang X, Barone FC. 1998. Cytokines in brain ischemia—the role of TNF alpha. *Cell Mol Neurobiol.* 18:695–701.

Florio P, Gazzolo D, Luisi S, Petraglia F. 2007. Activin A in brain injury. *Adv Clin Chem.* 43:117–130.

Floyd RA, Hensley K. 2000. Nitrone inhibition of age-associated oxidative damage. *Ann N Y Acad Sci.* 899:222–237.

Forster C, Clark HB, Ross ME, Iadecola C. 1999. Inducible nitric oxide synthase expression in human cerebral infarcts. *Acta Neuropathol (Berl).* 97:215–220.

Fowler JC. 1990. Adenosine antagonists alter the synaptic response to in vitro ischemia in the rat hippocampus. *Brain Res.* 509:331–334.

Fowler JC, Gervitz LM, Hamilton ME, Walker JA. 2003. Systemic hypoxia and the depression of synaptic transmission in rat hippocampus after carotid artery occlusion. *J Physiol.* 550:961–972.

Franklin A, Parmentier-Batteur S, Walter L, Greenberg DA, Stella N. 2003. Palmitoylethanolamide increases after focal cerebral ischemia and potentiates microglial cell motility. *J Neurosci.* 23:7767–7775.

Frijns CJ, Kappelle LJ. 2002. Inflammatory cell adhesion molecules in ischemic cerebrovascular disease. *Stroke.* 33:2115–2122.

Frisen J, Johansson CB, Torok C, Risling M, Lendahl U. 1995. Rapid, widespread, and longlasting induction of nestin contributes to the generation of glial scar tissue after CNS injury. *J Cell Biol.* 131:453–464.

Garcia JH, Liu KF, Yoshida Y, Lian J, Chen S, del Zoppo GJ. 1994. Influx of leukocytes and platelets in an evolving brain infarct (Wistar rat). *Am J Pathol.* 144:188–199.

Garcia JH, Liu KF, Relton JK. 1995. Interleukin-1 receptor antagonist decreases the number of necrotic neurons in rats with middle cerebral artery occlusion. *Am J Pathol.* 147:1477–1486.

Gendron TF, Brunette E, Tauskela JS, Morley P. 2005. The dual role of prostaglandin e(2) in excitotoxicity and preconditioning-induced neuroprotection. *Eur J Pharmacol.* 517:17–27.

Gerzanich V, Ivanova S, Simard JM. 2003. Early pathophysiological changes in cerebral vessels predisposing to stroke. *Clin Hemorheol Microcirc.* 29:291–294.

Ginis I, Jaiswal R, Klimanis D, Liu J, Greenspon J, Hallenbeck JM. 2002. TNF-alpha-induced tolerance to ischemic injury involves differential control of NF-KappaB transactivation: the role of NFkappaB association with P300 adaptor. *J Cereb Blood Flow Metab.* 22:142–152.

Ginsberg MD, Busto R. 1998. Combating hyperthermia in acute stroke: a significant clinical concern. *Stroke.* 29:529–534.

Ginsberg MD. 2007. Life after cerovive: a personal perspective on ischemic neuroprotection in the post-NXY-059 Era. *Stroke.* 38:1967–1972.

Godoy D, Boccio A, Hugo N. 2002. Systemic inflammatory response syndrome and primary of spontaneous intracerebral haemorrhage. *Rev Neurol.* 35:1101–1105.

Gonzalez-Scarano F, Baltuch G. 1999. Microglia as mediators of inflammatory and degenerative diseases. *Annu Rev Neurosci.* 22:219–240.

Gottschall PE, Yu X, Bing B. 1995. Increased production of gelatinase B (matrix metalloproteinase-9) and Interleukin-6 by activated rat microglia in culture. *J Neurosci Res.* 42:335–342.

Gould E, A Beylin, Tanapat P, Reeves A, Shors TJ. 1999. Learning enhances adult neurogenesis in the hippocampal formation. *Nat Neurosci.* 2:260–265.

Gozal D, Row BW, Kheirandish L et al. 2003. Increased susceptibility to intermittent hypoxia in aging rats: changes in proteasomal activity, neuronal apoptosis and spatial function. *J Neurochem.* 86:1545–1552

Grady CL, Craik FI. 2000. Changes in memory processing with age. *Curr Opin Neurobiol.* 10:224–231.

Green AR, Ashwood T, Odergren T, Jackson DM. 2003. Nitrones as neuroprotective agents in cerebral ischemia, with particular reference to NXY-059. *Pharmacol Ther.* 100:195–214.

Haag P, Schneider T, Schabitz W, Hacke W. 2000. Effect of Propentofylline (HWA 285) on focal ischemia in rats: effect of treatment and posttreatment duration on infarct size. *J Neurol Sci.* 175:52–56.

Hajdu MA, Heistad DD, Siems JE, Baumbach GL. 1990. Effects of aging on mechanics and composition of cerebral arterioles in rats. *Circ Res.* 66:1747–1754.

Hallenbeck JM. 2002. The many faces of tumor necrosis factor in stroke. *Nat Med.* 8:1363–1368.

Han HS, Yenari MA. 2003. Cellular targets of brain inflammation in stroke. *Curr Opin Investig Drugs.* 4:522–529.

Han HS, Karabiyikoglu M, Kelly S, Sobel RA, Yenari MA. 2003. Mild hypothermia inhibits Nuclear Factor-KappaB translocation in experimental stroke. *J Cereb Blood Flow Metab.* 23:589–598.

Haqqani AS, Nesic M, Preston E, Baumann E, Kelly J, Stanimirovic D. 2005. Characterization of vascular protein expression patterns in cerebral ischemia/reperfusion using laser capture microdissection and ICAT-NanoLC-MS/MS. *FASEB J.* 19:1809–1821.

Hara H, Huang PL, Panahian N, Fishman MC, Moskowitz MA. 1996. Reduced brain edema and infarction volume in mice lacking the neuronal isoform of nitric oxide synthase after transient MCA occlusion. *J Cereb Blood Flow Metab.* 16:605–611.

Haring HP, Berg EL, Tsurushita N, Tagaya M, del Zoppo GJ. 1996. E-selectin appears in nonischemic tissue during experimental focal cerebral ischemia. *Stroke.* 27:1386–1391.

Hartl R, Schurer L, Schmid-Schonbein GW, del Zoppo GJ. 1996. Experimental antileukocyte interventions in cerebral ischemia. *J Cereb Blood Flow Metab.* 16:1108–1119.

Hattiangady B, AK Shetty. 2008. Aging does not alter the number or phenotype of putative stem/progenitor cells in the neurogenic region of the hippocampus. *Neurobiol Aging.* 29:129–147. Epub 2006 Nov 7.

He Z, Crook JE, Meschia JF, Brott TG, Dickson DW, McKinney M. 2005. Aging blunts ischemic-preconditioning-induced neuroprotection following transient global ischemia in rats *Curr Neurovasc Res.* 2:365–374.

Heo JH, Lucero J, Abumiya T, Koziol JA, Copeland BR, del Zoppo GJ. 1999. Matrix metalloproteinases increase very early during experimental focal cerebral ischemia. *J Cereb Blood Flow Metab.* 19:624–633.

Herrera DG, AG Yague, Johnsen-Soriano M, Romero FJ, Garcia-Verdugo JM. 2003. Selective impairment of hippocampal neurogenesis by chronic alcoholism: protective effects of an antioxidant. *Proc Natl Acad Sci U S A.* 100:7919–7924.

Herrmann O, Tarabin V, Suzuki S et al. 2003. Regulation of body temperature and neuroprotection by endogenous Interleukin-6 in cerebral ischemia. *J Cereb Blood Flow Metab.* 23:406–415.

Hess DC, Hill WD, Carroll JE, Borlongan CV. 2004. Do bone marrow cells generate neurons? *Arch Neurol.* 61:483–485

Hiona A, Leeuwenburgh C. 2004. Effects of age and caloric restriction on brain neuronal cell death/survival. *Ann N Y Acad Sci.* 1019:96–105.

Hoane MR, Lasley LA, Akstulewicz SL. 2004. Middle age increases tissue vulnerability and impairs sensorimotor and cognitive recovery following traumatic brain injury in the rat. *Behav Brain Res.* 153:189–197.

Holley JE, Gveric D, Newcombe J, Cuzner ML, Gutowski NJ. (2003) Astrocyte characterization in the multiple sclerosis glial scar. *Neuropathol Appl Neurobiol.* 29:434–444.

Hossmann KA. 2006. Pathophysiology and therapy of experimental stroke. *Cell Mol Neurobiol.* 26:1057–1083.

Hu J, Van den Steen PE, Sang QX, Opdenakker G. 2007. Matrix metalloproteinase inhibitors as therapy for inflammatory and vascular diseases. *Nat Rev Drug Discov.* 6:480–498.

Huang J, Kim LJ, Mealey R et al. 1999. Neuronal protection in stroke by an SLex-glycosylated complement inhibitory protein. *Science.* 285:595–599.

Huang J, Upadhyay UM, Tamargo RJ. 2006. Inflammation in stroke and focal cerebral ischemia. *Surg Neurol.* 66:232–245.

Huang Z, Huang PL, Ma J et al. 1996. Enlarged infarcts in endothelial nitric oxide synthase knockout mice are attenuated by Nitro-L-Arginine. *J Cereb Blood Flow Metab.* 16:981–987.

Iadecola C, Zhang F, Xu S, Casey R, Ross ME. 1995. Inducible nitric oxide synthase gene expression in brain following cerebral ischemia. *J Cereb Blood Flow Metab.* 15:378–384.

Iadecola C, Forster C, Nogawa S, Clark HB, Ross ME. 1999. Cyclooxygenase-2 immunoreactivity in the human brain following cerebral ischemia. *Acta Neuropathol (Berl).* 98:9–14.

Iadecola C, Alexander M. 2001. Cerebral ischemia and inflammation. *Curr Opin Neurol.* 14:89–94.

Iadecola C, Niwa K, Nogawa S et al. 2001a. Reduced susceptibility to ischemic brain injury and N-methyl-D-aspartate-mediated neurotoxicity in cyclooxygenase-2-deficient mice. *Proc Natl Acad Sci U S A.* 98:1294–1299.

Iadecola C, Sugimoto K, Niwa K, Kazama K, Ross ME. 2001b. Increased susceptibility to ischemic brain injury in cyclooxygenase-1-deficient mice. *J Cereb Blood Flow Metab.* 21:1436–1441.

Ilie A, Ciocan D, Zagrean AM, Nita DA, Zagrean L, Moldovan M. 2006. Endogenous activation of adenosine A(1) receptors accelerates ischemic suppression of spontaneous electrocortical activity. *J Neurophysiol.* 96:2809–2814.

Irving EA, Bamford M. 2002. Role of mitogen- and stress-activated kinases in ischemic Injury. *J Cereb Blood Flow Metab.* 22:631–647.

Jain, RK. 2003. Molecular regulation of vessel maturation. *Nat Med.* 9:685–693.

Jander S, Schroeter M, Saleh A. 2007. Imaging inflammation in acute brain ischemia. *Stroke.* 38:642–645.

Jialal I, Devaraj S, Venugopal SK. 2004. C-reactive protein: risk marker or mediator in atherothrombosis? *Hypertension.* 44:6–11.

Jiang N, Moyle M, Soule HR, Rote WE, Chopp M. 1995. Neutrophil inhibitory factor is neuroprotective after focal ischemia in rats. *Ann Neurol.* 38:935–942.

Jin K, M Minami, Xie L et al. 2001. Neurogenesis in dentate subgranular zone and rostral subventricular zone after focal cerebral ischemia in the rat. *Proc Natl Acad Sc U S A.* 98:4710–4715.

Jin K, Y Sun, Xie L et al. 2003. Neurogenesis and aging: FGF-2 and HB-EGF restore neurogenesis in hippocampus and subventricular zone of aged mice. *Aging Cell.* 2:175–183.

Jin K, Minami M, Xie L et al. 2004. Ischemia-induced neurogenesis is preserved but reduced in the aged rodent brain. *Aging Cell.* 3:373–377.

Jin K, Wang X, Xie L et al. 2006. Evidence for stroke-induced neurogenesis in the human brain. *Proc Natl Acad Sci USA.* 103:13198–13202.

Jucker M, Walker LC, Schwab P et al. 1994. Age-related deposition of glia-associated fibrillar material in brains of C57BL/6 mice. *Neuroscience.* 60:875–889.

Justicia C, Martin A, Rojas S et al. 2005. Anti-VCAM-1 antibodies did not protect against ischemic damage either in rats or in mice. *J Cereb Blood Flow Metab.* 26:421–432.

Kalinowska A, Losy J. 2006. PECAM-1, a key player in neuroinflammation. *Eur J Neurol.* 13:1284–1290.

Kariko K, Weissman D, Welsh FA. 2004. Inhibition of Toll-like receptor and cytokine signaling—a unifying theme in ischemic tolerance. *J Cereb Blood Flow Metab.* 24:1288–1304.

Karin M, Yamamoto Y, Wang QM. 2004. The IKK NF-Kappa B system: a treasure trove for drug development. *Nat Rev Drug Discov.* 3:17–26.

Kato H, Kogure K, Liu XH, Araki T, Itoyama Y. 1996. Progressive expression of immunomolecules on activated microglia and invading leukocytes following focal cerebral ischemia in the rat. *Brain Res.* 734:203–212.

Kawano T, Anrather J, Zhou P et al. 2006. Prostaglandin E2 EP1 receptors: downstream effectors of COX-2 neurotoxicity. *Nat Med.* 12:225–229.

Kee N J, E Preston, Woittowicz JM. 2001. Enhanced neurogenesis after transient global ischemia in the dentate gyrus of the rat. *Exp Brain Res.* 136:313–320.

Kelly KM, Jukkola PI, Kharamov EA et al. 2006. Long-term video-EEG recordings following transient unilateral middle cerebral and common carotid artery occlusion in Long-Evans rats. *Exp Neurol.* 201:495–506.

Kelly S, Bliss T M, Shah A K et al. 2004. Transplanted human fetal neural stem cells survive, migrate, and differentiate in ischemic rat cerebral cortex. *Proc Natl Acad Sci U S A.* 101:11839–11844.

Kempermann G, HG Kuhn, Gage FH. 1997. More hippocampal neurons in adult mice living in an enriched environment. *Nature.* 386:493–495.

Kempermann G, HG Kuhn, Gage FH. 1998. Experience-induced neurogenesis in the senescent dentate gyrus. *J Neurosci.* 18:3206–3212.

Kempermann G, D Gast, Gage FH. 2002. Neuroplasticity in old age: sustained fivefold induction of hippocampal neurogenesis by long-term environmental enrichment. *Ann Neurol.* 52:135–143.

Kempermann G, Gast D, Kronenberg G, Yamaguchi M, Gage FH. 2003. Early determination and long-term persistence of adult-generated new neurons in the hippocampus of mice. *Development.* 130:391–399.

Khaja AM, Grotta JC. 2007. Established treatments for acute ischaemic stroke. *Lancet.* 369:319–330.

Khan M, Sekhon B, Giri S et al. 2005. S-nitrosoglutathione reduces inflammation and protects brain against focal cerebral ischemia in a rat model of experimental stroke. *J Cereb Blood Flow Metab.* 25:177–192.

Khan M, Jatana M, Elango C, Paintlia AS, Singh AK, Singh I. 2006. Cerebrovascular protection by various nitric oxide donors in rats after experimental stroke. *Nitric Oxide.* 15:114–124.

Kim JB, Piao CS, Lee KW et al. 2004. Delayed genomic responses to transient middle cerebral artery occlusion in the rat. *J Neurochem.* 89:1271–1282.

Kim JB, Yu Y M, Kim S W, Lee J K. 2005. Anti-inflammatory mechanism is involved in ethyl pyruvate-mediated efficacious neuroprotection in the postischemic brain. *Brain Res.* 1060:188–192.

Kim JS, Gautam S C, Chopp M et al. 1995. Expression of monocyte chemoattractant protein-1 and macrophage inflammatory protein-1 after focal cerebral ischemia in the rat. *J Neuroimmunol.* 56:127–134.

Kirino T, Tsujita Y, Tamura A. 1991. Induced tolerance to ischemia in gerbil hippocampal neurons. *J Cereb Blood Flow Metab.* 11:299–307.

Kitagawa K, Matsumoto M, Mabuchi T et al. 1998. Deficiency of intercellular adhesion molecule 1 attenuates microcirculatory disturbance and infarction size in focal cerebral ischemia. *J Cereb Blood Flow Metab.* 18:1336–1345.

Kochanek PM, Hallenbeck JM. 1992. Polymorphonuclear leukocytes and monocytes/macrophages in the pathogenesis of cerebral ischemia and stroke. *Stroke.* 23:1367–1379.

Koistinaho M, Kettunen MI, Holtzman DM, Kauppinen RA, Higgins LS, Koistinaho J. 2002. Expression of human apolipoprotein E downregulates amyloid precursor protein-induced ischemic susceptibility. *Stroke.* 33:1905–1910.

Komitova M, E Perfilieva Mattsson B, Eriksson PS, Johansson BB. 2002. Effects of cortical ischemia and postischemic environmental enrichment on hippocampal cell genesis and differentiation in the adult rat. *J Cereb Blood Flow Metab.* 22:852–860.

Kostulas N, Kivisakk P, Huang Y, Matusevicius D, Kostulas V, Link H. 1998. Ischemic stroke is associated with a systemic increase of blood mononuclear cells expressing interleukin-8 MRNA. *Stroke.* 29:462–466.

Kostulas N, Pelidou S H, Kivisakk P, Kostulas V, Link H. 1999. Increased IL-1beta, IL-8, and IL-17 mRNA expression in blood mononuclear cells observed in a prospective ischemic stroke study. *Stroke.* 30:2174–2179.

Kouwenhoven M, Carlstrom C, Ozenci V, Link H. 2001. Matrix metalloproteinase and cytokine profiles in monocytes over the course of stroke. *J Clin Immunol.* 21:365–375.

Krams M, Lees KR, Hacke W, Grieve AP, Orgogozo JM, Ford GA. 2003. Acute Stroke Therapy by Inhibition of Neutrophils (ASTIN): an adaptive dose-response study of UK-279,276 in acute ischemic stroke. *Stroke.* 34:2543–2548.

Kuhn HG, Dickinson-Anson H, Gage FH. 1996. Neurogenesis in the dentate gyrus of the adult rat: age-related decrease of neuronal progenitor proliferation. *J Neurosci.* 16:2027–2033.

Kuhn HG, Winkler J, Kempermann G, Thal LJ, Gage FH. 1997. Epidermal growth factor and fibroblast growth factor-2 have different effects on neural progenitors in the adult rat brain. *J Neurosci.* 17:5820–5829.

Kuluz JW, Prado RHD, Zhao W, Dietrich WD, Watson B. 2007. New pediatric model of ischemic stroke in infant piglets by photothrombosis: acute changes in cerebral blood flow, microvasculature, and early histopathology. *Stroke.* 38:1932–1937.

Kuta AE, Baum LL. 1986. C-reactive protein is produced by a small number of normal human peripheral blood lymphocytes. *J Exp Med.* 164:321–326.

Lai AY, Todd KG. 2006a. Hypoxia-activated microglial mediators of neuronal survival are differentially regulated by tetracyclines. *Glia.* 53:809–816.

Lai AY, Todd KG. 2006b. Microglia in cerebral ischemia: molecular actions and interactions. *Can J Physiol Pharmacol.* 84:49–59.

Lambeth JD. 2004. NOX enzymes and the biology of reactive oxygen. *Nat Rev Immunol.* 4:181–189.

Lapchak PA, Araujo DM. 2001. Reducing bleeding complications after thrombolytic therapy for stroke: clinical potential of metalloproteinase inhibitors and spin trap agents. *CNS Drugs.* 15:819–829.

Lavine SD, Hofman FM, Zlokovic BV. 1998. Circulating antibody against tumor necrosis factor-alpha protects rat brain from reperfusion injury. *J Cereb Blood Flow Metab.* 18:52–58.

Lee JC, Cho GS, Choi BO et al. 2006. Intracerebral hemorrhage-induced brain injury is aggravated in senescence-accelerated prone mice. *Stroke.* 37:216–222.

Lee JK, Park MS, Kim YS et al. 2007. Photochemically induced cerebral ischemia in a mouse model. *Surg Neurol.* 67:620–625.

Lee MY, Kuan YH, Chen HY et al. 2007. Intravenous administration of melatonin reduces the intracerebral cellular inflammatory response following transient focal cerebral ischemia in rats. *J Pineal Res.* 42:297–309.

Lehrmann E, Christensen T, Zimmer J, Diemer NH, Finsen B. 1997. Microglial and macrophage reactions mark progressive changes and define the penumbra in the rat neocortex and striatum after transient middle cerebral artery occlusion. *J Comp Neurol.* 386:461–476.

Lehrmann E, Kiefer R, Christensen T et al. 1998. Microglia and macrophages are major sources of locally produced transforming growth factor-beta1 after transient middle cerebral artery occlusion in rats. *Glia.* 24:437–448.

Leira R, Rodriguez-Yanez M, Castellanos M et al. 2006. Hyperthermia is a surrogate marker of inflammation-mediated cause of brain damage in acute ischaemic stroke. *J Intern Med.* 260:343–349.

Lewington S, Clarke R, Qizilbash N, Peto R, Collins R. 2002. Age-specific relevance of usual blood pressure to vascular mortality: a meta-analysis of individual data for one million adults in 61 prospective studies. *Lancet.* 360:1903–1913.

Li GZ, Zhong D, Yang LM et al. 2005. Expression of Interleukin-17 in ischemic brain tissue. *Scand J Immunol.* 62:481–486.

Li S, Zheng J, Carmichael ST. 2006. Increased oxidative protein and DNA damage but decreased stress response in the aged brain following experimental stroke. *Neurobiology of Disease.* 18:432–440.

Li WW, Penderis J, Zhao C, Schumacher M, Franklin RJ. 2006. Females remyelinate more efficiently than males following demyelination in the aged but not young adult CNS. *Exp Neurol.* 202:250–254.

Li Y, Chopp M. 1999. Temporal profile of nestin expression after focal cerebral ischemia in adult rat. *Brain Res.* 14:1–10.

Lin CH, Cheng FC, Lu YZ, Chu LF, Wang CH, Hsueh CM. 2006a. Protection of ischemic brain cells is dependent on astrocyte-derived growth factors and their receptors. *Exp Neurol.* 201:225–233.

Lin TN, Cheung WM, Wu JS et al. 2006b. 15d-Prostaglandin J2 protects brain from ischemia-reperfusion injury. *Arterioscler Thromb Vasc Biol.* 26:481–487.

Lindner MD, Gribkoff VK, Donlan NA, Jones TA. 2003. Long-lasting functional disabilities in middle-aged rats with small cerebral infarcts. *J Neurosci.* 23:10913–10922.

Lindsberg PJ, Carpen O, Paetau A, Karjalainen-Lindsberg ML, Kaste M. 1996a. Endothelial ICAM-1 expression associated with inflammatory cell response in human ischemic stroke. *Circulation.* 94:939–945.

Lindsberg PJ, Ohman J, Lehto T et al. 1996b. Complement activation in the central nervous system following blood-brain barrier damage in man. *Ann Neurol.* 40:587–596.

Lipton P. 1999. Ischemic cell death in brain neurons. *Physiol Rev.* 79:1431–1568.

Liu J, K Solway, Messing RO, Sharp FR. 1998. Increased neurogenesis in the dentate gyrus after transient global ischemia in gerbils. *J Neurosci.* 18:7768–7778.

Liu R, Wang X, Liu Q, Yang SH, Simpkins JW. 2007. Dose dependence and therapeutic window for the neuroprotective effects of 17beta-estradiol when administered after cerebral ischemia. *Neurosci Lett.* 415:237–241.

Liu T, McDonnell PC, Young PR et al. 1993a. Interleukin-1 Beta MRNA expression in ischemic rat cortex. *Stroke.* 24:1746–1750.

Liu T, Young PR, McDonnell PC, White RF, Barone FC, Feuerstein GZ. 1993b. Cytokine-induced neutrophil chemoattractant MRNA expressed in cerebral ischemia. *Neurosci Lett.* 164:125–128.

Liu T, Clark RK, McDonnell PC et al. 1994. Tumor necrosis factor-alpha expression in ischemic neurons. *Stroke.* 25:1481–1488.

Losy J, Zaremba J. 2001. Monocyte chemoattractant protein-1 is increased in the cerebrospinal fluid of patients with ischemic stroke. *Stroke.* 32:2695–2696.

Lovering F, Zhang Y. 2005. Therapeutic potential of TACE inhibitors in stroke. *Curr Drug Targets CNS Neurol Disord.* 4:161–168.

Lu MXC, Williams AJ, Tortella FC. 2001. Quantitative electroencephalography spectral analysis and topographic mapping in a rat model of middle cerebral artery occlusion. *Neuropathology and Applied Neurobiology.* 27:481–495.

Lu XC, Williams AJ, Yao C et al. 2004. Microarray analysis of acute and delayed gene expression profile in rats after focal ischemic brain injury and reperfusion. *J Neurosci Res.* 77:843–857.

Lu YZ, Lin CH, Cheng FC, Hsueh CM. 2005. Molecular mechanisms responsible for microglia-derived protection of sprague-dawley rat brain cells during in vitro ischemia. *Neurosci Lett.* 373:159–164.

Lucius R, Sievers J. 1996. Postnatal retinal ganglion cells in vitro: protection against reactive oxygen species (ROS)-induced axonal degeneration by cocultured astrocytes. *Brain Res.* 743:65–62.

Luo J, SB Daniels, Lennington JB, Notti RQ, Conover JC. 2006. The aging neurogenic subventricular zone. *Aging Cell.* 5:139–152.

Luo JL, Kamata H, Karin M. 2005. The anti-death machinery in IKK/NF-KappaB signaling. *J Clin Immunol.* 25:541–550.

Luo Y, Yin W, Signore AP et al. 2006. Neuroprotection against focal ischemic brain injury by the peroxisome proliferator-activated receptor-gamma agonist rosiglitazone. *J Neurochem.* 97:435–448.

Lyden PD, Shuaib A, Lees KR et al. 2007. Safety and tolerability of NXY-059 for acute intracerebral hemorrhage: the CHANT Trial. *Stroke.* 38:2262–2269.

Lynch NJ, Willis CL, Nolan CC et al. 2004. Microglial activation and increased synthesis of complement component

C1q precedes blood-brain barrier dysfunction in rats. *Mol Immunol.* 40:709–716.

Macas J, Nern C, Plate KH, Momma S. 2006. Increased generation of neuronal progenitors after ischemic injury in the aged adult human forebrain. *J Neurosci.* 26:13114–13119.

Mackiewicz A, Schooltink H, Heinrich PC, Rose-John S. 1992. Complex of soluble human IL-6-receptor/ IL-6 up-regulates expression of acute-phase proteins. *J Immunol.* 149:2021–2027.

Manabe Y, Anrather J, Kawano T et al. 2004. Prostanoids, not reactive oxygen species, mediate COX-2-dependent neurotoxicity. *Ann Neurol.* 55:668–675.

Marchiori PE, Lino AM, Hirata MT, Carvalho NB, Brotto MW, Scaff M. 2006. Occurrence of nervous system involvement in SIRS. *J Neurol Sci.* 250:147–152.

Markakis EA, FH Gage. 1999. Adult-generated neurons in the dentate gyrus send axonal projections to field CA3 and are surrounded by synaptic vesicles. *J Comp Neurol.* 406:449–460.

Markus TM, Tsai SY, Bollnow MR et al. 2005. Recovery and brain reorganization after stroke in adult and aged rats. *Ann Neurol.* 58:950–953.

Martinez-Lara E, Canuelo AR, Siles E et al. 2005. Constitutive nitric oxide synthases are responsible for the nitric oxideproduction in the ischemic aged cerebral cortex. *Brain Res.* 1054:88–94.

Maslov AY, TA Barone, Plunkett RJ, Pruitt SC. 2004. Neural stem cell detection, characterization, and age-related changes in the subventricular zone of mice. *J Neurosci.* 24:1726–1733.

Matsuda T, Arakawa N, Takuma K et al. 2001. SEA0400, a novel and selective inhibitor of the Na+-Ca2+ exchanger, attenuates reperfusion injury in the in vitro and in vivo cerebral ischemic models. *J Pharmacol Exp Ther.* 298:249–256.

Matsumoto T, Ikeda K, Mukaida N et al. 1997. Prevention of cerebral edema and infarct in cerebral reperfusion injury by an antibody to interleukin-8. *Lab Invest.* 77:119–125.

Matsuo Y, Onodera H, Shiga Y et al. 1994. Role of cell adhesion molecules in brain injury after transient middle cerebral artery occlusion in the rat. *Brain Res.* 656:344–352.

Mattson MP, Cheng B, Baldwin SA et al. 1995. Brain injury and tumor necrosis factors induce calbindin D-28k in astrocytes: evidence for a cytoprotective response. *J Neurosci Res.* 42:357–370.

Mattson MP, Camandola S. 2001. NF-KappaB in neuronal plasticity and neurodegenerative disorders. *J Clin Invest.* 107:247–254.

McColl BW, Rothwell NJ, Allan SM. 2007. Systemic inflammatory stimulus potentiates the acute phase and CXC chemokine responses to experimental stroke and exacerbates brain damage via interleukin-1- and neutrophil-dependent mechanisms. *J Neurosci.* 27:4403–4412.

Meiner Z, Arber N, Liberman E, Leibovitz E, Seltzer D, Berliner S. 1997. Increased leukocyte adhesiveness/ aggregation in patients with recurrent TIA. *Acta Neurol Scand.* 96:123–126.

Merkle FT, A Alvarez-Buylla. 2006. Neural stem cells in mammalian development. *Curr Opin Cell Biol.* 18:704–709.

Mesches MH, Gemma C, Veng LM et al. 2004. Sulindac improves memory and increases NMDA receptor subunits in aged Fischer 344 rats. *Neurobiol Aging.* 25:315–324.

Milne SA, McGregor AL, McCulloch J, Sharkey J. 2005. Increased expression of macrophage receptor with collagenous structure (MARCO) in mouse cortex following middle cerebral artery occlusion. *Neurosci Lett.* 383:58–62.

Min KJ, Yang MS, Kim SU, Jou I, Joe EH. 2006. Astrocytes induce hemeoxygenase-1 expression in microglia: a feasible mechanism for preventing excessive brain inflammation. *J Neurosci.* 26:1880–1887.

Mocco J, Mack WJ, Ducruet AF et al. 2006a. Complement component C3 mediates inflammatory injury following focal cerebral ischemia. *Circ Res.* 99:209–217.

Mocco J, Sughrue ME, Ducruet AF, Komotar RJ, Sosunov SA, Connolly ES, Jr. 2006b. The complement system: a potential target for stroke therapy. *Adv Exp Med Biol.* 586:189–201.

Mocco J, Wilson DA, Komotar RJ et al. 2006c. Alterations in plasma complement levels after human ischemic stroke. *Neurosurgery.* 59:28–33.

Moldovan M, Munteanu AM, Nita DAl, Popa DP, Spulber St, Zagrean L. 2000. Ischemic electrocortical suppression— an active mechanism? *J Med Biochem.* 4:103–111.

Molofsky AV, SG Slutsky, Joseph NM et al. 2006. Increasing p16INK4a expression decreases forebrain progenitors and neurogenesis during ageing. *Nature.* 443:448–452.

Montaner J, Alvarez-Sabin J, Molina C et al. 2001. Matrix metalloproteinase expression after human cardioembolic stroke: temporal profile and relation to neurological impairment. *Stroke.* 32:1759–1766.

Montaner J, Molina CA, Monasterio J et al. 2003a. Matrix metalloproteinase-9 pretreatment level predicts intracranial hemorrhagic complications after thrombolysis in human stroke. *Circulation.* 107:598–603.

Montaner J, Rovira A, Molina CA et al. 2003b. Plasmatic level of neuroinflammatory markers predict the extent of diffusion-weighted image lesions in hyperacute stroke. *J Cereb Blood Flow Metab.* 23:1403–1407.

Montaron MF, KG Petry, Rodriguez JJ et al. 1999. Adrenalectomy increases neurogenesis but not PSA-NCAM expression in aged dentate gyrus. *Eur J Neurosci.* 11:1479–1485.

Montaron MF, Drapeau E, Dupret D et al. 2006. Lifelong corticosterone level determines age-related decline in neurogenesis and memory. *Neurobiol Aging.* 27:645–654.

Montfort MJ, Olivares CR, Mulcahy JM, Fleming WH. 2002. Adult blood vessels restore host hematopoiesis following lethal irradiation. *Exp Hematol.* 30:950–956.

Morikawa E, Zhang SM, Seko Y, Toyoda T, Kirino T. 1996. Treatment of focal cerebral ischemia with synthetic oligopeptide corresponding to lectin domain of selectin. *Stroke.* 27:951–955.

Moyanova SG, Kortenska LV, Rumiana-Mitreva RG, Pashova VD, Ngomba RT, Nicoletti F. 2007. Multimodal assessment of neuroprotection applied to the use of MK-801 in the endothelin-1 model of transient focal brain ischemia. *Brain research*. 1153:58–67.

Muckart DJ, Bhagwanjee S. 1997. American College of Chest Physicians/Society of Critical Care Medicine Consensus Conference definitions of the systemic inflammatory response syndrome and allied disorders in relation to critically injured patients. *Crit Care Med*. 25:1789–1795.

Muir KW, Tyrrell P, Sattar N, Warburton E. 2007. Inflammation and ischaemic stroke. *Curr Opin Neurol*. 20:334–342.

Mulcahy NJ, Ross J, Rothwell NJ, Loddick SA. 2003. Delayed administration of interleukin-1 receptor antagonist protects against transient cerebral ischaemia in the rat. *Br J Pharmacol*. 140:471–476.

Mulholland PJ, Stepanyan TD, Self RL et al. 2005. Cortico-sterone and dexamethasone potentiate cytotoxicity associated with oxygen-glucose deprivation in organo-typic cerebellar slice cultures. *Neuroscience*. 136:259–267.

Murphy EJ, Owada Y, Kitanaka N, Kondo H, Glatz JF. 2005. Brain arachidonic acid incorporation is decreased in heart fatty acid binding protein gene-ablated mice. *Biochemistry*. 44:6350–6360.

Nadareishvili ZG, Li H, Wright V et al. 2004. Elevated pro-inflammatory CD4+. *Neurology*. 63:1446–1451.

Nakatomi H, T Kuriu, Okabe S et al. 2002. Regeneration of hippocampal pyramidal neurons after ischemic brain injury by recruitment of endogenous neural progeni-tors. *Cell*. 110:429–441.

Nakayama H, Jørgensen HS, Raaschou HO, Olsen TS. 1994. The influence of age on stroke outcome. The Copenhagen Stroke Study. *Stroke*. 25:808–813.

Napolitano LM, Ferrer T, McCarter RJ Jr, Scalea TM. 2000. Systemic inflammatory response syndrome score at admission independently predicts mortality and length of stay in trauma patients. *J Trauma*. 49:647–652.

Navarro Ana, Carmen Gomez, Maria-Jesus Sanchez-Pino et al. 2005. Vitamin E at high doses improves survival, neurological performance, and brain mitochondrial function in aging male mice. *Am J Physiol Regul Integr Comp Physiol*. 289:1392–1399.

Newman MB, Willing AE, Manresa JJ, Davis-Sanberg C, Sanberg PR. 2005. Stroke-induced migration of human umbilical cord blood cells: time course and cytokines. *Stem Cells Dev*. 14:576–586.

Ng YK, Ling EA. 2001. Microglial reaction in focal cerebral ischaemia induced by intra-carotid homologous clot injection. *Histol Histopathol*. 16:167–174.

Nishimura I, Uetsuki T, Dani SU et al. 1998. Interaction between inducible nitric oxide synthase and cyclo-oxygenase-2 after cerebral ischemia. *Proc Natl Acad Sci U S A*. 95:10966–10971.

Nogawa S, Zhang F, Ross ME, Iadecola C. 1997. Cyclo-oxygenase-2 gene expression in neurons contributes to ischemic brain damage. *J Neurosci*. 17:2746–2755.

Noor R, Wang CX, Shuaib A. 2003. Effects of hyperthermia on infarct volume in focal embolic model of cerebral ischemia in rats. *Neurosci Lett*. 349:130–132.

Noto D, Barbagallo CM, Cavera G et al. 2001. Leukocyte count, diabetes mellitus and age are strong predictors

of stroke in a rural population in southern Italy: an 8-year follow-up. *Atherosclerosis*. 157:225–231.

Offner H, Subramanian S, Parker SM, Afentoulis ME, Vandenbark AA, Hurn PD. 2006. Experimental stroke induces massive, rapid activation of the peripheral immune system. *J Cereb Blood Flow Metab*. 26:654–665.

Okada Y, Copeland BR, Mori E, Tung MM, Thomas WS, del Zoppo GJ. 1994. P-selectin and Intercellular adhesion molecule-1 expression after focal brain ischemia and reperfusion. *Stroke*. 25:202–211.

Olariu A, KM Cleaver Cameron HA. 2007. Decreased neu-rogenesis in aged rats results from loss of granule cell precursors without lengthening of the cell cycle. *J Comp Neurol*. 501:659–67.

O'Neill MJ, Murray TK, McCarty DR et al. 2000. ARL 17477, a Selective nitric oxide synthase inhibitor, with neuro-protective effects in animal models of global and focal cerebral ischaemia. *Brain Res*. 871:234–244.

Ooboshi H, Ibayashi S, Heistad DD, Fujishima M. 2000. Adenovirus-mediated gene transfer to cerebral circu-lation. *Mech Ageing Dev*. 116:95–101.

Oster-Granite ML, McPhie DL, Greenan J, Neve RL. 1996. Age-dependent neuronal and synaptic degeneration in mice transgenic for the C terminus of the amyloid pre-cursor protein. *J Neurosci*. 16:6732–6741.

Pan J, Konstas AA, Bateman B, Ortolano GA, Pile-Spellman J. 2007. Reperfusion injury following cerebral ische-mia: pathophysiology, mr imaging, and potential ther-apies. *Neuroradiology*. 49:93–102.

Pang L, Ye W, Che XM, Roessler BJ, Betz AL, Yang GY. 2001. Reduction of inflammatory response in the mouse brain with adenoviral-mediated transforming growth factor-Ss1 expression. *Stroke*. 32:544–552.

Panickar KS, Norenberg MD. 2005. Astrocytes in cerebral ischemic injury: morphological and general consider-ations. *Glia*. 50:287–298.

Pantoni L, Sarti C, Inzitari D. 1998. Cytokines and cell adhesion molecules in cerebral ischemia: experimental bases and therapeutic perspectives. *Arterioscler Thromb Vasc Biol*. 18:503–513.

Parent JM, Yu TW, Leibowitz RT, Geschwind DH, Sloviter RS, Lowenstein DH. 1997. Dentate granule cell neu-rogenesis is increased by seizures and contributes to aberrant network reorganization in the adult rat hip-pocampus. *J Neurosci*. 17:3727–3738.

Parent JM, Vexler ZS, Gong C, Derugin N, Ferriero DM. 2002. Rat forebrain neurogenesis and striatal neu-ron replacement after focal stroke. *Ann Neurol*. 52:802–813.

Paulson OB. 2002. Blood-brain barrier, brain metabolism and cerebral blood flow. *Eur. Neuropharmacol*. 12:495–501.

Pedersen ED, Waje-Andreassen U, Vedeler CA, Aamodt G, Mollnes TE. 2004. Systemic complement activa-tion following human acute ischaemic stroke. *Clin Exp Immunol*. 137:117–122.

Pekny M, Nilsson M. 2005. Astrocyte activation and reactive gliosis. *Glia*. 50:427–434.

Pekny M, Wilhelmsson U, Bogestal YR, Pekna M. 2007. The role of astrocytes and complement system in neural plasticity. *Int Rev Neurobiol*. 82:95–111.

Pelidou SH, Kostulas N, Matusevicius D, Kivisakk P, Kostulas V, Link H. 1999. High levels of IL-10 secreting cells are present in blood in cerebrovascular diseases. *Eur J Neurol.* 6:437–442.

Pepys MB, Hirschfield GM. 2003. C-reactive protein: a critical update. *J Clin Invest.* 111:1805–1812.

Pepys MB, Hirschfield GM, Tennent GA et al. 2006. Targeting C-reactive protein for the treatment of cardiovascular disease. *Nature.* 440:1217–1221.

Pereira MP, Hurtado O, Cardenas A et al. 2006. Rosiglitazone and 15-deoxy-delta12,14-prostaglandin J2 cause potent neuroprotection after experimental stroke through noncompletely overlapping mechanisms. *J Cereb Blood Flow Metab.* 26:218–229.

Perini F, Morra M, Alecci M, Galloni E, Marchi M, Toso V. 2001. Temporal profile of serum anti-inflammatory and pro-inflammatory interleukins in acute ischemic stroke patients. *Neurol Sci.* 22:289–296.

Perkins ND. 2000. The Rel/NF-Kappa B family: friend and foe. *Trends Biochem Sci.* 25:434–440.

Persson M, Brantefjord M, Hansson E, Ronnback L. 2005. Lipopolysaccharide increases microglial GLT-1 expression and glutamate uptake capacity in vitro by a mechanism dependent on TNF-alpha. *Glia.* 51:111–120.

Peters A. 2002. Structural changes that occur during normal aging of primate cerebral hemispheres. *Neurosci Biobehav Rev.* 26:733–741.

Peterson JT. 2004. Matrix metalloproteinase inhibitor development and the remodeling of drug discovery. *Heart Fail Rev.* 9:63–79.

Pinteaux E, Rothwell NJ, Boutin H. 2006. Neuroprotective actions of endogenous interleukin-1 receptor antagonist (IL-1ra) are mediated by glia. *Glia.* 53:551–556.

Plaschke K, Grant M, Weigand MA, Zuchner J, Martin E, Bardenheuer HJ. 2001. Neuromodulatory effect of propentofylline on rat brain under acute and long-term hypoperfusion. *Br J Pharmacol.* 133:107–116.

Polavarapu R, Gongora MC, Winkles JA, Yepes M. 2005. Tumor necrosis factor-like weak inducer of apoptosis increases the permeability of the neurovascular unit through nuclear factor-kappa B pathway activation. *J Neurosci.* 25:10094–10100.

Popa-Wagner A, Schroder E, Walker LC, Kessler Ch. 1998. Beta-amyloid precursor protein and ss-amyloid peptide immunoreactivity in the rat brain after middle cerebral artery occlusion: effect of age. *Stroke.* 29:2196–2202.

Popa-Wagner A, Schröder E, Schmoll H, Walker LC, Kessler Ch. 1999. Upregulation of MAP1B and MAP2 in the rat brain following middle cerebral artery occlusion: effect of age. *J Cereb Blood Flow Metab.* 19:425–434.

Popa-Wagner A, Dinca I, Suofu Y, Walker L, Kroemer H, Kessler C. 2006. Accelerated delimitation of the infarct zone by capillary-derived nestin-positive cells in aged rats. *Curr Neurovasc Res.* 3:3–13.

Popa-Wagner A, Badan I, Walker L, Groppa S, Patrana N, Kessler Ch. 2007. Accelerated infarct development, cytogenesis and apoptosis following transient cerebral ischemia in aged rats. *Acta Neuropathol Berlin.* 113:277–293.

Popa-Wagner A, Carmichael ST, Kokaia Z, Kessler Ch, Walker LC. 2007. The response of the aged brain to stroke: too much, too soon? *Curr Neurovasc Res.* 4:216–277.

Popa-Wagner A, Badan I, Walker L, Groppa S, Patrana N, Kessler C. 2007a. Accelerated infarct development, cytogenesis and apoptosis following transient cerebral ischemia in aged rats. *Acta Neuropathol (Berl).* 113:277–293.

Popa-Wagner A, Carmichael ST, Kokaia Z, Kessler C, Walker LC. 2007b. The response of the aged brain to stroke: too much, too soon? *Curr Neurovasc Res.* 4:216–227.

Potrovita I, Zhang W, Burkly L et al. 2004. Tumor necrosis factor-like weak inducer of apoptosis-induced neurodegeneration. *J Neurosci.* 24:8237–8244.

Pozzilli C, Lenzi GL, Argentino C et al. 1985. Peripheral white blood cell count in cerebral ischemic infarction. *Acta Neurol Scand.* 71:396–400.

Prasad KV, Ao Z, Yoon Y et al. 1997. CD27, a member of the tumor necrosis factor receptor family, induces apoptosis and binds to Siva, a proapoptotic protein. *Proc Natl Acad Sci U S A.* 94:6346–6351.

Prentice RL, Szatrowski TP, Kato H, Mason MW. 1982. Leukocyte counts and cerebrovascular disease. *J Chronic Dis.* 35:703–714.

Price CJ, Menon DK, Peters AM et al. 2004. Cerebral neutrophil recruitment, histology, and outcome in acute ischemic stroke: an imaging-based study. *Stroke.* 35:1659–1664.

Price CJ, Crinion J. 2005. The latest on functional imaging studies of aphasic stroke. *Curr Opin Neurol.* 18:429–434.

Price CJ, Wang D, Menon DK et al. 2006. Intrinsic activated microglia map to the peri-infarct zone in the subacute phase of ischemic stroke. *Stroke.* 37:1749–1753.

Priller J, Persons DA, Klett FF, Kempermann G, Kreutzberg GW, Dirnagl U. 2001. Neogenesis of cerebellar purkinje neurons from gene-marked bone marrow cells in vivo. *J Cell Biol.* 155:733–738.

Pulsinelli WA, Brierley JB. 1979. A new model of bilateral hemispheric ischemia in the unanesthetized rat. *Stroke.* 10:267–272.

Pulsinelli WA, Levy DE, Duffy TE. 1982. Regional cerebral blood flow and glucose metabolism following transient forebrain ischemia. *Ann Neurol.* 11:499–509.

Pulsinelli WA, Buchan AM. 1988. The four-vessel occlusion rat model: method for complete occlusion of vertebral arteries and control of collateral circulation (comments). *Stroke.* 19:913–914.

Pyo H, Yang MS, Jou I, Joe EH. 2003. Wortmannin enhances lipopolysaccharide-induced inducible nitric oxide synthase expression in microglia in the presence of astrocytes in rats. *Neurosci Lett.* 346:141–144.

Raber J, Y Fan, Matsumori Z et al. 2004. Irradiation attenuates neurogenesis and exacerbates ischemia-induced deficits. *Ann Neurol.* 55:381–389.

Raffin CN, Harrison M, Sick TJ, Rosenthal M. 1991. EEG suppression and anoxic depolarization: influences on cerebral oxygenation during ischemia. *J Cereb Blood Flow Metab.* 11:407–415.

Rallidis LS, Vikelis M, Panagiotakos DB et al. 2006. Inflammatory markers and in-hospital mortality in acute ischaemic stroke. *Atherosclerosis.* 189:193–197.

Rao AM, Hatcher JF, Kindy MS, Dempsey RJ. 1999. Arachidonic acid and leukotriene C4: role in transient cerebral ischemia of gerbils. *Neurochem Res.* 24:1225–1232.

Redon J, Cea-Calvo L. 2007. Blood pressure control and stroke mortality across populations. *Curr Hypertens Rep.* 9:440-441.

Reith J, Jorgensen HS, Pedersen P, Mez et al. 1996. Body temperature in acute stroke: relation to stroke severity, infarct size, mortality, and outcome. *Lancet.* 347:422–425.

Riddle DR, Sonntag WE, Lichtenwalner RJ. 2003. Microvascular plasticity in aging. *Ageing Res Rev.* 2:149–168.

Rochefort C, G Gheusi Vincent JD, Lledo PM. 2002. Enriched odor exposure increases the number of newborn neurons in the adult olfactory bulb and improves odor memory. *J Neurosci.* 22:2679–2689.

Rochester MA, Riedemann J, Hellawell GO, Brewster SF, Macaulay VM. 2005. Silencing of the IGF1R gene enhances sensitivity to DNA-damaging agents in both PTEN wild-type and mutant human prostate cancer. *Cancer Gene Ther.* 12:90–100.

Romanic AM, White RF, Arleth AJ, Ohlstein EH, Barone FC. 1998. Matrix metalloproteinase expression increases after cerebral focal ischemia in rats: inhibition of matrix metalloproteinase-9 reduces infarct Size. *Stroke.* 29:1020–1030.

Roos-Mattjus P, Vroman BT, Burtelow MA, Rauen M, Eapen AK, Karnitz LM. 2002. Genotoxin-induced Rad9-Husl-Rad1 (9-1-1) chromatin association is an early checkpoint signaling event. *J Biol Chem.* 277:43809–43812.

Rosen CL, Dinapoli VA, Nagamine T, Crocco T. 2005. Influence of age on stroke outcome following transient focal ischemia. *J Neurosurg.* 103:687–694.

Rosenblum WI, El-Sabban F. 1977. Effects of combined parenchymal and vascular injury on platelet aggregation in pial arterioles of living mice: evidence for release of aggregate-inhibiting materials. *Stroke.* 8:691–693.

Rost NS, Wolf PA, Kase CS et al. 2001. Plasma concentration of C-reactive protein and risk of ischemic stroke and transient ischemic attack: the Framingham study. *Stroke.* 32:2575–2579.

Rothoerl RD, Schebesch KM, Kubitza M, Woertgen C, Brawanski A, Pina AL. 2006. ICAM-1 and VCAM-1 expression following aneurysmal subarachnoid hemorrhage and their possible role in the pathophysiology of subsequent ischemic deficits. *Cerebrovasc Dis.* 22:143–149.

Rozovsky I, Wei M, Morgan TE, Finch CE. 2005. Reversible age impairments in neurite outgrowth by manipulations of astrocytic GFAP. *Neurobiol Aging* 26:705–715.

Rus H, Cudrici C, David S, Niculescu F. 2006. The complement system in central nervous system diseases. *Autoimmunity.* 39:395–402.

Rygg M, Uhlar CM, Thorn C et al. 2001. In vitro evaluation of an enhanced human serum amyloid A (SAA2) promoter-regulated soluble TNF receptor fusion protein for anti-inflammatory gene therapy. *Scand J Immunol.* 53:588–595.

Saas P, Boucraut J, Walker PR et al. 2000. TWEAK stimulation of astrocytes and the proinflammatory consequences. *Glia.* 32:102–107.

Sacco RL, Chong JY, Prabhakaran S, Elkind MS. 2007. Experimental treatments for acute ischemic stroke. *Lancet.* 369:331–341.

Sairanen T, Carpen O, Karjalainen-Lindsberg ML et al. 2001. Evolution of cerebral Tumor necrosis factor-alpha production during human ischemic stroke. *Stroke.* 32:1750–1758.

Sairanen TR, Lindsberg PJ, Brenner M, Siren AL. 1997. Global forebrain ischemia results in differential cellular expression of Interleukin-1beta (IL-1beta) and its receptor at MRNA and protein level. *J Cereb Blood Flow Metab.* 17:1107–1120.

Sanai N, AD Tramontin, Quinones-Hinojosa A et al. 2004. Unique astrocyte ribbon in adult human brain contains neural stem cells but lacks chain migration. *Nature.* 427:740–744.

Sanchez-Moreno C, Dashe JF, Scott T, Thaler D, Folstein MF, Martin A. 2004. Decreased levels of plasma Vitamin C and increased concentrations of inflammatory and oxidative stress markers after stroke. *Stroke.* 35:163–168.

Santos-Silva A, Rebelo I, Castro E et al. 2002. Erythrocyte damage and leukocyte activation in ischemic stroke. *Clin Chim Acta.* 320:29–35.

Savitz SI, Fisher M. 2007. Future of neuroprotection for acute stroke: in the aftermath of the SAINT Trials. *Ann Neurol.* 61:396–402.

Schafer MK, Schwaeble WJ, Post C et al. 2000. Complement C1q is dramatically up-regulated in brain microglia in response to transient global cerebral ischemia. *J Immunol.* 164:5446–5452.

Schilling M, Besselmann M, Muller M, Strecker JK, Ringelstein EB, Kiefer R. 2005. Predominant phagocytic activity of resident microglia over hematogenous macrophages following transient focal cerebral ischemia: an investigation using green fluorescent protein transgenic bone marrow chimeric mice. *Exp Neurol.* 196:290–297.

Schmedtje JF Jr., Ji YS, Liu WL, DuBois RN, Runge MS. 1997. Hypoxia induces cyclooxygenase-2 via the NF-KappaB P65 transcription factor in human vascular endothelial cells. *J Biol Chem.* 272:601–608.

Schroeter M, Jander S, Witte OW, Stoll G. 1994. Local immune responses in the rat cerebral cortex after middle cerebral artery occlusion. *J Neuroimmunol.* 55:195–203.

Schumacher HC, Khaw AV, Meyers PM, Gupta R, Higashida RT. 2004. Intracranial revascularization therapy: angioplasty and stenting. *Curr Treat Options Cardiovasc Med.* 6:193–198.

Schwab JM, Beschorner R, Meyermann R, Gozalan F, Schluesener HJ. 2002. Persistent accumulation of cyclooxygenase-1-expressing microglial cells and macrophages and transient upregulation by endothelium in human brain injury. *J Neurosurg.* 96:892–899.

Schwaninger M, Inta I, Herrmann O. 2006. NF-KappaB signalling in cerebral ischaemia. *Biochem Soc Trans.* 34:1291–1294.

Seki T, Arai Y. 1995. Age-related production of new granule cells in the adult dentate gyrus. *Neuroreport.* 6:2479–2482.

Seri B, Garcia-Verdugo JM, BS McEwen, A Alvarez-Buylla. 2001. Astrocytes give rise to new neurons in the adult mammalian hippocampus. *J Neurosci.* 21(18):7153–7160.

Seri B, Garcia-Verdugo JM, Collado-Morente L, McEwen BS, Alvarez-Buylla A. 2004. Cell types, lineage, and architecture of the germinal zone in the adult dentate gyrus. *J Comp Neurol.* 478:359–378.

Seshadri S, Beiser A, Kelly-Hayes M et al. 2006. The lifetime risk of stroke: estimates from the Framingham Study. *Stroke.* 37:345–350.

Shainkin-Kestenbaum R, Zimlichman S, Lis M et al. 1996. Effect of serum amyloid A, HDL-apolipoprotein, on endothelial cell proliferation. Implication of an enigmatic protein to atherosclerosis. *Biomed Pept Proteins Nucleic Acids.* 2:79–84.

Sharkey J, Ritchie IM, Kelly PAT. 1993. Perivascular microapplication of Endothelin-1: a new model of focal cerebral ischaemia in the rat. *J Cereb Blood Flow Metab.* 13:865–871.

Sharkey J, Butcher SP, Kelly JS. 1994. Endothelin-1 induced middle cerebral artery occlusion: pathological consequences and neuroprotective effects of MK801. *J Auton Nerv Syst.* 49:177–185.

Shetty AK, Hattiangady B, Shetty GA. 2005. Stem/progenitor cell proliferation factors FGF-2, IGF-1, and VEGF exhibit early decline during the course of aging in the hippocampus: role of astrocytes. *Glia.* 51:173–186.

Shimakura A, Kamanaka Y, Ikeda Y, Kondo K, Suzuki Y, Umemura K. 2000. Neutrophil elastase inhibition reduces cerebral ischemic damage in the middle cerebral artery occlusion. *Brain Res.* 858:55–60.

Shors TJ, G Miesegaes, Beylin A, Zhao MR, Rydel T, Gould E. 2001. Neurogenesis in the adult is involved in the formation of trace memories. *Nature.* 410:372–376.

Shuaib A, Lees KR, Lyden P et al. 2007. NXY-059 for the treatment of acute ischemic stroke. *N Engl J Med.* 357:562–571.

Simard JM, Kent TA, Chen M, Tarasov KV, Gerzanich V. 2007. Brain oedema in focal ischaemia: molecular pathophysiology and theoretical implications. *Lancet Neurol.* 6:258–268.

Simundic AM, Basic V, Topic E et al. 2004. Soluble adhesion molecules in acute ischemic stroke. *Clin Invest Med.* 27:86–92.

Slowik A, Turaj W, Pankiewicz J, Dziedzic T, Szermer P, Szczudlik A. 2002. Hypercortisolemia in acute stroke is related to the inflammatory response. *J Neurol Sci.* 196:27–32.

Smith CJ, Emsley HC, Gavin CM et al. 2004. Peak plasma Interleukin-6 and other peripheral markers of inflammation in the first week of ischaemic stroke correlate with brain infarct volume, stroke severity and long-term outcome. *BMC Neurol.* 4:2.

Smith M-L, Bendek G, Dalhgren N, Rosen I, Wieloch T, Siesjo BK. 1984. Models for studying long-term recovery following forebrain ischemia in the rat. 2. A 2-vessel occlusion model. *Acta Neurol. Scand.* 69:385–401.

Somjen GG. 2004. *Ions in the Brain- Normal function, Sezures, and Stroke.* New York: Oxford University Press.

Somogyvari-Vigh A, Reglodi D. 2004. Pituitary adenylate cyclase activating polypeptide: a potential neuroprotective peptide. *Curr Pharm Des.* 10:2861–2889.

Soriano SG, Lipton SA, Wang YF et al. 1996. Intercellular adhesion molecule-1-deficient mice are less susceptible to cerebral ischemia-reperfusion injury. *Ann Neurol.* 39:618–624.

Sornas R, Ostlund H, Muller R. 1972. Cerebrospinal fluid cytology after stroke. *Arch Neurol.* 26:489–501.

Sotgiu S, Zanda B, Marchetti B et al. 2006. Inflammatory biomarkers in blood of patients with acute brain ischemia. *Eur J Neurol.* 13:505–513.

Stamatovic SM, Shakui P, Keep RF et al. 2005. Monocyte chemoattractant protein-1 regulation of blood-brain barrier permeability. *J Cereb Blood Flow Metab.* 25:593–606.

Stephenson D, Yin T, Smalstig EB et al. 2000. Transcription factor nuclear factor-Kappa B is activated in neurons after focal cerebral ischemia. *J Cereb Blood Flow Metab.* 20:592–603.

Stephenson DT, Schober DA, Smalstig EB, Mincy RE, Gehlert DR, Clemens JA. 1995. Peripheral benzodiazepine receptors are colocalized with activated microglia following transient global forebrain ischemia in the rat. *J Neurosci.* 15:5263–5274.

Stevens SL, Bao J, Hollis J, Lessov NS, Clark WM, Stenzel-Poore MP. 2002. The use of flow cytometry to evaluate temporal changes in inflammatory cells following focal cerebral ischemia in mice. *Brain Res.* 932:110–119.

Stoll G, Jander S, Schroeter M. 1998. Inflammation and glial responses in ischemic brain lesions. *Prog Neurobiol.* 56:149–171.

Strle K, Zhou JH, Shen WH et al. 2001. Interleukin-10 in the brain. *Crit Rev Immunol.* 21:427–449.

Subramanyam B, Pond SM, Eyles DW, Whiteford HA. 1999. Fouda Stroke therapy academic industry roundtable (STAIR–1999) recommendations for standards regarding preclinical neuroprotective andrestorative drug development. *Stroke.* 30:2752–2758.

Sughrue ME, Mehra A, Connolly ES, Jr, D'Ambrosio AL. 2004. Anti-adhesion molecule strategies as potential neuroprotective agents in cerebral ischemia: a critical review of the literature. *Inflamm Res.* 53:497–508.

Sugimoto K, Iadecola C. 2003. Delayed effect of administration of COX-2 inhibitor in mice with acute cerebral ischemia. *Brain Res.* 960:273–276.

Suk K, Park JH, Lee WH. 2004. Neuropeptide PACAP inhibits hypoxic activation of brain microglia: a protective mechanism against microglial neurotoxicity in ischemia. *Brain Res.* 1026:151–156.

Sutherland GR, Dix GA, Auer RN. 1996. Effect of age in rodent models of focal and forebrain ischemia. *Stroke.* 27:1663–1667.

Suzuki Y, Takagi Y, Nakamura R, Hashimoto K, Umemura K. 2003. Ability of NMDA and non-NMDA receptor antagonists to inhibit cerebral ischemic damage in middle aged rats. *Brain Res.* 964:116–120.

Svedin P, Hagberg H, Savman K, Zhu C, Mallard C. 2007. Matrix metalloproteinase-9 gene knock-out protects the immature brain after cerebral hypoxia-ischemia. *J Neurosci.* 27:1511–1518.

Swanson RA, Ying W, Kauppinen TM. 2004. Astrocyte influences on ischemic neuronal death. *Curr Mol Med.* 4:193–205.

Sydserff SG, Borelli AR, Green AR, Cross AJ. 2002. Effect of NXY-059 on infarct volume after transient or permanent middle cerebral artery occlusion in the rat; studies on dose, plasma concentration and therapeutic time window. *Br J Pharmacol.* 135:103–112.

Takagi Y, Nozaki K, Takahashi J, Ishikawa M, Hashimoto N. 1999. Proliferation of neuronal precursor cells in the dentate gyrus is accelerated after transient forebrain ischemia in mice. *Brain Res.* 831:283–287.

Takasawa K, Kitagawa K, Yagita Y et al. 2002. Increased proliferation of neural progenitor cells but reduced survival of newborn cells in the contralateral hippocampus after focal cerebral ischemia in rats. *J Cereb Blood Flow Metab.* 22:299–307.

Tamas A, Reglodi D, Szanto Z, Borsiczky B, Nemeth J, Lengvari I. 2002. Comparative neuroprotective effects of preischemic PACAP and VIP administration in permanent occlusion of the middle cerebral artery in rats. *Neuro Endocrinol Lett.* 23:249–254.

Tang H, Wang Y et al. 2007. Effect of neural precursor proliferation level on neurogenesis in rat brain during aging and after focal ischemia. *Neurobiol Aging.* [Epub ahead of print].

Tang Y, Xu H, Du X et al. 2006. Gene expression in blood changes rapidly in neutrophils and monocytes after ischemic stroke in humans: a microarray study. *J Cereb Blood Flow Metab.* 26:1089–1102.

Tarkowski E, Rosengren L, Blomstrand C et al. 1997. Intrathecal release of pro- and anti-inflammatory cytokines during stroke. *Clin Exp Immunol.* 110:492–499.

Ten VS, Sosunov SA, Mazer SP et al. 2005. C1q-deficiency is neuroprotective against hypoxic-ischemic brain injury in neonatal mice. *Stroke.* 36:2244–2250.

The RANTTAS Investigators. 1996. A randomized trial of tirilazad mesylate in patients with acute stroke (RANTTAS). *Stroke.* 27:1453–1458.

Theodorsson A, Theodorsson E. 2005. Estradiol increases brain lesions in the cortex and lateral striatum after transient occlusion of the middle cerebral artery in rats: no effect of ischemia on galanin in the stroke area but decreased levels in the hippocampus. *Peptides.* 26:2257–2264.

Tirilazad International Steering Committee. 2000. Tirilazad mesylate in acute ischemic stroke: a systematic review. *Stroke.* 31:2257–2265.

Tolonen U, Sulg IA. 1981. Comparison of quantitative EEG parameters from four different analysis techniques in evaluation of relationships between EEG and CBF in brain infarction. *Electroencephalogr Clin Neurophysiol.* 51:177–185.

Tomimoto H, Shibata M, Ihara M, Akiguchi I, Ohtani R, Budka H. 2002. A comparative study on the expression of cyclooxygenase and 5-lipoxygenase during cerebral ischemia in humans. *Acta Neuropathol (Berl).* 104:601–607.

Tropepe V, Craig CG, CM Morshead, D van der Kooy. 1997. Transforming growth factor-alpha null and senescent mice show decreased neural progenitor cell proliferation in the forebrain subependyma. *J Neurosci.* 17:7850–7859.

Tu Y, Hou ST, Huang Z, Robertson GS, MacManus JP. 1998. Increased Mdm2 expression in rat brain after transient middle cerebral artery occlusion. *J Cereb Blood Flow Metab.* 18:658–669.

Tureyen K, Kapadia R, Bowen KK et al. 2007. Peroxisome proliferator-activated receptor-gamma agonists induce neuroprotection following transient focal ischemia in normotensive, normoglycemic as well as hypertensive and type-2 diabetic Rodents. *J Neurochem.* 101:41–56.

Uchida Y, S Nakano, Gomi F, Takahashi H. 2007. Differential regulation of basic helix-loop-helix factors Mash1 and Olig2 by beta-amyloid accelerates both differentiation and death of cultured neural stem/progenitor cells. *J Biol Chem.* 282:19700–19709.

Uhlar CM, Whitehead AS. 1999. Serum amyloid a, the major vertebrate acute-phase reactant. *Eur J Biochem.* 265:501–523.

Vallieres L, Sawchenko PE. 2003. Bone marrow-derived cells that populate the adult mouse brain preserve their hematopoietic identity. *J Neurosci.* 23:5197–5207.

van Breda EJ, van der Worp HB, van Gemert HM et al. 2005. PAIS: paracetamol (acetaminophen) in stroke; protocol for a randomized, double blind clinical trial [ISCRTN 74418480]. *BMC Cardiovasc Disord.* 5:24.

van Exel E, Gussekloo J, de Craen AJ, Bootsma-van der Wiel A, Frolich M, Westendorp RG. 2002. Inflammation and stroke: the leiden 85-plus study. *Stroke.* 33:1135–1138.

van Praag H, Kempermann G et al. (1999) Running increases cell proliferation and neurogenesis in the adult mouse dentate gyrus. *Nat Neurosci.* 2:266–270.

van Praag H, AF Schinder, BR Christie, Toni N, Palmer TD, Gage FH. 2002. Functional neurogenesis in the adult hippocampus. *Nature.* 415:1030–1034.

Van Remmen H, Qi W, Sabia M et al. 2004. Multiple deficiencies in antioxidant enzymes in mice result in a compound increase in sensitivity to oxidative stress. *Free Radic Biol Med.* 36:1625–1634.

Vargas M, Horcajada JP, Obach V et al. 2006. Clinical consequences of infection in patients with acute stroke: is it prime time for further antibiotic trials? *Stroke.* 37:461–465.

Vasthare US, Barone FC, Sarau HM et al. 1998. Complement depletion improves neurological function in cerebral ischemia. *Brain Res Bull.* 45:413–419.

Vaughan CJ, Delanty N. 1999. Neuroprotective properties of statins in cerebral ischemia and stroke. *Stroke.* 30:1969–1973.

Vaughan DW, Peters A. 1974. Neuroglial cells in the cerebral cortex of rats from young adulthood to old age: an electron microscope study. *J Neurocytol.* 3:405–429.

Vedder NB, Winn RK, Rice CL, Chi EY, Arfors KE, Harlan JM. 1990. Inhibition of leukocyte adherence by anti-CD18 monoclonal antibody attenuates reperfusion injury in the rabbit ear. *Proc Natl Acad Sci U S A.* 87:2643–2646.

Verret L, Jankowsky JL, Xu GM, Borchelt DR, Rampon C. 2007. Alzheimer's-type amyloidosis in transgenic mice impairs survival of newborn neurons derived from adult hippocampal neurogenesis. *J Neurosci.* 27(25):6771–6780.

Vila N, Castillo J, Davalos A, Chamorro A. 2000. Proinflammatory cytokines and early neurological worsening in ischemic stroke. *Stroke.* 31:2325–2329.

Vuorte J, Lindsberg PJ, Kaste M et al. 1999. Anti-ICAM-1 monoclonal antibody R6.5 (Enlimomab) promotes activation of neutrophils in whole blood. *J Immunol.* 162:2353–2357.

Wang L, Li Y, Chen J, Gautam SC, Zhang Z, Lu M, Chopp M. 2002a. Ischemic cerebral tissue and MCP-1 enhance rat bone marrow stromal cell migration in interface culture. *Exp Hematol.* 30:831–836.

Wang L, Li Y, Chen X et al. 2002b. MCP-1, MIP-1, IL-8 and ischemic cerebral tissue enhance human bone marrow stromal cell migration in interface culture. *Hematology.* 7:113–117.

Wang LC, Futrell N, Wang DZ, Chen FJ, Zhai QH, Schulz LR. 1995. A reproducible model of middle cerebral infarcts, compatible with long-term survival, in aged rats. *Stroke.* 26:2087–2090

Wang PY, Kao CH, Mui MY, Wang SJ. 1993. Leukocyte infiltration in acute hemispheric ischemic stroke. *Stroke.* 24:236–240.

Wang X, Yue TL, Barone FC, White RF, Gagnon RC, Feuerstein GZ. 1994. Concomitant cortical expression of TNF-Alpha and IL-1 beta MRNAs follows early response gene expression in transient focal ischemia. *Mol Chem Neuropathol.* 23:103–114.

Wang X, Yue TL, Barone FC, Feuerstein GZ. 1995a. Monocyte chemoattractant protein-1 messenger rna expression in rat ischemic cortex. *Stroke.* 26:661–665.

Wang X, Yue TL, Young PR, Barone FC, Feuerstein GZ. 1995b. Expression of Interleukin-6, C-Fos, and Zif268 MRNAs in rat ischemic cortex. *J Cereb Blood Flow Metab.* 15:166–171.

Ward NS. 2007. Future perspectives in functional neuroimaging in stroke recovery. *Eura Medicophys.* 43:285–294.

Watanabe T, Zhang N, Liu M, Tanaka R, Mizuno Y, Urabe T. 2006. Cilostazol protects against brain white matter damage and cognitive impairment in a rat model of chronic cerebral hypoperfusion. *Stroke.* 37:1539–1545.

Watson BD, Dietrich WD, Busto R. 1985. Induction of reproducible brain infarction by photochemically initiated thrombosis. *Ann Neurol.* 17:497–504.

Welin AK, Svedin P, Lapatto R et al. 2007. Melatonin reduces inflammation and cell death in white matter in the mid-gestation fetal sheep following umbilical cord occlusion. *Pediatr Res* 61:153–158.

Weng YC, Kriz J. 2007. Differential neuroprotective effects of a minocycline-based drug cocktail in transient and permanent focal cerebral ischemia. *Exp Neurol.* 204:433–442.

Whicher J, Biasucci L, Rifai N. 1999. Inflammation, the acute phase response and atherosclerosis. *Clin Chem Lab Med.* 37:495–503.

Williams AJ, Dave JR, Tortella FC. 2006. Neuroprotection with the proteasome inhibitor MLN519 in focal ischemic brain injury: relation to Nuclear Factor KappaB (NF-KappaB), inflammatory gene expression, and leukocyte infiltration. *Neurochem Int.* 49:106–112.

Willmot MR, Bath PM. 2003. The potential of nitric oxide therapeutics in stroke. *Expert Opin Investig Drugs.* 12:455–470.

Winbeck K, Poppert H, Etgen T, Conrad B, Sander D. 2002. Prognostic relevance of early serial C-reactive protein measurements after first ischemic stroke. *Stroke.* 33:2459–2464.

Winner B, Rockenstein E, Lie DC et al. 2008. Mutant alpha-synuclein exacerbates age-related decrease of neurogenesis. *Neurobiol Aging.* 6:913–925.

Wojcik C, Di Napoli M. 2004. Ubiquitin-proteasome system and proteasome inhibition: new strategies in stroke therapy. *Stroke.* 35:1506–1518.

Wood PL. 1995. Microglia as a unique cellular target in the treatment of stroke: potential neurotoxic mediators produced by activated microglia. *Neurol Res.* 17:242–248.

Xiong ZG, Chu XP, Simon RP. 2007. Acid sensing ion channels—novel therapeutic targets for ischemic brain injury. *Front Biosci.* 12:1376–1386.

Yagita Y, Kitagawa K, Ohtsuki T et al. 2001. Neurogenesis by progenitor cells in the ischemic adult rat hippocampus. *Stroke.* 32:1890–1896.

Yamagami S, Tamura M, Hayashi M et al. 1999. Differential production of MCP-1 and cytokine-induced neutrophil chemoattractant in the ischemic brain after transient focal ischemia in rats. *J Leukoc Biol.* 65:744–749.

Yamasaki Y, Matsuo Y, Matsuura N, Onodera H, Itoyama Y, Kogure K. 1995. Transient increase of cytokine-induced neutrophil chemoattractant, a member of the interleukin-8 family, in ischemic brain areas after focal ischemia in rats. *Stroke.* 26:318–322.

Yamashima T, Tonchev AB, Vachkov IH et al. 2004. Vascular adventitia generates neuronal progenitors in the monkey hippocampus after ischemia. *Hippocampus.* 14(7):861–75.

Yang GY, Zhao YJ, Davidson BL, Betz AL. 1997. Overexpression of Interleukin-1 receptor antagonist in the mouse brain reduces ischemic brain injury. *Brain Res.* 751:181–188.

Yenari MA, Kunis D, Sun GH et al. 1998. Hu23F2G, an antibody recognizing the leukocyte CD11/CD18 integrin, reduces injury in a rabbit model of transient focal cerebral ischemia. *Exp Neurol.* 153:223–233.

Yepes M, Brown SA, Moore EG, Smith EP, Lawrence DA, Winkles JA. 2005. A soluble Fn14-Fc decoy receptor reduces infarct volume in a murine model of cerebral ischemia. *Am J Pathol.* 166:511–520.

Yoshimoto Y, Tanaka Y, Hoya K. 2001. Acute systemic inflammatory response syndrome in subarachnoid hemorrhage. *Stroke.* 32:1989–1993.

Yrjanheikki J, Keinanen R, Pellikka M, Hokfelt T, Koistinaho J. 1998. Tetracyclines inhibit microglial activation and are neuroprotective in global brain ischemia. *Proc Natl Acad Sci U S A.* 95:15769–15774.

Yrjanheikki J, Tikka T, Keinanen R, Goldsteins G, Chan PH, Koistinaho J. 1999. A tetracycline derivative, minocycline, reduces inflammation and protects against focal cerebral ischemia with a wide therapeutic window. *Proc Natl Acad Sci U S A.* 96:13496–13500.

Yu WH, Go L, Guinn BA, Fraser PE, Westaway D, McLaurin J. 2002. Phenotypic and functional changes in glial cells as a function of age. *Neurobiol Aging.* 23:105–115.

Zagrean L, Moldovan M, Munteanu AM, Spulber S, Voiculescu BA, Popescu BO. 2000. Early electrocortical changes consistent with ischemic preconditioning in rat. *J Cell Mol Med.* 4:215–223.

Zausinger S, Westermaier T, Plesnila N, Steiger HJ, Schmid-Elsaesser R. 2003. Neuroprotection in transient focal cerebral ischemia by combination drug therapy and mild hypothermia: comparison with customary therapeutic regimen. *Stroke.* 34:1526–1532.

Zawadzka M, Kaminska B. 2005. A novel mechanism of FK506-mediated neuroprotection: downregulation of cytokine expression in glial cells. *Glia.* 49:36–51.

Zazulia AR. 2002. Stroke. In Ramachandran VS, ed. *Encyclopedia of the Human Brain.* San Diego, CA: Academic Press/Elsevier Science, 475–492.

Zhang F, Iadecola C. 1998. Temporal characteristics of the protective effect of aminoguanidine on cerebral ischemic damage. *Brain Res.* 802:104–110.

Zhang L, Zhang ZG, Liu X et al. 2006. Treatment of embolic stroke in rats with bortezomib and recombinant human tissue plasminogen activator. *Thromb Haemost.* 95:166–173.

Zhang N, Komine-Kobayashi M, Tanaka R, Liu M, Mizuno Y, Urabe T. 2005. Edaravone reduces early accumulation of oxidative products and sequential inflammatory responses after transient focal ischemia in mice brain. *Stroke.* 36:2220–2225.

Zhang RL, Chopp M, Chen H, Garcia JH. 1994a. Temporal profile of ischemic tissue damage, neutrophil response, and vascular plugging following permanent and transient (2H) middle cerebral artery occlusion in the rat. *J Neurol Sci.* 125:3–10.

Zhang RL, Chopp M, Li Y et al. 1994b. Anti-ICAM-1 antibody reduces ischemic cell damage after transient middle cerebral artery occlusion in the rat. *Neurology.* 44:1747–1751.

Zhang RL, Chopp M, Jiang N et al. 1995a. Anti-intercellular adhesion molecule-1 antibody reduces ischemic cell damage after transient but not permanent middle cerebral artery occlusion in the wistar rat. *Stroke.* 26:1438–1442.

Zhang RL, Chopp M, Zaloga C et al. 1995b. The temporal profiles of ICAM-1 protein and MRNA expression after transient MCA occlusion in the rat. *Brain Res.* 682:182–188.

Zhang RL, Zhang ZG, Zhang L, Chopp M. 2001. Proliferation and differentiation of progenitor cells in the cortex and the subventricular zone in the adult rat after focal cerebral ischemia. *Neuroscience.* 105:33–41.

Zhang ZG, Chopp M, Tang WX, Jiang N, Zhang RL. 1995c. Postischemic treatment (2–4 H) with anti-CD11b and anti-CD18 monoclonal antibodies are neuroprotective after transient (2 H) focal cerebral ischemia in the rat. *Brain Res.* 698:79–85.

Zhao CS, Puurunen K, Schallert T, Sivenius J, Jolkkonen J. 2005a. Effect of cholinergic medication, before and after focal photothrombotic ischemic cortical injury, on histological and functional outcome in aged and young adult rats. Behav *Brain Res.* 156:85–94.

Zhao X, Haensel C, Araki E, Ross ME, Iadecola C. 2000. Gene-dosing effect and persistence of reduction in ischemic brain injury in mice lacking inducible nitric oxide synthase. *Brain Res.* 872:215–218.

Zheng L, Fisher G, Miller RE, Peschon J, Lynch DH, Lenardo MJ. 1995. Induction of apoptosis in mature T cells by tumour necrosis factor. *Nature.* 377:348–351.

Zivin JA, DeGirolami U, Kochhar A, Lyden PD, Mazzarella V, Hemenway CC. 1987. A model for quantitative evaluation of embolic stroke therapy. *Brain Res.* 435:305–309.

Chapter 18

PROTEIN MISFOLDING, MITOCHONDRIAL DISTURBANCES, AND KYNURENINES IN THE PATHOGENESIS OF NEURODEGENERATIVE DISORDERS

Gabriella Gárdián, Katalin Sas, József Toldi, and László Vécsei

ABSTRACT

As a population ages, neurodegenerative diseases become increasingly prevalent. These are different clinical entities, though they display many common features in their clinical, biochemical, and morphological appearance. The majority of them have both genetic and environmental components in their pathomechanism. The genetic background involves a single gene mutation (e.g., *spinocerebellar ataxias 1, 2,* and *3* and *Huntington's disease* [PD]), heterozygote gene modifications following the patterns of the Mendelian laws (e.g., *familial Parkinson's disease* [PD] and *familial Alzheimer's disease* [AD]), multiple predisposing genes (e.g., *sporadic PD and sporadic AD*), or mitochondrial DNA (mtDNA) defects. Protein misfolding, mitochondrial impairment, oxidative stress, endoplasmic reticulum stress (ERS), excitotoxicity, caspase cascade activation, and apoptosis are common mechanisms acknowledged to lead to cell death in the different neurodegenerative disorders.

Keywords: protein misfolding, endoplasmic reticulum stress, apoptosis, molecular chaperones, ubiquitin proteasome system, protein aggregation, free radicals, oxidative stress, kynurenic acid, quinolinic acid.

PROTEIN MISFOLDING

The pathological hallmark of human neurodegenerative diseases, including Parkinson's disease (PD), Alzheimer's disease (AD), amyotrophic lateral sclerosis, polyglutamine extension disorders, and prion diseases, is the deposition of abnormally folded protein aggregates in different regions of the brain (Chaudhuri, Paul 2006). These diseases, which are known to result from or be associated with misfolding of the cellular protein, can occur sporadically or result from mutations to the gene that encodes the accumulated protein. The transgenic and toxin animal

Table 18.1 Mechanisms Against Misfolded Proteins

Chaperones sequester damaged, unfolded proteins and transfer the proteins to the proteasomal system

The ubiquitin-proteasomal system degrades misfolded, unwanted proteins

Aggregation is a multistep process, involving aggresomes and inclusion bodies

models of neurodegenerative diseases are capable of providing considerable information about the cellular process. However, little is known concerning the roles of the encoded proteins. It appears likely that misfolded soluble intermediates, the protofibrillar forms of aggregates, activate cell death pathways and cause neurotoxicity (Taylor, Hardy, Fischbeck 2002; Arrasate, Mitra, Schweitzer et al. 2004). On the other hand, the segregation of misfolded proteins into aggregates can be protective and is merely an adaptive stress response. The accumulation of misfolded proteins must result from an inability of the cells either to refold them or to degrade them. Cells have adaptive mechanisms whereby they can avoid the accumulation of incorrectly folded proteins, although their adequacy to deal with these proteins progresses with aging. The neurodegenerative disorders usually exhibit a late onset. The mechanisms of protein degradation involve molecular chaperones that fold proteins; the ubiquitin-proteasome system (UPS), which degrades the misfolded proteins; and some special enzymes (superoxide dismutase [SOD], catalase, γ-glutamylcysteine synthetase, methionin sulfoxide reductase) that maintain the appropriate redox potential in the cytosol (Goldberg 2003; Ciechanover 2005) (Table 18.1).

Endoplasmic Reticulum

Impairment of the endoplasmic reticulum (ER) function may play a role in the pathomechanism of neurodegenerative disorders. The functions of the ER include the folding and processing of newly synthesized proteins, Ca^{2+} storage, and cell signaling. The mutant and misfolded proteins are transported from the ER back into the cytosol, where they are rapidly degraded. A malfunction in the processes of the ER is termed endoplasmic reticulum stress (ERS) (Paschen, Mengesdorf 2005). Impairment of the processes of the ER results in misfolded proteins, which are usually resistant to degradation and can induce oxidative stress, mitochondrial and proteasomal dysfunctions and apoptosis, leading ultimately to neuronal cell death (Sitia, Braakman 2003). Depletion of the ER Ca^{2+} pool plays an important part in ERS, because the protein folding machinery requires a considerable amount of Ca^{2+}. To prevent

the accumulation of unwanted proteins in the ER, the cells respond by activating a transcriptional program. This unfolded protein response increases the production of a group of molecular chaperones in the ER, which is analogous to the heat shock response in the cytosol. Molecular chaperones assist proteins to enhance the folding efficiency, achieve active three-dimensional structures, prevent the formation of misfolded structures, and translocate to different cellular compartment. The ER, the molecular chaperones, the proteasome system, and the lysosomes are together responsible for protein processing and the degradation of most cytosolic, nuclear, and damaged proteins (Sherman, Goldberg 2001). Correctly folded proteins are transported to the Golgi apparatus, while misfolded proteins are translocated from the ER to the cytosol, where they are polyubiquitinated by specific enzymes and then targeted to the UPS for degradation. Secretory and internalized proteins are cleared by lysosomes (Fig. 18.1).

Ubiquitin–Proteasome System

The generation of abnormal proteins is part of the normal cell cycle. It is a special task in the brain because of the high utilization of O_2, the elevated rates of metabolism and enzymatic oxidation, and the fact that the neurons do not turn over and have a limited ability for repair and regeneration. The abnormal proteins comprise a potential risk factor in the cell because they can misfold, aggregate, interfere with intracellular processes, and induce cytotoxicity (Bennett, Bence, Jayakumar et al. 2005). Thus, it is important to limit the accumulation of abnormal proteins by rapid clearance. The UPS is involved in numerous cellular processes, including protein trafficking, cell cycling and signaling, gene transcription, DNA repair, and apoptosis (Ciechanover, Brundin 2003). The UPS plays the main role in the degradation of abnormal proteins and in the turnover of short-lived regulatory proteins. UPS-mediated processes occur diffusely throughout the cell, including the cytoplasm, nucleus, and ER. Misfolded proteins are targeted to a degradation pathway. This is referred to as a protein "quality control" system. The process occurs in two sequential steps: (1) ubiquitination/deubiquitination and (2) proteolysis (Fig. 18.1).

In the first step, unwanted proteins are tagged for degradation via polyubiquitin molecules attached to the internal Lys residue of the substrate protein (at least four molecules). This is an adenosine triphosphate (ATP)-dependent process. The ubiquitination is mediated by ubiquitin-activating enzyme, ubiquitin-conjugating enzyme, and ubiquitin ligases. Each of the several ligases is specific for one or a limited

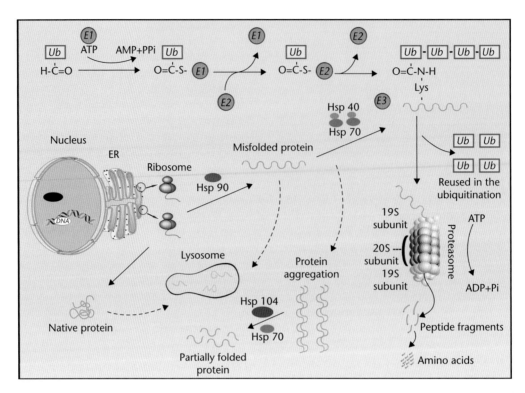

Figure 18.1 Intracellular protein handling. E1, ubiquitin-activating enzyme; E2, ubiquitin-conjugating enzyme; E3, ubiquitin ligase; ER, endoplasmic reticulum; Ub, ubiquitin.

number of different proteins, whereas there is merely a single ubiquitin-activating enzyme.

In the second step, the polyubiquitinated proteins are transported to the proteasomes for degradation; they are first deubiquitinated and then translocated into the core of the 26S proteasome complex. The 26S proteasome consists of two 19S regulatory complexes situated at either or both ends of the 20S core proteasome. The 20S proteasome contains three active proteolytic sites to mediate the hydrolysis of proteins at the C-terminus of hydrophobic, basic, and acidic residues. The 19S complex recognizes polyubiquitinated proteins, allows them entry into the catalytic core, and opens the channel through the 20S proteasome, where proteins are degraded into small peptides. Here, the unwanted proteins are degraded in an ATP-dependent process. The products are small peptide fragments (3 to 25 amino acids long) that undergo hydrolysis by cytosolic peptidases to produce their constituent amino acids (Pickart 2001; Petrucelli, Dawson 2004). It is noteworthy that short peptides, some oxidatively damaged proteins, and possibly α-synuclein can be degraded by the 20S proteasome without prior ubiquitination and in an ATP-independent manner. The proteasome lacks the capacity to hydrolyze within repeated sequences of glutamine, which may be a factor in the pathomechanism of some neurodegenerative disorders (Bence, Sampat, Kopito 2001). Thus, the relatively insoluble

polyQ sequences may aggregate and form inclusion bodies.

Chaperones

Chaperones are ubiquitous, highly conserved proteins (mostly heat shock proteins [HSPs]). Normally, the expression of heat shock genes is inhibited by the presence of molecular chaperones. The transcription of HSPs is induced by the accumulation of unwanted proteins in the cytosol, ER, or nucleus, and they bind preferentially to Hsp 90 and Hsp 70, in this way preventing these chaperones from inhibiting the expression of heat shock genes. HSPs protect against proteolytic stress by promoting the refolding of proteins to their native state and facilitating protein degradation by acting as chaperones to transport abnormal proteins to the proteasomes (Muchowski, Wacker 2005). The chaperones Hsp 90, Hsp 70 and Hsp 40 are essential for ubiquitination and rapid degradation. The HSPs activate phosphatases to prevent the formation of proapoptotic proteins (Hartl, Hayer-Hartl 2002; Soti, Csermely 2003; Chaudhuri, Paul 2006) (Table 18.2).

Protein Aggregation

Unwanted protein aggregates bind HSPs and block them to exert protective effects. The formation of

Table 18.2 Roles of Molecular Chaperones

Facilitation of protein folding

Prevention of protein aggregation

Regulation of autophagy

Regulation of vesicle fusion

Regulation of signal transduction

Regulation of apoptosis

Regulation of proteasomal degradation

oligomers and aggregates occurs in a cell when a critical concentration of misfolded protein is reached. A common feature of almost all protein conformational diseases is the formation of an aggregate caused by destabilization of the α-helical structure and the simultaneous formation of a β-sheet. Abnormal protein accumulation and aggregation activate the creation of inclusions known as aggresomes. Inclusion body formation is a complex process, in which the cellular machinery appears to be actively involved. Undegraded proteins and aggregates are transported by the microtubular system to the centrosomes, which form inclusion bodies/aggresomes to sequester proteins (Lyubchenko, Sherman, Shlyakhtenko et al. 2006). The formation of inclusions is a multistep process. The UPS and chaperones are recruited to the centrosomes/aggresomes to facilitate the clearance of abnormal proteins. The proteins in the inclusions appear to be in a dynamic state, continually turning over and being replaced by other unfolded molecules as the cell strives to maintain its viability. The proteasomal activity tends to decrease with increasing age, that is, at the same time as the proportion of damaged proteins is increasing (Kopito 2000). Proteolytic stress is a disturbance of the balance between the production of unwanted proteins and their clearance. Undegraded proteins tend to aggregate with each other and with normal proteins, promoting oxidative stress, destroying physiological intracellular processes, and facilitating apoptosis (Shastry 2003).

MITOCHONDRIA

The mitochondria are intracellular organelles that are ubiquitous among eukaryotic cells. They are responsible for the energy supply of cells and play critical roles in signaling processes, Ca^{2+} homeostasis, cell cycle regulation, apoptosis, free radical generation, and aging. The mitochondria are the sites where the lipid metabolism, the citric acid cycle, the respiratory chain, and oxidative phosphorylation take place. The term mitochondrion was introduced in 1898 by Benda, but mitochondria were first physically separated from disrupted cells by Kölliker. mtDNA was

first identified by Nass and Nass in 1963–1964, and the complete nucleotide sequence of human mtDNA had been established by 1981. mtDNA is inherited along maternal lines. It was an important finding that mtDNA undergoes mutation at a rate 5 to 10 times higher than that for nuclear DNA (nDNA). There is evidence that the "normal" aging process is accompanied by the accumulation of oxidatively damaged molecules, including mtDNA.

Structure of the Mitochondria

The mitochondria are double-membraned organelles that are composed of four distinct compartments, all of which have their own unique compositions and functions (Fig. 18.2). The porous outer membrane, which encompasses the whole organelle, contains many important enzymes and receptors. It is freely permeable to small molecules and ions. The convoluted and invaginated inner mitochondrial membrane contains the enzymes of oxidative phosphorylation, the cofactor coenzyme Q10 (ubiquinone Q), ATP synthase, and some carrier proteins. It is rich in cardiolipin and is impermeable to most small molecules and ions, including H^+. Between the outer and inner membranes is the intermembrane space, with specialized proteins. In the matrix, bordered by the inner membrane, there are many enzymes for different metabolic pathways, including the citric acid cycle (Krebs cycle), fatty acid oxidation (β-oxidation), and the urea cycle, and also mtDNA, peptidases, and chaperones. The high-conductance mitochondrial permeability transition pore (mtPTP) is a pathway involving certain inner membrane proteins, mostly adenine nucleotide translocator, a voltage-dependent anion channel (in the outer membrane), and cyclophilin D (in the matrix) (Chavez, Melendez, Zazueta et al. 1997). Members of the Bcl-2 family and peripheral benzodiazepine receptors are associated with the outer face of the pore (Crompton 2000), which can open in response to certain stimuli, for example, oxidative stress, a Ca^{2+} overload or ATP depletion, leading to loss of the mitochondrial membrane potential, and consequently to the release of cytochrome c (cyt c) to induce apoptosis (Krieger, Duchen 2002). The conformational change of the adenine nucleotide carrier can be catalyzed by cyclophilin D and inhibited by cyclosporine A.

The mitochondrial respiratory chain, consisting of several enzyme complexes and cofactors (complexes I–IV, and an enzyme often referred to as complex V: I: nicotinamide adenine dehydrogenase (NADH) ubiquinone oxidoreductase, II: succinate ubiquinone oxidoreductase, III: ubiquinone cytochrome c reductase, IV: cytochrome c oxidase (COX), V: ATP

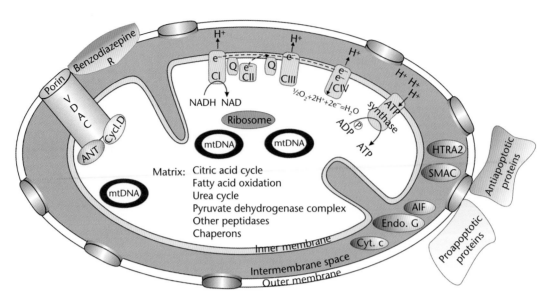

Figure 18.2 Structure of the mitochondria. CI: NADH ubiquinone oxidoreductase; CII: succinate ubiquinone oxidoreductase; CIII: ubiquinone cytochrome c reductase; CIV: cytochrome c oxidase; mtPTP: mitochondrial permeability transition pore; ANT: adenine nucleotide translocator; VDAC: voltage-dependent anion channel; Cycl. D: cyclophilin D; Cyt. c: cytochrome c; AIF: apoptosis-inducing factor; Endo G: endonuclease G; HTRA2: inhibit cytosolic inhibitor of apoptosis proteins; Smac: second mitochondrial activator of caspases.

synthase) is embedded in the inner mitochondrial membrane, arranged functionally according to the electrochemical hierarchy based on their redox potentials. These large oligomers are built up from approximately 85 subunits, 72 being encoded by nDNA and 13 by mtDNA. The enzymes of complexes I, III, and IV are encoded by both nDNA and mtDNA, while for complex II this is carried out exclusively by nDNA (Papa 1996; Orth, Schapira 2001). The tricarboxylic acid cycle maintains the coenzymes NADH and flavoproteins in a reduced state to supply reducing equivalents for the electron transport chain. Together with the latter, the transfer of electrons originating from the oxidation of $NADH_2$ (at complex I) or $FADH_2$ (at complex III) by ubiquinone to complex IV occurs where they react with O_2 to reduce it to H_2O. COX (complex IV) consists of a dimer linked by two cardiolipin molecules. The transfer of electrons along the respiratory chain provides the energy to pump protons from the matrix into the intermembrane space at complexes I, III, and IV, generating the proton gradient known as the membrane potential (negative inside: $\Delta\Psi_m$: −150 to −180 mV) and an electrochemical gradient (ΔpH, alkaline inside). As the inner membrane is impermeable to H^+, it can reenter the matrix only through ATP-ase, inducing a conformational change in the active site of the enzyme that favors adenosine diphosphate (ADP) phosphorylation and hence ATP synthesis (Dykens 1997). Briefly, the redox energy is used to generate a proton gradient, the energy then being converted into high-energy macromolecules.

The brain has high-energy requirements: it accounts for about 20% of the total O_2 consumption in resting humans, though it furnishes only 2% of the body weight.

Mitochondrial Genome

The mitochondrion is the only cellular organelle under the dual control of both the nuclear and its own genomes. The matrix contains mtDNA, a multicopy, circular, double-stranded molecule containing 37 genes (16,569 base pairs), encoding for 13 polypeptides (all of them parts of the respiratory chain complexes), 22 transfer RNAs, and 2 ribosomal RNAs (12S and 16S). The 13 mtDNA-encoded proteins account for only a small fraction of the mitochondrial proteins. The principles of the genetics differ greatly from the Mendelian inheritance of nuclear mutations (Chan 2006). As mentioned above, the mitochondria are inherited maternally, due to the transmission of mitochondria from the egg to the zygote. Paternal mitochondria from the sperm are targeted for degradation. During cell divisions, mitochondria are distributed to the daughter cells in a more or less random manner. However, under special circumstances, such as during early oogenesis, there can be a drastic reduction in the total number of copies of mtDNA, which results in a genetic bottleneck. This dramatically affects the ratio of mutant to wild-type mtDNA and can result in the segregation of mutant mtDNA to some offspring. Because of the nature of mitochondrial segregation, mtDNA diseases can have variable outcomes and an unpredictable course. The clinical symptoms of mtDNA diseases progress with aging. This feature is due to the accumulation of mtDNA mutations and an increased ROS level (ROS: superoxide, hydrogen peroxide and hydroxyl free radical). mtDNA mutations that reduce the accuracy of electron transfer increase the likelihood of ROS production and further mtDNA damage, leading to a vicious circle. In the nonsynaptic mitochondria, complex I has to be inhibited by approximately 60%, in contrast with the synaptosomes, where a 25% decrease in the activity of the complex is sufficient to compromise ATP formation (Davey, Canevari, Clark et al. 1997). While a reduction in the activity of one or more complexes has been reported in the majority of neurodegenerative diseases, it should be mentioned that in certain cases increases have been detected (e.g., complex IV in active multiple sclerosis plaque), perhaps as a compensatory reaction for the lowered complex I activity (Lu, Selak, O'Connor et al. 2000). Platelets can be used as biomarkers of mitochondrial lesions, as their energy supply is based exclusively on glycolysis and mitochondrial oxidative phosphorylation (Holmsen, Robkin 1980).

The mitochondrial genome regularly replicates in postmitotic cells, about once per month. The mitochondria divide mainly in response to the energy needs of the cell, that is, independently of the cell cycle phases. When a cell needs high-energy, the mitochondria grow and divide, and when the cell utilizes relatively low energy, they are destroyed or become inactive. Moreover, in consequence of mitochondrial fusion and fission, the mitochondria in heteroplasmic cells are highly intermixed, and contain both wild-type and modified mitochondrial genes. Through this continuous action of the mitochondria, the deleterious effects of mitochondrial mutations are reduced, and the potential for the removal of modified mtDNA by autophagy increases. A given mitochondrion contains several copies of its genome (2 to 15 copies, "polyplasmia"), either the wild-type or the mutant variant ("heteroplasmia"). As heteroplasmic cells divide, the ratio of pathogenic to wild-type mtDNA genomes can vary in the different tissues and in the individual cells within the tissues. This is due to the random distribution of mtDNA during cell division. Symptoms appear above a certain threshold (threshold effect). It is generally thought that tissues such as the muscle, brain, liver, heart, and endocrine glands are particularly dependent on the respiratory function and have a lower bioenergetic threshold (Chan 2006). There is a complex interplay between the mitochondria and the host cells, as many proteins in the mitochondria are encoded by the nDNA (including the enzymes of the complexes and of regulators of mtDNA processing) and these proteins are then imported into the mitochondria through a complex receptor and transport system. mtDNA is more vulnerable to oxidative stress (Yakes, Van Houten 1997): its mutation rate is about 5 to 10 times higher than that of nDNA. Although mtDNA lacks protective histones, it possesses the DNA repair machinery (which is entirely nuclear encoded) required to protect against oxidative and nitrative/nitrosative (i.e. caused by nitric oxide radicals [NO^-] and peroxynitrite anion [$ONOO^-$]) damage.

Free Radicals, Oxidative Stress

Free radicals are atoms or molecules with unpaired electrons in their outer orbit. This state makes them chemical species that are highly reactive toward organic macromolecules, leading to cell and tissue damage. Free radicals can extract electrons from neighboring molecules to complete the electron requirements of their own orbitals. This leads to the oxidation of molecules, that is, oxidative damage. The biochemistry of organic oxidative injury is complex.

Although most of the O_2 consumed by the mitochondria is reduced fully to water at complex IV, some (1% to 2%) O_2 is reduced only incompletely, to O_2^-. In the event of a damaged function of one or more respiratory chain complexes, the enhanced production of free radicals further worsens the mitochondrial function by causing oxidative damage and by opening the mtPTPs, thereby inducing apoptosis.

The mitochondrial respiratory chain is one of the major sources of damage-inducing free radicals in the human organism (Delanty, Dichter 1998). Unpaired electrons escaping from the respiratory complexes (mainly from complexes I and III) can lead to the formation of O_2^- by the interaction with O_2. O_2^- itself is moderately damaging, but highly reactive (Beckman, Beckman, Chen et al. 1990). O_2^- undergoes spontaneous dismutation to form H_2O_2. The reaction is catalyzed by SOD. H_2O_2 is subsequently removed by the action of catalase (Beal 1997; Delanty, Dichter 1998).

In response to physiological or pathological stimuli, the activation of excitatory amino acid receptors (*N*-methyl-D-aspartate, NMDA) leads to intracellular Ca^{2+} accumulation and nitric oxide synthase (NOS) activation, with the formation of NO. NO is known to compete with O_2 for the O_2-binding site in complex IV. In this way, NO inhibits electron transfer to O_2 and increases the rate of production of O_2^- and H_2O_2 (Poderoso, Carreras, Lisdero et al. 1996; Stewart,

Heales 2003). An increasing amount of O_2^- interacts with NO to yield the very toxic $ONOO^-$. This reaction occurs at an extremely high rate, 3 times faster than the rate of dismutation of O_2^- by SOD.

$$O_2^- + NO \longrightarrow ONOO^-$$

$$O_2^- \xrightarrow{SOD} H_2O_2 + O_2$$

$$(2O_2^- + 2H \longrightarrow H_2O_2 + O_2)$$

The mitochondrial respiratory chain is particularly sensitive to both NO and $ONOO^-$-mediated damage. Besides causing damage to the respiratory chain complexes (mostly complexes I and IV), $ONOO^-$ may exert a toxic effect through the induction of mtPTP and the activation of caspase-dependent and/or caspase-independent pathways (Bolanos, Heales, Land et al. 1995; Chavez, Melendez, Zazueta et al. 1997). In contrast, NO itself can either induce or inhibit mtPTP (Balakirev, Khramtsov, Zimmer 1997). $ONOO^-$ also causes damage to the DNA and the subsequent overactivation of poly(ADP-ribose) polymerase (PARP) in order to repair the genetic fault. The function of the latter enzyme is a double-edged sword, as it simultaneously involves the consumption of ATP and NAD^+, depletion of which can contribute to cell death. Whereas the activation of PARP-1 by mild genotoxic stimuli may facilitate DNA repair and cell survival, irreparable DNA damage triggers apoptotic or necrotic cell death. In apoptosis, early PARP activation may assist the apoptotic cascade (e.g., by mediating the translocation of the apoptosis-inducing factor [AIF] from the mitochondria to the nucleus or by inhibiting the early activation of DNases). However, in more severe oxidative stress situations, excessive DNA damage causes the overactivation of PARP-1, which incapacitates the apoptotic machinery and switches the mode of cell death from apoptosis to necrosis (Virág 2005).

Under physiological condition, H_2O_2 is broken down by glutathione peroxidase, but if it is formed in excess, it can react with transition metal ions (Fe^{2+} or Cu^{2+}) in the *Fenton reaction*, to generate the highly reactive, toxic radical $OH^\bullet$:

$$H_2O_2 + Fe^{2+} \longrightarrow Fe^{3+} + OH^- + OH^\bullet$$

These reactive radicals destroy cellular macromolecules, including lipids, proteins, and DNA. Free radicals can react with the lipid bilayer of cell membranes, alter their membrane fluidity characteristics, and also lead to the release of potentially toxic by-products. Protein oxidation and nitration may be of crucial importance in the cell cycle (Brookes, Yoon, Robotham et al. 2004). Oxidized and nitrated proteins preferentially undergo rapid proteolytic

degradation. Free radicals also react with DNA and RNA, leading to somatic mutations and to disturbances of transcription and translation.

The mitochondria (the electron transport chain) are one of the major sources of free radicals, but other pathways are also known (e.g., involving xanthine oxidase, monoamine oxidase, cytochrome P450, NOS, myeloperoxidase, and nicotinamide adenine dinucleotide phosphate oxidase [NADPH]).

Cells possess an adaptive, restorative repertoire against oxidative stress, such as the enhanced production of defensive enzymes, an increase in glycolysis, and the activation of genes encoding transcription factors and structural proteins. Antioxidant mechanisms are available to protect against oxidative injury. Mechanisms that protect cells include the compartmentalization of cellular processes (e.g., the action of lysosomes); enzyme systems, such as SOD, glutathione peroxidase, catalase, peroxidase, peroxiredoxin, and some supporting enzymes; specific transport proteins and binding molecules for iron and other metal ions, to maintain them in a nonreactive state (e.g., transferrin, ferritin, and coeruloplasmin); endogenous antioxidant compounds and low molecular weight antioxidants such as the indirect-acting antioxidants (e.g., chelating agents) and direct-acting compounds (e.g., glutathione [GSH] and NADPH); and exogenous agents from dietary sources such as ascorbic acid, lipoic acid, polyphenols, and carotenoids (Sies 1993; Gilgun-Sherki, Melamed, Offen 2001) (Table 18.3).

However, these protective mechanisms are not particularly efficient. Astrocytes are more resistant than neurons to $ONOO^-$, which may be due to their higher GSH content, which functions as a defensive tool in neutralizing NO^-. They can increase glycolysis to maintain their energy homeostasis, as opposed to neurons. Moreover, astrocytes even donate GSH precursors to neurons. They are presumed to release a factor, termed "extracellular SOD" to protect released GSH from degradation (Heales, Bolanos, Stewart et al. 1999).

Overall, it may be assumed that the redox states of the mitochondria are the key components in the regulation of various basic cellular functions, such as mitogen-activated protein kinase cascade activation, ion transport, Ca^{2+} homeostasis, and apoptosis program activation.

Table 18.3 Antioxidant Mechanisms

Compartmentalization

Enzyme systems

Specific transport proteins

Endogenous antioxidant compounds

Exogenous agents from dietary sources

APOPTOSIS

The mitochondria play a central role in both cell life and death. The latter can be necrotic or apoptotic cell death, depending on the severity of the initial insult (Beal 2000). They differ both morphologically and biochemically. Apoptosis is favored in the event of mild insults and relatively preserved ATP production of the cell, while necrosis occurs when the cell suffers a severe, toxic insult. Under certain conditions, of course, the borders between the two forms are not sharp, and the characteristics of both forms can be recognized. In recent years, other forms of cell death have also been described, including autophagy, paraptosis, necroptosis, and oncosis (Leist, Jaattela 2001). The hallmarks of apoptosis, also known as programmed cell death, are nuclear and cytoplasmic shrinkage, fragmentation, and condensation with blebbing of the plasma membrane, which later fragments into several membrane-enclosed particles, termed *apoptotic bodies.* These bodies are recognized, ingested, and degraded by specialized phagocytes (macrophages and immature dendritic cells) and neighboring cells (fibroblasts and endothelial cells). Apoptosis, which is typically not accompanied by an inflammatory reaction (Fadeel, Orrenius 2005), is an important mechanism in the normal cell turnover in growth and development (embryogenesis), in the differentiation of immune cells, and in eliminating redundant or abnormal cells from the organism. Both the failure and the exaggeration of apoptosis in the human organism can lead to diseases, for example, cancer and autoimmune and neurodegenerative disorders, respectively.

Apoptosis means that certain stimuli (the release of proapoptotic members of the Bcl-2 family) set in several biochemical cascade to commit the cells' own suicide program and/or to destroy essential molecules required for cell survival (Emerit, Edeas, Bricaire 2004). The process is mediated by caspases, a family of 14 cysteine proteases. Caspase-2, 8, 9, and 10 constitute the apoptosis activator group, caspase-3, 6, and 7 the apoptosis executioner group, and caspase-1, 4, 5, 11, 12, 13, and 14 the inflammatory mediator group. The executioner caspases are known to cleave more than 280 nuclear and cytoplasmic proteins that are essential components of the cell. Inactivation of these enzymes leads to morphological and biochemical changes (described above) that ultimately cause cell death. The caspases are synthesized and stored as inactive proenzymes.

There are two pathways through which caspases can be activated: one is the death receptor-mediated (extrinsic) pathway; the other is the stress-induced, mitochondrion-mediated (intrinsic) pathway. Intrinsic stimuli can be evoked, for example, by growth-factor deprivation, or by oxidative/mitochondrial or ERS. ERS-induced apoptosis is also driven through the internal pathway, but interestingly without cyt c release (Fan, Han, Cong et al. 2005; Nagata 2005). Following intrinsic stimuli (e.g., moderately decreased levels of ATP), proapoptotic members of the Bcl-2 family become activated and the mitochondrial outer membrane becomes permeable to cyt c, which is subsequently released from the inner membrane into the cytoplasm to trigger caspase activation. This can be inhibited by release of the antiapoptotic members of the Bcl-2 family. Other mitochondrial proteins, such as the AIF and endonuclease G, are liberated from the intermembrane space; they translocate to the nucleus and augment caspase-independent DNA fragmentation (Kluck, Bossy-Wetzel, Green et al. 1997; Bredesen, Rao, Mehlen 2006). In the cytosol, cyt c interacts with an adaptor, Apaf-1 (apoptotic protease-activating factor-1), and procaspase-9, forming a massive complex (containing procaspase-9, cyt c, oligomerized Apaf-1, and dATP) called *apoptosome.* This complex then activates caspase-9, which in turn activates procaspase-3 and leads to the induction of apoptosis (Crompton 2000). Caspase-3 cleaves ICAD (inhibitor of caspase-activated DNase) from CAD (released from the mitochondria), thereby activating the former to a functioning enzyme which, together with others, is responsible for DNA degradation. Substrates of caspases further downstream are lamin A (a component of the nuclear skeleton), the activation of which can lead to the condensation of chromatins and decomposition of the nuclear membrane, and fodrin, which contributes to apoptotic body formation. With the cleavage of PARP, the possibility of DNA repair is diminished. Moreover, the mitochondrial outer membrane is associated with a family of antiapoptotic (such as Bcl-2, Bcl-x_L, Bcl-w, and Bcl-B) and proapoptotic proteins (including Bid, Bax, Bak, Bok, Bad, Puma, Noxa, etc.); these members of the Bcl-2 protein family regulate the permeability of the outer mitochondrial membrane to cyt c and control the responses of the mitochondria to apoptotic signals. Another group of caspase regulators is the inhibitor of apoptosis protein (IAP) family, which can inhibit the process of apoptosis. X-linked IAP (XIAP) binds and inhibits caspase-3 and caspase-9. Smac/Diablo (the second mitochondrial activator of the caspases) is a mitochondrial XIAP antagonist. It can bind to IAP (hence its alternative name, Diablo [direct IAP binding protein of low PI]), thereby preventing the inhibitory effect of IAP on caspase activation (Crompton 2000).

The extrinsic pathway of apoptosis is triggered by the binding of death factors, such as Fas ligand (also termed CD95 ligand) and tumor necrosis factor (TNF) to their receptors (TNFR1). These complexes, together with procaspase-8, which contains two death effector domain-like molecules, constitute the death-inducing signaling complex and activate procaspase-8. The activated complex then activates other caspases, either directly (e.g., procaspase-3) or indirectly, by cleaving Bid. Activated Bid acts as a signal to facilitate the release of cyt c in the intrinsic pathway (Bredesen, Rao, Mehlen 2006).

Evidence is accumulating that suggests that apoptosis is involved in the neuronal death in various acute and chronic central nervous system (CNS) diseases. Caspases and other proteins involved in apoptosis are therapeutic targets in a variety of neurodegenerative disorders. The preclinical evidence is promising, but clinical studies have not yet been performed.

THE KYNURENINE SYSTEM

Tryptophan is metabolized in a number of pathways. The most widely known is the serotonergic pathway, which yields 5-hydroxytryptophan and then serotonin, this route being active in platelets and neurons. Tryptophan is also the precursor of a pineal hormone, melatonin. A less well-known pathway, but actually the main alternative route for the tryptophan metabolism, is through the L-kynurenine (KYN) pathway. This was recognized in 1947. The metabolic cascade was originally known as a source of its end products, nicotinic acid and the two ubiquitous coenzymes of basic cellular processes, NAD^+ and NADP (Moroni 1999). Interest in the importance of the KYN family in neurobiology grew when it emerged that two metabolites of the pathway, quinolinic acid (QUIN) and kynurenic acid (KYNA), act on glutamate receptors. QUIN was shown to be an agonist at the NMDA receptors, whereas KYNA proved to be antagonist of excitatory amino acid receptors. Since excitatory amino acid receptor overactivation is implicated in stroke, epilepsy, and neurodegenerative disorders, considerable drug development research has been focused on the NMDA antagonists. Glutamate-binding site antagonists have certain adverse effects that have limited their clinical usefulness. Accordingly, metabolites of the KYN pathway provide an attractive target for influencing excitatory amino acid receptor functions (Sas, Robotka, Toldi et al. 2007).

Kynurenine Pathway

The enzymatic machinery for the catabolism of tryptophan (Fig. 18.3) exists both in the brain and in the periphery, although it has a much higher capacity in the latter. Under physiological conditions, the vast majority of the brain KYN comes from the periphery; after systemic immunostimulation, it stems exclusively from the blood. In contrast, during CNS-localized immune activation, more than 98% of the KYN and QUIN originates from local synthesis in the brain (Kita, Morrison, Heyes et al. 2002). Tryptophan is converted by indoleamine 2,3-dioxygenase (IDO) to N-formyl-KYN, which is further degraded by formamidase to L-KYN. Bacterial lipopolysaccharides, or some pro-inflammatory cytokines such as interferon γ, are stimulants, while others such as interleukin 4 or 10 (Chiarugi, Calvani, Meli et al. 2001) or SOD (Hirata, Hayaishi 1971), inhibit IDO activity. L-KYN is metabolized in three distinct ways. It serves as a substrate for kynureninase, yielding anthranilic acid; as a substrate for KYN-aminotransferases (KATs), forming KYNA; and as a substrate for KYN-3-hydroxylase, giving rise to 3-OH-KYN. There are two types of KATs within the brain (Okuno, Nakamura, Schwarcz 1991). KAT-I and KAT-II have substantially different pH optima and substrate specificities. KAT-I has an optimal pH of 9.5 to 10, whereas KAT-II is active at neutral pH. Under physiological conditions, they are localized mainly in the astrocytes (Du, Schmidt, Okuno et al. 1992), but they are also present in a few neurons in the hippocampus and in the striatum (Knyihar-Csillik, Okuno, Vécsei 1999) as well as in most of the neurons in the medulla and spinal cord (Kapoor, Okuno, Kido et al. 1997). KAT-II is more specific for L-KYN as a substrate. Thus, large amounts of newly produced KYNA in the brain can be attributed to KAT-II activity (Kiss, Ceresoli-Borroni, Guidetti et al. 2003). 3-OH-KYN is further metabolized by kynureninase, leading to 3-hydroxyanthranilic acid formation. 3-Hydroxyanthranilic acid oxygenase then converts it to α-amino-ω-carboxymuconoic acid semialdehyde, which rearranges itself nonenzymatically to QUIN. Finally, QUIN is degraded by phosphoribosyl transferase to nicotinamide and NAD^+, the end products of the pathway. Within the CNS, the enzymatic machinery for the KYN pathways is within the glial cells. Noticeably though, the astrocytes contain hardly any KYN-3-hydroxylase, and are responsible primarily for KYNA synthesis, while the microglial cells harbor little KAT and in response to certain stimuli can produce large amounts of QUIN. Thus, KYNA synthesis occurs primarily in the astrocytes and QUIN synthesis in the microglial cells (Guillemin, Kerr, Smythe et al. 2001; Lehrmann, Molinari, Speciale et al. 2001).

Kynurenine Pathway Metabolites

A major compound in the pathway is L-KYN, the physiological concentration of which in the brain is 2 μM

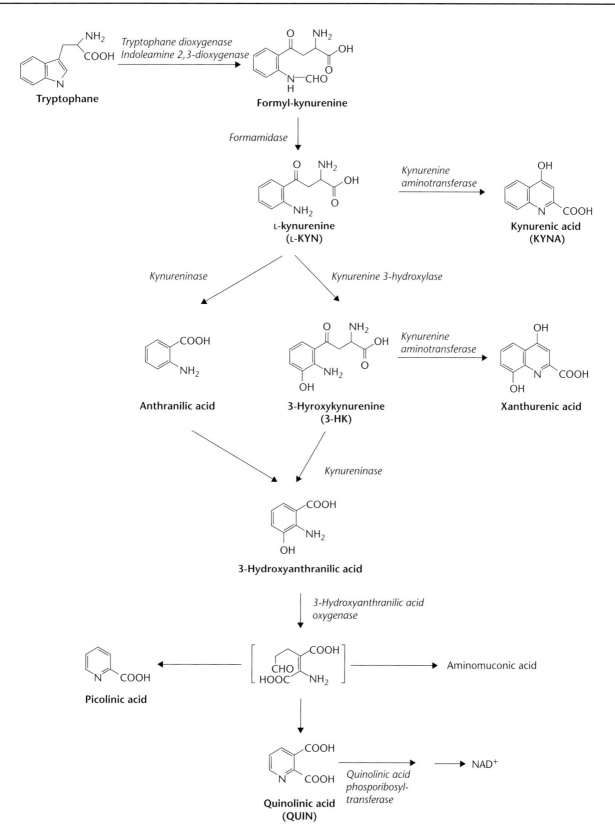

Figure 18.3 The kynurenine pathway.

(Joseph, Baker, Lawson 1978). L-KYN can be metabolized to other components of the pathway: the neuroprotective KYNA, or the neurotoxic 3-OH-KYN and then QUIN. L-KYN, 3-OH-KYN, and anthranilic acid cross the blood–brain barrier well, whereas KYNA, QUIN, and 3-hydroxyanthranilic acid penetrate it poorly (Fukui, Schwarcz, Rapoport et al. 1991). These three metabolites are commonly referred to as neuroactive KYNs. KYN metabolites are also present in comparatively high concentrations in the serum. The cellular uptake of KYN occurs rapidly, predominantly in the astrocytes and microglial cells. While KYNA production is regulated by sophisticated mechanisms, no reuptake or catabolic process for the removal of extracellular KYNA and QUIN has so far been identified. The synaptic effect of QUIN might be long lasting (unlike that of glutamate), which can contribute to the high in vivo potency of this agent (Foster, Schwarcz 1989). The result is that even minor changes in QUIN levels can be potentially dangerous to the neurons.

KYNURENIC ACID

The tissue concentrations of KYNA in the human brain have been estimated to be 0.2 to 1.5 μM (Moroni, Russi, Lombardi et al. 1988; Turski, Nakamura, Todd et al. 1988). KYNA has proved to be a broad-spectrum endogenous antagonist of ionotropic excitatory amino acid receptors (Stone, Connick 1985). KYNA exhibits a particularly high affinity for the glycine-binding site of the NMDA receptor, blocking its activity in low micromolar concentrations (IC50 ≈7.9 μM to 15 μM). Blockade of the glutamate-binding site of the NMDA receptor complex requires concentrations 10 to 20 times higher than those for the glycine site (EC50 ≈200 to 500 μM) (Kessler et al. 1989), whereas KYNA exhibits a weak antagonistic effect on the α-amino-3-hydroxy-5-methylisoxazolepropionate (AMPA) and kainate receptors (Perkins et al. 1985). However, a previously unrecognized higher-affinity positive modulatory binding site at the AMPA receptor has recently been discovered (Prescott, Weeks, Staley et al. 2006). The presynaptic α7-nicotinic acetylcholine receptor is a confirmed site of action for KYNA in a noncompetitive manner (Hilmas, Pereira, Alkondon et al. 2001). It has been concluded that there is a functional connection between the glutamatergic–cholinergic system and the KYN pathway in the brain. NMDA receptors have been found to be substantially less sensitive than α7-nicotinic receptors to KYNA. The local administration of KYNA (30 to 100 nM) into the rat caudal nucleus significantly reduced the glutamate output. This supported the idea that the KYNA-induced inhibition of glutamate release is not mediated by glutamate, but rather via the nicotinic acetylcholine receptors (Carpenedo, Pittaluga, Cozzi et al. 2001). High concentrations of KYNA are anticonvulsant and neuroprotective, and provide protection against excitotoxic injury. The intracerebroventricular administration of KYNA to rats resulted in acute behavioral changes (ataxia and stereotypia, which are characteristics of NMDA open channel blockers) in a dose-dependent manner, while equimolar doses of KYN had only slight behavioral effects (Vécsei, Beal 1990). KYNA can protect against both kainic acid and QUIN neurotoxicity in the adult rat striatum (Foster, Miller, Oldendorf et al. 1984). A reduction in KYNA level enhances the vulnerability to excitotoxic insults and, conversely, a modest elevation of KYNA inhibits glutamate release (Carpenedo, Pittaluga, Cozzi et al. 2001). It has been proposed that, by shifting the KYN metabolism toward KYNA formation, it is possible to reduce glutamate receptor activation and excitotoxic neuronal damage. Peripherally administered L-KYN has been found to increase the cerebral concentrations of KYNA dose-dependently, prompting the suggestion of the existence of a functional, inducible KYN pathway in the CNS (Swartz, During, Freese et al. 1990; Vécsei, Miller, MacGarvey et al. 1992). It is now known that astrocytes generally lack KYN-3-hydroxylase and therefore favor KYNA synthesis, whereas microglial cells contain only a little KAT and preferentially produce intermediates of the QUIN branch of the pathway (Guillemin, Kerr, Smythe et al. 2001). Thus, it appears likely that astrocytes alone are neuroprotective with respect to the KYN balance by minimizing QUIN production and maximizing the synthesis of KYNA. However, in the presence of macrophages and/or microglia, astrocytes can be neurotoxic by producing large quantities of KYN that can be metabolized by neighboring monocytic cells to QUIN (Guillemin, Smith, Kerr et al. 2000). In some neurodegenerative diseases or other pathological states, the changes in the KYN pathway metabolites are modest and balanced with regard to the two KYN branches, probably depending on whether astrocytes or microglia cells are preferentially taking part in the process (Stone 2001; Nemeth, Robotka, Kis et al. 2004; Nemeth, Toldi, Vécsei 2005).

In the early 1990s, focus centered on the effects of peripheral precursor (KYN) loading, in consequence of the poor blood–brain barrier penetration ability of KYNA itself. Accordingly, research attention in the past few years has been directed toward enzyme inhibitors, and particularly the specific and more potent KYN-3-hydroxylase inhibitors, which simultaneously increase KYNA production and block QUIN formation (Stone 2001). Another possibility by which to increase brain KYNA levels is to use analogs of KYNA that can easily penetrate the blood–brain barrier (Stone 2001; Schwarcz 2004). One possible example is the newly synthesized glucoseamine-KYNA, which potently antagonizes the NMDA-receptor-mediated evoked activity of the CA1 region of the rat hippocampus after intraperitoneal administration (Robotka, Nemeth, Somlai et al. 2005).

QUINOLINIC ACID

QUIN is a weak, though specific, competitive agonist of the NMDA receptor subgroup containing the NR2A and NR2B subunits (Stone, Perkins 1981; de Carvalho, Bochet, Rossier 1996), with low receptor affinity (ED50> 100 μM). The QUIN concentrations in the brain tissue are in the nanomolar range (50 to 100 nM) (Moroni 1999), while those in the serum are approximately one order of magnitude higher. Examinations conducted over recent years have revealed that the neurotoxic properties of QUIN involve several mechanisms. In addition to NMDA receptor agonism, it also induces lipid peroxidation (Rios, Santamaria 1991), and produces ROS (Rodriguez-Martinez, Camacho, Maldonado et al. 2000; Santamaría, Galván-Arzate, Lisý et al. 2001). NO, a free radical itself and a precursor of potent toxic radicals such as $ONOO^-$, may contribute to QUIN toxicity, since L-arginine, a well-known NO precursor, enhances QUIN-induced lipid peroxidation in rat striatal slices. The enhanced release of synaptosomal glutamate, as a consequence of the inhibition of glutamate uptake into the astrocytes by QUIN, can be a further factor in its neurotoxicity, by increasing the extracellular glutamate concentrations, which will lead to overstimulation of these receptors (Tavares, Tasca, Santos et al. 2002).

In certain pathological conditions, in which microglial activation occurs at the same time, elevated QUIN levels were measured in the brain or cerebrospinal fluid (CSF) with the result that the accumulation of this compound was implicated in the etiology or pathology of a broad spectrum of human neurological diseases. By virtue of the excitotoxic and free radical generating properties of this compound, the injection of QUIN into the rat striatum leads to excitotoxic damage duplicating the neurochemical features of Huntington's disease [HD] (Schwarcz, Foster, French et al. 1984; Beal, Kowall, Ellison et al. 1986; Beal, Ferrante, Swartz et al. 1991). Many human diseases have been identified in which minor alterations in different KYN pathway metabolites have been observed. However, the numerous experimental data that have accumulated indicate that these multiple imbalances of the KYN pathway metabolism may disturb the normal brain function.

PARKINSON'S DISEASE

PD is the second most common neurodegenerative disorder after AD. The incidence and prevalence rates increase in parallel with aging, about 1% of the population being affected by the age of 65 years. PD is characterized clinically by resting tremor, rigidity, bradykinesia, and postural instability. The pathological hallmarks are a preferential loss of dopaminergic neurons in the substantia nigra pars compacta and the presence of intracytoplasmic inclusions (Lewy bodies) containing α-synuclein, ubiquitin, ubiquitinated protein, neurofilaments, and HSPs. Current modes of therapy for PD are based on the replacement of dopamine, which improves the symptoms but does not modify the progression of the degeneration. An obvious target would be a stop at any point of the pathogenic mechanism of neurodegeneration (McNaught, Olanow 2003, 2006). The important question is to determine whether there is one common pathway in sporadic PD.

Evidence of a mitochondrial dysfunction in idiopathic PD comes from a significant decrease in complex I activity in the substantia nigra and platelets, but this defect does not affect any other part of the respiratory chain (Schapira, Cooper, Dexter et al. 1989). In PD, there is abundant evidence of the occurrence of mitochondrial damage and oxidative stress, both in the clinical setting and in experimental models. Chronic infusions of the complex I inhibitor rotenone produce an animal model of PD in rats. Exposure to the environmental toxin 1-methyl-4-phenyl-1,2,3, 4-tetrahydropyridine (MPTP) results in a Parkinsonian syndrome. Studies of the mechanism of MPTP neurotoxicity have demonstrated that 1-methyl-4-phenylpyridinium (MPP^+), the major metabolite of MPTP, is responsible for the neuronal injury. MPP^+ formation in astrocytes is catalyzed by monoamine oxidase B. MPP^+ is taken up into the dopaminergic neurons by the synaptic dopamine transporter and concentrated in the mitochondria, where it inhibits complex I of the electron transport chain (Tipton, Singer 1993). A 30% reduction in complex I activity has been described in the brain, muscle, and platelets of idiopathic PD patients (Schapira, Cooper, Dexter et al. 1990). This has two major consequences: the depletion of ATP, and the generation of free radicals that cause oxidative stress, as indicated by findings of reduced levels of antioxidants and GSH, an increased level of pro-oxidant iron, and evidence of oxidative damage to proteins, lipids, and DNA. mtDNA itself may also be implicated in PD, but no specific mutations in mtDNA protein coding regions have been found so far. However, specific mtDNA polymorphisms or haplotypes have been proposed to be implicated in PD. There is a reduced risk of PD

Table 18.4 Summary of Genetic Causes of PD

α-Synuclein	Cytosolic protein	Polymeropoulos et al. 1997
Parkin	Ubiquitin E3 ligase	Kitada et al. 1998
DJ-1	Redox sensor	Bonifati et al. 2003
PINK1	Nuclear-encoded mitochondrial kinase	Valente et al. 2004
OMI/HTRA2	Proapoptotic serine protease	Strauss et al. 2005
LRRK2	Kinase interacts with parkin	Zimprich et al. 2004
UCHL1	Ubiquitin carboxyl-terminal esterase L1	Leroy et al. 1998

in individuals with haplotypes J and K (Van der Walt, Nicodemus, Martin et al. 2003), and haplotype cluster UKJT (Pyle et al. 2005), whereas the supercluster JTIWX increases the risk of PD (Autere et al. 2004). The dopaminergic neurons in the substantia nigra preferentially accumulate high levels of deletions in mtDNA with aging, resulting in a loss of respiratory chain activity (Bender et al. 2006; Kraytsberg et al. 2006).

Genetic causes of PD affect the mitochondrial function (Table 18.4). Mutations in α-synuclein are associated with autosomal dominant familial PD and the increased formation of oligomeric or fibrillar aggregates, damaging the mitochondria directly (Polymeropoulos et al. 1997; Martin, Pan, Price et al. 2006).

Mutations in parkin are associated with autosomal recessive juvenile PD (Kitada et al. 1998). Parkin encodes a ubiquitin E3 ligase, which is involved in the UPS (Betarbet, Sherer, Greenamyre 2005). Parkin can associate with the outer mitochondrial membrane and prevent mitochondrial swelling, cyt c release, and caspase activation. The S-nitrosylation of parkin, an oxidative modification, compromises its protective function (Darios, Corti, Lucking et al. 2003). Parkin interacts with mitochondrial transcription factor A and enhances mtDNA transcription and replication (Kuroda, Mitsui, Kunishige et al. 2006).

Mutations in DJ-1 are associated with autosomal recessive juvenile PD (Bonifati et al. 2003). DJ-1 is localized in both the mitochondrial matrix and intermembrane space. Its function is to modulate the oxidative stress response (Zhang, Shimoji, Thomas et al. 2005). The overexpression of DJ-1 appears to protect cells against mitochondrial complex I inhibitors and the oxidative stress induced by H_2O_2 (Yang, Gehrke, Haque et al. 2005).

Mutations in PINK1 are also associated with autosomal recessive juvenile PD. PINK1 is a kinase localized to the mitochondria, which protects against cell death via decreases in cyt c release and caspase

activation (Valente, Abou-Sleiman, Caputo et al. 2004; Petit, Kawarai, Paitel et al. 2005).

OMI/Htra2 is a ubiquitously expressed serine protease that shares functional properties with Smac/Diablo. It is localized to the mitochondrial intermembrane space, but is released to the cytosol by proapoptotic stimuli. It then interacts with cytosolic IAP proteins and hence promotes apoptosis (Suzuki, Imai, Nakayama et al. 2001; Strauss et al. 2005).

Mutations in LRRK2 cause late-onset autosomal dominant PD. LRRK2 encodes for a protein called *dardarin*. This is a member of a novel family of protein kinases that exhibit sequence similarity to both tyrosine and serine/threonine kinases. The protein is associated with the outer mitochondrial membrane. It has been found to interact with parkin (Zimprich et al. 2004).

UCHL1 is a neuron-specific protein that belongs to a family of deubiquitinating enzymes. Reduced UCHL1 activity might impair the efficiency of the UPS by reducing the availability of free ubiquitin monomers. It leads to potentially deleterious protein accumulation (Leroy et al. 1998).

Endogenous excitotoxins have also been implicated in the degeneration of the nigral dopaminergic neurons in PD. Activation of the NMDA receptors has been shown to be toxic to substantia nigra pars compacta dopamine-containing neurons in vitro (Kikuchi et al. 1989). The activation of the NMDA receptors leads to intracellular Ca^{2+} accumulation and NOS (mtNOS or nNOS) activation, with the production of NO. The levels of 3-OH-KYN are elevated in the putamen and substantia nigra of brains for patients with PD. The ratio KYN/3-OH-KYN is reduced from the control levels in the substantia nigra, frontal cortex, and putamen (KYN can be metabolized toward the NMDA receptor agonist QUIN through 3-OH-KYN, and toward KYNA, the excitotoxin antagonist) (Ogawa, Matson, Beal et al. 1992). This would imply not only an increased synthesis of the toxic metabolite 3-OH-KYN but also a reduced proportion of KYN being available, which would contribute to the susceptibility of these neurons to damage.

The intracerebroventricular administration of nicotinylalanine, an inhibitor of kynureninase and KYN-3-hydroxylase (inhibiting the QUIN metabolic pathway and turning the metabolism of KYN toward KYNA synthesis), together with systemic KYN and probenecid, an inhibitor of organic acid transport (to prevent KYNA excretion), elevated the brain KYNA levels and prevented QUIN toxicity (Miranda, Boegman, Beninger et al. 1997). It also diminished the turning behavior of animals with QUIN-induced partial lesions of the substantia nigra. It was concluded that the protective effect may be due to a combination of an increase in KYNA and the prevention of endogenous QUIN production (Miranda, Sutton, Beninger et al. 1999).

Mitochondrial toxins, some of them found in the environment, are thought to be involved in the pathogenesis of certain neurodegenerative diseases. Treatment with MPTP, a complex I inhibitor used to model PD, resulted in decreased numbers of KAT-I-immunoreactive neurons in the pars compacta and certain microglial cells in the pars reticularis of the substantia nigra in mice (Knyihar-Csillik, Csillik, Pakaski et al. 2004), and in a reduced level of available ATP, ultimately leading to a cellular energy deficit. MPTP has been shown to inhibit KYNA synthesis via interference with KAT-I and KAT-II (Luchowski, Luchowska, Turski et al. 2002). FK506 is a neuroimmunophilin ligand that belongs in a relatively new class of drugs, nowadays used in the clinical setting as immunosuppressants. It was recently recognized that some of its derivatives display neurotrophic and neuroreparative activity, although the precise mechanisms are not yet clear. Experimentally, FK506 not only enhanced the formation of KYNA in cortical slices but even abolished the inhibition of KYNA synthesis evoked by MPP$^+$ and 3-nitropropionic acid (Luchowska, Luchowski, Wielosz et al. 2003). It was concluded that the protective effect of this compound against the mitochondrial toxin-related inhibition of KYNA synthesis may result from the restoration of ATP levels, and FK506 may be the first drug with the ability to enhance the formation of KYNA, an endogenous glutamate receptor antagonist ligand. Pharmacological manipulation of KYNA formation in the brain, as a novel therapeutic approach to modulate basic glutamatergic responses in target brain

areas, may be of promise as a better mode of treatment of PD (Fig. 18.4).

ALZHEIMER'S DISEASE

AD, the most common form of dementia in the elderly, is a chronic, progressive, irreversible degenerative neurological disorder. AD is characterized clinically by an impairment of the cognitive functions and changes in behavior and personality. The neuropathological hallmarks of the disorder are synaptic loss, neuronal cell death, reactive astrogliosis, extracellular amyloid plaques, and intracellular neurofibrillary tangles. The major constituent of the amyloid plaques is β-amyloid peptide (Aβ), while that of the neurofibrillary tangles is the hyperphosphorylated tau protein (Rosenberg 2000). The abnormal deposition of amyloid peptides is caused by the altered processing of the amyloid precursor protein (APP) (Selkoe 2001). Aβ is the primary molecule in the pathogenic cascade for AD, and the tau dysfunction and tangle formation are downstream events in the process.

There are five principal risk factors for AD: age; mutations in the presenilin 1 (*PS1*) gene on chromosome 14 (Sherrington, Rogaev, Liang et al. 1995); mutations in the presenilin 2 (*PS2*) gene on chromosome 1 (Rogaev, Sherrington, Rogaeva et al. 1995; Levy-Lahad, Wasco, Poorkaj et al. 1995); mutations in the *APP* gene on chromosome 21 (Goate, Chartier-Harlin, Mullan et al. 1991); and APOE alleles positioned on the proximal long arm of chromosome 19 (Farrer, Cupples, Haines et al. 1997). AD is genetically

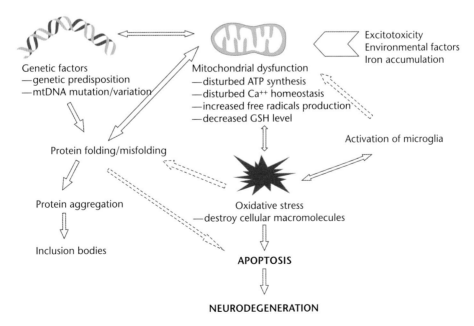

Figure 18.4 Pathomechanism of sporadic Parkinson's disease.

complex: most AD cases are nonfamilial, sporadic late-onset forms, and only approximately 2% to 3% of the cases of AD are inherited in an autosomal dominant manner.

A mitochondrial dysfunction is widely implicated in the pathogenesis of AD. Oxidative damage occurs early in the AD brain, before the onset of significant plaque pathology (Nunomura, Perry, Aliev et al. 2001). The reduction in the metabolism of the temporoparietal cortices precedes the clinical symptoms by decades (Small, Mazziotta, Collins et al. 1995). Impaired activities of the enzyme complexes pyruvate dehydrogenase, isocitrate dehydrogenase, and α-ketoglutarate dehydrogenase in the tricarboxylic acid cycle (the Krebs cycle) have been found in postmortem AD brain samples (Bubber, Haroutunian, Fisch et al. 2005). All the changes observed in the tricarboxylic acid cycle activities are correlated with the clinical state. The mitochondrial enzyme for which a defect in activity is reported most consistently in AD is cyt c oxidase (complex IV). Deficient complex IV activity has been reported in different brain regions, platelets, and fibroblasts (Kish, Bergeron, Rajput et al. 1992). The degree of the deficiency in the cortex has been assessed to be 25% to 30% (Mutisya, Bowling, Beal 1994). This may result in ATP depletion, an increased production of ROS, and an increase in Aβ production, thereby augmenting the pathological cascade (de Vrij et al. 2004). Moreover, it has been shown that Aβ could directly inhibit the activity of complex IV in the nonsynaptic brain mitochondria (Canevari, Clark, Bates 1999). Thus, Aβ can be viewed as a direct mitochondrial toxin, leading to a vicious circle of mitochondrial compromise (Maccioni, Munoz, Barbeito 2001). Involvement of other mitochondrial electron transport chain complexes is more controversial.

While it is clear that mtDNA mutations accumulate with aging, AD has not been found to be associated with specific point mutations in mtDNA. Moreover, mtDNA polymorphisms have been presumed to have a role in the pathogenesis of AD. While haplogroup J seems to be overrepresented, haplogroup T is underrepresented in AD patients (Chagnon, Gee, Filion et al. 1999); the exact roles of the haplogroups remain to be clarified.

The role of Aβ in the neuropathology of AD is to cause free radical injury and excitotoxicity. A high concentration of Aβ increases the vulnerability of the neurons to glutamate-induced cell death through the inhibition of astrocytic glutamate transporters (Harris, Wang, Pedigo et al. 1996). Aβ binds to a mitochondrial matrix protein termed *Aβ-binding alcohol dehydrogenase*. Blockade of this interaction suppresses free radical generation and Aβ-induced apoptosis in neurons (Takuma, Yao, Huang et al. 2005).

Alterations in the KYN pathway have been implicated in the pathogenesis of AD. Postmortem studies of AD brains revealed elevated brain KYNA concentrations in the putamen and caudate nucleus, which was accompanied by a significant increase in KAT-I activity in both nuclei (Baran, Jellinger, Deecke 1999). It was concluded that the marked increase in KYNA in these brain regions may reflect a compensatory mechanism whereby the striatofrontal loop becomes hyperactivated as a response to neuronal loss in the cortical target areas. Elevated KYNA concentrations may exert an inhibitory effect on NMDA receptor activation, and thus may serve as a pathogenic factor in a neuronal dysfunction causing a cognitive deterioration in AD. On the other hand, QUIN can also be involved in the pathogenesis of AD. Recent data provide evidence that the KYN–QUIN pathway is upregulated in the AD brain. It has been reported that the plasma level of tryptophan falls with aging in humans and is further lowered in AD, with elevation of the KYN levels. These alterations in the KYN pathways may be associated with the induction of IDO, the catalyst of the initial step of the metabolic pathway, induced by the chronic inflammation that accompanies both disease processes (Widner, Leblhuber, Walli et al. 1999). Guillemin and colleagues also found the microglial and astrocytic expressions of IDO and QUIN production in the AD hippocampus, which were highest in the perimeter of the senile plaques (Guillemin, Brew, Noonan et al. 2005). These results may open up new avenues in the treatment of AD patients. Nevertheless, neurons exposed to Aβ exhibit an increased vulnerability to excitotoxicity, and the slow form of excitotoxicity is known to be one of the underlying pathological processes of AD. Aβ induces the production of QUIN by the microglia and macrophages so that it can reach neurotoxic concentrations. Besides the NMDA agonistic effect, QUIN exerts a marked toxic effect by inducing lipid peroxidation and consequently the generation of toxic free radicals, which are known to have a great impact on the pathogenesis of AD (Guillemin, Brew 2002).

HUNTINGTON'S DISEASE

HD is an autosomal dominantly inherited progressive neurodegenerative disorder. The main symptoms are choreiform, involuntary movements, personality changes, and dementia. The symptoms usually appear in mid-life and the progression of the disease inevitably leads to death within 15 to 20 years.

HD is a member of a group of diseases caused by cytosine–adenine–guanine (CAG) repeat expansions. The mutant gene causing HD has been localized to chromosome 4p16.3 and is named IT 15 (interesting transcript). It codes a protein, huntingtin, which is widely distributed in both neurons and extraneuronal tissues. Wild-type huntingtin may act as a molecular scaffold, regulating several cellular processes, including endocytosis, vesicle transport, excitatory synapses, transcriptional events, and the mitochondrial function. The mutation in the HD gene involves the expansion of a trinucleotide (CAG) repeat encoding glutamine, resulting in a polyglutamine stretch in huntingtin. Expanded polyglutamine domains in the mutant protein are postulated to promote cytoplasmic and nuclear protein–protein interactions (Perutz, Johnson, Suzuki et al. 1994). Elongation of the glutamine repeats beyond a certain length may lead to conformational change, oligomerization, and then amyloid-like aggregate formation (Valera et al. 2005).

The aggregates do not contain the entire huntingtin, but only N-terminal fragments. Cleavage seems to be a precondition for the translocation of polyglutamine-containing fragments into the nucleus (DiFiglia, Sapp, Chase et al. 1997). There, huntingtin interacts with a number of transcription factors themselves containing polyglutamine-rich regions (e.g. CBP, p53, TAF$_{II}$130, and Sp1). Consequently, the mutant huntingtin alters numerous forms of the gene expression by changing the functions of the transcriptional factors (Walton, Dragunow 2000; Wyttenbach, Swartz, Kita H et al. 2001). Thus, there is change in neuronal function (Gárdián, Vécsei 2004; Gárdián, Browne, Choi et al. 2005).

One research aim is to determine the earliest molecular changes associated with HD. There is no possibility for this in humans, but various early changes have been identified in an animal model of HD. They involve an excitotoxin causing striatal lesions, or mitochondrial toxins inducing energy impairment, or the generation of transgenic mice. Marked decreases in the activities of mitochondrial complexes II and III, and a smaller reduction in that of complex IV, have been detected in the caudate and putamen of postmortem HD brain samples (Gu, Gash, Mann et al. 1996; Browne, Bowling, MacGarvey et al. 1997). Malonate and 3-NP are mitochondrial toxins that act as inhibitors of complex II of the respiratory chain. The administration of 3-NP (local intrastriatal or chronic systematic) causes a chronic encephalopathy characterized by late-onset basal ganglia degeneration, motor disturbances (dystonia), and frontal-type cognitive deficits, all resembling Huntington's chorea. Besides ATP depletion, 3-NP causes additional oxidative damage and NMDA receptor activation, so that systemic administration of the toxin can replicate many of the characteristic histological, biochemical, and behavioral features of HD, but with the exception of the expanded polyglutamine repeat of huntingtin (Beal, Brouillet, Jenkins et al. 1993; Brouillet, Conde,

Beal et al. 1999). There is evidence that excitotoxicity may play a role in the pathogenesis of HD (Coyle, Schwarcz 1976; McGeer, McGeer 1976; DiFiglia 1990). It has been demonstrated that the injection of QUIN produces a lesion that is a reliable model of HD (Schwarcz, Whetsell, Mangano 1983; Beal, Kowall, Ellison et al. 1986; Vécsei, Beal 1996; Vécsei, Dibo, Kiss 1998). An impairment of the mitochondrial energy metabolism can result in decreased ATP production, with an accompanying reduction of the Na$^+$–K$^+$ ATPase activity. Partial cell depolarization may occur, leading to alleviation of the voltage-dependent Mg^{2+} blockade of NMDA receptor-associated channels. Accordingly, endogenous levels of glutamate activate NMDA receptors. The concomitant increase in Ca^{2+} influx into the neurons may trigger further free radical production (Beal 1992). Huntingtin-mediated aggregation might induce the initiation of programmed cell death (apoptosis) via activation of the initiator caspase-8, 9, and 10. A mitochondrial dysfunction, excitotoxicity, and apoptosis have been implicated in the pathogenesis of HD, but they could be secondary (Manfredi, Beal 2000).

As mentioned above, a part has long been attributed to QUIN in the pathophysiology of HD, because the intrastriatal injection of QUIN duplicates many of the distinct neuropathological features of the striatum in patients with HD. The CSF and blood QUIN levels do not differ in HD patients as compared with controls (Reynolds, Pearson, Halket et al. 1988; Schwarcz, Tamminga, Kurlan et al. 1988; Stoy, Mackay, Forrest et al. 2005). The level of KYNA in the striatum has been reported to be reduced in HD patients (Beal, Matson, Storey et al. 1992), although others found it to be elevated (Jauch, Sethy, Weick et al. 1993). Nevertheless, the CSF level of KYNA does not appear to change in HD (Heyes, Saito, Crowley et al. 1992).

The accumulated evidence allows the assumption that an expansion of the CAG trinucleotide repeat in the gene encoding polyglutamine repeats in the protein named huntingtin is the primary cause of the disease. This mutated protein can alter several cellular processes, among others gene transcription, and can induce a mitochondrial dysfunction. It may be assumed that mitochondrial energy impairment sensitizes the neurons to the excitotoxic effects of glutamate released tonically from the corticostriatal afferents and ultimately causes selective neuronal cell death by apoptosis.

ACKNOWLEDGMENTS Thanks are due to D. Durham from England for the linguistic correction of manuscript. This work was supported by grants ETT 215/2006 and RET-08/2004.

REFERENCES

Arrasate M, Mitra S, Schweitzer ES, Segal MR, Finkbeiner S. 2004. Inclusion body formation reduces levels of mutant huntington and the risk of neuronal death. *Nature*. 431:805–810.

Autere J, Moilanen JS, Finnila S, Soininen H et al. 2004. Mitochondrial DNA polymorphisms as risk factors for Parkinson's disease and Parkinson's disease dementia. *Hum Genet*. 115:29–35.

Balakirev MY, Khramtsov VV, Zimmer G. 1997. Modulation of the mitochondrial permeability transition by nitric oxide. *Eur J Biochem*. 246:710–718.

Baran H, Jellinger K, Deecke L. 1999. Kynurenine metabolism in Alzheimer's disease. *J Neural Transm*. 106:165–181.

Beal MF. 1992. Does impairment of energy metabolism result in excitotoxic neuronal death in neurodegenerative illnesses? *Ann Neurology*. 31:119–130.

Beal MF. 1997. Oxidative damage in neurodegenerative diseases. *Neuroscientist*. 3:21–27.

Beal MF. 2000. Energetics in the pathogenesis of neurodegenerative diseases. *Trends Neurosci*. 23:298–304.

Beal MF, Kowall NW, Ellison DW, Mazurek MF, Swartz KJ, Martin JB. 1986. Replication of the neurochemical characteristics of Huntington's disease by quinolinic acid. *Nature*. 321:168–171.

Beal MF, Ferrante RJ, Swartz KJ, Kowall NW. 1991. Chronic quinolinic acid lesions in rats closely resemble Huntington's disease. *J Neurosci*. 11:1649–1659.

Beal MF, Matson WR, Storey E et al. 1992. Kynurenic acid concentrations are reduced in Huntington's disease cerebral cortex. *J Neurol Sci*. 108:80–87.

Beal MF, Brouillet E, Jenkins BG et al. 1993. Neurochemical and histologic characterization of striatal excitotoxic lesions produced by the mitochondrial toxin 3-nitropropionic acid. *J Neurosci*. 13:4181–4192.

Beckman JS, Beckman TW, Chen J, Marshall PA, Freeman BA. 1990. Apparent hydroxyl radical production by peroxynitrite: implications for endothelial injury from nitric oxide and superoxide. *Proc Natl Acad Sci USA*. 87:1620–1624.

Bence NF, Sampat RM, Kopito RR. 2001. Impairment of the ubiquitin-proteasome system by protein aggregation. *Science*. 292:1552–1555.

Bender A, Krishnan KJ, Morris CM et al. 2006. High levels of mitochondrial DNA deletions in substantia nigra neurons in aging and Parkinson disease. *Nat Genet*. 38:515–517.

Bennett EJ, Bence NF, Jayakumar R, Kopito RR. 2005. Global impairment of the ubiquitin-proteasome system by nuclear or cytoplasmic protein aggregates precedes inclusion body formation. *Mol Cell*. 17:351–365.

Betarbet R, Sherer TB, Greenamyre JT. 2005. Ubiquitin-proteasome system and Parkinson's diseases. *Exp Neurol*. 191(Suppl 1):S17–S27.

Bolanos JP, Heales SJ, Land JM, Clark JB. 1995. Effect of peroxynitrite on the mitochondrial respiratory chain: differential susceptibility of neurones and astrocytes in primary culture. *J Neurochem*. 64:1965–1972.

Bonifati V, Rizzu P, van Baren MJ et al. 2003. Mutations in the DJ-1 gene associated with autosomal recessive early-onset parkinsonism. *Science*. 299:256–259.

Bredesen DE, Rao RV, Mehlen P. 2006. Cell death in the nervous system. *Nature*. 443:796–802.

Brookes PS, Yoon Y, Robotham JL, Anders MW, Sheu SS. 2004. Calcium, ATP, and ROS: a mitochondrial love-hate triangle. *Am J Physiol Cell Physiol*. 287:C817–C833.

Brouillet E, Conde F, Beal MF, Hantraye P. 1999. Replicating Huntington's disease phenotype in experimental animals. *Prog Neurobiol*. 59:427–468.

Browne SE, Bowling AC, MacGarvey U et al. 1997. Oxidative damage and metabolic dysfunction in Huntington's disease: selective vulnerability of the basal ganglia. *Ann Neurol*. 41:646–653.

Bubber P, Haroutunian V, Fisch G, Blass JP, Gibson GE. 2005. Mitochondrial abnormalities in Alzheimer brain: mechanistic implications. *Ann Neurol*. 57:695–703.

Canevari L, Clark JB, Bates TE. 1999. Beta-amyloid fragment 25–35 selectively decreases complex IV activity in isolated mitochondria. *FEBS Lett*. 457:131–134.

Carpenedo R, Pittaluga A, Cozzi A et al. 2001. Presynaptic kynurenate-sensitive receptors inhibit glutamate release. *Eur J Neurosci*. 13:2141–2147.

Chagnon P, Gee M, Filion M, Robitaille Y, Belouchi M, Gauvreau D. 1999. Phylogenetic analysis of the mitochondrial genome indicates significant differences between patients with Alzheimer's disease and controls in a French–Canadian founder population. *Am J Med Genet*. 85:20–30.

Chan DC. 2006. Mitochondria: dynamic organelles in disease, aging, and development. *Cell*. 125:1241–1252.

Chaudhuri TK, Paul S. 2006. Protein-misfolding diseases and chaperone-based therapeutic approaches. *FEBS J*. 273:1331–1349.

Chavez E, Melendez E, Zazueta C, Reyes-Vivas H, Perales SG. 1997. Membrane permeability transition as induced by dysfunction of the electron transport chain. *Biochem Mol Biol Int*. 41:961–968.

Chiarugi A, Calvani M, Meli E, Traggiai E, Moroni F. 2001. Synthesis and release of neurotoxic kynurenine metabolites by human monocyte-derived macrophages. *J Neuroimmunol*. 120:190–198.

Ciechanover A. 2005. Proteolysis: from the lysosome to ubiquitin and the proteasome. *Nat Rev Mol Cell Biol*. 6:79–87.

Ciechanover A, Brundin P. 2003. The ubiquitin proteasome system in neurodegenerative diseases: sometimes the chicken, sometimes the egg. *Neuron*. 40:427–446.

Coyle JT, Schwarcz R. 1976. Lesion of striatal neurons with kainic acid provides a model of Huntington's chorea. *Nature*. 263:244–246.

Crompton M. 2000. Mitochondrial intermembrane junctional complexes and their role in cell death. *J Physiol*. 529:11–21.

Darios F, Corti O, Lucking CB et al. 2003. Parkin prevents mitochondrial swelling and cytochrome c release in mitochondria-dependent cell death. *Hum Mol Genet*. 12:517–526.

Davey GP, Canevari L, Clark JB. 1997. Threshold effects in synaptosomal and nonsynaptic mitochondria from hippocampal CA1 and paramedian neocortex brain regions. *J Neurochem*. 69:2564–2570.

de Carvalho LP, Bochet P, Rossier J. 1996. The endogenous agonist quinolinic acid and the nonendogenous homoquinolinic acid discriminate between NMDAR2 receptor subunits. *Neurochem Int.* 28:445–452.

Delanty N, Dichter MA. 1998. Oxidative injury in the nervous system. *Acta Neurol Scand.* 98:145–153.

de Vrij FM, Fischer DF, van Leeuwen FW, Hol EM. 2004. Protein quality control in Alzheimer's disease by the ubiquitin-proteasome system. *Prog Neurobiol.* 74:249–270.

DiFiglia M. 1990. Excitotoxic injury of the neostriatum: a model for Huntington's disease. *Trends Neurosci.* 13:286–289.

DiFiglia M, Sapp E, Chase KO et al. 1997. Aggregation of huntingtin in neuronal intranuclear inclusions and dystrophic neuritis in brain. *Science.* 277:1990–1993.

Du F, Schmidt W, Okuno E, Kido R, Köhler C, Schwarcz R. 1992. Localization of kynurenine aminotransferase immunoreactivity in the rat hippocampus. *J Comp Neurol.* 321:477–487.

Dykens JA. 1997. Mitochondrial free radical production and oxidative pathophysiology: implications for neurodegenerative disease. In Beal MF, Howell N, Bódis-Wollner I, eds. *Mitochondria and Free Radicals in Neurodegenerative Diseases.* New York: John Wiley-Liss, Inc, 29–56.

Emerit J, Edeas M, Bricaire F. 2004. Neurodegenerative diseases and oxidative stress. *Biomed Pharmacother.* 58:39–46.

Fadeel B, Orrenius S. 2005. Apoptosis: a basic biological phenomenon with wide-ranging implications in human disease. *J Intern Med.* 258:479–517.

Fan TJ, Han LH, Cong RS, Liang J. 2005. Caspase family proteases and apoptosis. *Acta Biochim Biophys Sin (Shanghai).* 37:719–727.

Farrer LA, Cupples LA, Haines JL et al. 1997. Effects of age, sex, and ethnicity on the association between apolipoprotein E genotype and Alzheimer disease. A meta-analysis APOE and Alzheimer disease meta Analysis Consortium. *JAMA.* 278:1349–1356.

Foster AC, Miller LP, Oldendorf WH, Schwarcz R. 1984. Studies on the disposition of quinolinic acid after intracerebral or systemic administration in the rat. *Exp Neurol.* 84:428–440.

Foster AC, Schwarcz R. 1989. Neurotoxic effects of quionolinic acid in the central nervous system. In Stone TW, ed. *Quinolinic Acid and Other Kynurenines.* Boca Raton, FL: CRC Press, 173–192.

Fukui S, Schwarcz R, Rapoport SI, Takada Y, Smith QR. 1991. Blood–brain barrier transport of kynurenines: implications for brain synthesis and metabolism. *J Neurochem.* 56:2007–2017.

Gárdián G, Vécsei L. 2004. Huntington's disease: pathomechanism and therapeutic perspectives. *J Neural Transm.* 111:1485–1494.

Gárdián G, Browne SE, Choi DK et al. 2005. Neuroprotective effects of phenylbutyrate in the N171–82Q transgenic mouse model of Huntington's disease. *J Biol Chem.* 280:556–563.

Gilgun-Sherki Y, Melamed E, Offen D. 2001. Oxidative stress induced-neurodegenerative diseases: the need for antioxidants that penetrate the blood brain barrier. *Neuropharmacology.* 40:959–975.

Goate A, Chartier-Harlin MC, Mullan M et al. 1991. Segregation of a missense mutation in the amyloid precursor protein gene with familial Alzheimer's disease. *Nature.* 349:704–706.

Goldberg AL. 2003. Protein degradation and protection against misfolded or damaged proteins. *Nature.* 426:895–899.

Gu M, Gash MT, Mann VM, Javoy-Agid F, Cooper JM, Schapira AH. 1996. Mitochondrial defect in Huntington's disease caudate nucleus. *Ann Neurol.* 39:385–389.

Guillemin GJ, Smith DG, Kerr SJ et al. 2000. Characterisation of kynurenine pathway metabolism in human astrocytes and implications in neuropathogenesis. *Redox Rep.* 5:108–111.

Guillemin GJ, Kerr SJ, Smythe GA et al. 2001. Kynurenine pathway metabolism in human astrocytes: a paradox for neuronal protection. *J Neurochem.* 78:842–853.

Guillemin GJ, Brew BJ. 2002. Implications of the kynurenine pathway and quinolinic acid in Alzheimer's disease. *Redox Rep.* 7:199–206.

Guillemin GJ, Brew BJ, Noonan CE, Takikawa O, Cullen KM. 2005. Indoleamine 2,3 dioxygenase and quinolinic acid immunoreactivity in Alzheimer's disease hippocampus. *Neuropathol Appl Neurobiol.* 31:395–404.

Harris ME, Wang Y, Pedigo NW Jr, Hensley K, Butterfield DA, Carney JM. 1996. Amyloid beta peptide (25–35) inhibits Na$^+$-dependent glutamate uptake in rat hippocampal astrocyte cultures. *J Neurochem.* 67:277–286.

Hartl FU, Hayer-Hartl M. 2002. Molecular chaperones in the cytosol: from nascent chain to folded protein. *Science.* 295:1852–1858.

Heales SJ, Bolanos JP, Stewart VC, Brookes PS, Land JM, Clark JB. 1999. Nitric oxide, mitochondria and neurological disease. *Biochim Biophys Acta.* 1410:215–228.

Heyes MP, Saito K, Crowley JS et al. 1992. Quinolinic acid and kynurenine pathway metabolism in inflammatory and non-inflammatory neurologic disease. *Brain.* 115:1249–1273.

Hilmas C, Pereira EFR, Alkondon M, Rassoulpour A, Schwarcz R, Albuquerque EX. 2001. The brain metabolite kynurenic acid inhibits α7 nicotinic receptor activity and increases non-α7 nicotinic receptor expression: physiological implications. *J Neurosci.* 21:7463–7473.

Hirata F, Hayaishi O. 1971. Possible participation of superoxide anion in the intestinal tryptophan 2,3-dioxygenase reaction. *J Biol Chem.* 246:7825–7826.

Holmsen H, Robkin L. 1980. Effects of antimycin A and 2-deoxyglucose on energy metabolism in washed human platelets. *Thromb Haemost.* 42:1460–1472.

Jauch DA, Sethy VH, Weick BG, Chase TN, Schwarcz R. 1993. Intravenous administration of L-kynurenine to rhesus monkeys: effect on quinolinate and kynurenate levels in serum and cerebrospinal fluid. *Neuropharmacology.* 32:467–472.

Joseph MH, Baker HF, Lawson AM. 1978. Positive identification of kynurenine in rat and human brain. *Biochem Soc Trans.* 6:123–126.

Kapoor R, Okuno E, Kido R, Kapoor V. 1997. Immunolocalization of kynurenine aminotransferase (KAT) in the rat medulla and spinal cord. *Neuroreport.* 8:3619–3623.

Kessler M, Terramani T, Lynch G, Boundary M. 1989. A glycine site associated with N-methyl-D-aspartic acid receptors: characterization and identification of a new class of antagonists. *J Neurochem.* 52:1319–1328.

Kikuchi S, Kim SU. 1993. Glutamate neurotoxicity in mesencephalic dopaminergic neurons in culture. *J Neurosci Res*. 36:558–569.

Kish SJ, Bergeron C, Rajput A et al. 1992. Brain cytochrome oxidase in Alzheimer's disease. *J Neurochem*. 59:776–779.

Kiss C, Ceresoli-Borroni C, Guidetti P, Zielke CL, Zielke HR, Schwarcz R. 2003. Kynurenate production by cultured human astrocytes. *J Neural Transm*. 110:1–14.

Kita T, Morrison PF, Heyes MP, Markey SP. 2002. Effects of systemic and central nervous system localized inflammation on the contributions of metabolic precursors of the L-kynurenine and quinolinic acid pools in brain. *J Neurochem*. 82:258–268.

Kitada T, Asakawa S, Hattori N et al. 1998. Mutations in the parkin gene cause autosomal recessive juvenile parkinsonism. *Nature*. 392:605–608.

Kluck RM, Bossy-Wetzel E, Green DR, Newmeyer DD. 1997. The release of cytochrome c from mitochondria: a primary site for Bcl-2 regulation of apoptosis. *Science*. 275:1132–1136.

Knyihar-Csillik E, Okuno E, Vécsei L. 1999. Effects of in vivo sodium azide administration on the immunohistochemical localization of kynurenine aminotransferase in the rat brain. *Neuroscience*. 94:269–277.

Knyihar-Csillik E, Csillik B, Pakaski M et al. 2004. Decreased expression of kynurenine aminotransferase-I (KAT-I) in the substantia nigra of mice after 1-methyl-4-phenyl-1,2,3,6-tetrahydropyridine (MPTP) treatment. *Neuroscience*. 126:899–914.

Kopito RR. 2000. Aggresomes, inclusion bodies and protein aggregation. *Trends Cell Biol*. 10:524–530.

Kraytsberg Y, Kudryavtseva E, McKee AC et al. 2006. Mitochondrial DNA deletions are abundant and cause functional impairment in aged human substantia nigra neurons. *Nat Genet*. 38:518–520.

Krieger C, Duchen MR. 2002. Mitochondria, Ca^{2+} and neurodegenerative disease. *Eur J Pharmacol*. 447:177–188.

Kuroda Y, Mitsui T, Kunishige M et al. 2006. Parkin enhances mitochondrial biogenesis in proliferating cells. *Hum Mol Genet*. 15:883–895.

Lehrmann E, Molinari A, Speciale C, Schwarcz R. 2001. Immunohistochemical visualisation of newly formed quinolinate in the normal and excitotoxically lesioned rat striatum. *Exp Brain Res*. 141:389–397.

Leist M, Jaattela M. 2001. Four deaths and a funeral: from caspases to alternative mechanisms. *Nat Rev Mol Cell Biol*. 2:589–598.

Leroy E, Boyer R, Auburger G et al. 1998. The ubiquitin pathway in Parkinson's disease. Nature. 395:451–452.

Levy-Lahad E, Wasco W, Poorkaj P et al. 1995. Candidate gene for the chromosome 1 familial Alzheimer's disease locus. *Science*. 269:973–977.

Lu F, Selak M, O'Connor J et al. 2000. Oxidative damage to mitochondrial DNA and activity of mitochondrial enzymes in chronic active lesions of multiple sclerosis. *J Neurol Sci*. 177:95–103.

Luchowski P, Luchowska E, Turski WA, Urbanska EM. 2002. 1-Methyl-4-phenylpyridinium and 3-nitropropionic acid diminish cortical synthesis of kynurenic acid via interference with kynurenine aminotransferases in rats. *Neurosci Lett*. 330:49–52.

Luchowska E, Luchowski P, Wielosz M, Turski WA, Urbanska EM. 2003. FK506 attenuates 1-methyl-4-phenylpyridinium- and 3-nitropropionic acid-evoked inhibition of kynurenic acid synthesis in rat cortical slices. *Acta Neurobiol Exp (Wars)*. 63:101–108.

Lyubchenko YL, Sherman S, Shlyakhtenko LS, Uversky VN. 2006. Nanoimaging for protein misfolding and related diseases. *J Cell Biochem*. 99:52–70.

Maccioni RB, Munoz JP, Barbeito L. 2001. The molecular bases of Alzheimer's disease and other neurodegenerative disorders. *Arch Med Res*. 32:367–381.

Manfredi G, Beal F. 2000. The role of mitochondria in the pathogenesis of neurodegenerative diseases. *Brain Pathol*. 10:462–472.

Martin LJ, Pan Y, Price AC et al. 2006. Parkinson's disease alpha-synuclein transgenic mice develop neuronal mitochondrial degeneration and cell death. *J Neurosci*. 26:41–50.

McGeer EG, McGeer PL. 1976. Duplication of biochemical changes of Huntington's chorea by intrastriatal injection of glutamic and kainic acids. *Nature*. 263:517–519.

McNaught KS, Olanow CW. 2003. Proteolytic stress. A unifying concept in the etiopathogenesis of familial and sporadic Parkinson's disease. *Ann Neurol*. 53(Suppl 3): S73–S84.

McNaught KS, Olanow CW. 2006. Protein aggregation in the pathogenesis of familial and sporadic Parkinson's disease. *Neurobiol Aging*. 27:530–545.

Miranda AF, Boegman RJ, Beninger RJ, Jhamadas K. 1997. Protection against quinolinic acid-mediated excitotoxicity in nigrostriatal dopaminergic neurons by endogenous kynurenic acid. *Neuroscience*. 78:967–975.

Miranda AF, Sutton MA, Beninger RJ, Jhamadas K, Boegman RJ. 1999. Quinolinic acid lesion of the nigrostriatal pathway: effect on turning behaviour and protection by elevation of endogenous kynurenic acid in *Rattus norvegicus*. *Neurosci Lett*. 262:81–84.

Moroni F. 1999. Tryptophan metabolism and brain function: focus on kynurenine and other indol metabolites. *Eur J Pharmacol*. 375:87–100.

Moroni F, Russi G, Lombardi G, Beni M, Carla V. 1988. Presence of kynurenic acid in the mammalian brain. *J Neurochem*. 51:177–180.

Muchowski PJ, Wacker JI. 2005. Modulation of neurodegeneration by molecular chaperones. *Nat Rev Neurosci*. 6:11–22.

Mutisya EM, Bowling AC, Beal MF. 1994. Cortical cytochrome oxidase activity is reduced in Alzheimer's disease. *J Neurochem*. 63:2179–2184.

Nagata S. 2005. DNA degradation in development and programmed cell death. *Annu Rev Immunol*. 23:853–875.

Nass S, Nass MM. 1963. Intramitochondrial fibers and DNA characteristics. II. Enzymatic and other hydrolytic treatments. *J Cell Biol*. 19:613–629.

Nemeth H, Robotka H, Kis Z et al. 2004. Kynurenine administered together with probenecid markedly inhibits pentylenetetrazol-induced seizures. An electrophysiological and behavioural study. *Neuropharmacology*. 47:916–925.

Nemeth H, Toldi J, Vécsei L. 2005. Role of kynurenines in the central and peripheral nervous systems. *Curr Neurovasc Res.* 2:249–260.

Nunomura A, Perry G, Aliev G et al. 2001. Oxidative damage is the earliest event in Alzheimer disease. *J Neuropathol Exp Neurol.* 60:759–767.

Ogawa T, Matson WR, Beal MF et al. 1992. Kynurenine pathway abnormalities in Parkinson's disease. *Neurology.* 42:1702–1706.

Okuno E, Nakamura M, Schwarcz R. 1991. Two kynurenine aminotransferases in human brain. *Brain Res.* 542:307–312.

Orth M, Schapira AH. 2001. Mitochondria and degenerative disorders. *Am J Med Genet.* 106:27–36.

Papa S. 1996. Mitochondrial oxidative phosphorylation changes in the life span. Molecular aspects and physiopathological implications. *Biochim Biophys Acta.* 1276:87–105.

Paschen W, Mengesdorf T. 2005. Endoplasmic reticulum stress response and neurodegeneration. *Cell Calcium.* 38:409–415.

Perkins MN, Stone TW. 1985. Actions of kynurenic acid and quinolinic acid in the rat hippocampus in vivo. *Exp Neurol.* 88:570–579.

Perutz MF, Johnson T, Suzuki M, Finch JT. 1994. Glutamine repeats as polar zippers: their possible role in inherited neurodegenerative diseases. *Proc Natl Acad Sci U S A.* 91:5355–5358.

Petit A, Kawarai T, Paitel E et al. 2005. Wild-type PINK1 prevents basal and induced neuronal apoptosis, a protective effect abrogated by Parkinson's disease-related mutations. *J Biol Chem.* 280:34025–34032.

Petrucelli I, Dawson TM. 2004. Mechanism of neurodegenerative disease: role of the ubiquitin proteasome system. *Ann Med.* 36:315–320.

Pickart CM. 2001. Mechanisms underlying ubiquitination. *Annu Rev Biochem.* 70:503–533.

Poderoso JJ, Carreras MC, Lisdero C, Riobo N, Schopfer F, Boveris A. 1996. Nitric oxide inhibits electron transfer and increases superoxide radical production in rat heart mitochondria and submitochondrial particles. *Arch Biochem Biophys.* 328:85–92.

Polymeropoulos MH, Lavedan C, Leroy E, Ide SE et al. 1997. Mutation in the alpha-synuclein gene identified in families with Parkinson's disease. *Science.* 276:2045–2047.

Prescott C, Weeks AM, Staley KJ, Partin KM. 2006. Kynurenic acid has a dual action on AMPA receptor responses. *Neurosci Lett.* 402:108–112.

Pyle A, Foltynie T, Tiangyou W et al. 2005. Mitochondrial DNA haplogroup cluster UKJT reduces the risk of PD. *Ann Neurol.* 57:564–567.

Reynolds GP, Pearson SJ, Halket J, Sandler M. 1988. Brain quinolinic acid in Huntington's disease. *J Neurochem.* 50:1959–1960.

Rios C, Santamaria A. 1991. Quinolinic acid is a potent lipid peroxidant in rat brain homogenates. *Neurochem Res.* 16:1139–1143.

Robotka H, Nemeth H, Somlai C, Vécsei L, Toldi J. 2005. Systemically administered glucosamine-kynurenic acid, but not pure kynurenic acid, is effective in decreasing the evoked activity in area CA1 of the rat hipocampus. *Eur J Pharmacol.* 513:75–80.

Rodriguez-Martinez E, Camacho A, Maldonado PD et al. 2000. Effect of quinolinic acid on endogenous antioxidants in rat corpus striatum. *Brain Res.* 858:436–439.

Rogaev EI, Sherrington R, Rogaeva EA et al. 1995. Familiar Alzheimer's disease in kindreds with missense mutations in a gene on chromosome 1 related to the Alzheimer's disease type 3 gene. *Nature.* 376:775–778.

Rosenberg RN. 2000. The molecular and and genetic basis of Alzheimer's disease: the end of the beginning. *Neurology.* 54:2045–2054.

Santamaría A, Galván-Arzate S, Lisý V et al. 2001. Quinolinic acid induces oxidative stress in rat brain synaptosomes. *Neuroreport.* 12:871–874.

Sas K, Robotka H, Toldi J, Vécsei L. 2007. Mitochondria, metabolic disturbances, oxidative stress and the kynurenine system, with focus on neurodegenerative disorders. *J Neur Sci.* 257:221–239.

Schapira AH, Cooper JM, Dexter D, Jenner P, Clark JB, Marsden CD. 1989. Mitochondrial complex I deficiency in Parkinson's disease. *Lancet.* 1:1269.

Schapira AH, Cooper JM, Dexter D, Clark JB, Jenner P, Marsden CD. 1990. Mitochondrial complex I deficiency in Parkinson's disease. *J Neurochem.* 54:823–827.

Schwarcz R. 2004. The kynurenine pathway of tryptophan degradation as a drug target. *Curr Opin Pharmacol.* 4:12–17.

Schwarcz R, Whetsell WO Jr, Mangano RM. 1983. Quinolinic acid an endogenous metabolite that produces axon-sparing lesion in rat brain. *Science.* 219:316–318.

Schwarcz R, Foster AC, French ED, Whetsell WO Jr, Kohler C. 1984. Excitotoxic models for neurodegenerative disorders. *Life Sci.* 35:19–32.

Schwarcz R, Tamminga CA, Kurlan R, Shoulson I. 1988. Cerebrospinal fluid levels of quinolinic acid in Huntington's disease and schizophrenia. *Ann Neurol.* 24:580–582.

Selkoe DJ. 2001. Alzheimer's disease: genes, proteins, and therapy. *Physiol Rev.* 81:741–766.

Shastry BS. 2003. Neurodegenerative disorders of protein aggregation. *Neurochem Int.* 43:1–7.

Sherman MY, Goldberg AL. 2001. Cellular defenses against unfolded proteins a cell biologist thinks about neurodegenerative diseases. *Neuron.* 29:15–32.

Sherrington R, Rogaev EI, Liang Y et al. 1995. Cloning of the gene bearing missense mutations in early-onset familial Alzheimer's disease. *Nature.* 375:754–760.

Sies H. 1993. Strategies of antioxidant defense. *Eur J Biochem.* 215:213–219.

Sitia R, Braakman I. 2003. Quality control in the endoplasmic reticulum protein factory. *Nature.* 426:891–894.

Small GW, Mazziotta JC, Collins MT et al. 1995. Apolipoprotein E type 4 allele and cerebral glucose metabolism in relatives at risk for familial Alzheimer disease. *JAMA.* 273:942–947.

Soti C, Csermely P. 2003. Aging and molecular shaperones. *Exp Gerontol.* 38:1037–1040.

Stewart VC, Heales SJ. 2003. Nitric oxide-induced mitochondrial dysfunction: implications for neurodegeneration. *Free Radic Biol Med.* 34:287–303.

Stone TW. 2001. Kynurenic acid antagonists and kynurenine pathway 45. *Exp Opin Invest Drugs.* 10:633.

Stone TW. 2001. Kynurenines in the CNS: from endogenous obscurity to therapeutic importance. *Progr Neurobiol.* 64:185–218.

Stone TW, Perkins MN. 1981. Quinolinic acid: A potent endogenous excitant at amino acid receptors in CNS. *Eur J Pharmacol.* 72:411–412.

Stone TW, Connick JH. 1985. Quinolinic acid and other kynurenines in the central nervous system. *Neuroscience.* 15:597–617.

Stoy N, Mackay GM, Forrest CM et al. 2005. Tryptophan metabolism and oxidative stress in patients with Huntington's disease. *J Neurochem.* 93:611–623.

Strauss KM, Martins LM, Plun-Favreau H et al. 2005. Loss of function mutations in the gene encoding Omi/HtrA2 in Parkinson's disease. *Hum Mol Genet.* 14:2099–2111.

Suzuki Y, Imai Y, Nakayama H, Takahashi K, Takio K, Takahashi R. 2001. A serine protease, HtrA2, is released from the mitochondria and interacts with XIAP, inducing cell death. *Mol Cell.* 8:613–621.

Swartz KJ, During MJ, Freese A, Beal MF. 1990. Cerebral synthesis and release of kynurenic acid: an endogenous antagonist of excitatory amino acid receptors. *J Neurosci.* 10:2965–2973.

Takuma K, Yao J, Huang J et al. 2005. ABAD enhances Abeta-induced cell stress via mitochondrial dysfunction. *FASEB J.* 19:597–598.

Tavares RG, Tasca CI, Santos CE et al. 2002. Quinolinic acid stimulates synaptosomal glutamate release and inhibits glutamate uptake into astrocytes. *Neurochem Int.* 40:621–627.

Taylor JP, Hardy J, Fischbeck KH. 2002. Toxic proteins in neurodegenerative disease. *Science.* 296:1991–1995.

Tipton KF, Singer TP. 1993. Advances in our understanding of the mechanisms of the neurotoxicity of MPTP and related compounds. *J Neurochem.* 61:1191–1206.

Turski WA, Nakamura M, Todd WP, Carpenter BK, Whetsell WO Jr, Schwarcz R. 1988. Identification and quantification of kynurenic acid in human brain tissue. *Brain Res.* 454:164–169.

Valente EM, Abou-Sleiman PM, Caputo V et al. 2004. Hereditary early-onset Parkinson's disease caused by mutations in PINK1. *Science.* 304:1158–1160.

Valera AG, Diaz-Hernandez M, Hernandez F, Ortega Z, Lucas JJ. 2005. The ubiquitin-proteasome system in Huntington's disease. *Neuroscientist.* 11:583–594.

van der Walt JM, Nicodemus KK, Martin ER et al. 2003. Mitochondrial polymorphisms significantly reduce the risk of Parkinson's disease. *Am J Hum Genet.* 72:804–811.

Van Houten B, Woshner V, Santos JH. 2006. Role of mitochondrial DNA in toxic responses to oxidative stress. *DNA Repair (Amst).* 5:145–152.

Vécsei L, Beal MF. 1990. Intracerebroventricular injection of kynurenic acid, but not kynurenine, induces ataxia and stereotyped behavior in rats. *Brain Res Bull.* 25:623–627.

Vécsei L, Beal MF. 1991. Comparative behavioral and pharmacological studies with centrally administered kynurenine and kynurenic acid in rats. *Eur J Pharmacol.* 196:239–246.

Vécsei L, Miller J, MacGarvey U, Beal MF. 1992. Kynurenine and probenecid inhibit pentylentetrazol- and NMDLA-induced seizures and increase kynurenic acid concentrations in the brain. *Brain Res Bull.* 28:233–238.

Vécsei L, Beal MF. 1996. Huntington's disease, behavioral disturbances, and kynurenines: preclinical findings and therapeutic perspectives. *Biol Psychiatry.* 39:1061–1063.

Vécsei L, Dibo G, Kiss C. 1998. Neurotoxins and neurodegenerative disorders. *Neurotoxicology.* 19:511–514.

Virág L. 2005. Structure and function of poly(ADP-ribose) polymerase-1: role in oxidative stress-related pathologies. *Curr Vasc Pharmacol.* 3:209–214.

Walton MR, Dragunow I. 2000. Is CREB a key to neuronal survival? *Trends Neurosci.* 23:48–53.

Widner B, Leblhuber F, Walli J, Tilz GP, Demel U, Fuchs D. 1999. Degradation of tryptophan in neurodegenerative disorders. *Adv Exp Med Biol.* 467:133–138.

Wyttenbach A, Swartz J, Kita H et al. 2001. Polyglutamine expansions cause decreased CREB-mediated transcription and early gene expression changes prior to cell death in an inducible cell model of Huntington's disease. *Hum Mol Genet.* 10:1829–1845.

Yakes FM, Van Houten B. 1997. Mitochondrial DNA damage is more extensive and persists longer than nuclear DNA damage in human cells following oxidative stress. *Proc Natl Acad Sci U S A.* 94:514–519.

Yang Y, Gehrke S, Haque ME et al. 2005. Inactivation of Drosophila DJ-1 leads to impairments of oxidative stress response and phosphatidylinositol 3-kinase/Akt signaling. *Proc Natl Acad Sci U S A.* 102:13670–13675.

Zhang L, Shimoji M, Thomas B et al. 2005. Mitochondrial localization of the Parkinson's disease related protein DJ-1: implications for pathogenesis. *Hum Mol Genet.* 14:2063–2073.

Zimprich A, Biskup S, Leitner P et al. 2004. Mutations in LRRK2 cause autosomal-dominant parkinsonism with pleomorphic pathology. *Neuron.* 44:601–607.

Chapter *19*

REDOX SIGNALING AND VASCULAR FUNCTION

J. Will Langston, Magdalena L. Circu, and Tak Yee Aw

ABSTRACT

Over the last two decades, redox signaling has emerged as an important regulator of cell function, and it is now well appreciated that reactive oxygen and nitrogen species act as second messengers that modulate vascular activity via direct interactions with specific enzymes, proteins, and transcription factors to regulate cell signaling and/or gene expression. The growing interest in the role of redox signaling in the vasculature stems primarily from evidence that oxidative stress-induced endothelial dysfunction underlies a number of cardiovascular pathologies including hypertension, atherosclerosis, and diabetes, and that antioxidant intervention may be an important treatment modality in these vascular disorders. Of interest is the thiol antioxidant, reduced glutathione (GSH), a crucial regulator of cellular redox potential, and whose synthesis is transcriptionally upregulated under conditions of cellular oxidative stress. The transcriptional upregulation of the rate-limiting enzyme of GSH synthesis, glutamate cysteine ligase (GCL), under oxidative conditions by the transcription factor Nrf2 represents an important area of investigation in terms of its role in redox regulation of endothelial function, its role in vascular pathology, and its potential as a therapeutic target for treatment of cardiovascular disorders that involve vascular oxidative stress.

Keywords: GSH redox status and signaling, GSH and vascular function, redox regulation of GSH synthesis, mechanisms of redox signaling.

Redox signaling and posttranslational redox modifications of protein thiols are emerging to be fundamentally important signaling mechanisms in the regulation of mammalian cell function. In addition to redox regulation of cell signaling being a modulator of normal function, a disturbance of redox signaling has also been suggested to underpin a variety of pathologies, including vascular diseases. The current chapter will first focus on a general discussion of the concept of cellular redox status, the compartmentation of cellular redox systems, and the mechanisms of redox signaling and its targets. The rest of the chapter will be devoted to coverage of the specific role of vascular-derived reactive oxygen and nitrogen species, the involvement of the glutathione redox system and Nrf2 in the pathways of redox signaling in vascular function and dysfunction, specific oxidative stress–associated vascular diseases, and antioxidant therapy in treatment of vascular disorders.

GENERAL CONSIDERATION OF THE REDOX STATE OF A CELL AND ITS SIGNIFICANCE

The redox state of a cell is defined by the ratio of the interconvertible reduced and oxidized forms of the different cellular redox couples. More generally, the term *redox environment* has been used to describe the state of the cellular redox pairs (Schafer, Buettner 2001).

The intracellular thiol redox pairs are represented by the reduced glutathione/glutathione disulfide (GSH/GSSG), and the reduced and oxidized thioredoxin (Trx/TrxSS) systems, while the cysteine/cystine (Cys/CySS) redox couple plays an important role in maintaining the redox state of the plasma. The pyridine nucleotide couples include nicotinamide adenine dinucleotide/reduced nicotinamide adenine dinucleotide (NAD^+/NADH) and NAD phosphate/reduced NAD phosphate ($NADP^+$/NADPH). The oxidation–reduction status of the redox components is responsible for creating an optimal redox environment within the cell, which directly affects the activity of different cellular proteins. Recently, Hansen et al. proposed that the cellular redox systems are differentially compartmentalized among different organelles, where the distribution of redox systems is independently controlled in the plasma membrane, cytosol, nucleus, mitochondria, and endoplasmic reticulum (ER) (Hansen, Go, Jones 2006). Thus, depending on the concentrations of the respective redox couples and their fluxes, the compartmentation of specific redox systems may, in fact, represent a crucial and generalized mechanism for optimizing cell activity within mammalian cells. We have, in recent years established a paradigm that an oxidative shift in the cellular GSH/GSSG redox couple is an important determinant of cell fate; the phenotypic endpoint of proliferation, growth arrest or apoptosis is a function of the extent of GSH/GSSG imbalance (Aw 1999, 2003; Noda, Iwakiri, Fujimoto et al. 2001; Gotoh, Noda, Iwakiri et al. 2002). In various cell types, the loss of GSH/GSSG redox balance preceding cell apoptosis is an early event that occurred within a relatively narrow time window (30 minutes) post–oxidant challenge and is preventable by pretreatment with the thiol antioxidant, *N*-acetylcysteine (NAC) (Wang, Gotoh, Jennings et al. 2000; Pias, Aw 2002a, 2002b; Pias, Ekshyyan, Rhoads et al. 2003; Ekshyyan, Aw 2005; Okouchi, Okayama, Aw 2005). These findings suggest that GSH/GSSG redox signaling may represent a generalized mechanism in oxidative cell killing in mammalian cells. The control of cellular apoptosis by mucosal GSH/GSSG redox status has been demonstrated in vivo (Tsunada, Iwakiri R, Noda et al. 2003).

The current understanding of redox signaling is that it is a regulatory process in which the signal occurs through redox reactions induced by reactive oxygen species (ROS) or reactive nitrogen species (RNS) that results in posttranslational modification of proteins in various signal transduction pathways. Many proteins contain cysteine residues that provide a redox-sensitive switch for regulating protein function, and ROS-induced oxidation of cysteine-SH can result in the formation of intra- and/or interchain disulfide bonds. Moreover, the direct addition of GSSG leads

to S-glutathionylation of the thiol moiety. In addition, nitric oxide ($NO^•$) can induce S-nitrosylation of specific cysteine thiols in proteins such as soluble guanylate cyclase (sGC) and the newly discovered mitochondrial $NO^•$/cytochrome c oxidase signaling pathway (Shiva, Huang, Grubina et al. 2007; Landar, Darley-Usmar 2007). These redox signal transduction processes are important in various physiological and biological activities including vascular function.

CONCEPT OF OXIDATIVE AND NITROSATIVE STRESS AND REDOX SIGNALING

In redox signaling, modifications of targeted proteins are initiated by ROS and RNS. The common ROS are superoxide anions ($O_2^{•-}$), hydrogen peroxide (H_2O_2), and hydroxyl radicals (HO•) while RNS comprise $NO^•$ and its derivatives, peroxynitrite ($ONOO^-$) or dinitrogen trioxide (N_2O_3) (Fig. 19.1). Endogenous sources of $O_2^{•-}$ include the mitochondrial respiratory chain, NADPH oxidase, xantine oxidase, and NADPH cytochrome P450 (Cross, Jones 1991). Intracellular derived $O_2^{•-}$ is readily dismutated to H_2O_2 by cytosolic or mitochondrial superoxide dismutases (SOD). In the presence of metal ions, H_2O_2 and $O_2^{•-}$ are converted to HO•, a highly potent oxidant that induces oxidative damage to cellular proteins, lipids, or DNA. Exogenous sources such as xenobiotics or UV/γ-radiations are known ROS generators that contribute to the overall oxidant burden of a cell. $O_2^{•-}$ can further react with $NO^•$ to form the reactive $ONOO^-$ that oxidizes cellular lipids or DNA, resulting in nitrosative stress (for review see Pacher, Beckman, Liaudet 2007). $NO^•$ is generated by NO synthases (NOS), of which three isoforms exist in mammalian cells; these are endothelial NOS (eNOS), neuronal NOS (nNOS), and inducible NOS (iNOS). In the vasculature, eNOS is the predominant isoform and is responsible for maintaining vascular $NO^•$ homeostasis and vascular tone. Oxidation of the essential NOS cofactor by $ONOO^-$ transforms eNOS into an ROS producer (Forstermann, Closs, Pollock et al. 1994). Another RNS derivative with a potential role in cellular signaling is N_2O_3, which participates in the nitrosation of thiol groups to form nitrosothiols, an important class of redox signaling molecules. Endothelial ROS and RNS generation and their specific roles in vascular function are discussed in sections on cellular sources of endothelial ROS and ROS and vascular signaling.

It is well recognized that different concentrations of ROS/RNS mediate distinct cellular responses. While high ROS/RNS concentration induces oxidative damage to macromolecules that lead to oxidative/

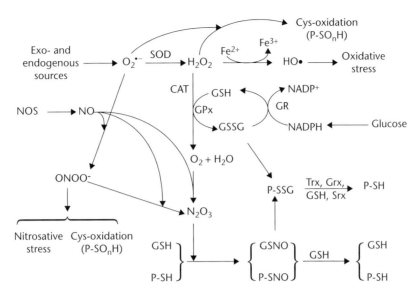

Figure 19.1 Metabolic pathways of ROS/RNS formation and the interactions with antioxidant systems. ROS are formed from exogenous and endogenous sources. While highly reactive HO• induces oxidative stress, $O_2^{\cdot-}$ and H_2O_2 are either substrates for antioxidant enzymes or induce sequential oxidation of Cys residues of target proteins of various signaling pathways. The formation of GSSG can participate in the S-glutathionylation of proteins (P-SSG). NO radicals produced by NOS isoenzymes can form diverse RNS intermediates that either participate in S-nitrosylation of Cys residues of proteins to form GSNO/P-SNO derivatives or induce nitrosative stress and the formation of tyrosine nitrosative derivatives. The redox status of proteins is restored by the GSH, Trx, Grx, and the newly discovered Srx redox systems. CAT, catalase; GSH, glutathione; GPx, GSH peroxidase; GR, GSH reductase; Grx, glutaredoxin; GSSG, glutathione disulfide; NO• nitric oxide radical; NOS, nitric oxide synthases; N_2O_3, dinitrogen trioxide; ONOO⁻, peroxynitrite; SOD, superoxide dismutase; Srx, sulfiredoxin; Trx, thioredoxin.

nitrosative stress, low-to-moderate levels are important in cell signaling and the regulation of various biological processes. The balance of detrimental and beneficial actions caused by ROS/RNS is achieved through "redox regulation" mechanisms; this refers to enzymatic reactions with specific roles in maintaining the redox homeostasis of targeted proteins that are essential for cell function and survival (Droge 2002). The cytotoxic effects of ROS/RNS are ameliorated by intracellular antioxidant mechanisms that maintain a balance of the reduced and oxidized species (Fig. 19.1). For example, H_2O_2 and hydroperoxides are eliminated by GSH peroxidase at the expense of cellular GSH, and the resultant increase in GSSG is reduced by glutathione reductase with NADPH as the reductant. Peroxiredoxin (Prx) is another example of antioxidant redox proteins that are involved in the breakdown of cellular toxic hydroperoxides. Previous studies have demonstrated that these cysteine-specific peroxidases can function as molecular switches sensitive to different levels of H_2O_2 (Bozonet, Findlay, Day et al. 2005). The Trx/Trx reductase and glutaredoxin (Grx)/GSH system also contribute to cellular antioxidant defense against redox imbalance as do the sulfiredoxins (Srx) in the reduction of oxidized proteins (Fig. 19.1; section on redox proteins and cell signaling).

COMPARTMENTATION OF CELLULAR REDOX SYSTEMS AND REDOX PROTEINS IN CELL SIGNALING

GSH/GSSG Redox System and its Subcellular Compartmentation

Given its cellular abundance and its role in protein thiol modification, the status of the GSH/GSSG redox system reflects the redox buffering capacity of a cell. Indeed, an oxidative shift in the GSH-to-GSSG ratio is often used as an indicator of cellular oxidative stress.

GSH/GSSG and Cellular Redox Balance

GSH (γ-glutamylcysteinyl glycine) is the most abundant low-molecular-weight thiol in cells that exhibits important roles in the control of the thiol–disulfide redox state of cellular proteins (Meister, Anderson 1983; Sies 1999). Additionally, GSH is involved in redox activation of transcription factors as part of an adaptive mechanism that participates in cell signaling and stress responses (Kamata, Hirata 1999). Within cells, GSH exists mainly in its biologically active, thiol-reduced form, and oxidation of GSH results in the formation of glutathione disulfide, GSSG. The ratio of GSH and GSSG is maintained in favor of the reduced state (>90% reduced), which is accomplished by three mechanisms: GSH synthesis, GSSG reduction, and GSH uptake. *De novo* synthesis of GSH from precursor amino acids (glutamate, cysteine, and glycine) occurs in the cytosol and is catalyzed by two ATP-dependent enzymatic reactions, γ-glutamate cysteine ligase (GCL) and GSH synthetase (GS) (Fig. 19.2). GCL activity is rate limiting in GSH synthesis and is regulated by GSH and the availability of cysteine. GSSG reduction is catalyzed by glutathione reductase, and uptake of extracellular GSH occurs through specific carriers localized at the plasma membrane (Lash, Putt, Xu et al. 2007).

Intracellular Compartmentation of GSH

In mammalian cells, GSH is present in millimolar concentrations and is differentially distributed among various cellular compartments, such as the cytosol, mitochondria, ER, and nucleus where it forms separate and distinct redox pools (Fig. 19.2). Within the cytosol, GSH concentrations are maintained between 5 mM and 10 mM (Meister, Anderson 1983) and the redox pool is highly reduced; for example, the GSH-to-GSSG ratio under normal conditions is maintained

in excess of 100-to-1 in liver cells, and this ratio significantly decreases to less than 4 to 1 during oxidative stress.

The mitochondria maintain a distinct GSH pool that is supported through GSH transport from the cytosolic compartment via the dicarboxylate and 2-oxoglutarate GSH carriers located in the mitochondrial inner membrane (Chen, Lash 1998). This GSH redox compartment is metabolically separate from the cytosol with regard to synthetic rate, turnover, and sensitivity to chemical depletion. Matrix GSH concentrations are between 5 and 10 mM and varies from 10% to 15% of the total GSH in the liver (Jocelyn, Kamminga 1974) to 15% to 30% of total GSH pool in the renal proximal tubule (Schnellmann 1991). Functionally, mitochondrial GSH preserves the integrity of mitochondrial proteins and lipids and controls mitochondrial generation of ROS. Early studies demonstrated that the status of mitochondrial GSH is a determining factor in oxidative vulnerability; in this regard, mitochondrial GSH loss has been linked to cytotoxicity induced by aromatic hydrocarbons (Hallberg, Rydstrom 1989), hypoxia (Lluis, Morales, Blasco et al. 2005), *tert*-butylhydroperoxide (*t*BH) (Olafsdottir, Reed 1988), and ethanol intoxication

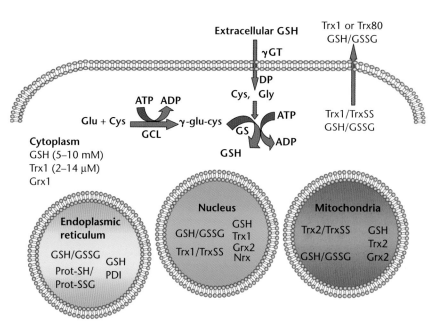

Figure 19.2 GSH synthesis and compartmentation of thiol/disulfide redox state and redox proteins. Synthesis of GSH from its constituent amino acids (glutamate, cysteine, glycine) takes place in the cytosol and is catalyzed by glutamate cysteine ligase (GCL) and glutathione synthase (GS) at the expense of two moles of ATP. Some cells can export GSH or Trx1 which, once outside the cells, can contribute to maintaining the redox environment of the plasma. Extracellular GSH is hydrolyzed to its component amino acids by γ-glutamyltransferase (γ-GT) and dipeptidase (DP). The main redox couples that participate in maintaining the cellular reduced-to-oxidized environment include GSH/GSSG and Trx/TrxSS. The cysteine residues in cellular proteins are maintained in the reduced state by GSH and thiol reductases, namely, Trx, Grx, Nrx, or PDI that have different cellular localization in the cytoplasm, mitochondria, endoplasmic reticulum, and nucleus. Cys, cysteine; Grx, glutaredoxin; GSH, glutathione; GSSG, glutathione disulfide; Nrx, nucleoredoxin; PDI, protein disulfide isomerase; PrSH, reduced protein; Pr-SSG, oxidized protein; Trx, thioredoxin; TrxSS, oxidized thioredoxin; Trx80, truncated form of Trx.

(Fernandez-Checa, Garcia-Ruiz, Ookhtens et al. 1991). Our recent studies validated that oxidant-induced apoptosis is triggered by a loss of mitochondrial GSH/GSSG balance (Circu, Rodriguez, Maloney et al. 2008). Mechanistically, oxidative susceptibility is associated with an increase in mitochondrial ROS production secondary to matrix GSH decrease (Lluis, Buricchi, Chiarugi et al. 2007).

The existence of a distinct GSH pool in the ER has been described and its concentration (6 mM to 10 mM) mirrors those in the cytosolic and mitochondrial compartments (Fig. 19.2). Notably, the GSH redox environment in ER is highly oxidized (GSH-to-GSSG ratio of 3:1–1:1), a state that favors the oxidative folding of proteins (Bass, Ruddock, Klappa et al. 2004). The luminal GSSG concentration is, indeed, optimal for disulfide bond formation (Lyles, Gilbert 1991), and appears to be generated through an oxidative pathway catalyzed by the oxidoreductase enzyme, ErO1 (Tu, Weissman 2004). Also notable is that less than 50% of the ER thiol pool (GSH + GSSG) is free; the majority of GSH is reversibly bound to proteins as protein-mixed disulfides formed through thiol oxidation by GSSG. Functionally, it is believed that high concentrations of protein-mixed disulfides serve as GSH reserve within the ER, in the maintenance of oxidoreductase catalytic function, or as a redox buffer against ER-generated ROS (Jessop, Bulleid 2004; Chakravarthi, Jessop, Bulleid 2006). Elevated levels of reduced GSH disrupt ER function and activate the unfolded protein response (UPR) that triggers cellular apoptosis (Frand, Kaiser 2000).

An independent nuclear GSH pool functions in DNA synthesis and protection against oxidative and ionizing radiation induced DNA damage (Cotgreave 2003). The size of the nuclear GSH pool is unknown, and recent evidence suggests that the cytosolic and nuclear redox pools are not in equilibrium. Bellomo and coworkers (Bellomo, Palladini, Vairetti 1997) demonstrated a GSH ratio of 3:1 between the nuclear and cytosolic compartments, while Thomas et al. (1995) and Soderdahl et al. (2003) reported lower ratios. Moreover, nuclear proteins are more prone to thiol oxidation (Soderdahl, Enoksson, Lundberg et al. 2003). Interestingly, nuclear GSH distribution is dynamic and directly correlates with cell cycle progression where nuclear GSH was 4-fold higher than cytosolic GSH in the proliferative state, but was equally distributed between the two compartments when cells reached confluency (Chen, Delannoy, Odwin et al. 2003; Markovic, Borras, Ortega et al. 2007). These results suggest a specific role for nuclear GSH in preserving nuclear proteins in a reducing environment that is essential for gene transcription during cell cycle progression (Chen, Delannoy, Odwin et al. 2003). The mechanism for nuclear GSH transport is unresolved;

current evidence suggests a passive diffusion of GSH from the cytosol into the nucleus via nuclear pores (Ho, Guenthner 1997).

Redox Proteins and Cell Signaling

Members of the Trx family of proteins are active in the redox regulation of cysteine residues of specialized proteins that significantly impact cell signaling and function. Among the better-studied redox proteins are Trx, Grx, peroxiredoxin, and protein disulfide isomerase (PDI).

Thioredoxins

Thioredoxins (Trx) are small ubiquitous redox proteins that contain two redox-active cysteine residues in the catalytic site (Cys-X-X-Cys). The intracellular concentrations of Trx are between 2 μM and 14 μM, which is three orders of magnitude lower than that of GSH (2 mM to 10 mM) (Nakamura, Nakamura, Yodoi 1997). Trx, together with NADPH and Trx reductase, functions to maintain the thiol/disulfide redox state of proteins in mammalian cells. Trx catalyzes the reversible reduction of disulfide bonds in oxidized proteins at the expense of cysteine residues in its active motif site; the active reduced Trx is regenerated by Trx reductase and NADPH.

Mammalian cells contain two forms of Trx, Trx1, and Trx2, which are localized in different cellular compartments, cytosol, mitochondria, or nucleus. Trx 1 is expressed ubiquitously and is a cytosolic enzyme that can translocate to the nucleus during oxidative stress. Cytosolic Trx1 can function as a cofactor, binding partner, or reductant. For example, as a cofactor for Prx, Trx1 functions in hydroperoxide elimination. The binding of Trx1 with the apoptosis signal–regulated kinase 1 (ASK-1) plays an anti-apoptotic role (Saitoh, Nishitoh, Fujii et al. 1998). As a reductant, Trx1 and Trx-like protein (TRP14) reactivate the protein tyrosine phosphatase (PTP), phosphatase-like tensin homolog (PTEN), which reverses phosphoinositide 3-kinase (PI3K) signaling (Lee, Yang, Kwon et al. 2002). Through reduction of protein disulfides, Trx functions in redox-sensitive signaling and the activation of transcriptional factors (for review see Watson, Yang, Choi et al. 2004). During oxidative challenge, Trx1 translocates to the nucleus where it participates in the redox regulation of transcription factors such as activator protein 1 (AP-1), p53, and nuclear transcription factor kappa B (NF-κB). Trx1 involvement in redox control of transcriptional activity is supported by the observation that the redox state of nuclear Trx1 is more reduced than that of the cytosolic protein (Watson, Jones 2003). Several studies have reported the secretion of Trx1 extracellularly from various cell types such as lymphocytes, hepatocytes, fibroblasts, and endothelial cells (Kondo, Ishii, Kwon et al. 2004) where it contributes to intracellular redox signaling and redox homeostasis in neighboring cells. There is evidence that extracellular Trx1 may also function as a cytokine or a chemokine (Pekkari, Holmgren 2004).

Trx2 is localized exclusively in the mitochondria and is expressed strongly in the heart, skeletal muscle, cerebellum, adrenal gland, and testis. Compared to cytosolic Trx1, mitochondrial Trx2 is relatively more oxidized (Watson, Jones 2003). Mammalian Trx2 possesses a conserved Trx-active site, Trp-Cys-Gly-Pro-Cys, that is involved in antioxidant protection and preservation of mitochondrial redox homeostasis. Trx2 overexpression in HEK-293 cells plays an important role in the regulation of the mitochondrial membrane potential (Damdimopoulos, Miranda-Vizuete, Pelto-Huikko et al. 2002). Trx2 in human umbilical vein endothelial cells functions as a redox sensor and inhibitor of the mitochondrial ASK-1–mediated apoptotic signaling pathway (Zhang, Al-Lamki, Bai et al. 2004). Additionally, Trx2–Prx3 interaction functions in parallel with the GSH system to protect mitochondria from low level oxidative challenge (Zhang, Go, Jones 2007). A novel role for Trx2 has been reported in the protection against high ambient glucose concentrations (Liang, Pietrusz 2007). In the ER, transmembrane Trx-related protein (TXM) (Matsuo, Akiyama, Nakamura et al. 2001) is involved in attenuating ER-mediated oxidative stress.

Thioredoxin reductase (TrxR) is a selenoprotein that participates in the reduction of oxidized Trx via electrons transferred from NADPH. Mammalian TrxR is a dimeric NADPH-dependent, FAD-containing disulfide reductase with the sequence Cys-Secys-Gly at the C terminus of each subunit. In mammalian cells there are three isoforms of TrxR: cytosolic TrxR1; mitochondrial TrxR2 and testis-specific TGR (Trx GSH reductase) (Zhong, Arner, Holmgren 2000). The importance of the Trx system in the control of cell function is evidenced by the observation that mice deficient in Trx1 and Trx2 (Trx1/2$^{-/-}$ null) die during embryogenesis (Nakamura 2005). Several other oxidoreductases belonging to the Trx family of proteins catalyze the reduction of disulfides in oxidized proteins. Among these are Grx and PDIs. These proteins share a common structural motif called the *thioredoxin fold* represented by a four-stranded β-sheet and three surrounding α-helices (Lillig, Holmgren 2007).

Trx redox proteins

GLUTAREDOXINS Glutaredoxins (Grx) are cellular enzymes that share common functions with Trx in preserving sulfhydryl groups of redox-sensitive proteins. Similar to Trx, Grx utilizes the two redox-active cysteine of its conserved Cys-X-X-Cys catalytic site to reduce proteins, but differs from Trx in that it is a GSH-dependent oxidoreductase. The reduction of oxidized Grx is catalyzed by GSH with the formation of GSSG; the regeneration of GSH is coupled to GR activity and NADPH consumption. Functionally, Grx is more active in the reduction of S-glutathionylated substrates than Trx (Johansson, Lillig, Holmgren 2004). Three Grx isoenzymes exist in mammalian cells with different cellular localization and catalytic properties. Cytosolic and nuclear Grx1 contains a common Cys-Pro-Tyr-Cys active site motif and is involved in redox control of transcription factors and protection against oxidant-induced apoptosis. Mitochondrial Grx2 is derived from alternative splicing of the primary Grx RNA transcript (Fernandes, Holmgren 2004). Human mitochondrial Grx2 has a Cys-Ser-Tyr-Cys sequence in the catalytic site and is the first iron-sulfur protein belonging to the Trx family of proteins discovered so far (Lillig, Berndt, Vergnolle et al. 2005). It functions as a redox sensor in the activation of Grx2 during oxidative stress (Lillig, Berndt, Vergnolle et al. 2005). In unstressed cells, the inactive enzyme, consisting of Grx2 holoenzyme formed from 2-FeS clusters, two Grx2 monomers and two molecules of GSH that are noncovalently bound to proteins, is in equilibrium with GSH in solution. Under oxidizing conditions, when the mitochondrial GSH concentration decreases, the holo-Grx2 complex dissociates and yields enzymatically active Grx2.

The structural difference between Grx1 and Grx2 has important implications for regulation of their activity under oxidative/nitrosative conditions. While cytosolic/nuclear Grx1 are inactivated by S-nitrosylation and oxidation, mitochondrial Grx2 activity is not inhibited. Within the mitochondria, nitrosylation causes the dissociation of the dimeric iron sulfur/Grx2 cluster and activation of the enzyme. The mechanism of reduction catalyzed by these two isoforms is also different. While Grx1 utilizes only GSH in its reductive reaction, mitochondrial Grx2 can reduce oxidized substrates either using GSH or by coupling to TrxR (Gladyshev, Liu, Novoselov et al. 2001; Johansson, Lillig, Holmgren 2004). The direct reduction of Grx2 by TrxR enables Grx2 to reduce glutathionylated proteins under conditions of oxidative stress and low mitochondrial GSH (Johansson, Lillig, Holmgren 2004). It is recently suggested that the differences in regulation between Grx1 and Grx2 is an adaptation to their subcellular compartmentation (Hashemy, Johansson, Berndt et al. 2007) and that they have different regulatory functions in redox signaling. The biological function of a recently discovered third Grx isoenzyme, Grx5, has yet to be characterized (Wingert, Galloway, Barut et al. 2005).

OTHER REDOX-ACTIVE TRX PROTEINS

Mammalian nucleoredoxin. Nucleoredoxin (Nrx) is a ubiquitously distributed thiol reductase that belongs to the Trx family of proteins with a cytosolic localization. During oxidative stress, Nrx can translocate to the nucleus (Funato, Michiue, Asashima et al. 2006), but its involvement in redox control and cell signaling is unclear at present. Current literature evidence suggests that Nrx can participate in redox regulation of nuclear transcription factors (Hirota, Matsui, Murata et al. 2000) and suppression of the Wnt-catenin signaling pathway through its redox-sensitive association with disheveled (Dvl) (Funato, Michiue, Asashima et al. 2006).

Protein disulfide isomerase. PDI is a member of the Trx family that is located in the ER. PDI is a multidomain and multifunctional protein involved in all steps of disulfide bond formation in nascent proteins; the reaction of thiol–disulfide oxidation, reduction, and isomerization takes place at the two thiredoxin-like catalytic domains of PDI (Schwaller, Wilkinson, Gilbert 2003). While the exact mechanism of PDI action is not defined, it is suggested that the reoxidation of PDI by the GSH redox buffer (GSH + GSSG) is rate limiting in PDI-catalyzed disulfide bond formation. To date, eighteen PDI-family members are found in human ER with possible overlapping functions in disulfide bond formation (Ellgaard, Ruddock 2005).

Proteins with Redox-Active Cys Active Sites

Peroxiredoxins. Peroxiredoxins (Prxs) are a group of non-seleno thiol-specific peroxidases with an oxidizable cysteine-active site and a role in antioxidant defense that involves the breakdown of organic hydroperoxides and H_2O_2 (Rhee, Chae, Kim 2005). Prx are divided into three classes: typical 2-Cys Prx, atypical 2-Cys Prx, and 1-Cys Prx, but all classes share the same catalytic mechanism when an active cysteine (peroxidatic cysteine) is oxidized to Cys-SOH by the peroxide substrate. In mammalian cells six isoforms (PrxI to PrxVI) have been identified: PrxI and II are located in the cytosol, Prx III in the mitochondria, Prx IV in the extracellular space, and Prx V in the mitochondria and the microsomes (Fujii, Ikeda 2002; Hofmann, Hecht, Flohe 2002). Prx I to Prx IV belong to the 2-Cys Prx subgroup, Prx V to the atypical 2-Cys subgroup, and Prx VI to the 1-Cys subgroup. In eukaryotic cells, 2-Cys Prx enzymes are abundant and susceptible to reversible peroxidation to cysteine sulfinic acid during catalysis. It is recently proposed that overoxidation of the peroxidatic cysteine from the catalytic

site of 2-Cys Prx functions as a molecular switch in transcriptional activity in response to low and high levels of H_2O_2 (Bozonet, Findlay, Day et al. 2005). The regeneration of the thiol status of the active cysteine differs among the Prx classes; thiol regeneration of the typical and atypical 2-Cys Prx classes is catalyzed by a disulfide reductase and the Trx/TrxR system while reduction of 1-Cys Prx requires a thiol-containing reductant (Wood, Schroder, Robin Harris et al. 2003). Different biological roles have been attributed to these Prx members, notably cell cycle arrest or cell proliferation in response to superoxidation or reduction of the active site cysteine, respectively (Phalen, Weirather, Deming et al. 2006). Despite being less efficient than catalase, Prxs are important in cytoprotection against oxidative stress, given their cellular abundance and high affinity for peroxide substrates.

Sulfiredoxins. Sulfiredoxins (Srxs) are cytosolic enzymes that contain a highly conserved active site cysteine residue and function in the reduction of sulfinic and sulfonic acid derivatives of oxidized proteins such as Prxs (Biteau, Labarre, Toledano 2003) of which the 2-Cys Prx class are excellent substrates (Woo, Jeong, Chang et al. 2005). Srx is the first protein identified in the reduction of de-glutathionylation of proteins mediated by the one cysteine residue in the active catalytic site (Findlay, Townsend, Morris et al. 2006), and the reduction mechanism involves ATP hydrolysis and requires Mg^{2+} and thiols (such as GSH or Trx) as electron donors (Chang, Jeong, Woo et al. 2004). Specific examples of proteins de-glutathionylated by Srx include actin and protein tyrosine phosphatase 1B (PTP1B), a regulator of insulin signaling (Findlay, Townsend, Morris et al. 2006).

MECHANISMS OF REDOX SIGNALING

Many cellular proteins contain cysteine residues as redox-sensitive switches where the reversible oxidation of cysteine of targeted proteins is an important posttranslational redox mechanism in the regulation of protein function. ROS-induced oxidation of cysteine-SH group results in the formation of intra- and/or inter-chain disulfide bonds, while reactions with GSH disulfide and NO• result in S-glutathionylation and S-nitrosylation of cysteine thiols, respectively (Biswas, Chida, Rahman 2006). The sulfur atom of cysteine can exist in several oxidation states (Fig. 19.3): the sulfhydryl group (–SH, a –2 state, the disulfide (–S–S–, a –1 state), and the sulfenic acid (–SOH, a 0 state), all of which participate in reversible redox reactions. Disulfide formation is reversed by the action of the GSH or Trx redox systems. The higher oxidation states of sulfinic acid (–SO$_2$H, a +2 state) and sulfonic acid (–SO$_3$H, a + 4 state) are

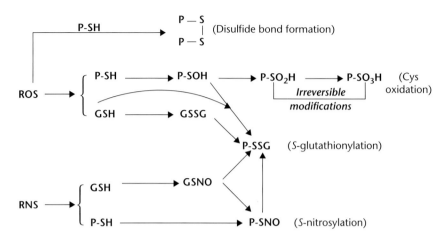

Figure 19.3 Redox modification of protein thiols with role in cellular signaling. Cysteine residues from target proteins can undergo reversible and irreversible modifications by reactions with ROS and RNS. ROS can mediate intra- or intermolecular disulfide bridge formation to yield protein disulfide cross-links or S-hydroxylation of protein thiols or GSH to form sulfenic acids (Pr-S-OH) or GSSG (glutathione disulfide), respectively. NO•, through its higher nitrogen species (e.g., N_2O_3) can cause S-nitrosylation of GSH or protein thiols to form nitrosothiols (GSNO/Pr-S-NO). GSSG can induce S-glutathionylation of protein thiols through the exchange of disulfide bonds with protein thiols to form mixed disulfides (Pr-SSG). As secondary reactions, GSH reacts with nitrosothiols and/or sulfenic acids to induce S-glutathionylation. In addition, GSNO can induce both S-nitrosylation and S-glutathionylation of protein thiols.

generally irreversible and associated with oxidant burden. However, recent studies demonstrated that cysteine sulfinic acid produced during the catalytic cycle of peroxiredoxins can be reduced by Srxs (Woo, Chae, Hwang et al. 2003).

Redox Regulation by S-Glutathionylation

S-glutathionylatioin is a process where protein-containing accessible thiol groups form mixed disulfides with low-molecular-weight thiols, such as GSH. The reversible covalent addition of GSH to cysteine within proteins results in an S-glutathionylated protein. The formation of glutathionylated protein occurs through thiol–disulfide exchange between free protein-SH (PrSH) and GSSG, through reactions of cysteine oxidation products, such as sulfenic acid (protein-SOH) or sulfinic acid (protein-SO_2H) with GSH, through formation of protein S-nitrosothiols (protein-SNO) and subsequent reaction with GSH, or through reactions of thiyl radical (RS•) formed by oxidized proteins that form mixed disulfide adduct with cellular GSH (Ghezzi 2005). The formation of GSH sulfenic acid (GSOH), GSSG-monoxide [GS(O)SG], or the GSH thiyl radical following interaction with HO• can also contribute to S-glutathionylation of targeted proteins (Giustarini, Milzani, Aldini et al. 2005). In the absence of GSH, the redox-active cysteine moieties can be oxidize to the irreversible sulfinic or sulfonic states, resulting in loss of protein function (Poole, Karplus, Claiborne 2004).

The growing number of cellular proteins that are found to be reversibly S-glutathionylated indicates that

this process is an important mechanism in regulation of protein activity. Protein S-glutathionylation can occur under physiological and oxidative conditions, and in the context of cell signaling, S-glutathionylation acts as an intracellular redox sensor during mild oxidative and nitrosative stress (Biswas, Chida, Rahman 2006; Dalle-Donne, Rossi, Giustarini et al. 2007). The involvement and effectiveness of S-glutathionylation in cellular signaling is attributed to its reversibility, a process that has been compared to phosphorylation/dephosphorylation reactions. De-glutathionylation, which represents the removal of the GSH from protein-mixed disulfides, can occur nonenzymatically in a reducing GSH/GSSG environment or enzymatically in the reactions catalyzed by Trx/TrxR, Grx/GrxR or Srx (Shelton, Chock, Mieyal 2005; Holmgren, Johansson, Berndt et al. 2005; Findlay, Townsend, Morris et al. 2006). While Trx and Srx induce the reduction of their substrates, Grx can catalyze the S-glutathionylation of several other proteins. For Grx, S-glutathionylation involves participation of only one of the essential cysteine residues in the catalytic site of Grx, whereas de-glutathionylation involves both cysteine moieties (Xiao, Lundstrom-Ljung, Holmgren et al. 2005).

During oxidative stress, GSH S-glutathionylation can be viewed as a strategy to conserve cell GSH since GSSG formed from GSH oxidation could be lost to the extracellular space through efflux (Sies, Akerboom 1984). In addition, S-glutathionylation also function in protection of redox-sensitive cysteine residues of proteins such as α-ketoglutarate dehydrogenase (Nulton-Persson, Starke, Mieyal et al. 2003) against overoxidation and the formation of sulfinic or sulfonic acid derivatives (Mallis, Buss, Thomas 2001; Mallis, Hamann, Zhao et al. 2002).

Redox Regulation by S-Nitrosylation

Similar to ROS, NO• plays an important role in the regulation of cell function through formation of S-nitroso derivatives of cysteine residues of targeted proteins (Gaston, Carver, Doctor et al. 2003; Sun, Steenbergen, Murphy 2006). S-nitrosylation refers to the covalent binding of an NO• residue to the sulfhydryl moieties of proteins in the presence of an electron acceptor to form an S–NO bond that results in the formation of SNOs. The mechanism of SNO formation is unclear and could involve nitrogen dioxide (N_2O_3) as a nitrosating agent that is formed intracellularly in a reaction between NO_2 and NO• (Kharitonov, Sundquist, Sharma 1995). Other mechanisms of SNO production include reactions of NO• with a thiyl radical (Karoui, Hogg, Frejaville et al. 1996) or of ONOO⁻ with thiols (Kharitonov, Sundquist, Sharma 1995). A growing body of evidence indicates that SNO formation is a crucial posttranslational protein modification in the redox control of signal transduction. Under mild oxidative challenge, the formation of SNOs appears to be a regulatory mechanism that assures reversible protein oxidation against further oxidative modification by ROS. During increased oxidative stress the disequilibrium of NO•-mediated nitrosylation induces nitrosative stress, such as in the scenario of elevated ONOO⁻ formation that results in irreversible oxidation of cysteine or nitration of protein tyrosine. Since NO• is short-lived in vivo, it has been suggested that the formation of SNOs serves as "NO• carriers" for NO• storage and transport (Muller, Kleschyov, Alencar et al. 2002). One example is GSNO, a proposed storage and transport form of NO• in the regulation of cardiac function (Muller, Kleschyov, Alencar et al. 2002). Intracellularly, GSNO is formed by the reaction of NO• with GSH (Sarr, Lobysheva, Diallo et al. 2005) and functions in the reversible modification of protein thiols through transnitrosylation or S-glutathionylation, depending on the cellular redox environment. Examples of proteins shown to react with GSNO include the cystic fibrosis transmembrane regulatory gene, *CFTR*, hypoxia inducible factor-1 (HIF-1), and the nuclear transcription factor, NF-κB (Zaman, Palmer, Doctor et al. 2004). Cellular SNOs have a short half-life and are readily reduced by GSH or Trx through transnitrosation and subsequent de-nitrosylation (Freedman, Frei, Welch et al. 1995).

S-nitrosylation regulates the activity of a variety of proteins in different cellular compartments, including a role in mitochondrial apoptotic signaling. It has been demonstrated that S-nitrosylated inactive caspases are localized within the mitochondrial intermembrane space, and upon apoptotic stimulation, the inactive caspases undergo de-nitrosylation and activation in the cytosol (Mannick, Schonhoff, Papeta et al. 2001). Trx1-catalyzed inactivation of procaspase-3 through a transnitrosylation reaction that leads to inhibition of apoptosis has been demonstrated in Jurkat cells; this involvement of Trx1 in transnitrosylation reaction was suggested to be a general mechanism of protein–protein interaction subjected to cellular redox modulation (Mitchell, Morton, Fernhoff et al. 2007). Apart from apoptosis signaling, the interaction of NO• with cytochrome *c* oxidase is an important regulatory mechanism of mitochondrial respiration, wherein NO• binding to cytochrome oxidase active site inhibits respiration, which has been suggested to have a role in hypoxic cell death (Liu, Miller, Joshi et al. 1998; Thomas, Liu, Kantrow et al. 2001).

Membrane receptors (Eu, Sun, Xu et al. 2000), kinases (Park, Huh, Kim et al. 2000), G proteins (Raines, Bonini, Campbell 2007), and transcription factors (Tabuchi, Sano, Oh et al. 1994; Palmer, Gaston, Johns 2000; Marshall, Stamler 2001; Zaman, Palmer, Doctor et al. 2004;) are other examples of proteins whose functions are regulated by S-nitrosylation. Functionally, S-nitrosylation can lead to activation (e.g., p21ras or Trx) or inhibition (e.g., caspases) of protein activity, and only specific protein thiols are targeted. For instance, NO• selectively targets Cys[69] in Trx (Haendeler, Hoffmann, Tischler et al. 2002), and Cys[3635] among the 50 residues in the ryanodine-responsive calcium channel of the skeletal muscle (Sun, Xin, Eu et al. 2001) for S-nitrosylation. The reason for this targeted selectivity is unclear. S-nitrosylation also exhibits stereoselectivity in that the L-, but not D-isomer of SNOs is bioactive.

TARGETS OF REDOX REGULATION IN CELL SIGNALING

Redox Modulation of Protein Tyrosine Kinases and Phosphatases

The binding of cytokines or growth factors to their membrane receptors can generate ROS at the receptor level that activates a cascade of intracellular signaling pathways. Protein tyrosine kinase (PTK) and PTP are among the direct targets of ROS, and signaling by PTK/PTP phosphorylation/dephosphorylation controls many biological processes. PTK belongs to the transmembrane receptor family or the cytosolic nonreceptor tyrosine kinases with a functional role in regulating cell metabolism, growth, migration, and differentiation (Chiarugi, Buricchi 2007). PTP, which catalyzes the dephosphorylation of tyrosine residues, represents an effective mechanism by which cells enhance or terminate receptor tyrosine kinase signaling at the level of the receptor. The deprotonated cysteine in the catalytic site of PTP is susceptible to oxidation by ROS to a sulfenic derivative (Tonks, Neel 2001; Salmeen, Barford 2005); the loss of phosphatase activity results in hyperphosphorylation of PTK (Minetti, Mallozzi, Di Stasi 2002). This mechanism of PTK regulation has been referred to as "indirect PTK redox regulation through reversible PTP oxidation" (Chiarugi, Buricchi 2007).

The control of tyrosine kinase activity has been described for platelet-derived growth factor receptor (PDGFR); the two PTPs involved in regulation are the low-molecular-weight PTP (LMW-PTP) and SHP2 (Chiarugi, Fiaschi, Taddei et al. 2001; Meng, Fukada, Tonks 2002). LMW-PTP contains two cysteine residues in the catalytic site that forms a disulfide bond during oxidation and is thereby protected against irreversible inactivation due to the formation of sulfinic and sulfonic derivatives (Caselli, Marzocchini, Camici et al. 1998). PTEN is another dual specificity phosphatase where, upon oxidation, Cys^{124} and Cys^{71} are involved in disulfide bond formation (Lee, Yang, Kwon et al. 2002). It has been proposed that redox modulation of PTEN is attributed to Trx1; one study demonstrated that oxidized PTEN is reduced by Trx1, which restores activity (Lee, Yang, Kwon et al. 2002; Meuillet, Mahadevan, Berggren et al. 2004), while another study showed that Trx 1, by forming covalent disulfide bonds with PTEN, in fact inhibits PTEN activity (Lee, Yang, Kwon et al. 2002; Meuillet, Mahadevan, Berggren et al. 2004). At present, the role of Trx1 in PTEN regulation is unresolved. Better known is the fact that the activity of PTEN and its capacity to be recruited in protein complexes is negatively regulated by the phosphorylation of Ser^{380}, Thr^{382}, and Thr^{383} of the PTEN tail (Vazquez, Ramaswamy, Nakamura et al. 2000; Vazquez, Grossman, Takahashi et al. 2001).

Another well-studied example of redox regulation of PTK activity is the insulin tyrosine kinase receptor. Insulin stimulation has been shown to generate $O_2^{\bullet-}$ and H_2O_2 via Nox4, which oxidatively inhibit the PTP, PTP1B, as well as PTEN (Mahadev, Motoshima, Wu et al. 2004; Seo, Ahn, Lee et al. 2005). The inhibition of PTP1B increases insulin receptor autophosphorylation, thereby extending receptor activation time, while inhibition of PTEN facilitates PI3K signaling, which is responsible for many of the cellular effects of insulin. In each instance, S-glutathionylation of cysteine thiol oxidation at phosphatase-active sites protects the enzyme from further, irreversible oxidation. For PTP1B, the cyclic sulfonamide derivative is the intermediate of cysteine oxidation (Meng, Buckley, Galic et al. 2004). Redox regulation of other intracellular kinases such as Src tyrosine kinase, focal adhesion kinase, as well as serine/threonine kinases or dual specific tyrosine/threonine mitogen-activated protein kinases (MAPK), or protein kinase B (Akt/PKB) and apoptosis signal–regulating kinases (ASK) have all been demonstrated to be through oxidation of redox-active cysteine in their catalytic sites (Chiarugi, Cirri 2003; Giannoni, Buricchi, Raugei et al. 2005).

Redox Regulation of Serine/Threonine Kinases

Protein Kinase C

Protein kinase C (PKC) is a serine/threonine kinase whose redox regulation is well documented. In contrast to PTK whose activities are indirectly controlled by redox regulation of PTP, serine/threonine kinases are directly modified by cysteine oxidation or thiolation. In purified PKC, high concentrations of H_2O_2 inactivate the enzyme while lower oxidant levels modify the regulatory subunit that activates the enzyme in the absence of classical PKC stimulators such as Ca^{2+} and diacylglycerol (Gopalakrishna, Anderson 1989). The mechanism for oxidative activation involves cysteine thiol oxidation and release of zinc (Knapp, Klann 2000); glutathionylation of critical cysteine inhibits enzyme activity (Chu, Ward, O'Brian 2001). As with S-glutathionylation of protein cysteines, specific cysteine residues of PKC are targeted, such as PKC_ε Cys^{452} (Chu, Koomen, Kobayashi et al. 2005). Functionally, thiol modification of PKC plays an important role in endothelial homeostasis.

Mitogen-Activated Protein Kinase (MAPK) and Apoptosis Signal-Regulating Kinase 1

MAPKs are key players in the signaling cascades involved in proliferation, differentiation, gene expression, mitosis, or apoptosis. MAPK phosphorylates specific serine and threonine residues of target proteins and can be activated by ROS. The transduction of signal involves a cascade of phosphorylation in which upstream MAPK kinase kinase (MAPKKK) activates MAPK kinase (MAPKK), which in turn activates MAPK (Kyriakis, Avruch 2001). On the basis of structural differences, mammalian MAPK has been divided into three classes: extracellular signal–regulated protein kinase (ERK), c-Jun NH2-terminal kinase (JNK), and p38 MAPK. MAPK cascades are involved in ROS-induced cellular response and have a role in redox signaling, often in association with apoptosis signal–regulating kinase 1 (ASK-1), another serine/threonine protein kinase that is activated by stress signals such as cytokines, ROS, ER stress, serum withdrawal, and Ca^{2+}. It has been shown that on activation, ASK-1 signaling leads to the activation of p38 and JNK pathways (Nishitoh, Saitoh, Mochida et al. 1998).

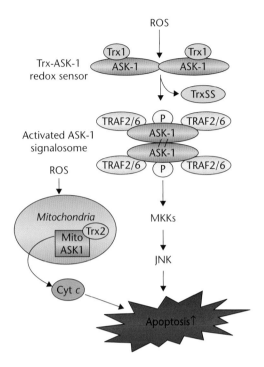

Figure 19.4 ROS-mediated ASK-1 signaling and apoptosis. ROS generated from different sources induce the oxidation of sulphydryl groups in the redox active site of thioredoxin 1 (Trx1) causing its dissociation from the redox complex with apoptosis signaling–regulating kinase 1 (ASK-1). After Trx1 dissociation, the activated "ASK-1 signalosome" is stabilized through covalent bond formation among its subunits and other proteins such as tumor necrosis factor receptor–associated factor 2 and 6 (TRAF 2/6) that are recruited to the signalosome. In addition, ASK-1 can autophosphorylate. The signalosome signals the activation of JNK, resulting in cell apoptosis. Similarly, ROS can induce the oxidation and dissociation of mitochondrial thioredoxin (Trx2) from its complex with ASK-1 that results in apoptosis through a JNK-independent mechanism.

Oxidative stress is one of the most potent activator of ASK-1–mediated signaling and cell death (Fig. 19.4). Human ASK-1 is a protein of ≈1300 amino acids that contains three domains: the N-terminal regulatory domain, a serine/threonine kinase domain in the middle of the molecule, and a C-terminal regulatory domain (Nishitoh, Saitoh, Mochida et al. 1998). In nonstressed cells, ASK-1 forms homo-oligomers of ≈1500 kDa to 2000 kDa that are noncovalently associated through N-terminal domains. The binding of Trx1 through cysteine residues directly to the N-terminal domain inhibits the kinase activity (Saitoh, Nishitoh, Fujii et al. 1998). This high molecular weight complex exists in an inactive form and is known as the *ASK signalosome* (Fig. 19.4). The interaction of Trx1-ASK-1 is dependent on the redox state of Trx1, and only reduced Trx1 will bind (Liu, Min 2002). Thus, the Trx1/ASK-1 couple can be regarded as an intracellular redox switch that can be turned on

or off under oxidative conditions (Fujino, Noguchi, Takeda et al. 2006). Under oxidizing conditions, the cysteine oxidation and disulfide bond formation result in Trx1 dissociation from the signalosome; subsequent complex rearrangement permits the autophosphorylation and activation of ASK-1 (Noguchi, Takeda, Matsuzawa et al. 2005). ASK-1 signaling activates downstream MAPK kinases (MKK3/MKK6 and MKK4/MKK7) that promote activation of the JNK and p38 signaling pathways and induces cell apoptosis (Fig. 19.4). Depending on cell types, ASK-1 activation can exert other biological effects including cell differentiation, cytokine induction, cardiac remodeling, and neurite outgrowth (Nagai, Noguchi, Takeda et al. 2007). A modification to the existing model of ASK-1 activation was recently proposed by Nadeau et al. (2007). These investigators propose that exposure of cells to H_2O_2 promoted rapid ASK-1 oxidation and ASK-1 multimerization through inter-chain disulfide bonds formation. The formation of such covalently associated homodimers is a requisite for downstream activation of JNK-mediated apoptosis. Additionally, the stable multimer complex is able to recruit new proteins (TRAF2/6 and PKD) that enhance its competence for downstream signaling. Through reduction of oxidized ASK-1, Trx1 can negatively regulate ASK-1 signaling.

ASK-1 interacts with Trx2 within the mitochondria, and an increase in mitochondrial ROS induces ASK-1 dissociation, cytochrome *c* release, and cellular apoptosis independent of JNK activation (Zhang, Al-Lamki, Bai et al. 2004). Apart from Trx1/Trx2, other proteins such as TRAF2 and death domain-associated protein (Daxx) are shown to be enhancers of ASK-1 activation, while Grx, the phosphoserine/phosphothreonine-binding protein (14–3-3), and protein serine/threonine phosphatase 5 (PP5) are among notable inhibitors of ASK-1. Mechanistically, Grx1 inhibits ASK-1 through reduction of oxidized ASK-1 (Song, Lee 2003), whereas 14–3-3 mediates ASK-1 inhibition through Ser[967] phosphorylation (Fujii, Goldman, Park et al. 2004) and PP5 through Thr[845] dephosphorylation (Morita, Saitoh, Tobiume et al. 2001). S-nitrosylation of specific cysteine residues of ASK-1 (Cys[869]) or Trx1 (Cys[31], Cys[35], Cys[69]) interferes with the propagation of ASK signaling (Park, Yu, Cho et al. 2004).

Redox Control of Transcription Factors

Activator Protein 1

AP-1 belongs to a family of basic leucine zipper (bZIP) transcription factors that regulates the expression of various enzymes involved in cellular survival, proliferation, differentiation, and death. AP-1 exists as a heterodimer consisting of subunits from the Fos, Jun, Maf, and ATF subfamilies, but mostly, AP-1 is a heterodimer of c-Fos and c-Jun that binds TPA response elements (TREs) in the promoters of target genes, and is sensitive to redox regulation. Oxidative stress is shown to promote c-Fos and c-Jun transcription (Wenk, Brenneisen, Wlaschek et al. 1999), and AP-1 binding to DNA is enhanced by the reduction of the cysteine residue located in the DNA-binding domain of each monomer (Abate, Patel, Rauscher et al. 1990). The redox state of AP-1 is controlled by apurinic/apyrimidinic endonuclease (APE), also known as redox factor-1 (Ref-1), and the redox state of APE is in turn controlled by Trx1 (Hirota, Matsui, Iwata et al. 1997). It has been demonstrated that DNA binding of AP-1 is attenuated by S-glutathionylation of the cysteine residue in the AP-1 catalytic site in response to decreased cellular GSH/GSSG ratio (Klatt, Molina, De Lacoba et al. 1999). Similarly, NO$^\bullet$ modulates AP-1 DNA-binding by reversible S-nitrosylation (Cys^{272} of c-Jun), but this modification is cell-type specific (Morris 1995; Klatt, Molina, Lamas 1999). Indirectly, ROS stimulates AP-1 activity through regulation of JNK and PKC-mediated activation of a c-Jun phosphatase and the dephosphorylation of serine and threonine residues.

Nuclear Factor Kappa B

NF-κB is a transcription factor that is composed of homo- or heterodimers of the Rel protein family and is involved in the expression of genes that govern cell survival, inflammation, and proliferation. In nonstimulated cells, NF-κB is sequestered in the cytoplasm by inhibitory IκB protein, and its dissociation promoted by oxidative stimuli such as tumor necrosis factor-α, ionizing radiation, and ROS leads to NF-κB activation (Baeuerle 1998). It is well recognized that NF-κB activation and DNA binding are sensitive to the cellular redox status. For example, NF-κB/DNA binding is decreased by thiol oxidants such as diamide and increased by thiol-reducing compounds such as dithiothreitol and β-mercaptoethanol (Hayashi, Ueno, Okamoto 1993). Cytosolic NF-κkB activation and nuclear DNA binding are differentially modulated by Trx1. In the cytosol, Trx1 inhibits the dissociation and degradation of IκB resulting in inhibition of NF-κB activation (Hirota, Murata, Sachi et al. 1999) whereas within the nucleus, Trx1 reduces Cys^{62} of the p50 subunit of NF-κB, resulting in increased binding to DNA (Matthews, Wakasugi, Virelizier et al. 1992). S-glutathionylation is another mode of redox control of NF-κB activity. S-glutathionylation of Cys^{62} of the p50 subunit has been shown to inhibit NF-κB binding to DNA (Pineda-Molina, Klatt, Vazquez et al. 2001), while S-glutathionylation of Cys^{179} of the β-subunit of

IκB under oxidizing conditions represses its kinase activity, which can be prevented by Grx1. Indeed, the de-glutathionylation of IκB is currently regarded as a highly sensitive physiological redox mechanism in the modulation of the magnitude of NF-κB activation (Reynaert, van der Vliet, Guala et al. 2006).

Nuclear Factor Erythroid 2-Related Factor (Nrf2) and Cellular Redox Maintenance

Nrf2 is a member of the cap and collar (cnc) family of bZIP transcription factors that plays an important role in cellular oxidative stress and redox homeostasis. Under normal conditions, Nrf2 is kept sequestered in the cytosol by a homodimer of the actin-associated protein Kelch-associated protein 1 (Keap1). In this arrangement, Nrf2 and Keap1 are part of a larger protein complex that includes the scaffolding protein Cul-3 as well as an E3 ubiquitin ligase, and the interaction between Nrf2 and Keap1 ensures the ubiquitylation and proteasomal degradation of Nrf2 (Kobayashi, Kang, Watai et al. 2006). It is known that ROS causes the dissociation of Nrf2 from Keap1, which determines the steady state levels of Nrf2 and its nuclear translocation. ROS can directly induce Nrf2 dissociation via oxidation of specific cysteine residues on Keap1. It has also been shown that oxidative stress–induced activation of PI3K and PKC facilitates Nrf2 nuclear translocation. Within the nucleus, Nrf2 binds to specific DNA sequences called *antioxidant response elements* (AREs, also called electrophillic response elements or EpREs) in the promoters of various genes that are involved in response to oxidative and xenobiotic stress. A notable example is the catalytic subunit of GCL (GCLc), the rate-limiting enzyme in GSH synthesis; thus, by regulating GCL expression and cellular GSH concentrations, Nrf2 exerts a significant impact on cellular redox signaling. Our recent studies uncovered a unique influence of Nrf2 signaling on vascular endothelial GSH redox balance and cytoprotection against hyperglycemic stress (Okouchi, Okayama, Alexander et al. 2006; section on Nrf2 and redox regulation of vascular function).

ROS, REDOX REGULATION, AND CELL SIGNALING IN THE VASCULATURE

The vascular endothelium comprises the innermost lining of blood vessels, and serves as a selective permeable barrier between blood and tissue. Once thought of as a relatively "benign" tissue, it is now well recognized that the endothelium is a dynamic structure that plays integral roles in a number of vascular functions including regulation of vascular tone, permeability, tissue perfusion, inflammation, and angiogenesis. An emerging common feature in the regulation of these complex vascular processes is the involvement of ROS in cell signaling. Endothelial ROS, generated in response to acute humoral (i.e. growth factors and cytokines) and mechanical (i.e. sheer) stimuli (Fig. 19.5), can participate in redox signaling. Chronic, dysregulated overproduction of ROS, however, causes oxidative stress, which underpins a variety of vascular pathologies. Increased ROS production during oxidative stress is often accompanied by decreased levels of antioxidants, and as it is in other cell types, GSH is a primary intracellular antioxidant with an important role in the regulation of endothelial cell redox status.

CELLULAR SOURCES OF ENDOTHELIAL ROS

In recent studies, we have demonstrated that the mitochondria is an important source of $O_2^{\bullet-}$ in endothelial cells (Ichikawa, Kokura, Aw 2004). Under physiological conditions, as much as 1% to 3% of mitochondrial O_2 consumption is reduced to $O_2^{\bullet-}$ by electron leak from the electron transport chain (Halliwell 1999), and mitochondrial sites of electron leak and $O_2^{\bullet-}$ formation have been localized to complexes I and III. In the pathophysiological states of hypoxia (Guzy, Hoyos, Robin et al. 2005), hyperoxia (Brueckl, Kaestle, Kerem et al. 2006), ischemia-reperfusion (Kim, Kondo, Noshita et al. 2002), and hyperglycemia

(Nishikawa, Kukidome, Sonoda et al. 2007), mitochondria derived ROS is a significant contributor to cellular oxidative stress. In addition, mitochondrial ROS plays an important role in mitochondrial redox signaling, which is an integral component of apoptotic regulation.

Several oxidases are important enzymatic sources of ROS in the endothelium. These include xanthine oxidase (XO) and NADPH oxidase (Nox). Under physiological conditions, XO functions as a dehydrogenase that couples the reduction of NAD^+ to the oxidation of xanthine and hypoxanthine. During oxidative stress, however, the enzyme is converted to an oxidase that donates electrons to O_2 to produce $O_2^{\bullet-}$. Similar to the mitochondria, XO-derived ROS is a significant contributor to oxidative stress during hypoxia when ATP levels are low and hypoxanthine levels are high. Involvement of XO in pro-inflammatory signaling has been suggested; ROS generation upon endothelial ICAM-1 cross-linking, which mimics leukocyte adhesion, can be blocked with the XO inhibitor, allopurinol (Wang, Pfeiffer, Gaarde 2003).

The Nox family of enzymes consists of a number of multisubunit protein complexes that catalyze the reduction of O_2 to $O_2^{\bullet-}$ using NADPH as an electron source. Originally discovered as $O_2^{\bullet-}$-producing bactericidal enzymes in phagocytic leukocytes, Nox has recently been characterized in nonphagocytic cells such as endothelial cells. The catalytic subunit of the phagocytic Nox, gp91phox, is expressed in endothelial cells to a lesser extent, which accounts

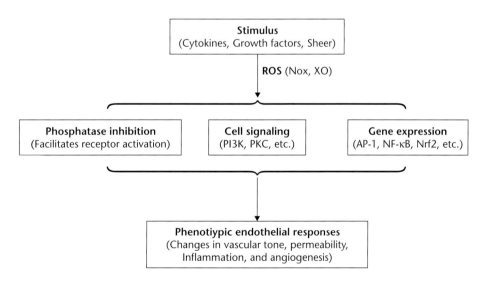

Figure 19.5 ROS signaling on endothelial function. ROS generated in response to a variety of mechanical and chemical stimuli activate receptor tyrosine kinase activity facilitated by tyrosine phosphatase inactivation. Activation of various signal transduction pathways occurs through direct oxidative modification of PKC or indirectly through phosphatase inactivation (PI3K and PTEN) and transcription factor-mediated endothelial gene. These signaling events result in changes in endothelial function (i.e., induction of inflammation, angiogenesis, altered vascular tone, etc.).

for the decreased $O_2^{\bullet-}$ production by endothelial Nox enzymes. Several Nox isoforms are important in endothelial cell signaling in a wide range of vascular functions, including regulation of vascular tone, inflammation, and angiogenesis. As examples, the vasoconstrictive effects of angiotensin II (Ang II) are mediated in part by Nox generated $O_2^{\bullet-}$, which reacts with and scavenges $NO^{\bullet}$, and vascular endothelial growth factor (VEGF)-induced endothelial growth and migration is mediated by $O_2^{\bullet-}$ generated by Nox2 (a gp91phox containing Nox) (Ushio-Fukai, Tang, Fukai et al. 2002; Colavitti, Pani, Bedogni et al. 2002). VEGF angiogenesis is attenuated in gp91phox knockout mice (Ushio-Fukai, Tang, Fukai et al. 2002). There is a well-established role for Nox in vascular diseases such as hypertension and diabetes; evidence shows that ischemia-induced retinal angiogenesis is inhibited in gp91phox knockout mice (Al-Shabrawey, Bartoli, El-Remessy et al. 2005), and Nox inhibition restores neovascularization in the hindlimbs of diabetic mice after femoral artery ligation (Ebrahimian, Heymes, You et al. 2006).

Research over the past decade has implicated uncoupled eNOS as an unexpected source of endothelial $O_2^{\bullet-}$. While generally known for its role in constitutive $NO^{\bullet}$ production in the regulation of vascular tone and inflammation, recent evidence suggests that eNOS can become "uncoupled" in the absence of its cofactor, tetrahydrobiopterin (BH$_4$), and can generate $O_2^{\bullet-}$ and H_2O_2 instead of $NO^{\bullet}$. Validation that eNOS is a source of ROS in vivo comes from findings that BH$_4$ supplementation attenuated oxidative stress and restored $NO^{\bullet}$ bioavailability and vascular reactivity in animal models of vascular oxidative stress (Landmesser, Dikalov, Price et al. 2003).

ROS and Vascular Signaling

ROS in Physiological Function

Regulation of vascular tone. Current evidence indicates that ROS can mediate vasodilatory as well as vasoconstrictive effects, depending on the ROS species, its concentration, and the target vascular bed. For instance, $O_2^{\bullet-}$, through interaction with $NO^{\bullet}$ inhibits acetylcholine-mediated aortic ring relaxation (Gryglewski, Palmer, Moncada 1986) while in cerebral vasculature, XO-derived $O_2^{\bullet-}$, H_2O_2, and $ONOO^-$ induce vasodilation of cerebral arterioles (Wei, Kontos, Beckman 1996). In general, physiological concentrations of ROS mediate vasodilation, whereas at concentrations that induce oxidative stress, ROS causes vasoconstriction, presumably via $NO^{\bullet}$ scavenging. This notion is consistent with observations of increased oxidative stress and decreased $NO^{\bullet}$ levels in

the vasculature of hypertensive animals (Landmesser, Dikalov, Price et al. 2003). Similar to $NO^{\bullet}$, H_2O_2-induced vasodilation is mediated through activation of sGC and cGMP formation (Burke, Wolin 1987). In the vascular smooth muscle (VSM), activation of cGMP-dependent protein kinase (PKG), and Ca^{2+}-activated K^+ (K_{Ca}^{2+}) channels results in VSM hyperpolarization and vasodilation (Wei, Kontos, Beckman 1996; Sobey, Heistad, Faraci 1997). It is suggested that H_2O_2 is the mediator of $O_2^{\bullet-}$-induced vasodilation (Rubanyi, Vanhoutte 1986), and $ONOO^-$-mediated glutathionylation and activation of the sarcoplasmic/ER Ca^{2+} ATPase (SERCA) in the inhibition of VSM contraction has recently been reported (Adachi, Weisbrod, Pimentel et al. 2004). An interesting relation exists between O_2 and $NO^{\bullet}$ in red blood cells where the binding of O_2 to hemoglobin (Hb) promotes S-nitrosylation at the Cys^{93} of the β chain (Jia, Bonaventura, Bonaventura et al. 1996). The deoxygenated form of Hb releases $NO^{\bullet}$ into the microcirculation and promotes regulation of vascular tone (Datta, Tufnell-Barrett, Bleasdale et al. 2004). In this manner, a fluctuation in O_2 tension can influence the vascular response to Hb-released $NO^{\bullet}$ (Foster, Pawloski, Singel et al. 2005).

ROS in Endothelial Dysfunction

ROS and endothelial permeability. ROS such as $O_2^{\bullet-}$, $HO^{\bullet}$, and H_2O_2 have all been shown to increase endothelial permeability (Del Maestro 1982). H_2O_2-stimulated increase in endothelial permeability is Ca^{2+} dependent (Yamada, Yokota, Furumichi et al. 1990; Siflinger-Birnboim, Lum, Del Vecchio et al. 1996), which is interesting considering that H_2O_2 stimulates Ca^{2+} efflux from VSM. ROS-induced endothelial permeability is likely to have important pathophysiological significance for the paracellular and transcellular transport of solutes and macromolecules across the endothelial barrier.

Paracellular transport is the movement of solutes between endothelial cells across interendothelial junctions (IEJs), and the width of these junctions creates a selectively permeable barrier based on molecular size. The width of IEJs is regulated by different endothelial junctional complexes, namely tight junctions (TJs), adherens junctions (AJs), and gap junctions (GJs). H_2O_2 at millimolar concentrations (1 mM) is implicated in the increase in endothelial permeability through rearrangement of specific proteins within these junctional complexes, such as vascular endothelial cadherin (VE-cadherin), an important component of endothelial AJs (Alexander, Alexander, Eppihimer et al. 2000). Additionally, millimolar concentrations of H_2O_2 (1 mM) also stimulate the removal of occludin from endothelial TJs, which is associated with its dissociation from zona occludin 1 (ZO-1), an intracellular protein responsible for linking occludin to the actin cytoskeleton (Kevil, Oshima, Alexander et al. 2000). These junctional protein responses to H_2O_2 could be significant for the cerebral microcirculation and vascular beds with high occludin expression and well-developed TJs. Transcellular transport across the endothelium involves receptor-mediated vesicular transport through the cell. In endothelial cells, H_2O_2 exposure induces the phosphorylation of caveolin 1, an important structural component of caveolae, and vesicular transport (Vepa, Scribner, Natarajan 1997).

ROS in inflammatory response and angiogenesis. It is well-established that exposure of endothelial monolayers to ROS elicits an inflammatory response involving leukocyte adhesion and extravasation. Acute ROS exposure enhances the adhesive interactions between leukocyte ligands and endothelial adhesion molecules as evidenced by increased adhesion of polomorphonuclear neutrophils to human umbilical vein endothelial cells at 15 minutes after treatment with xanthine and XO (Sellak, Franzini, Hakim et al. 1994). Acute $O_2^{\bullet-}$ and H_2O_2 exposure also mediates a rapid upregulation of surface expression of endothelial adhesion molecules such as glycoprotein granule membrane protein 140 (GMP 140) (Patel, Zimmerman, Prescott et al. 1991) and P-selectin, as well as the translocation of adhesion molecule such as ICAM-1 and PECAM-1 to basal endothelial surfaces (Bradley, Thiru, Pober 1995) that facilitates leukocyte extravasation. This is followed over the next few hours by transcriptional upregulation of various pro-inflammatory molecules such as ICAM-1 (Lo, Janakidevi, Lai et al. 1993). In contrast to ROS, $NO^{\bullet}$ exerts anti-inflammatory actions that include inhibition of adhesion molecule expression, platelet aggregation, leukocyte adhesion, and VSM proliferation. $NO^{\bullet}$ scavenging by $O_2^{\bullet-}$ quenches its anti-inflammatory activity.

Angiogenesis is a complex process that involves concerted proliferation, movement, and tube formation by endothelial cells, all of which are enhanced by H_2O_2. Experimentally, the induction of tube formation, proliferation, and motility in bovine aortic endothelial cells seeded on collagen gel was shown to be elicited at micromolar H_2O_2 concentrations (1 μM) (Yasuda, Ohzeki, Shimizu et al. 1999). Coincidentally, many of the cytokines and growth factors that induce angiogenesis and inflammation also generate $O_2^{\bullet-}$ and H_2O_2 as part of their intracellular signaling process (Colavitti, Pani, Bedogni et al. 2002). In fact, VEGF angiogenesis is blunted in mice deficient in gp91phox, a subunit of the $O_2^{\bullet-}$-producing Nox (Ushio-Fukai, Tang, Fukai et al. 2002). Furthermore, H_2O_2 has been shown to increase the production of endothelial growth factor, including VEGF, PDGF, and fibroblast growth factor (FGF).

Endothelial oxidative stress. It is clear that ROS not only play a physiological role in normal endothelial function but are also major contributors to endothelial dysfunction and vascular oxidative stress. Of particular importance to vascular physiology and pathophysiology is the fact that overproduction of $O_2^{\bullet-}$ decreases $NO^{\bullet}$ bioavailability, which attenuates the vascular effects of $NO^{\bullet}$ in vascular tone homeostasis. eNOS knockout mice are hypertensive (Shesely, Maeda, Kim et al. 1996), and endothelial cells isolated from these mice exhibit enhanced ROS production (Kuhlencordt, Rosel, Gerszten et al. 2004). Given the proinflammatory and proangiogenic effects of ROS, vascular oxidative stress is implicated as an underlying cause in various vascular disorders, such as atherosclerosis (Ohara, Peterson, Harrison 1993), diabetic retinopathy (Ellis, Grant, Murray et al. 1998), and inflammatory bowel disease (IBD) (Segui, Gil, Gironella et al. 2005). Antioxidants such as ascorbate, α-tocopherol, and GSH have been shown to inhibit inflammation and angiogenesis and improve endothelial function in vitro and in vivo (Ashino, Shimamura, Nakajima et al. 2003; Chade, Bentley, Zhu et al. 2004; Kevil, Oshima, Alexander et al. 2004; Langston, Chidlow, Booth et al. 2007). However, despite the successes of antioxidant therapy in attenuating vascular dysfunction in a number of animal models of vascular diseases, results from human trials utilizing antioxidants as therapy for vascular diseases have not been as promising.

GSH AND VASCULAR REDOX SIGNALING

Transcriptional Expression of GCL in Control of Cell GSH

As discussed in the section on GSH/GSSG and cellular redox balance, the maintenance of cellular GSH is critical to cell redox homeostasis and is achieved by the integration of *de novo* GSH synthesis, GSSG reduction, and GSH transport. The importance of *de novo* synthesis in GSH homeostasis is underscored by the fact that inhibition of synthesis with buthionine sulfoximine can essentially completely deplete the cellular GSH pool (Sun, Ragsdale, Benson et al. 1985). Since GCL-catalyzed formation of γ-glutamylcysteine is the rate-limiting step in GSH synthesis, its activity is tightly regulated, at both the transcriptional and posttranslational levels. GCL is a heterodimer composed of the modulatory subunit of GCL (GCLm) and GCLc subunit. While GCLc possesses essential catalytic activity of the enzyme, dimerization with GCLm enhances enzyme activity and effectively increases the concentration of GSH that is necessary for feedback inhibition.

Regulation of GCL activity at the posttranscriptional level is redox-dependent and is thought to occur via disulfide bond formation between cysteines on the two subunits, which enhances holoenzyme formation. Evidence also suggests that GCL is constitutively phosphorylated on serine and threonine residues that inhibit enzyme activity independent of holoenzyme formation. There are consensus phosphorylation sites for PKA, PKC, and Ca^{2+}/calmodulin-dependent protein kinase II (CaMKII) within GCLc, each of which can phosphorylate the holoenzyme (Sun, Huang, Lu 1996). Additionally, GCLc can be autophosphorylated (Sekhar, Freeman 1999). By far, the most common and best-studied means of increasing GCL activity is through transcriptional upregulation of its subunits. While the basic information on transcriptional regulation of GCL to date are derived from studies in nonvascular tissues such as the liver, the fundamental regulatory mechanisms briefly summarized in the following section are likely to be applicable in vascular tissues as well.

Transcriptional Regulation of GCLc Expression

The promoters of GCL subunits contain consensus binding sites for the redox-regulated transcription factors, NF-κB, AP-1, and Nrf2. Evidence of tight regulation of GCLc expression is underscored by the findings that transgenic overexpression and genetic deletion of GCLc are embryonic lethal, and conditional liver-specific overexpression of GCLc yielded no more than a twofold increase in protein levels (Dalton, Dieter, Yang et al. 2000; Botta, Shi, White et al. 2006). Furthermore, stimuli for transcriptional upregulation of GCLc rarely increase enzyme expression more than twofold; in tissues with high GSH content such as alveolar epithelium and liver, expression levels can be threefold. These findings are consistent with a tight regulation of the GCLc promoter activity. First cloned in 1995 (Mulcahy, Gipp 1995), the human GCLc promoter notably contained consensus sites for AP-1, AP-2, SP-1, and Nrf2. Four AREs are uncovered (Mulcahy, Wartman, Bailey et al. 1997), of which the most distal ARE4 is responsible for constitutive and β-naphthflavone (β-NF)–induced GCLc promoter activity; specifically, a TRE within ARE4 controls constitutive GCLc promoter activity (Wild, Gipp, Mulcahy 1998). Further characterization of ARE4 revealed Nrf2 binding in response to β-NF (Wild, Moinova, Mulcahy 1999). The rat liver GClc promoter was cloned in 2001 and was found to contain consensus binding sites for C/EBP, AP-1, myeloid zinc finger 1, NF-κB, heat shock transcription factors 1 and 2 (HSF 1 and 2), c-Myc, and nuclear factor-1 (Yang, Wang, Huang et al. 2001). In contrast to the human promoter, there were no consensus AREs in the rat GCLc promoter; GCLc expression mediated by Nrf2 or oxidative stress was controlled indirectly through AP-1 and NF-κB (Yang, Magilnick, Lee et al. 2005).

Transcriptional Regulation of GCLm Expression

GCLm knockout mice do not exhibit the lethal phenotype of GCLc knockouts; nevertheless, these mice exhibit profound tissue oxidative stress (Yang, Dieter, Chen et al. 2002). The GCLm promoter shares common elements with the GCLc promoter in that it possesses elements of housekeeping genes, including high GC content, consensus SP-1 binding sites, and multiple transcription start sites. An ARE regulates β-NF induction of the GCLm promoter, while an AP-1 binding site regulates constitutive promoter activity (Moinova, Mulcahy 1998). The cloned rat GCLm promoter contains consensus sites for AP-1, NF-κB, and HSFs (Yang, Wang, Ou et al. 2001), and AP-1 was found to be responsible for constitutive and *tert*-butylhydroquinone (tBHQ) induction of GCLm promoter activity (Yang, Zeng, Lee et al. 2002). A mouse GCLm promoter has been cloned and characterized (Solis, Dalton, Dieter et al. 2002).

GSH and Redox Regulation of Vascular Function and Cell Signaling

The role of GSH on endothelial function is inextricably tied to the role of ROS and vascular oxidative stress. As an antioxidant, GSH plays a protective role in the pathological states of hypertension and dysregulation of inflammation and angiogenesis; indeed vascular tissues obtained from animal models of hypertension, atherosclerosis, and diabetes all display decreased levels of GSH. Other notable vascular activity of GSH include inhibition of vascular growth (Ashino, Shimamura, Nakajima et al. 2003), endothelial motility, constitutive and agonist-induced adhesion molecule expression, as well as leukocyte adhesion–endothelial cell interaction (Kevil, Oshima, Alexander et al. 2004). In scavenging ROS, GSH maintains endothelial barrier function and attenuates H_2O_2 mediated decreases in transendothelial resistance (Usatyuk, Vepa, Watkins et al. 2003).

As discussed previously in the section on redox modulation of protein tyrosine kinases and phosphatases, GSH-dependent protein S-glutathionylation is a redox mechanism in posttranslational regulation of enzyme activity, and a growing body of evidence supports S-glutathionylation as an important mechanism in redox regulation of vascular function. A direct role for glutathionylation has been demonstrated in endothelial apoptosis. The activation/cleavage of procaspase-3 is an effector of TNF-α induced apoptosis, and evidence shows that Grx-induced caspase-3 de-glutathionylation facilitates enzyme cleavage and the apoptotic process (Pan, Berk 2007). The S-glutathionylation of actin has important consequences for endothelial biology. It has been shown that Grx-mediated de-glutathionylation increases actin polymerization by about sixfold; specifically actin de-glutathionylation at Cys^{374} promotes f-actin formation in response to EGF signaling (Wang, Boja, Tan et al. 2001). Vascular endothelial protein tyrosine phosphatase (VE-PTP) is a recently identified endothelial specific tyrosine phosphatase, and has been shown to interact with and dephosphorylate the angiopoietin receptor Tie2 (Fachinger, Deutsch, Risau 1999). Given that a common mechanism for reversible inhibition of many PTPs is glutathionylation of the catalytic cysteine residues, it may be postulated that oxidative activation of the Tie2 receptor subscribes to reversible VE-PTP glutathionylation and inactivation. NO$^{•}$-induced vasodilatation and VSM relaxation involves S-glutathionylation of Cys^{674} of the sarcoplasmic reticulum Ca^{2+} ATPase (SERCA). Pathophysiological conditions such as hyperlipidemia, hyperglycemia, and hypertension determine the oxidation of Cys^{674} and result in impairment of vasodilatation regulation and consequent cardiovascular complication (Cohen, Adachi 2006).

Among the various signaling pathways, current evidence shows that vascular PI3K signaling is positively regulated by ROS. In VSM cells, H_2O_2 was found to stimulate Akt phosphorylation in a PI3K-dependent manner (Ushio-Fukai, Alexander, Akers et al. 1999); the mechanism of H_2O_2-induced PI3K activation was through oxidative inactivation of the endogenous PI3K inhibitor, PTEN (Lee, Yang, Kwon et al. 2002). In addition, it has been demonstrated that downstream activation of Src, PI3K, MAP kinases, and Akt that leads to endothelial cell migration and proliferation is mediated by ROS-induced VEGF autophosphorylation (Griendling, Sorescu, Lassegue et al. 2000). Moreover, following VEGF stimulation, the Nox subunit, p47phox, associates with two proteins, Rac1 and PAK1, that result in p47phox phosphorylation, ROS production, and membrane ruffles formation. Thus, Nox-produced localized ROS contributed to redox-stimulated directional cell migration (Ushio-Fukai 2006). Ang II participates in another redox signaling pathway in endothelial cells. For instance, Ang II increases production of ROS by endothelial Nox and induces vascular hypertrophy, a process that was mediated through redox-dependent as well as redox-independent activation of p38 and Akt in vascular smooth muscle cells (VSMC) (Ushio-Fukai, Alexander, Akers et al. 1999). A more recent

study by Adachi et al. found that the activation of Ras by S-glutathionylation of Cys^{118} was a critical step in redox-sensitive signaling that leads to Ras activation, p38 and Akt phosphorylation and to Ang II-induced hypertrophy (Adachi, Pimentel, Heibeck et al. 2004).

Nrf2 and Redox Regulation of Vascular Function

Physiological Role of Nrf2

Activation and nuclear transport of Nrf2. The control Nrf2 signaling in the transcriptional regulation of GSH synthesis will have significant impact on the cellular GSH homeostatic state. Figure 19.6 illustrates some of the better-understood aspects of the signaling pathways that regulate Nrf2 activity. H_2O_2 stimulation of upstream PI3K and PKC signaling represents two major pathways in Nrf2 activation. In response to insulin stimulation, PI3K mediates the downstream activation of Akt/mTOR/p70S6K in Nrf2 phosphorylation and nuclear translocation in human cerebral

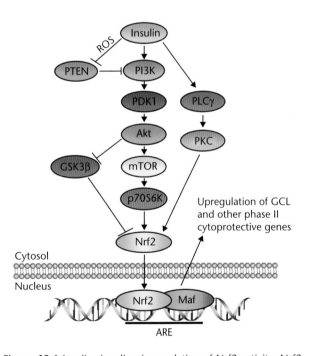

Figure 19.6 Insulin signaling in regulation of Nrf2 activity. Nrf2 nuclear translocation and activation occurs by two main signaling pathways. Activation of PI3K mediates Akt, mTOR, p70S6K signaling, and Nrf2 phosphorylation, while activation of PKC directly phosphorylates Nrf2 on Ser40 and induces nuclear accumulation and DNA binding. In addition, activated Akt also phosphorylates and inactivates GSK3β, which prevents Nrf2 phosphorylation, and thereby inhibits Nrf2 activity. Insulin has been shown to induce endothelial Nrf2 activity via PI3K/Akt/mTOR/p70S6K signaling; although insulin stimulation does activate PKC, the role of this PKC signaling in insulin-mediated endothelial Nrf2 activation has not been demonstrated.

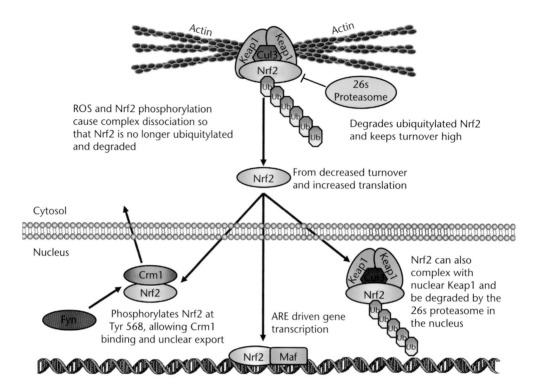

Figure 19.7 Regulation of Nrf2 nuclear translocation and activity. Under normal conditions, Nrf2 exists in a complex with the homodimeric actin-binding protein Keap1 in the cytoplasm. This Nrf2–Keap1 interaction permits Nrf2 ubiquitylation by a Cul-3 containing E3 ubiquitin ligase, which keeps Nrf2 expression low. On stimuli from growth factors, sheer stress, and oxidative stress, and so on, Nrf2 dissociates from the complex and promotes Nrf2 nuclear translocation. Under these conditions, Nrf2 translation is increased as well. Within the nucleus, Nrf2 heterodimerizes with small Maf proteins and induces gene transcription. Nrf2 can also complex with Keap1 in the nucleus, which induces its ubiquitylation and proteasomal degradation. The phosphorylation of nuclear Nrf2 by Fyn kinase at tyrosine residues induces its interaction with the nuclear export protein, Crm1. In some hepatic cell lines, Nrf2 consititutively expressed in the nucleus forms a distinct nuclear Nrf2 pool, the turnover of which is mediated by transient shuttling of Keap1 between the cytoplasm. At present, the existence of a separate Nrf2 pool in vascular cells is unknown.

microvascular endothelial cells (Okouchi, Okayama, Alexander et al. 2006). Although the mechanism is not entirely clear, Akt itself plays a pivotal role in the phosphorylation/inhibition of glycogen synthase kinase 3β (GSK3β), which prevents Nrf2 phosphorylation (Salazar, Rojo, Velasco et al. 2006). PKC activation directly phosphorylates Nrf2 at Ser[40], which promotes Nrf2 dissociation from Keap1 and Nrf2 translocation into the nucleus (Bloom, Jaiswal 2003). Regulation of Nrf2 activity also occurs at the level of the nucleus; Nrf2 contains several different nuclear import and export signals that regulate its nuclear access (Jain, Bloom, Jaiswal 2005; Li, Jain, Chen et al. 2005; Li, Yu, Kong 2006). In particular, phosphorylation of Tyr[568] promotes Nrf2 nuclear export through its interaction with the nuclear export protein Crm1 (Fig. 19.7). Mutation of this tyrosine residue to alanine essentially traps Nrf2 within the nucleus. Studies using siRNA further identified the Fyn kinase as the enzyme responsible for Tyr[568] phosphorylation (Fig. 19.7; Jain, Jaiswal 2006).

Within the nucleus, activated Nrf2 heterodimerizes with small Maf proteins; heterodimer binding to specific DNA sequences leads to increased promoter activity and gene transcription of a number of enzymes, including those involved in GSH synthesis, namely GCLc and GCLm (Fig. 19.7). Thus, by controlling the transcriptional expression of GCL, Nrf2 exerts an influence on redox signaling. Interestingly, in several hepatocyte cell lines, Nrf2 is found to be consititutively expressed in the nucleus, indicating the existence of a distinct nuclear Nrf2 pool (Nguyen, Sherratt, Nioi et al. 2005). The control of this nuclear Nrf2 pool appears to be mediated by a transient shuttling of Keap 1 between the cytoplasm and nucleus, which regulates proteosomal degradation of Nrf2 within the nucleus (Fig. 19.7). It is unknown whether a distinct nuclear Nrf2 pool exists in vascular cells.

Tissue oxidative stress and biological importance of Nrf2. Insights into the physiological importance of Nrf2 are largely derived from studies in the Nrf2 null

(Nrf2$^{-/-}$) mouse. The susceptibility of Nrf2$^{-/-}$ mice to butylated hydroxytoluene–induced lung injury is associated with significant decreases in mRNA levels of the cytoprotective enzymes, GCLm, SOD 1, heme oxygenase 1 (HO-1), NAD(P)H:quinine oxidoreductase 1 (NQ01), and catalase (Chan, Kan 1999). Hyperoxic lung injury was also observed to be exacerbated in Nrf2$^{-/-}$ mice concomitant with decreased Nrf2-mediated expression of antioxidant and cytoprotective genes, a finding that was similar to bleomycin-induced pulmonary fibrosis in Nrf2$^{-/-}$ mice (Cho, Jedlicka, Reddy et al. 2002; Cho, Reddy, Yamamoto et al. 2004). At doses that are generally tolerated in WT mice, Nrf2$^{-/-}$ mice are highly sensitive to acetaminophen-induced hepatocellular injury (Enomoto, Itoh, Nagayoshi et al. 2001). A recent finding that GSH supplementation can reverse the decrease in proliferative capacity of type II alveolar cells in Nrf2$^{-/-}$ mice (Reddy, Kleeberger, Cho et al. 2007) is consistent with an antioxidant property associated with Nrf2.

Nrf2 Signaling in Vascular Function and Pathology

It is not until recently that the role of Nrf2 in vascular function and pathology is being better appreciated. While literature evidence remains scanty, prevailing evidence support an anti-inflammatory function for the transcription factor. For instance, the anti-inflammatory effect of laminar blood flow in inhibiting leukocyte adhesion and recruitment is associated with Nrf2-mediated gene expression that is prevented by Nrf2-specific siRNA or overexpression of a dominant negative Nrf2 mutant (Chen, Varner, Rao et al. 2003). Additionally, TNF-α–mediated VCAM-1 expression is inhibited by Nrf2 overexpression (Chen, Varner, Rao et al. 2003). A protective role for Nrf2 in vascular pathologies such as atherosclerosis is evidenced by its anti-inflammatory and antiatherogenic effects. The finding of induction of GCL acitivity and GSH production associated with NO• signaling and atheroprotection (Moellering, Mc Andrew, Patel et al. 1999) is suggestive of enhanced Nrf2 activity. This suggestion is supported by the finding that NO• does, in fact, increase the steady state protein levels of Nrf2 and its nuclear accumulation (Buckley, Marshall, Whorton 2003). In addition, the observation that decreases in aortic GCL mRNA expression and GSH content preceded atherogenesis in ApoE$^{-/-}$ mice (Biswas, Newby, Rahman et al. 2005) further supports an atheroprotective role of Nrf2.

Recent evidence from our laboratory suggests that Nrf2 may play an important protective role in neurovascular degeneration associated with diabetic encephalopathy (Okouchi, Ekshyyan, Maracine et al. 2007). We demonstrated that insulin-Nrf2 signaling

afforded cytoprotection against chronic hyperglycemic stress in human microvascular brain endothelial cells through the upregulation of GCL activity and restoration of cellular GSH levels (Okouchi, Okayama, Alexander et al. 2006). Insulin-induced phosphorylation/activation of Nrf2 was mediated by the PI3K/Akt/mTOR/p70S6K pathway (Fig. 19.6) (Okouchi, Okayama, Alexander et al. 2006). Our results agree with previous findings that PI3K/Akt/mTOR/p70S6K signaling mediates insulin-induced GCLc induction under normoglycemic conditions in hepatocytes (Lu, Ge, Kuhlenkamp et al. 1992; Park, Yu, Cho et al. 2004). Given that insulin receptors are widespread in the brain and that insulin responsiveness is attenuated in the diabetic endothelium, this result has important implications for understanding hyperglycemic challenge and insulin protection in diabetes-associated neurovascular dysfunction. At present, the generality of Nrf2 redox signaling in vascular health and disease is unknown. There is no compelling evidence that Nrf2 is an integral player, directly or indirectly, in the various vascular processes that are responsive to GSH modulation; it can only be speculated that Nrf2 could influence these redox-sensitive vascular processes through its transcriptional control of GSH synthesis.

Redox Activation of Transcription Factors in Vascular Disorders

It is widely accepted that ROS play major roles in the development of diabetic, atherosclerotic, or chronic vascular diseases. ROS promotion of endothelial dysfunction was associated with activation of signaling pathways that enhance transcription factor activation and protein synthesis. Nrf2, NF-κB, and AP-1 are among the better-studied redox-sensitive transcription factors that play important roles in vascular redox signaling and gene expression. The major cellular pathways that induce redox activation of these transcription factors in different vascular diseases are summarized in Tables 19.1 to 19.3 and are discussed in the following sections.

Nrf2. Accumulating evidence show that physiological or pathological ROS and RNS production mediates the activation of different vascular signaling pathways, which results in downstream redox activation of the transcription factor, Nrf2 (Table 19.1). Subsequent Nrf2 nuclear translocation promotes the transcription of ARE-responsive genes that are associated with antioxidant protection in different vascular diseases. At least three major signaling pathways that are associated with endothelial activity and antioxidative and/or antiatherogenic effects are linked to redox activation of Nrf2: (1) activation of the JNK signaling by moderately oxidized LDL augmented

Table 19.1 Cellular Pathways That Induce Redox-Activation of Nrf2 in Different Vascular Diseases

Cellular Pathway	Disease or Disorder	References
MoxLDL/↑JNK/↑Nrf2/↑HO-1 and cellular GSH levels	Atherosclerosis	Anwar et al. 2005
Laminar shear stress/↑ROS-RNS/Keap1 dissociation/ Nrf2 activation/↑ expression of Nrf2-regulated gene		Warabi et al. 2007
ROS/↑p38 MAPK/↑ expression of Nrf2-regulated gene		Chen et al. 2006; Lim et al. 2007
Hyperglycemia/cellular redox imbalance/ actin-Keap1 S-glutathionylation/↑Nrf2 activation	Neurodegenerative disorders in diabetes	Okouchi et al. 2006
Cyclic stretch/↑ROS/EGFR/↑PI3K-Akt/↑Nrf2-ARE mediated transcription	Lung injury and inflammation	Papaiahgari et al. 2007
NO/↑ ERK and p38 MAPK/Keap1 dissociation /↑Nrf2–ARE-driven genes	Vascular homeostasis	Buckley et al. 2003
NO/Keap1 dissociation/ Nrf2 nuclear translocation and ↑ gene expression	Vascular survival during nitrosative stress	Liu et al. 2007
LNO$_2$/Keap1 dissociation/↑Nrf2/ARE-responsive genes	Vascular proliferation	Villacorta et al. 2007

EGFR, epidermal growth factor receptor; ERK, extracellular signal-regulated kinase; HO-1, heme oxygenase 1; JNK, c-Jun N-terminal kinase; Keap1, Kelch-like ECH-associated protein 1; LNO$_2$, nitro-linoleic acids; moxLDL, moderately oxidized LDL; MAPK, mitogen-activated protein kinase; NO, nitric oxide.

Table 19.2 Cellular Pathways That Induce Redox-Activation of NF-κB in Different Vascular Diseases

Cellular Pathway	Disease or Disorder	References
↑ NO/↑ p50 or p65 nitrosylation/↓NF-κB	Reduced vascular inflammation in response to acute injury or laminar shear stress	Marshall, Stamler 2001; Grumbach et al. 2005; Ckless et al. 2007; Mitchell et al. 2007
ONOO$^-$/↓IKKβ phosphorylation/↓NF-κB nuclear translocation	Cardiovascular inflammation	Levrand et al. 2005
Ang II /↑ROS/↑NF-κB	Atherosclerosis	Costanzo et al. 2003; Browatzki et al. 2005
Mito ROS (O$_2^-$)/↑ NF-κB	Vascular aging	Ungvari et al. 2007
↑NADPH oxidase/↑ROS/↑NF-κB	Vascular inflammation	Csiszar et al. 2005
↑ Low shear stress /↑ ROS/↑NF-κB	Atherosclerosis, typically at the level of branching arteries	Mohan et al. 2007

Ang II, angiotensin II; IKK, inhibitory κB kinase; NF-κB, nuclear transcription factor kappa B; NO, nitric oxide; NOS, NO synthase; O$_2^-$, superoxide anion; ONOO$^-$, peroxinitrite; ROS, reactive oxygen species; RNS, reactive nitrogen species.

Nrf2-dependent expression of HO-1 (Anwar, Li, Leake et al. 2005); (2) laminar shear stress induced-ROS and RNS generation via X/XO or NADPH oxidase mediated Keap1 dissociation and Nrf2 activation (Warabi, Takabe, Minami et al. 2007); (3) elevated endothelial ROS-mediated the activation of p38 MAPK and the increase in *Nrf2* gene expression (Chen, Dodd, Thomas et al. 2006; Lim, Lee, Lee et al. 2007). In addition, Nrf2-mediated antioxidant gene transcription was shown to confer protection against oxidative stress in diabetes-associated neuron degeneration wherein hyperglycemia-induced cytosolic/mitochondrial redox imbalance and S-glutathionylation of Keap 1 resulted in Nrf2 activation and upregulation of GSH synthesis (Okouchi, Okayama, Alexander et al. 2006). Moreover, in lung inflammation and injury, cyclic stretch-mediated ROS resulted in EGFR activation and PI3K-Akt signaling that induced Nrf2 activation (Papaiahgari, Yerrapureddy, Hassoun et al. 2007). NO•–mediated signaling and Nrf2 activation have been demonstrated. Adaptive response in vascular homeostasis was conferred by NO• via activated ERK and p38 MAPK signaling pathways that promoted Keap 1 oxidation and Nrf2 nuclear translocation (Buckley, Marshall, Whorton 2003). Induction of antioxidant genes during nitrosative stress in the vasculature promotes vascular survival; for example, endothelial-derived NO• directly induces redox-dependent modification of Keap1, resulting in nuclear translocation of Nrf2 and increased gene

Table 19.3 Cellular Pathways That Result in Redox-Activation of AP-1 in Different Vascular Diseases

Cellular Pathway	Disease or Disorder	References
Glycated albumin/↑NADPH oxidase/↑ROS/ ↑PKB-IKK/JNK activation/↑NF-κB and AP-1	Vascular complication of diabetes	Higai et al. 2006
↑NADPH oxidase/↑ROS/JNK1 and p38 MAPK activation/↑ c-Fos, c-Jun and JunB expression, ↑AP-1 activity	Mitogenesis associated with atherosclerosis, aging, or cancer	Rao et al. 1999
↑ROS-RNS/↑AP-1 activity/↑MMP-2/cardiac remodeling	Response to I/R injury	Alfonso-Jaume et al. 2006
↑I/R-ROS/NF-κB and AP-1 activation/ICAM-1 upregulation/acute inflammation	Acute inflammation in postischemic myocardium	Fan et al. 2002; Toledo-Pereyra et al. 2006
↑NADPH oxidase-mediated ROS/ JNK activation/↑AP-1/ Proliferation	Vascular muscle cell proliferation	Kyaw et al. 2001; Kyaw et al. 2002
NADPH oxidase-mediated ROS/↑AP-1/vessel remodeling	Vascular remodeling	Renault et al. 2005
Ang II/↑NADPH oxidase/↑ROS/JNK and p38 activation/↑AP-1	Pathogenesis of atherosclerosis	Viedt et al. 2000
↑X/XO-driven ROS/JNK-p38 MAPK activation/↑AP-1/ endothelial dysfunction	Chronic vascular disease	Matesanz et al. 2007
GD3/VSMC-mediated ROS production/↓NF-κB and AP-1/change in VSMC response	VSMC phenotypic changes associated with plaque instability in atherosclerosis	Moon et al. 2006

Ang II, angiotensin II; AP-1, activator protein 1; GD3, disialoganglioside; JNK, c-Jun N-terminal kinase; MAPK, mitogen-activated protein kinase; NF-κB, nuclear transcription factor kappa B; PKB, protein kinase B; ROS, reactive oxygen species; VSMC, vascular smooth muscle cells; X/XO, xanthine/xanthine oxidase system.

expression (Liu, Peyton, Ensenat et al. 2007). In addition, the antiproliferative effect of nitroalkenes was shown to occur through S-nitrosylation of Keap1 and increased transcription of Nrf2-responsive genes (Villacorta, Zhang, Garcia-Barrio et al. 2007).

NF-κB. Recent studies revealed that vascular ROS and RNS can mediate NF-κB redox activation through several signaling pathways associated with both anti- and pro-inflammatory effects in different vascular diseases (Table 19.2). For example, eNOS regulates S-nitrosylation of either p50 or p65 subunit of NF-κB that results in decreased inflammatory gene expression (Grumbach, Chen, Mertens et al. 2005; Ckless, van der Vliet, Janssen-Heininger 2007; Mitchell, Morton, Fernhoff et al. 2007). Another anti-inflammatory mechanism mediated by ONOO⁻ involves redox inhibition of NF-κB activation by blocking inhibitory κB (IκB) kinase β (IKKβ) phosphorylation and NF-κB nuclear translocation, which decrease inflammation in cardiovascular diseases (Levrand, Pesse, Feihl et al. 2005). Pro-inflammatory effects of NF-κB redox activation are associated with atherosclerosis, vascular aging, or a shift in vascular phenotype. One mechanism of NF-κB redox activation is promoted by Ang II–mediated ROS that increases expression of pro-inflammatory mediators with proatherogenic effects (Costanzo, Moretti, Burgio et al. 2003; Browatzki, Larsen, Pfeiffer et al. 2005). In vascular aging, mitochondrial-derived $O_2^{\bullet-}$ mediated endothelial NF-κB activation and an increase in inflammatory gene expression that contributed to pro-inflammatory phenotypic alterations

in the aged vessels (Ungvari, Orosz, Labinskyy et al. 2007). Additionally, TNF-α and vascular high pressure are activators of the NAD(P)H oxidase-ROS signaling pathway that mediates NF-κB induction in vascular inflammation and atherosclerosis (Csiszar, Smith, Koller et al. 2005). More recently, Mohan et al. (2007) demonstrated that low shear stress associated with atheroslerosis selectively enhances ROS production that results in NF-κB activation.

AP-1. AP-1 is an important endothelial transcription factor that responds to redox changes in association with different vascular diseases (Table 19.3). Increases in DNA synthesis and vascular proliferation in atherosclerosis, aging, or cancer have been reported to occur through AP-1 activation. Specifically, mitogenesis as mediated by NAPDH oxidase–derived ROS involves activation of JNK and p38 MAPK signaling that increases expression of c-Fos, c-Jun and JunB, and activity of AP-1 (Rao, Katki, Madamanchi et al. 1999). Studies of Kyaw et al. (2001, 2002) provide additional evidence that induction of VSMC proliferation by ROS occurs through activation of JNK signaling and increased AP-1–DNA binding and activity. Interestingly, in the pathogenesis of atherosclerosis, the same signaling pathway is invoked by Ang II, namely, ROS generation at the level of vascular NADPH oxidase, JNK and p38 MAPK activation, and increased AP-1 activity, in mediating a pro-atherogenic effect in VSMC (Viedt, Soto, Krieger-Brauer et al. 2000). In vascular remodeling, NADPH oxidase–derived ROS can directly promote AP-1 activation in VSMC to upregulate the remodeling associated gene, *osteopontine*

(Renault, Jalvy, Potier et al. 2005). More recently, Matesanz et al. (2007) demonstrated that MAPK (JNK, p38) signaling in AP-1 activation and vascular remodeling can be mediated by ROS produced by the X/XO system. It is notable that in many instances, AP-1 activation occurs in parallel with activation of NF-κB. For instance, in vascular complication of diabetes, glycated albumin–induced ROS production via NADPH oxidase resulted in downstream nuclear translocation of AP-1 and NF-κB through PKB-IKK and JNK signaling (Higai, Shimamura, Matsumoto 2006). Suppression of AP-1 and NF-κB transcription resulted in VSMC phenotypic changes associated with plaque instability in atherosclerosis due to disialoganglioside (GD3)-mediated ROS production (Moon, Kang, Kim 2006). In other studies, I/R-induced vascular ROS generation promoted AP-1 and NF-κB activation that resulted in ICAM-1 upregulation and subsequent polymorphonuclear neutrophil (PMN) accumulation (Fan, Sun, Gu et al. 2002; Toledo-Pereyra, Lopez-Neblina, Lentsch et al. 2006). However, complication of I/R injury induced by endothelial-derived ROS and ONOO$^-$ was mediated by increased synthesis of FosB and JunB and AP-1 nuclear translocation (Alfonso-Jaume, Bergman, Mahimkar et al. 2006).

VASCULAR OXIDATIVE STRESS AND VASCULAR PATHOLOGY

Oxidative Stress–Associated Vascular Diseases

Among the better-studied examples of chronic vascular pathologies that involve endothelial oxidative stress and dysfunction are hypertension, atherosclerosis, and diabetes. In these disorders, oxidative stress–associated inflammation and angiogenesis facilitate the pathological process; in each instance, inhibition of vascular inflammatory and angiogenic complications attenuate disease progression (Aiello, Pierce, Foley et al. 1995; Moulton, Heller, Konerding et al. 1999; Moulton, Vakili, Zurakowski et al. 2003; Joussen, Poulaki, Le et al. 2004; Chidlow, Langston, Greer et al. 2006).

Hypertension. Hypertension is associated with a loss of normal vasodilatory function that results from increased vascular $O_2^{\bullet-}$ production and ONOO$^-$ formation through its reaction with NO$^\bullet$. In humans, hypertension is associated with the actions of the vasoconstrictors, Ang II and endothelin 1 (ET-1), which involve $O_2^{\bullet-}$ generation and NO$^\bullet$ scavenging. Notable enzymatic sources of $O_2^{\bullet-}$ include Nox, eNOS, and XO. Nox-derived $O_2^{\bullet-}$ are generated by a variety of vascular cell types such as leukocytes (Pettit, Wong, Lee et al. 2002), endothelial cells (Landmesser, Cai, Dikalov et al. 2002), VSM (Touyz, Schiffrin 2001),

fibroblasts (Pagano, Clark, Cifuentes-Pagano et al. 1997), and pericytes (Manea, Raicu, Simionescu 2005). In these cells, Ang II has been shown to activate Nox, while Ang II type 1 (AT1) receptor antagonists and Ang II converting enzyme (ACE) inhibitors attenuate Nox-mediated $O_2^{\bullet-}$ production (Williams, Griendling 2007). Though ET-1 also induces Nox activity (Li, Fink, Watts et al. 2003), its action has not been demonstrated in all vascular cell types. XO is present in the endothelium, VSM, macrophages, cardiac and skeletal muscle, and blood, the latter of which represents the most significant source of the enzyme. XO binds to endothelial cells extracellularly and generates $O_2^{\bullet-}$ at the plasma membrane. Enhanced liberation of XO from other tissues can further increase endothelial surface expression of XO and promote $O_2^{\bullet-}$ generation. Given that hypertension induces tissue injury, increased XO activity can perpetuate the hypertensive state once it has developed. In this regard, XO inhibition has been shown to inhibit ROS production and normalize blood pressure in spontaneously hypertensive rats (Suzuki, DeLano, Parks et al. 1998). Uncoupled eNOS during hypertension is another source of $O_2^{\bullet-}$. In mice with DOCA salt–induced hypertension, Landmesser et al. (2003) showed that Nox-derived $O_2^{\bullet-}$ induced eNOS uncoupling through BH4 oxidation; eNOS-induced aortic NO$^\bullet$ levels were restored by BH4 supplementation. Indeed, a significant portion of the vascular $O_2^{\bullet-}$ generated by Ang II and ET-1 has been suggested to originate from uncoupled eNOS via Nox-dependent oxidation of BH4 (Loomis, Sullivan, Osmond et al. 2005; Widder, Guzik, Mueller et al. 2007).

Atherosclerosis. Atherosclerosis is a chronic vascular inflammatory disease that is characterized by arterial vascular wall hardening, fat deposition, and oxidative stress. ROS-induced VSM proliferation and leukocyte recruitment cause plaque formation, vessel wall thickening, and subsequent occlusion of blood flow that result in ischemic tissue injury. It is now generally accepted that the etiology of atherosclerosis lies in a localized endothelial dysfunction, most prominently in areas of turbulent blood flow at vessel bifurcations. Oscillatory sheer stress (which mimics turbulent flow) activates endothelial Nox and promotes $O_2^{\bullet-}$ formation (De Keulenaer, Chappell, Ishizaka et al. 1998), thus, causing a preferential localization of endothelial oxidative stress at points of aortic and arterial branching. Accordingly, atherosclerotic plaque formation as driven by endothelial oxidative stress and increased serum lipid load promotes fatty streak deposition preferentially at vessel bifurcations in mouse models of atherosclerosis. Key among the many sources of ROS in atherosclerosis is leukocytes. During oxidative stress, increased endothelial surface expression of adhesion molecules (E-selectin,

ICAM-1 and VCAM-1) serve to tether circulating leukocytes to the endothelium which increased $O_2^{\bullet-}$ and H_2O_2 formation. For instance, endothelial VCAM-1 and ICAM-1 cross-linking respectively stimulates Nox-dependent (Matheny, Deem, Cook-Mills 2000) and XO-dependent $O_2^{\bullet-}$ production (section VII.1). Additional sources of $O_2^{\bullet-}$, H_2O_2, and $NO^{\bullet}$ are derived from infiltrating monocytes, lymphocytes, and macrophages, the latter of which also express myeloperoxidase (MPO) and produces hypochlorous acid (HOCl) with pro-atherogenic properties.

Other oxidants, such as oxidized low-density lipoproteins (ox-LDLs) have been implicated in plaque formation and development. Ox-LDLs can induce NF-κB–dependent expression of endothelial adhesion molecules, increase formation of monocyte chemoattractant protein 1 (MCP-1) and macrophage colony-stimulating factor (M-CSF) (Halliwell 1999), and promote apoptosis of macrophage and VSM, which advances atherosclerotic lesion formation. Ox-LDLs are internalized by macrophages and endothelial cells via their respective distinct receptors, the macrophage scavenger receptors (which are also found on VSM), and the endothelial lectin-like oxidized LDL receptors (LOXs). Macrophage uptake of ox-LDLs is responsible for their conversion into foam cells and perpetuation of leukocyte recruitment to the lesion. Binding of ox-LDL to LOX-1 induces Nox4-dependent $O_2^{\bullet-}$ and H_2O_2 production (Thum, Borlak 2004) and activates NF-κB (Matsunaga, Hokari, Koyama et al. 2003). Markedly smaller atherosclerotic lesions are associated with double knockout of the LOX-1/LDL receptors (Mehta, Sanada, Hu et al. 2007). Oxidation of LDLs can occur in a variety of ways: within macrophages (Rosenblat, Coleman, Aviram 2002), mediated by endothelial cells and VSM (Parthasarathy, Steinberg, Witztum, 1992), or chemically modified by MPO-derived HOCl within atherosclerotic lesions. HOCl modified LDLs are taken up by macrophages via class B scavenger receptors and contribute to foam cell formation (Marsche, Zimmermann, Horiuchi et al. 2003). Additional evidence implicates mitochondrial respiration and transition metals as ROS sources (Stocker, Keaney 2004), and a role for 15-lipoxygenase in oxidant-induced atherosclerotic lesions in ApoE$^{-/-}$ and LDLR$^{-/-}$ mouse models of atherosclerosis.

Diabetes Mellitus. Diabetes Mellitus is a major risk factor for the onset of cardiovascular diseases (CVDs), which accounts for 66% of diabetic fatalities. Therefore, the ROS sources that are responsible for hypertension and atherosclerosis are also important contributors to diabetes-associated CVD, namely, Nox, XO, uncoupled eNOS, and the mitochondrial respiratory chain, which represent significant sources of $O_2^{\bullet-}$ and H_2O_2 in the diabetic vascular wall. Other vascular-derived ROS contributors include cyclooxygenase I and II (COXI and II), cytochrome P450 enzymes, thromboxane synthase (TXS), and iNOS. MPO, iNOS, and Nox are important leukocyte sources of ROS in the diabetic vasculature (Spitaler, Graier 2002). Of significance to diabetes is the contribution of hyperglycemia to ROS production in diabetic vessels. Hyperglycemia has been shown to promote endothelial production of $O_2^{\bullet-}$ and H_2O_2 by complex II of the mitochondrial electron transport chain and ROS-mediated activation of PKC and formation of advanced glycation end products (AGEs) in the diabetic endothelium. Moreover, the consumption of NADPH in the conversion of glucose to sorbitol, and of GSH in NADPH regeneration from NADP$^+$ can deplete cellular reductant pools and promote oxidative stress. Accordingly, inhibition of mitochondrial ROS production in hyperglycemic endothelial cells restores normal PKC activity and attenuates AGE generation and glucose to sorbitol conversion. Apart from inducing ROS generation, hyperglycemia also exerts effects on $NO^{\bullet}$ bioavailability and eNOS activity. Although eNOS expression was shown to increase (Cosentino, Hishikawa, Katusic et al. 1997), hyperglycemia is better associated with decreased eNOS activity and endothelial $NO^{\bullet}$ levels (Kimura, Oike, Koyama et al. 2001).

Antioxidants in the Treatment of Vascular Diseases

The involvement of endothelial dysfunction and oxidative stress in hypertension, atherosclerosis, and diabetes has spurred investigations into the therapeutic benefits of antioxidants. Inhibitors of enzymatic sources of ROS, small-molecule antioxidant enzyme mimetics, inhibitors of the renin–angiotensin system, antioxidant vitamins, thiazolidinediones, and statins have all been shown to have beneficial effects against endothelial dysfunction and vascular oxidative stress.

Nox inhibitors. Experimental evidence suggests that Nox inhibition provides a promising therapeutic target for vascular diseases. The 18 amino acid–peptide inhibitor gp91ds-tat, which specifically inhibits the interaction between p47- and gp91phox, has been shown to reduce aortic $O_2^{\bullet-}$ levels and normalize systolic blood pressure in mice when coinfused with Ang II (Rey, Cifuentes, Kiarash et al. 2001). However, its clinical utility at this point is limited due to low bioavailability after oral administration. Several small-molecule Nox inhibitors such as apocynin, S17834, and diphenylene iodonium (DPI) all show promise in animal models. In particular, apocynin was reported to decrease oxidative stress and endothelial dysfunction and blood pressure in various experimental genetic and pharmacological models of hypertension

(Williams, Griendling 2007) and to inhibit ischemia-induced retinopathy in mice, a classical symptom of advanced diabetes (Al-Shabrawey, Bartoli, El-Remessy et al. 2005). However, its therapeutic potential has yet to be tested in humans. S17834, originally identified as a small-molecule inhibitor of TNF-α–induced VCAM-1, ICAM-1, and E-selectin expression, was shown to inhibit aortic $O_2^{\bullet-}$ production and atherosclerotic lesion formation in ApoE$^{-/-}$ mice. DPI was shown to inhibit vascular $O_2^{\bullet-}$ production and reduce systolic blood pressure in DOCA salt, Ang II, and ET-1 infusion models of hypertension (Williams, Griendling 2007), but its lack of specificity for Nox (DPI also inhibits other flavin-containing proteins), makes its clinical efficacy doubtful. The utility of S17834 and DPI in the treatment of human CVD has not been assessed.

Given the role of Nox involvement in atherosclerosis, antihypertensive medications such as ACE inhibitors and Ang II type 1 (AT1) receptor antagonists have shown efficacy in animal models and human studies. For instance, treatment with the AT1 receptor antagonist, telmisartan, decreased vascular $O_2^{\bullet-}$ levels and atherosclerotic lesion size in ApoE$^{-/-}$ mice (Takaya, Kawashima, Shinohara et al. 2006). Similarly, treatment with either ACE inhibitors or AT1 receptor antagonists reduced vascular $O_2^{\bullet-}$ levels (Berry, Anderson, Kirk et al. 2001) and improved endothelial dysfunction (Mancini, Henry, Macaya et al. 1996; Hornig Landmesser, Kohler et al. 2001) in patients with coronary artery disease (CAD), and prevented heart attack and stroke in patients with vascular diseases (Yusuf, Sleight, Pogue et al. 2000). Results from clinical trials also show that AT1 receptor antagonists can improve endothelial function in type 2 diabetics (Cheetham et al. 2000). These observations are consistent with inhibitory drug effects on Ang II–mediated Nox activation; however, other evidence in patients suggests that ACE inhibitors and AT1 receptor antagonists can also increase extracellular SOD activity (Hornig, Landmesser, Kohler et al. 2001).

Other inhibitors of ROS and vascular oxidative stress. *SOD and GPx mimetics* have received considerable attention for their ROS-scavenging abilities. The GPx mimetic and ONOO$^-$ scavenger, ebselen, was shown to alleviate vascular dysfunction in a rat model of type 2 diabetes (Brodsky, Gealekman, Chen et al. 2004; Gealekman, Brodsky, Zhang et al. 2004) and reduce blood pressure in various rodent models of hypertension (Sui, Wang, Wang et al. 2005; Wang, Chabrashvili, Borrego et al. 2006). In clinical trials for the treatment of stroke, ebselen exhibited beneficial effects if given within 24 hours of the ischemic event (Yamaguchi, Sano, Takakura et al. 1998); its therapeutic potential in other cardiovascular-related disorders has not been examined. SOD mimetics such as tempol

show promise in attenuating endothelial dysfunction in animal models (Wang, Chabrashvili, Borrego et al. 2006), but its potential efficacy in humans remains to be tested. *Statins*, which are HMG-CoA reductase inhibitors, exhibit pleiotropic beneficial effects on vascular dysfunction. Apart from inhibition of cholesterol synthesis, statins were shown to attenuate Nox activation in VSM via inhibition of Rac1 geranylgeranylation at the plasma membrane (Negre-Aminou, van Leeuwen, van Thiel et al. 2002; Wassmann, Laufs, Muller et al. 2002). It is probably through this mechanism that statins decrease hypertension and $O_2^{\bullet-}$ production in mice and rats that were independent of their effects on plasma cholesterol levels (Wassmann, Laufs, Baumer et al. 2001). However, results from clinical trials in use of statins for hypertension to date have been mixed (Wierzbicki 2006). Other roles of statins include increased eNOS activity and NO$^{\bullet}$ bioavailability, and as direct antioxidants (Davignon, Jacob, Mason 2004), as in the inhibition of LDL oxidation by simvastatin in a dose-dependent manner in vitro (Girona, La Ville, Sola et al. 1999). Statins are commonly prescribed to diabetics to attenuate the cardiovascular complications of the disease. *Insulin-sensitizing medications* developed for the treatment of diabetes have been shown to possess antioxidant properties. Thiazolidinediones, such as troglitazone and piglitazone, are peroxisome proliferator-activated receptor (PPAR) agonists, and together with the biguanide, metformin can reduce vascular oxidative stress and increase vascular reactivity that is independent of their glycemic lowering effects (Garg, Kumbkarni, Aljada et al. 2000; Mather, Verma, Anderson 2001). Specifically, troglitazone decreases the expression of leukocyte Nox subunits and ROS generation in type 2 diabetics (Aljada, Garg, Ghanim et al. 2001), while metformin increases the expression of SOD in erythrocytes and plasma GSH levels (Fenster, Tsao, Rockson 2003).

An emerging field of redox physiology that could contribute significantly to our future understanding of the relationship between vascular oxidative stress and vascular pathophysiology is the redox state of the plasma. In recent years, Jones (2006a, 2006b) has forwarded the hypothesis that the plasma redox state is a useful measure of oxidative stress in humans based on results from a series of clinical studies that examine, at the systemic level, plasma GSH and/or cysteine redox in relation to oxidative stress associated with aging and chronic disease states. The intriguing proposal that plasma redox states may serve as predictive markers of health and pathology is supported by evidence that plasma GSH and cysteine redox are oxidized in association with age, age-related diseases, and disease risk in smokers and patients with type 2 diabetes (Samiec, Drews-Botsch, Flagg et al. 1998; Moriarty, Shah, Lynn et al. 2003) and by the link between GSH/GSSG redox potential and carotid intima media thickening in early atherosclerosis (Ashfaq, Abramson, Jones et al. 2006). The finding that antioxidants such as vitamin E, vitamin C, and β-carotene can reverse age-associated cysteine oxidation in human plasma (Moriarty-Craige, Adkison, Lynn et al. 2005) further supports a relationship between maintenance of plasma redox homeostasis and human health.

SUMMARY AND PERSPECTIVE

The recent advances in our understanding of vascular redox signaling and homeostasis are likely to present new and exciting avenues and directions for future clinical research. If, for instance, oxidative stress–associated vascular pathologies are, in fact, closely correlated with an oxidized redox state in human plasma, a routine determination of the plasma GSH and/or cysteine redox status could provide a simple and relatively noninvasive clinical assessment of vascular health or disease in the affected patient populations. Moreover, the recent findings that bioactive polyphenols in green tea and/or red wine can reverse endothelial dysfunction and improve vascular activity in animal models (Sarr, Chatoigneau, Martins et al. 2006; Potenza, Marasciulo, Tarquinio et al. 2007) and patients with coronary artery disease (Widlansky, Hamburg, Anter et al. 2007) hold promise for a new class of naturally occurring compounds in antioxidant therapy, despite the mixed successes of current conventional antioxidants such as ascorbate and vitamin E. Finally, since GSH is a potent antioxidant and plays a central role in vascular redox signaling and homeostasis, future interventions that specifically target Nrf2 signaling in the transcriptional regulation of the vascular GSH redox state could prove to be an effective strategy in the therapeutic treatment of a variety of oxidative stress–associated vascular disorders.

ACKNOWLEDGMENT Research in the authour's laboratory was supported by an NIH grant DK44510.

REFERENCES

Abate C, Patel L, Rauscher FJ 3rd, Curran T. 1990. Redox regulation of fos and jun DNA-binding activity in vitro. *Science.* 249(4973):1157–1161.

Adachi T, Pimentel DR, Heibeck T et al. 2004. S-glutathiolation of Ras mediates redox-sensitive signaling by angiotensin II in vascular smooth muscle cells. *J Biol Chem.* 279(28):29857–29862.

Adachi T, Weisbrod RM, Pimentel DR et al. 2004. S-Glutathiolation by peroxynitrite activates SERCA during arterial relaxation by nitric oxide. *Nat Med.* 10(11):1200–1207.

Aiello LP, Pierce EA, Foley ED et al. 1995. Suppression of retinal neovascularization in vivo by inhibition of vascular endothelial growth factor (VEGF) using soluble VEGF-receptor chimeric proteins. *Proc Natl Acad Sci U S A.* 92(23):10457–10461.

Alexander JS, Alexander BC, Eppihimer LA et al. 2000. Inflammatory mediators induce sequestration of VE-cadherin in cultured human endothelial cells. *Inflammation.* 24(2):99–113.

Alfonso-Jaume MA, Bergman MR, Mahimkar R et al. 2006. Cardiac ischemia-reperfusion injury induces matrix metalloproteinase-2 expression through the AP-1 components FosB and JunB. *Am J Physiol Heart Circ Physiol.* 291(4):H1838–H1846.

Aljada A, Garg R, Ghanim H et al. 2001. Nuclear factor-kappaB suppressive and inhibitor-kappaB stimulatory effects of troglitazone in obese patients with type 2 diabetes: evidence of an antiinflammatory action? *J Clin Endocrinol Metab.* 86(7):3250–3256.

Al-Shabrawey M, Bartoli M, El-Remessy AB et al. 2005. Inhibition of NAD(P)H oxidase activity blocks vascular endothelial growth factor overexpression and neovascularization during ischemic retinopathy. *Am J Pathol.* 167(2):599–607.

Anwar AA, Li FY, Leake DS, Ishii T, Mann GE, Siow RC. 2005. Induction of heme oxygenase 1 by moderately oxidized low-density lipoproteins in human vascular smooth muscle cells: role of mitogen-activated protein kinases and Nrf2. *Free Radic Biol Med.* 39(2):227–236.

Ashfaq S, Abramson JL, Jones DP et al. 2006. The relationship between plasma levels of oxidized and reduced thiols and early atherosclerosis in healthy adults. *J Am Col Cardiol.* 47:1005–1011.

Ashino H, Shimamura M, Nakajima H et al. 2003. Novel function of ascorbic acid as an angiostatic factor. *Angiogenesis.* 6(4):259–269.

Aw TY. 1999. Molecular and cellular responses to oxidative stress and changes in oxidation-reduction imbalance in the intestine. *Am J Clin Nutr.* 70(4):557–565.

Aw TY. 2003. Cellular redox: a modulator of intestinal epithelial cell proliferation. *News Physiol Sci.* 18:201–204.

Baeuerle PA. 1998. IkappaB-NF-kappaB structures: at the interface of inflammation control. *Cell.* 95(6):729–731.

Bass R, Ruddock LW, Klappa P, Freedman RB. 2004. A major fraction of endoplasmic reticulum-located glutathione is present as mixed disulfides with protein. *J Biol Chem.* 279(7):5257–5262.

Bellomo G, Palladini G, Vairetti M. 1997. Intranuclear distribution, function and fate of glutathione and glutathione-S-conjugate in living rat hepatocytes studied by fluorescence microscopy. *Microsc Res Tech.* 36(4):243–252.

Berry C, Anderson N, Kirk AJ, Dominiczak AF, McMurray JJ. 2001. Renin angiotensin system inhibition is associated with reduced free radical concentrations in arteries of patients with coronary heart disease. *Heart.* 86(2):217–220.

Biswas S, Chida AS, Rahman I. 2006. Redox modifications of protein-thiols: emerging roles in cell signaling. *Biochem Pharmacol.* 71(5):551–564.

Biswas SK, Newby DE, Rahman I, Megson IL. 2005. Depressed glutathione synthesis precedes oxidative stress and atherogenesis in Apo-E(-/-) mice. *Biochem Biophys Res Commun.* 338(3):1368–1373.

Biteau B, Labarre J, Toledano MB. 2003. ATP-dependent reduction of cysteine-sulphinic acid by S. cerevisiae sulphiredoxin. *Nature.* 425(6961):980–984.

Bloom DA, Jaiswal AK. 2003. Phosphorylation of Nrf2 at Ser40 by protein kinase C in response to antioxidants leads to the release of Nrf2 from INrf2, but is not required for Nrf2 stabilization/accumulation in the nucleus and transcriptional activation of antioxidant response element-mediated NAD(P)H:quinone oxidoreductase-1 gene expression. *J Biol Chem.* 278(45):44675–44682.

Botta D, Shi S, White CC et al. 2006. Acetaminophen-induced liver injury is attenuated in male glutamate-cysteine ligase transgenic mice. *J Biol Chem.* 281(39):28865–28875.

Bozonet SM, Findlay VJ, Day AM, Cameron J, Veal EA, Morgan BA. 2005. Oxidation of a eukaryotic 2-Cys peroxiredoxin is a molecular switch controlling the transcriptional response to increasing levels of hydrogen peroxide. *J Biol Chem.* 280(24):23319–23327.

Bradley JR, Thiru S, Pober JS. 1995. Hydrogen peroxide-induced endothelial retraction is accompanied by a loss of the normal spatial organization of endothelial cell adhesion molecules. *Am J Pathol.* 147(3):627–641.

Brodsky SV, Gealekman O, Chen J et al. 2004. Prevention and reversal of premature endothelial cell senescence and vasculopathy in obesity-induced diabetes by ebselen. *Circ Res.* 94(3):377–384.

Browatzki M, Larsen D, Pfeiffer CA et al. 2005. Angiotensin II stimulates matrix metalloproteinase secretion in human vascular smooth muscle cells via nuclear factor-kappaB and activator protein 1 in a redox-sensitive manner. *J Vasc Res.* 42(5):415–423.

Brueckl C, Kaestle S, Kerem A et al. 2006. Hyperoxia-induced reactive oxygen species formation in pulmonary capillary endothelial cells in situ. *Am J Respir Cell Mol Biol.* 34(4):453–463.

Buckley BJ, Marshall ZM, Whorton AR. et al. 2003. Nitric oxide stimulates Nrf2 nuclear translocation in vascular endothelium. *Biochem Biophys Res Commun.* 307(4):973–979.

Burke TM, Wolin MS. 1987. Hydrogen peroxide elicits pulmonary arterial relaxation and guanylate cyclase activation. *Am J Physiol.* 252(4 Pt 2):H721–H732.

Caselli A, Marzocchini R, Camici G et al. 1998. The inactivation mechanism of low molecular weight phosphotyrosine-protein phosphatase by H2O2. *J Biol Chem.* 273(49):32554–32560.

Chade AR, Bentley MD, Zhu X et al. 2004. Antioxidant intervention prevents renal neovascularization in hypercholesterolemic pigs. *J Am Soc Nephrol.* 15(7):1816–1825.

Chakravarthi S, Jessop CE, Bulleid NJ. 2006. The role of glutathione in disulphide bond formation and endoplasmic-reticulum-generated oxidative stress. *EMBO Rep.* 7(3):271–275.

Chan K, Kan YW. 1999. Nrf2 is essential for protection against acute pulmonary injury in mice. *Proc Natl Acad Sci U S A.* 96(22):12731–12736.

Chang TS, Jeong W, Woo HA, Lee SM, Park S, Rhee SG. 2004. Characterization of mammalian sulfiredoxin

and its reactivation of hyperoxidized peroxiredoxin through reduction of cysteine sulfinic acid in the active site to cysteine. *J Biol Chem.* 279(49):50994–51001.

Cheetham C, Collis J, O'Driscoll G, Stanton K, Taylor R, Green D. 2000. Losartan, an angiotensin type 1 receptor antagonist, improves endothelial function innon-insulin-dependent diabetes. *J Am Coll Cardiol.* 36(5):1461–1466.

Chen J, Delannoy M, Odwin S, He P, Trush MA, Yager JD. 2003. Enhanced mitochondrial gene transcript, ATP, bcl-2 protein levels, and altered glutathione distribution in ethinyl estradiol-treated cultured female rat hepatocytes. *Toxicol Sci.* 75(2):271–278.

Chen XL, Varner SE, Rao AS et al. 2003. Laminar flow induction of antioxidant response element-mediated genes in endothelial cells. A novel anti-inflammatory mechanism. *J Biol Chem.* 278(2):703–711.

Chen XL, Dodd G, Thomas S et al. 2006. Activation of Nrf2/ARE pathway protects endothelial cells from oxidant injury and inhibits inflammatory gene expression. *Am J Physiol Heart Circ Physiol.* 290(5):H1862–H1870.

Chen Z, Lash LH. 1998. Evidence for mitochondrial uptake of glutathione by dicarboxylate and 2-oxoglutarate carriers. *J Pharmacol Exp Ther.* 285(2):608–618.

Chiarugi P, Fiaschi T, Taddei ML et al. 2001. Two vicinal cysteines confer a peculiar redox regulation to low molecular weight protein tyrosine phosphatase in response to platelet-derived growth factor receptor stimulation. *J Biol Chem.* 276(36):33478–33487.

Chiarugi P, Cirri P. 2003. Redox regulation of protein tyrosine phosphatases during receptor tyrosine kinase signal transduction. *Trends Biochem Sci.* 28(9):509–514.

Chiarugi P, Buricchi F. 2007. Protein tyrosine phosphorylation and reversible oxidation: two cross-talking posttranslation modifications. *Antioxid Redox Signal.* 9(1):1–24.

Chidlow JH Jr, Langston W, Greer JJ et al. 2006. Differential angiogenic regulation of experimental colitis. *Am J Pathol.* 169(6):2014–2030.

Cho HY, Jedlicka AE, Reddy SP et al. 2002. Role of NRF2 in protection against hyperoxic lung injury in mice. *Am J Respir Cell Mol Biol.* 26(2):175–182.

Cho HY, Reddy SP, Yamamoto M, Kleeberger SR. 2004. The transcription factor NRF2 protects against pulmonary fibrosis. *FASEB J.* 18(11):1258–1260.

Chu F, Ward NE, O'Brian CA. 2001. Potent inactivation of representative members of each PKC isozyme subfamily and PKD via S-thiolation by the tumor-promotion/progression antagonist glutathione but not by its precursor cysteine. *Carcinogenesis.* 22(8):1221–1229.

Chu F, Koomen JM, Kobayashi R, O'Brian CA. 2005. Identification of an inactivating cysteine switch in protein kinase Cepsilon, a rational target for the design of protein kinase Cepsilon-inhibitory cancer therapeutics. *Cancer Res.* 65(22):10478–10485.

Circu ML, Rodriguez C, Maloney R, Moyer MP, Aw TY. 2008. Contribution of mitochondrial GSH transport to matrix GSH status and colonic epithelial cell apoptosis. *Free Rad Biol Med.* 44(5):768–778.

Ckless K, van der Vliet A, Janssen-Heininger Y. 2007. Oxidative-nitrosative stress and post-translational protein modifications: implications to lung structure-function relations. Arginase modulates NF-kappaB activity via a nitric oxide-dependent mechanism. *Am J Respir Cell Mol Biol.* 36(6):645–653.

Cohen RA, Adachi T. 2006. Nitric-oxide-induced vasodilatation: regulation by physiologic s-glutathiolation and pathologic oxidation of the sarcoplasmic endoplasmic reticulum calcium ATPase. *Trends Cardiovasc Med.* 16(4):109–114.

Colavitti R, Pani G, Bedogni B et al. 2002. Reactive oxygen species as downstream mediators of angiogenic signaling by vascular endothelial growth factor receptor-2/KDR. *J Biol Chem.* 277(5):3101–3108.

Cosentino F, Hishikawa K, Katusic ZS, Luscher TF. 1997. High glucose increases nitric oxide synthase expression and superoxide anion generation in human aortic endothelial cells. *Circulation.* 96(1):25–28.

Costanzo A, Moretti F, Burgio VL et al. 2003. Endothelial activation by angiotensin II through NFkappaB and p38 pathways: involvement of NFkappaB-inducible kinase (NIK), free oxygen radicals, and selective inhibition by aspirin. *J Cell Physiol.* 195(3):402–410.

Cotgreave IA. 2003. Analytical developments in the assay of intra- and extracellular GSH homeostasis: specific protein S-glutathionylation, cellular GSH and mixed disulphide compartmentalisation and interstitial GSH redox balance. *Biofactors.* 17(1–4):269–277.

Cross AR, Jones OT. 1991. Enzymic mechanisms of superoxide production. *Biochim Biophys Acta.* 1057(3):281–298.

Csiszar A, Smith KE, Koller A, Kaley G, Edwards JG, Ungvari Z. 2005. Regulation of bone morphogenetic protein-2 expression in endothelial cells: role of nuclear factor-kappaB activation by tumor necrosis factor-alpha, H202, and high intravascular pressure. *Circulation.* 111(18):2364–2372.

Dalle-Donne I, Rossi R, Giustarini D, Colombo R, Milzani A. 2007. S-glutathionylation in protein redox regulation. *Free Radic Biol Med.* 43(6):883–898.

Dalton TP, Dieter MZ, Yang Y, Shertzer HG, Nebert DW. 2000. Knockout of the mouse glutamate cysteine ligase catalytic subunit (Gclc) gene: embryonic lethal when homozygous, and proposed model for moderate glutathione deficiency when heterozygous. *Biochem Biophys Res Commun.* 279(2):324–329.

Damdimopoulos AE, Miranda-Vizuete A, Pelto-Huikko M, Gustafsson JA, Spyrou G. 2002. Human mitochondrial thioredoxin. Involvement in mitochondrial membrane potential and cell death. *J Biol Chem.* 277(36):33249–33257.

Datta B, Tufnell-Barrett T, Bleasdale RA et al. 2004. Red blood cell nitric oxide as an endocrine vasoregulator: a potential role in congestive heart failure. *Circulation.* 109(11):1339–1342.

Davignon J, Jacob RF, Mason RP. 2004. The antioxidant effects of statins. *Coron Artery Dis.* 15(5):251–258.

De Keulenaer GW, Chappell DC, Ishizaka N, Nerem RM, Alexander RW, Griendling KK. 1998. Oscillatory and steady laminar shear stress differentially affect human endothelial redox state: role of a superoxide-producing NADH oxidase. *Circ Res.* 82(10):1094–1101.

Del Maestro RF. 1982. Role of superoxide anion radicals in microvascular permeability and leukocyte behaviour. *Can J Physiol Pharmacol.* 60(11):1406–1414.

Droge W. 2002. Free radicals in the physiological control of cell function. *Physiol Rev.* 82(1):47–95.

Ebrahimian TG, Heymes C, You D et al. 2006. NADPH oxidase-derived overproduction of reactive oxygen species impairs postischemic neovascularization in mice with type 1 diabetes. *Am J Pathol.* 169(2):719–728.

Ekshyyan O, Aw TY. 2005. Decreased susceptibility of differentiated PC12 cells to oxidative challenge: relationship to cellular redox and expression of apoptotic protease activator factor-1. *Cell Death Differ.* 12(8):1066–1077.

Ellgaard L, Ruddock LW. 2005. The human protein disulphide isomerase family: substrate interactions and functional properties. *EMBO Rep.* 6(1):28–32.

Ellis EA, Grant MB, Murray FT, et al. 1998. Increased NADH oxidase activity in the retina of the BBZ/Wor diabetic rat. *Free Radic Biol Med.* 24(1):111–120.

Enomoto A, Itoh K, Nagayoshi E et al. 2001. High sensitivity of Nrf2 knockout mice to acetaminophen hepatotoxicity associated with decreased expression of ARE-regulated drug metabolizing enzymes and antioxidant genes. *Toxicol Sci.* 59(1):169–177.

Eu JP, Sun J, Xu L, Stamler JS, Meissner G. 2000. The skeletal muscle calcium release channel: coupled 02 sensor and NO signaling functions. *Cell.* 102(4):499–509.

Fachinger G, Deutsch U, Risau W. 1999. Functional interaction of vascular endothelial-protein-tyrosine phosphatase with the angiopoietin receptor Tie-2. *Oncogene.* 18(43):5948–5953.

Fan H, Sun B, Gu Q, Lafond-Walker A, Cao S, Becker LC. 2002. Oxygen radicals trigger activation of NF-kappaB and AP-1 and upregulation of ICAM-1 in reperfused canine heart. *Am J Physiol Heart Circ Physiol.* 282(5):H1778–H1786.

Fenster BE, Tsao PS, Rockson SG. 2003. Endothelial dysfunction: clinical strategies for treating oxidant stress. *Am Heart J.* 146(2):218–226.

Fernandes AP, Holmgren A. 2004. Glutaredoxins: glutathione-dependent redox enzymes with functions far beyond a simple thioredoxin backup system. *Antioxid Redox Signal.* 6(1):63–74.

Fernandez-Checa JC, Garcia-Ruiz C, Ookhtens M, Kaplowitz N. 1991. Impaired uptake of glutathione by hepatic mitochondria from chronic ethanol-fed rats. Tracer kinetic studies in vitro and in vivo and susceptibility to oxidant stress. *J Clin Invest.* 87(2):397–405.

Findlay VJ, Townsend DM, Morris TE, Fraser JP, He L, Tew KD. 2006. A novel role for human sulfiredoxin in the reversal of glutathionylation. *Cancer Res.* 66(13):6800–6806.

Forstermann U, Closs EI, Pollock JS et al. 1994. Nitric oxide synthase isozymes. Characterization, purification, molecular cloning, and functions. *Hypertension.* 23(6 Pt 2):1121–1131.

Foster MW, Pawloski JR, Singel DJ, Stamler JS. 2005. Role of circulating S-nitrosothiols in control of blood pressure. *Hypertension.* 45(1):15–17.

Frand AR, Kaiser CA. 2000. Two pairs of conserved cysteines are required for the oxidative activity of Er01p in protein disulfide bond formation in the endoplasmic reticulum. *Mol Biol Cell.* 11(9):2833–2843.

Freedman JE, Frei B, Welch GN, Loscalzo J. 1995. Glutathione peroxidase potentiates the inhibition of platelet function by S-nitrosothiols. *J Clin Invest.* 96(1):394–400.

Fujii J, Ikeda Y. 2002. Advances in our understanding of peroxiredoxin, a multifunctional, mammalian redox protein. *Redox Rep.* 7(3):123–130.

Fujii K, Goldman EH, Park HR, Zhang L, Chen J, Fu H. 2004. Negative control of apoptosis signal-regulating kinase 1 through phosphorylation of Ser-1034. *Oncogene.* 23(29):5099–5104.

Fujino G, Noguchi T, Takeda K, Ichijo H. 2006. Thioredoxin and protein kinases in redox signaling. *Semin Cancer Biol.* 16(6):427–435.

Funato Y, Michiue T, Asashima M, Miki H. 2006. The thioredoxin-related redox-regulating protein nucleoredoxin inhibits Wnt-beta-catenin signalling through dishevelled. *Nat Cell Biol.* 8(5):501–508.

Garg R, Kumbkarni Y, Aljada A et al. 2000. Troglitazone reduces reactive oxygen species generation by leukocytes and lipid peroxidation and improves flow-mediated vasodilatation in obese subjects. *Hypertension.* 36(3):430–435.

Gaston BM, Carver J, Doctor A, Palmer LA. 2003. S-nitrosylation signaling in cell biology. *Mol Interv.* 3(5):253–263.

Gealekman O, Brodsky SV, Zhang F et al. 2004. Endothelial dysfunction as a modifier of angiogenic response in Zucker diabetic fat rat: amelioration with Ebselen. *Kidney Int.* 66(6):2337–2347.

Ghezzi P. 2005. Regulation of protein function by glutathionylation. *Free Radic Res.* 39(6):573–580.

Giannoni E, Buricchi F, Raugei G, Ramponi G, Chiarugi P. 2005. Intracellular reactive oxygen species activate Src tyrosine kinase during cell adhesion and anchorage-dependent cell growth. *Mol Cell Biol.* 25(15):6391–6403.

Girona J, La Ville AE, Sola R, Plana N, Masana L. 1999. Simvastatin decreases aldehyde production derived from lipoprotein oxidation. *Am J Cardiol.* 83(6):846–851.

Giustarini D, Milzani A, Aldini G, Carini M, Rossi R, Dalle-Donne I. 2005. S-nitrosation versus S-glutathionylation of protein sulfhydryl groups by S-nitrosoglutathione. *Antioxid Redox Signal.* 7(7–8):930–939.

Gladyshev VN, Liu A, Novoselov SV et al. 2001. Identification and characterization of a new mammalian glutaredoxin (thioltransferase), Grx2. *J Biol Chem.* 276(32):30374–30380.

Gopalakrishna R, Anderson WB. 1989. Ca2+- and phospholipid-independent activation of protein kinase C by selective oxidative modification of the regulatory domain. *Proc Natl Acad Sci U S A.* 86(17):6758–6762.

Gotoh Y, Noda T, Iwakiri R, Fujimoto K, Rhoads CA, Aw TY. 2002. Lipid peroxide-induced redox imbalance differentially mediates CaCo-2 cell proliferation and growth arrest. *Cell Prolif.* 35(4):221–235.

Griendling KK, Sorescu D, Lassegue B, Ushio-Fukai M. 2000. Modulation of protein kinase activity and gene expression by reactive oxygen species and their role in vascular physiology and pathophysiology. *Arterioscler Thromb Vasc Biol.* 20(10):2175–2183.

Grumbach IM, Chen W, Mertens SA, Harrison DG. 2005. A negative feedback mechanism involving nitric oxide and nuclear factor kappa-B modulates endothelial nitric oxide synthase transcription. *J Mol Cell Cardiol.* 39(4):595–603.

Gryglewski RJ, Palmer RM, Moncada S. 1986. Superoxide anion is involved in the breakdown of endothelium-derived vascular relaxing factor. *Nature.* 320(6061):454–456.

Guzy RD, Hoyos B, Robin E et al. 2005. Mitochondrial complex III is required for hypoxia-induced ROS production and cellular oxygen sensing. *Cell Metab.* 1(6):401–408.

Haendeler J, Hoffmann J, Tischler V, Berk BC, Zeiher AM, Dimmeler S. 2002. Redox regulatory and anti-apoptotic functions of thioredoxin depend on S-nitrosylation at cysteine 69. *Nat Cell Biol.* 4(10):743–749.

Hallberg E, Rydstrom J. 1989. Selective oxidation of mitochondrial glutathione in cultured rat adrenal cells and its relation to polycyclic aromatic hydrocarbon-induced cytotoxicity. *Arch Biochem Biophys.* 270(2):662–671.

Halliwell B, Gutterridge JMC. 1999. *Free Radicals in Biology and Medicine.* 3rd ed: New York, NY: Oxford University Press.

Hansen JM, Go YM, Jones DP. 2006. Nuclear and mitochondrial compartmentation of oxidative stress and redox signaling. *Annu Rev Pharmacol Toxicol.* 46:215–234.

Hashemy SI, Johansson C, Berndt C, Lillig CH, Holmgren A. 2007. Oxidation and S-nitrosylation of cysteines in human cytosolic and mitochondrial glutaredoxins: effects on structure and activity. *J Biol Chem.* 282(19):14428–14436.

Hayashi T, Ueno Y, Okamoto T. 1993. Oxidoreductive regulation of nuclear factor kappa B. Involvement of a cellular reducing catalyst thioredoxin. *J Biol Chem.* 268(15):11380–11388.

Higai K, Shimamura A, Matsumoto K. 2006. Amadori-modified glycated albumin predominantly induces E-selectin expression on human umbilical vein endothelial cells through NADPH oxidase activation. *Clin Chim Acta.* 367(1–2):137–143.

Hirota K, Matsui M, Iwata S, Nishiyama A, Mori K, Yodoi J. 1997. AP-1 transcriptional activity is regulated by a direct association between thioredoxin and Ref-1. *Proc Natl Acad Sci U S A.* 94(8):3633–3638.

Hirota K, Murata M, Sachi Y et al. 1999. Distinct roles of thioredoxin in the cytoplasm and in the nucleus. A two-step mechanism of redox regulation of transcription factor NF-kappaB. *J Biol Chem.* 274(39):27891–27897.

Hirota K, Matsui M, Murata M et al. 2000. Nucleoredoxin, glutaredoxin, and thioredoxin differentially regulate NF-kappaB, AP-1, and CREB activation in HEK293 cells. *Biochem Biophys Res Commun.* 274(1):177–182.

Ho YF, Guenthner TM. 1997. Isolation of liver nuclei that retain functional trans-membrane transport. *J Pharmacol Toxicol Methods.* 38(3):163–168.

Hofmann B, Hecht HJ, Flohe L. 2002. Peroxiredoxins. *Biol Chem.* 383(3–4):347–364.

Holmgren A, Johansson C, Berndt C, Lonn ME, Hudemann C, Lillig CH. 2005. Thiol redox control via thioredoxin and glutaredoxin systems. *Biochem Soc Trans.* 33(Pt 6):1375–1377.

Hornig B, Landmesser U, Kohler C et al. 2001. Comparative effect of ace inhibition and angiotensin II type 1 receptor antagonism on bioavailability of nitric oxide in patients with coronary artery disease: role of superoxide dismutase. *Circulation.* 103(6):799–805.

Ichikawa H, Kokura S, Aw TY. 2004. Role of endothelial mitochondria in oxidant production and modulation of neutrophil adherence. *J Vasc Res.* 41:432–444.

Jain AK, Bloom DA, Jaiswal AK. 2005. Nuclear import and export signals in control of Nrf2. *J Biol Chem.* 280(32):29158–29168.

Jain AK, Jaiswal AK. 2006. Phosphorylation of tyrosine 568 controls nuclear export of Nrf2. *J Biol Chem.* 281(17):12132–12142.

Jessop CE, Bulleid NJ. 2004. Glutathione directly reduces an oxidoreductase in the endoplasmic reticulum of mammalian cells. *J Biol Chem.* 279(53):55341–55347.

Jia L, Bonaventura C, Bonaventura J, Stamler JS. 1996. S-nitrosohaemoglobin: a dynamic activity of blood involved in vascular control. *Nature.* 380(6571):221–226.

Jocelyn PC, Kamminga A. 1974. The non-protein thiol of rat liver mitochondria. *Biochim Biophys Acta.* 343(2):356–362.

Johansson C, Lillig CH, Holmgren A. 2004. Human mitochondrial glutaredoxin reduces S-glutathionylated proteins with high affinity accepting electrons from either glutathione or thioredoxin reductase. *J Biol Chem.* 279(9):7537–7543.

Jones DP. 2006a. Extracellular redox state: refining the definition of oxidative stress in aging. *Rejuvenation Res.* 9:169–181.

Jones DP. 2006b. Redefining oxidative stress. *Antiox Redox Signaling.* 8:1865–1879.

Joussen AM, Poulaki V, Le ML et al. 2004. A central role for inflammation in the pathogenesis of diabetic retinopathy. *FASEB J.* 18(12):1450–1452.

Kamata H, Hirata H. 1999. Redox regulation of cellular signalling. *Cell Signal.* 11(1):1–14.

Karoui H, Hogg N, Frejaville C, Tordo P, Kalyanaraman B. 1996. Characterization of sulfur-centered radical intermediates formed during the oxidation of thiols and sulfite by peroxynitrite. ESR-spin trapping and oxygen uptake studies. *J Biol Chem.* 271(11):6000–6009.

Kevil CG, Oshima T, Alexander B, Coe LL, Alexander JS. 2000. H(2)O(2)-mediated permeability: role of MAPK and occludin. *Am J Physiol Cell Physiol.* 279(1):C21–C30.

Kevil CG, Pruitt H, Kavanagh TJ et al. 2004. Regulation of endothelial glutathione by ICAM-1: implications for inflammation. *FASEB J.* 18(11):1321–1323.

Kharitonov VG, Sundquist AR, Sharma VS. 1995. Kinetics of nitrosation of thiols by nitric oxide in the presence of oxygen. *J Biol Chem.* 270(47):28158–28164.

Kim GW, Kondo T, Noshita N, Chan PH. 2002. Manganese superoxide dismutase deficiency exacerbates cerebral infarction after focal cerebral ischemia/reperfusion in mice: implications for the production and role of superoxide radicals. *Stroke.* 33(3):809–815.

Kimura C, Oike M, Koyama T, Ito Y. 2001. Impairment of endothelial nitric oxide production by acute glucose overload. *Am J Physiol Endocrinol Metab.* 280(1):E171–E178.

Klatt P, Molina EP, De Lacoba MG et al. 1999. Redox regulation of c-Jun DNA binding by reversible S-glutathiolation. *FASEB J.* 13(12):1481–1490.

Klatt P, Molina EP, Lamas S. 1999. Nitric oxide inhibits c-Jun DNA binding by specifically targeted S-glutathionylation. *J Biol Chem.* 274(22):15857–15864.

Knapp LT, Klann E. 2000. Superoxide-induced stimulation of protein kinase C via thiol modification and modulation of zinc content. *J Biol Chem.* 275(31):24136–24145.

Kobayashi A, Kang MI, Watai Y et al. 2006. Oxidative and electrophilic stresses activate Nrf2 through inhibition of ubiquitination activity of Keap1. *Mol Cell Biol.* 26(1):221–229.

Kondo N, Ishii Y, Kwon YW et al. 2004. Redox-sensing release of human thioredoxin from T lymphocytes with negative feedback loops. *J Immunol.* 172(1):442–448.

Kuhlencordt PJ, Rosel E, Gerszten RE et al. 2004. Role of endothelial nitric oxide synthase in endothelial activation: insights from eNOS knockout endothelial cells. *Am J Physiol Cell Physiol.* 286(5):C1195–C1202.

Kyaw M, Yoshizumi M, Tsuchiya K, Kirima K, Tamaki T. 2001. Antioxidants inhibit JNK and p38 MAPK activation but not ERK 1/2 activation by angiotensin II in rat aortic smooth muscle cells. *Hypertens Res.* 24(3):251–261.

Kyaw M, Yoshizumi M, Tsuchiya K et al. 2002. Antioxidants inhibit endothelin-1 (1–31)-induced proliferation of vascular smooth muscle cells via the inhibition of mitogen-activated protein (MAP) kinase and activator protein-1 (AP-1). *Biochem Pharmacol.* 64(10):1521–1531.

Kyriakis JM, Avruch J. 2001. Mammalian mitogen-activated protein kinase signal transduction pathways activated by stress and inflammation. *Physiol Rev.* 81(2):807–869.

Landar A, Darley-Usmar VM. 2007. Evidence for oxygen as the master regulator of the responsiveness of soluble guanylate cyclase and cytochrome c oxidase to nitric oxide. *Biochem J.* 405(2):e3–e4.

Landmesser U, Cai H, Dikalov S et al. 2002. Role of p47(phox) in vascular oxidative stress and hypertension caused by angiotensin II. *Hypertension.* 40(4):511–515.

Landmesser U, Dikalov S, Price SR et al. 2003. Oxidation of tetrahydrobiopterin leads to uncoupling of endothelial cell nitric oxide synthase in hypertension. *J Clin Invest.* 111(8):1201–1219.

Langston W, Chidlow JH Jr, Booth BA et al. 2007. Regulation of endothelial glutathione by ICAM-1 governs VEGF-A-mediated eNOS activity and angiogenesis. *Free Radic Biol Med.* 42(5):720–729.

Lash LH, Putt DA, Xu F, Matherly LH. 2007. Role of rat organic anion transporter 3 (Oat3) in the renal basolateral transport of glutathione. *Chem Biol Interact.* 170(2):124–134.

Lee SR, Yang KS, Kwon J, Lee C, Jeong W, Rhee SG. 2002. Reversible inactivation of the tumor suppressor PTEN by H2O2. *J Biol Chem.* 277(23):20336–20342.

Levrand S, Pesse B, Feihl F et al. 2005. Peroxynitrite is a potent inhibitor of NF-{kappa}B activation triggered by inflammatory stimuli in cardiac and endothelial cell lines. *J Biol Chem.* 280(41):34878–34887.

Li L, Fink GD, Watts SW et al. 2003. Endothelin-1 increases vascular superoxide via endothelin(A)-NADPH oxidase pathway in low-renin hypertension. *Circulation.* 107(7):1053–1058.

Li W, Jain MR, Chen C et al. 2005. Nrf2 possesses a redox-insensitive nuclear export signal overlapping with the leucine zipper motif. *J Biol Chem.* 280(31):28430–28438.

Li W, Yu SW, Kong AN. 2006. Nrf2 possesses a redox-sensitive nuclear exporting signal in the Neh5 transactivation domain. *J Biol Chem.* 281(37):27251–27263.

Liang M, Pietrusz JL. 2007. Thiol-related genes in diabetic complications: a novel protective role for endogenous thioredoxin 2. *Arterioscler Thromb Vasc Biol.* 27(1):77–83.

Lillig CH, Berndt C, Vergnolle O et al. 2005. Characterization of human glutaredoxin 2 as iron-sulfur protein: a possible role as redox sensor. *Proc Natl Acad Sci U S A.* 102(23):8168–8173.

Lillig CH, Holmgren A. 2007. Thioredoxin and related molecules--from biology to health and disease. *Antioxid Redox Signal.* 9(1):25–47.

Lim HJ, Lee KS, Lee S et al. 2007. 15d-PGJ2 stimulates HO-1 expression through p38 MAP kinase and Nrf-2 pathway in rat vascular smooth muscle cells. *Toxicol Appl Pharmacol.* 223(1):20–27.

Liu X, Miller MJ, Joshi MS, Thomas DD, Lancaster JR Jr. 1998. Accelerated reaction of nitric oxide with 02 within the hydrophobic interior of biological membranes. *Proc Natl Acad Sci U S A.* 95(5):2175–2179.

Liu XM, Peyton KJ, Ensenat D et al. 2007. Nitric oxide stimulates heme oxygenase-1 gene transcription via the Nrf2/ARE complex to promote vascular smooth muscle cell survival. *Cardiovasc Res.* 75(2):381–389.

Liu Y, Min W. 2002. Thioredoxin promotes ASK1 ubiquitination and degradation to inhibit ASK1-mediated apoptosis in a redox activity-independent manner. *Circ Res.* 90(12):1259–1266.

Lluis JM, Morales A, Blasco C et al. 2005. Critical role of mitochondrial glutathione in the survival of hepatocytes during hypoxia. *J Biol Chem.* 280(5):3224–3232.

Lluis JM, Buricchi F, Chiarugi P, Morales A, Fernandez-Checa JC. 2007. Dual role of mitochondrial reactive oxygen species in hypoxia signaling: activation of nuclear factor-{kappa}B via c-SRC and oxidant-dependent cell death. *Cancer Res.* 67(15):7368–7377.

Lo SK, Janakidevi K, Lai L, Malik AB. 1993. Hydrogen peroxide-induced increase in endothelial adhesiveness is dependent on ICAM-1 activation. *Am J Physiol.* 264(4 Pt 1):L406–L412.

Loomis ED, Sullivan JC, Osmond DA, Pollock DM, Pollock JS. 2005. Endothelin mediates superoxide production and vasoconstriction through activation of NADPH oxidase and uncoupled nitric-oxide synthase in the rat aorta. *J Pharmacol Exp Ther.* 315(3):1058–1064.

Lu SC, Ge JL, Kuhlenkamp J, Kaplowitz N. 1992. Insulin and glucocorticoid dependence of hepatic gamma-glutamylcysteine synthetase and glutathione synthesis in the rat. Studies in cultured hepatocytes and in vivo. *J Clin Invest.* 90(2):524–532.

Lyles MM, Gilbert HF. 1991. Catalysis of the oxidative folding of ribonuclease A by protein disulfide isomerase: pre-steady-state kinetics and the utilization of the oxidizing equivalents of the isomerase. *Biochemistry.* 30(3):619–625.

Mahadev K, Motoshima H, Wu X et al. 2004. The NAD(P)H oxidase homolog Nox4 modulates insulin-stimulated generation of H202 and plays an integral role in insulin signal transduction. *Mol Cell Biol.* 24(5):1844–1854.

Mallis RJ, Buss JE, Thomas JA. 2001. Oxidative modification of H-ras: S-thiolation and S-nitrosylation of reactive cysteines. *Biochem J.* 355(Pt 1):145–153.

Mallis RJ, Hamann MJ, Zhao W, Zhang T, Hendrich S, Thomas JA. 2002. Irreversible thiol oxidation in carbonic anhydrase III: protection by S-glutathiolation and detection in aging rats. *Biol Chem.* 383(3–4):649–662.

Mancini GB, Henry GC, Macaya C et al. 1996. Angiotensin-converting enzyme inhibition with quinapril improves endothelial vasomotor dysfunction in patients with coronary artery disease. The TREND (Trial on Reversing Endothelial Dysfunction) Study. *Circulation.* 94(3):258–265.

Manea A, Raicu M, Simionescu M. 2005. Expression of functionally phagocyte-type NAD(P)H oxidase in pericytes: effect of angiotensin II and high glucose. *Biol Cell.* 97(9):723–734.

Mannick JB, Schonhoff C, Papeta N et al. 2001. S-Nitrosylation of mitochondrial caspases. *J Cell Biol.* 154(6):1111–1116.

Markovic J, Borras C, Ortega A, Sastre J, Vina J, Pallardo FV. 2007. Glutathione is recruited into the nucleus in early phases of cell proliferation. *J Biol Chem.* 282(28):20416–20424.

Marsche G, Zimmermann R, Horiuchi S, Tandon NN, Sattler W, Malle E. 2003. Class B scavenger receptors CD36 and SR-BI are receptors for hypochlorite-modified low density lipoprotein. *J Biol Chem.* 278(48):47562–47570.

Marshall HE, Stamler JS. 2001. Inhibition of NF-kappa B by S-nitrosylation. *Biochemistry.* 40(6):1688–1693.

Matesanz N, Lafuente N, Azcutia V et al. 2007. Xanthine oxidase-derived extracellular superoxide anions stimulate activator protein 1 activity and hypertrophy in human vascular smooth muscle via c-Jun N-terminal kinase and p38 mitogen-activated protein kinases. *J Hypertens.* 25(3):609–618.

Matheny HE, Deem TL, Cook-Mills JM. 2000. Lymphocyte migration through monolayers of endothelial cell lines involves VCAM-1 signaling via endothelial cell NADPH oxidase. *J Immunol.* 164(12):6550–6559.

Mather KJ, Verma S, Anderson TJ. 2001. Improved endothelial function with metformin in type 2 diabetes mellitus. *J Am Coll Cardiol.* 37(5):1344–1350.

Matsunaga T, Hokari S, Koyama I, Harada T, Komoda T. 2003. NF-kappa B activation in endothelial cells treated with oxidized high-density lipoprotein. *Biochem Biophys Res Commun.* 303(1):313–319.

Matsuo Y, Akiyama N, Nakamura H, Yodoi J, Noda M, Kizaka-Kondoh S. 2001. Identification of a novel thioredoxin-related transmembrane protein. *J Biol Chem.* 276(13):10032–10038.

Matthews JR, Wakasugi N, Virelizier JL, Yodoi J, Hay RT. 1992. Thioredoxin regulates the DNA binding activity of NF-kappa B by reduction of a disulphide bond involving cysteine 62. *Nucleic Acids Res.* 20(15):3821–3830.

Mehta JL, Sanada N, Hu CP et al. 2007. Deletion of LOX-1 reduces atherogenesis in LDLR knockout mice fed high cholesterol diet. *Circ Res.* 100(11):1634–1642.

Meister A, Anderson ME. 1983. Glutathione. *Annu Rev Biochem.* 52:711–60.

Meng TC, Fukada T, Tonks NK. 2002. Reversible oxidation and inactivation of protein tyrosine phosphatases in vivo. *Mol Cell.* 9(2):387–399.

Meng TC, Buckley DA, Galic, Tiganis T, Tonks NK. 2004. Regulation of insulin signaling through reversible oxidation of the protein-tyrosine phosphatases TC45 and PTP1B. *J Biol Chem.* 279(36):37716–37725.

Meuillet EJ, Mahadevan D, Berggren M, Coon A, Powis G. 2004. Thioredoxin-1 binds to the C2 domain of PTEN inhibiting PTEN's lipid phosphatase activity and membrane binding: a mechanism for the functional loss of PTEN's tumor suppressor activity. *Arch Biochem Biophys.* 429(2):123–133.

Minetti M, Mallozzi C, Di Stasi AM. 2002. Peroxynitrite activates kinases of the src family and upregulates tyrosine phosphorylation signaling. *Free Radic Biol Med.* 33(6):744–754.

Mitchell DA, Morton SU, Fernhoff NB, Marletta MA. 2007. Thioredoxin is required for S-nitrosation of procaspase-3 and the inhibition of apoptosis in Jurkat cells. *Proc Natl Acad Sci U S A.* 104(28):11609–11614.

Moellering D, Mc Andrew J, Patel RP et al. 1999. The induction of GSH synthesis by nanomolar concentrations of NO in endothelial cells: a role for gamma-glutamylcysteine synthetase and gamma-glutamyl transpeptidase. *FEBS Lett.* 448(2–3):292–296.

Mohan S, Koyoma K, Thangasamy A, Nakano H, Glickman RD, Mohan N. 2007. Low shear stress preferentially enhances IKK activity through selective sources of ROS for persistent activation of NF-kappaB in endothelial cells. *Am J Physiol Cell Physiol.* 292(1):C362–C371.

Moinova HR, Mulcahy RT. 1998. An electrophile responsive element (EpRE) regulates beta-naphthoflavone induction of the human gamma-glutamylcysteine synthetase regulatory subunit gene. Constitutive expression is mediated by an adjacent AP-1 site. *J Biol Chem.* 273(24):14683–14689.

Moon SK, Kang SK, Kim CH. 2006. Reactive oxygen species mediates disialoganglioside GD3-induced inhibition of ERK1/2 and matrix metalloproteinase-9 expression in vascular smooth muscle cells. *FASEB J.* 20(9):1387–1395.

Moriarty SE, Shah JH, Lynn M et al. 2003. Oxidation of glutathione and cysteine in human plasma associated with smoking. *Free Rad Biol Med.* 35:1582–1588.

Moriarty-Craige SE, Adkison J, Lynn M et al. 2005. Antioxidant supplements prevent oxidation of cysteine/cystine redox in patients with age-related macular degeneration. *Am J Opthalmol.* 140(6):1020–1026.

Morita K, Saitoh M, Tobiume K et al. 2001. Negative feedback regulation of ASK1 by protein phosphatase 5 (PP5) in response to oxidative stress. *EMBO J.* 20(21):6028–6036.

Morris BJ. 1995. Stimulation of immediate early gene expression in striatal neurons by nitric oxide. *J Biol Chem.* 270(42):24740–24744.

Moulton KS, Heller E, Konerding MA, Flynn E, Palinski W, Folkman J. 1999. Angiogenesis inhibitors endostatin or TNP-470 reduce intimal neovascularization and plaque growth in apolipoprotein E-deficient mice. *Circulation.* 99(13):1726–1732.

Moulton KS, Vakili K, Zurakowski D et al. 2003. Inhibition of plaque neovascularization reduces macrophage accumulation and progression of advanced atherosclerosis. *Proc Natl Acad Sci U S A.* 100(8):4736–4741.

Mulcahy RT, Gipp JJ. 1995. Identification of a putative antioxidant response element in the 5'-flanking region of the human gamma-glutamylcysteine synthetase heavy subunit gene. *Biochem Biophys Res Commun.* 209(1):227–233.

Mulcahy RT, Wartman MA, Bailey HH, Gipp JJ. 1997. Constitutive and beta-naphthoflavone-induced expression of the human gamma-glutamylcysteine synthetase heavy subunit gene is regulated by a distal antioxidant response element/TRE sequence. *J Biol Chem.* 272(11):7445–7454.

Muller B, Kleschyov AL, Alencar JL, Vanin A, Stoclet JC. 2002. Nitric oxide transport and storage in the cardiovascular system. *Ann N Y Acad Sci.* 962:131–139.

Nadeau PJ, Charette SJ, Toledano MB, Landry J. 2007. Disulfide bond-mediated multimerization of Ask1 and its reduction by thioredoxin-1 regulate H2O2-induced JNK activation and apoptosis. *Mol Biol Cell.* 18(10):3903–3913.

Nagai H, Noguchi T, Takeda K, Ichijo H. 2007. Pathophysiological roles of ASK1-MAP kinase signaling pathways. *J Biochem Mol Biol.* 40(1):1–6.

Nakamura H. 2005. Thioredoxin and its related molecules: update 2005. *Antioxid Redox Signal.* 7(5–6):823–828.

Nakamura H, Nakamura K, Yodoi J. 1997. Redox regulation of cellular activation. *Annu Rev Immunol.* 15:351–369.

Negre-Aminou P, van Leeuwen RE, van Thiel GC et al. 2002. Differential effect of simvastatin on activation of Rac(1) vs. activation of the heat shock protein 27-mediated pathway upon oxidative stress, in human smooth muscle cells. *Biochem Pharmacol.* 64(10):1483–1491.

Nguyen T, Sherratt PJ, Nioi P, Yang CS, Pickett CB. 2005. Nrf2 controls constitutive and inducible expression of ARE-driven genes through a dynamic pathway involving nucleocytoplasmic shuttling by Keap1. *J Biol Chem.* 280(37):32485–32492.

Nishikawa T, Kukidome D, Sonoda K et al. 2007. Impact of mitochondrial ROS production on diabetic vascular complications. *Diabetes Res Clin Pract.* 77(Suppl 1): 541–545.

Nishitoh H, Saitoh M, Mochida Y et al. 1998. ASK1 is essential for JNK/SAPK activation by TRAF2. *Mol Cell.* 2(3):389–395.

Noda T, Iwakiri R, Fujimoto K, Aw TY. 2001. Induction of mild intracellular redox imbalance inhibits proliferation of CaCo-2 cells. *FASEB J.* 15(12):2131–2139.

Noguchi T, Takeda K, Matsuzawa A et al. 2005. Recruitment of tumor necrosis factor receptor-associated factor family proteins to apoptosis signal-regulating kinase 1 signalosome is essential for oxidative stress-induced cell death. *J Biol Chem.* 280(44):37033–37040.

Nulton-Persson AC, Starke DW, Mieyal JJ, Szweda LI. 2003. Reversible inactivation of alpha-ketoglutarate dehydrogenase in response to alterations in the mitochondrial glutathione status. *Biochemistry.* 42(14):4235–4242.

Ohara Y, Peterson TE, Harrison DG. 1993. Hypercholesterolemia increases endothelial superoxide anion production. *J Clin Invest.* 91(6):2546–2551.

Okouchi M, Okayama N, Aw TY. 2005. Differential susceptibility of naïve and differentiated PC12 cells to methylglyoxal-induced apoptosis: influence of cellular redox. *Curr Neurovasc Res.* 2(1):13–22.

Okouchi M, Okayama N, Alexander JS, Aw TY. 2006. Nrf2-dependent glutamate-L-cysteine ligase catalytic subunit expression mediates insulin protection against hyperglycemia-induced brain endothelial cell apoptosis. *Curr Neurovasc Res.* 3(4):249–261.

Okouchi M, Ekshyyan O, Maracine M, Aw TY. 2007. Neuronal apoptosis in neurodegeneration. *Antiox Redox Signal.* 9(8):1059–1096.

Olafsdottir K, Reed DJ. 1988. Retention of oxidized glutathione by isolated rat liver mitochondria during hydroperoxide treatment. *Biochim Biophys Acta.* 964(3):377–382.

Pacher P, Beckman JS, Liaudet L. 2007. Nitric oxide and peroxynitrite in health and disease. *Physiol Rev.* 87(1):315–424.

Pagano PJ, Clark JK, Cifuentes-Pagano ME et al. 1997. Localization of a constitutively active, phagocyte-like NADPH oxidase in rabbit aortic adventitia: enhancement by angiotensin II. *Proc Natl Acad Sci U S A.* 94(26):14483–14488.

Palmer LA, Gaston B, Johns RA. 2000. Normoxic stabilization of hypoxia-inducible factor-1 expression and activity: redox-dependent effect of nitrogen oxides. *Mol Pharmacol.* 58(6):1197–1203.

Pan S, Berk BC. 2007. Glutathiolation regulates tumor necrosis factor-alpha-induced caspase-3 cleavage and apoptosis: key role for glutaredoxin in the death pathway. *Circ Res.* 100(2):213–219.

Papaiahgari S, Yerrapureddy A, Hassoun PM, Garcia JG, Birukov KG, Reddy SP. 2007. EGFR-activated signaling and actin remodeling regulate cyclic stretch-induced NRF2-ARE activation. *Am J Respir Cell Mol Biol.* 36(3):304–312.

Park HS, Huh SH, Kim MS, Lee SH, Choi EJ. 2000. Nitric oxide negatively regulates c-Jun N-terminal kinase/stress-activated protein kinase by means of S-nitrosylation. *Proc Natl Acad Sci U S A.* 97(26):14382–14387.

Park HS, Yu JW, Cho JH et al. 2004. Inhibition of apoptosis signal-regulating kinase 1 by nitric oxide through a thiol redox mechanism. *J Biol Chem.* 279(9):7584–7590.

Parthasarathy S, Steinberg D, Witztum JL. 1992. The role of oxidized low-density lipoproteins in the pathogenesis of atherosclerosis. *Annu Rev Med.* 43:219–225.

Patel KD, Zimmerman GA, Prescott SM, McEver RP, McIntyre TM. 1991. Oxygen radicals induce human endothelial cells to express GMP-140 and bind neutrophils. *J Cell Biol.* 112(4):749–759.

Pekkari K, Holmgren A. 2004. Truncated thioredoxin: physiological functions and mechanism. *Antioxid Redox Signal.* 6(1):53–61.

Pettit AI, Wong RK, Lee V, Jennings S, Quinn PA, Ng LL. 2002. Increased free radical production in hypertension due to increased expression of the NADPH oxidase subunit p22(phox) in lymphoblast cell lines. *J Hypertens.* 20(4):677–683.

Phalen TJ, Weirather K, Deming PB et al. 2006. Oxidation state governs structural transitions in peroxiredoxin II that correlate with cell cycle arrest and recovery. *J Cell Biol.* 175(5):779–789.

Pias EK, Aw TY. 2002a. Early redox imbalance mediates hydroperoxide-induced apoptosis in mitotic competent undifferentiated cells. *Cell Death Differ.* 9(9):1007–1016.

Pias EK, Aw TY. 2002b. Apoptosis in mitotic competent undifferentiated cells is induced by redox imbalance independently of reactive oxygen species production. *FASEB J.* 16(8):781–790.

Pias EK, Ekshyyan OY, Rhoads CA, Fuseler JW, Harrison L, Aw TY. 2003. Differential effects of superoxide dismutase isoform expression on hydroperoxide-induced apoptosis in PC12 cells. *J Biol Chem.* 278(15):13294–13301.

Pineda-Molina E, Klatt P, Vazquez J et al. 2001. Glutathionylation of the p50 subunit of NF-kappaB: a mechanism for redox-induced inhibition of DNA binding. *Biochemistry.* 40(47):14134–14142.

Poole LB, Karplus PA, Claiborne A. 2004. Protein sulfenic acids in redox signaling. *Annu Rev Pharmacol Toxicol.* 44:325–347.

Potenza MA, Marasciulo FL, Tarquinio M et al. 2007. EGCG, a green tea polyphenol, improves endothelial function and insulin sensitivity, reduces blood pressure, and protects against myocardial I/R injury in SHR. *Am J Physiol Endocrinol Metab.* 292(5):E1378–E1387.

Raines KW, Bonini MG, Campbell SL. 2007. Nitric oxide cell signaling: S-nitrosation of Ras superfamily GTPases. *Cardiovasc Res.* 75(2):229–239.

Rao GN, Katki KA, Madamanchi NR, Wu Y, Birrer MJ. 1999. JunB forms the majority of the AP-1 complex and is a target for redox regulation by receptor tyrosine kinase and G protein-coupled receptor agonists in smooth muscle cells. *J Biol Chem.* 274(9):6003–6010.

Reddy NM, Kleeberger SR, Cho HY et al. 2007. Deficiency in Nrf2-GSH signaling impairs type II cell growth and enhances sensitivity to oxidants. *Am J Respir Cell Mol Biol.* 37(1):3–8.

Renault MA, Jalvy S, Potier M et al. 2005. UTP induces osteopontin expression through a coordinate action of NFkappaB, activator protein-1, and upstream stimulatory factor in arterial smooth muscle cells. *J Biol Chem.* 280(4):2708–2713.

Rey FE, Cifuentes ME, Kiarash A, Quinn MT, Pagano PJ. 2001. Novel competitive inhibitor of NAD(P)H oxidase assembly attenuates vascular O(2)(-) and systolic blood pressure in mice. *Circ Res.* 89(5):408–414.

Reynaert NL, van der Vliet A, Guala AS et al. 2006. Dynamic redox control of NF-kappaB through glutaredoxin-regulated S-glutathionylation of inhibitory kappaB kinase beta. *Proc Natl Acad Sci U S A.* 103(35):13086–13091.

Rhee SG, Chae HZ, Kim K. 2005. Peroxiredoxins: a historical overview and speculative preview of novel mechanisms and emerging concepts in cell signaling. *Free Radic Biol Med.* 38(12):1543–1552.

Rosenblat M, Coleman R, Aviram M. 2002. Increased macrophage glutathione content reduces cell-mediated oxidation of LDL and atherosclerosis in apolipoprotein E-deficient mice. *Atherosclerosis.* 163(1):17–28.

Rubanyi GM, Vanhoutte PM. 1986. Superoxide anions and hyperoxia inactivate endothelium-derived relaxing factor. *Am J Physiol.* 250(5 Pt 2):H822–H827.

Saitoh M, Nishitoh H, Fujii M et al. 1998. Mammalian thioredoxin is a direct inhibitor of apoptosis signal-regulating kinase (ASK) 1. *EMBO J.* 17(9):2596–2606.

Salazar M, Rojo AI, Velasco D, de Sagarra RM, Cuadrado A. 2006. Glycogen synthase kinase-3beta inhibits the xenobiotic and antioxidant cell response by direct phosphorylation and nuclear exclusion of the transcription factor Nrf2. *J Biol Chem.* 281(21):14841–14851.

Salmeen A, Barford D. 2005. Functions and mechanisms of redox regulation of cysteine-based phosphatases. *Antioxid Redox Signal.* 7(5–6):560–577.

Samiec PS, Drews-Botsch C, Flagg EW et al. 1998. Glutathione in human plasma: decline in association with aging, age-related macular degeneration, and diabetes. *Free Rad Biol Med.* 24:699–704.

Sarr M, Lobysheva I, Diallo AS, Stoclet JC, Schini-Kerth VB, Muller B. 2005. Formation of releasable NO stores by S-nitrosoglutathione in arteries exhibiting tolerance to glyceryl-trinitrate. *Eur J Pharmacol.* 513(1–2):119–123.

Sarr M, Chataigneau M, Martins S et al. 2006. Red wine polyphenols prevent angiotensin II-induced hypertension and endothelial dysfunction in rats: role of NADPH oxidase. *Cardiovasc Res.* 71(4):794–802.

Schafer FQ, Buettner GR. 2001. Redox environment of the cell as viewed through the redox state of the glutathione disulfide/glutathione couple. *Free Radic Biol Med.* 30(11):1191–1212.

Schnellmann RG. 1991. Renal mitochondrial glutathione transport. *Life Sci.* 49(5):393–398.

Schwaller M, Wilkinson B, Gilbert HF. 2003. Reduction-reoxidation cycles contribute to catalysis of disulfide isomerization by protein-disulfide isomerase. *J Biol Chem.* 278(9):7154–7159.

Segui J, Gil F, Gironella M et al. 2005. Down-regulation of endothelial adhesion molecules and leukocyte adhesion by treatment with superoxide dismutase is beneficial in chronic immune experimental colitis. *Inflamm Bowel Dis.* 11(10):872–882.

Sekhar KR, Freeman ML. 1999. Autophosphorylation inhibits the activity of gamma-glutamylcysteine synthetase. *J Enzyme Inhib.* 14(4):323–330.

Sellak H, Franzini E, Hakim J, Pasquier C. 1994. Reactive oxygen species rapidly increase endothelial ICAM-1 ability to bind neutrophils without detectable upregulation. *Blood.* 83(9):2669–2677.

Seo JH, Ahn Y, Lee SR, Yeol Yeo C, Chung Hur K. 2005. The major target of the endogenously generated reactive oxygen species in response to insulin stimulation is phosphatase and tensin homolog and not phosphoinositide-3 kinase (PI-3 kinase) in the PI-3 kinase/Akt pathway. *Mol Biol Cell.* 16(1):348–357.

Shelton MD, Chock PB, Mieyal JJ. 2005. Glutaredoxin: role in reversible protein s-glutathionylation and regulation of redox signal transduction and protein translocation. *Antioxid Redox Signal.* 7(3–4):348–366.

Shesely EG, Maeda N, Kim HS et al. 1996. Elevated blood pressures in mice lacking endothelial nitric oxide synthase. *Proc Natl Acad Sci U S A.* 93(23):13176–13181.

Shiva S, Huang Z, Grubina R et al. 2007. Deoxymyoglobin is a nitrite reductase that generates nitric oxide and regulates mitochondrial respiration. *Circ Res.* 100(5):654–661.

Sies H. 1999. Glutathione and its role in cellular functions. *Free Radic Biol Med.* 27(9–10):916–921.

Sies H, Akerboom TP. 1984. Glutathione disulfide (GSSG) efflux from cells and tissues. *Methods Enzymol.* 105:445–451.

Siflinger-Birnboim A, Lum H, Del Vecchio PJ, Malik AB. 1996. Involvement of Ca2+ in the H202-induced increase in endothelial permeability. *Am J Physiol.* 270(6 Pt 1):L973–L978.

Sobey CG, Heistad DD, Faraci FM. 1997. Mechanisms of bradykinin-induced cerebral vasodilatation in rats. Evidence that reactive oxygen species activate K+ channels. *Stroke.* 28(11):2290–2294; discussion 2295.

Soderdahl T, Enoksson M, Lundberg M et al. 2003. Visualization of the compartmentalization of glutathione and protein-glutathione mixed disulfides in cultured cells. *FASEB J.* 17(1):124–126.

Solis WA, Dalton TP, Dieter MZ et al. 2002. Glutamate-cysteine ligase modifier subunit: mouse Gclm gene structure and regulation by agents that cause oxidative stress. *Biochem Pharmacol.* 63(9):1739–1754.

Song JJ, Lee YJ. 2003. Differential role of glutaredoxin and thioredoxin in metabolic oxidative stress-induced activation of apoptosis signal-regulating kinase 1. *Biochem J.* 373(Pt 3):845–853.

Spitaler MM, Graier WF. 2002. Vascular targets of redox signalling in diabetes mellitus. *Diabetologia.* 45(4):476–494.

Stocker R, Keaney JF Jr. 2004. Role of oxidative modifications in atherosclerosis. *Physiol Rev.* 84(4):1381–1478.

Sui H, Wang W, Wang PH, Liu LS. 2005. Effect of glutathione peroxidase mimic ebselen (PZ51) on endothelium and vascular structure of stroke-prone spontaneously hypertensive rats. *Blood Press.* 14(6):366–372.

Sun JD, Ragsdale SS, Benson JM, Henderson RF. 1985. Effects of the long-term depletion of reduced glutathione in mice administered L-buthionine-S, R-sulfoximine. *Fundam Appl Toxicol.* 5(5):913–919.

Sun J, Xin C, Eu JP, Stamler JS, Meissner G. 2001. Cysteine-3635 is responsible for skeletal muscle ryanodine receptor modulation by NO. *Proc Natl Acad Sci U S A.* 98(20):11158–11162.

Sun J, Steenbergen C, Murphy E. 2006. S-nitrosylation: NO-related redox signaling to protect against oxidative stress. *Antioxid Redox Signal.* 8(9–10):1693–1705.

Sun WM, Huang ZZ, Lu SC. 1996. Regulation of gamma-glutamylcysteine synthetase by protein phosphorylation. *Biochem J.* 320(Pt 1):321–328.

Suzuki H, DeLano FA, Parks DA et al. 1998. Xanthine oxidase activity associated with arterial blood pressure in spontaneously hypertensive rats. *Proc Natl Acad Sci U S A.* 95(8):4754–4759.

Tabuchi A, Sano K, Oh E, Tsuchiya T, Tsuda M. 1994. Modulation of AP-1 activity by nitric oxide (NO) in vitro: NO-mediated modulation of AP-1. *FEBS Lett.* 351(1):123–127.

Takaya T, Kawashima S, Shinohara M et al. 2006. Angiotensin II type 1 receptor blocker telmisartan suppresses superoxide production and reduces atherosclerotic lesion formation in apolipoprotein E-deficient mice. *Atherosclerosis.* 186(2):402–410.

Thomas DD, Liu X, Kantrow SP, Lancaster JR Jr. 2001. The biological lifetime of nitric oxide: implications for the perivascular dynamics of NO and 02. *Proc Natl Acad Sci U S A.* 98(1):355–360.

Thomas M, Nicklee T, Hedley DW. 1995. Differential effects of depleting agents on cytoplasmic and nuclear non-protein sulphydryls: a fluorescence image cytometry study. *Br J Cancer.* 72(1):45–50.

Thum T, Borlak J. 2004. Mechanistic role of cytochrome P450 monooxygenases in oxidized low-density lipoprotein-induced vascular injury: therapy through LOX-1 receptor antagonism? *Circ Res.* 94(1):e1–e13.

Toledo-Pereyra LH, Lopez-Neblina F, Lentsch AB, Anaya-Prado R, Romano SJ, Ward PA. 2006. Selectin inhibition modulates NF-kappa B and AP-1 signaling after liver ischemia/reperfusion. *J Invest Surg.* 19(5):313–322.

Tonks NK, Neel BG. 2001. Combinatorial control of the specificity of protein tyrosine phosphatases. *Curr Opin Cell Biol.* 13(2):182–195.

Touyz RM, Schiffrin EL. 2001. Increased generation of superoxide by angiotensin II in smooth muscle cells from resistance arteries of hypertensive patients: role of phospholipase D-dependent NAD(P)H oxidase-sensitive pathways. *J Hypertens.* 19(7):1245–1254.

Tsunada S, Iwakiri R, Noda T, Fujimoto K, Fuseler JW, Aw TY. 2003. Chronic exposure to subtoxic levels of peroxidized lipids suppresses mucosal cell turnover in rat small intestine and the reversal by glutathione. *Dig Dis Sci.* 48(1):210–222.

Tu BP, Weissman JS. 2004. Oxidative protein folding in eukaryotes: mechanisms and consequences. *J Cell Biol.* 164(3):341–346.

Ungvari Z, Orosz Z, Labinskyy N et al. 2007. Increased mitochondrial H_2O_2 production promotes endothelial NF-kappaB activation in aged rat arteries. *Am J Physiol Heart Circ Physiol.* 293(1):H37–H47.

Usatyuk PV, Vepa S, Watkins T, He D, Parinandi NL, Natarajan V. 2003. Redox regulation of reactive oxygen species-induced p38 MAP kinase activation and barrier dysfunction in lung microvascular endothelial cells. *Antioxid Redox Signal.* 5(6):723–730.

Ushio-Fukai M. 2006. Localizing NADPH oxidase-derived ROS. *Sci STKE.* 2006(349):re8.

Ushio-Fukai M, Alexander RW, Akers M et al. 1999. Reactive oxygen species mediate the activation of Akt/protein kinase B by angiotensin II in vascular smooth muscle cells. *J Biol Chem.* 274(32):22699–22704.

Ushio-Fukai M, Tang Y, Fukai T et al. 2002. Novel role of gp91(phox)-containing NAD(P)H oxidase in vascular endothelial growth factor-induced signaling and angiogenesis. *Circ Res.* 91(12):1160–1167.

Vazquez F, Ramaswamy S, Nakamura N, Sellers WR. 2000. Phosphorylation of the PTEN tail regulates protein stability and function. *Mol Cell Biol.* 20(14):5010–5018.

Vazquez F, Grossman SR, Takahashi Y, Rokas MV, Nakamura N, Sellers WR. 2001. Phosphorylation of the PTEN tail acts as an inhibitory switch by preventing its recruitment into a protein complex. *J Biol Chem.* 276(52):48627–48630.

Vepa S, Scribner WM, Natarajan V. 1997. Activation of protein phosphorylation by oxidants in vascular endothelial cells: identification of tyrosine phosphorylation of caveolin. *Free Radic Biol Med.* 22(1–2):25–35.

Viedt C, Soto U, Krieger-Brauer HI et al. 2000. Differential activation of mitogen-activated protein kinases in smooth muscle cells by angiotensin II: involvement of p22phox and reactive oxygen species. *Arterioscler Thromb Vasc Biol.* 20(4):940–948.

Villacorta L, Zhang J, Garcia-Barrio MT et al. 2007. Nitrolinoleic acid inhibits vascular smooth muscle cell proliferation via the Keap1/Nrf2 signaling pathway. *Am J Physiol Heart Circ Physiol.* 293(1):H770–H776.

Wang D, Chabrashvili T, Borrego L, Aslam S, Umans JG. 2006. Angiotensin II infusion alters vascular function in mouse resistance vessels: roles of O and endothelium. *J Vasc Res.* 43(1):109–119.

Wang J, Boja ES, Tan W et al. 2001. Reversible glutathionylation regulates actin polymerization in A431 cells. *J Biol Chem.* 276(51):47763–47766.

Wang Q, Pfeiffer GR 2nd, Gaarde WA. 2003. Activation of SRC tyrosine kinases in response to ICAM-1 ligation in pulmonary microvascular endothelial cells. *J Biol Chem.* 278(48):47731–47743.

Wang TG, Gotoh Y, Jennings MH, Rhoads CA, Aw TY. 2000. Cellular redox imbalance induced by lipid hydroperoxide promotes apoptosis in human colonic CaCo-2 cells. *FASEB J.* 14:1567–1576.

Warabi E, Takabe W, Minami T et al. 2007. Shear stress stabilizes NF-E2-related factor 2 and induces antioxidant genes in endothelial cells: role of reactive oxygen/nitrogen species. *Free Radic Biol Med.* 42(2):260–269.

Wassmann S, Laufs U, Baumer AT et al. 2001. HMG-CoA reductase inhibitors improve endothelial dysfunction in normocholesterolemic hypertension via reduced production of reactive oxygen species. *Hypertension.* 37(6):1450–1457.

Wassmann S, Laufs U, Muller K et al. 2002. Cellular antioxidant effects of atorvastatin in vitro and in vivo. *Arterioscler Thromb Vasc Biol.* 22(2):300–305.

Watson WH, Jones DP. 2003. Oxidation of nuclear thioredoxin during oxidative stress. *FEBS Lett.* 543(1–3):144–147.

Watson WH, Yang X, Choi YE, Jones DP, Kehrer JP. 2004. Thioredoxin and its role in toxicology. *Toxicol Sci.* 78(1):3–14.

Wei EP, Kontos HA, Beckman JS. 1996. Mechanisms of cerebral vasodilation by superoxide, hydrogen peroxide, and peroxynitrite. *Am J Physiol.* 271(3 Pt 2):H1262–H1266.

Wenk J, Brenneisen P, Wlaschek M et al. 1999. Stable overexpression of manganese superoxide dismutase in mitochondria identifies hydrogen peroxide as a major oxidant in the AP-1-mediated induction of matrix-degrading metalloprotease-1. *J Biol Chem.* 274(36):25869–25876.

Widder JD, Guzik TJ, Mueller CF et al. 2007. Role of the multidrug resistance protein-1 in hypertension and vascular dysfunction caused by angiotensin II. *Arterioscler Thromb Vasc Biol.* 27(4):762–768.

Widlansky ME, Hamburg NM, Anter E et al. 2007. Acute EGCG supplementation reverses endothelial dysfunction in patients with coronary artery disease. *J Am Coll Nutr.* 26(2):95–102.

Wierzbicki AS. 2006. Statins and hypertension. *J Hum Hypertens.* 20(8):554–556.

Wild AC, Gipp JJ, Mulcahy T. 1998. Overlapping antioxidant response element and PMA response element sequences mediate basal and beta-naphthoflavone-induced expression of the human gamma-glutamylcysteine synthetase catalytic subunit gene. *Biochem J.* 332(Pt 2):373–381.

Wild AC, Moinova HR, Mulcahy RT. 1999. Regulation of gamma-glutamylcysteine synthetase subunit gene expression by the transcription factor Nrf2. *J Biol Chem.* 274(47):33627–33636.

Williams HC, Griendling KK. 2007. NADPH oxidase inhibitors: new antihypertensive agents? *J Cardiovasc Pharmacol.* 50(1):9–16.

Wingert RA, Galloway JL, Barut B et al. 2005. Deficiency of glutaredoxin 5 reveals Fe-S clusters are required for vertebrate haem synthesis. *Nature.* 436(7053):1035–1039.

Woo HA, Chae HZ, Hwang SC et al. 2003. Reversing the inactivation of peroxiredoxins caused by cysteine sulfinic acid formation. *Science.* 300(5619):653–656.

Woo HA, Jeong W, Chang TS et al. 2005. Reduction of cysteine sulfinic acid by sulfiredoxin is specific to 2-cys peroxiredoxins. *J Biol Chem.* 280(5):3125–3128.

Wood ZA, Schroder E, Robin Harris J, Poole LB. 2003. Structure, mechanism and regulation of peroxiredoxins. *Trends Biochem Sci.* 28(1):32–40.

Xiao R, Lundstrom-Ljung J, Holmgren A, Gilbert HF. 2005. Catalysis of thiol/disulfide exchange. Glutaredoxin 1 and protein-disulfide isomerase use different mechanisms to enhance oxidase and reductase activities. *J Biol Chem.* 280(22):21099–21106.

Yamada Y, Yokota M, Furumichi T, Furui H, Yamauchi K, Saito H. 1990. Protective effects of calcium channel blockers on hydrogen peroxide induced increases in endothelial permeability. *Cardiovasc Res.* 24(12):993–997.

Yamaguchi T, Sano K, Takakura K et al. 1998. Ebselen in acute ischemic stroke: a placebo-controlled, double-blind clinical trial. Ebselen Study Group. *Stroke.* 29(1):12–17.

Yang H, Wang J, Huang ZZ, Ou X, Lu SC. 2001. Cloning and characterization of the 5'-flanking region of the rat glutamate-cysteine ligase catalytic subunit. *Biochem J.* 357(Pt 2):447–455.

Yang H, Wang J, Ou X, Huang ZZ, Lu SC. 2001. Cloning and analysis of the rat glutamate-cysteine ligase modifier subunit promoter. *Biochem Biophys Res Commun.* 285(2):476–482.

Yang H, Zeng Y, Lee TD et al. 2002. Role of AP-1 in the coordinate induction of rat glutamate-cysteine ligase and glutathione synthetase by tert-butylhydroquinone. *J Biol Chem.* 277(38):35232–35239.

Yang H, Magilnick N, Lee C et al. 2005. Nrf1 and Nrf2 regulate rat glutamate-cysteine ligase catalytic subunit transcription indirectly via NF-kappaB and AP-1. *Mol Cell Biol.* 25(14):5933–5946.

Yang Y, Dieter MZ, Chen Y, Shertzer HG, Nebert DW, Dalton TP. 2002. Initial characterization of the glutamate-cysteine ligase modifier subunit Gclm(-/-) knockout mouse. Novel model system for a severely compromised oxidative stress response. *J Biol Chem.* 277(51):49446–49452.

Yasuda M, Ohzeki Y, Shimizu S et al. 1999. Stimulation of in vitro angiogenesis by hydrogen peroxide and the relation with ETS-1 in endothelial cells. *Life Sci.* 64(4):249–258.

Yusuf S, Sleight P, Pogue J, Bosch J, Davies R, Dagenais G. 2000. Effects of an angiotensin-converting-enzyme inhibitor, ramipril, on cardiovascular events in high-risk patients. The Heart Outcomes Prevention Evaluation Study Investigators. *N Engl J Med.* 342(3):145–153.

Zaman K, Palmer LA, Doctor A, Hunt JF, Gaston B. 2004. Concentration-dependent effects of endogenous S-nitrosoglutathione on gene regulation by specificity proteins Sp3 and Sp1. *Biochem J.* 380(Pt 1):67–74.

Zhang H, Go YM, Jones DP. 2007. Mitochondrial thioredoxin-2/peroxiredoxin-3 system functions in parallel with mitochondrial GSH system in protection against oxidative stress. *Arch Biochem Biophys.* 465(1):119–126.

Zhang R, Al-Lamki R, Bai L et al. 2004. Thioredoxin-2 inhibits mitochondria-located ASK1-mediated apoptosis in a JNK-independent manner. *Circ Res.* 94(11):1483–1491.

Zhong L, Arner ES, Holmgren A. 2000. Structure and mechanism of mammalian thioredoxin reductase: the active site is a redox-active selenolthiol/selenenylsulfide formed from the conserved cysteine-selenocysteine sequence. *Proc Natl Acad Sci U S A.* 97(11):5854–5849.

Chapter 20

GENE THERAPY TOWARD CLINICAL APPLICATION IN THE CARDIOVASCULAR FIELD

Hironori Nakagami, Mariana Kiomy Osako, and Ryuichi Morishita

ABSTRACT

Gene therapy is emerging as a potential strategy for the treatment of cardiovascular diseases, such as peripheral arterial disease, ischemic heart disease, restenosis after angioplasty, vascular bypass graft occlusion, and transplant coronary vasculopathy, for which no known effective therapy exists. The strategy of therapeutic angiogenesis was developed more than 10 years ago, and the first human trial in peripheral arterial disease (PAD) was conducted utilizing vascular endothelial growth factor. After that, many different potent angiogenic growth factors have been tested in clinical trials for the treatment of peripheral arterial disease. The results from these clinical trials have exceeded expectations; improvement in the clinical symptoms of PAD and ischemic heart disease has been reported. We identified the potential of hepatocyte growth factor as a powerful angiogenic factor and performed a clinical study for treating PAD. We designed another strategy for combating the disease processes, targeting the transcriptional process, utilizing transfection of cis-element double-stranded oligodeoxynucleotide (ODN), which was named as *decoy*. Transfection of decoy attenuates the authentic cis–trans interaction, leading to removal of trans-factors from the endogenous cis-elements and subsequent modulation of gene expression. We developed decoy for nuclear factor kappa B (NF-κB) that resulted in the inhibition of NF-κB–dependent gene activation including several kind of cytokines, chemokines, and adhesion molecules. In animal experiments, the transfection of NF-κB decoy into coronary artery decreased the infarction size in the ischemic-reperfusion rat myocardial infarction model, and also reduced the neointimal formation after balloon injury of rat carotid artery. Taken together with the results from other animal models, ODN decoy strategy has a great potential in gene therapy for cardiovascular disease.

Keywords: hepatocyte growth factor, angiogenesis, NF-κB, decoy ODN strategy.

HEPATOCYTE GROWTH FACTOR IN CARDIOVASCULAR SYSTEM

Hepatocyte growth factor (HGF) is a mesenchyme-derived pleiotropic factor that regulates growth, motility, and morphogenesis of various types of cells, and is thus considered a humoral mediator of the epithelial–mesenchymal interactions responsible for morphogenic tissue interactions during embryonic development and organogenesis (Nakamura, Nishizawa, Hagiya et al. 1989). Although HGF was originally identified as a potent mitogen for hepatocytes, the mitogenic action of HGF on human ECs was most potent among growth factors (Nakamura, Morishita, Higaki et al. 1996b; Van Belle, Witzenbichler, Chen et al. 1998). Moreover, the presence of a local HGF system (HGF and its specific receptor, c-met) was observed in vascular cells and cardiac myocytes in vitro as well as in vivo (Nakamura, Morishita, Higaki et al. 1995). Production of local HGF in vascular cells is regulated by various cytokines including transforming growth factor (TGF)-β and angiotensin II (Ang II) (Nakano, Moriguchi, Morishita et al. 1997). Interestingly, exogenously expressed HGF also stimulated endogenous HGF expression through induction of ets activity, which plays important roles in regulating gene expression in response to multiple developmental and mitogenic signals. The promoter region of HGF contains a number of putative regulatory elements, such as a B cell- and a macrophage-specific transcription factor–binding site (PU.1/ets), as well as an interleukin-6 response element (IL-6 RE), a TGF-β inhibitory element (TIE), and a cAMP response element (CRE) (Liu, Michalopoulos, Zarnegar 1994). On the other hand, serum HGF concentration was significantly correlated with blood pressure. These results suggest that HGF secretion might be elevated in response to high blood pressure as a countersystem against endothelial dysfunction, and may be considered as an index of severity of hypertension (Nakamura, Morishita, Nakamura et al. 1996a).

Signaling Pathway of HGF in Endothelial Cells

HGF acts as a mitogen, dissociation factor, and motility factor for many epithelial cells in culture through its tyrosine kinase receptor, c-met (Bussolino, Di Renzo, Ziche et al. 1992) (Nakamura, Morishita, Higaki et al. 1996b). Various intracellular signaling pathways have been shown to be activated by tyrosine kinases linked to c-met. As shown in Figure 20.1, the biological responses mediated by c-met are triggered by tyrosine phosphorylation of a single multifunctional docking site located at the carboxy terminal of the receptor tail (Ponzetto, Bardelli, Zhen et al. 1994). This sequence, containing two phosphotyrosines, interacts with several cytoplasmic signal transducers either directly or indirectly through molecular adapters such as Grb2, Shc, and Gab1 (Pelicci, Giordano, Zhen et al. 1995; Weidner, Di Cesare, Sachs et al. 1996). After HGF stimulation, c-met binds and activates phosphatidylinositol-3-OH kinase (PI3K) and recruits the Grb-SOS complex, stimulating the Ras-MAP kinase cascade (Graziani,Gramaglia, Cantley et al. 1991; Graziani,

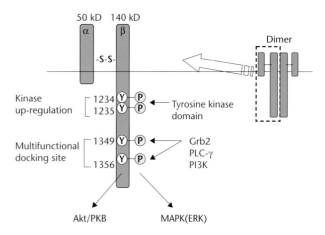

Figure 20.1 Scheme of c-met (HGF receptor) structure. The HGF receptor (c-met) consists of alpha (50 kDa) and beta (140 kDa) chains, which form a heterodimer. The biological responses mediated by c-met are triggered by tyrosine phosphorylation of a single multifunctional docking site located in the carboxy terminal tail of the alpha chain (Ponzetto, Bardelli, Zhen et al. 1994). This sequence, containing two phosphotyrosines, interacts with several cytoplasmic signal transducers either directly or indirectly through molecular adapters such as Grb2, Shc, and Gab1 (Pelicci, Giordano, Zhen et al. 1995; Weidner, Di Cesare, Sachs et al. 1996). After HGF stimulation, c-met binds and activates phosphatidylinositol-3-OH kinase (PI3K) and recruits the Grb-SOS complex, stimulating the Ras-MAP kinase cascade (Graziani, Gramaglia, Cantley et al. 1991; Graziani, Gramaglia, dalla Zonca et al. 1993). In addition, the induction of epithelial tubules by HGF is dependent on activation of the STAT pathway, and importantly, c-met, the HGF tyrosine receptor, can bind and directly phosphorylate STAT3 (Boccaccio, Ando, Tamagnone et al. 1998).

Gramaglia, dalla Zonca et al. 1993). In addition, the induction of epithelial tubules by HGF is dependent on activation of the signal transducer and activator of transcription (STAT) pathway, and importantly, c-met/the HGF tyrosine receptor can bind and directly phosphorylate STAT3 (Boccaccio, Ando, Tamagnone et al. 1998). We also demonstrated that HGF stimulated cell proliferation through the ERK-STAT3 pathway and had an antiapoptotic action through the PI3K-Akt pathway in human aortic ECs (Nakagami, Morishita, Yamamoto et al. 2001). Interestingly, HGF also increases bcl-2 protein, an antiapoptotic gene, and inhibits translocation of bax protein from the cytosol to the mitochondrial membrane, a trigger of apoptosis (Nakagami, Morishita, Yamamoto et al. 2002). It has also been reported that HGF can protect against cell death through inhibition of bad translocation, which is regulated by phosphorylation, and bax translocation, which is regulated by a conformational change resulting in the exposure of its BH3 domain via PI3K (Gilmore, Metcalfe, Romer et al. 2000) (Fig. 20.2).

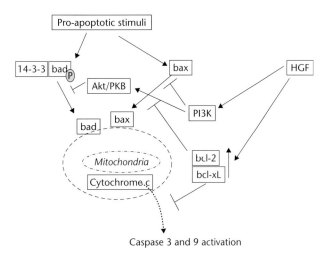

Figure 20.2 Potential mechanisms of antiapoptotic action of HGF. A pro-apoptotic stimulus increases pro-apoptotic genes, such as bax, and also stimulates translocation of bax and/or bad to the mitochondrial heavy membrane. This bad translocation is regulated by binding to 14-3-3 protein through phosphorylation of bad via the PI3K-Akt/PKB pathway (Gilmore, Metcalfe, Romer et al. 2000). Since HGF can activate the PI3K-Akt/PKB pathway and significantly increase bcl-2 and/or bcl-xL protein, it can block the translocation of bax and/or bad (Nakagami, Morishita, Yamamoto et al. 2002). These changes in bax and/or bad protein release cytochrome c from mitochondria, resulting in activation of the caspase cascade. Therefore, HGF can block the release of cytochrome c through both a direct action on mitochondria and blockade of bax and/or bad translocation.

PRECLINICAL STUDY OF ANGIOGENIC THERAPY FOR ISCHEMIC DISEASES

Critical limb ischemia is estimated to develop in 500 to 1000 individuals per million per year. In a large proportion of these patients, the anatomic extent and the distribution of arterial occlusive disease make the patients unsuitable for operative or percutaneous revascularization. Thus, the disease frequently follows an inexorable downhill course (Dormandy, Mahir, Ascady et al. 1989). Of importance, there is no optimal medical therapy for critical limb ischemia, as concluded by the Consensus Document of the European Working Group on Critical Limb Ischemia. Therefore, novel therapeutics are required to treat these patients. Pathophysiology of the disease suggests that in the event of obstruction of a major artery, blood flow to the ischemic tissue is often dependent on collateral vessels. When spontaneous development of collateral vessels is insufficient to allow normal perfusion of the tissue at risk, residual ischemia occurs. Preclinical studies have demonstrated that angiogenic growth factors can stimulate the development of collateral arteries in animal models of peripheral and myocardial ischemia

(Bauters, Asahara, Zheng et al. 1994, 1995), a concept called *therapeutic angiogenesis*. Most of the studies have used vascular endothelial growth factor (VEGF), also known as vascular permeability factor as well as a secreted endothelial cell mitogen. The endothelial cell specificity of VEGF has been considered to be an important advantage for therapeutic angiogenesis, as ECs represent the critical cellular element responsible for new vessel formation. More recently, the efficacy of therapeutic angiogenesis with *VEGF* gene transfer has been reported in human patients with critical limb ischemia (Isner, Pieczek, Schainfeld et al. 1996). Thus, a strategy for therapeutic angiogenesis using angiogenic growth factors should be considered for the treatment of patients with critical limb ischemia (Fig. 20.3).

We have confirmed that intra-arterial administration of recombinant HGF induced angiogenesis in a rabbit hindlimb ischemia model (Morishita, Nakamura, Hayashi et al. 1999), and examined the feasibility of gene therapy using HGF to treat peripheral arterial disease (PAD) rather than recombinant therapy because of its disadvantages. Intramuscular injection of "naked" human HGF plasmid resulted in a significant increase in blood flow as assessed by laser Doppler imaging, accompanied by the detection of human HGF protein and a significant increase in capillary density. Importantly, at 5 weeks after transfection, the degree of angiogenesis induced by transfection of HGF plasmid was significantly greater than that caused by a single injection of recombinant HGF. As a preclinical study of human gene therapy, intramuscular injection of HGF plasmid once on day 10 after surgery produced significant augmentation of collateral vessel development on day 30 in a rabbit hindlimb ischemia model, as assessed by angiography. Serial angiograms revealed progressive linear extension of collateral arteries from the origin stem artery to the distal point of the reconstituted parent vessel in HGF-transfected animals. In addition, a significant increase in blood flow, assessed by a Doppler flow wire and the ratio of blood pressure in the ischemic limb to that in the normal limb, was observed in rabbits transfected with HGF plasmid (Fig. 20.3) (Taniyama, Morishita, Aoki et al. 2001).

It could be assumed that overexpression of angiogenic growth factors may enhance tumor growth. To resolve this issue, we examined the overexpression of HGF in tumor-bearing mice. Tumors on their backs were induced by intradermal inoculation of A431, human epidermoid cancer cells expressing c-met. These mice were intramuscularly injected with human HGF plasmid or control plasmid into the femoral muscle. Human HGF concentration was increased only in the femoral muscle, but not in blood. Although recombinant HGF stimulated the growth of A431 cells

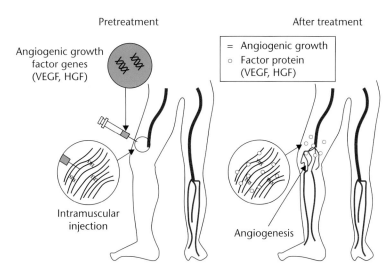

Figure 20.3 The concept of therapeutic angiogenesis by angiogenic growth factor for peripheral arterial diseases. In the pathophysiology of the disease, in the presence of obstruction of a major artery, blood flow to the ischemic tissue is often dependent on collateral vessels. When spontaneous development of collateral vessels is insufficient to allow normal perfusion of the tissue at risk, residual ischemia occurs. Preclinical studies have demonstrated that angiogenic growth factors can stimulate the development of collateral arteries in peripheral arterial diseases, a concept called *therapeutic angiogenesis*. The endothelial cell specificity of VEGF has been considered to be an important advantage for therapeutic angiogenesis, as endothelial cells represent the critical cellular element responsible for new vessel formation. We also identified the therapeutic potential of hepatocyte growth factor (HGF) as a powerful angiogenic growth factor. Thus, a strategy for therapeutic angiogenesis using angiogenic growth factors should be considered for the treatment of patients with critical limb ischemia.

in vitro, temporally and locally, HGF elevation in the hindlimb had no effect on tumor growth in mice (Matsuki, Yamamoto, Nakagami et al. 2004).

CLINICAL TRIAL OF ANGIOGENIC THERAPY FOR ISCHEMIC DISEASES

Therapeutic angiogenesis using angiogenic growth factors is expected to be a new effective treatment for patients with critical limb ischemia. We investigated the safety and efficacy of HGF plasmid DNA in patients with critical limb ischemia in a prospective open-labeled clinical trial (Morishita, Yamamoto, Nakagami et al. 2004). Patients could be enrolled if they (a) had had chronic critical limb ischemia, including rest pain or a nonhealing ischemic ulcer, for a minimum of 4 weeks; (b) had been resistant to conventional drug therapy for at least 4 weeks after hospitalization; (c) were not candidates for surgical or percutaneous revascularization based on usual practice standards; (d) did not have cancer or a history of cancer; and (e) did not have severe unstable retinopathy. Objective documentation of ischemia, including a resting ankle brachial index (ABI) of less that 0.6 in the affected limb on two consecutive examinations performed 1 week apart, was necessary. Patients were observed for 4 weeks under conventional drug therapy to confirm that their clinical symptoms and objective parameters were not improved. The selection criteria

were confirmed by an independent committee for assessment and evaluation of clinical gene therapy at Osaka University, Japan, which was approved by the Ministry of Welfare and the Ministry of Education (Science and Culture).

Intramuscular injection of naked plasmid DNA was performed in the ischemic limbs of six patients with critical limb ischemia with arteriosclerosis obliterans (*n* = 3) or Buerger disease (*n* = 3) graded as Fontaine III or IV. First, a test intramuscular injection of a small dose (0.4 mg plasmid DNA) was performed to examine for acute or subacute allergy to plasmid DNA. After confirming that there is no allergic reaction or anaphylaxis, a therapeutic dose (2 mg) of naked HGF plasmid DNA was intramuscularly injected 2 weeks after the test injection. Four injection sites were selected, according to the angiographic findings and the available muscle mass. Four weeks after the initial injection, a second injection (2 mg) was similarly administered, giving a total dose of 4 mg plasmid DNA per patient.

The primary end points were side effects and improvement of ischemic symptoms at 12 weeks after transfection. For safety evaluation, we focused on the (a) allergic reaction against plasmid DNA, (b) the incidence of angiogenesis-related disease such as tumor, and (c) other severe complications. To identify an allergic reaction, we used a test injection of a small amount of plasmid DNA. However, neither the test nor the initial or second therapeutic injection of human HGF plasmid DNA induced an allergic or anaphylactic reaction. Throughout the gene therapy period, there were no signs of systemic or local inflammatory reactions, and no critical side effects related to gene therapy were seen. To date, no development of tumors or progression of diabetic retinopathy has been observed in any patient transfected with HGF plasmid DNA during the trial. Two-month follow-up studies showed no evidence of development of neoplasm or hemangioma. In addition, no significant increase in serum HGF concentration was observed throughout the gene therapy period. We also measured the plasma level of plasmid HGF DNA. As expected, at 1 week after transfection, plasmid DNA could not be detected in the plasma, whereas at 1 day after transfection, a low level of plasmid DNA could be detected by polymerase chain reaction. Although one patient developed signs of cerebral infarction immediately after angiography during the trial period, the committee determined that this incident was related to the angiography catheter, and there was no relationship with the gene therapy. To date, no change in visual acuity has been observed in any patient treated with plasmid *HGF* gene transfer. It is noteworthy that no edema was observed in this trial, although transient lower-extremity edema was reported with clinical gene therapy using the *VEGF* gene, because of an increase in vascular permeability.

For efficacy evaluation, a reduction of pain scale of more than 1 cm on a visual analog pain scale was observed in five of six patients. An increase in ankle pressure index of more than 0.1 was observed in five of five patients. The long diameter of 8 of 11 ischemic ulcers in four patients was reduced by more than 25%. Thus, intramuscular injection of naked HGF plasmid is safe, feasible, and can achieve successful improvement of ischemic limbs. The efficacy of angiogenesis induction by plasmid DNA was also evaluated, although the patient number was small in this open-labeled trial. Unfortunately, it is difficult to detect distinct angiogenesis because angiography cannot visualize vessels less than 200 μm in diameter. Nevertheless, an improvement in digital subtraction angiography (DSA) findings was shown in two of six treated ischemic limbs. A large vessel was newly observed. Although it is not clear whether this vessel was new or not, it is possible that an increase of new microvessels led to recanalization. This recanalization was also confirmed by serial magnetic resonance angiograms. DSA in another patient with Buerger disease showed a marked increase in peripheral blood flow and formation of new blood vessels. To evaluate the functional improvement by *HGF* gene therapy, we also measured ankle brachial index (ABI) during gene therapy. Although ABI could not be measured in one patient because of uncompressible severely

calcified vessels, ABI was significantly increased from 0.426 ± 0.046 ($n = 5$) at baseline (before administration) to 0.626 ± 0.071 ($P = 0.0155$; $n = 5$) at 4 weeks after the second injection and to 0.596 ± 0.046 ($P = 0.0360$; $n = 5$) at 8 weeks after the second injection. The absolute value of systolic ankle pressure was significantly increased in five limbs after gene transfer, whereas ankle pressures of untreated limbs were not significantly changed. Also, toe pressure index (TPI), which could be measured only in two patients, tended to increase, accompanied by an improvement of ABI. However, TPI was not measured in four patients because of ischemic ulcers on the great toes of their ischemic legs. When an increase in ABI of >0.1 was assumed to be an improvement, according to the standard of Rutherford, five of five patients (100%) showed a positive response. In addition, as transcutaneous Po_2 (T_cPo_2) is an indicator of the effectiveness in terms of angiogenesis and increase in blood supply in targeted ischemic lesions, we also measured $TcPo_2$. The change in $TcPo_2$ after O_2 stimulation was significantly increased at 8 weeks compared with baseline ($P < 0.05$). To evaluate the effects of *HGF* gene therapy on clinical symptoms, we used the change in ischemic ulcers and visual analogue scale. In this trial, a total of 11 ischemic ulcers were found in 4 patients. Two of 11 ulcers completely disappeared. Considering an improvement of ischemic ulcers of more than 25% as positive, 8 of 11 ulcers (72%) improved. Three of four patients demonstrated an improvement of the ischemic ulcer of the longest diameter of $>25\%$ (efficacy rate = 75%). Also, we evaluated resting pain using a visual analog scale, as a standard method for the evaluation of pain, where 0.0 cm means "pain free" or no pain, and 10 cm means most severe pain. Pain was significantly improved in a time-dependent manner.

Although the present data were obtained to demonstrate the safety in a phase I/early phase IIa trial, the initial clinical outcome with *HGF* gene transfer seems to indicate its usefulness as sole therapy for critical limb ischemia. Randomized placebo-controlled clinical trials of alternative dosing regimens of gene therapy will be required to define the efficacy of this therapy.

NEXT 5 YEARS PERSPECTIVE—FUTURE DIRECTION OF "HGF" THERAPY

Here, we introduce a new strategy, therapeutic angiogenesis using cotransfection of the *HGF* and *prostacyclin synthase* genes, as gene therapy for the treatment of patients with critical limb ischemia (Koike, Morishita, Iguchi et al. 2003). The reason we chose prostacyclin synthase was the utility of vasodilator agents such as prostaglandins and phosphodiesterase type III inhibitors to treat human patients with peripheral artery disease. The combination of angiogenesis induced by HGF and vasodilation of newly generated blood vessels induced by prostacyclin would enhance blood flow recovery and maintain new vessel formation. As expected, severe peripheral neuropathy in diabetic animals, characterized by significant slowing of nerve conduction velocity compared with nondiabetic control animals, was ameliorated. Cotransfection of the *prostacyclin synthase* and *HGF* genes was more effective to stimulate angiogenesis than single-gene transfection, and it significantly improved neuropathy. Peripheral neuropathy is common and ultimately accounts for significant morbidity in diabetics. However, there are currently no therapeutic options for patients with diabetic neuropathy. Earlier work using animal models of hind limb ischemia also documented favorable effects of *VEGF* gene transfer on ischemic peripheral neuropathy (Simovic, Isner, Ropper et al. 2001). It is intriguing to note that the neurological and neurophysiological findings in a prospective study of diabetic patients undergoing *phVEGF$_{165}$* gene transfer for critical limb ischemia showed clinical improvement in electrophysiological measurements. Although the model used in the present study was more severe compared with the previous work, cotransfection of the *HGF* and *prostacyclin synthase* genes was able to improve the electrophysiological findings. As HGF has been reported to have direct effects on nerve cells, the results of these experiments do not exclude the possible contribution of direct effects of HGF on nerve integrity. In addition, the therapeutic angiogenesis may have the contribution for this neuronal improvement because neovascularization in ischemic limb can also support the survival of neurons (Fig. 20.3).

HGF also acts as a neurotrophic factor (Ebens, Brose, Leonardo et al. 1996; Korhonen, Sjoholm, Takei et al. 2000). We examined the therapeutic effects of HGF on brain injury in a rat permanent middle cerebral artery occlusion model, because an ideal therapeutic approach to treat ischemia might have both aspects of enhancement of collateral formation and prevention of neuronal death (Shimamura, Sato, Oshima et al. 2004). Gene transfer into the brain was performed by injection of human *HGF* gene into the cerebrospinal fluid via the cisterna magna. Overexpression of the *HGF* gene resulted in a significant decrease in the infarcted brain area as assessed by triphenyltetrazolium chloride staining after 24 hours of ischemia (Fig. 20.4). Consistently, the decrease in neurological deficit was significantly attenuated in rats transfected with the *HGF* gene at 24 hours after the ischemic event. Stimulation of angiogenesis was also detected in rats transfected with the *HGF* gene compared with controls. No cerebral edema or destruction

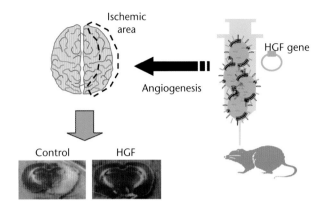

Figure 20.4 Effect of HGF on cerebral infarction model. We examined the therapeutic effects of HGF on brain injury in a rat permanent middle cerebral artery occlusion model, because an ideal therapeutic approach to treat ischemia might have both aspects of enhancement of collateral formation and prevention of neuronal death (Shimamura, Sato, Oshima et al. 2004). Gene transfer into the brain was performed by injection of human *HGF* gene into the cerebrospinal fluid via the cisterna magna. Overexpression of the *HGF* gene resulted in a significant decrease in the infarcted brain area as assessed by triphenyltetrazolium chloride staining after 24 hours of ischemia compared to control group.

of the blood–brain barrier was observed in rats transfected with the *HGF* gene. In particular, the reduction of brain injury by HGF may provide a new therapeutic option to treat cerebrovascular disease.

Gene therapy in the field of cardiovascular disease will be useful for the treatment of many diseases, including peripheral arterial disease, myocardial infarction, restenosis after angioplasty, and rejection in heart transplantation. The first federally approved human gene therapy protocol started on September 14, 1990 for adenosine deaminase deficiency patients, and more than 4000 patients have been treated with gene therapy. Although there are still many unresolved issues in the clinical application of gene therapy, it now appears to be not far from reality and it is time to take a hard look at practical issues that will determine its real clinical potential; for example, (a) further innovations in gene transfer methods, (b) well-defined disease targets, (c) cell-specific targeting strategies, and (d) effective and safe delivery systems.

TRANSCRIPTIONAL FACTOR, NF-κB, AS THERAPEUTIC TARGET UTILIZING "DECOY"

Gene therapy based on oligodeoxynucleotides (ODNs) offers a novel approach for the prevention and treatment of cardiovascular diseases. We focused on the regulation of powerful transcriptional factors, which could be mainly involved in the process of atherosclerosis, myocardial infarction, vascular remodeling, and so on.

Nuclear factor kappa B (NF-κB) is a transcription factor and it was so named because its first identified binding site is located within an enhancer in the *Ig κ light-chain* gene in mature B cells. The functional NF-κB is a homo or heterodimer of homologous proteins that share a common structure motif called *rel domain*. The Rel family in the vertebrate includes five cellular proteins: p50 (NF-κB1), p52 (NF-κB2), p65 (RelA), RelB, and c-Rel. The most common NF-κB consists of a p65:p50 heterodimer.

NF-κB activation is triggered by signal-induced phosphorylation of specific serine residues in the inhibitor κB (IκB) proteins by an enzymatic complex called *IκB kinase (IKK)*, which is activated by tumor necrosis factor receptor (TNFR), T-cell receptor (TCR), or cytokines receptors and involves TNF receptor-activated factor (TRAF) family adapter proteins. The phosphorylation targets the inhibitor for ubiquitination and rapid degradation by proteasome, and as a consequence of the release from IκB, NF-κB translocates into the nucleus and binds to specific sequences in the promoter region, called *κB-sites*, regulating the expression of target genes. The gene expression controlled by NF-κB regulates cell growth and differentiation, inflammatory responses, apoptosis, and neoplastic transformation.

NF-κB is activated by a variety of stimulants: reactive oxygen intermediates; hypoxia; hyperoxia; cytokines; protein kinase C activators; mitogen-activated protein kinase (MAPK) activators; bacterial or viral products, such as lipopolysaccharide (LPS); dsRNA; and UV-radiation.

Owing to the role of NF-κB as a convergent point for the pathways of different stimulants, this transcription factor has a key role in many pathologies, specially the cardiovascular diseases, since it orchestrates the response of EC, myocytes, and vascular smooth muscle cells (VSMC) in face of hypoxia, tissue injury, and inflammation.

Effects of NF-κB Activation in the Cardiovascular System

Myocardial ischemia-reperfusion injury, balloon-injured vessels, vasculopathy in cardiac transplantation, aorta aneurism, and vein bypass graft failure are examples of pathologies extremely difficult to treat because of the lack of effective pharmacological agents. The pathophysiology involved is complex, with numerous cytokines including interleukin (IL)-1, -2, -6, -8 and TNF-α, to name a few, regulating the process. However, NF-κB has been reported to regulate the

signaling pathway of these pro-inflammatory cytokines, and to upregulate their expression in a positive feedback. NF-κB activation also leads to intercellular adhesion molecule (ICAM), vascular cell adhesion molecule (VCAM), and E-selectin expression, which facilitate neutrophils, macrophages, and leukocytes adhesion with subsequent release of cytotoxic molecules. Other important NF-κB–regulated genes expressed in cardiovascular disease are *matrix metalloproteinases* (*MMP*), *cyclooxygenase-2*, and *inducible nitric oxide synthase* (*iNOS*).

The numerous gene products that are regulated by NF-κB coordinate not only the cell response following stress but also the balance between cell survival and cell death; this apparent contradiction can be explained when the molecules upstream of NF-κB activation are considered. TNFR family, for example, has a cytoplasmic domain with structural motifs that function as docking sites for signaling molecules. Signaling from this receptor passes through two principal classes of cytoplasmic adaptor proteins: the death domain (DD) molecules and TRAFs.

DD can bind to other cytoplasmic and adaptor molecules such as TNF receptor–activated death domain (TRADD), and Fas-associated death domain (FADD), which ultimately cause caspase 8 activation and apoptosis. TRAF2 and receptor interacting protein (RIP) can also bind to TRADD, and activate NF-κB–dependent gene expression that eventually may lead to cell survival through the induction of antiapoptotic factors, in particular, the mitochondrial antiapoptotic factor Bcl-2.

Despite its protective role in specific situations, the acute NF-κB activation is responsible for a great part of the pathophysiology of most cardiovascular diseases. Strategies to specifically inhibit NF-κB in a certain organ or tissue and consequent suppression of multiple gene expression have been largely pursued. With the recent progress in molecular biology, new techniques for inhibiting target gene expression have emerged, and in particular, decoy ODN strategy has been reported to successfully target and inhibit NF-κB signaling.

Decoy Oligodeoxynucleotide Strategy

The principle of the transcription factor decoy ODN approach consists in promoter activity reduction as a result of the inhibition of transcription factor binding to its specific sequence in the promoter region (Bielinska, Shivdasani, Zhang et al. 1990). Synthetic double-stranded ODN act as decoy cis-elements that block the binding of nuclear factors to promoter regions of targeted genes, resulting in the inhibition of gene transactivation (Fig. 20.4).

- Gene expression

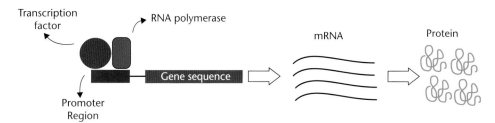

- Gene expression after decoy ODN transfection

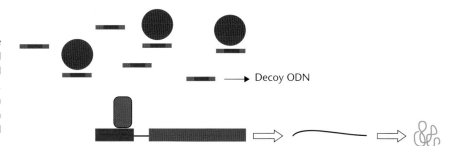

Figure 20.5 Illustrative scheme of decoy ODN concept and strategy. Decoy ODN transfected into the cells act as cis-elements, bind to the target transcription factors, and prevent them from binding to the promoter and activate the gene expression.

The decoy ODN strategy is particularly attractive for several reasons: potential drug targets (transcription factors) are plentiful and readily identifiable; knowledge of the exact molecular structure of the target transcription factor is unnecessary; the synthesis of a sequence-specific decoy is relatively simple and can be targeted to specific tissues.

The therapeutic effectiveness of synthetic double-stranded ODN in modulating specific gene expression largely depends on many factors, including stability, specificity, and efficient cellular and tissue ODN uptake. One of the obstacles to use of the decoy ODN strategy as a pharmaceutical drug is related to its stability in cells and the blood. Since phosphodiester ODNs, the natural type (N-ODN), are precluded because of their instability under physiological conditions, chemical modifications of ODN have been employed to decrease their susceptibility to degradation by exo- and endonucleases (Miller, McParland, Jayaraman et al. 1981; Eckestein 1983).

The first generation of chemical modified decoy is the phosphorothioated ODN (S-ODN), which consists of the replacement of a nonbridging oxygen for sulfur in the phosphate group of the deoxynucleotide backbone (Fig. 20.5). Although their efficacy in inhibiting a large variety of transcription factors has been reported (Morishita, Gibbons, Horiuchi et al. 1995; Morishita, Sugimoto, Aoki et al. 1997; Kume, Komori, Matsumoto et al. 2002), the use of S-ODN has brought other problems such as safety and the cost of production resulting from chemical modification (Gao, Han, Storm et al. 1992; Brown, Kang, Gryaznov et al. 1994;

Burgess, Fisher, Ross et al. 1995; Hosoya, Takeuchi, Kanesaka et al. 1999). One of the major concerns is the nonspecific effect, particularly those attributed to the polyanionic nature of S-ODN. Non–sequence-specific inhibition may operate through blockade of cell surface receptor activity or interference with other proteins (Gibson 1996). The toxicity of phosphorothioate ODN may also be relevant. Although low dosage administration does not seem to cause any toxicity, bolus infusions may be dangerous. High doses over prolonged periods of time may cause kidney damage, as evidenced by proteinuria and leukocytes in urine in animals; liver enzymes may also be increased in animals treated with moderate to high doses. (Henry, Bolte, Auletta et al. 1997a). Several S-ODN have been shown to cause acute hypotensive events in monkeys (Srinivasan, Iversen 1995; Iversen, Cornish, Iversen et al. 1999), probably due to complement activation (Henry, Giclas, Leeds et al. 1997b). More recently, prolongation of prothrombin, partial thromboplastin, and bleeding times has been reported in monkeys (Crooke 1995). Although these effects are transient if managed properly, and are relatively uncommon, this toxicity might be avoided by using a construction that chemically resembles the natural DNA oligomer.

Therefore, to overcome the nonspecific effects caused by chemical modifications, a new construction called *Ribbon-type ODN* was designed. It is a non–chemical-modified decoy ODN with a dumbbell-shaped structure formed by ligation of the extremities of two single phosphodiester strands. Such construction significantly increased the stability of

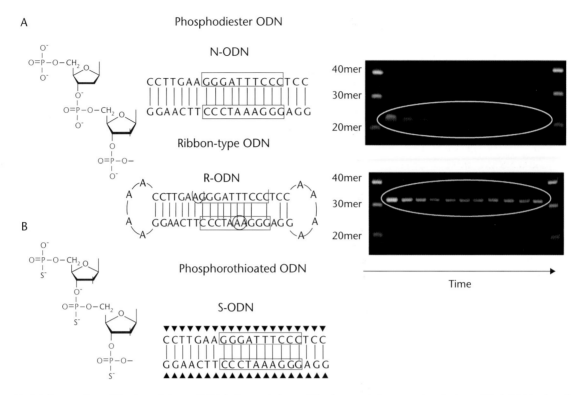

Figure 20.6 Scheme of modification of decoy ODN. Left panel shows (A) scheme of the non–chemical-modified ODN: phosphodiester ODN and ribbon-type ODN, and (B) the phosphorothioated ODN (S-ODN). The NF-kB binding sequence is marked by rectangles. The symbol ▲ in the S-ODN represents the replacement of one nonbridging oxygen by sulfur in the phosphate group. The circles in the R-ODN sequence indicate the nucleotides involved in the ligation reaction. Right panel shows the ODN stability against nucleases: (A) stability test of nonmodified ODN, and (B) ribbon-type ODN after treatment with exonuclease III for 0 to 10 hours at 37°C. ODN were analyzed in 20% denaturing polyacrylamide gel.

the phosphodiester backbone against nucleases compared to N-ODN, and showed to be as efficient as S-ODN in inhibiting the transcription factor NF-κB (Osako, Tomita, Nakagami et al. 2007) (Fig. 20.6). Development and optimization of ODN construction is a growing field, with new constructions emerging fast and with justified expectations for therapeutic applications.

In the next section there are descriptions of successful use of decoy ODN targeting NF-κB in a variety of animal models. Further studies may improve this therapeutic device for using in cardiovascular pathologies.

NF-κB Decoy ODN in Cardiovascular Diseases

Myocardial Infarction

Myocardial reperfusion injury develops mostly as a result of severe damage of myocytes and endothelial cells (ECs), probably induced by the complex interaction of multiple cytokines and adhesion molecules activated by reperfusion. Increased NF-κB binding activity was confirmed in hearts with myocardial

infarction, and transfection of NF-κB decoy ODNs into rat coronary arteries before left anterior descending coronary artery occlusion markedly reduced the damaged area of myocytes 24 hours after reperfusion, whereas no difference was observed between scrambled decoy ODN-treated and untransfected rats. The therapeutic efficacy of this strategy via intracoronary administration immediately after reperfusion, similar to the clinical situation, was also confirmed (Morishita, Sugimoto, Aoki et al. 1997). The selectivity of the NF-κB decoy ODN effect was shown further by the demonstration that reduction of the damaged myocardial area was not observed in rats treated with antisense ODN directed against the rat *iNOS* gene. The specificity of the NF-κB decoy in the inhibition of cytokine and adhesion molecule expression was also confirmed by in vitro experiments using human and rat coronary artery EC. Transfection of NF-κB decoy ODNs markedly inhibited the protein expression of cytokines (IL-6 and IL-8) and adhesion molecules (VCAM, ICAM, and E-selectin) in response to TNF-α stimulation in human aortic EC. In contrast, the control scrambled decoy ODN failed to inhibit the induction of these protein expressions. Cell numbers after transfection were not changed, indicating that the NF-κB decoy induces a specific inhibitory effect rather than nonspecific cytotoxicity.

Vascular Bypass Graft Occlusion

Coronary bypass graft failure is another example of potential application of NF-κB decoy strategy. Autologous vein is commonly used for the surgical treatment of coronary artery disease and peripheral artery disease. Although bypass grafts are highly successful in relieving symptoms in patients with severe ischemic arterial disease, the long-term survival of vein grafts is still a critical problem. Acute vein graft failure is mainly due to thrombosis, and late failure is associated with progressive graft atherosclerosis. Another important process involved is the progression of neointimal hyperplasia. It is mainly caused by endothelial injury and migration and accumulation of blood-derived cells such as macrophages, which express numerous growth factors, cytokines, and proteases regulated by NF-κB activation, ultimately leading to VSMC migration and proliferation from media into intima. In the vein graft of a rabbit hypercholesterolemic model, transfection of NF-κB decoy, but not scrambled ODN, significantly inhibited the migration and accumulation of macrophages in the subendothelial layer, and the VSMC growth by induction of VSMC apoptosis (Miyake, Aoki, Shiraya et al. 2006a). Moreover, there was an inhibition of the transformation of MMP-9 into active MMP-9 and reduced MMP-2 activity, and the transfection of NF-κB decoy ODN resulted in the preservation of acetylcholine-mediated vasorelaxation. Inhibition of NF-κB activity by decoy ODN in vein grafts protected the surviving ECs from hemodynamic stress and ischemic injury at the time of surgery. This study raises the possibility of further studies in clinical situations for prevention of graft failure by decoy ODN targeting NF-κB.

Restenosis after Angioplasty

NF-κB decoy ODN has also been reported as a potential device in the treatment of restenosis after balloon angioplasty. Intimal hyperplasia, as mentioned above, develops largely as a result of VSMC proliferation and migration induced by the complex interaction of multiple growth factors activated by vascular injury. Transfection of NF-κB decoy ODN into balloon-injured rat carotid artery or porcine coronary artery markedly reduced neointimal formation, whereas no difference was observed between scrambled decoy ODN-treated and untransfected blood vessels (Yoshimura, Morishita, Hayashi et al. 2001; Yamasaki, Asai, Shimizu et al. 2003). In addition to VSMC proliferation, endothelial damage also contributes to the

development of restenosis. Interestingly, transfection of NF-κB decoy ODN inhibited EC death, and consequently decreased the vascular inflammation, since EC plays an important role in suppression of VSMC growth, maintenance of vascular tonus, and protection from monocyte and platelet adhesion. On the basis of the therapeutic efficacy of this strategy shown in those animal models, we obtained permission for a second clinical trial using the decoy strategy to treat restenosis from 2002. In this trial, NF-κB decoy ODN was delivered to the vessel wall through a hydrogel-coated catheter without any viral or nonviral vector. Efficient ODN transfection was confirmed with FITC-labeled ODN. The hydrogel-coated catheter was able to deliver the ODN not only to the coronary endothelium but also to the vascular wall (Jun-Ichi ,Hiroshi, Ryo et al. 2004). On the basis of this high transfection efficiency, an efficient NF-κB inhibition and decrease in the restenosis incidence are expected.

Cardiac Transplant Rejection and Vasculopathy

Acute rejection and graft arteriopathy limit the long-term survival of recipients after cardiac transplantation. Acute rejection is enhanced by several cytokines, adhesion molecules, and major histocompatibility complex (MHC) expression, and the arteriopathy is characterized by intimal thickening comprised of proliferative VSMC. NF-κB decoy ODN was infused into donor hearts in a complex with hemmagglutinating virus of Japan (HVJ)-liposome and transplanted into murine recipients. Strikingly, nontreated ($n = 6$; 7.8 ± 0.4 days) or scrambled decoy ($n = 6$; 8.0 ± 0.6 days) transfected allografts were acutely rejected, while NF-κB decoy transfection significantly prolonged allograft survival ($n = 6$; 13.7 ± 2.4 days, $P < 0.05$). In addition, NF-κB decoy not only attenuated myocardial cell infiltration but also inhibited arterial neointimal formation in cardiac allografts (Suzuki, Morishita, Amano et al. 2000).

Abdominal Aorta Aneurism

NF-κB inhibition by decoy ODN has also been reported in rat model for abdominal aorta aneurism (AAA) using a chimeric decoy ODN with binding sites for two transcription factors: NF-κB and ets. Destruction of elastin is considered to be one of the major causes of AAA. Elastic fibers normally maintain the structure of the vascular wall against hemodynamic stress; proteolytic degradation induces remodeling of extracellular matrix, resulting in aneurysmal development and finally rupture. MMP secreted by invasive macrophages, migrating VSMC, and EC play important roles in such mechanisms of AAA. NF-κB regulates the transcription of MMP-1, MMP-2, MMP-3, and MMP-9. Ets family activates the transcription of genes encoding MMP-1, MMP-3, MMP-9 and urokinase plasminogen activator; all are proteases involved in extracellular matrix degradation. Because of the similar roles in MMP expression, use of a chimeric decoy ODN targeting both NF-κB and ets is proposed in the treatment for AAA.

AAA was induced in rats by transient aortic perfusion with elastase, and the decoy ODN was transfected by wrapping a delivery sheet containing the chimeric decoy ODN around the aorta (Miyake, Aoki, Nakashima et al. 2006b). Ultrasound and angiographic analysis demonstrated that treatment with chimeric decoy ODN significantly prevented the progression of elastase-induced aortic dilatation. It was confirmed by histological studies and the progression of AAA was inhibited by the chimeric ODN even 4 weeks after transfection. There were marked inhibition of the elastin proteolysis and suppression of *VCAM-1* and *MCP-1* gene expression, leading to inhibition of macrophage infiltration in the adventitia and decrease of *MMP* gene expression as compared with the scrambled decoy ODN and nontransfected group.

As discussed throughout the examples, NF-κB has a crucial role in the molecular mechanism behind the development of cardiovascular diseases, and decoy ODN has been shown to successfully inhibit the NF-κB transcriptional activity. Together, they show great potential of NF-κB decoy ODN strategy for the treatment of cardiovascular diseases.

PERSPECTIVES FOR DECOY ODN STRATEGY IN CARDIOVASCULAR DISEASES

Recent progress in molecular and cellular biology has led to the development of numerous effective cardiovascular drugs. However, there are still a number of diseases, such as ischemic heart disease, restenosis after angioplasty, vascular bypass graft occlusion, and aorta aneurism, for which no known effective therapy exists. Despite its limitations, gene therapy is emerging as a potential strategy for the treatment of cardiovascular disease, and ODN offers a novel approach for the prevention and treatment of cardiovascular diseases.

Decoy ODN targeting NF-κB, a transcription factor common to pathways involved in the pathophysiologic process, has been reported as a successful strategy in a variety of animal models for cardiovascular diseases, and its application has crossed the barrier to other disease models such as rheumatoid arthritis and glomerular nephritis, eventually reaching the phase II of clinical trial in atopic dermatitis.

However, ODN-based gene therapy still shows some unsolved issues. Further modifications on ODN will facilitate the potential clinical utility of these agents by, for example, (a) increasing its half-life, which will allow a shorter intraluminal incubation time to preserve organ perfusion and prolong the duration of biological action; (b) improving uptake of ODN by a specific target cell using efficient vehicles or innovations in the gene transfer methods, in a way that the nonspecific effects of high doses can be avoided; and (c) improving ODN resistance against nucleases by chemical or structural modifications because the site of decoy ODN effects is at the nucleus, and bypassing the endocytotic pathway and translocation from the cytoplasm are a critical point for the therapeutic efficiency. In the future, ODN-based gene therapy might overcome present limitations to treat unmet cardiovascular diseases.

In summary, it is clearly evident that the gene therapy approach for cardiovascular diseases is experimentally sound, intellectually exciting, and technically feasible and holds promise for the long-term control. Although gene therapy has a great potential in cardiovascular disease, many important issues must first be resolved before this strategy is deemed ready for clinical trials. Some of these issues include the following: (a) the development of a vector system that can regulate transgene expression to match for individual degrees of disease severity and that can switch off transgene expression in case of adverse effects; (b) the discovery and/or general consensus for an ideal gene target for cardiovascular diseases; and (c) the extensive safety evaluation of viral gene delivery systems.

REFERENCES

Bauters C, Asahara T, Zheng LP et al. 1994. Physiological assessment of augmented vascularity induced by VEGF in ischemic rabbit hindlimb. *Am J Physiol.* 267:H1263–1271.

Bauters C, Asahara T, Zheng LP et al. 1995. Site-specific therapeutic angiogenesis after systemic administration of vascular endothelial growth factor. *J Vasc Surg.* 21:314–324; discussion 324–315.

Bielinska A, Shivdasani RA, Zhang LQ, Nabel GJ. 1990. Regulation of gene expression with double-stranded phosphorothioate oligonucleotides. *Science.* 250:997–1000.

Boccaccio C, Ando M, Tamagnone L et al. 1998. Induction of epithelial tubules by growth factor HGF depends on the STAT pathway. *Nature.* 391:285–288.

Brown DA, Kang SH, Gryaznov SM et al. 1994. Effect of phosphorothioate modification of oligodeoxynucleotides on specific protein binding. *J Biol Chem.* 269:26801–26805.

Burgess TL, Fisher EF, Ross SL et al. 1995. The anti-proliferative activity of c-myb and c-myc antisense oligonucleotides in smooth muscle cells is caused by a nonantisense mechanism. *Proc Natl Acad Sci U S A.* 92:4051–4055.

Bussolino F, Di Renzo MF, Ziche M et al. 1992. Hepatocyte growth factor is a potent angiogenic factor which stimulates endothelial cell motility and growth. *J Cell Biol.* 119:629–641.

Crooke ST. 1995. Progress in antisense therapeutics. *Hematol Pathol.* 9:59–72.

Dormandy J, Mahir M, Ascady G et al. 1989. Fate of the patient with chronic leg ischaemia. A review article. *J Cardiovasc Surg.* 30:50–57.

Ebens A, Brose K, Leonardo ED et al. 1996. Hepatocyte growth factor/scatter factor is an axonal chemoattractant and a neurotrophic factor for spinal motor neurons. *Neuron.* 17:1157–1172.

Eckstein F. 1983. Phosphorothioate analogues of nucleotides—Tools for the investigation of biochemical processes. *Angew Chem Int Ed Engl.* 22:423–439.

Gao WY, Han FS, Storm C, Egan W, Cheng YC. 1992. Phosphorothioate oligonucleotides are inhibitors of human DNA polymerases and RNase H: implications for antisense technology. *Mol Pharmacol.* 41:223–229.

Gibson I. 1996. Antisense approaches to the gene therapy of cancer–'Recnac'. *Cancer Metastasis Rev.* 15:287–299.

Gilmore AP, Metcalfe AD, Romer LH, Streuli CH. 2000. Integrin-mediated survival signals regulate the apoptotic function of Bax through its conformation and subcellular localization. *J. Cell Biol.* 149:431–446.

Graziani A, Gramaglia D, Cantley LC, Comoglio PM. 1991. The tyrosine-phosphorylated hepatocyte growth factor/scatter factor receptor associates with phosphatidylinositol 3-kinase. *J Biol Chem.* 266:22087–22090.

Graziani A, Gramaglia D, dalla Zonca P, Comoglio PM. 1993. Hepatocyte growth factor/scatter factor stimulates the Ras-guanine nucleotide exchanger. *J Biol Chem.* 268:9165–9168.

Henry SP, Bolte H, Auletta C, Kornbrust DJ. 1997a. Evaluation of the toxicity of ISIS 2302, a phosphorothioate oligonucleotide, in a four-week study in cynomolgus monkeys. *Toxicology.* 120:145–155.

Henry SP, Giclas PC, Leeds J et al. 1997b. Activation of the alternative pathway of complement by a phosphorothioate oligonucleotide: potential mechanism of action. *J Pharmacol Exp Ther.* 281:810–816.

Hosoya T, Takeuchi H, Kanesaka Y et al. 1999. Sequence-specific inhibition of a transcription factor by circular dumbbell DNA oligonucleotides. *FEBS Lett.* 461:136–140.

Isner JM, Pieczek A, Schainfeld R et al. 1996. Clinical evidence of angiogenesis after arterial gene transfer of phVEGF165 in patient with ischaemic limb. *Lancet.* 348:370–374.

Iversen PL, Cornish KG, Iversen LJ, Mata JE, Bylund DB. 1999. Bolus intravenous injection of phosphorothioate oligonucleotides causes hypotension by acting as alpha(1)-adrenergic receptor antagonists. *Toxicol Appl Pharmacol.* 160:289–296.

Jun-Ichi S, Hiroshi I, Ryo G, Ryuichi M, Kensuke E, Mitsuaki I. 2004. Initial clinical cases of the use of a NF-kappaB decoy at the site of coronary stenting for the prevention of restenosis. *Circ J.* 68:270–271.

Koike H, Morishita R, Iguchi S et al. 2003. Enhanced angiogenesis and improvement of neuropathy by cotransfection of human hepatocyte growth factor and prostacyclin synthase gene. *FASEB J.* 17:779–781.

Korhonen L, Sjoholm U, Takei N et al. 2000. Expression of c-Met in developing rat hippocampus: evidence for HGF as a neurotrophic factor for calbindin D-expressing neurons. *Eur J Neurosci.* 12:3453–3461.

Kume M, Komori K, Matsumoto T et al. 2002. Administration of a decoy against the activator protein-1 binding site suppresses neointimal thickening in rabbit balloon-injured arteries. *Circulation.* 105:1226–1232.

Liu Y, Michalopoulos GK, Zarnegar R. 1994. Structural and functional characterization of the mouse hepatocyte growth factor gene promoter. *J Biol Chem.* 269:4152–4160.

Matsuki A, Yamamoto S, Nakagami H et al. 2004. No influence of tumor growth by intramuscular injection of hepatocyte growth factor plasmid DNA: safety evaluation of therapeutic angiogenesis gene therapy in mice. *Biochem Biophys Res Commun.* 315:59–65.

Miller PS, McParland KB, Jayaraman K, Ts'o PO. 1981. Biochemical and biological effects of nonionic nucleic acid methylphosphonates. *Biochemistry.* 20:1874–1880.

Miyake T, Aoki M, Shiraya S et al. 2006a. Inhibitory effects of NFkappaB decoy oligodeoxynucleotides on neointimal hyperplasia in a rabbit vein graft model. *J Mol Cell Cardiol.* 41:431–440.

Miyake T, Aoki M, Nakashima H et al. 2006b. Prevention of abdominal aortic aneurysms by simultaneous inhibition of NFkappaB and ets using chimeric decoy oligonucleotides in a rabbit model. *Gene Ther.* 13:695–704.

Morishita R, Gibbons GH, Horiuchi M et al. 1995. A gene therapy strategy using a transcription factor decoy of the E2F binding site inhibits smooth muscle proliferation in vivo. *Proc Natl Acad Sci U S A.* 92:5855–5859.

Morishita R, Sugimoto T, Aoki M et al. 1997. In vivo transfection of cis element "decoy" against nuclear factor-kappaB binding site prevents myocardial infarction. *Nat Med.* 3:894–899.

Morishita R, Nakamura S, Hayashi S et al. 1999. Therapeutic angiogenesis induced by human recombinant hepatocyte growth factor in rabbit hind limb ischemia model as cytokine supplement therapy. *Hypertension.* 33:1379–1384.

Morishita R, Aoki M, Hashiya N et al. 2004. Safety evaluation of clinical gene therapy using hepatocyte growth factor to treat peripheral arterial disease. *Hypertension.* 44:203–209.

Nakagami H, Morishita R, Yamamoto K et al. 2001. Mitogenic and antiapoptotic actions of hepatocyte growth factor through ERK, STAT3, and AKT in endothelial cells. *Hypertension.* 37:581–586.

Nakagami H, Morishita R, Yamamoto K et al. 2002. Hepatocyte growth factor prevents endothelial cell death through inhibition of bax translocation from cytosol to mitochondrial membrane. *Diabetes.* 51:2604–2611.

Nakamura T, Nishizawa T, Hagiya M et al. 1989. Molecular cloning and expression of human hepatocyte growth factor. *Nature.* 342:440–443.

Nakamura Y, Morishita R, Higaki J et al. 1995. Expression of local hepatocyte growth factor system in vascular tissues. *Biochem Biophys Res Commun.* 215:483–488.

Nakamura Y, Morishita R, Nakamura S et al. 1996a. A vascular modulator, hepatocyte growth factor, is associated with systolic pressure. *Hypertension.* 28:409–413.

Nakamura Y, Morishita R, Higaki J et al. 1996b. Hepatocyte growth factor is a novel member of the endothelium-specific growth factors: additive stimulatory effect of hepatocyte growth factor with basic fibroblast growth factor but not with vascular endothelial growth factor. *J Hypertens.* 14:1067–1072.

Nakano N, Moriguchi A, Morishita R et al. 1997. Role of angiotensin II in the regulation of a novel vascular modulator, hepatocyte growth factor (HGF), in experimental hypertensive rats. *Hypertension.* 30:1448–1454.

Osako MK, Tomita N, Nakagami H et al. 2007. Increase in nuclease resistance and incorporation of NF-kappaB decoy oligodeoxynucleotides by modification of the 3'-terminus. *J Gene Med.* 9:812–819.

Pelicci G, Giordano S, Zhen Z et al. 1995. The motogenic and mitogenic responses to HGF are amplified by the Shc adaptor protein. *Oncogene.* 10:1631–1638.

Ponzetto C, Bardelli A, Zhen Z et al. 1994. A multifunctional docking site mediates signaling and transformation by the hepatocyte growth factor/scatter factor receptor family. *Cell.* 77:261–271.

Shimamura M, Sato N, Oshima K et al. 2004. Novel therapeutic strategy to treat brain ischemia: overexpression of hepatocyte growth factor gene reduced ischemic injury without cerebral edema in rat model. *Circulation.* 109:424–431.

Simovic D, Isner JM, Ropper AH, Pieczek A, Weinberg DH. 2001. Improvement in chronic ischemic neuropathy after intramuscular phVEGF165 gene transfer in patients with critical limb ischemia. *Arch Neurol.* 58:761–768.

Srinivasan SK, Iversen P. 1995. Review of in vivo pharmacokinetics and toxicology of phosphorothioate oligonucleotides. *J Clin Lab Anal.* 9:129–137.

Suzuki J, Morishita R, Amano J, Kaneda Y, Isobe M. 2000. Decoy against nuclear factor-kappa B attenuates myocardial cell infiltration and arterial neointimal formation in murine cardiac allografts. *Gene Ther.* 7:1847–1852.

Taniyama Y, Morishita R, Aoki M et al. 2001. Therapeutic angiogenesis induced by human hepatocyte growth factor gene in rat and rabbit hindlimb ischemia models: preclinical study for treatment of peripheral arterial disease. *Gene Ther.* 8:181–189.

Van Belle E, Witzenbichler B, Chen D et al. 1998. Potentiated angiogenic effect of scatter factor/hepatocyte growth factor via induction of vascular endothelial growth factor: the case for paracrine amplification of angiogenesis. *Circulation.* 97:381–390.

Weidner KM, Di Cesare S, Sachs M, Brinkmann V, Behrens J, Birchmeier W. 1996. Interaction between Gab1 and the c-Met receptor tyrosine kinase is responsible for epithelial morphogenesis. *Nature.* 384:173–176.

Yamasaki K, Asai T, Shimizu M et al. 2003. Inhibition of NFkappaB activation using cis-element 'decoy' of NFkappaB binding site reduces neointimal formation in porcine balloon-injured coronary artery model. *Gene Ther.* 10:356–364.

Yoshimura S, Morishita R, Hayashi K et al. 2001. Inhibition of intimal hyperplasia after balloon injury in rat carotid artery model using cis-element 'decoy' of nuclear factor-kappaB binding site as a novel molecular strategy. *Gene Ther.* 8:1635–1642.

Chapter 21

ROLE OF ADVANCED GLYCATION END PRODUCTS, OXIDATIVE STRESS, AND INFLAMMATION IN DIABETIC VASCULAR COMPLICATIONS

Sho-ichi Yamagishi, Takanori Matsui, and Kazuo Nakamura

ABSTRACT

Diabetic vascular complication is a leading cause of end-stage renal failure, acquired blindness, a variety of neuropathies, and accelerated atherosclerosis, which could account for disabilities and high mortality rates in patients with diabetes. Recent large prospective clinical studies have shown that intensive glucose control effectively reduces microvascular complications among patients with diabetes. However, strict control of blood glucose is often difficult to maintain with current therapeutic options. Therefore, to develop a novel therapeutic strategy that specially targets diabetic vascular complications is actually desired for patients with diabetes. Nonenzymatic modification of proteins by reducing sugars, a process that is also known as Maillard reaction, leads to the formation of advanced glycation end products (AGEs) in vivo. It is now well established that formation and accumulation of AGEs progress during normal aging, and at an extremely accelerated rate under diabetes, thus being implicated in diabetic vascular complications. Further, there is accumulating evidence that AGE and the receptor for AGE (RAGE) interaction elicits oxidative stress generation and subsequently evokes inflammation in vascular wall cells. In addition, digested food-derived AGEs are found to play an important role in the pathogenesis of diabetic vascular complications as well. These observations suggest that the AGE–RAGE axis and other hyperglycemia-related metabolic derangements are interrelated to each other, being involved in diabetic vascular complications. This chapter summarizes the molecular mechanisms of diabetic vascular complications, especially focusing on endogenously formed and food-derived AGEs. We further discuss here the potential therapeutic interventions that could prevent these devastating disorders.

Keywords: AGEs, oxidative stress, RAGE.

Diabetic vascular complication is a leading cause of end-stage renal failure, acquired blindness, a variety of neuropathies, and accelerated atherosclerosis, which could account for disabilities and high mortality rates in diabetic patients. Indeed, cardiovascular diseases (CVDs) account for about 70% of total mortality, and all of their manifestations such as coronary heart disease, stroke, and peripheral vascular disease are substantially more common in patients with diabetes (Laakso 1999; Brownlee 2001). Two recent large prospective clinical studies, the Diabetes Control and Complications Trial (DCCT) and the United Kigdom Prospective Diabetes Study (UKPDS), have shown that intensive blood glucose control effectively reduces microvascular complications among patients with diabetes (DCCT Research Group 1993; UKPDS Group 1998) (Table 21.1). Further, there is a growing body of evidence to conclude that tight blood glucose control has no more than a marginal impact on CVD in general, and on coronary heart disease in particular, regardless of the type of diabetes (Winocour 2003). However, control of hyperglycemia to strict levels is often very difficult to maintain with current therapeutic options and may increase the risk of severe hypoglycemia in diabetic patients (DCCT Research Group 1993; UKPDS Group 1998). Therefore, to develop novel therapeutic strategies that specifically target diabetic vascular complications may be helpful for most patients with diabetes.

Various hyperglycemia-induced metabolic and hemodynamic derangements, including increased advanced glycation end product (AGE) formation, enhanced production of reactive oxygen species (ROS), activation of protein kinase C (PKC), and stimulation of the polyol pathway and the renin–angiotensin system (RAS), contribute to the characteristic histopathological changes observed in diabetic vascular complications (Brownlee 2001). However, a recent clinical study, the Diabetes Control and Complications Trial–Epidemiology of Diabetes Interventions and Complications (DCCT-EDIC) Research, has shown that the reduction in the risk of progressive retinopathy and nephropathy resulting from intensive therapy in patients with type 1 diabetes persisted for at least several years, despite increasing hyperglycemia (DCCT-EDIC Research Group 2000; Writing Team for DCCT-EDIC Research Group 2003). Intensive therapy during the DCCT resulted in decreased progression of intima-media thickness and subsequently reduced the risk of nonfatal myocardial infarction, stroke, or death from cardiovascular disease by 57%, 11 years after the end of the trials (Nathan, Lachin, Cleary et al. 2003; Nathan, Cleary, Backlund et al. 2005). These findings indicate that intensive diabetes therapy has long-term beneficial effects on the risk of diabetic retinopathy, nephropathy, and CVD in patients with type 1 diabetes, strongly suggesting that so-called hyperglycemic memory causes chronic abnormalities in diabetic vessels that are not easily reversed, even by subsequent, relatively good control of blood glucose. Among various pathways activated under diabetes, biochemical nature of AGEs and their mode of action are the most compatible with the theory "hyperglycemic memory" (Brownlee, Cerami, Vlassara 1988).

Reducing sugars can react nonenzymatically with the amino groups of proteins to form reversible Schiff bases, and then Amadori products (Brownlee, Cerami, Vlassara 1988; Dyer, Blackledge, Thorpe et al. 1991; Grandhee, Monnier 1991). These early glycation products undergo further complex reactions such as rearrangement, dehydration, and condensation to become irreversibly cross-linked, heterogeneous fluorescent derivatives termed AGEs (Brownlee, Cerami, Vlassara 1988; Dyer, Blackledge, Thorpe et al. 1991; Grandhee, Monnier 1991). The formation and accumulation of AGEs have been reported to progress under normal aging and at an accelerated rate under diabetes. The pathological role of the nonenzymatic glycation of proteins has become increasingly evident in various types of disorders including diabetic microangiopathy and atherosclerotic CVD (Bucala, Cerami 1992; Vlassara, Bucala, Striker 1994; Brownlee 1995; Yamagishi, Nakamura, Takeuchi et al. 2004; Abe, Shimizu, Sugawara et al. 2004; Takeuchi, Yamagishi 2004; Yamagishi, Imaizumi 2005; Yamagishi, Nakamura, Inoue 2005; Yamagishi, Nakamura, Inoue et al. 2005; Sato, Iwaki, Shimogaito et al. 2006; Sato, Shimogaito, Wu et al. 2006; Takenaka, Yamagishi, Matsui et al. 2006). Furthermore, there is a growing body of evidence that RAGE is a signal-transducing

Table 21.1 Summary of Clinical Trials

Clinical Trials	Results
DCCT	Intensive blood glucose control reduces the risk for diabetic microangiopathies in patients with type 1 diabetes
UKPDS	Intensive blood glucose control reduces the risk for diabetic microangiopathies in patients with type 2 diabetes
DCCT-EDIC	Beneficial effects of intensive therapy on the risk for diabetic vascular complications persist several years after the end of the DCCT trials
EUCLID	An inhibitor of angiotensin converting enzyme inhibits the development and progression of diabetic nephropathy and retinopathy in patients with type 1 diabetes
ACTION I	Pimagedine reduces the decrease in glomerular filtration rate and inhibits proteinuria in patients with type 1 diabetes

receptor for AGEs and that the engagement of RAGE with AGEs evokes oxidative stress, vascular inflammation, thrombogenesis, and pathological angiogenesis, thereby being involved in the pathogenesis of various AGE-related disorders (Bierhaus, Hofmann, Ziegler et al. 1998; Schmidt, Stern 2000; Yamagishi, Takeuchi, Inagaki 2003; Yamagishi, Nakamura, Matsui 2006). In addition, diet is a major environmental source of pro-inflammatory AGEs, thus playing an important role in the pathogenesis of diabetic vascular complications as well (Vlassara 2005). This chapter summarizes the molecular mechanisms of diabetic vascular complications, especially focusing on endogenously formed and food-derived AGEs. We further discuss here the potential therapeutic interventions that could prevent these devastating disorders even in the presence of hyperglycemia.

ENDOGENOUSLY FORMED AGEs

Reactive derivatives from nonenzymatic glucose–protein condensation reactions, as well as lipids and nucleic acids exposed to reducing sugars, form a heterogeneous group of irreversible adducts called "AGEs." AGEs were originally characterized by a yellow-brown fluorescent color and by an ability to form cross-links with and between amino groups, but the term is now used for a broad range of advanced products of the glycation process (also called the *Maillard reaction*), including N-carboxymethyllysine (CML) and pyrraline, which show neither color nor fluorescence and do not cross-link proteins (Brownlee, Cerami, Vlassara 1988; Dyer, Blackledge, Thorpe et al. 1991; Grandhee, Monnier 1991). CML can be formed from the precursors glyoxal and glycolaldehyde by an intramolecular Cannizzaro reaction, a process that is largely independent of glucose autoxidation (Glomb, Monnier 1995). The concept that CML is a marker of oxidation rather than glycation has recently attracted support.

The formation of AGEs in vitro and in vivo is dependent on the turnover rate of the chemically modified target, the time available, and the sugar concentration. The structures of the various cross-linked AGEs that are generated in vivo have not yet been completely determined. Because of their heterogeneity and the complexity of the chemical reactions involved, only some AGEs have been structurally characterized in vivo. The structural identity of AGEs with cytotoxic properties remains unknown.

AGEs are formed by the Maillard process, a non-enzymatic reaction between ketone group of the glucose molecule or aldehydes and the amino groups of proteins that contributes to the aging of proteins and to the pathological complications of diabetes (Bucala,

Cerami 1992; Vlassara, Bucala, Striker 1994; Brownlee 1995; Abe, Shimizu, Sugawara et al. 2004; Takeuchi, Yamagishi 2004; Yamagishi, Nakamura, Takeuchi et al. 2004; Yamagishi, Imaizumi 2005; Yamagishi, Nakamura, Inoue 2005; Yamagishi, Nakamura, Inoue et al. 2005; Sato, Iwaki, Shimogaito et al. 2006; Sato, Shimogaito, Wu et al. 2006; Takenaka, Yamagishi, Matsui et al. 2006). In the hyperglycemia elicited by diabetes, this process begins with the conversion of reversible Schiff base adducts to more stable, covalently bound Amadori rearrangement products. Over the course of days to weeks, these Amadori products undergo further rearrangement reactions to form the irreversibly bound moieties known as AGEs. Recent studies have suggested that AGEs can arise not only from sugars but also from carbonyl compounds derived from the autoxidation of sugars and other metabolic pathways (Takeuchi, Yamagishi 2004).

FOOD-DERIVED AGEs

Heat processing of food containing sugars and/or lipids and proteins may generate AGEs (Uribarri, Cai, Sandu et al. 2005). Nutrient composition, temperature, and method of cooking can affect the formation of AGEs in foods; fats or meat-derived products processed by high heat such as broiling and oven-frying contain more AGEs than carbohydrates boiled for longer periods (Goldberg, Cai, Peppa et al. 2004; Uribarri, Cai, Sandu et al. 2005). That is, in the absence of lipids and proteins or heat, sugar content does not necessarily correlate with AGEs values in the food. The absence of sugars does not necessarily predict low AGE content, as in preparations containing pre-formed AGE-like caramel additives (Koschinsky, He, Mitsuhashi et al. 1997). Further, recent human studies revealed that approximately 10% of diet-derived AGEs were absorbed, two-thirds of which remained in the body and only one-third of the absorbed AGEs was excreted into the urine within 3 days from ingestion (Koschinsky, He, Mitsuhashi et al. 1997; He, Sabol, Mitsuhashi et al. 1999). Indeed, ingestion of the AGE-rich meal (threefold higher in AGE content compared with a regular diet) is reported to increase serum levels of AGEs by about 1.5-folds. In diabetic patients, especially those with advanced renal disease, urinary elimination of absorbed food-derived AGEs is markedly impaired and the elevation of serum AGEs persists beyond 48 hours postingestion (Koschinsky, He, Mitsuhashi et al. 1997). The increase in serum AGE levels after a single AGE-rich meal is in direct proportion to the amount of AGEs ingested (Koschinsky, He, Mitsuhashi et al. 1997). Moreover, the in vitro exposure of serum fractions after a single AGE-rich meal formed covalently linked complexes with fibronectin, a matrix protein, and subsequently resulted in two-fold increase in fibronectin aggregation, which was blocked by aminoguanidine, an inhibitor of AGE cross-linking (Koschinsky, He, Mitsuhashi et al. 1997; He, Sabol, Mitsuhashi et al. 1999). These observations suggest that food-derived AGEs play a role in the pathogenesis of various AGE-related disorders and that inhibition of absorption of dietary AGEs may be a therapeutic target for these devastating disorders.

ROLE OF AGEs IN DIABETIC RETINOPATHY

Diabetic retinopathy is one of the most important microvascular complications in diabetes and is a leading cause of acquired blindness among the people of occupational age (L'Esperance, James, Judson et al. 1990). The earliest histopathological hallmark of diabetic retinopathy is loss of pericytes (Cogan, Toussaint, Kuwabara 1961) (Fig. 21.1). In parallel with loss of pericytes, several characteristic changes including thickening of the basement membrane, hyperpermeability, and formation of microaneurysm are observed (Frank 1991; Mandarino 1992). These structural and functional abnormalities are followed by microvascular occlusion in the retinas, which ultimately progresses to proliferative changes associated with neovascularization (Frank 1991; Mandarino 1992). It has been postulated that many of these changes are a consequence of the loss of pericytes.

Pericytes are elongated cells of the mesodermal origin, wrapping around and along endothelial cells (ECs) of small vessels (Sims 1991). As pericytes contain contractile muscle filaments on their EC side, they have been regarded for a long time just as microvascular counterparts of smooth muscle cells and implicated in the maintenance of capillary tone (Herman,

D'Amore 1985; Joyce, Haire, Palade 1985). In 1983, Gitlin and D'Amore developed a procedure for isolating pericytes from small vessels; this procedure enabled us to elucidate the functional roles and biological characteristics of pericytes. By using pericyte-EC coculture systems, we found that pericytes not only regulate the growth but also preserve the prostacyclin-producing ability and protect against lipid-peroxide-induced injury of ECs, thus playing an important role in the maintenance of microvascular homeostasis (Yamagishi, Hsu, Kobayashi et al. 1993; Yamagishi, Kobayashi, Yamamoto 1993). Therefore, the loss of pericytes could predispose the vessels to angiogenesis, thrombogenesis, and EC injury, leading to full clinical expression of diabetic retinopathy. Signals that mediate these functional interactions between pericytes and ECs might involve cell surface molecules, because the EC overgrowth inhibition and stimulation of prostacyclin production were accomplished by direct contact of ECs to pericytes (Fig. 21.2). D'Amore et al. demonstrated that an active form of transforming growth factor-β (TGF-β) was produced by cocultures of ECs and pericytes and that antibodies against TGF-β added to the coculture systems abolished the growth inhibitory effects of pericytes on neighboring ECs (Antonelli-Orlidge, Saunders, Smith et al. 1989). These observations suggest that a candidate molecule that would mediate the functional interactions between pericytes and ECs is TGF-β.

Recently, Hammes et al. (2002) investigated the role of capillary coverage with pericytes in early diabetic retinopathy and the contribution to proliferative retinopathy using mice with a single functional allele of platelet-derived growth factor-B (PDGF-B(+/−) mice). They demonstrated in their studies that retinal capillary coverage with pericytes is crucial for the survival of ECs, particularly under stress conditions such as diabetes, and that pericyte deficiency leads to reduced inhibition of EC proliferation, thus promoting angiogenesis in the retinopathy of prematurity model. Our in vitro and their recent in vivo observations provide a basis for understanding why diabetic

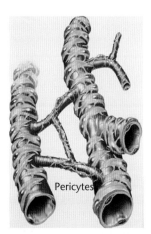
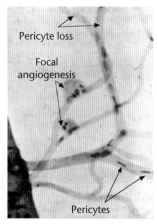

Figure 21.1 A clinical color image of early diabetic retinopathy of the retina.

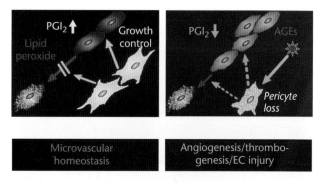

Figure 21.2 An image of EC coculture system.

retinopathy develops consequent to pericyte loss, the earliest histopathological hallmarks of diabetic retinopathy.

Retinal pericytes accumulate AGEs during diabetes (Stitt, Li, Gardiner et al. 1997), which would be expected to have a detrimental influence on pericyte survival and function (Sharma, Gardiner, Archer 1985). AGEs are toxic to retinal pericytes in vitro (Yamagishi, Hsu, Taniguchi et al. 1995; Yamagishi, Amano, Inagaki et al. 2002). We have found that AGEs not only induce growth retardation and apoptotic cell death of cultured retinal pericytes, but also cause immediate toxicity to these cells (Yamagishi, Hsu, Taniguchi et al. 1995; Yamagishi, Amano, Inagaki et al. 2002). Antisense DNA complementary mRNA coding for RAGE reversed the AGE-induced decrease in viable cell number of pericytes, while overexpression of RAGE augmented the proapoptotic effects of AGEs. Further, an antioxidant *N*-acetylcysteine (NAC) completely reversed the toxic effects of AGEs (Yamagishi, Inagaki, Amano et al. 2002). These results suggest that the RAGE-induced ROS generation mediated these deleterious effects of AGEs on pericytes. Moreover, AGEs upregulated RAGE mRNA levels in pericytes through the intracellular ROS generation as well (Yamagishi, Okamoto, Amano et al. 2002). These positive feedback loops transduced the AGE signals, further exacerbating the cytotoxic effects of AGEs on retinal pericytes.

We have recently found that beraprost sodium, a prostacyclin analogue, or forskolin, an activator of adenylate cyclase, protects against the AGE-induced injury in retinal pericytes by suppressing ROS generation: 10 nM beraprost sodium or 1 μM forskolin completely blocked the AGE-induced superoxide generation in cultured retinal pericytes (Fig. 21.3) (Yamagishi, Amano, Inagaki et al. 2002). Since cyclic AMP-elevating agents were known to block ROS generation in neutrophils by inhibiting reduced nicotinamide adenine dinucleotide phosphate (NADPH) oxidase activity (Ottonello, Morone, Dapino et al. 1995), NADPH oxidase might be a source of ROS production elicited by AGEs and also be a target of beraprost sodium.

Pericyte dysfunction has also been considered to be one of the characteristic changes of the early phase of diabetic retinopathy. AGEs act on pericytes to stimulate vascular endothelial growth factor (VEGF) expression (Yamagishi, Amano, Inagaki et al. 2002). VEGF is a specific mitogen to ECs, also known as vascular permeability factor, and is generally thought to be involved in the pathogenesis of proliferative diabetic retinopathy. Indeed, some clinical observations have demonstrated that VEGF level in ocular fluid is positively correlated with the activity of neovascularization in diabetic retinopathy (Adamis, Miller, Bernal et al. 1994; Aiello, Avery, Arrigg et al. 1994).

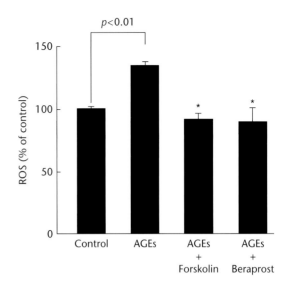

Figure 21.3 Effects of cyclic AMP-elevating agents on AGE-induced ROS generation in pericytes. Pericytes were treated with 100 μg/ml of AGE-BSA or non-glycated BSA (control) in the presence or absence of 10 nM beraprost sodium or 1 μM forskolin for 24 hours, and then ROS were quantitatively analyzed. *, $P<0.01$ compared to the value of with AGE-BSA alone.

Recently, VEGF level was also found to be associated with the breakdown of the blood–retinal barrier, thus being involved in microvascular hyperpermeability in background retinopathy (Murata, Ishibashi, Khalil et al. 1995). These observations suggest that the AGE–RAGE axis might be involved in the development and progression of diabetic retinopathy by inducing VEGF overexpression in pericytes as well.

There has been increasing interest in the role of inflammatory reaction in diabetic retinopathy (Schroder, Palinski, Schmid-Schonbein 1991). AGEs are implicated in the process of vascular inflammation as well. Indeed, AGEs have been recently shown to increase leukocyte adhesion to cultured retinal microvascular ECs by inducing intracellular cell adhesion molecule-1 (ICAM-1) expression (Moore, Moore, Kaji et al. 2003). This phenomenon is also apparent in nondiabetic mice infused with preformed AGEs, which results in significant leukostasis and blood–retinal barrier dysfunction in these mice (Moore, Moore, Kaji et al. 2003). Recently, retinal VEGF has been found to induce ICAM-1 expression, thus leading to leukostasis and breakdown of blood–retinal barrier in vivo (Lu, Perez, Ma et al. 1999; Joussen, Poulaki, Qin et al. 2002; Ishida, Usui, Yamashiro et al. 2003). Therefore, it is conceivable that the AGE-elicited pro-inflammatory reaction could be partly mediated by VEGF. Further, AGEs are known to induce monocyte chemoattractant protein-1 (MCP-1) in microvascular ECs through intracellular ROS generation (Inagaki, Yamagishi, Okamoto et al. 2003). Since the levels of MCP-1 in vitreous fluids are correlated with the severity of proliferative diabetic retinopathy (Mitamura, Takeuchi, Matsuda et al. 2000), AGEs may be one of the key pro-inflammatory factors for progression of diabetic retinopathy.

Microthrombosis formation contributes to capillary obliteration and retinal ischemia, thus being involved in the progression of diabetic retinopathy (Boeri, Maiello, Lorenzi 2001). AGEs inhibit prostacyclin production and induce plasminogen activator inhibitor-1 (PAI-1) in microvascular ECs through an interaction with RAGE (Yamagishi, Yamamoto, Harada et al. 1996; Yamagishi, Fujimori, Yonekura et al. 1998). These observations suggest that AGE have the ability to cause platelet aggregation and fibrin stabilization, resulting in a predisposition to thrombogenesis and thereby contributing to the promotion of diabetic retinopathy. Retinal ischemia due to microthrombus formation may trigger VEGF expression in retinal cells, thus further promoting diabetic retinopathy (Nomura, Yamagishi, Harada et al. 1995; Yamagishi, Kawakami, Fujimori et al. 1999; Yamagishi, Yonekura, Yamamoto et al. 1999). Since AGEs decrease the intracellular cyclic AMP concentrations in ECs and that cyclic AMP agonists such as beraprost sodium and forskolin reduce the AGE-induced PAI-1 production, cyclic AMP-elevating agents may have a therapeutic potential in the treatment of diabetic retinopathy.

Exposure of retinal cells to preformed AGEs is known to cause significant upregulation of VEGF both in vitro and in vivo (Yamagishi, Yonekura, Yamamoto et al. 1997; Lu, Kuroki, Amano et al. 1998; Segawa, Shirao, Yamagishi et al. 1998; Stitt, Bhaduri, McMullen et al. 2000; Okamoto, Yamagishi, Inagaki et al. 2002; Okamoto, Yamagishi, Inagaki et al. 2002; Yamagishi, Amano, Inagaki et al. 2002; Yamagishi, Nakamura, Matsui et al. 2006; Yamagishi, Nakamura, Matsui et al. 2007). AGEs directly stimulate growth and tube formation of microvascular ECs, the key steps of angiogenesis, through the interaction with RAGE (Okamoto, Yamagishi, Inagaki et al. 2002; Okamoto, Yamagishi, Inagaki et al. 2002; Yamagishi, Nakamura, Matsui et al. 2006; Yamagishi, Nakamura, Matsui et al. 2007). We found that it was autocrine VEGF production in ECs that mainly mediated the angiogenic activity of AGEs. Although the molecular mechanisms of VEGF overexpression elicited by AGEs are not fully understood, our recent investigation has shown that the AGE–RAGE interaction might increase VEGF gene transcription in microvascular ECs by NADPH oxidase-mediated ROS generation and subsequent nuclear factor-κB (NF-κB) activation via Ras-mitogen activated protein kinase (MAPK) pathway (Okamoto, Yamagishi, Inagaki et al. 2002; Okamoto, Yamagishi, Inagaki et al. 2002; Yamagishi, Nakamura, Matsui et al. 2006; Yamagishi, Nakamura, Matsui et al. 2007).

Angiopoietin (ang)-Tie receptor interaction plays an important role in both physiological and pathological angiogenesis as well (Folkman, D'Aore 1996). Engagement of Tie-2 by ang-1 has been known to promote recruitment of pericytes, thereby supporting the establishment and maintenance of vascular integrity; while ang-2 is a naturally occurring antagonist of ang-1, and induces the loosening of contacts between ECs and pericytes (Folkman, D'Aore 1996; Maisonpierre, Suri, Jones et al. 1997; Jonnes, Iljin, Dumont et al. 2001). AGEs increase a ratio of ang-2 to ang-1 mRNA level and simultaneously upregulate VEGF mRNA levels in microvascular ECs. A plastic window for blood vessel remodeling is defined by pericyte coverage of the preformed endothelial network (Benjamin, Hemo, Keshet 1998). Therefore, the AGE-induced pericyte apoptosis and increased ratio of ang-2/ang-1 in ECs could disrupt the pericyte-EC interactions, thus promoting neoangiogeneis by acting in concert with VEGF.

The above-mentioned in vitro and in vivo properties of AGEs strongly suggest a pathological role for these senescent macroproteins in diabetic retinopathy. Further, serum levels of AGEs are correlated to the severity of diabetic retinopathy with both type 1 and type 2 diabetes (Koga, Yamagishi, Okamoto et al. 2002; Miura, Yamagishi, Uchigata et al. 2003). In addition, vitreous levels of AGEs and VEGF are significantly higher in type 2 diabetic patients than in control subjects, and there is a significant correlation between the vitreous AGE and VEGF levels (Yokoi, Yamagishi, Takeuchi et al. 2005; Yokoi, Yamagishi, Takeuchi et al. 2007). Total antioxidant status is decreased in vitreous in patients with diabetes compared with the controls (Yokoi, Yamagishi, Takeuchi et al. 2005). Furthermore, both AGE and VEGF levels are inversely correlated with the total antioxidant status (Yokoi, Yamagishi, Takeuchi et al. 2005). Since VEGF is considered to be involved in various steps of diabetic retinopathy (Yamagishi, Nakamura, Matsui et al. 2006; Yamagishi, Nakamura, Matsui et al. 2007), the observations suggest that AGEs and decreased total antioxidant status may contribute to the development and progression of diabetic retinopathy via induction of VEGF. Therefore, the inhibition of AGE formation, blockade of AGE–RAGE interactions, or the downstream signaling pathways has been supposed to be potential therapeutic strategies in the prevention of diabetic retinopathy.

The hydrazine compound aminoguanidine is the first AGE inhibitor that was discovered (Brownlee, Vlassara, Kooney et al. 1986). Treatment of diabetic rats for 26 weeks with aminoguanidine prevented a 2.6-fold accumulation of these products at branching sites of precapillary arterioles and thereby prevented abnormal EC proliferation and significantly diminished pericyte dropout (Hammes, Martin, Federlin et al. 1991). A multicenter clinical trial revealed that pimagedine[R] (aminoguanidine) slowed the progression of diabetic retinopathy, although it was terminated early due to safety concerns (Vasan, Foiles, Founds 2001; Thornalley 2003).

Amadorins have an ability to scavenge dicarbonyls and therefore inhibit the conversion of Amadori intermediates to AGEs (Khalifah, Baynes, Hudson 1999; Voziyan, Metz, Baynes et al. 2002). The derivative of vitamin B_6, pyridoxamine, has shown to be an efficacious and specific post-Amadori inhibitor, with the ability to prevent upregulation of retinal basement membrane-associated genes and capillary dropout (Stitt, Gardiner, Alderson et al. 2002).

Studies in rodent models of diabetes have demonstrated that the blockade of the AGE–RAGE axis by administration of soluble form of RAGE (sRAGE) ameliorates neuronal dysfunction and reduces the development of acellular capillaries and pericyte ghosts in hyperglycemic, hyperlipidemic mice (Barile, Pachydaki, Tari et al. 2005). Furthermore, recently, Kaji et al. (2007) have also shown that attenuation of the RAGE axis with sRAGE inhibits retinal leukostasis and blood–retinal barrier breakdown in the diabetic C57/BJ6 and RAGE-transgenic mice that are accompanied by decreased expression of VEGF and ICAM-1 in the retina, thus suggesting that antagonism of the RAGE axis by sRAGE is a novel therapeutic target for early diabetic retinopathy

Compared to the strategy of preventing AGEs formation or the blockade of AGE–RAGE interactions, the manipulation of the AGE signaling pathway as a therapeutic option in diabetic retinopathy remains much less developed. However, recently, we have found that pigment epithelium-derived factor (PEDF), one of the superfamily of serine protease inhibitors with potent neuronal differentiating activity in human retinoblastoma cells (Tombran-Tink, Chader, Johnson 1991), inhibits the AGE-induced pericyte apoptosis and EC proliferation and activation through its antioxidative properties (Yamagishi, Inagaki, Amano et al. 2002; Inagaki, Yamagishi, Okamoto et al. 2003; Yamagishi, Nakamura, Matsui et al. 2006; Yamagishi, Nakamura, Matsui et al. 2007). Administration of PEDF or pyridoxal phosphate, an AGE inhibitor, was found to decrease retinal levels of 8-hydroxydeoxyguanosine and suppress *ICAM-1* gene expression and retinal leukostasis in diabetic rats (Yamagishi, Matsui, Nakamura et al. 2006; Yamagishi, Matsui, Nakamura et al. 2007). Further, intravenous administration of AGEs to normal rats increased ICAM-1 and *VEGF gene* expression and subsequently induced retinal leukostasis and hyperpermeability, all of which were blocked by the simultaneous treatment of PEDF (Yamagishi, Nakamura, Matsui et al. 2006;

Yamagishi, Matsui, Nakamura et al. 2006; Yamagishi, Matsui, Nakamura et al. 2007). PEDF also inhibited the AGE-induced T cell adhesion to ECs and vascular hyperpermeability in vitro by suppressing ICAM-1 and VEGF expression, respectively, via suppression of NADPH oxidase-mediated ROS generation (Yamagishi, Nakamura, Matsui et al. 2006; Yamagishi, Matsui, Nakamura et al. 2006; Yamagishi, Matsui, Nakamura et al. 2007). Since PEDF levels in vitreous fluid or aqueous humor are decreased in angiogenic eye diseases such as proliferative diabetic retinopathy and positively associated with total antioxidant capacity (Spranger, Osterhoff, Reimann et al. 2002; Boehm, Lang, Volpert et al. 2003; Yokoi, Yamagishi, Sato et al. 2006; Yoshida, Yamagishi, Matsui et al. 2007), substitution of PEDF may disrupt inappropriate retinal cell responses to AGEs, thus being a promising strategy for treatment of patients with diabetic retinopathy.

Cross talk between the AGE–RAGE Axis and Other Metabolic Pathways in Diabetic Retinopathy

The polyol pathway consists of two enzymes, aldose reductase (AR) and sorbitol dehydrogenase (SDH); the former is the first enzyme in the polyol pathway that catalyzes reduction of glucose to sorbitol, while the latter is the second enzyme that converts sorbitol into fructose using NAD+ as a cofactor (Yabe-Nishimura 1998). The polyol pathway is activated under hyperglycemic conditions, and increased flux through SDH can lead to an increased ratio of nicotinamide adenine dinucleotide (NADH)/NAD that may alter lipid metabolism and increase production of ROS, thus contributing to the development of diabetic vascular complications (pseudohypoxia hypothesis) (Williamson, Chang, Frangos et al. 1993). This redox imbalance may be associated with impaired regulation of retinal blood flow in humans with diabetes and in nondiabetic acutely hyperglycemic animals (Van den Enden, Nyengaard, Ostrow et al. 1995). In order to further examine a functional role of SDH in diabetic retinopathy, we studied effects of SDH overexpression on glucose toxicity to cultured retinal pericytes (Amano, Yamagishi, Kato et al. 2002). High glucose modestly increased ROS generation, decreased DNA synthesis and upregulated VEGF mRNA levels in retinal pericytes. SDH overexpression was found to significantly stimulate ROS generation in high glucose–exposed pericytes and subsequently augment the cytotoxic effects of glucose. An antioxidant NAC, completely prevented these deleterious effects of SDH overexpression on pericytes. Further, blockade of the polyol pathway was found to significantly prevent vascular hyperpermeability, the characteristic changes of the early phase of diabetic retinopathy, in streptozotocin-induced diabetic rats. These observations suggest that SDH-mediated conversion of sorbitol into fructose and the resultant ROS generation may play a role in the pathogenesis of diabetic retinopathy. Since fructose is a stronger glycating agent than glucose, intracellular AGEs formation via the SDH pathway might be involved in glucose toxicity to retinal pericytes (Rosen, Nawroth, King et al. 2001).

There is a growing body of evidence that generation of ROS is increased in diabetes. High glucose concentrations, via various mechanisms such as glucose autoxidation, increased the production of AGEs, activation of PKC, and stimulation of the polyol pathway, and it enhanced ROS generation (Rosen, Nawroth, King et al. 2001; Bonnefont-Rousselot 2002). Increased ROS generation has been found to regulate vascular inflammation, altered gene expression of growth factors and cytokines, and platelet and macrophage activation, thus playing a central role in the pathogenesis of diabetic vascular complications (Yamagishi, Edelstein, Du et al. 2001; Yamagishi, Edelstein, Du et al. 2001; Yamagishi, Okamoto, Amano et al. 2002; Spitaler, Graier 2002; Yamagishi, Inagaki, Amano et al. 2002; Yamagishi S, Amano S, Inagaki et al. 2003). Further, we have recently found that high glucose–induced mitochondrial overproduction of superoxide serves as a causal link between elevated glucose and hyperglycemic vascular damage in ECs (Nishikawa, Edelstein, Du et al. 2000; Brownlee 2001). Normalizing levels of mitochondrial ROS prevent glucose-induced formation of AGEs, activation of PKC, sorbitol accumulation, and NF-κB activation. These observations suggest that the three main mechanisms implicated in the pathogenesis of diabetic vascular complications might reflect a single hyperglycemia-induced process, thus providing a novel therapeutic target for diabetic angiopathies. Recently, Hammes et al. (Hammes, Du, Edelstein et al. 2003) have discovered that the lipid-soluble thiamine derivative benfotiamine can inhibit the three major biochemical pathways as well as hyperglycemia-associated NF-κB activation (Hammes, Du, Edelstein et al. 2003). They showed that benfotiamine prevented experimental diabetic retinopathy by activating the pentose phosphate pathway enzyme, transketolase, in the retinas, which converts glyceraldehyde-3-phosphate and fructose-6-phosphate into pentose-5-phosphates and other sugars (Hammes, Du, Edelstein et al. 2003). Thiamine and benfotiamine therapy is reported to prevent streptozotocin-induced incipient diabetic nephropathy as well (Babaei-Jadidi, Karachalias, Ahmed et al. 2003).

The local RAS is activated under diabetes (Anderson 1997). We have recently found that angiotensin II (Ang II) stimulated intracellular ROS generation in retinal pericytes through an interaction with type 1 receptor. Further, Ang II decreased DNA synthesis and simultaneously upregulated VEGF mRNA levels in pericytes, both of which were blocked by treatment with telmisartan, a commercially available Ang II type 1 receptor blocker, or an antioxidant NAC (Yamagishi, Amano, Inagaki et al. 2003; Amano, Yamagishi, Inagaki et al. 2003). These results suggest that Ang II-type 1 receptor interaction could induce pericyte loss and dysfunction through intracellular ROS generation, thus being involved in diabetic retinopathy. Since Ang II induces the VEGF receptor, KDR, expression in retinal microvascular ECs, the retinal RAS might augment the permeability- and angiogenesis-inducing activity of VEGF, thus implicated in the progression of diabetic retinopathy as well (Otani, Takagi, Suzuma et al. 1998).

Blockade of the RAS by inhibitors of angiotensin converting enzyme or Ang II type 1 receptor antagonists can reduce retinal overexpression of VEGF and hyperpermeability and neovascularization in experimental diabetes (Babaei-Jadidi, Karachalias, Ahmed et al. 2003; Anderson 1997; Yamagishi, Amano, Inagaki et al. 2003). Funatsu et al. (Funatsu, Yamashita, Nakanishi et al. 2002) recently found that the vitreous fluid level of Ang II was significantly correlated with that of VEGF, and both of them were significantly higher in patients with active proliferative diabetic retinopathy than in those with quiescent proliferative diabetic retinopathy (Amano, Yamagishi, Inagaki et al. 2003). These findings further support the concept that Ang II contributes to development and progression of proliferative diabetic retinopathy in combination with VEGF. In the EUCLID Study, the angiotensin-converting enzyme inhibitor, lisinopril, reduced the risk of progression of retinopathy by approximately 50% and also significantly reduced the risk of progression to proliferative retinopathy although retinopathy was not a primary end point and the study was not sufficiently powered for eye-related outcomes (Otani, Takagi, Suzuma et al. 1998). The interaction of the RAS and AGE–RAGE system has also been proposed. We have found that Ang II potentiates the deleterious effects of AGEs on pericytes by inducing RAGE protein expression (Yamagishi, Takeuchi, Matsui et al. 2005). In vivo, AGE injection stimulated RAGE expression in the eye of spontaneously hypertensive rats, which was blocked by telmisartan. In vitro, Ang II-type 1 receptor-mediated ROS generation elicited *RAGE* gene expression in retinal pericytes through NF-κB

Table 21.2 Diabetic Retinopathy

Etiology	Cellular Pathway	Treatment Regimen
AGE–RAGE	VEGF	Pimagedine
ROS	ICAM-1	Amadorins
Polyol pathway	MCP-1	OPB-9195
PKC	PAI-1	sRAGE
RAS	Angiopoietins	PEDF
		Benfotiamine
		Telmisartan

activation. Further, Ang II augmented AGE-induced pericyte apoptosis, the earliest hallmark of diabetic retinopathy. Further, we have recently found that telmisartan blocks the Ang II-induced RAGE expression in ECs as well (Nakamura, Yamagishi, Nakamura et al. 2005). Telmisartan could decrease endothelial RAGE levels in patients with essential hypertension. Taken together, these observations provide the functional interaction between the AGE–RAGE system and the RAS in the pathogenesis of diabetic retinopathy, thus suggesting a novel beneficial aspect of telmisartan on the devastating disorder. We posit a table that presents the etiologies of diabetic retinopathy and its possible therapeutic agents (Table 21.2).

ROLE OF AGEs IN DIABETIC NEPHROPATHY

Diabetic nephropathy is a leading cause of ESRD and accounts for disabilities and the high mortality rate in patients with diabetes (Krolewski, Warram, Valsania et al. 1991). Development of diabetic nephropathy is characterized by glomerular hyperfiltration and thickening of glomerular basement membranes, followed by an expansion of extracellular matrix in mesangial areas and increased urinary albumin excretion rate (UAER). Diabetic nephropathy ultimately progresses to glomerular sclerosis associated with renal dysfunction (Sharma, Ziyadeh 1995). Further, it has recently been recognized that changes within tubulointerstitium, including proximal tubular cell atrophy and tubulointerstitial fibrosis, are also important in terms of renal prognosis in diabetic nephropathy (Ziyadeh, Goldfarb 1991; Lane, Steffes, Fioretto et al. 1993; Taft, Nolan, Yeung et al. 1994; Jones, Saunders, Qi et al. 1999; Gilbert, Cooper 1999). Such tubular changes have been reported to be the dominant lesion in about one-third of patients with type 2 diabetes (Fiorreto, Mauer, Brocco et al. 1996). It appears that both metabolic and hemodynamic factors interact to stimulate the expression of cytokines and growth factors in glomeruli and tubules from the diabetic kidney

(Cooper, Bonnet, Oldfield et al. 2001). Evidence has implicated the TGF-β system as a major etiologic agent in the pathogenesis of glomerulosclerosis and tubulointerstitial fibrosis in diabetic nephropathy (Sharma, Ziyadeh 1995; Aoyama, Shimokata, Niwa 2000; Wang, LaPage, Hirschberg 2000).

AGEs induce apoptotic cell death and VEGF expression in human-cultured mesangial cells, as the case in pericytes (Yamagishi, Inagaki, Okamoto et al. 2002). Mesangial cells occupy a central anatomical position in the glomerulus, playing crucial roles in maintaining structure and function of glomerular capillary tufts (Dworkin, Ichikawa, Brenner 1983). They actually provide structural support for capillary loops and modulate glomerular filtration by its smooth muscle activity (Dworkin, Ichikawa, Brenner 1983; Kreisberg, Venkatachalam, Troyer 1985; Schlondorff 1987). Therefore, it is conceivable that the AGE-induced mesangial apoptosis and dysfunction may contribute in part to glomerular hyperfiltration, an early renal dysfunction in diabetes. Several experimental and clinical studies support the pathological role for VEGF in diabetic nephropathy. Indeed, antibodies against VEGF have been found to improve hyperfiltration and albuminuria in streptozotocin-induced diabetic rats (De Vriese, Tilton, Elger et al. 2001). Inhibition of VEGF also prevents glomerular hypertrophy in a model of obese type 2 diabetes, the Zucker diabetic fatty rat (Schrijvers, Flyvbjerg, Tilton et al. 2006). Further, urinary VEGF levels are positively correlated with the urinary albumin to creatinine ratio and negatively correlated with creatinine clearance in type 2 diabetic patients (Kim, Oh, Seo et al. 2005). These observations suggest that urinary VEGF might be used as a sensitive marker of diabetic nephropathy. VEGF overproduction elicited by AGEs may be involved in diabetic nephropathy.

Moreover, we have recently found that AGE–RAGE interaction stimulates MCP-1 expression in mesangial cells through ROS generation (Yamagishi, Inagaki, Okamoto et al. 2002). Increased MCP-1 expression associated with monocyte infiltration in mesangium has been observed in the early phase of diabetic nephropathy as well (Banba, Nakamura, Matsumura et al. 2000). Plasma MCP-1 was positively correlated with urinary albumin excretion rate in type 1 diabetic patients (Chiarelli, Cipollone, Mohn et al. 2002). AGE accumulation in glomerulus could also be implicated in the initiation of diabetic nephropathy by promoting the secretion of MCP-1.

AGE formation on extracellular matrix proteins alters both matrix–matrix and cell–matrix interactions, involved in the pathogenesis of diabetic glomerulosclerosis. For example, nonenzymatic glycations of type IV collagen and laminin reduce their ability to interact with negatively charged proteoglycans, increasing vascular permeability to albumin (Silbiger, Crowley, Shan et al. 1993). Furthermore, AGE formation on various types of matrix proteins impairs their degradation by matrix metalloproteinases, contributing to basement membrane thickening and mesangial expansion, hallmarks of diabetic nephropathy (Brownlee 1993; Mott, Khalifah, Nagase et al. 1997). AGEs formed on the matrix components can trap and covalently cross-link with the extravasated plasma proteins such as lipoproteins, thereby exacerbating diabetic glomerulosclerosis (Brownlee 1993).

AGEs stimulate insulin-like growth factor-I, -II, PDGF and TGF-β in mesangial cells, which in turn mediate production of type IV collagen, laminin, and fibronectin (Matsumura, Yamagishi, Brownlee 2000; Yamagishi, Takeuchi, Makita 2001). AGEs induce TGF-β overexpression in both podocytes and proximal tubular cells as well (Wendt TM, Tanji N, Guo J, et al. 2003; Yamagishi, Inagaki, Okamoto et al. 2003). Recently, Ziyadeh et al. (2000) reported that long-term treatment of type 2 diabetic model mice with blocking antibodies against TGF-β suppressed excess matrix gene expression, glomerulosclerosis, and prevented the development of renal insufficiency. These observations suggest that AGE-induced TGF-β expression plays an important role in the pathogenesis of glomerulosclerosis and tubulointerstitial fibrosis in diabetic nephropathy (Raj, Choudhury, Welbourne et al. 2000; Yamagishi, Koga, Inagaki et al. 2002).

In vivo, the administration of AGE-albumin to normal healthy mice for 4 weeks has been found to induce glomerular hypertrophy with overexpression of type IV collagen, laminin B1, and TGF-β genes (Yang, Vlassara, Peten et al. 1994). Furthermore, chronic infusion of AGE-albumin to otherwise healthy rats leads to focal glomerulosclerosis, mesangial expansion, and albuminuria (Vlassara H, Striker LJ, Teichberg et al. 1994). Recently, RAGE-overexpressing diabetic mice have been found to show progressive glomerulosclerosis with renal dysfunction, compared with diabetic littermates lacking the RAGE transgene (Yamamoto, Kato, Doi et al. 2001). Further, diabetic homozygous RAGE null mice failed to develop significantly increased mesangial matrix expansion or thickening of the glomerular basement membrane (Wendt, Tanji, Guo et al. 2003). Taken together, these findings suggest that the activation of AGE–RAGE axis contributes to expression of VEGF and enhanced attraction/activation of inflammatory cells in the diabetic glomerulus, thereby setting the stage for mesangial activation and TGF-β production; processes that converge to cause albuminuria and glomerulosclerosis.

AGEs including glycoxidation or lipoxidation products such as Nᵋ-(carboxymethyl)lysine, pentosidine, malondialdehyde-lysine accumulate in the expanded mesangial matrix and thickened glomerular basement membranes of early diabetic nephropathy, and in nodular lesions of advanced disease, further suggesting the active role of AGEs for diabetic nephropathy (Suzuki, Miyata, Saotome et al. 1999).

A number of studies have demonstrated that aminoguanidine decreased AGE accumulation and plasma protein trapping in the glomerular basement membrane (Matsumura, Yamagishi, Brownlee 2000). In streptozocin-induced diabetic rats, aminoguanidine treatment for 32 weeks dramatically reduced the level of albumin excretion and prevented the development of mesangial expansion (Soulis-Liparota Cooper, Papazoglou et al. 1991). Furthermore, aminoguanidine treatment was found to prevent albuminuria in diabetic hypertensive rats without affecting blood pressure (Edelstein, Brownlee 1992). Whether inhibition by aminoguanidine of inducible nitric oxide synthase (iNOS) could contribute to these renoprotective effects remains to be elucidated. However, methylguanidine, which inhibits iNOS but not AGE formation, was reported not to retard the development of albuminuria in diabetic rats (Soulis, Cooper, Sastra et al. 1997). These observations suggest that the beneficial effects of aminoguanidine could be mediated predominantly by decreased AGE formation rather than by iNOS inhibition. A recent randomized, double-masked, placebo-controlled study (ACTION I trial) revealed that pimagedineᴿ (aminoguanidine) reduced the decrease in glomerular filtration rate and 24-hour total proteinuria in type 1 diabetic patients (Bolton, Cattran, Williams et al. 2004). Although the time for doubling of serum creatinine, a primary end point of this study, was not significantly improved by pimagedineᴿ treatment ($P = 0.099$), the trial provided the first clinical proof of the concept that blockade of AGE formation could result in a significant attenuation of diabetic nephropathy.

We have found that OPB-9195, a synthetic thiazolidine derivative and novel inhibitor of AGEs, prevented the progression of diabetic nephropathy by lowing serum concentrations of AGEs and their deposition of glomeruli in Otsuka–Long–Evans–Tokushima–Fatty rats, a type 2 diabetes mellitus model animal (Tsuchida, Makita, Yamagishi et al. 1999). OPB-9195 was also found to retard the progression of diabetic nephropathy by blocking type IV collagen production and suppressing overproduction of two growth factors, TGF-β and VEGF.

Recently, Degenhardt and Baynes et al. (Degenhardt, Alderson, Arrington et al. 2002) reported that pyridoxamine inhibited the progression of renal disease and decreases hyperlipidemia and apparent redox imbalances in diabetic rats. Pyridoxamine and aminoguanidine had similar effects on parameters measured, supporting a mechanism of action involving AGE inhibition (Degenhardt, Alderson, Arrington et al. 2002). Although the results of AGE inhibitors in animal models of diabetic nephropathy are promising, effectiveness of these AGE inhibitors must be confirmed by multicenter, randomized, double-blind clinical studies.

Cross Talk between the AGE–RAGE Axis and the RAS in Diabetic Nephropathy

Recent experiments have focused on the interaction of the AGE–RAGE axis and the RAS thought to be critical to the development of diabetic nephropathy. Indeed, angiotensin converting enzyme inhibition reduces the accumulation of renal and serum AGEs, probably via effects on oxidative pathways (Forbes, Cooper, Thallas et al. 2002). Long-term treatment with Ang II receptor 1 antagonist may exert salutary effects on AGEs levels in the rat remnant kidney model, probably due to improved renal function (Sebekova, Schinzel, Munch et al. 1999). Ramipril administration has been recently shown to result in a mild decline of fluorescent non-carboxymethyllysine-AGEs and malondialdehyde concentrations in nondiabetic nephropathy patients (Sebekova, Gazdikova, Syrova et al. 2003). Further, we have recently found that the AGE–RAGE-mediated ROS generation activates TGF-β-Smad signaling and subsequently induces mesangial cell hypertrophy and fibronectin synthesis by autocrine production of Ang II (Fukami, Ueda, Yamagishi et al. 2004). In addition, AGEs induce mitogenesis and collagen production in renal interstitial fibroblasts as well via Ang II-connective tissue growth factor pathway (Lee, Guh, Chen et al. 2005). Moreover, olmesartan medoxomil, an Ang II type 1 receptor blocker, protects against glomerulosclerosis and renal tubular injury in AGE-injected rats, thus further supporting the concept that AGEs could induce renal damage in diabetes partly via the activation of RAS (Yamagishi, Takeuchi, Inoue et al. 2005). We posit a table that presents the etiologies of diabetic nephropathy and its possible therapeutic agents (Table 21.3).

Table 21.3 Diabetic Nephropathy

Etiology	Cellular Pathway	Treatment Regimen
AGE–RAGE	VEGF	Pimagedine
ROS	MCP-1	Pyridoxamine
PKC	TGF-β	OPB-9195
RAS	Smad	Olmesartan
Hyperfiltration		

ROLE OF AGEs IN CVD

Atherosclerotic arterial disease may be manifested clinically as CVD. Deaths from CVD predominate in patients with diabetes of over 30 years' duration and in those diagnosed after 40 years of age. CVD is responsible for about 70% of all causes of death in patients with type 2 diabetes (Laakso 1999). In Framingham study, the incidence of CVD was 2 to 4 times greater in diabetic patients than in general polulation (Haffner, Lehto, Ronnemaa et al. 1998). Conventional risk factors, including hyperlipidemia, hypertension, smoking, obesity, lack of exercise, and a positive family history, contribute similarly to macrovascular complications in type 2 diabetic patients and nondiabetic subjects (Laakso 1999). The levels of these factors in diabetic patients were certainly increased, but not enough to explain the exaggerated risk for macrovascular complications in diabetic population (Standl, Balletshofer, Dahl et al. 1996). Therefore, specific diabetes-related risk factors should be involved in the excess risk in diabetic patients.

A variety of molecular mechanisms underlying the actions of AGEs and their contribution to diabetic macrovascular complications have been proposed (Stitt, Bucala, Vlassara 1997; Bierhaus, Hofmann, Ziegler et al. 1998; Schmidt, Stern 2000; Vlassara, Palace 2002; Wendt, Bucciarelli, Qu et al. 2002). AGEs formed on the extracellular matrix results in decreased elasticity of vasculatures, and quench nitric oxide, which could mediate defective endothelium-dependent vasodilatation in diabetes (Bucala, Tracey, Cerami 1991). AGE modification of low-density lipoprotein (LDL) exhibits impaired plasma clearance and contributes significantly to increased LDL in vivo, thus being involved in atherosclerosis (Bucala, Mitchell, Arnold et al. 1995). Binding of AGEs to RAGE results in generation of intracellular ROS generation and subsequent activation of the redox-sensitive transcription factor NF-κB in vascular wall cells, which promotes the expression of a variety of atherosclerosis-related genes, including ICAM-1, vascular cell adhesion molecule-1, MCP-1, PAI-1, tissue factor, VEGF, and RAGE (Stitt, Bucala, Vlassara 1997; Bierhaus, Hofmann, Ziegler et al. 1998; Schmidt, Stern 2000; Tanaka, Yonekura, Yamagishi et al. 2000; Vlassara, Palace 2002; Wendt, Bucciarelli, Qu et al. 2002). AGEs have the ability to induce osteoblastic differentiation of microvascular pericytes, which would contribute to the development of vascular calcification in accelerated atherosclerosis in diabetes as well (Yamagishi, Fujimori, Yonekura et al. 1999). The interaction of the RAS and AGEs in the development of diabetic macrovascular complications has also been proposed. AGE–RAGE interaction augments

Ang II-induced smooth muscle cell proliferation and activation, thus being involved in accelerated atherosclerosis in diabetes (Shaw, Schmidt, Banes et al. 2003). AGEs have been actually detected within atherosclerotic lesions in both extra- and intracellular locations (Nakamura, Horii, Nishino et al. 1993; Niwa, Katsuzaki, Miyazaki et al. 1997; Sima, Popov, Starodub et al. 1997).

In animal models, Park et al. (1998) has demonstrated that diabetic apolipoprotein E (apoE) null animals receiving soluble RAGE (sRAGE) display a dose-dependent suppression of accelerated atherosclerosis in these mice. Lesions that formed in animals receiving sRAGE appeared largely arrested at the fatty streak stage; the number of complex atherosclerotic lesions was strikingly reduced in diabetic apoE null mice. The tissue and plasma AGE burden was suppressed in diabetic apoE null mice receiving sRAGE, suggesting that the AGE–RAGE-induced oxidative stress generation might participate in AGEs formation themselves. Treatment with sRAGE did not affect the levels of established risk factors in these mice. These observations suggest the active involvement of AGE–RAGE interaction in the pathogenesis in accelerated atherosclerosis in diabetes. The same group has recently reported that the AGE–RAGE system contributes to the atherosclerotic lesion progression as well, and RAGE blockade stabilizes the lesions in these mice (Bucciarelli, Wendt, Qu et al. 2002). Another study shows a correlation between AGE levels and the degree of atheroma in cholesterol-fed rabbits, and aminoguanidine has an antiatherogenic effect in these rabbits by inhibiting AGEs formation (Panagiotopoulos, O'Brien, Bucala et al. 1998). In humans, RAGE overexpression is associated with enhanced inflammatory reaction and cyclooxygenase-2 and prostaglandin E synthase-1 expression in diabetic plaque macrophages, and this effect may contribute to plaque destabilization by inducing culprit metalloproteinase expression (Cipollone, Iezzi, Fazia et al. 2003).

Recently, food-derived AGEs are reported to induce oxidative stress and promote inflammatory signals (Cai, Gao, Zhu et al. 2002). Dietary glycotoxins promote diabetic atherosclerosis in apoE-deficient mice (Lin, Reis, Dore et al. 2002; Lin, Choudhury, Cai et al. 2003). Further, an AGE-poor diet that contained four- to fivefold lower AGE contents for 2 months also decreased serum levels of AGEs and markedly reduced tissue AGE and RAGE expression, numbers of inflammatory cells, tissue factor, VCAM-1, and MCP-1 levels in diabetic apolipoprotein E-deficient mice (Lin, Choudhury, Cai et al. 2003).

Diet is a major environmental source of pro-inflammatory AGEs in humans as well (Vlassara, Cai, Crandall et al. 2002). In diabetic patients, diets with fivefold lower AGE content significantly decreased serum levels of AGEs, soluble form of VCAM-1 and C-reactive protein (CRP), compared to equivalent regular diets (Vlassara, Cai, Crandall et al. 2002). AGE-poor diets also reduced peripheral mononuclear cell tumor necrosis factor-α (TNF-α) expression at both mRNA and protein levels (Vlassara, Cai, Crandall et al. 2002). Further, LDL pooled from diabetic patients on a standard diet for 6 weeks (high AGE-LDL) was more glycated and oxidized than that from diabetic patients on an AGE-poor diet (low AGE-LDL) (Cai, He, Zhu et al. 2004). High AGE-LDL significantly induced soluble form of VCAM-1 expression in human umbilical vein ECs via redox-sensitive MAPK activation, compared to native LDL or low AGE-LDL (Cai, He, Zhu et al. 2004). In addition, AGE pronyl-glycine, a food-derived AGE, was reported to elicit inflammatory response to cellular proliferation in an intestinal cell line, Caco-2, through the RAGE-mediated MAPK activation (Zill, Bek, Hofmann et al. 2003). These observations suggest the causal link between dietary intake of AGEs and proinflammation and vascular injury, thus providing the clinical relevance of dietary AGE restriction in the prevention of accelerated atherosclerosis in diabetes. We have very recently found that PAI-1 and fibrinogen levels are positively associated with serum AGE levels in nondiabetic general population. Food-derived AGEs may also be associated with thrombogenic tendency in nondiabetic subjects (Enomoto, Adachi, Yamagishi et al. 2006).

CONCLUSION

In the DCCT-EDIC, the reduction in the risk of progressive diabetic micro- and macroangipathies resulting from intensive therapy in patients with type 1 diabetes persisted for at least several years, despite increasing hyperglycemia (DCCT-EDIC Research Group 2000; Writing Team for DCCT-EDIC Research Group 2003; Nathan, Lachin, Cleary et al. 2003; Nathan, Cleary, Backlund et al. 2005). These clinical studies strongly suggest that so-called *hyperglycemic memory* is involved in the pathogenesis of diabetic vascular complications, AGE hypothesis seems to be most compatible with this theory. Moreover, large clinical investigations will be needed to clarify whether the inhibition of AGE formation or the blockade of their downstream signaling could prevent the development and progression of vascular complications in diabetes. Until the specific remedy that targets diabetic vascular complications are developed, multifactorial intensified intervention will be a promising therapeutic strategy for the prevention of these devastating disorders.

REFERENCES

Abe R, Shimizu T, Sugawara H et al. 2004. Regulation of human melanoma growth and metastasis by AGE-AGE receptor interactions. *J Invest Dermatol.* 122:461–467.

Adamis AP, Miller JW, Bernal MT et al. 1994. Increased vascular endothelial growth factor levels in the vitreous of eyes with proliferative diabetic retinopathy. *Am J Ophthalmol.* 118:445–450.

Aiello LP, Avery RL, Arrigg PG et al. 1994. Vascular endothelial growth factor in ocular fluid of patients with diabetic retinopathy and other retinal disorders. *N Engl J Med.* 331:1480–1487.

Amano S, Yamagishi S, Kato N et al. 2002. Sorbitol dehydrogenase overexpression potentiates glucose toxicity to cultured retinal pericytes. *Biochem Biophys Res Commun.* 299:183–188.

Amano S, Yamagishi S, Inagaki Y, Okamoto T. 2003. Angiotensin II stimulates platelet-derived growth factor-B gene expression in cultured retinal pericytes through intracellular reactive oxygen species generation. *Int J Tissue React.* 25:51–55.

Amano S, Yamagishi S, Koda Y et al. 2003. Polymorphisms of sorbitol dehydrogenase (SDH) gene and susceptibility to diabetic retinopathy. *Med Hypotheses.* 60:550–551.

Anderson S. 1997. Role of local and systemic angiotensin in diabetic renal disease. *Kidney Int Suppl.* 63:S107–S110.

Antonelli-Orlidge A, Saunders KB, Smith SR, D'Amore PA. 1989. An active form of transforming growth factor-β was produced by co-cultures of ECs and pericytes. *Proc Natl Acad Sci U S A.* 86:4544–4548.

Aoyama I, Shimokata K, Niwa T. 2000. Oral adsorbent AST-120 ameliorates interstitial fibrosis and transforming growth factor-beta(1) expression in spontaneously diabetic (OLETF) rats. *Am J Nephrol.* 20:232–241.

Babaei-Jadidi R, Karachalias N, Ahmed N, Battah S, Thornalley PJ. 2003. Prevention of incipient diabetic nephropathy by high-dose thiamine and benfotiamine. *Diabetes.* 52:2110–2120.

Banba N, Nakamura T, Matsumura M, Kuroda H, Hattori Y, Kasai K. 2000. Possible relationship of monocyte chemoattractant protein-1 with diabetic nephropathy. *Kidney Int.* 58:684–690.

Barile GR, Pachydaki SI, Tari SR et al. 2005. The RAGE axis in early diabetic retinopathy. *Invest Ophthalmol Vis Sci.* 46:2916–2924.

Benjamin LE, Hemo I, Keshet E. 1998. A plasticity window for blood vessel remodelling is defined by pericyte coverage of the preformed endothelial network and is regulated by PDGF-B and VEGF. *Development.* 125:1591–1598.

Bierhaus A, Hofmann MA, Ziegler R, Nawroth PP. 1998. AGEs and their interaction with AGE-receptors in vascular disease and diabetes mellitus. I. The AGE concept. *Cardiovasc Res.* 37:586–600.

Boehm BO, Lang G, Volpert O et al. 2003. Low content of the natural ocular anti-angiogenic agent pigment epithelium-derived factor (PEDF) in aqueous humor predicts progression of diabetic retinopathy. *Diabetologia.* 46:394–400.

Boeri D, Maiello M, Lorenzi M. 2001. Increased prevalence of microthromboses in retinal capillaries of diabetic individuals. *Diabetes.* 50:1432–1439.

Bolton WK, Cattran DC, Williams ME et al. 2004. ACTION I Investigator Group. Randomized trial of an inhibitor of formation of advanced glycation end products in diabetic nephropathy. *Am J Nephrol.* 24:32–40.

Bonnefont-Rousselot D. 2002. Glucose and reactive oxygen species. *Curr Opin Clin Nutr Metab Care.* 5:561–568.

Brownlee M, Vlassara H, Kooney A, Ulrich P, Cerami A. 1986. Aminoguanidine prevents diabetes-induced arterial wall protein cross-linking. *Science.* 232:1629–1632.

Brownlee M, Cerami A, Vlassara H. 1988. Advanced glycosylation end products in tissue and the biochemical basis of diabetic complications. *N Engl J Med.* 318:1315–1321.

Brownlee M. 1994. Lilly Lecture 1993. Glycation and diabetic complications. *Diabetes.* 43:836–841.

Brownlee M. 1995. Advanced protein glycosylation in diabetes and aging. *Ann Rev Med.* 46:223–234.

Brownlee M. 2001. Biochemistry and molecular cell biology of diabetic complications. *Nature.* 414:813–820.

Bucala R, Tracey KJ, Cerami A. 1991. Advanced glycosylation products quench nitric oxide and mediate defective endothelium-dependent vasodilatation in experimental diabetes. *J Clin Invest.* 87:432–438.

Bucala, Cerami A. 1992. Advanced glycosylation: chemistry, biology, and implications for diabetes and aging. *Adv Pharmacol.* 23:1–34.

Bucala R, Mitchell R, Arnold K, Innerarity T, Vlassara H, Cerami, A. 1995. Identification of the major site of apolipoprotein B modification by advanced glycosylation end products blocking uptake by the low density lipoprotein receptor. *J Biol Chem.* 270:10828–10832.

Bucciarelli LG, Wendt T, Qu W et al. 2002. RAGE blockade stabilizes established atherosclerosis in diabetic apolipoprotein E-null mice. *Circulation.* 106:2827–2835.

Cai W, Gao QD, Zhu L, Peppa M, He C, Vlassara H. 2002. Oxidative stress-inducing carbonyl compounds from common foods: novel mediators of cellular dysfunction. *Mol Med.* 8:337–346.

Cai W, He JC, Zhu L et al. 2004. High levels of dietary advanced glycation end products transform low-density lipoprotein into a potent redox-sensitive mitogen-activated protein kinase stimulant in diabetic patients. *Circulation.* 110:285–291.

Chiarelli F, Cipollone F, Mohn A et al. 2002. Circulating monocyte chemoattractant protein-1 and early development of nephropathy in type 1 diabetes. *Diabetes Care.* 25:1829–1834.

Cipollone F, Iezzi A, Fazia M et al. 2003. The receptor RAGE as a progression factor amplifying arachidonate-dependent inflammatory and proteolytic response in human atherosclerotic plaques: role of glycemic control. *Circulation.* 108:1070–1077.

Cogan DG, Toussaint D, Kuwabara T. 1961. Retinal vascular patterns. IV. Diabetic retinopathy. *Arch Ophthalmo.* 66:366–378.

Cooper ME, Bonnet F, Oldfield M, Jandeleit-Dahm K. 2001. Mechanisms of diabetic vasculopathy: an overview. *Am J Hypertens.* 14:475–486.

De Vriese AS, Tilton RG, Elger M, Stephan CC, Kriz W, Lameire. 2001. Antibodies against vascular endothelial growth factor improve early renal dysfunction in experimental diabetes. *J Am Soc Nephrol.* 12:993–1000.

Degenhardt TP, Alderson NL, Arrington DD et al. 2002. Pyridoxamine inhibits early renal disease and dyslipidemia in the streptozotocin-diabetic rat. *Kidney Int.* 6:939–950.

Dworkin LD, Ichikawa I, Brenner BM. 1983. Hormonal modulation of glomerular function. *Am J Physiol.* 244:F95–F104.

Dyer DG, Blackledge JA, Thorpe SR, Baynes JW. 1991. Formation of pentosidine during nonenzymatic browning of proteins by glucose. Identification of glucose and other carbohydrates as possible precursors of pentosidine in vivo. *J Biol Chem.* 266:11654–11660.

Edelstein D, Brownlee M. 1992. Aminoguanidine ameliorates albuminuria in diabetic hypertensive rats. *Diabetologia.* 35:96–97.

Enomoto M, Adachi H, Yamagishi S et al. 2006. Positive association of serum levels of advanced glycation end products with thrombogenic markers in humans. *Metabolism.* 55:912–917.

Fiorreto P, Mauer M, Brocco E et al. 1996. Patterns of renal injury in NIDDM patients with microalbuminuria. *Diabetologia.* 39:1569–1576.

Folkman J, D'Amore PA. 1996. Blood vessel formation: what is its molecular basis? *Cell.* 87:1153–1155.

Forbes JM, Cooper ME, Thallas V et al. 2002. Reduction of the accumulation of advanced glycation end products by ACE inhibition in experimental diabetic nephropathy. *Diabetes.* 51:3274–3282.

Frank RN. 1991. On the pathogenesis of diabetic retinopathy. A 1990 update. *Ophthalmology.* 98:586–593.

Fukami K, Ueda S, Yamagishi S et al. 2004. AGEs activate mesangial TGF-beta-Smad signaling via an angiotensin II type I receptor interaction. *Kidney Int.* 66:2137–2147.

Funatsu H, Yamashita H, Nakanishi Y, Hori S. 2002. Angiotensin II and vascular endothelial growth factor in the vitreous fluid of patients with proliferative diabetic retinopathy. *Br J Ophthalmol.* 86: 311–315.

Gilbert RE, Cooper ME. 1999. The tubulointerstitium in progressive diabetic kidney disease: more than an aftermath of glomerular injury? *Kidney Int.* 56:1627–1637.

Gitlin JD, D'Amore PA. 1983. Culture of retinal capillary cells using selective growth media. *Microvasc Res.* 26:1455–1462.

Glomb MA, Monnier VM. 1995. Mechanism of protein modification by glyoxal and glycolaldehyde, reactive intermediates of the Maillard reaction. *J Biol Chem.* 70:10017–10026.

Goldberg T, Cai W, Peppa M et al. 2004. Advanced glycoxidation end products in commonly consumed foods. *J Am Diet Assoc.* 104:1287–1291.

Grandhee SK, Monnier VM. 1991. Mechanism of formation of the Maillard protein cross-link pentosidine. Glucose, fructose, and ascorbate as pentosidine precursors. *J Biol Chem.* 266:11649–11653.

Haffner SM, Lehto S, Ronnemaa T, Pyorala K, Laakso M. 1998. Mortality from coronary heart disease in subjects with type 2 diabetes and in nondiabetic subjects with

and without prior myocardial infarction. *N Engl J Med.* 339:229–234.

Hammes HP, Martin S, Federlin K, Geisen K, Brownlee M. 1991. Aminoguanidine treatment inhibits the development of experimental diabetic retinopathy. *Proc Natl Acad Sci U S A.* 88:11555–11558.

Hammes HP, Lin J, Renner O et al. 2002. Pericytes and the pathogenesis of diabetic retinopathy. *Diabetes.* 51:3107–3112.

Hammes HP, Du X, Edelstein D et al. 2003. Benfotiamine blocks three major pathways of hyperglycemic damage and prevents experimental diabetic retinopathy. *Nat Med.* 9:294–299.

He C, Sabol J, Mitsuhashi T, Vlassara H. 1999. Dietary glycotoxins: inhibition of reactive products by aminoguanidine facilitates renal clearance and reduces tissue sequestration. *Diabetes.* 48:1308–1315.

Herman IM, D'Amore PA. 1985. Microvascular pericytes contain muscle and nonmuscle actins. *J Cell Biol.* 101:43–52.

Inagaki Y, Yamagishi S, Okamoto T, Takeuchi M, Amano S. 2003. Pigment epithelium-derived factor prevents advanced glycation end products-induced monocyte chemoattractant protein-1 production in microvascular endothelial cells by suppressing intracellular reactive oxygen species generation. *Diabetologia.* 46:284–287.

Ishida S, Usui T, Yamashiro K et al. 2003. VEGF164 is proinflammatory in the diabetic retina. *Invest Ophthalmol Vis Sci.* 44:2155–2162.

Jones SC, Saunders HJ, Qi W, Pollock CA. 1999. Intermittent high glucose enhances cell growth and collagen synthesis in cultured human tubulointerstitial cells. *Diabetologia.* 42:1113–1119.

Jonnes N, Iljin K, Dumont DJ, Alitalo K. 2001. Tie receptors: new modulators of angiogenic and lymphangiogenic responses. *Nat Rev Mol Cell Biol.* 2:257–267.

Joussen AM, Poulaki V, Qin W et al. 2002. Retinal vascular endothelial growth factor induces intercellular adhesion molecule-1 and endothelial nitric oxide synthase expression and initiates early diabetic retinal leukocyte adhesion in vivo. *Am J Pathol.* 160:501–509.

Joyce NC, Haire MF, Palade GE. 1985. Contractile proteins in pericytes. II. Immunocytochemical evidence for the presence of two isomyosins in graded concentrations. *J Cell Biol.* 100:1387–1395.

Kaji Y, Usui T, Ishida S et al. 2007. Inhibition of diabetic leukostasis and blood-retinal barrier breakdown with a soluble form of a receptor for advanced glycation end products. *Invest Ophthalmol Vis Sci.* 48:858–865.

Khalifah RG, Baynes JW, Hudson BG. 1999. Amadorins: novel post-Amadori inhibitors of advanced glycation reactions. *Biochem Biophys Res Commun.* 257:251–258.

Kim NH, Oh JH, Seo JA et al. 2005. Vascular endothelial growth factor (VEGF) and soluble VEGF receptor FLT-1 in diabetic nephropathy. *Kidney Int.* 67:167–177.

Koga K, Yamagishi S, Okamoto T et al. 2002. Serum levels of glucose-derived advanced glycation end products are associated with the severity of diabetic retinopathy in type 2 diabetic patients without renal dysfunction. *Int J Clin Pharmacol Res.* 22:13–17.

Koschinsky T, He CJ, Mitsuhashi T et al. 1997. Orally absorbed reactive glycation products (glycotoxins): an environmental risk factor in diabetic nephropathy. *Proc Natl Acad Sci U S A.* 94:6474–6479.

Kreisberg JI, Venkatachalam M, Troyer D. 1985. Contractile properties of cultured glomerular mesangial cells. *Am J Physiol.* 249:F457–F463.

Krolewski AS, Warram JH, Valsania P et al. 1991. Evolving natural history of coronary artery disease in diabetes mellitus. *Am J Med.* 90:56S–61S.

L'Esperance FA, James WA, Judson PH. 1990. The eye and diabetes mellitus. In Lifkin H, Porte D, ed. *Ellenberg and Rifkin's Diabetes Mellitus, Theory and Practice.* New York: Elsevier. 661–683.

Laakso M. 1999. Hyperglycemia and cardiovascular disease in type 2 diabetes. *Diabetes.* 48:937–942.

Lane PH, Steffes MW, Fioretto P, Mauer SM. 1993. Renal interstitial expansion in insulin-dependent diabetes mellitus. *Kidney Int.* 43:661–667.

Lee CI, Guh JY, Chen HC, Hung WC, Yang YL, Chuang LY. 2005. Advanced glycation end-product-induced mitogenesis and collagen production are dependent on angiotensin II and connective tissue growth factor in NRK-49F cells. *J Cell Biochem.* 95:281–292.

Lin RY, Reis ED, Dore AT et al. 2002. Lowering of dietary advanced glycation endproducts (AGE) reduces neointimal formation after arterial injury in genetically hypercholesterolemic mice. *Atherosclerosis.* 163:303–311.

Lin RY, Choudhury RP, Cai W et al. 2003. Dietary glycotoxins promote diabetic atherosclerosis in apolipoprotein E-deficient mice. *Atherosclerosis.* 68:213–220.

Lu M, Kuroki M, Amano S et al. 1998. Advanced glycation end products increase retinal vascular endothelial growth factor expression. *J Clin Invest.* 101:1219–1224.

Lu M, Perez VL, Ma N et al. 1999. VEGF increases retinal vascular ICAM-1 expression in vivo. *Invest Ophthalmol Vis Sci.* 40:1808–1812.

Maisonpierre PC, Suri C, Jones PF et al. 1997. Angiopoietin-2, a natural antagonist for Tie2 that disrupts in vivo angiogenesis. *Science.* 277:55–60.

Mandarino LJ. 1992. Current hypotheses for the biochemical basis of diabetic retinopathy. *Diabetes Care.* 15:1892–1901.

Matsumura T, Yamagishi S, Brownlee M. 2000. Advanced glycation end products and the pathogenesis of diabetic complications. In Leroith D, Taylor SI, Olefsky JM, ed. *Diabetes Mellitus: a Fundamental and Clinical Text.* New York: Lippincott-Raven Publishers. 983–991.

Mitamura Y, Takeuchi S, Matsuda A, Tagawa, Y Mizue, J Nishihira. 2000. Monocyte chemotactic protein-1 in the vitreous of patients with proliferative diabetic retinopathy. *Ophthalmologica.* 215:415–418.

Miura J, Yamagishi S, Uchigata Y et al. 2003. Serum levels of non-carboxymethyllysine advanced glycation endproducts are correlated to severity of microvascular complications in patients with Type 1 diabetes. *J Diabetes Complications.* 17:16–21.

Moore TC, Moore JE, Kaji Y et al. 2003. The role of advanced glycation end products in retinal microvascular leukostasis. *Invest Ophthalmol Vis Sci.* 44:4457–4464.

Mott JD, Khalifah RG, Nagase H, Shield CF III, Hudson JK, Hudson BG. 1997. Nonenzymatic glycation of type IV collagen and matrix metalloproteinase susceptibility. *Kidney Int.* 52:1302–1312.

Murata T, Ishibashi T, Khalil A et al. 1995. Vascular endothelial growth factor plays a role in hyperpermeability of diabetic retinal vessels. *Ophthalmic Res.* 27:48–52.

Nakamura Y, Horii Y, Nishino T et al. 1993. Immunohistochemical localization of advanced glycosylation end products in coronary atheroma and cardiac tissue in diabetes mellitus. *Am J Pathol.* 143:1649–1656.

Nakamura K, Yamagishi S, Nakamura Y, et al. 2005. Telmisartan inhibits expression of a receptor for advanced glycation end products (RAGE) in angiotensin-II-exposed endothelial cells and decreases serum levels of soluble RAGE in patients with essential hypertension. *Microvasc Res.* 70:137–141.

Nathan DM, Lachin J, Cleary P et al. 2003. Intensive diabetes therapy and carotid intima-media thickness in type 1 diabetes mellitus. *N Engl J Med.* 348:2294–2303.

Nathan DM, Cleary PA, Backlund JY et al. 2005. Intensive diabetes treatment and cardiovascular disease in patients with type 1 diabetes. *N Engl J Med.* 353:2643–2653.

Nishikawa T, Edelstein D, Du XL et al. 2000. Normalizing mitochondrial superoxide production blocks three pathways of hyperglycaemic damage. *Nature.* 404:787–790.

Niwa T, Katsuzaki T, Miyazaki S et al. 1997. Immunohistochemical detection of imidazolone, a novel advanced glycation end product, in kidneys and aortas of diabetic patients. *J Clin Invest.* 99:1272–1280.

Nomura M, Yamagishi S, Harada S et al. 1995. Possible participation of autocrine and paracrine vascular endothelial growth factors in hypoxia-induced proliferation of endothelial cells and pericytes. *J Biol Chem.* 270:28316–28324.

Okamoto T, Yamagishi S, Inagaki Y et al. 2002. Angiogenesis induced by advanced glycation end products and its prevention by cerivastatin. *FASEB J.* 16:1928–1930.

Okamoto T, Yamagishi S, Inagaki Y et al. 2002. Incadronate disodium inhibits advanced glycation end products-induced angiogenesis in vitro. *Biochem Biophys Res Commun.* 297:419–424.

Otani A, Takagi H, Suzuma K, Honda Y. 1998. Angiotensin II potentiates vascular endothelial growth factor-induced angiogenic activity in retinal microcapillary endothelial cells. *Circ Res.* 82:619–628.

Ottonello L, Morone MP, Dapino P, Dallegri F. 1995. Tumor necrosis factor-alpha-induced oxidative burst in neutrophils adherent to fibronectin: effects of cyclic AMP-elevating agents. *Br J Haematol.* 91:566–570.

Panagiotopoulos S, O'Brien RC, Bucala R, Cooper ME, Jerums G. 1998. Aminoguanidine has an anti-atherogenic effect in the cholesterol-fed rabbit. *Atherosclerosis.* 136:125–131.

Park L, Raman KG, Lee KJ et al. 1998. Suppression of accelerated diabetic atherosclerosis by the soluble receptor for advanced glycation endproducts. *Nat Med.* 4:1025–1031.

Raj DS, Choudhury D, Welbourne TC, Levi M. 2000. Advanced glycation end products: a Nephrologist's perspective. *Am J Kidney Dis.* 35:365–380.

Rosen P, Nawroth PP, King G, Moller W, Tritschler HJ, Packer L. 2001. The role of oxidative stress in the onset and progression of diabetes and its complications: a summary of a Congress Series sponsored by UNESCO-MCBN, the American Diabetes Association and the German Diabetes Society. *Diabetes Metab Res Rev.* 17:189–212.

Sato T, Iwaki M, Shimogaito N, X. Wu, S. Yamagishi, M. Takeuchi. 2006. TAGE (toxic AGEs) theory in diabetic complications. *Curr Mol Med.* 6:351–358.

Sato T, Shimogaito N, Wu X, Kikuchi, S.-i. Yamagishi, M. Takeuchi. 2006. Toxic advanced glycation end products (TAGE) theory in Alzheimer's disease. *Am J Alzheimers Dis Other Demen.* 21:197–208.

Schlondorff D. 1987. The glomerular mesangial cell: an expanding role for a specialized pericyte. *FASEB J.* 1:272–281.

Schmidt AM, Stern D. 2000. Atherosclerosis and diabetes: the RAGE connection. *Curr Atheroscler Rep.* 2:430–436.

Schrijvers BF, Flyvbjerg A, Tilton RG, Lameire NH, De Vriese AS. 2006. A neutralizing VEGF antibody prevents glomerular hypertrophy in a model of obese type 2 diabetes, the Zucker diabetic fatty rat. *Nephrol Dial Transplant.* 21:324–329.

Schroder S, Palinski W, Schmid-Schonbein GW. 1991. Activated monocytes and granulocytes, capillary nonperfusion, and neovascularization in diabetic retinopathy. *Am J Pathol.* 139:81–100.

Sebekova K, Schinzel R, Munch G, Krivosikova Z, Dzurik R, Heidland A. 1999. Advanced glycation end-product levels in subtotally nephrectomized rats: beneficial effects of angiotensin II receptor 1 antagonist losartan. *Miner Electrolyte Metab.* 25:380–383.

Sebekova K, Gazdikova K, Syrova D et al. 2003. Effects of ramipril in nondiabetic nephropathy: improved parameters of oxidatives stress and potential modulation of advanced glycation end products. *J Hum Hypertens.* 17:265–270.

Segawa Y, Shirao Y, Yamagishi S et al. 1998. Upregulation of retinal vascular endothelial growth factor mRNAs in spontaneously diabetic rats without ophthalmoscopic retinopathy. A possible participation of advanced glycation end products in the development of the early phase of diabetic retinopathy. *Ophthalmic Res.* 30:333–339.

Sharma K, Ziyadeh FN. 1995. Hyperglycemia and diabetic kidney disease. The case for transforming growth factor-beta as a key mediator. *Diabetes.* 44:1139–1146.

Sharma NK, Gardiner TA, Archer DB. 1985. A morphologic and autoradiographic study of cell death and regeneration in the retinal microvasculature of normal and diabetic rats. *Am J Ophthalmol.* 100:51–60.

Shaw SS, Schmidt AM, Banes AK, Wang X, Stern DM, Marrero MB. 2003. S100B-RAGE-mediated augmentation of angiotensin II-induced activation of JAK2 in vascular smooth muscle cells is dependent on PLD2. *Diabetes.* 52:2381–2388.

Silbiger S, Crowley S, Shan Z, Brownlee M, Satriano J, Schlondorff D. 1993. Nonenzymatic elevated glucose reduces collagen synthesis and proteoglycan charge. *Kidney Int.* 43:853–864.

Sima A, Popov D, Starodub O et al. 1997. Pathobiology of the heart in experimental diabetes: immunolocalization of lipoproteins, immunoglobulin G, and advanced glycation endproducts proteins in diabetic and/or hyperlipidemic hamster. *Lab Invest.* 77:3–18.

Sims DE. 1991. Recent advances in pericyte biology–implications for health and disease. *Can J Cardiol.* 7:431–443.

Soulis T, Cooper ME, Sastra S et al. 1997. Relative contributions of advanced glycation and nitric oxide synthase inhibition to aminoguanidine-mediated renoprotection in diabetic rats. *Diabetologia.* 40:1141–1151.

Soulis-Liparota T, Cooper M, Papazoglou D, Clarke B, Jerums G. 1991. Retardation by aminoguanidine of development of albuminuria, mesangial expansion, and tissue fluorescence in streptozocin-induced diabetic rat. *Diabetes.* 40:1328–1334.

Spitaler MM, Graier WF. 2002. Vascular targets of redox signalling in diabetes mellitus. *Diabetologia.* 45:476–494.

Spranger J, Osterhoff M, Reimann M et al. 2002. Loss of the antiangiogenic pigment epithelium-derived factor in patients with angiogenic eye disease. *Diabetes.* 50:2641–2645.

Standl E, Balletshofer B, Dahl B et al. 1996. Predictors of 10-year macrovascular and overall mortality in patients with NIDDM: the Munich General Practitioner Project. *Diabetologia.* 39:1540–1545.

Stitt A, Gardiner TA, Alderson NL et al. 2002. The AGE inhibitor pyridoxamine inhibits development of retinopathy in experimental diabetes. *Diabetes.* 51:2826–2832.

Stitt AW, Bucala R, Vlassara H. 1997. Atherogenesis and advanced glycation: promotion, progression, and prevention. *Ann N Y Acad Sci.* 811:115–127.

Stitt AW, Li YM, Gardiner TA, et al. 1997. Advanced glycation end products (AGEs) co-localize with AGE receptors in the retinal vasculature of diabetic and AGE-infused rats. *Am J Pathol.* 150:523–531.

Stitt AW, Bhaduri T, McMullen CB, Gardiner TA, Archer DB. 2000. Advanced glycation end products induce blood-retinal barrier dysfunction in normoglycemic rats. *Mol Cell Biol Res Commun.* 3:380–388.

Suzuki D, Miyata T, Saotome N et al. 1999. Immunohistochemical evidence for an increased oxidative stress and carbonyl modification of proteins in diabetic glomerular lesions. *J Am Soc Nephrol.* 10:822–832.

Taft J, Nolan CJ, Yeung SP, Hewitson TD, Martin FI. 1994. Clinical and histological correlations of decline in renal function in diabetic patients with proteinuria. *Diabetes.* 43:1046–1051.

Takenaka K, Yamagishi S, Matsui T, Nakamura K, Imaizumi T. 2006. Role of advanced glycation end products (AGEs) in thrombogenic abnormalities in diabetes. *Curr Neurovasc Res.* 3:73–77.

Takeuchi M, Yamagishi S. 2004. Alternative routes for the formation of glyceraldehyde-derived AGEs (TAGE) in vivo. *Med Hypotheses.* 63:453–455.

Takeuchi M, Yamagishi S. 2004. TAGE (toxic AGEs) hypothesis in various chronic diseases. *Med Hypotheses.* 63:449–452.

Tanaka N, Yonekura H, Yamagishi S et al. 2000. The receptor for advanced glycation end products is induced by the glycation products themselves and tumor necrosis factor-alpha through nuclear factor-kappa B, and by 17beta-estradiol through Sp-1 in human vascular endothelial cells. *J Biol Chem.* 275:25781–25790.

The Diabetes Control and Complications Trial Research Group. 1993. The effect of intensive treatment of diabetes on the development and progression of long-term complications in insulin-dependent diabetes mellitus. *N Engl J Med.* 329:977–986.

The Diabetes Control and Complications Trial/Epidemiology of Diabetes Interventions and Complications Research Group. 2000. Retinopathy and nephropathy in patients with type 1 diabetes four years after a trial of intensive therapy. *N Engl J Med.* 342:381–389.

Thornalley PJ. 2003. Use of aminoguanidine (Pimagedine) to prevent the formation of advanced glycation endproducts. *Arch Biochem Biophys.* 419:31–40.

Tombran-Tink J, Chader CG, Johnson LV. 1991. PEDF: Pigment epithelium-derived factor with potent neuronal differentiative activity. *Exp Eye Res.* 53:411–414.

Tsuchida K, Makita Z, Yamagishi S et al. 1999. Suppression of transforming growth factor beta and vascular endothelial growth factor in diabetic nephropathy in rats by a novel advanced glycation end product inhibitor, OPB-9195. *Diabetologia.* 4:579–588.

UK Prospective Diabetes Study (UKPDS) Group. 1998. Intensive blood-glucose control with sulphonylureas or insulin compared with conventional treatment and risk complications in patients with type 2 diabetes (UKPS 33). *Lancet.* 352:837–853.

Uribarri J, Cai W, Sandu O, Peppa M, Goldberg T, Vlassarah H. 2005. Diet-derived advanced glycation end products are major contributors to the body's AGE pool and induce inflammation in healthy subjects. *Ann N Y Acad Sci.* 1043:461–466.

Van den Enden MK, Nyengaard JR, Ostrow E, Burgan JH, Williamson JR. 1995. Elevated glucose levels increase retinal glycolysis and sorbitol pathway metabolism. Implications for diabetic retinopathy. *Invest Ophthalmol Vis Sci.* 36:1675–1685.

Vasan S, Foiles PG, Founds HW. 2001. Therapeutic potential of AGE inhibitors and breakers of AGE protein cross-links. *Expert Opin Investig Drugs.* 10:1977–1987.

Vlassara H, Bucala R, Striker L. 1994. Pathogenic effects of advanced glycosylation: biochemical, biologic, and clinical implications for diabetes and aging. *Lab Invest.* 70:138–151.

Vlassara H, Striker LJ, Teichberg S et al. 1994. Advanced glycation end products induce glomerular sclerosis and albuminuria in normal rats. *Proc Natl Acad Sci U S A.* 91:11704–11708.

Vlassara H, Cai W, Crandall J et al. 2002. Inflammatory mediators are induced by dietary glycotoxins, a major risk factor for diabetic angiopathy. *Proc Natl Acad Sci U S A.* 99:15596–15601.

Vlassara H, Palace MR. 2002. Diabetes and advanced glycation endproducts. *J Intern Med.* 251:87–101.

Vlassara H. 2005. Advanced glycation in health and disease: role of the modern environment. *Ann N Y Acad Sci.* 1043:452–460.

Voziyan PA, Metz TO, Baynes JW, Hudson BG. 2002. A post-Amadori inhibitor pyridoxamine also inhibits chemical modification of proteins by scavenging carbonyl intermediates of carbohydrate and lipid degradation. *J Biol Chem.* 277:3397–3403.

Wang SN, LaPage J, Hirschberg R. 2000. Role of glomerular ultrafiltration of growth factors in progressive interstitial fibrosis in diabetic nephropathy. *Kidney Int.* 57:1002–1014.

Wendt T, Bucciarelli L, Qu W, Lu Y, Yan SF et al. 2002. Receptor for advanced glycation endproducts (RAGE) and vascular inflammation: insights into the pathogenesis of macrovascular complications in diabetes. *Curr Atheroscler Rep.* 4:228–237.

Wendt TM, Tanji N, Guo J et al. 2003. RAGE drives the development of glomerulosclerosis and implicates podocyte activation in the pathogenesis of diabetic nephropathy. *Am J Pathol.* 162:1123–1137.

Williamson JR, Chang K, Frangos M et al. 1993. Hyperglycemic pseudohypoxia and diabetic complications. *Diabetes.* 42:801–813.

Winocour PH. 2003. In Fisher M, ed. *Heart Disease and Diabetes.* London: Martin Dunitz Ltd. 121–170.

Writing Team For The Diabetes Control And Complications Trial/Epidemiology Of Diabetes Interventions And Complications Research Group. 2003. Sustained effect of intensive treatment of type 1 diabetes mellitus on development and progression of diabetic nephropathy: the Epidemiology of Diabetes Interventions and Complications (EDIC) study. *JAMA.* 290:2159–2167.

Yabe-Nishimura C. 1998. Aldose reductase in glucose toxicity: a potential target for the prevention of diabetic complications. *Pharmacol Rev.* 50:21–33.

Yamagishi S, Hsu CC, Kobayashi K, Yamamoto H. 1993. Endothelin 1 mediates endothelial cell-dependent proliferation of vascular pericytes. *Biochem Biophys Res Commun.* 191:840–846.

Yamagishi S, Kobayashi K, Yamamoto H. 1993. Vascular pericytes not only regulate growth, but also preserve prostacyclin-producing ability and protect against lipid peroxide-induced injury of co-cultured endothelial cells. *Biochem Biophys Res Commun.* 190:418–425.

Yamagishi S, Hsu CC, Taniguchi M et al. 1995. Receptor-mediated toxicity to pericytes of advanced glycosylation end products: a possible mechanism of pericyte loss in diabetic microangiopathy. *Biochem Biophys Res Commun.* 213:681–687.

Yamagishi S, Yamamoto Y, Harada S, Hsu CC, Yamamoto H. 1996. Advanced glycosylation end products stimulate the growth but inhibit the prostacyclin-producing ability of endothelial cells through interactions with their receptors. *FEBS Lett.* 384:103–106.

Yamagishi S, Yonekura H, Yamamoto Y et al. 1997. Advanced glycation end products-driven angiogenesis in vitro. Induction of the growth and tube formation of human microvascular endothelial cells through autocrine vascular endothelial growth factor. *J Biol Chem.* 272:8723–8730.

Yamagishi S, Fujimori H, Yonekura H, Yamamoto Y, Yamamoto H. 1998. Advanced glycation endproducts inhibit prostacyclin production and induce plasminogen activator inhibitor-1 in human microvascular endothelial cells. *Diabetologia.* 41:1435–1441.

Yamagishi S, Fujimori H, Yonekura H, Tanaka N, Yamamoto H. 1999. Advanced glycation endproducts accelerate calcification in microvascular pericytes. *Biochem Biophys Res Commun.* 258:353–357.

Yamagishi S, Kawakami T, Fujimori H et al. 1999. Insulin stimulates the growth and tube formation of human microvascular endothelial cells through autocrine vascular endothelial growth factor. *Microvasc Res.* 57:329–339.

Yamagishi S, Yonekura H, Yamamoto Y et al. 1999. Vascular endothelial growth factor acts as a pericyte mitogen under hypoxic conditions. *Lab Invest.* 79:501–509.

Yamagishi S, Edelstein D, Du XL, Brownlee M. 2001. Hyperglycemia potentiates collagen-induced platelet activation through mitochondrial superoxide overproduction. *Diabetes.* 50:1491–1494.

Yamagishi S, Edelstein D, Du XL, Kaneda Y, Guzman M, Brownlee M. 2001. Leptin induces mitochondrial superoxide production and monocyte chemoattractant protein-1 expression in aortic endothelial cells by increasing fatty acid oxidation via protein kinase A. *J Biol Chem.* 276:25096–25100.

Yamagishi S, Takeuchi M, Makita Z. 2001. Advanced glycation end products and the pathogenesis of diabetic nephropathy. In Tomino Y, ed. *Type-2 Diabetic Nephropathy in Japan, from Bench to Bedside.* Basel: Karger. 30–35.

Yamagishi S, Amano S, Inagaki Y et al. 2002. Advanced glycation end products-induced apoptosis and over-expression of vascular endothelial growth factor in bovine retinal pericytes. *Biochem Biophys Res Commun.* 290:973–978.

Yamagishi S, Amano S, Inagaki Y, Okamoto T, Takeuchi M, Makita Z. 2002. Beraprost sodium, a prostaglandin I_2 analogue, protects against advanced glycation end products-induced injury in cultured retinal pericytes. *Mol Med.* 8:546–550.

Yamagishi S, Inagaki Y, Amano S, Okamoto T, Takeuchi M. 2002. Up-regulation of vascular endothelial growth factor and down-regulation of pigment epithelium-derived factor messenger ribonucleic acid levels in leptin-exposed cultured retinal pericytes. *Int J Tissue React.* 24:137–142.

Yamagishi S, Inagaki Y, Amano S, Okamoto T, Takeuchi M, Makita Z. 2002. Pigment epithelium-derived factor protects cultured retinal pericytes from advanced glycation end product-induced injury through its antioxidative properties. *Biochem Biophys Res Commun.* 296:877–882.

Yamagishi S, Inagaki Y, Okamoto T et al. 2002. Advanced glycation end product-induced apoptosis and overexpression of vascular endothelial growth factor and monocyte chemoattractant protein-1 in human-cultured mesangial cells. *J Biol Chem.* 277:20309–20315.

Yamagishi S, Koga K, Inagaki Y et al. 2002. Dilazep hydrochloride, an antiplatelet drug, prevents progression of diabetic nephropathy in Otsuka Long-Evans Tokushima fatty rats. *Drugs Exp Clin Res.* 28:221–227.

Yamagishi S, Okamoto T, Amano S et al. 2002. Palmitate-induced apoptosis of microvascular endothelial cells and pericytes. *Mol Med.* 8:178–183.

Yamagishi S, Amano S, Inagaki Y, Okamoto T, Takeuchi M, Inoue H. 2003. Pigment epithelium-derived factor inhibits leptin-induced angiogenesis by suppressing vascular endothelial growth factor gene expression through anti-oxidative properties. *Microvasc Res.* 65:186–190.

Yamagishi S, Amano S, Inagaki Y et al. 2003. Angiotensin II-type 1 receptor interaction upregulates vascular endothelial growth factor messenger RNA levels in retinal pericytes through intracellular reactive oxygen species generation. *Drugs Exp Clin Res.* 29:75–80.

Yamagishi S, Inagaki Y, Okamoto T et al. 2003. Advanced glycation end products inhibit de novo protein synthesis and induce TGF-beta overexpression in proximal tubular cells. *Kidney Int.* 63:464–473.

Yamagishi S, Takeuchi M, Inagaki Y, Nakamura K, Imaizumi T. 2003. Role of advanced glycation end products (AGEs) and their receptor (RAGE) in the pathogenesis of diabetic microangiopathy. *Int J Clin Pharmacol Res.* 23:129–134.

Yamagishi S, Nakamura K, Takeuchi M, Imaizumi T. 2004. Molecular mechanism for accelerated atherosclerosis in diabetes and its potential therapeutic intervention. *Int J Clin Pharmacol Res.* 24:129–134.

Yamagishi S, Imaizumi T. 2005. Diabetic vascular complications: pathophysiology, biochemical basis and potential therapeutic strategy. *Curr Pharm Des.* 11:2279–2299.

Yamagishi S, Nakamura K, Inoue H. 2005. Possible participation of advanced glycation end products in the pathogenesis of osteoporosis in diabetic patients. *Med Hypotheses.* 65:1013–1015.

Yamagishi S, Nakamura K, Inoue H, Kikuchi S, Takeuchi M. 2005. Serum or cerebrospinal fluid levels of glyceraldehyde-derived advanced glycation end products (AGEs) may be a promising biomarker for early detection of Alzheimer's disease. *Med Hypotheses.* 64:1205–1207.

Yamagishi S, Takeuchi M, Matsui T et al. 2005. Angiotensin II augments advanced glycation end product-induced pericyte apoptosis through RAGE overexpression. *FEBS Lett.* 579:4265–4270.

Yamagishi S, Takeuchi M, Inoue H. 2005. Olmesartan medoxomil, a newly developed angiotensin II type 1 receptor antagonist, protects against renal damage in advanced glycation end product (age)-injected rats. *Drugs Exp Clin Res.* 31:45–51.

Yamagishi S, Matsui T, Nakamura K, et al. 2006. Pigment epithelium-derived factor (PEDF) prevents diabetes- or advanced glycation end products (AGE)-elicited retinal leukostasis. *Microvasc Res.* 72:86–90.

Yamagishi S, Nakamura K, Matsui T. 2006. Advanced glycation end products (AGEs) and their receptor (RAGE) system in diabetic retinopathy. *Curr Drug Discov Technol.* 3:83–88.

Yamagishi S, Nakamura K, Matsui T et al. 2006. Pigment epithelium-derived factor inhibits advanced glycation end product-induced retinal vascular hyperpermeability by blocking reactive oxygen species-mediated vascular endothelial growth factor expression. *J Biol Chem.* 281:20213–20220.

Yamagishi S, Matsui T, Nakamura K et al. 2007. Pigment-epithelium-derived factor suppresses expression of receptor for advanced glycation end products in the eye of diabetic rats. *Ophthalmic Res.* 39:92–97.

Yamagishi SI, Nakamura K, Matsui T, et al. 2007. Pigment epithelium-derived factor (PEDF) blocks advanced glycation end product (AGE)-induced angiogenesis in vitro. *Horm Metab Res.* 39:233–235.

Yamamoto Y, Kato I, Doi T et al. 2001. Development and prevention of advanced diabetic nephropathy in RAGE-overexpressing mice. *J Clin Invest.* 108:261–268.

Yang CW, Vlassara H, Peten EP et al. 1994. Advanced glycation end products up-regulate gene expression found in diabetic glomerular disease. *Proc Natl Acad Sci U S A.* 91:9436–9440.

Yokoi M, Yamagishi S, Takeuchi M et al. 2005. Elevations of AGE and vascular endothelial growth factor with decreased total antioxidant status in the vitreous fluid of diabetic patients with retinopathy. *Br J Ophthalmol.* 89:673–675.

Yoshida Y, Yamagishi S, Matsui T et al. 2007. Positive correlation of pigment epithelium-derived factor (PEDF) and total anti-oxidant capacity in aqueous humor of patients with uveitis and proliferative diabetic retinopathy. *Br J Ophthalmol.* 91:1133–1134.

Yokoi M, Yamagishi S, Sato A et al. 2007. Positive association of pigment epithelium-derived factor (PEDF) with total anti-oxidant capacity in the vitreous fluid of patients with proliferative diabetic retinopathy. *Br J Ophthalmol.* 91:885–887.

Yokoi M, Yamagishi S, Takeuchi M et al. 2007. Positive correlation between vitreous levels of advanced glycation end products and vascular endothelial growth factor in patients with diabetic retinopathy sufficiently treated with photocoagulation. *Br J Ophthalmol.* 91:397–398.

Zill H, Bek S, Hofmann T et al. 2003. RAGE-mediated MAPK activation by food-derived AGE and non-AGE products. *Biochem Biophys Res Commun.* 300:311–315.

Ziyadeh FN, Goldfarb S. 1991. The renal tubulointerstitium in diabetes mellitus. *Kidney Int.* 39:464–475.

Ziyadeh FN, Hoffman BB, Han DC et al. 2000. Long-term prevention of renal insufficiency, excess matrix gene expression, and glomerular mesangial matrix expansion by treatment with monoclonal antitransforming growth factor-beta antibody in db/db diabetic mice. *Proc Natl Acad Sci U S A.* 97:8015–8020.

Chapter 22

REDUCING OXIDATIVE STRESS AND ENHANCING NEUROVASCULAR LONGEVITY DURING DIABETES MELLITUS

Kenneth Maiese, Zhao Zhong Chong, and Faqi Li

ABSTRACT

Our book *Neurovascular Medicine: Pursuing Cellular Longevity for Healthy Aging* provides a unique perspective from a diverse group of internationally recognized investigators with a broad range of experience in neuronal, vascular, and immune-mediated disease processes to translate basic cellular mechanisms into viable therapeutic measures. Yet, as with any form of published literature, the work presented is not all encompassing and intends to not only highlight and explore new avenues to extend cell longevity for healthy aging but also outline the potential concerns and limitations of novel treatment approaches for patients. With this in mind, this concluding chapter of the book serves to exemplify the raves and risks of novel therapeutic strategies that are translational in nature by focusing upon the complications of oxidative stress and diabetes mellitus in the neuronal and vascular systems.

Both type 1 and type 2 diabetes mellitus (DM) can lead to significant disability in the nervous and cardiovascular systems, such as cognitive loss and cardiac insufficiency. Intimately connected to these disorders in the nervous and vascular systems are the pathways of oxidative stress. Furthermore, oxidative stress is a principal pathway for the destruction of cells in several disease entities including diabetes mellitus. As a result, innovative strategies that directly target oxidative stress to preserve neuronal and vascular longevity could offer viable therapeutic options to diabetic patients in addition to the more conventional treatments that are designed to control serum glucose levels. Here we discuss the novel applications of nicotinamide, Wnt signaling, and erythropoietin (EPO) that modulate cellular oxidative stress and offer significant promise for the prevention of diabetic complications in the nervous and vascular systems. Essential to this process is the precise focus upon the cellular pathways governed by nicotinamide, Wnt signaling, and EPO to avoid detrimental clinical complications and offer the development of effective and safe future therapy for patients.

Keywords: endothelial, neurodegeneration, oxidative stress, erythropoietin, Wnt, FoxO, forkhead, nicotinamide, diabetes, cardiovascular.

THE CLINICAL RELEVANCE OF DM IN THE NEUROVASCULAR SYSTEMS

DM is a significant health concern in the clinical population (Maiese, Chong, Shang 2007a). The disease is present in at least 16 million individuals in the United States and in more than 165 million individuals worldwide (Quinn 2001). Furthermore, by the year 2030, it is predicted that more than 360 million individuals will be affected by DM (Wild, Roglic, Green et al. 2004). At least 80% of all diabetic patients have type 2 DM, which is increasing in incidence as a result of changes in human behavior relating to diet and daily exercise (Laakso 2001). Although type 1 (insulin-dependent) DM accounts for only 5% to 10% of all diabetic patients (Maiese, Morhan, Chong 2007c), its incidence is increasing in adolescent minority groups (Dabelea, Bell, D'Agostino et al. 2007). Of potentially greater concern is the incidence of undiagnosed diabetes that consists of impaired glucose tolerance and fluctuations in serum glucose levels that can increase the risk for the development of DM (Jacobson, Musen, Ryan et al. 2007). Individuals with impaired glucose tolerance have a more than two times the risk for the development of diabetic complications than individuals with normal glucose tolerance (Harris, Eastman 2000).

Both acute and long-term occurrence of type 1 and type 2 DM can result in complications of the neuronal and vascular systems. For example, DM can impair vascular integrity and alter cardiac output (Donahoe, Stewart, McCabe et al. 2007), which eventually diminish the capacity of sensitive cognitive regions of the brain, leading to functional impairment and dementia (Schnaider Beeri, Goldbourt, Silverman et al. 2004; Chong, Li, Maiese 2005b; Li, Chong, Maiese 2006a). Disease of the nervous system can become the most debilitating complication for DM and affect the sensitive cognitive regions of the brain, such as the hippocampus that modulates memory function, resulting in significant functional impairment and dementia (Awad, Gagnon, Messier 2004). DM has also been found to increase the risk for vascular dementia in elderly subjects (Schnaider Beeri, Goldbourt, Silverman et al. 2004; Xu, Qiu, Wahlin et al. 2004), as well as potentially alter the course of Alzheimer's disease. Although some studies have found that diabetic patients may have less neuritic plaques and neurofibrillary tangles than nondiabetic patients (Beeri, Silverman, Davis et al. 2005), contrasting work suggests the modest adjusted relative risk of Alzheimer's disease in patients with diabetes as compared with those without diabetes to be 1.3 (Luchsinger, Tang, Stern et al. 2001). Furthermore,

costs to care for cognitive impairments resulting from diabetes that can mimic Alzheimer's disease can approach $100 billion a year (McCormick, Hardy, Kukull et al. 2001; Mendiondo, Kryscio, Schmitt 2001; Maiese, Chong 2004).

OXIDATIVE PATHWAYS AND DM

Closely tied to the development of insulin resistance and the complications of DM in the nervous and vascular systems is the presence of cellular oxidative stress and the release of reactive oxygen species (Maiese, Morhan, Chong 2007c). Oxidative stress occurs as a result of the development of reactive oxygen species that consist of oxygen free radicals and other chemical entities. Oxygen consumption in organisms, or at least the rate of oxygen consumption in organisms, has intrigued a host of investigators and may have had some of its origins in the work of Pearl. Pearl proposed that increased exposure to oxygen through an increased metabolic rate could lead to a shortened lifespan (Pearl, 1928). Subsequent work by multiple investigators has furthered this hypothesis by demonstrating that increased metabolic rates could be detrimental to animals in an environment of elevated oxygen (Muller, Lustgarten, Jang et al. 2007). When one moves to more current work, oxygen free radicals and mitochondrial DNA mutations have become associated with oxidative stress injury, aging mechanisms, and accumulated toxicity in an organism (Yui, Matsuura 2006).

Oxidative stress represents a significant mechanism for the destruction of cells that can involve apoptotic neuronal and vascular cell injury (Lin, Maiese 2001; Chong, Li, Maiese 2006b; De Felice, Velasco, Lambert et al. 2007). In fact, it has recently been shown that genes involved in the apoptotic process are replicated early during processes that involve cell replication and transcription, suggesting a much broader role for these genes than originally anticipated (Cohen, Cordeiro-Stone, Kaufman 2007). Apoptotic-induced oxidative stress in conjunction with processes of mitochondrial dysfunction can contribute to a variety of disease states such as diabetes, ischemia, general cognitive loss, Alzheimer's disease, and trauma (Chong, Li, Maiese 2005b, 2005d; Harris, Fox, Wright et al. 2007; Leuner, Hauptmann, Abdel-Kader et al. 2007; Okouchi, Ekshyyan, Maracine et al. 2007). Oxidative stress can lead to apoptosis in a variety of cell types including neurons, endothelial cells (ECs), cardiomyocytes, and smooth muscle cells through multiple cellular pathways (Kang, Chong, Maiese 2003b; Chong, Kang, Maiese 2004a; Harris, Fox, Wright et al. 2007; Karunakaran, Diwakar, Saeed et al. 2007; Verdaguer, Susana Gde, Clemens et al. 2007; Chong Li, Maiese et al. 2007c).

Membrane phosphatidylserine (PS) externalization is an early event during cell apoptosis (Maiese, Vincent, Lin et al. 2000; Mari, Karabiyikoglu, Goris et al. 2004) and can signal the phagocytosis of cells (Lin, Maiese 2001; Chong, Kang, Li et al. 2005e; Li, Chong, Maiese 2006c). The loss of membrane phospholipid asymmetry leads to the externalization of membrane PS residues and assists microglia to target cells for phagocytosis (Maiese, Chong 2003; Kang, Chong, Maiese 2003a, 2003b; Chong, Kang, Maiese 2003c; Mallat, Marin-Teva, Cheret 2005). This process occurs with the expression of the phosphatidylserine receptor (PSR) on microglia during oxidative stress (Li, Chong, Maiese 2006a, 2006b), since blockade of PSR function in microglia prevents the activation of microglia (Kang, Chong, Maiese 2003a; Chong, Kang, Maiese 2003b). As an example, externalization of membrane PS residues occurs in neurons during anoxia (Maiese, Boccone 1995; Vincent, Maiese 1999b; Maiese 2001), during nitric oxide exposure (Maiese, TenBroeke, Kue 1997; Chong, Lin, Kang et al. 2003e), and during the administration of agents that induce the production of reactive oxygen species, such as 6-hydroxydopamine (Salinas, Diaz, Abraham et al. 2003). Membrane PS externalization on platelets has also been associated with clot formation in the vascular system (Leytin, Allen, Mykhaylov et al. 2006).

The cleavage of genomic DNA into fragments (Maiese, Ahmad, TenBroeke et al. 1999; Maiese, Vincent 2000a, 2000b) is considered to be a later event during apoptotic injury (Chong, Kang Maiese 2004c). Several enzymes responsible for DNA degradation have been differentiated and include the acidic, cation-independent endonuclease (DNase II), cyclophilins, and the 97-kDa magnesium-dependent endonuclease (Chong, Li, Maiese 2005b; Chong, Maiese 2007b). Three separate endonuclease activities are present in neurons that include a constitutive acidic cation-independent endonuclease, a constitutive calcium-/magnesium-dependent endonuclease, and an inducible magnesium-dependent endonuclease (Vincent, Maiese 1999a; Vincent, TenBroeke, Maiese 1999a).

During oxidative stress, the mitochondrial membrane transition pore permeability is also increased (Lin, Vincent, Shaw 2000; Di Lisa, Menabo, Canton et al. 2001; Chong, Kang, Maiese 2003a; Kang, Chong, Maiese 2003b), a significant loss of mitochondrial nicotinamide adenine dinucleotide (NAD^+) stores occurs, and further generation of superoxide radicals leads to cell injury (Maiese, Chong 2003; Chong, Lin, Li et al. 2005f). In addition, mitochondria are a significant source of superoxide radicals that are associated with oxidative stress (Maiese, Chong 2004; Chong, Li, Maiese 2005b). Blockade of the electron transfer chain at the flavin mononucleotide group of complex I or at the ubiquinone site of complex III results in the active generation of free radicals that can impair mitochondrial electron transport and enhance free radical production (Li, Chong, Maiese 2006a; Chong, Maiese 2007b). Furthermore, mutations in the mitochondrial genome have been associated with the potential development of a host of disorders, such as hypertension, hypercholesterolemia, and hypomagnesemia (Wilson, Hariri, Farhi et al. 2004; Li, Chong, Maiese 2004b). Reactive oxygen species may also lead to the induction of acidosis-induced cellular toxicity and subsequent mitochondrial failure (Chong, Li, Maiese 2005d). Disorders, such as hypoxia (Roberts, Chih 1997), diabetes (Cardella 2005; Kratzsch, Knerr, Galler et al. 2006), and excessive free radical production (Ito, Bartunek, Spitzer et al. 1997; Vincent, TenBroeke, Maiese 1999a, 1999b), can result in the disturbance of intracellular pH.

In disorders such as DM, elevated levels of ceruloplasmin have been suggested to represent increased concentration of reactive oxygen species (Memisogullari, Bakan 2004) and acute glucose fluctuations have been described as a potential source of oxidative stress (Monnier, Mas, Ginet et al. 2006). Elevated serum glucose levels have also been shown to lead to increased production of reactive oxygen species in ECs, but prolonged duration of hyperglycemia is not necessary to lead to oxidative stress injury, since even short periods of hyperglycemia can generate reactive oxygen species in vascular cells (Yano, Hasegawa, Ishii et al. 2004). Recent clinical correlates support these experimental studies to show that acute glucose swings in addition to chronic hyperglycemia can trigger oxidative stress mechanisms during type 2 DM, illustrating the importance of therapeutic interventions during acute and sustained hyperglycemic episodes (Monnier, Mas, Ginet et al. 2006).

The maintenance of cellular energy reserves and mitochondrial integrity also becomes a significant factor in DM (Newsholme, Haber, Hirabara et al. 2007). During DM, fatty acid accumulation leads to both the generation of reactive oxygen species and mitochondrial DNA damage (Rachek, Thornley, Grishko et al. 2006). A decrease in the levels of mitochondrial proteins and mitochondrial DNA in adipocytes has been correlated with the development of type 2 DM (Choo, Kim, Kwon et al. 2006). In addition, insulin resistance in the elderly has been linked to fat accumulation and reduction in mitochondrial oxidative and phosphorylation activity (Petersen, Befroy, Dufour et al. 2003; Pospisilik, Knauf, Joza et al. 2007).

INNOVATIVE DIRECTIONS FOR NEUROVASCULAR PROTECTION DURING DM

Possible pathways that may decrease neuronal and vascular longevity during DM are broad in scope and involve multiple precipitating factors. Yet, oxidative stress-induced cellular signaling is believed to be a significant factor responsible for cell injury that is initially set in motion following hyperglycemia. For example, studies have shown that administration of insulin or insulin growth factor at concentrations that were insufficient to reverse hyperglycemia could nevertheless reduce oxidative stress injury to cells and maintain mitochondrial inner membrane potential (Maiese, Chong, Shang 2007a; Maiese, Morhan, Chong 2007c). As a result, innovative strategies that directly target the reduction of oxidative stress toxicity to neuronal and vascular cells could offer viable therapeutic options to patients with DM in addition to the more conventional treatments that are targeted to control serum glucose levels.

A Growth Factor and Cytokine

EPO is a 30.4-kDa glycoprotein with approximately 50% of its molecular weight derived from carbohydrates (Maiese, Li, Chong 2005b). As a growth factor and cytokine, EPO is considered to be ubiquitous in the body (Maiese, Chong, Shang 2007a; Maiese, Morhan, Chong 2007c), since it can be detected in the breath of healthy individuals (Schumann, Triantafilou, Krueger et al. 2006). EPO may also provide developmental cognitive support in humans, with the recent observations that elevated EPO concentrations during infant maturation have been correlated with increased Mental Development Index scores (Bierer, Peceny, Hartenberger et al. 2006). Although EPO is currently approved for the treatment of anemia, the role of EPO has become far more reaching beyond the need for erythropoiesis in other organs and tissues, such as the brain, heart, and vascular system (Chong, Kang, Maiese 2002b, 2003b; Moon, Krawczyk, Paik et al. 2006; Mikati, Hokayem, Sabban 2007; Um, Gross, Lodish 2007; Chong, Maiese 2007a).

It is the discovery of EPO and the EPO receptor (EPOR) in the nervous and vascular systems that has resulted in a heightened level of interest and enthusiasm in the potential clinical applications of EPO, such as in Alzheimer's disease, cardiac insufficiency (Palazzuoli, Silverberg, Iovine et al. 2006; Assaraf, Diaz, Liberman et al. 2007), and cardiac transplantation (Gleissner, Klingenberg, Staritz et al. 2006; Mocini, Leone, Tubaro et al. 2007). The primary organs of EPO production and secretion are the kidney, liver, brain, and uterus. EPO production and secretion occurs foremost in the kidney (Fliser, Haller 2007). The kidney peritubular interstitial cells are responsible for the production and secretion of EPO (Fisher 2003). With the use of cDNA probes derived from the *EPO* gene, peritubular ECs, tubular epithelial cells, and nephron segments in the kidney have also been demonstrated to be vital cells for the production and secretion of EPO (Lacombe, Da Silva, Bruneval et al. 1991; Mujais, Beru, Pullman et al. 1999). During periods of acute renal failure, EPO may provide assistance for the protection of nephrons (Sharples, Thiemermann, Yaqoob 2005; Sharples, Yaqoob 2006). Secondary sites of EPO production and secretion are the liver and the uterus (Chong, Kang, Maiese 2002c). Hepatocytes, hepatoma cells, and Kupffer cells of the liver can produce EPO (Fisher 2003), and in turn, EPO may provide a protective environment for these cells (Schmeding, Neumann, Boas-Knoop et al. 2007). In regards to the uterine production of EPO, it is believed that neonatal anemia that can occur in the early weeks after birth may partly result from the loss of EPO production and secretion by the placenta (Davis, Widness, Brace 2003). In the nervous system, the major sites of EPO production and secretion are in the hippocampus, internal capsule, cortex, midbrain, cerebral ECs, and astrocytes (Chong, Kang, Maiese 2002c; Li, Chong, Maiese 2004a). Further work has revealed several other organs as secretory tissues for EPO that include peripheral ECs (Anagnostou, Liu, Steiner et al. 1994), myoblasts (Ogilvie, Yu, Nicolas-Metral et al. 2000), insulin-producing cells (Fenjves, Ochoa, Cabrera et al. 2003), and cardiac tissue (Maiese, Li, Chong 2005b; Fliser, Haller 2007).

As a strong cytoprotectant against oxidative stress, EPO can enhance the survival of a number of cells in the nervous system (Maiese, Li, Chong 2004, 2005b; Lykissas, Korompilias, Vekris et al. 2007) (Table 22.1). In cells of the brain or the retina, EPO can prevent injury from hypoxic ischemia (Chong, Kang, Maiese 2002b, 2003b; Yu, Xu, Zhang et al. 2005; Liu, Suzuki, Guo et al. 2006; Meloni, Tilbrook, Boulos et al. 2006), excitotoxicity (Yamasaki, Mishima, Yamashita et al. 2005; Montero, Poulsen, Noraberg et al. 2007), infection (Kaiser, Texier, Ferrandiz et al. 2006), free radical exposure (Chong, Kang, Maiese 2003a; Chong, Lin, Kang et al. 2003d; Yamasaki, Mishima, Yamashita et al. 2005), amyloid exposure (Chong, Li, Maiese 2005c), staurosporine (Pregi, Vittori, Perez et al. 2006), and dopaminergic cell injury (McLeod, Hong, Mukhida et al. 2006). In addition, administration of EPO also represents a viable option for the prevention of retinal cell injury during glutamate toxicity (Zhong, Yao, Deng et al. 2007) and glaucoma (Tsai, Song, Wu

Table 22.1 Therapeutic Potential and Adverse Effects of Erythropoietin

Therapeutic Potential	Outcomes	Selected References
Diabetes mellitus	Cytoprotection Cardiac function improvement	Silverberg et al. 2006; Chong et al. 2007b
Alzheimer's disease	Neuroprotection	Chong et al. 2005c; Assaraf et al. 2007
Epilepsy	Decrease epileptic activity	Mikati et al. 2007; Nadam et al. 2007
Parkinson's disease	Reduce functional diability	McLeod et al. 2006
Cardiac transplantation	Resolution of anemia	Gleissner et al. 2006
Congestive heart failure or anemia	Functional tolerance is increased, improvement in left ventricular function and renal function	Maiese et al., 2005b; Palazzuoli et al. 2006, 2007
Chronic heart failure	Functional capacity is increased	Goldberg et al. 1992; Mancini et al. 2003
Acute renal failure	Nephron protection	Sharples et al. 2005; Sharples, Yaqoob 2006
Cerebral ischemia	Neuroprotection	Yu et al. 2005; Zhang et al. 2006
Subarachnoid hemorrhage	Autoregulation of cerebral blood flow, basilar artery dilation, and neuroprotection	Olsen 2003
Neurotrauma	Neuroprotection and functional improvement	King et al. 2007; Okutan et al. 2007; Verdonck et al. 2007; Cherian et al. 2007
Adverse effects		
Vascular intima hyperplasia	Excessive neointima formation	Reddy et al. 2007
Thrombosis	Increase in mortality	Corwin et al. 2007
Cardiac dysfunction	Potential impaired prognosis with elevated erythropoietin levels	van der Meer et al. 2007
Cancer progression	Tumor cell growth is increased, progression of metastases, survival of cancer patients is decreased	Leyland-Jones et al. 2005; Hardee et al. 2006; Lai, Grandis 2006

et al. 2007). Systemic application of EPO also can improve functional outcome and reduce cell loss during spinal cord injury (King, Averill, Hewazy et al. 2007; Okutan, Solaroglu, Beskonakli et al. 2007), traumatic cerebral edema (Verdonck, Lahrech, Francony et al. 2007), cortical trauma (Cherian, Goodman, Robertson 2007), and epileptic activity (Mikati, Hokayem, Sabban 2007; Nadam, Navarro, Sanchez et al. 2007). In direct relation to the potential cerebroprotective effects of EPO, enhanced survival by EPO also extends to afford protection to the neurovascular unit during cerebral vascular disease (Maiese, Chong 2004; Keogh, Yu, Wei 2007). In addition, EPO can protect sensitive hippocampal neurons from both focal and global ischemic brain injury (Yu, Xu, Zhang et al. 2005; Zhang, Signore, Zhou et al. 2006). Systemic administration of EPO also represents a viable option for several other disorders. EPO administration for retinal cell injury can protect retinal ganglion cells from apoptosis (Grimm, Wenzel, Groszer et al. 2002); EPO can also improve functional outcome and reduce lipid peroxidation during spinal cord injury (Kaptanoglu, Solaroglu, Okutan et al. 2004), and can maintain autoregulation of cerebral blood flow, reverse basilar artery

vasoconstriction, and enhance neuronal survival and functional recovery following subarachnoid hemorrhage (Olsen 2003).

EPO also plays a significant role in the cardiovascular system (Maiese, Li, Chong 2004, 2005b) and in the renal system (Sharples, Yaqoob 2006) to limit injury from oxidative stress that can ultimately affect the function of the nervous system (Table 22.1). For example, in patients with anemia, EPO administration can increase left ventricular ejection fraction and stroke volume (Goldberg, Lundin, Delano et al. 1992). More recent studies have shown that patients with acute myocardial infarction have increased plasma EPO levels within 7 days of a cardiac insult, suggesting a possible protective response from the body (Ferrario, Massa, Rosti et al. 2007). In addition, EPO administration in patients with anemia and congestive heart failure can improve exercise tolerance, renal function, and left ventricular systolic function (Palazzuoli, Silverberg, Iovine et al. 2006, 2007). Tightly integrated with cardiac performance, pulmonary function is also believed to be enhanced during EPO administration, especially in the setting of ischemic reperfusion injury of the lung (Wu, Ren, Zhu et al. 2006). Serum levels of EPO may also function as a biomarker of cardiovascular injury (Fu, Van Eyk 2006). Work from experimental studies illustrates that EPO plays a critical role in the vascular and renal systems by maintaining erythrocyte (Foller, Kasinathan, Koka et al. 2007) and podocyte (Eto Wada, Inagi et al. 2007) integrity , regulating the survival of ECs (Chong, Kang, Maiese 2002b, 2003a), and acting as a powerful endogenous protectant during cardiac injury (Asaumi, Kagaya, Takeda et al. 2007).

In light of the fact that during elevated glucose concentrations antioxidants can block free radical production and prevent the production of advanced glycation end-products known to produce reactive oxygen species and oxidative stress during DM (Giardino, Edelstein, Brownlee 1996), EPO may

offer an attractive alternative therapy to maintain proper cellular metabolism and mitochondrial membrane potential ($\Delta\Psi_m$) during DM (Fig. 22.1). In clinical studies with DM, plasma EPO level is often low in diabetic patients with anemia (Mojiminiyi, Abdella, Zaki et al. 2006) or without anemia (Symeonidis, Kouraklis-Symeonidis, Psiroyiannis et al. 2006). Furthermore, the failure of these individuals to produce EPO in response to a declining hemoglobin level suggests an impaired EPO response in diabetic patients (Thomas, Cooper, Tsalamandris et al. 2005). Yet, increased EPO secretion during diabetic pregnancies may represent the body's attempt at endogenous protection against the complications of DM (Teramo, Kari, Eronen et al. 2004). Similar to the

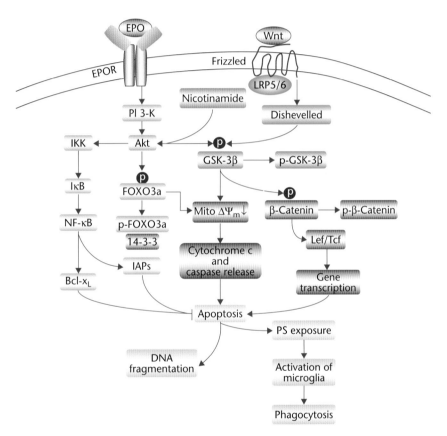

Figure 22.1 Erythropoietin (EPO), nicotinamide, and Wnt use diverse as well as common pathways to foster cellular longevity. EPO and the EPO receptor (EPOR) can increase cellular longevity through protein kinase B (Akt), the forkhead transcription factor family member FOXO3a, glycogen synthase kinase-3β (GSK-3β), nuclear factor-κB (NF-κB), and Bcl-xL. Similar to EPO, nicotinamide modulates the activity of FOXO3a through phosphorylation (p) along with 14–3-3 protein and can maintain cellular integrity and prevent inflammatory activation of microglia that ultimately can lead to apoptosis through the maintenance of mitochondrial membrane potential (ΔΨm), the release of cytochrome c, and the prevention of caspase activation. Wnt signaling begins with Frizzled receptors resulting in the activation of Dishevelled followed by the inhibition of glycogen synthase kinase (GSK-3β) through phosphorylation (p). The suppressed GSK-3β along with other Wnt signaling complexes prevents phosphorylation (p) of β-catenin and leads to the accumulation of β-catenin. β-catenin enters into cellular nucleus and contributes to the formation of lymphocyte enhancer factor/T cell factor (Lef/Tcf) and the β-catenin complex that leads to gene transcription, resulting in cellular proliferation, differentiation, survival, and apoptosis. Interconnected pathways with EPO, nicotinamide, and Wnt involve IκB kinase (IKK), IκB, inhibitors of apoptotic protein (IAPs), GSK-3β, NF-κB, mitochondrial membrane potential (ΔΨm), and cytochrome c. Ultimately, these pathways converge upon early apoptotic injury with phosphatidylserine (PS) exposure and later apoptotic DNA degradation that can impact the activation of microglia. PI3-K, phosphatidylinositol-3-kinase.

potential protective role of insulin (Duarte, Proenca, Oliveira et al. 2006), EPO administration has been shown both in diabetic and nondiabetic patients with severe, resistant congestive heart failure to decrease fatigue, increase left ventricular ejection fraction, and significantly decrease the number of hospitalization days (Silverberg, Wexler, Iaina et al. 2006). In studies that examine the toxic effects of elevated glucose levels upon vascular cells, EPO was found to be protective and prevent early apoptotic membrane PS exposure and late DNA degradation at concentrations that were clinically relevant (Chong, Kang, Maiese 2002b) to cellular protection in patients with cardiac or renal disease (Mason-Garcia, Beckman, Brookins et al. 1990; Namiuchi, Kagaya, Ohta et al. 2005).

Also relevant to cellular metabolism and DM management, cellular protection by EPO is closely tied to protein kinase B (Akt) to prevent cell injury and the subsequent induction of the apoptotic cascades (Chong, Kang, Maiese 2002b; Mikati, Hokayem, Sabban 2007; Chong, Maiese 2007a) (Fig. 22.1). Phosphorylation of Akt leads to its activation and protects cells against genomic DNA degradation and membrane PS exposure (Chong, Kang, Maiese 2003a, 2003b; Chong, Lin, Kang et al. 2003d). Upregulation of Akt activity during multiple injury paradigms, such as vascular and cardiomyocyte ischemia (Parsa, Matsumoto, Kim et al. 2003; Miki, Miura, Yano et al. 2006), free radical exposure (Matsuzaki, Tamatani, Mitsuda et al. 1999; Chong, Kang, Maiese 2003b), N-methyl-D-aspartate toxicity (Dzietko, Felderhoff-Mueser, Sifringer et al. 2004), hypoxia (Chong, Kang, Maiese 2002b; Zhang, Park, Gidday et al. 2007), β-amyloid toxicity (Nakagami, Nishimura, Murasugi et al. 2002; Du, Ohmichi, Takahashi et al. 2004; Chong, Li, Maiese 2005c), DNA damage (Henry, Lynch, Eapen et al. 2001; Chong, Kang, Maiese 2002b; Kang, Chong, Maiese 2003a; Chong, Kang, Maiese

2004a), heat-acclimation protection (Shein, Tsenter, Alexandrovich et al. 2007), metabotropic receptor signaling (Maiese, Chong, Li 2005a; Chong, Kang Li et al. 2005e; Chong, Li, Maiese 2006a), cell metabolic pathways (Maiese, Chong 2003; Chong, Lin, Li et al. 2005f), and oxidative stress (Kang, Chong, Maiese 2003a, 2003b; Chong, Kang, Maiese 2004a), increases cell survival and protects against these toxic insults. Cytoprotection through Akt also can involve control of inflammatory cell activation (Chong, Kang, Maiese 2003a; Kang, Chong, Maiese 2003a, 2003b), transcription factor regulation (Chong, Maiese 2007a), maintenance of mitochondrial membrane potential ($\Delta\Psi_m$), prevention of cytochrome c release (Chong, Kang, Maiese 2003a, 2003b; Chong, Lin, Kang et al. 2003d), and blockade of caspase activity (Chong, Kang, Maiese 2002b, 2003a, 2003b), each of which is relevant to the protection offered by EPO (Maiese, Chong, Kang 2003) (Table 22.2).

Other studies suggest that EPO interfaces with the mammalian forkhead transcription factor family that oversees processes that can involve cell metabolism, hormone modulation, and apoptosis (Cuesta, Zaret, Santisteban 2007; Maiese, Chong, Shang 2007a; Maiese, Chong, Shang 2007b). The first member of this family was the *Drosophila melanogaster* gene *Forkhead*. Since this time, more than 100 *forkhead* genes and 19 human subgroups extending from FOXA to FOXS have been discovered (Maiese, Chong, Shang 2007b). The forkhead box (*FOX*) family of genes is characterized by a conserved forkhead domain commonly noted as a "forkhead box" or a "winged helix" as a result of the butterfly-like appearance on X-ray crystallography (Clark, Halay, Lai et al. 1993) and nuclear magnetic resonance (Jin, Marsden, Chen et al. 1998). All Fox proteins contain the 100-amino acid winged helix domain, but it should be noted that not all winged helix domains are Fox proteins (Larson, Eilers, Menon et al. 2007).

Table 22.2 Cellular Pathways Modulated by Erythropoietin

Cellular Mechanisms	Possible Biological and Clinical Effects	Selected References
Akt activation and maintenance of mitochondrial potential	Inhibition of cytochrome c release and apoptosis; increase in cell survival	Chong et al. 2002b; Parsa et al. 2003; Miki et al. 2006; Chong, Maiese 2007; Mikati et al. 2007
	Inhibition of inflammatory cell activation	Chong et al. 2003d
	Blockade of caspase activation	Chong et al. 2002b, 2003a, 2003b, 2003d
FOXO3a inactivation	Inhibition of FOXO3a activation, maintenance of FOXO3a in the cytoplasm	Chong, Maiese 2007a
Nuclear factor (NF)-κB activation	Inhibition of apoptosis against oxidative stress	Bittorf et al 2001; Chong et al. 2005c; Spandou et al. 2006; Li et al. 2006c
Wnt signaling	Increase of Wnt expression, cytoprotection of vascular cells during elevated glucose	Chong et al. 2007b
GSK-3β inactivation	Inhibition of cell injury, potential benefits with exercise against diabetes mellitus	Howlett et al. 2006; Li et al. 2006c; Wu et al. 2007; Chong et al. 2007b

Of the forkhead transcription factors, FOXO3a is one member that exemplifies the ability to function as a versatile component during normal physiological conditions as well as during disorders such as DM (Maiese, Chong, Shang 2007b). The nomenclature for human Fox proteins places all letters in uppercase, otherwise only the initial letter is listed as uppercase for the mouse, and for all other chordates the initial and subclass letters are in uppercase. FOXO3a appears to be involved in several pathways responsible for cell metabolism, DM onset, and diabetic complications (Maiese, Li, Chong 2004; Maiese, Chong, Li 2005a; Maiese, Li, Chong 2005b; Chong, Maiese 2007b). A clinical study of 734 individuals that examined all exons of the *FOXO* genes—*FOXO1a, FOXO3a*, and *FOXO4*—found one promoter single nucleotide polymorphism in the 5' flanking region of *FOXO3a* that displayed a significant association with body mass index such that the highest body mass index was present in individuals who were homozygous for this allele (Kim, Jung, Bae et al. 2006). Although other studies have reported that haplotype analyses of *FOXO1a* rather than *FOXO3a* in individuals is associated with higher HbA_{1c} levels to suggest evidence of at least an association with disorders of glucose intolerance, *FOXO3a* haplotypes also have been associated with an increased risk for stroke (Kuningas, Magi, Westendorp et al. 2007). In addition, the human immunodeficiency virus (HIV) 1 accessory protein Vpr has been reported to contribute to insulin resistance in HIV patients by interfering with FoxO3a signaling with protein 14–3–3 (Kino, De Martino, Charmandari et al. 2005).

Experimental work on DM has indicated that administration of a high-fat diet in animals that lead to hyperinsulinemic insulin-resistant obesity was associated with an increased expression of FoxO3a (Relling, Esberg, Fang et al. 2006). Some studies have suggested that FoxO3a may be beneficial during elevated glucose exposure and DM. For example, interferon γ–driven expression of tryptophan catabolism by cytotoxic T-lymphocyte antigen 4 may activate FoxO3a to protect dendritic cells from injury in nonobese diabetic mice (Fallarino, Bianchi, Orabona et al. 2004). Yet, the role of forkhead transcription factors can vary among different cell types and tissues. Mice overexpressing FoxO1 in skeletal muscle suffer from reduced skeletal muscle mass and poor glycemic control (Kamei, Miura, Suzuki et al. 2004). Additional investigations have linked diabetic nephropathy to FoxO3a by demonstrating that phosphorylation of FoxO3a increases in rat and mouse renal cortical tissues 2 weeks after the induction of diabetes by streptozotocin (Kato, Yuan, Xu et al. 2006). Furthermore, enteric neurons can be protected from hyperglycemia by glial cell line–derived neurotrophic factors that

can affect Akt signaling and prevent FoxO3a activation and nuclear translocation (Anitha, Gondha, Sutliff et al. 2006). Interestingly, the ability of Akt to also inhibit pyruvate dehydrogenase kinase 4 expression, a protein that conserves gluconeogenic substrates during DM, requires the inhibition of FoxO3a activity (Kwon, Huang, Unterman et al. 2004).

As a result, FoxO3a has emerged as an important target for DM. Akt can phosphorylate FoxO3a and inhibit its activity to sequester FoxO3a in the cytoplasm by association with 14–3–3 proteins (Brunet, Kanai, Stehn et al. 2002; Kino, De Martino, Charmandari et al. 2005; Dong, Kang, Gu et al. 2007; Munoz-Fontela, Marcos-Villar, Gallego et al. 2007; Chong, Maiese 2007a) (Fig. 22.1). In the absence of inhibitory Akt1 phosphorylation, FoxO3a is active, can translocate to the nucleus, and controls a variety of functions that involve cell cycle progression, cell longevity, and apoptosis (Lehtinen, Yuan, Boag et al. 2006; Li, Chong, Maiese 2006a; Maiese, Chong, Shang 2007a). Control of FoxO3a is considered to be a viable therapeutic target for agents such as metabotropic glutamate receptors (Chong, Li, Maiese 2006a), neurotrophins (Zheng, Kar, Quirion 2002), and cytokines such as EPO (Chong, Maiese 2007a) to increase cell survival (Table 22.2). EPO controls the phosphorylation and degradation of FoxO3a to retain it in the cytoplasm through binding to 14–3–3 protein and to foster vascular cell protection during oxidative stress (Chong, Maiese 2007a) (Fig. 22.2).

Cytoprotection by EPO also is mediated through the activation of nuclear factor-κB (NF-κB) tied to Akt (Fig. 22.1). NF-κB proteins are composed of several homo- and heterodimer proteins that can bind to common DNA elements. It is the phosphorylation of IκB proteins by the IκB kinase (IKK) and their subsequent degradation that lead to the release of NF-κB for its translocation to the nucleus to initiate gene transcription (Hayden, Ghosh 2004). Dependent upon Akt-controlled pathways, the transactivation domain of the p65 subunit of NF-κB is activated by IKK and the IKKα catalytic subunit to lead to the induction of protective antiapoptotic pathways (Chong, Li, Maiese 2005a). Increased expression of NF-κB during injury can occur in cells, such as inflammatory microglial cells (Chong, Li, Maiese 2005c; Guo, Bhat 2006; Chong, Li, Maiese 2007c) and neurons (Sanz, Acarin, Gonzalez et al. 2002). NF-κB represents a critical pathway that is responsible for the activation of inhibitors of apoptotic proteins (IAPs), the maintenance of Bcl-x_L expression (Chen, Edelstein, Gelinas 2000; Chong, Li, Maiese 2005d), and protection against cell injury during oxidative stress (Chong, Li, Maiese 2005c). EPO employs NF-κB to prevent apoptosis through the enhanced expression and translocation of NF-κB to the nucleus to

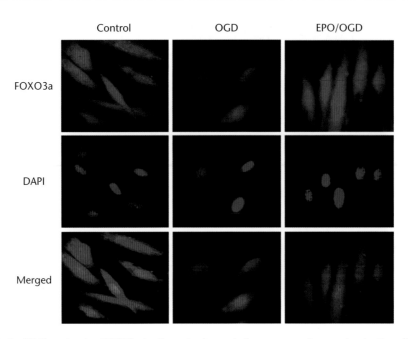

	Control	OGD	EPO/OGD
FOXO3a			
DAPI			
Merged			

Figure 22.2 Erythropoietin (EPO) maintains FOXO3a in the cytoplasm during oxygen-glucose deprivation (OGD). Administration of EPO (10 ng/ml) with an 8 hour period of OGD, OGD alone, or untreated cells (Control) was followed at 6 hours with immunofluorescent staining for FOXO3a (Texas-red) in endothelial cells (ECs). The nuclei of ECs were counterstained with DAPI. In merged images, control cells or cells with combined EPO and OGD show EC nuclei with minimal FOXO3a staining (control, blue/white, EPO/OGD, green/white) and show EC cytoplasm with significant FOXO3a staining (red). This is in contrast to cells with OGD alone with significant FOXO3a staining in both the cytoplasm and the nuclei of ECs, demonstrating the ability of EPO to maintain FOXO3a in the cytoplasm.

elicit antiapoptotic gene activation (Bittorf, Buchse, Sasse et al. 2001; Chong, Li, Maiese 2005c; Spandou, Tsouchnikas, Karkavelas et al. 2006; Li, Chong, Maiese 2006c) (Table 22.2).

A Precursor for the Coenzyme β-Nicotinamide Adenine Dinucleotide

As the amide form of niacin or vitamin B_3, nicotinamide plays a critical role in cellular metabolism and can offer significant neuronal and vascular cell protection during a wide range of disorders that include DM. Nicotinamide is the precursor for the coenzyme β-NAD^+ and is essential for the synthesis of nicotinamide adenine dinucleotide phosphate ($NADP^+$) (Maiese, Chong 2003; Li, Chong, Maiese 2004b). Nicotinamide and nicotinic acid can be obtained either through synthesis in the body, such as in the liver, or through a dietary source that is rapidly absorbed through the gastrointestinal epithelium. Once nicotinamide is available to the body, it is utilized to synthesize NAD^+ (Li, Chong, Maiese 2006a).

In clinical studies for DM, oral nicotinamide protects β-cell function, prevents clinical disease in islet cell–antibody-positive first-degree relatives of type 1 DM (Olmos, Hodgson, Maiz et al. 2005), and in combination therapy with insulin reduces HbA_{1c} levels (Crino, Schiaffini, Ciampalini et al. 2005). Potentially

relevant to diabetic patients with renal failure, nicotinamide has been shown to also reduce intestinal absorption of phosphate and prevent the development of hyperphosphatemia and progressive renal dysfunction (Eto, Miyata, Ohno et al. 2005). In animal and cell culture studies, nicotinamide can also maintain normal fasting blood glucose in animals with streptozotocin-induced diabetes (Reddy, Bibby, Wu et al. 1995b; Hu, Wang, Wang et al. 1996), reduce peripheral nerve injury during elevated glucose (Stevens, Li, Drel et al. 2007), lead to the remission of type 1 DM in mice with acetyl-1-carnitine (Cresto, Fabiano de Bruno, Cao et al. 2006), and inhibit oxidative stress pathways that lead to apoptosis (Chong, Lin, Maiese 2002a; Chong, Lin, Li et al. 2005f; Ieraci, Herrera 2006; Chlopicki, Swies, Mogielnicki et al. 2007; Hara, Yamada, Shibata et al. 2007) (Table 22.3).

Nicotinamide can exert protean endocrine effects in the body (Aoyagi, Archer 2008) and derive its protective capacity through a number of cellular pathways. In addition to the neuroprotective attributes of nicotinamide (Chong, Lin, Maiese 2004b; Anderson, Bradbury, Schneider 2006; Feng, Paul, LeBlanc 2006), one potential pathway to consider for the protective capacity of nicotinamide in DM involves the maintenance of vascular integrity (Maiese, Chong 2003; Li, Chong, Maiese 2004b, 2006a). For example, nicotinamide can protect the function of the blood–brain barrier (Hoane, Kaplan,

Table 22.3 Therapeutic Potential of Nicotinamide

Diseases	Function	Selected References
Diabetes mellitus	May prevent clinical disease	Olmos et al. 2005
	Reduces HbA$_{1C}$ levels	Crino et al. 2005
	Maintains normal fasting blood glucose levels in animal models with streptozotocin	Reddy et al. 1995b; Hu et al. 1996
	Reduces peripheral nerve injury during elevated glucose	Stevens et al. 2007
Traumatic brain injury	Maintains the integrity of the BBB	Hoane et al. 2006a
	Reduces cortical neuronal death and edema	Hoane et al. 2006b
Atherosclerotic diseases	Increases arteriolar dilation and blood flow	Giulumian et al. 2000
	Decreases atherosclerotic plaque	Oumouna-Benachour et al. 2007
	Promotes platelet production	Giammona et al. 2006
Oxidative stress	Maintains EC viability	Autor et al. 1984; Lin et al. 2001; Maiese, Chong 2003
	Inhibits PARP and protects human cardiac blasts and endocardial ECs	Bowes et al. 1998; Cox et al. 2002
	Maintains mitochondrial membrane potential	Lin et al. 2000; Chong et al. 2002a
Inflammation	Inhibits microglial activation	Lin et al. 2001; Chong et al. 2004b
	Inhibits the release of interleukin-1β, -6, and -8, and TNF	Reddy et al. 2001; Chen et al. 2001a; Maiese, Chong 2003; Moberg et al. 2003; Ungerstedt et al. 2003
Cytokine modulation	Alters major histocompatibility complexes	Fukuzawa et al. 1997
	Inhibits the expression of intracellular adhesion molecules	Hiromatsu et al. 1992
	Modulates the production of TNF Reduces demyelination	Fukuzawa et al. 1997; Kaneko et al. 2006

BBB, blood–brain barrier; EC, endothelial cell; PARP, poly(ADP-ribose) polymerase; TNF, tumor necrosis factor.

Ellis et al. 2006a; Hoane, Gilbert, Holland et al. 2006b), influence arteriolar dilatation and blood flow (Giulumian, Meszaros, Fuchs 2000), potentially lead to decreased atherosclerotic plaque through inhibition of poly(ADP-ribose) polymerase (Oumouna-Benachour, Hans, Suzuki et al. 2007), and promote platelet production through megakaryocyte maturation (Giammona, Fuhrken, Papoutsakis et al. 2006) (Table 22.3). Nicotinamide can also maintain EC viability during reactive oxygen species exposure (Autor, Bonham, Thies 1984; Lin, Chong, Maiese 2001; Chong, Lin, Maiese 2002a; Maiese, Chong 2003). Nicotinamide is believed to be responsible for the preservation of cerebral (Sadanaga-Akiyoshi, Yao, Tanuma et al. 2003) and endocardial (Bowes, Piper, Thiemermann 1998; Cox, Sood, Hunt et al. 2002) ECs during models of oxidative stress. Interestingly, during periods of ischemia and oxidative stress, acidosis-induced cellular toxicity may ensue (Chong, Li, Maiese 2005d) and lead to subsequent mitochondrial failure (Sensi, Jeng 2004). Yet, nicotinamide cannot prevent cellular injury during intracellular acidification paradigms (Lin, Vincent, Shaw 2000).

An alternative mechanism for nicotinamide may require the maintenance of the mitochondrial membrane potential ($\Delta\Psi_m$) to protect cells from injury (Fig. 22.1). Nicotinamide can preserve mitochondrial NAD-linked respiration and block the depolarization of the mitochondrial membrane (Lin, Vincent,

Shaw 2000; Chong, Lin, Maiese 2002a) (Table 22.3). Interestingly, nicotinamide appears to act directly at the level of mitochondrial membrane pore formation to prevent cytochrome c release (Lin, Vincent, Shaw 2000; Chong, Lin, Maiese 2002a).

Nicotinamide can also prevent inflammatory cell demise through the maintenance of membrane asymmetry, the activation of Akt, and the inhibition of cytokine release (Maiese, Chong 2003; Li, Chong, Maiese 2004b, 2006a). Nicotinamide blocks membrane PS externalization during a variety of insults that involve anoxia, free radical exposure, and oxygen-glucose deprivation (Lin, Vincent, Shaw 2000; Lin, Chong, Maiese 2001; Chong, Lin, Maiese 2002a). Nicotinamide regulates membrane PS exposure and microglial activation through activation of Akt, a central pathway for cytoprotection (Chong, Lin, Maiese 2004b) (Fig. 22.1).

In addition to targeting the activity of membrane PS exposure and microglial activation, nicotinamide inhibits several proinflammatory cytokines, such as interleukin-1β, interleukin-6, interleukin-8, tissue factor, and tumor necrosis factor α (TNF-α) (Reddy, Young, Ginn 2001; Chen, Wang, Hwang et al. 2001a; Moberg, Olsson, Berne et al. 2003; Ungerstedt, Blomback, Soderstrom 2003). Nicotinamide also can alter major histocompatibility complexes (Fukuzawa, Satoh, Muto et al. 1997), inhibit intracellular adhesion molecule expression

(Hiromatsu, Sato, Yamada et al. 1992), and modulate the production of TNF in vascular cells (Fukuzawa, Satoh, Muto et al. 1997) that may be responsible for the ability of nicotinamide to reduce demyelination in models of multiple sclerosis (Kaneko, Wang, Kaneko et al. 2006). However, translation of these experimental studies to clinical efficacy appears to require further work, since some studies show that oral nicotinamide administration following endotoxin challenge in healthy volunteers did not demonstrate a significant effect upon serum cytokine levels (Soop, Albert, Weitzberg et al. 2004).

Similar to EPO, nicotinamide may also require other substrates of the Akt pathway, such as the forkhead transcription factorFoxO3a, to prevent cell injury (Fig. 22.1). FoxO3a interfaces with several pathways that regulate cellular lifespan (Lehtinen, Yuan, Boag et al. 2006) and function to control neoplastic growth (Li, Wang, Kong et al. 2007). Given the potential treatment advantages of nicotinamide in DM, it should be of interest that nicotinamide may be cytoprotective through two separate mechanisms of posttranslational modification of FoxO3a. Nicotinamide can not only maintain phosphorylation of FoxO3a and inhibit its activity but also preserve the integrity of the FoxO3a protein (Chong, Lin, Maiese 2004b) to block FoxO3a proteolysis that can yield potentially proapoptotic amino-terminal (Nt) fragments (Charvet, Alberti, Luciano et al. 2003).

Cysteine-Rich Glycosylated Wnt Proteins

Wnt proteins are secreted cysteine-rich glycosylated proteins that can be dependent upon Akt signaling and oversee embryonic cell proliferation, differentiation, survival, and death (Li, Chong, Maiese 2006b; Speese, Budnik 2007; Chong, Li, Maiese 2007a; Chong, Shang, Maiese 2007b). More than 80 target genes of Wnt signaling pathways have been demonstrated in humans, mouse, *Drosophila*, Xenopus, and zebrafish. This representation encompasses several cellular populations, such as neurons, cardiomyocytes, endothelial cells, cancer cells, and preadipocytes (Chong, Maiese 2004; Li, Chong, Maiese 2005). In addition, at least 19 of 24 Wnt genes that express Wnt proteins have been identified in humans.

In general, all Wnt signaling pathways are initiated by interaction of Wnt proteins with Frizzled (FZD) receptors and by the binding of the Wnt protein to the FZD transmembrane receptor in the presence of the co-receptor LRP-5/6 (Mao, Wang, Liu et al. 2001) (Fig. 22.1). Once Wnt protein binds to the FZD transmembrane receptor and the co-receptor LRP-5/6, Dishevelled, a cytoplasmic multifunctional phosphoprotein, is recruited (Salinas 1999;

Table 22.4 Cellular Expression of Wnt Protein and the Biological Response

Cellular Expression of Wnt	Biological Response
Neurons	Brain development and resistance to injury
Astrocytes	Brain development and protection
Endothelial cells	Angiogenesis
Vascular smooth muscle cells	Angiogenesis, vascular remodeling, and cytoprotection
Progenitor cardiac stem cells	Cardiomyogenesis
Endocardial cells	Endocardial cushion formation
Cardiomyocytes	Cardiac remodeling and cytoprotection
Adipocytes, bone cells	Adipogenesis, metabolism, bone formation
Cancer cells	Cell growth

Patapoutian, Reichardt 2000; Li, Chong, Maiese 2005). The Wnt-FZD transduction pathway plays a significant role in the control of the pattern of the body axis as well as in the development and maturation of the central nervous system (Augustine, Liu, Sadler 1993; Ikeya, Lee, Johnson et al. 1997), cardiovascular system (Marvin, Di Rocco, Gardiner et al. 2001; Naito, Shiojima, Akazawa et al. 2006; Palpant, Yasuda, MacDougald et al. 2007; Singh, Li, Hamazaki et al. 2007), and the limbs (Kengaku, Twombly, Tabin 1997) (Table 22.4). During embryological development, alternations of the Wnt-FZD pathway can lead to abnormal morphogenesis in animal models (Stark, Vainio, Vassileva et al. 1994; Ikeya, Lee, Johnson et al. 1997; Liu, Wakamiya, Shea et al. 1999) and congenital defects in humans (Jordan, Mohammed, Ching et al. 2001; Rodova, Islam, Maser et al. 2002; Niemann, Zhao, Pascu et al. 2004). In mature tissues, the Wnt-FZD pathway is involved in the self-renewal of pluripotent embryonic stem cells (Bakre, Hoi, Mong et al. 2007) and bone formation (Canalis, Giustina, Bilezikian 2007), and may be responsible for the maintenance of many normal tissues (Ross, Hemati, Longo et al. 2000; Reya, Duncan, Ailles et al. 2003; Willert, Brown, Danenberg et al. 2003; He, Zhang, Tong et al. 2004) as well as cellular senescence (Liu, Fergusson, Castilho et al. 2007) (Table 22.4). Other studies have revealed that dysfunction of the Wnt-FZD pathway can lead to neurodegenerative disorders, such as Alzheimer's disease (Soriano, Kang, Fu et al. 2001; Marambaud, Shioi, Serban et al. 2002; Morin, Medina, Semenov et al. 2004; Balaraman, Limaye, Levey et al. 2006; Chong, Li, Maiese 2007a) and heart failure (Barandon, Couffinhal, Ezan et al. 2003; Barandon, Dufourcq, Costet et al. 2005; Li, Chong, Maiese 2006b; van de Schans, van den Borne, Strzelecka et al. 2007).

Wnt signaling can prevent cell injury through β-catenin/Tcf transcription-mediated pathways (Chen, Guttridge, You et al. 2001b) and against c-myc-induced apoptosis through cyclooxygenase-2- and Wnt-induced secreted protein (You, Saims, Chen et al. 2002). However, more recent work has linked Wnt cytoprotection in neuronal and vascular cells with more unconventional pathways of Wnt that involve Akt (Fig. 22.1). For example, neuronal cell differentiation that is dependent upon Wnt signaling and trophic factor induction is blocked during the repression of Akt activity (Fukumoto, Hsieh, Maemura et al. 2001) and Wnt differentiation of cardiomyocytes does not proceed without Akt activation (Naito, Akazawa, Takano et al. 2005). Soluble secreted FZD-related proteins, which can modulate Wnt signaling, also employ Akt for cardiac tissue repair (Mirotsou, Zhang, Deb et al. 2007) (Table 22.5). Reduction in tissue injury through Wnt signaling during pressure overload cardiac hypertrophy is linked to Akt activation (van de Schans, van den Borne, Strzelecka et al. 2007), and the benefits of cardiac ischemic preconditioning appear to rely upon Akt (Barandon, Dufourcq, Costet et al. 2005). In the neuronal system, Wnt overexpression can independently increase the phosphorylation and activation of Akt to promote neuronal protection

(Chong, Li, Maiese 2007a). Inhibition of the phosphatidylinositol-3-kinase (PI 3-K) pathway or gene silencing of Akt expression prevents Wnt from blocking apoptotic injury and microglial activation (Chong, Li, Maiese 2007a).

Abnormalities in the Wnt signaling pathways, such as with *transcription factor 7-like 2* gene, may lead to increased risk for type 2 DM in some populations (Grant, Thorleifsson, Reynisdottir et al. 2006; Scott, Bonnycastle, Willer et al. 2006; Lehman, Hunt, Leach et al. 2007), as well as have increased association with obesity (Guo, Xiong, Shen et al. 2006) (Table 22.5). Additional work has described the expression of Wnt5b in adipose tissue, the pancreas, and the liver in diabetic patients, suggesting a potential regulation of adipose cell function (Kanazawa, Tsukada, Sekine et al. 2004). Clinical observations in patients with coronary artery disease and the combined metabolic syndrome with hypertension, hyperlipidemia, and DM have indicated impaired Wnt signaling through a missense mutation in LRP-6 (Mani, Radhakrishnan, Wang et al. 2007). Experimental studies in mice that develop hyperglycemia through a high-fat diet also demonstrate increased expression of some Wnt family members, such as Wnt3a and Wnt7a (Al-Aly, Shao, Lai et al. 2007). Yet, intact Wnt family members may

Table 22.5 Wnt Signaling Pathways in Disease

Physiological and Pathological Entities	Wnt Signaling Components	Outcome	Selected References
Development and maturation	Wnt-Frizzled activation	Control of body pattern; normal morphogenesis; self-renewal of pluripotent embryonic stem cells; bone formation	Augustine et al. 1993; Kengaku et al. 1997; Ikeya et al. 1997; Marvin et al. 2001; Natio et al. 2006; Palpant et al. 2007; Singh et al. 2007; Canalis et al. 2007
		Maintenance of normal tissues	Ross et al. 2000; Reya et al. 2003; Willert et al. 2003; He et al. 2004
		Cellular senescence	Liu et al. 2007
Alzheimer's disease	Wnt-Frizzled dysfunction; increased production of Aβ	Decrease in amyloid production and toxicity; increase in β-catenin degradation; increase in GSK-3β activity and decrease in β-catenin activity; increase in microglial activation	Soriano et al. 2001; Marambaud et al. 2002; Morin et al. 2004; Li et al. 2005; Balaraman et al. 2006; Chong et al. 2007a
Diabetes mellitus	Increased expression of Wnt5b, Wnt3a, Wnt7a Abnormalities of transcription factor 7-like 2 gene Wnt expression	Association with obesity Increased risk for type 2 diabetes mellitus Decreased obesity High glucose-induced injury in ECs reduced with inhibition of GSK-3β; mesangial cells protected	Guo et al. 2006; Al-Aly et al. 2007 Grant et al. 2006; Scott et al. 2006; Lehman et al. 2007; Wright et al. 2007; Lin et al. 2006; Chong et al. 2007b
Myocardial infarction	Over-expression of Frizzled A Wnt-Frizzled signaling modulation	Reduced cardiac infarction; enhanced ischemic preconditioning; influenced Akt activation; reduction in pressure overload–induced cardiac hypertrophy	Barandon et al. 2003; Barandon et al. 2005; Li et al. 2006b; Van de Schans et al. 2007
Cardiac repair	Release of SFRP modulates Wnt signaling	Akt activation with cardiac repair	Mirotsou et al. 2007

Aβ, beta-amyloid; EC, endothelial cell; GSK-3β, glycogen synthase kinase-3β; SFRP, secreted Frizzled-related protein.

offer glucose tolerance and increased insulin sensitivity (Wright, Longo, Dolinsky et al. 2007), as well as protect glomerular mesangial cells from elevated glucose–induced apoptosis (Lin, Wang. Huang 2006) (Table 22.5). Animals that overexpressed Wnt10b and were placed on a high-fat diet had a reduction in body weight, hyperinsulinemia, and triglyceride plasma levels, and improved glucose homeostasis (Aslanidi, Kroutov, Philipsberg et al. 2007).

These clinical and experimental investigations for the Wnt pathway suggest a potentially protective cellular mechanism for Wnt during DM. Recent in vitro studies demonstrate that the Wnt1 protein is necessary and sufficient to provide cellular protection during elevated glucose exposure (Chong, Shang, Maiese 2007b) (Table 22.2). Administration of exogenous Wnt1 protein can significantly prevent apoptotic EC injury during elevated glucose exposure. Interestingly, this protection by Wnt1 can be regulated by the growth factor and cytokine EPO (Maiese, Li, Chong 2004, 2005b; Nangaku, Fliser 2007). Through the Wnt pathway, EPO may offer an attractive therapy to maintain proper cellular metabolism and mitochondrial membrane potential ($\Delta\Psi_m$) during conditions of oxidative stress and DM. In cell culture and animal studies, EPO is cytoprotective during elevated glucose levels (Chong, Shang, Maiese 2007b), and it has the capacity to prevent the depolarization of the mitochondrial membrane, which also affects the release of cytochrome c (Chong, Kang, Maiese 2002b; Chong, Lin, Kang et al. 2003d; Miki, Miura, Yano et al. 2006). With the Wnt pathway, EPO maintains the expression of Wnt1 during elevated glucose exposure and prevents the loss of Wnt1 expression that would normally occur in the absence of EPO during elevated glucose levels. In addition, blockade of Wnt1 with a Wnt1 antibody can neutralize the protective capacity of EPO, illustrating that Wnt1 is a critical component in the cytoprotection of EPO during elevated glucose exposure (Chong, Shang, Maiese 2007b) (Table 22.5).

Interestingly, Wnt also can protect cells during oxidative stress (Chong, Maiese 2004) and other toxic injuries such as β-amyloid toxicity (Chong, Maiese 2004) through the modulation of glycogen synthase kinase-3β (GSK-3β) and β-catenin (Chong, Li, Maiese 2007a) (Fig. 22.1). Inhibition of GSK-3β activity can increase cell survival during oxidative stress, and as a result, GSK-3β is considered to be a therapeutic target for some neurodegenerative disorders (Chong, Li, Maiese 2005b; Balaraman, Limaye, Levey et al. 2006; Nurmi, Goldsteins, Narvainen et al. 2006; Qin, Peng, Ksiezak-Reding et al. 2006). GSK-3β also may influence inflammatory cell survival (Chong, Li, Maiese 2007c) and activation (Tanuma, Sakuma, Sasaki et al. 2006). In metabolic disease, inactivation of GSK-3β by small molecule inhibitors or RNA interference

prevents toxicity from high concentrations of glucose and increases rat β-cell replication, suggesting a possible target of GSK-3β for pancreatic β-cell regeneration (Mussmann, Geese, Harder et al. 2007). Clinical applications for Wnt that involve GSK-3β are attractive (Rowe, Wiest, Chuang 2007), especially in concert with EPO (Table 22.2). For example, both the potential benefits of EPO to improve cardiovascular function in diabetic patients (Silverberg, Wexler, Sheps et al. 2001; Silverberg, Wexler, Iaina et al. 2006) and the positive effects of exercise to improve glycemic control during DM (Maiorana, O'Driscoll, Goodman et al. 2002) appear to rely upon the inhibition of GSK-3β activity. EPO blocks GSK-3β activity (Li, Chong, Maiese 2006c; Wu, Shang, Sun et al. 2007; ChongShang, Maiese 2007b), and when combined with exercise, it may offer synergistic benefits, since physical exercise has also been shown to phosphorylate and inhibit GSK-3β activity (Howlett, Sakamoto, Yu et al. 2006) (Table 22.2).

RAVES AND RISKS FOR FUTURE CLINICAL APPLICATIONS

As basic experimental studies and clinical trials continue to outline the advantageous effects of EPO, nicotinamide, and Wnt signaling, raves for these innovative agents and their novel pathways for enhancement of cell longevity will continue to unfold at a surprisingly rapid pace. Yet, these therapeutic approaches can present with significant risks for some patients and ultimately lead to disease progression or other consequences. For example, with annual sale revenues in the United States for EPO reported to approach 9 billion dollars (Donohue, Cevasco, Rosenthal 2007), adverse effects or lack of efficacy during treatment with EPO is also becoming increasingly evident (Table 22.1). Some cardiac injury experimental models do not consistently demonstrate a benefit with EPO (Olea, Vera Janavel, De Lorenzi et al. 2006), and elevated plasma levels of EPO independent of hemoglobin concentration can be associated with increased severity of disease in individuals with congestive heart failure (van der Meer, Voors, Lipsic et al. 2004) or can contribute to vascular stenosis with intima hyperplasia (Reddy, Vasir, Hegde et al. 2007). Other adverse conditions associated with EPO include increased incidence of thrombotic vascular effects, elevation in mean arterial pressure, and increased metabolic rate and blood viscosity (Maiese, Li, Chong 2005b; Corwin, Gettinger, Fabian et al. 2007). The potential progression of cancer has been another significant concern raised with EPO administration (Maiese, Li, Chong 2005c; Kokhaei, Abdalla, Hansson et al. 2007). Not only has both EPO and its receptor been demonstrated in tumor specimens, but under some conditions EPO expression has also been suggested to block tumor cell apoptosis through Akt (Hardee, Rabbani, Arcasoy et al. 2006), enhance tumor progression, increase metastatic disease (Lai, Grandis 2006), decrease survival in cancer patients (Leyland-Jones, Semiglazov, Pawlicki et al. 2005), and negate the effects of radiotherapy by assisting with tumor angiogenesis (Ceelen, Boterberg, Smeets et al. 2007). When evaluating the possible tumor-promoting ability of EPO (Rades, Golke, Schild et al. 2007), a number of competing factors must be considered including the possible benefits of EPO administration in patients with cancer that involve the synergistic effects of EPO with chemotherapeutic modalities (Sigounas, Sallah, Sigounas 2004; Ning, Hartley, Molineux et al. 2005), potential protection against chemotherapy tissue injury (Joyeux-Faure 2007), and the treatment of cancer-related anemia.

Nicotinamide also has been reported to have diverse biological roles that include cellular lifespan reduction. Prolonged exposure to nicotinamide in some studies can lead to impaired β-cell function and reduction in cell growth (Reddy, Salari-Lak, Sandler 1995a; Liu, Green, Flatt et al. 2004). Nicotinamide may also inhibit P450 and hepatic metabolism (Gaudineau, Auclair 2004) and play a role in the progression of Parkinson's disease if cellular compartmentation is abruptly changed (Williams, Cartwright, Ramsden 2005). Under other conditions, nicotinamide has been described as an agent that limits cell growth and promotes cell injury. Nicotinamide in the presence of transforming growth factor β-1 can block hepatic cell proliferation and lead to apoptosis with caspase 3 activation (Traister, Breitman, Bar-Lev et al. 2005). During moderate temperature hyperthermia or carbogen breathing, nicotinamide can also result in enhanced solid tumor radiosensitivity and assist with tumor load reduction (Griffin, Ogawa, Williams et al. 2005). In addition, nicotinamide offers cellular protection in millimole concentrations against oxidative stress, but in relation to cell longevity, lower concentrations of nicotinamide can function as an inhibitor of sirtuins, which are necessary for the promotion of increased lifespan in yeast and metazoans (Porcu, Chiarugi 2005; Li, Chong, Maiese 2006a; Saunders, Verdin 2007). Interestingly, it has been postulated that sirtuins may prevent nicotinamide from assisting with DNA repair by altering the accessibility of DNA-damaged sites for repair enzymes (Kruszewski, Szumiel 2005). Given the intimate and inverse relationship of sirtuins with nicotinamide and the latter's ability to alter cell longevity, alternative approaches for the protection of neuronal and vascular cells during DM may be required that may involve the tight modulation of intracellular nicotinamide accumulation.

In the Wnt pathway, Wnt signaling can either facilitate or prevent apoptosis depending upon the environmental stimuli. For example, Wnt proteins can enhance apoptosis within rhombomeres 3 and 5 in the developing hindbrain and in limb buds during vertebrate limb development to control growth of the hindbrain and limbs (Ellies, Church, Francis-West et al. 2000; Grotewold, Ruther 2002a, 2002b). Wnt signaling has also been closely linked to tumorigenesis for a number of years (Li, Chong, Maiese 2006b; Emami, Corey 2007). Furthermore, in studies that involve DM, neuronal disorders, or vascular disease, it is not consistently clear whether mutations in genes of the Wnt pathway or alterations in protein expression of the Wnt pathway components during these disorders confer protective or detrimental effects.

For innovative strategies to effectively and safely work against a variety of disorders, future investigations that utilize data from basic and clinical research must translate and integrate this knowledge to effectively balance the potential for high impact clinical success with the avoidance of treatment complications. Paramount to achieving these goals is the targeted focus upon intricate and often common cellular pathways governed by potential strategies, such as EPO, nicotinamide, and Wnt signaling, to overcome the present challenges and controversies of existing or developing therapies. With such an approach, the fruitful development of new therapeutic agents to preserve neuronal and vascular longevity during debilitating conditions such as DM will continue to grow at an exponential pace to yield substantial benefits for clinical care.

Acknowledgment This work was supported by the following grants (KM): American Diabetes Association, American Heart Association (National), Bugher Foundation Award, Janssen Neuroscience Award, LEARN Foundation Award, MI Life Sciences Challenge Award, Nelson Foundation Award, NIH NIEHS (P30 ES06639), and NIH NINDS/NIA.

REFERENCES

Al-Aly Z, Shao JS, Lai CF et al. 2007. Aortic Msx2-Wnt calcification cascade is regulated by TNF-alpha-dependent signals in diabetic Ldlr−/−mice. *Arterioscler Thromb Vasc Biol.* 27:2589–2596.

Anagnostou A, Liu Z, Steiner M et al. 1994. Erythropoietin receptor mRNA expression in human endothelial cells. *Proc Natl Acad Sci U S A.* 91:3974–3978.

Anderson DW, Bradbury KA, Schneider JS. 2006. Neuroprotection in Parkinson models varies with toxin administration protocol. *Eur J Neurosci.* 24:3174–3182.

Anitha M, Gondha C, Sutliff R et al. 2006. GDNF rescues hyperglycemia-induced diabetic enteric neuropathy through activation of the PI3K/Akt pathway. *J Clin Invest.* 116:344–356.

Aoyagi S, Archer TK. 2008. Nicotinamide uncouples hormone-dependent chromatin remodeling from transcription complex assembly. *Mol Cell Biol.* 28:30–39.

Asaumi Y, Kagaya Y, Takeda M et al. 2007. Protective role of endogenous erythropoietin system in nonhematopoietic cells against pressure overload-induced left ventricular dysfunction in mice. *Circulation.* 115:2022–2032.

Aslanidi G, Kroutov V, Philipsberg G et al. 2007. Ectopic expression of Wnt10b decreases adiposity and improves glucose homeostasis in obese rats. *Am J Physiol Endocrinol Metab.* 293:E726–E736.

Assaraf MI, Diaz Z, Liberman A et al. 2007. Brain erythropoietin receptor expression in Alzheimer disease and mild cognitive impairment. *J Neuropathol Exp Neurol.* 66:389–398.

Augustine K, Liu ET, Sadler TW. 1993. Antisense attenuation of Wnt-1 and Wnt-3a expression in whole embryo culture reveals roles for these genes in craniofacial, spinal cord, and cardiac morphogenesis. *Dev Genet.* 14:500–520.

Autor AP, Bonham AC, Thies RL. 1984. Toxicity of oxygen radicals in cultured pulmonary endothelial cells. *J Toxicol Environ Health.* 13:387–395.

Awad N, Gagnon M, Messier C. 2004. The relationship between impaired glucose tolerance, type 2 diabetes, and cognitive function. *J Clin Exp Neuropsychol.* 26:1044–1080.

Bakre MM, Hoi A, Mong JC, Koh YY, Wong KY, Stanton LW. 2007. Generation of multipotential mesendodermal progenitors from mouse embryonic stem cells via sustained Wnt pathway activation. *J Biol Chem.* 282:31703–31712.

Balaraman Y, Limaye AR, Levey AI, Srinivasan S. 2006. Glycogen synthase kinase 3beta and Alzheimer's disease: pathophysiological and therapeutic significance. *Cell Mol Life Sci.* 63:1226–1235.

Barandon L, Couffinhal T, Ezan J et al. 2003. Reduction of infarct size and prevention of cardiac rupture in transgenic mice overexpressing FrzA. *Circulation.* 108:2282–2289.

Barandon L, Dufourcq P, Costet P et al. 2005. Involvement of FrzA/sFRP-1 and the Wnt/frizzled pathway in ischemic preconditioning. *Circ Res.* 96:1299–1306.

Beeri MS, Silverman JM, Davis KL et al. 2005. Type 2 diabetes is negatively associated with Alzheimer's disease neuropathology. *J Gerontol A Biol Sci Med Sci.* 60:471–475.

Bierer R, Peceny MC, Hartenberger CH, Ohls RK. 2006. Erythropoietin concentrations and neurodevelopmental outcome in preterm infants. *Pediatrics.* 118:e635–e640.

Bittorf T, Buchse T, Sasse T, Jaster R, Brock J. 2001. Activation of the transcription factor NF-kappaB by the erythropoietin receptor: structural requirements and biological significance. *Cell Signal.* 13:673–681.

Bowes J, Piper J, Thiemermann C. 1998. Inhibitors of the activity of poly (ADP-ribose) synthetase reduce the cell death caused by hydrogen peroxide in human cardiac myoblasts. *Br J Pharmacol.* 124:1760–1766.

Brunet A, Kanai F, Stehn J et al. 2002. 14–3–3 transits to the nucleus and participates in dynamic nucleocytoplasmic transport. *J Cell Biol.* 156:817–828.

Canalis E, Giustina A, Bilezikian JP. 2007. Mechanisms of anabolic therapies for osteoporosis. *N Engl J Med.* 357:905–916.

Cardella F. 2005. Insulin therapy during diabetic ketoacidosis in children. *Acta Biomed.* 76 (Suppl 3):49–54.

Ceelen W, Boterberg T, Smeets P et al. 2007. Recombinant human erythropoietin alpha modulates the effects of radiotherapy on colorectal cancer microvessels. *Br J Cancer.* 96:692–700.

Charvet C, Alberti I, Luciano F et al. 2003. Proteolytic regulation of Forkhead transcription factor FOXO3a by caspase-3-like proteases. *Oncogene.* 22:4557–4568.

Chen C, Edelstein LC, Gelinas C. 2000. The Rel/NF-kappaB family directly activates expression of the apoptosis inhibitor Bcl-x(L). *Mol Cell Biol.* 20:2687–2695.

Chen CF, Wang D, Hwang CP et al. 2001a. The protective effect of niacinamide on ischemia-reperfusion-induced liver injury. *J Biomed Sci.* 8:446–452.

Chen S, Guttridge DC, You Z et al. 2001b. Wnt-1 signaling inhibits apoptosis by activating beta-catenin/T cell factor-mediated transcription. *J Cell Biol.* 152:87–96.

Cherian L, Goodman JC, Robertson C. 2007. Neuroprotection with erythropoietin administration following controlled cortical impact injury in rats. *J Pharmacol Exp Ther.* 322:789–794.

Chlopicki S, Swies J, Mogielnicki A et al. 2007. 1-Methylnicotinamide (MNA), a primary metabolite of nicotinamide, exerts anti-thrombotic activity mediated by a cyclooxygenase-2/prostacyclin pathway. *Br J Pharmacol.* 152:230–239.

Chong ZZ, Lin SH, Maiese K. 2002a. Nicotinamide modulates mitochondrial membrane potential and cysteine protease activity during cerebral vascular endothelial cell injury. *J Vasc Res.* 39:131–147.

Chong ZZ, Kang JQ, Maiese K. 2002b. Erythropoietin is a novel vascular protectant through activation of Akt1 and mitochondrial modulation of cysteine proteases. *Circulation.* 106:2973–2979.

Chong ZZ, Kang JQ, Maiese K. 2002c. Angiogenesis and plasticity: role of erythropoietin in vascular systems. *J Hematother Stem Cell Res.* 11:863–871.

Chong ZZ, Kang JQ, Maiese K. 2003a. Apaf-1, Bcl-xL, Cytochrome c, and Caspase-9 form the critical elements for cerebral vascular protection by erythropoietin. *J Cereb Blood Flow Metab.* 23:320–330.

Chong ZZ, Kang JQ, Maiese K. 2003b. Erythropoietin fosters both intrinsic and extrinsic neuronal protection through modulation of microglia, Akt1, Bad, and caspase-mediated pathways. *Br J Pharmacol.* 138:1107–1118.

Chong ZZ, Kang JQ, Maiese K. 2003c. Metabotropic glutamate receptors promote neuronal and vascular plasticity through novel intracellular pathways. *Histol Histopathol.* 18:173–189.

Chong ZZ, Lin SH, Kang JQ, Maiese K. 2003d. Erythropoietin prevents early and late neuronal demise through modulation of Akt1 and induction of caspase 1, 3, and 8. *J Neurosci Res.* 71:659–669.

Chong ZZ, Lin SH, Kang JQ, Maiese K. 2003e. The tyrosine phosphatase SHP2 modulates MAP kinase p38 and caspase 1 and 3 to foster neuronal survival. *Cell Mol Neurobiol.* 23:561–578.

Chong ZZ, Maiese K. 2004. Targeting WNT, protein kinase B, and mitochondrial membrane integrity to foster cellular survival in the nervous system. *Histol Histopathol.* 19:495–504.

Chong ZZ, Kang JQ, Maiese K. 2004a. Akt1 drives endothelial cell membrane asymmetry and microglial activation through Bcl-x(L) and caspase 1, 3, and 9. *Exp Cell Res.* 296:196–207.

Chong ZZ, Lin SH, Maiese K. 2004b. The NAD+ precursor nicotinamide governs neuronal survival during oxidative stress through protein kinase B coupled to FOXO3a and mitochondrial membrane potential. *J Cereb Blood Flow Metab.* 24:728–743.

Chong ZZ, Kang JQ, Maiese K. 2004c. Essential cellular regulatory elements of oxidative stress in early and late phases of apoptosis in the central nervous system. *Antioxid Redox Signal.* 6:277–287.

Chong ZZ, Li F, Maiese K. 2005a. Activating Akt and the brain's resources to drive cellular survival and prevent inflammatory injury. *Histol Histopathol.* 20:299–315.

Chong ZZ, Li F, Maiese K. 2005b. Oxidative stress in the brain: novel cellular targets that govern survival during neurodegenerative disease. *Prog Neurobiol.* 75:207–246.

Chong ZZ, Li F, Maiese K. 2005c. Erythropoietin requires NF-kappaB and its nuclear translocation to prevent early and late apoptotic neuronal injury during beta-amyloid toxicity. *Curr Neurovasc Res.* 2:387–399.

Chong ZZ, Li F, Maiese K. 2005d. Stress in the brain: novel cellular mechanisms of injury linked to Alzheimer's disease. *Brain Res Brain Res Rev.* 49:1–21.

Chong ZZ, Kang J, Li F, Maiese K. 2005e. mGluRI targets microglial activation and selectively prevents neuronal cell engulfment Through Akt and caspase dependent pathways. *Curr Neurovasc Res.* 2:197–211.

Chong ZZ, Lin SH, Li F, Maiese K. 2005f. The sirtuin inhibitor nicotinamide enhances neuronal cell survival during acute anoxic injury through Akt, Bad, PARP, and mitochondrial associated "anti-apoptotic" pathways. *Curr Neurovasc Res.* 2:271–285.

Chong ZZ, Li F, Maiese K. 2006a. Group I Metabotropic receptor neuroprotection requires Akt and its substrates that govern FOXO3a, Bim, and beta-Catenin during oxidative stress. *Curr Neurovasc Res.* 3:107–117.

Chong ZZ, Li F, Maiese K. 2006b. Attempted cell cycle induction in post-mitotic neurons occurs in early and late apoptotic programs through Rb, E2F1, and Caspase 3. *Curr Neurovasc Res.* 3:25–39.

Chong ZZ, Li F, Maiese K. 2007a. Cellular demise and inflammatory microglial activation during beta-amyloid toxicity are governed by Wnt1 and canonical signaling pathways. *Cell Signal.* 19:1150–1162.

Chong ZZ, Shang YC, Maiese K. 2007b. Vascular injury during elevated glucose can be mitigated by erythropoietin and Wnt signaling. *Curr Neurovasc Res.* 4:194–204.

Chong ZZ, Li F, Maiese K. 2007c. The pro-survival pathways of mTOR and protein kinase B target glycogen synthase kinase-3beta and nuclear factor-kappaB to foster endogenous microglial cell protection. *Int J Mol Med.* 19:263–272.

Chong ZZ, Maiese K. 2007a. Erythropoietin involves the phosphatidylinositol 3-kinase pathway, 14–3–3 protein and FOXO3a nuclear trafficking to preserve endothelial cell integrity. *Br J Pharmacol.* 150:839–850.

Chong ZZ, Maiese K. 2007b. The Src homology 2 domain tyrosine phosphatases SHP-1 and SHP-2: diversified control of cell growth, inflammation, and injury. *Histol Histopathol.* 22:1251–1267.

Choo HJ, Kim JH, Kwon OB et al. 2006. Mitochondria are impaired in the adipocytes of type 2 diabetic mice. *Diabetologia.* 49:784–791.

Clark KL, Halay ED, Lai E, Burley SK. 1993. Co-crystal structure of the HNF-3/fork head DNA-recognition motif resembles histone H5. *Nature.* 364:412–420.

Cohen SM, Cordeiro-Stone M, Kaufman DG 2007. Early replication and the apoptotic pathway. *J Cell Physiol.* 213:434–439.

Corwin HL, Gettinger A, Fabian TC et al. 2007. Efficacy and safety of epoetin alfa in critically ill patients. *N Engl J Med.* 357:965–976.

Cox MJ, Sood HS, Hunt MJ et al. 2002. Apoptosis in the left ventricle of chronic volume overload causes endocardial endothelial dysfunction in rats. *Am J Physiol Heart Circ Physiol.* 282:H1197–H1205.

Cresto JC, Fabiano de Bruno LE, Cao GF et al. 2006. The association of acetyl-1-carnitine and nicotinamide remits the experimental diabetes in mice by multiple low-dose streptozotocin. *Pancreas.* 33:403–411.

Crino A, Schiaffini R, Ciampalini P et al. 2005. A two year observational study of nicotinamide and intensive insulin therapy in patients with recent onset type 1 diabetes mellitus. *J Pediatr Endocrinol Metab.* 18:749–754.

Cuesta I, Zaret KS, Santisteban P. 2007. The forkhead factor FoxE1 binds to the thyroperoxidase promoter during thyroid cell differentiation and modifies compacted chromatin structure. *Mol Cell Biol.* 27:7302–7314.

Dabelea D, Bell RA, D'Agostino RB Jr. et al. 2007. Incidence of diabetes in youth in the United States. *JAMA.* 297:2716–2724.

Davis LE, Widness JA, Brace RA. 2003. Renal and placental secretion of erythropoietin during anemia or hypoxia in the ovine fetus. *Am J Obstet Gynecol.* 189:1764–1770.

De Felice FG, Velasco PT, Lambert MP et al. 2007. Abeta oligomers induce neuronal oxidative stress through an N-methyl-D-aspartate receptor-dependent mechanism that is blocked by the Alzheimer drug memantine. *J Biol Chem.* 282:11590–11601.

Di Lisa F, Menabo R, Canton M, Barile M, Bernardi P. 2001. Opening of the mitochondrial permeability transition pore causes depletion of mitochondrial and cytosolic NAD+ and is a causative event in the death of myocytes in postischemic reperfusion of the heart. *J Biol Chem.* 276:2571–2575.

Donahoe SM, Stewart GC, McCabe CH et al. 2007. Diabetes and mortality following acute coronary syndromes. *JAMA.* 298:765–775.

Dong S, Kang S, Gu TL et al. 2007. 14-3-3 integrates pro-survival signals mediated by the AKT and MAPK pathways in ZNF198-FGFR1-transformed hematopoietic cells. *Blood.* 110:360–369.

Donohue JM, Cevasco M, Rosenthal MB. 2007. A decade of direct-to-consumer advertising of prescription drugs. *N Engl J Med.* 357:673–681.

Du B, Ohmichi M, Takahashi K et al. 2004. Both estrogen and raloxifene protect against beta-amyloid-induced neurotoxicity in estrogen receptor alpha-transfected PC12 cells by activation of telomerase activity via Akt cascade. *J Endocrinol.* 183:605–615.

Duarte AI, Proenca T, Oliveira CR, Santos MS, Rego AC. 2006. Insulin restores metabolic function in cultured cortical neurons subjected to oxidative stress. *Diabetes.* 55:2863–2870.

Dzietko M, Felderhoff-Mueser U, Sifringer M et al. 2004. Erythropoietin protects the developing brain against N-methyl-D-aspartate receptor antagonist neurotoxicity. *Neurobiol Dis.* 15:177–187.

Ellies DL, Church V, Francis-West P, Lumsden A. 2000. The WNT antagonist cSFRP2 modulates programmed cell death in the developing hindbrain. *Development.* 127:5285–5295.

Emami KH, Corey E. 2007. When prostate cancer meets bone: control by wnts. *Cancer Lett.* 253:170–179.

Eto N, Miyata Y, Ohno H, Yamashita T. 2005. Nicotinamide prevents the development of hyperphosphataemia by suppressing intestinal sodium-dependent phosphate transporter in rats with adenine-induced renal failure. *Nephrol Dial Transplant.* 20:1378–1384.

Eto N, Wada T, Inagi R et al. 2007. Podocyte protection by darbepoetin: preservation of the cytoskeleton and nephrin expression. *Kidney Int.* 72:455–463.

Fallarino F, Bianchi R, Orabona C et al. 2004. CTLA-4-Ig activates forkhead transcription factors and protects dendritic cells from oxidative stress in nonobese diabetic mice. *J Exp Med.* 200:1051–1062.

Feng Y, Paul IA, LeBlanc MH. 2006. Nicotinamide reduces hypoxic ischemic brain injury in the newborn rat. *Brain Res Bull.* 69:117–122.

Fenjves ES, Ochoa MS, Cabrera O et al. 2003. Human, non-human primate, and rat pancreatic islets express erythropoietin receptors. *Transplantation.* 75:1356–1360.

Ferrario M, Massa M, Rosti V et al. 2007. Early haemoglobin-independent increase of plasma erythropoietin levels in patients with acute myocardial infarction. *Eur Heart J.* 28:1805–1813.

Fisher JW. 2003. Erythropoietin: physiology and pharmacology update. *Exp Biol Med (Maywood).* 228:1–14.

Fliser D, Haller H. 2007. Erythropoietin and treatment of non-anemic conditions—cardiovascular protection. *Semin Hematol.* 44:212–217.

Foller M, Kasinathan RS, Koka S et al. 2007. Enhanced susceptibility to suicidal death of erythrocytes from transgenic mice overexpressing erythropoietin. *Am J Physiol Regul Integr Comp Physiol.* 293:R1127–R1134.

Fu Q, Van Eyk JE. 2006. Proteomics and heart disease: identifying biomarkers of clinical utility. *Expert Rev Proteomics.* 3:237–249.

Fukumoto S, Hsieh CM, Maemura K et al. 2001. Akt participation in the Wnt signaling pathway through Dishevelled. *J Biol Chem.* 276:17479–17483.

Fukuzawa M, Satoh J, Muto G et al. 1997. Inhibitory effect of nicotinamide on in vitro and in vivo production of tumor necrosis factor-alpha. *Immunol Lett.* 59:7–11.

Gaudineau C, Auclair K. 2004. Inhibition of human P450 enzymes by nicotinic acid and nicotinamide. *Biochem Biophys Res Commun.* 317:950–956.

Giammona LM, Fuhrken PG, Papoutsakis ET, Miller WM. 2006. Nicotinamide (vitamin B3) increases the polyploidisation and proplatelet formation of cultured primary human megakaryocytes. *Br J Haematol.* 135:554–566.

Giardino I, Edelstein D, Brownlee M. 1996. BCL-2 expression or antioxidants prevent hyperglycemia-induced formation of intracellular advanced glycation end-products in bovine endothelial cells. *J Clin Invest.* 97:1422–1428.

Giulumian AD, Meszaros LG, Fuchs LC. 2000. Endothelin-1-induced contraction of mesenteric small arteries is mediated by ryanodine receptor Ca2+ channels and cyclic ADP-ribose. *J Cardiovasc Pharmacol.* 36:758–763.

Gleissner CA, Klingenberg R, Staritz P et al. 2006. Role of erythropoietin in anemia after heart transplantation. *Int J Cardiol.* 112:341–347.

Goldberg N, Lundin AP, Delano B, Friedman EA, Stein RA. 1992. Changes in left ventricular size, wall thickness, and function in anemic patients treated with recombinant human erythropoietin. *Am Heart J.* 124:424–427.

Grant SF, Thorleifsson G, Reynisdottir I et al. 2006. Variant of transcription factor 7-like 2 (TCF7L2) gene confers risk of type 2 diabetes. *Nat Genet.* 38:320–323.

Griffin RJ, Ogawa A, Williams BW, Song CW. 2005. Hyperthermic enhancement of tumor radiosensitization strategies. *Immunol Invest.* 34:343–359.

Grimm C, Wenzel A, Groszer M et al. 2002. HIF-1-induced erythropoietin in the hypoxic retina protects against light-induced retinal degeneration. *Nat Med.* 8:718–724.

Grotewold L, Ruther U. 2002a. The Wnt antagonist Dickkopf-1 is regulated by Bmp signaling and c-Jun and modulates programmed cell death. *Embo J.* 21:966–975.

Grotewold L, Ruther U. 2002b. Bmp, Fgf and Wnt signalling in programmed cell death and chondrogenesis during vertebrate limb development: the role of Dickkopf-1. *Int J Dev Biol.* 46:943–947.

Guo G, Bhat NR. 2006. Hypoxia/Reoxygenation Differentially Modulates NF-kappaB Activation and iNOS Expression in Astrocytes and Microglia. *Antioxid Redox Signal.* 8:911–918.

Guo YF, Xiong DH, Shen H et al. 2006. Polymorphisms of the low-density lipoprotein receptor-related protein 5 (LRP5) gene are associated with obesity phenotypes in a large family-based association study. *J Med Genet.* 43:798–803.

Hara N, Yamada K, Shibata T, Osago H, Hashimoto T, Tsuchiya M. 2007. Elevation of cellular NAD levels by nicotinic acid and involvement of nicotinic acid phosphoribosyltransferase in human cells. *J Biol Chem.* 282:24574–24582.

Hardee ME, Rabbani ZN, Arcasoy MO et al. 2006. Erythropoietin inhibits apoptosis in breast cancer cells via an Akt-dependent pathway without modulating in vivo chemosensitivity. *Mol Cancer Ther.* 5:356–361.

Harris MI, Eastman RC. 2000. Early detection of undiagnosed diabetes mellitus: a US perspective. *Diabetes Metab Res Rev.* 16:230–236.

Harris SE, Fox H, Wright AF et al. 2007. A genetic association analysis of cognitive ability and cognitive ageing using 325 markers for 109 genes associated with oxidative stress or cognition. *BMC Genet.* 8:43.

Hayden MS, Ghosh S. 2004. Signaling to NF-kappaB. *Genes Dev.* 18:2195–2224.

He XC, Zhang J, Tong WG et al. 2004. BMP signaling inhibits intestinal stem cell self-renewal through suppression of Wnt-beta-catenin signaling. *Nat Genet.* 36:1117–1121.

Henry MK, Lynch JT, Eapen AK, Quelle FW. 2001. DNA damage-induced cell-cycle arrest of hematopoietic cells is overridden by activation of the PI-3 kinase/Akt signaling pathway. *Blood.* 98:834–841.

Hiromatsu Y, Sato M, Yamada K, Nonaka K. 1992. Inhibitory effects of nicotinamide on recombinant human interferon- gamma-induced intercellular adhesion molecule-1 (ICAM-1) and HLA-DR antigen expression on cultured human endothelial cells. *Immunol Lett.* 31:35–39.

Hoane MR, Kaplan SA, Ellis AL. 2006a. The effects of nicotinamide on apoptosis and blood-brain barrier breakdown following traumatic brain injury. *Brain Res.* 1125:185–193.

Hoane MR, Gilbert DR, Holland MA, Pierce JL. 2006b. Nicotinamide reduces acute cortical neuronal death and edema in the traumatically injured brain. *Neurosci Lett.* 408:35–39.

Howlett KF, Sakamoto K, Yu H, Goodyear LJ, Hargreaves M. 2006. Insulin-stimulated insulin receptor substrate-2-associated phosphatidylinositol 3-kinase activity is enhanced in human skeletal muscle after exercise. *Metabolism.* 55:1046–1052.

Hu Y, Wang Y et al. 1996. Effects of nicotinamide on prevention and treatment of streptozotocin-induced diabetes mellitus in rats. *Chin Med J (Engl).* 109:819–822.

Ieraci A, Herrera DG. 2006. Nicotinamide protects against ethanol-induced apoptotic neurodegeneration in the developing mouse brain. *PLoS Med.* 3:e101.

Ikeya M, Lee SM, Johnson JE, McMahon AP, Takada S. 1997. Wnt signalling required for expansion of neural crest and CNS progenitors. *Nature.* 389:966–970.

Ito N, Bartunek J, Spitzer KW, Lorell BH. 1997. Effects of the nitric oxide donor sodium nitroprusside on intracellular pH and contraction in hypertrophied myocytes. *Circulation.* 95:2303–2311.

Jacobson AM, Musen G, Ryan CM et al. 2007. Long-term effect of diabetes and its treatment on cognitive function. *N Engl J Med.* 356:1842–1852.

Jin C, Marsden I, Chen X, Liao X. 1998. Sequence specific collective motions in a winged helix DNA binding domain detected by 15N relaxation NMR. *Biochemistry.* 37:6179–6187.

Jordan BK, Mohammed M, Ching ST et al. 2001. Up-regulation of WNT-4 signaling and dosage-sensitive sex reversal in humans. *Am J Hum Genet.* 68:1102–1109.

Joyeux-Faure M. 2007. Cellular protection by erythropoietin: new therapeutic implications? *J Pharmacol Exp Ther.* 323:759–762.

Kaiser K, Texier A, Ferrandiz J et al. 2006. Recombinant human erythropoietin prevents the death of mice during cerebral malaria. *J Infect Dis.* 193:987–995.

Kamei Y, Miura S, Suzuki M et al. 2004. Skeletal muscle FOXO1 (FKHR) transgenic mice have less skeletal muscle mass, down-regulated Type I (slow twitch/red muscle) fiber genes, and impaired glycemic control. *J Biol Chem.* 279:41114–41123.

Kanazawa A, Tsukada S, Sekine A et al. 2004. Association of the gene encoding wingless-type mammary tumor virus integration-site family member 5B (WNT5B) with type 2 diabetes. *Am J Hum Genet.* 75:832–843.

Kaneko S, Wang J, Kaneko M et al. 2006. Protecting axonal degeneration by increasing nicotinamide adenine dinucleotide levels in experimental autoimmune encephalomyelitis models. *J Neurosci.* 26:9794–9804.

Kang JQ, Chong ZZ, Maiese K. 2003a. Akt1 protects against inflammatory microglial activation through maintenance of membrane asymmetry and modulation of cysteine protease activity. *J Neurosci Res.* 74:37–51.

Kang JQ, Chong ZZ, Maiese K. 2003b. Critical role for Akt1 in the modulation of apoptotic phosphatidylserine exposure and microglial activation. *Mol Pharmacol.* 64:557–569.

Kaptanoglu E, Solaroglu I, Okutan O, Surucu HS, Akbiyik F, Beskonakli E. 2004. Erythropoietin exerts neuroprotection after acute spinal cord injury in rats: effect on lipid peroxidation and early ultrastructural findings. *Neurosurg Rev.* 27:113–120.

Karunakaran S, Diwakar L, Saeed U et al. 2007. Activation of apoptosis signal regulating kinase 1 (ASK1) and translocation of death-associated protein, Daxx, in substantia nigra pars compacta in a mouse model of Parkinson's disease: protection by alpha-lipoic acid. *FASEB J.* 21:2226–2236.

Kato M, Yuan H, Xu ZG et al. 2006. Role of the Akt/ FoxO3a pathway in TGF-beta1-mediated mesangial cell dysfunction: a novel mechanism related to diabetic kidney disease. *J Am Soc Nephrol.* 17:3325–3335.

Kengaku M, Twombly V, Tabin C. 1997. Expression of Wnt and Frizzled genes during chick limb bud development. *Cold Spring Harb Symp Quant Biol.* 62:421–429.

Keogh CL, Yu SP, Wei L. 2007. The effect of recombinant human erythropoietin on neurovasculature repair after focal ischemic stroke in neonatal rats. *J Pharmacol Exp Ther.* 322:521–528.

Kim JR, Jung HS, Bae SW et al. 2006. Polymorphisms in FOXO gene family and association analysis with BMI. *Obesity (Silver Spring).* 14:188–193.

King VR, Averill SA, Hewazy D, Priestley JV, Torup L, Michael-Titus AT. 2007. Erythropoietin and carbamylated erythropoietin are neuroprotective following spinal cord hemisection in the rat. *Eur J Neurosci.* 26:90–100.

Kino T, De Martino MU, Charmandari E, Ichijo T, Outas T, Chrousos GP. 2005. HIV-1 accessory protein Vpr inhibits the effect of insulin on the Foxo subfamily of forkhead transcription factors by interfering with their binding to 14–3–3 proteins: potential clinical implications regarding the insulin resistance of HIV-1-infected patients. *Diabetes.* 54:23–31.

Kokhaei P, Abdalla AO, Hansson L et al. 2007. Expression of erythropoietin receptor and in vitro functional effects of epoetins in B-cell malignancies. *Clin Cancer Res.* 13:3536–3544.

Kratzsch J, Knerr I, Galler A et al. 2006. Metabolic decompensation in children with type 1 diabetes mellitus associated with increased serum levels of the soluble leptin receptor. *Eur J Endocrinol.* 155:609–614.

Kruszewski M, Szumiel I. 2005. Sirtuins (histone deacetylases III) in the cellular response to DNA damage-Facts and hypotheses. *DNA Repair (Amst).* 4(11):1306–1313.

Kuningas M, Magi R, Westendorp RG, Slagboom PE, Remm M, van Heemst D. 2007. Haplotypes in the human FoxO1a and FoxO3a genes; impact on disease and mortality at old age. *Eur J Hum Genet.* 15:294–301.

Kwon HS, Huang B, Unterman TG, Harris RA. 2004. Protein kinase B-alpha inhibits human pyruvate dehydrogenase kinase-4 gene induction by dexamethasone through inactivation of FOXO transcription factors. *Diabetes.* 53:899–910.

Laakso M. 2001. Cardiovascular disease in type 2 diabetes: challenge for treatment and prevention. *J Intern Med.* 249:225–235.

Lacombe C, Da Silva JL, Bruneval P et al. 1991. Erythropoietin: sites of synthesis and regulation of secretion. *Am J Kidney Dis.* 18:14–19.

Lai SY, Grandis JR. 2006. Understanding the presence and function of erythropoietin receptors on cancer cells. *J Clin Oncol.* 24:4675–4676.

Larson ET, Eilers B, Menon S et al. 2007. A winged-helix protein from sulfolobus turreted icosahedral virus points toward stabilizing disulfide bonds in the intracellular proteins of a hyperthermophilic virus. *Virology.* 368(2):249–261.

Lehman DM, Hunt KJ, Leach RJ et al. 2007. Haplotypes of transcription factor 7-like 2 (TCF7L2) gene and its upstream region are associated with type 2 diabetes and age of onset in Mexican Americans. *Diabetes.* 56:389–393.

Lehtinen MK, Yuan Z, Boag PR et al. 2006. A conserved MST-FOXO signaling pathway mediates oxidative-stress responses and extends life span. *Cell.* 125:987–1001.

Leuner K, Hauptmann S, Abdel-Kader R et al. 2007. Mitochondrial dysfunction: the first domino in brain aging and Alzheimer's disease? *Antioxid Redox Signal.* 9:1659–1675.

Leyland-Jones B, Semiglazov V, Pawlicki M et al. 2005. Maintaining normal hemoglobin levels with epoetin alfa in mainly nonanemic patients with metastatic breast cancer receiving first-line chemotherapy: a survival study. *J Clin Oncol.* 23:5960–5972.

Leytin V, Allen DJ, Mykhaylov S, Lyubimov E, Freedman J. 2006. Thrombin-triggered platelet apoptosis. *J Thromb Haemost.* 4:2656–2663.

Li F, Chong ZZ, Maiese K. 2004a. Erythropoietin on a Tightrope: balancing neuronal and vascular protection between intrinsic and extrinsic pathways. *Neurosignals.* 13:265–289.

Li F, Chong ZZ, Maiese K. 2004b. Navigating novel mechanisms of cellular plasticity with the NAD+ precursor and nutrient nicotinamide. *Front Biosci.* 9:2500–2520.

Li F, Chong ZZ, Maiese K. 2005. Vital elements of the wnt-frizzled signaling pathway in the nervous system. *Curr Neurovasc Res.* 2:331–340.

Li F, Chong ZZ, Maiese K. 2006a. Cell life versus cell longevity: the mysteries surrounding the NAD(+) precursor nicotinamide. *Curr Med Chem.* 13:883–895.

Li F, Chong ZZ, Maiese K. 2006b. Winding through the WNT pathway during cellular development and demise. *Histol Histopathol.* 21:103–124.

Li F, Chong ZZ, Maiese K. 2006c. Microglial integrity is maintained by erythropoietin through integration of Akt and its substrates of glycogen synthase kinase-3beta, beta-catenin, and nuclear factor-kappaB. *Curr Neurovasc Res.* 3:187–201.

Li Y, Wang Z, Kong D et al. 2007. Regulation of FOXO3a/beta-catenin/GSK-3beta signaling by 3,3'-diindolylmethane contributes to inhibition of cell proliferation and induction of apoptosis in prostate cancer cells. *J Biol Chem.* 282:21542–21550.

Lin CL, Wang JY, Huang YT, Kuo YH, Surendran K, Wang FS. 2006. Wnt/beta-catenin signaling modulates survival of high glucose-stressed mesangial cells. *J Am Soc Nephrol.* 17:2812–2820.

Lin SH, Vincent A, Shaw T, Maynard KI, Maiese K. 2000. Prevention of nitric oxide-induced neuronal injury through the modulation of independent pathways of programmed cell death. *J Cereb Blood Flow Metab.* 20:1380–1391.

Lin SH, Maiese K. 2001. The metabotropic glutamate receptor system protects against ischemic free radical programmed cell death in rat brain endothelial cells. *J Cereb Blood Flow Metab.* 21:262–275.

Lin SH, Chong ZZ, Maiese K. 2001. Nicotinamide: a nutritional supplement that provides protection against neuronal and vascular injury. *J Med Food.* 4:27–38.

Liu H, Fergusson MM, Castilho RM et al. 2007. Augmented Wnt signaling in a mammalian model of accelerated aging. *Science.* 317:803–806.

Liu HK, Green BD, Flatt PR, McClenaghan NH, McCluskey JT. 2004. Effects of long-term exposure to nicotinamide and sodium butyrate on growth, viability, and the function of clonal insulin secreting cells. *Endocr Res.* 30:61–68.

Liu P, Wakamiya M, Shea MJ, Albrecht U, Behringer RR, Bradley A. 1999. Requirement for Wnt3 in vertebrate axis formation. *Nat Genet.* 22:361–365.

Liu R, Suzuki A, Guo Z, Mizuno Y, Urabe T. 2006. Intrinsic and extrinsic erythropoietin enhances neuroprotection against ischemia and reperfusion injury in vitro. *J Neurochem.* 96:1101–1110.

Luchsinger JA, Tang MX, Stern Y, Shea S, Mayeux R. 2001. Diabetes mellitus and risk of Alzheimer's disease and dementia with stroke in a multiethnic cohort. *Am J Epidemiol.* 154:635–641.

Lykissas MG, Korompilias AV, Vekris MD, Mitsionis GI, Sakellariou E, Beris AE. 2007. The role of erythropoietin in central and peripheral nerve injury. *Clin Neurol Neurosurg.* 109:639–644.

Maiese K. 2001. The dynamics of cellular injury: transformation into neuronal and vascular protection. *Histol Histopathol.* 16:633–644.

Maiese K, Boccone L. 1995. Neuroprotection by peptide growth factors against anoxia and nitric oxide toxicity requires modulation of protein kinase C. *J Cereb Blood Flow Metab.* 15:440–449.

Maiese K, TenBroeke M, Kue I. 1997. Neuroprotection of lubeluzole is mediated through the signal transduction pathways of nitric oxide. *J Neurochem.* 68:710–714.

Maiese K, Ahmad I, TenBroeke M, Gallant J. 1999. Metabotropic glutamate receptor subtypes independently modulate neuronal intracellular calcium. *J Neurosci Res.* 55:472–485.

Maiese K, Vincent A, Lin SH, Shaw T. 2000. Group I and Group III metabotropic glutamate receptor subtypes provide enhanced neuroprotection. *J Neurosci Res.* 62:257–272.

Maiese K, Vincent AM. 2000a. Membrane asymmetry and DNA degradation: functionally distinct determinants of neuronal programmed cell death. *J Neurosci Res.* 59:568–580.

Maiese K, Vincent AM. 2000b. Critical temporal modulation of neuronal programmed cell injury. *Cell Mol Neurobiol.* 20:383–400.

Maiese K, Chong ZZ. 2003. Nicotinamide: necessary nutrient emerges as a novel cytoprotectant for the brain. *Trends Pharmacol Sci.* 24:228–232.

Maiese K, Chong ZZ, Kang J. 2003. Transformation into treatment: Novel therapeutics that begin within the cell. In: Maiese K, ed. *Neuronal and Vascular Plasticity: Elucidating Basic Cellular Mechanisms for Future Therapeutic Discovery.* Norwell, MA: Kluwer Academic Publishers, 1–26.

Maiese K, Chong ZZ. 2004. Insights into oxidative stress and potential novel therapeutic targets for Alzheimer disease. *Restor Neurol Neurosci.* 22:87–104.

Maiese K, Li F, Chong ZZ. 2004. Erythropoietin in the brain: can the promise to protect be fulfilled? *Trends Pharmacol Sci.* 25:577–583.

Maiese K, Chong ZZ, Li F. 2005a. Driving cellular plasticity and survival through the signal transduction pathways of metabotropic glutamate receptors. *Curr Neurovasc Res.* 2:425–446.

Maiese K, Li F, Chong ZZ. 2005b. New avenues of exploration for erythropoietin. *JAMA.* 293:90–95.

Maiese K, Li F, Chong ZZ. 2005c. Erythropoietin and cancer. *JAMA.* 293:1858–1859.

Maiese K, Chong ZZ, Shang YC. 2007a. Mechanistic insights into diabetes mellitus and oxidative stress. *Curr Med Chem.* 14:1689–1699.

Maiese K, Chong ZZ, Shang YC. 2007b. "Sly as a FOXO": new paths with forkhead signaling in the brain. *Curr Neurovasc Res.* 4:295–302.

Maiese K, Morhan SD, Chong ZZ. 2007c. Oxidative stress biology and cell injury during type 1 and type 2 diabetes mellitus. *Curr Neurovasc Res.* 4:63–71.

Maiorana A, O'Driscoll G, Goodman C, Taylor R, Green D. 2002. Combined aerobic and resistance exercise improves glycemic control and fitness in type 2 diabetes. *Diabetes Res Clin Pract.* 56:115–123.

Mallat M, Marin-Teva JL, Cheret C. 2005. Phagocytosis in the developing CNS: more than clearing the corpses. *Curr Opin Neurobiol.* 15:101–107.

Mani A, Radhakrishnan J, Wang H et al. 2007. LRP6 mutation in a family with early coronary disease and metabolic risk factors. *Science.* 315:1278–1282.

Mao J, Wang J, Liu B et al. 2001. Low-density lipoprotein receptor-related protein-5 binds to Axin and regulates the canonical Wnt signaling pathway. *Mol Cell.* 7:801–809.

Marambaud P, Shioi J, Serban G et al. 2002. A presenilin-1/gamma-secretase cleavage releases the E-cadherin intracellular domain and regulates disassembly of adherens junctions. *Embo J.* 21:1948–1956.

Mari C, Karabiyikoglu M, Goris ML, Tait JF, Yenari MA, Blankenberg FG. 2004. Detection of focal hypoxic-ischemic injury and neuronal stress in a rodent model of unilateral MCA occlusion/reperfusion using radiolabeled annexin V. *Eur J Nucl Med Mol Imaging.* 31:733–739.

Marvin MJ, Di Rocco G, Gardiner A, Bush SM, Lassar AB. 2001. Inhibition of Wnt activity induces heart formation from posterior mesoderm. *Genes Dev.* 15:316–327.

Mason-Garcia M, Beckman BS, Brookins JW et al. 1990. Development of a new radioimmunoassay for erythropoietin using recombinant erythropoietin. *Kidney Int.* 38:969–975.

Matsuzaki H, Tamatani M, Mitsuda N et al. 1999. Activation of Akt kinase inhibits apoptosis and changes in Bcl-2 and Bax expression induced by nitric oxide in primary hippocampal neurons. *J Neurochem.* 73:2037–2046.

McCormick WC, Hardy J, Kukull WA et al. 2001. Healthcare utilization and costs in managed care patients with Alzheimer's disease during the last few years of life. *J Am Geriatr Soc.* 49:1156–1160.

McLeod M, Hong M, Mukhida K, Sadi D, Ulalia R, Mendez I. 2006. Erythropoietin and GDNF enhance ventral mesencephalic fiber outgrowth and capillary proliferation following neural transplantation in a rodent model of Parkinson's disease. *Eur J Neurosci.* 24:361–370.

Meloni BP, Tilbrook PA, Boulos S, Arthur PG, Knuckey NW. 2006. Erythropoietin preconditioning in neuronal cultures: signaling, protection from in vitro ischemia, and proteomic analysis. *J Neurosci Res.* 83:584–593.

Memisogullari R, Bakan E. 2004. Levels of ceruloplasmin, transferrin, and lipid peroxidation in the serum of patients with Type 2 diabetes mellitus. *J Diabetes Complications.* 18:193–197.

Mendiondo MS, Kryscio RJ, Schmitt FA. 2001. Models of progression in Alzheimer's disease: predicting disability and costs. *Neurology.* 57:943–944.

Mikati MA, Hokayem JA, Sabban ME. 2007. Effects of a single dose of erythropoietin on subsequent seizure susceptibility in rats exposed to acute hypoxia at p10. *Epilepsia.* 48:175–181.

Miki T, Miura T, Yano T et al. 2006. Alteration in erythropoietin-induced cardioprotective signaling by postinfarct ventricular remodeling. *J Pharmacol Exp Ther.* 317:68–75.

Mirotsou M, Zhang Z, Deb A et al. 2007. Secreted frizzled related protein 2 (Sfrp2) is the key Akt-mesenchymal stem cell-released paracrine factor mediating myocardial survival and repair. *Proc Natl Acad Sci U S A.* 104:1643–1648.

Moberg L, Olsson A, Berne C et al. 2003. Nicotinamide inhibits tissue factor expression in isolated human pancreatic islets: implications for clinical islet transplantation. *Transplantation.* 76:1285–1288.

Mocini D, Leone T, Tubaro M, Santini M, Penco M. 2007. Structure, production and function of erythropoietin: implications for therapeutical use in cardiovascular disease. *Curr Med Chem.* 14:2278–2287.

Mojiminiyi OA, Abdella NA, Zaki MY, El Gebely SA, Mohamedi HM, Aldhahi WA. 2006. Prevalence and associations of low plasma erythropoietin in patients with type 2 diabetes mellitus. *Diabet Med.* 23:839–844.

Monnier L, Mas E, Ginet C et al. 2006. Activation of oxidative stress by acute glucose fluctuations compared with sustained chronic hyperglycemia in patients with type 2 diabetes. *JAMA.* 295:1681–1687.

Montero M, Poulsen FR, Noraberg J et al. 2007. Comparison of neuroprotective effects of erythropoietin (EPO) and carbamylerythropoietin (CEPO) against ischemia-like oxygen-glucose deprivation (OGD) and NMDA excitotoxicity in mouse hippocampal slice cultures. *Exp Neurol.* 204:106–117.

Moon C, Krawczyk M, Paik D et al. 2006. Erythropoietin, modified to not stimulate red blood cell production, retains its cardioprotective properties. *J Pharmacol Exp Ther.* 316:999–1005.

Morin PJ, Medina M, Semenov M, Brown AM, Kosik KS. 2004. Wnt-1 expression in PC12 cells induces exon 15 deletion and expression of L-APP. *Neurobiol Dis.* 16:59–67.

Mujais SK, Beru N, Pullman TN, Goldwasser E. 1999. Erythropoietin is produced by tubular cells of the rat kidney. *Cell Biochem Biophys.* 30:153–166.

Muller FL, Lustgarten MS, Jang Y, Richardson A, Van Remmen H. 2007. Trends in oxidative aging theories. *Free Radic Biol Med.* 43:477–503.

Munoz-Fontela C, Marcos-Villar L, Gallego P et al. 2007. Latent protein LANA2 from Kaposi's sarcoma-associated herpesvirus interacts with 14–3–3 proteins and inhibits FOXO3a transcription factor. *J Virol.* 81:1511–1516.

Mussmann R, Geese M, Harder F et al. 2007. Inhibition of glycogen synthase kinase (GSK) 3 promotes replication and survival of pancreatic beta cells. *J Biol Chem.* 282(16): 12030–12037.

Nadam J, Navarro F, Sanchez P et al. 2007. Neuroprotective effects of erythropoietin in the rat hippocampus after pilocarpine-induced status epilepticus. *Neurobiol Dis.* 25:412–426.

Naito AT, Akazawa H, Takano H et al. 2005. Phosphatidylinositol 3-kinase-Akt pathway plays a critical role in early cardiomyogenesis by regulating canonical Wnt signaling. *Circ Res.* 97:144–151.

Naito AT, Shiojima I, Akazawa H et al. 2006. Developmental stage-specific biphasic roles of Wnt/beta-catenin signaling in cardiomyogenesis and hematopoiesis. *Proc Natl Acad Sci U S A.* 103:19812–19817.

Nakagami Y, Nishimura S, Murasugi T et al. 2002. A novel compound RS-0466 reverses beta-amyloid-induced cytotoxicity through the Akt signaling pathway in vitro. *Eur J Pharmacol.* 457:11–17.

Namiuchi S, Kagaya Y, Ohta J et al. 2005. High serum erythropoietin level is associated with smaller infarct size in patients with acute myocardial infarction who undergo successful primary percutaneous coronary intervention. *J Am Coll Cardiol.* 45:1406–1412.

Nangaku M, Fliser D. 2007. Erythropoiesis-stimulating agents: past and future. *Kidney Int.* 107:Suppl:S1–S3.

Newsholme P, Haber EP, Hirabara SM et al. 2007. Diabetes associated cell stress and dysfunction: role of mitochondrial and non-mitochondrial ROS production and activity. *J Physiol.* 583:9–24.

Niemann S, Zhao C, Pascu F et al. 2004. Homozygous WNT3 mutation causes tetra-amelia in a large consanguineous family. *Am J Hum Genet.* 74:558–563.

Ning S, Hartley C, Molineux G, Knox SJ 2005. Darbepoietin alfa potentiates the efficacy of radiation therapy in mice with corrected or uncorrected anemia. *Cancer Res.* 65:284–290.

Nurmi A, Goldsteins G, Narvainen J et al. 2006. Antioxidant pyrrolidine dithiocarbamate activates Akt-GSK signaling and is neuroprotective in neonatal hypoxia-ischemia. *Free Radic Biol Med.* 40:1776–1784.

Ogilvie M, Yu X, Nicolas-Metral V et al. 2000. Erythropoietin stimulates proliferation and interferes with differentiation of myoblasts. *J Biol Chem.* 275:39754–39761.

Okouchi M, Ekshyyan O, Maracine M, Aw TY. 2007. Neuronal apoptosis in neurodegeneration. *Antioxid Redox Signal.* 9:1059–1096.

Okutan O, Solaroglu I, Beskonakli E, Taskin Y. 2007. Recombinant human erythropoietin decreases myeloperoxidase and caspase-3 activity and improves early functional results after spinal cord injury in rats. *J Clin Neurosci.* 14:364–368.

Olea FD, Vera Janavel G, De Lorenzi A et al.2006. High-dose erythropoietin has no long-term protective effects in sheep with reperfused myocardial infarction. *J Cardiovasc Pharmacol.* 47:736–741.

Olmos PR, Hodgson MI, Maiz A, et al. 2005. Nicotinamide protected first-phase insulin response (FPIR) and prevented clinical disease in first-degree relatives of type-1 diabetics. *Diabetes Res Clin Pract.* 71(3):320–333.

Olsen NV. 2003. Central nervous system frontiers for the use of erythropoietin. *Clin Infect Dis.* 37 (Suppl 4): S323–S330.

Oumouna-Benachour K, Hans CP, Suzuki Y et al. 2007. Poly(ADP-ribose) polymerase inhibition reduces atherosclerotic plaque size and promotes factors of plaque stability in apolipoprotein E-deficient mice: effects on macrophage recruitment, nuclear factor-kappaB nuclear translocation, and foam cell death. *Circulation.* 115:2442–2450.

Palazzuoli A, Silverberg D, Iovine F et al. 2006. Erythropoietin improves anemia exercise tolerance and renal function and reduces B-type natriuretic peptide and hospitalization in patients with heart failure and anemia. *Am Heart J.* 152:1096 e1099–e1015.

Palazzuoli A, Silverberg DS, Iovine F et al. 2007. Effects of beta-erythropoietin treatment on left ventricular remodeling, systolic function, and B-type natriuretic peptide levels in patients with the cardiorenal anemia syndrome. *Am Heart J.* 154:645 e649–e615.

Palpant NJ, Yasuda S, MacDougald O, Metzger JM. 2007. Non-canonical Wnt signaling enhances differentiation of Sca1+/c-kit+ adipose-derived murine stromal vascular cells into spontaneously beating cardiac myocytes. *J Mol Cell Cardiol.* 43:362–370.

Parsa CJ, Matsumoto A, Kim J et al. 2003. A novel protective effect of erythropoietin in the infarcted heart. *J Clin Invest.* 112:999–1007.

Patapoutian A, Reichardt LF. 2000. Roles of Wnt proteins in neural development and maintenance. *Curr Opin Neurobiol.* 10:392–399.

Pearl R. 1928. *The rate of living.* University of London Press, London.

Petersen KF, Befroy D, Dufour S et al. 2003. Mitochondrial dysfunction in the elderly: possible role in insulin resistance. *Science.* 300:1140–1142.

Porcu M, Chiarugi A. 2005. The emerging therapeutic potential of sirtuin-interacting drugs: from cell death to lifespan extension. *Trends Pharmacol Sci.* 26:94–103.

Pospisilik JA, Knauf C, Joza N et al. 2007. Targeted deletion of AIF decreases mitochondrial oxidative phosphorylation and protects from obesity and diabetes. *Cell.* 131:476–491.

Pregi N, Vittori D, Perez G, Leiros CP, Nesse A. 2006. Effect of erythropoietin on staurosporine-induced apoptosis and differentiation of SH-SY5Y neuroblastoma cells. *Biochim Biophys Acta.* 1763:238–246.

Qin W, Peng Y, Ksiezak-Reding H et al. 2006. Inhibition of cyclooxygenase as potential novel therapeutic strategy in N141I presenilin-2 familial Alzheimer's disease. *Mol Psychiatry.* 11:172–181.

Quinn L. 2001. Type 2 diabetes: epidemiology, pathophysiology, and diagnosis. *Nurs Clin North Am.* 36:175–192.

Rachek LI, Thornley NP, Grishko VI, LeDoux SP, Wilson GL. 2006. Protection of INS-1 cells from free fatty acid-induced apoptosis by targeting hOGG1 to mitochondria. *Diabetes.* 55:1022–1028.

Rades D, Golke H, Schild SE, Kilic E. 2007. The impact of tumor expression of erythropoietin receptors and erythropoietin on clinical outcome of esophageal cancer patients treated with chemoradiation. *Int J Radiat Oncol Biol Phys.* 71(1):152–159.

Reddy MK, Vasir JK, Hegde GV, Joshi SS, Labhasetwar V. 2007. Erythropoietin induces excessive neointima formation: a study in a rat carotid artery model of vascular injury. *J Cardiovasc Pharmacol Ther.* 12:237–247.

Reddy S, Salari-Lak N, Sandler S. 1995a. Long-term effects of nicotinamide-induced inhibition of poly (adenosine diphosphate-ribose) polymerase activity in rat pancreatic islets exposed to interleukin-1 beta. *Endocrinology.* 136:1907–1912.

Reddy S, Bibby NJ, Wu D, Swinney C, Barrow G, Elliott RB. 1995b. A combined casein-free-nicotinamide diet prevents diabetes in the NOD mouse with minimum insulitis. *Diabetes Res Clin Pract.* 29:83–92.

Reddy S, Young M, Ginn S. 2001. Immunoexpression of interleukin-1beta in pancreatic islets of NOD mice during cyclophosphamide-accelerated diabetes: co-localization in macrophages and endocrine cells and its attenuation with oral nicotinamide. *Histochem J.* 33:317–327.

Relling DP, Esberg LB, Fang CX et al. 2006. High-fat diet-induced juvenile obesity leads to cardiomyocyte dysfunction and upregulation of FoxO3a transcription factor independent of lipotoxicity and apoptosis. *J Hypertens.* 24:549–561.

Reya T, Duncan AW, Ailles L et al. 2003. A role for Wnt signalling in self-renewal of haematopoietic stem cells. *Nature.* 423:409–414.

Roberts E Jr, Chih CP. 1997. The influence of age of pH regulation in hippocampal slices before, during, and after anoxia. *J Cereb Blood Flow Metab.* 17:560–566.

Rodova M, Islam MR, Maser RL, Calvet JP. 2002. The polycystic kidney disease-1 promoter is a target of the beta-catenin/T-cell factor pathway. *J Biol Chem.* 277:29577–29583.

Ross SE, Hemati N, Longo KA et al. 2000. Inhibition of adipogenesis by Wnt signaling. *Science.* 289:950–953.

Rowe MK, Wiest C, Chuang DM. 2007. GSK-3 is a viable potential target for therapeutic intervention in bipolar disorder. *Neurosci Biobehav Rev.* 31:920–931.

Sadanaga-Akiyoshi F, Yao H, Tanuma S et al. 2003. Nicotinamide attenuates focal ischemic brain injury in rats: with special reference to changes in nicotinamide and NAD+ levels in ischemic core and penumbra. *Neurochem Res.* 28:1227–1234.

Salinas M, Diaz R, Abraham NG, Ruiz de Galarreta CM, Cuadrado A. 2003. Nerve growth factor protects against 6-hydroxydopamine-induced oxidative stress by increasing expression of heme oxygenase-1 in a phosphatidylinositol 3-kinase-dependent manner. *J Biol Chem.* 278:13898–13904.

Salinas PC. 1999. Wnt factors in axonal remodelling and synaptogenesis. *Biochem Soc Symp.* 65:101–109.

Sanz O, Acarin L, Gonzalez B, Castellano B. 2002. NF-kappaB and IkappaBalpha expression following traumatic brain injury to the immature rat brain. *J Neurosci Res.* 67:772–780.

Saunders LR, Verdin E. 2007. Sirtuins: critical regulators at the crossroads between cancer and aging. *Oncogene.* 26:5489–5504.

Schmeding M, Neumann UP, Boas-Knoop S, Spinelli A, Neuhaus P. 2007. Erythropoietin reduces ischemia-reperfusion injury in the rat liver. *Eur Surg Res.* 39:189–197.

Schnaider Beeri M, Goldbourt U, Silverman JM et al. 2004. Diabetes mellitus in midlife and the risk of dementia three decades later. *Neurology.* 63:1902–1907.

Schumann C, Triantafilou K, Krueger S et al. 2006. Detection of erythropoietin in exhaled breath condensate of nonhypoxic subjects using a multiplex bead array. *Mediators Inflamm.* 2006:18061.

Scott LJ, Bonnycastle LL, Willer CJ et al. 2006. Association of transcription factor 7-like 2 (TCF7L2) variants with type 2 diabetes in a finnish sample. *Diabetes.* 55:2649–2653.

Sensi SL, Jeng JM. 2004. Rethinking the excitotoxic ionic milieu: the emerging role of zn(2+) in ischemic neuronal injury. *Curr Mol Med.* 4:87–111.

Sharples EJ, Thiemermann C, Yaqoob MM. 2005. Mechanisms of disease: Cell death in acute renal failure and emerging evidence for a protective role of erythropoietin. *Nat Clin Pract Nephrol.* 1:87–97.

Sharples EJ, Yaqoob MM. 2006. Erythropoietin in experimental acute renal failure. *Nephron Exp Nephrol.* 104:e83–e88.

Shein NA, Tsenter J, Alexandrovich AG, Horowitz M, Shohami E. 2007. Akt phosphorylation is required for heat acclimation-induced neuroprotection. *J Neurochem.* 103:1523–1529.

Sigounas G, Sallah S, Sigounas VY. 2004. Erythropoietin modulates the anticancer activity of chemotherapeutic drugs in a murine lung cancer model. *Cancer Lett.* 214:171–179.

Silverberg DS, Wexler D, Sheps D et al. 2001. The effect of correction of mild anemia in severe, resistant congestive heart failure using subcutaneous erythropoietin and intravenous iron: a randomized controlled study. *J Am Coll Cardiol.* 37:1775–1780.

Silverberg DS, Wexler D, Iaina A, Schwartz D. 2006. The interaction between heart failure and other heart diseases, renal failure, and anemia. *Semin Nephrol.* 26:296–306.

Singh AM, Li FQ, Hamazaki T, Kasahara H, Takemaru K, Terada N. 2007. Chibby, an antagonist of the Wnt/beta-catenin pathway, facilitates cardiomyocyte differentiation of murine embryonic stem cells. *Circulation.* 115:617–626.

Soop A, Albert J, Weitzberg E, Bengtsson A, Nilsson CG, Sollevi A. 2004. Nicotinamide does not influence cytokines or exhaled NO in human experimental endotoxaemia. *Clin Exp Immunol.* 135:114–118.

Soriano S, Kang DE, Fu M et al. 2001. Presenilin 1 negatively regulates beta-catenin/T cell factor/lymphoid enhancer factor-1 signaling independently of beta-amyloid precursor protein and notch processing. *J Cell Biol.* 152:785–794.

Spandou E, Tsouchnikas I, Karkavelas G et al. 2006. Erythropoietin attenuates renal injury in experimental acute renal failure ischaemic/reperfusion model. *Nephrol Dial Transplant.* 21:330–336.

Speese SD, Budnik V. 2007. Wnts: up-and-coming at the synapse. *Trends Neurosci.* 30:268–275.

Stark K, Vainio S, Vassileva G, McMahon AP 1994. Epithelial transformation of metanephric mesenchyme in the developing kidney regulated by Wnt-4. *Nature.* 372:679–683.

Stevens MJ, Li F, Drel VR et al. 2007. Nicotinamide reverses neurological and neurovascular deficits in streptozotocin diabetic rats. *J Pharmacol Exp Ther.* 320:458–464.

Symeonidis A, Kouraklis-Symeonidis A, Psiroyiannis A et al. 2006. Inappropriately low erythropoietin response for the degree of anemia in patients with noninsulin-dependent diabetes mellitus. *Ann Hematol.* 85:79–85.

Tanuma N, Sakuma H, Sasaki A, Matsumoto Y. 2006. Chemokine expression by astrocytes plays a role in microglia/macrophage activation and subsequent neurodegeneration in secondary progressive multiple sclerosis. *Acta Neuropathol (Berl).* 112:195–204.

Teramo K, Kari MA, Eronen M, Markkanen H, Hiilesmaa V. 2004. High amniotic fluid erythropoietin levels are associated with an increased frequency of fetal and neonatal morbidity in type 1 diabetic pregnancies. *Diabetologia.* 47:1695–1703.

Thomas MC, Cooper ME, Tsalamandris C, MacIsaac R, Jerums G. 2005. Anemia with impaired erythropoietin response in diabetic patients. *Arch Intern Med.* 165:466–469.

Traister A, Breitman I, Bar-Lev E et al. 2005. Nicotinamide induces apoptosis and reduces collagen I and pro-inflammatory cytokines expression in rat hepatic stellate cells. *Scand J Gastroenterol.* 40:1226–1234.

Tsai JC, Song BJ, Wu L, Forbes M. 2007. Erythropoietin: a candidate neuroprotective agent in the treatment of glaucoma. *J Glaucoma.* 16:567–571.

Um M, Gross AW, Lodish HF. 2007. A "classical" homodimeric erythropoietin receptor is essential for the anti-apoptotic effects of erythropoietin on differentiated neuroblastoma SH-SY5Y and pheochromocytoma PC-12 cells. *Cell Signal.* 19:634–645.

Ungerstedt JS, Blomback M, Soderstrom T. 2003. Nicotinamide is a potent inhibitor of proinflammatory cytokines. *Clin Exp Immunol.* 131:48–52.

van de Schans VA, van den Borne SW, Strzelecka AE et al. 2007. Interruption of Wnt signaling attenuates the onset of pressure overload-induced cardiac hypertrophy. *Hypertension.* 49:473–480.

van der Meer P, Voors AA, Lipsic E, Smilde TD, van Gilst WH, van Veldhuisen DJ. 2004. Prognostic value of plasma erythropoietin on mortality in patients with chronic heart failure. *J Am Coll Cardiol.* 44:63–67.

Verdaguer E, Susana Gde A, Clemens A, Pallas M, Camins A. 2007. Implication of the transcription factor E2F-1 in the modulation of neuronal apoptosis. *Biomed Pharmacother.* 61:390–399.

Verdonck O, Lahrech H, Francony G et al. 2007. Erythropoietin protects from post-traumatic edema in the rat brain. *J Cereb Blood Flow Metab.* 27:1369–1376.

Vincent AM, Maiese K. 1999a. Nitric oxide induction of neuronal endonuclease activity in programmed cell death. *Exp Cell Res.* 246:290–300.

Vincent AM, Maiese K. 1999b. Direct temporal analysis of apoptosis induction in living adherent neurons. *J Histochem Cytochem.* 47:661–672.

Vincent AM, TenBroeke M, Maiese K. 1999a. Metabotropic glutamate receptors prevent programmed cell death through the modulation of neuronal endonuclease activity and intracellular pH. *Exp Neurol.* 155:79–94.

Vincent AM, TenBroeke M, Maiese K. 1999b. Neuronal intracellular pH directly mediates nitric oxide-induced programmed cell death. *J Neurobiol.* 40:171–184.

Wild S, Roglic G, Green A, Sicree R, King H. 2004. Global prevalence of diabetes: estimates for the year 2000 and projections for 2030. *Diabetes Care.* 27:1047–1053.

Willert K, Brown JD, Danenberg E et al. 2003. Wnt proteins are lipid-modified and can act as stem cell growth factors. *Nature.* 423:448–452.

Williams AC, Cartwright LS, Ramsden DB. 2005. Parkinson's disease: the first common neurological disease due to auto-intoxication? *Qjm.* 98:215–226.

Wilson FH, Hariri A, Farhi A et al. 2004. A cluster of metabolic defects caused by mutation in a mitochondrial tRNA. *Science.* 306:1190–1194.

Wright WS, Longo KA, Dolinsky VW et al. 2007. Wnt10b Inhibits Obesity in ob/ob and Agouti Mice. *Diabetes.* 56:295–303.

Wu H, Ren B, Zhu J et al. 2006. Pretreatment with recombined human erythropoietin attenuates ischemia-reperfusion-induced lung injury in rats. *Eur J Cardiothorac Surg.* 29:902–907.

Wu Y, Shang Y, Sun S, Liang H, Liu R. 2007. Erythropoietin prevents PC12 cells from 1-methyl-4-phenylpyridinium ion-induced apoptosis via the Akt/GSK-3beta/caspase-3 mediated signaling pathway. *Apoptosis.* 12:1365–1375.

Xu WL, Qiu CX, Wahlin A, Winblad B, Fratiglioni L. 2004. Diabetes mellitus and risk of dementia in the Kungsholmen project: a 6-year follow-up study. *Neurology.* 63:1181–1186.

Yamasaki M, Mishima HK, Yamashita H et al. 2005. Neuroprotective effects of erythropoietin on glutamate and nitric oxide toxicity in primary cultured retinal ganglion cells. *Brain Res.* 1050:15–26.

Yano M, Hasegawa G, Ishii M et al. 2004. Short-term exposure of high glucose concentration induces generation of reactive oxygen species in endothelial cells: implication for the oxidative stress associated with postprandial hyperglycemia. *Redox Rep.* 9:111–116.

You Z, Saims D, Chen S et al. 2002. Wnt signaling promotes oncogenic transformation by inhibiting c-Myc-induced apoptosis. *J Cell Biol.* 157:429–440.

Yu YP, Xu QQ, Zhang Q, Zhang WP, Zhang LH, Wei EQ. 2005. Intranasal recombinant human erythropoietin protects rats against focal cerebral ischemia. *Neurosci Lett.* 387:5–10.

Yui R, Matsuura ET. 2006. Detection of deletions flanked by short direct repeats in mitochondrial DNA of aging Drosophila. *Mutat Res.* 594:155–161.

Zhang F, Signore AP, Zhou Z, Wang S, Cao G, Chen J. 2006. Erythropoietin protects CA1 neurons against global cerebral ischemia in rat: potential signaling mechanisms. *J Neurosci Res.* 83:1241–1251.

Zhang Y, Park TS, Gidday JM. 2007. Hypoxic preconditioning protects human brain endothelium from ischemic apoptosis by Akt-dependent survivin activation. *Am J Physiol Heart Circ Physiol.* 292:H2573–H2581.

Zheng WH, Kar S, Quirion R. 2002. FKHRL1 and its homologs are new targets of nerve growth factor Trk receptor signaling. *J Neurochem.* 80:1049–1061.

Zhong Y, Yao H, Deng L, Cheng Y, Zhou X. 2007. Promotion of neurite outgrowth and protective effect of erythropoietin on the retinal neurons of rats. Graefes *Arch Clin Exp Ophthalmol.* 245:1859–1867.

Index

Note: Page numbers followed by *f* denote figures, while those followed by *t* denote tables.